Berek & Hacker's
Gynecologic Oncology

Fifth Edition

Jonathan S. Berek, MD, MMS

Professor and Chair
Department of Obstetrics and Gynecology
Stanford University School of Medicine
Director, Women's Cancer Program
Division of Gynecologic Oncology
Stanford Cancer Center
Stanford, California

Neville F. Hacker, MD

Professor of Gynaecologic Oncology
Conjoint, University of New South Wales
Director, Gynaecologic Cancer Centre
Royal Hospital for Women
Sydney, Australia

Illustrations and design by
Tim Hengst, CMI, FAMI
George Barile
Deborah Berek, MA

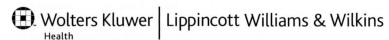

Philadelphia • Baltimore • New York • London
Buenos Aires • Hong Kong • Sydney • Tokyo

Acquisitions Editor: Sonya Seigafuse
Product Managers: Nicole Walz/Kerry Barrett
Vendor Manager: Alicia Jackson
Senior Manufacturing Manager: Benjamin Rivera
Marketing Manager: Kimberly Schonberger
Design Coordinator: Holly Reid McLaughlin
Production Service: Macmillan Publishing Solutions

Printed in China.

Library of Congress Cataloging-in-Publication Data

Berek & Hacker's gynecologic oncology / [edited by] Jonathan S. Berek,
Neville F. Hacker; illustrations and design by Tim Hengst, George Barile,
Deborah Berek. — 5th ed.
    p. ; cm.
 Rev. ed. of: Practical gynecologic oncology / [edited by] Jonathan S.
Berek, Neville F. Hacker. 4th ed. c2005.
 Includes bibliographical references and index.
 ISBN-13: 978-0-7817-9512-8 (alk. paper)
 ISBN-10: 0-7817-9512-5
 1. Generative organs, Female—Cancer. I. Berek, Jonathan S. II. Hacker,
Neville F. III. Practical gynecologic oncology. IV. Title: Berek and
Hacker's gynecologic oncology. V. Title: Gynecologic oncology.
 [DNLM: 1. Genital Neoplasms, Female. 2. Genitalia,
Female—physiopathology. WP 145 B487 2010]
 RC280.G5P73 2010
 616.99'465—dc22

                                                    2009028368

Care has been taken to confirm the accuracy of the information presented and to describe generally accepted practices. However, the authors, editors, and publisher are not responsible for errors or omissions or for any consequences from application of the information in this book and make no warranty, expressed or implied, with respect to the currency, completeness, or accuracy of the contents of the publication. Application of the information in a particular situation remains the professional responsibility of the practitioner.

The authors, editors, and publisher have exerted every effort to ensure that drug selection and dosage set forth in this text are in accordance with current recommendations and practice at the time of publication. However, in view of ongoing research, changes in government regulations, and the constant flow of information relating to drug therapy and drug reactions, the reader is urged to check the package insert for each drug for any change in indications and dosage and for added warnings and precautions. This is particularly important when the recommended agent is a new or infrequently employed drug.

Some drugs and medical devices presented in the publication have Food and Drug Administration (FDA) clearance for limited use in restricted research settings. It is the responsibility of the health care provider to ascertain the FDA status of each drug or device planned for use in their clinical practice.

To purchase additional copies of this book, call our customer service department at (800) 638-3030 or fax orders to (301) 223-2320. International customers should call (301) 223-2300.

Visit Lippincott Williams & Wilkins on the Internet: at LWW.com. Lippincott Williams & Wilkins customer service representatives are available from 8:30 am to 6 pm, EST.

10 9 8 7 6 5 4 3

RRS1212

To our wives, Deborah and Estelle; and to our patients whose courage in adversity inspires us to continue our work.

Foreword to the First Edition

Close to the beginning of this century, William Osler observed, "The practice of medicine is an art, based on science." That brief characterization of our profession rings true, even as we approach the next century in the midst of brilliant, accelerating scientific discovery.

Some aspects of the art—including compassion and the basic skills of history taking and physical examination—are, or should be, common to all physicians and remain largely unchanged by a century of research. In other ways, the "art," which can also be translated as "craft" from the original Greek work "techne," has been greatly enlarged and diversified by science and technology. Thus, the special skills required by a gynecologic oncologist derive not only from experience and practice, but also from the proliferation of knowledge in many branches of science. Indeed, it is mainly the developments of science in obstetrics and gynecology—and in some other disciplines—that have evolved the clinical subspeciality of gynecologic oncology.

The art and the science are connected not only by ancestry, however. Their relationship continues to be an interdependent one. One of the ever-expanding glories of medicine is that what is learned in the laboratory can enhance learning at the bedside and what is learned from experience with patients helps to shape and direct scientific inquiry.

Doctors who remain lifelong students are exhilarated by these interconnections and make the best teachers of clinical medicine. It is in the scholarly tradition that Jonathan S. Berek and Neville F. Hacker, with contributions from distinguished colleagues in their own discipline and in fields that bear upon it, have brought together the salient information required to develop the acumen and skills that enable clinicians to understand and to care for women suffering from tumors.

Practical Gynecologic Oncology reflects the indivisibility of art and science in medicine. The two editors—one in Los Angeles and one in Sydney—worked and studied together for 7 years in the same hospital and laboratories and remain mutually helpful intellectual allies on opposites shores of the Pacific Ocean.

Sherman M. Mellinkoff, MD
Dean Emeritus
Professor of Medicine
University of California, Los Angeles
School of Medicine
Los Angeles, California

Preface

Gynecologic oncology, as a subspecialty of Obstetrics and Gynecology, evolved slowly since the concept was first introduced in the United States in 1973. Canada, the United Kingdom, Australia, and New Zealand adopted the concept within the ensuing 15 years, and European countries followed later. Although gynecologic oncology was practiced by individuals in Western Europe for many years, official recognition of the subspecialty has been much more recent. Eastern Europe, India, and much of Asia have yet to officially recognize this discipline.

With subspecialization, research into gynecologic cancers flourished at both the clinical and molecular level, and accrual of knowledge expanded exponentially. The development of international collaborative groups like the Gynecologic Cancer Intergroup (GCIG) resulted in the recruitment of large numbers of patients for clinical trials within a relatively short period of time. Similarly, the multinational Human Genome Project paved the way for a better understanding of the genetic basis of cancer and facilitated the development of targeted therapies.

The first four editions of our book were titled *Practical Gynecologic Oncology,* and now, in recognition of its sustained utility, Lippincott Williams & Wilkins has renamed the fifth edition *Berek & Hacker's Gynecologic Oncology*. The previous edition was translated into Chinese and Spanish, an acknowledgment of the book's international appeal.

This edition preserves the basic format and style of the previous editions, being divided into four sections: general principles, disease sites, medical and surgical topics, and quality of life. All chapters have been thoroughly revised and incorporate a critical review of the recent literature. As with previous editions, where level I evidence is not available, we have injected our personal biases, but have tried to justify our position with adequate reference to the available literature. In this edition, a chapter on cancer in pregnancy has been added.

This book would not have been possible without the contributions of our co-authors, who are all acknowledged experts in their field. Dr. Michael Friedlander, an internationally recognized authority on the management of gynecologic cancer, has been recruited as an author. For the past two decades, he has served as the consultant medical oncologist at the Royal Hospital for Women in Sydney, Australia, and his inclusion gives added strength to the chapters on cervical, endometrial, and ovarian cancer. We are most grateful to Tim Hengst and George Barile for their outstanding illustrations and drawings, and to Deborah Berek for her valuable assistance with design and editing. We thank Estelle Hacker for her assistance with the manuscript. We gratefully acknowledge Kerry Garcia for her assistance at Stanford. We appreciate the important contribution of the Lippincott Williams & Wilkins staff, especially Sonya Seigafuse, Nicole Walz, Kerry Barrett, and of Daisy Sosa from Macmillan. Finally, we extend special thanks to Charley Mitchell who has been supportive of our book since its inception.

At Stanford, we acknowledge the generosity of our benefactors, especially Nicole Kidman and the Stanford Women's Cancer Program, as well as the support of our colleagues, Beverly Mitchell, the Director of the Stanford Cancer Center, and Dean Philip Pizzo of the Stanford University School of Medicine. In Sydney, we acknowledge the support of our Gynaecological Oncology (GO) Research Committee, especially Aleco Vrisakis, our Chairman, and Carmen Duncan, our Fund Raising Coordinator. At both institutions, the enduring support of our benefactors has been critical to our gynecologic oncology research and clinical programs.

Our book is written primarily for gynecologic oncologists and fellows undertaking training in gynecologic oncology and consultant gynecologists, as well as medical oncologists and radiation oncologists whose practices involve a significant component of gynecologic cancer care.

We offer this book to those who strive to improve the care of women with gynecologic malignancies.

Jonathan S. Berek

Neville F. Hacker

Contributors

Spencer R. Adams, MD

Assistant Clinical Professor
Department of Medicine
David Geffen School of Medicine at UCLA
Los Angeles, California
Santa Monica-UCLA and Orthopedic Hospital
Santa Monica, California

Barbara L. Anderson, PhD

Professor
Department of Psychology and Obstetrics and Gynecology
The Ohio State University
Columbus, Ohio

Walter F. Baile, MD

Professor
Department of Behavioral Science and Psychiatry
Psychiatrist and Director
Program for Interpersonal Communication and
    Relationship Enhancement (I*CARE)
Faculty Development
M.D. Anderson Cancer Center
University of Texas
Houston, Texas

Andrew Berchuck, MD

Professor and Director
Division of Gynecologic Oncology
Department of Obstetrics and Gynecology
Duke University School of Medicine
Durham, North Carolina

Ross S. Berkowitz, MD

William H. Baker Professor of Gynecology
Department of Obstetrics and Gynecology
Harvard Medical School
Director of Gynecologic Oncology
Co-Director, New England Trophoblastic Disease Center
Brigham and Women's Hospital
Dana Farber Cancer Institute
Boston, Massachusetts

Carlos A. Brun, MD

Department of Anesthesia
Stanford University School of Medicine
Stanford, California

Robert Buckman, MBBS, PhD

Professor
Department of Medicine
University of Toronto
Medical Oncologist, Consultant in Education
    and Communication
Princess Margaret Hospital
Toronto, Ontario

Michael Campion, MD

Director of Preinvasive Disease
Gynaecological Cancer Centre
Royal Hospital for Women
Randwick, New South Wales, Australia

Kristen M. Carpenter, PhD

Postdoctoral Fellow
Department of Psychology
The Ohio State University
Columbus, Ohio

Daniel W. Cramer, MD

Professor
Department of Obstetrics, Gynecology and
    Reproductive Biology
Harvard Medical School
Brigham and Women's Hospital
Boston, Massachusetts

Oliver Dorigo, MD, PhD

Assistant Professor
Division of Gynecologic Oncology
Department of Obstetrics and Gynecology
David Geffen School of Medicine at UCLA
Los Angeles, California

Maurize L. Druzin, MD

Charles B. and Ann L. Johnson Professor and Chief
Division of Maternal Fetal Medicine
Department of Obstetrics and Gynecology
Stanford University School of Medicine
Chief of Obstetrics
Lucile Packard Children's Hospital
Stanford, California

Patricia J. Eifel, MD

Professor
Department of Radiation Oncology
MD Anderson Cancer Center
University of Texas
Houston, Texas

Michael L. Friedlander MBChB, PhD

Conjoint Professor of Medicine
University of New South Wales
Director of Medical Oncology
The Prince of Wales Hospital
Randwick, Sydney, Australia

Donald P. Goldstein, MD

Professor of Obstetrics, Gynecology and
    Reproductive Medicine
Department of Obstetrics and Gynecology
Harvard Medical School
Senior Scientist
Brigham and Women's Hospital
Boston, Massachusetts

Richard Grady, MD

Associate Professor
Department of Urology
The University of Washington
Fellowship Program Director
Department of Surgery and Urology
Seattle Children's Hospital
Seattle, Washington

Armando E. Giuliano, MD

Chief of Science and Medicine
Department of Breast and Endocrine
John Wayne Cancer Institute
Director, John Wayne Cancer Institute Breast Center
Saint John's Health Center
Santa Monica, California

Kenneth D. Hatch, MD

Professor
Department of Obstetrics and Gynecology
University of Arizona School of Medicine
University Medical Center
Tucson, Arizona

Michael R. Hendrickson, MD

Professor
Department of Pathology
Stanford University School of Medicine
Director of Surgical Pathology
Stanford Hospital and Clinics
Stanford, California

Amreen Husain, MD

Associate Professor and Associate Director
Division of Gynecologic Oncology
Department of Obstetrics and Gynecology
Stanford University School of Medicine
Stanford Cancer Center
Stanford, California

Ian Jacobs, MBBS, MD

Dean and Professor
Faculty of Biomedical Sciences
University College London
Department of Gynaecological Oncology
Institute for Women's Health
Consultant, Gynaecological Oncology
University College Hospital London
London, England, United Kingdom

Margrit Juretzka, MD, MS

Assistant Professor
Division of Gynecologic Oncology
Department of Obstetrics and Gynecology
Stanford University School of Medicine
Stanford Cancer Center
Stanford, California

Christina S. Kong, MD

Associate Professor
Department of Pathology
Stanford University School of Medicine
Director of Cytopathology
Stanford Hospital and Clinics
Stanford, California

Laura Kruper, MD

Assistant Professor
Department of General and Oncologic Surgery
Breast Cancer Surgeon
Women's Health Center
City of Hope National Medical Center
Duarte, California

Roger M. Lee, MD

Assistant Clinical Professor
Department of Internal Medicine
David Geffen School of Medicine at UCLA
Los Angeles, California
Santa Monica-UCLA and Orthopedic
    Medical Center
Santa Monica, California

Anna O. Levin, BA

Graduate Research Associate
Department of Psychology
The Ohio State University
Columbus, Ohio

J. Norelle Lickiss, MD

Clinical Professor
Central Clinical School Sydney Medical School
University of Sydney
Senior Staff Specialist
Department of Palliative Care
Royal Prince Alfred Hospital
Sydney, New South Wales, Australia

Teri A. Longacre, MD

Professor
Department of Pathology
Stanford University School of Medicine
Associate Director of Surgical Pathology
Stanford Hospital and Clinics
Stanford, California

Maurie Markman, MD

Vice President for Clinical Research
M.D. Anderson Cancer Center
University of Texas
Houston, Texas

Ranjit Manchanda, MBBS

Clinical Research Fellow
Department of Gynaecological Oncology
Gynaecological Cancer Research Centre
Institute for Women's Health
University College London
London, England, United Kingdom

Otoniel Martínez-Maza, PhD

Professor
Department of Obstetrics and Gynecology, and
Microbiology, Immunology & Molecular Genetics
David Geffen School of Medicine at UCLA
Los, Angeles, California

Larry G. Maxwell, MD

Professor
Department of Obsterics and Gynecology
Uniformed Service University
Bethesda, Maryland
Chief, Division of Gynecology
Walter Reed Army Medical Center
Washington, DC

Usha Menon, MD

Head, Gynaecological Cancer Research Centre
Department of Gynaecological Oncology
Gynaecological Cancer Research Centre
Institute for Women's Health
University College London
Consultant Gynaecologist
University College London
London, England, United Kingdom

Jennifer A. M. Philip, PhD, MMed, MBBS

Deputy Director
Centre for Palliative Care Education & Research
Collaborative Centre of the University of Melbourne
Deputy Director, Palliative Medicine
Department of Medicine
St. Vincent's Hospital
Fitzroy, Victoria, Australia

Norman W. Rizk, MD

Berthold and Bell N. Guggenhime Professor in Medicine
Senior Dean of Clinical Affairs
Stanford University School of Medicine
Stanford, California

Samuel A. Skootsky, MD

Professor
Department of Medicine
David Geffen School of Medicine at UCLA
Los Angeles, California

Iain M. Smith, MD

Assistant Clinical Professor
Department of Medicine
David Geffen School of Medicine at UCLA
Los Angeles, California

Anil K. Sood, MD

Professor
Department of Gynecologic Oncology and
  Cancer Biology
M.D. Anderson Cancer Center
University of Texas
Houston, Texas

Contents

Section I
General Principles

GENERAL PRINCIPLES

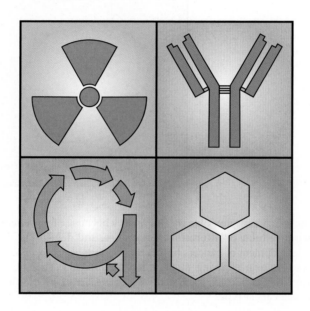

1

Biology and Genetics

G. Larry Maxwell
Anil Sood
Andrew Berchuck

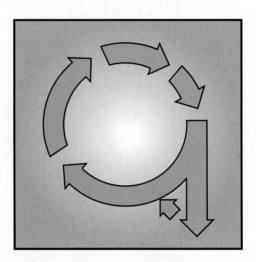

Cancer is a complex disease that arises because of genetic and epigenetic alterations that disrupt cellular proliferation, senescence, and death (Fig. 1.1). The alterations that underlie the development of cancers have a diverse etiology, and loss of DNA repair mechanisms often plays a role in allowing mutations to accumulate. Specific molecular changes that cause a normal cell to become malignant have been identified, but their spectrum varies considerably between cancer types.

The malignant phenotype is also characterized by its ability to invade surrounding tissues and metastasize. The development of a cancer elicits a considerable molecular response in the local microenvironment that is characterized by recruitment of stromal elements such as new blood vessels and by an active immunological response. These secondary events play a critical role in the evolution and progression of cancers. Although the molecular pathogenesis of gynecologic cancers has been only partially elucidated, advances in the understanding of these diseases are providing the opportunity for improvements in diagnosis, treatment, and prevention.

The initial sections of this chapter will outline what is known regarding the basic molecular mechanisms involved in the development of cancers and the evolution of the malignant phenotype. The molecular alterations characteristic of gynecologic cancers will be outlined in the latter sections.

Growth Regulation

Proliferation

The number of cells in normal tissues is tightly regulated by a balance between cellular proliferation and death. The final common pathway for cell division involves distinct molecular switches that control cell cycle progression from G_1 to the S phase of DNA synthesis. These include the retinoblastoma (*Rb*) and E2F proteins and their various regulatory cyclins, cyclin-dependent kinases (cdks), and cdk inhibitors. Likewise, the events that facilitate progression from G_2 to mitosis and cell division are regulated by other cyclins and cdks (Fig. 1.2).

In some tissues—such as the bone marrow, epidermis, and gastrointestinal tract—the life span of mature cells is relatively short, and high rates of proliferation by progenitor cells are required to maintain the population. In other tissues—such as liver, muscle, and brain—cells are long lived, and proliferation rarely occurs. Complex molecular mechanisms have evolved to closely

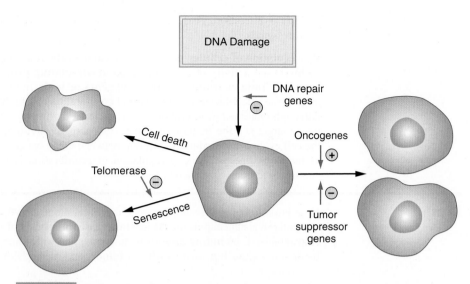

Figure 1.1 Role of proliferation, cell death, senescence, and DNA damage in cancer development.

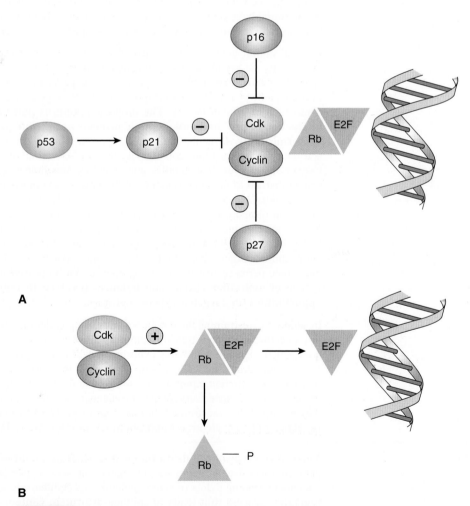

A

B

Figure 1.2 Regulation of cell cycle arrest in G₁ by cyclin-dependent kinase (cdk) inhibitors. (A) cell cycle arrest (B) cell cycle progression.

regulate proliferation. These involve a finely tuned balance between stimulatory and inhibitory growth signals.

Dysregulation of cellular proliferation is one of the main hallmarks of cancer. There may be increased activity of genes involved in stimulating proliferation (oncogenes) or loss of growth inhibitory (tumor suppressor) genes or both. In the past, it was thought that cancer might arise solely because of more rapid proliferation or a higher fraction of proliferating cells. Although increased proliferation is a characteristic of many cancers and is an appealing therapeutic target (1), the fraction of cancer cells actively dividing and the time required to transit the cell cycle is not strikingly different between many cancers and corresponding normal cells of the same lineage. Altered regulation of proliferation is only one of several factors that contribute to malignant transformation.

Cell Death

In addition to being driven by increased proliferation, growth of a cancer may be attributable to cellular resistance to death. **At least three distinct types of cell death pathways have been characterized, including apoptosis, necrosis, and autophagy** (2). **All three pathways may be ongoing simultaneously within a tumor**, and methods that distinguish between them are far from perfect.

Apoptosis

The term *apoptosis* derives from Greek and alludes to a process akin to leaves dying and falling off a tree. Apoptosis is an active, energy-dependent process that involves cleavage of the DNA by endonucleases and proteins by proteases called *caspases*. Morphologically, apoptosis is characterized by condensation of chromatin, nuclear and cytoplasmic blebbing, and cellular shrinkage. The molecular events that affect apoptosis in response to various stimuli are complex and have only been partially elucidated (3), but several reliable markers of apoptosis have been discovered including annexin V, caspase-3 activation, and DNA fragmentation (4).

External stimuli such as tumor necrosis factor, tumor necrosis factor-related apoptosis-inducing ligand, fatty acid synthase (Fas), and other death ligands that interact with cell surface receptors can induce activation of caspases and lead to apoptosis via an extrinsic pathway (Fig. 1.3). The intrinsic pathway is activated in response to a wide range of stresses including DNA damage and deprivation of growth factors. **The intrinsic apoptosis pathway is regulated by a complex interaction of pro- and antiapoptotic proteins in the mitochondrial membrane that affect its permeability.** Proteins that increase permeability allow release of cytochrome c, which activates the apoptosome complex leading to activation of caspases that affect apoptosis. Conversely, proteins that stabilize mitochondrial membranes inhibit apoptosis. The first major insight that led to the understanding of the intrinsic apoptosis pathway was the finding that an activating translocation of the *bcl-2* gene in B-cell lymphomas results in essentially complete inhibition of apoptosis (5). Subsequent studies demonstrated that the antiapoptotic effect of *bcl-2* is attributable to stabilization of the mitochondrial membrane. Additional genes related to *bcl-2* (such as *BAD, BCL-XL,* and others) also block apoptosis by inhibiting membrane permeability. Other genes in the *BCL* family (such as *BAX, BAK,* and others) increase membrane permeability and are proapoptotic. **An increased understanding of the complex system of molecular checks and balances involved in regulation of apoptosis provides opportunities for targeted cancer therapies;** several strategies are under development (6).

In addition to restraining the number of cells in a population, apoptosis serves an important role in preventing malignant transformation by allowing the elimination of cells that have undergone genetic damage. Following exposure of cells to mutagenic stimuli, including radiation and carcinogenic drugs, the cell cycle is arrested so that DNA damage may be repaired. If DNA repair is not sufficient, apoptosis occurs so that damaged cells do not survive (Fig. 1.1). This serves as an anticancer surveillance mechanism by which mutated cells are eliminated before they become fully transformed. In this regard, **the *TP53* tumor suppressor gene is a critical regulator of cell cycle arrest and apoptosis in response to DNA damage.**

Necrosis

Necrosis is a type of cell death that is distinct from apoptosis and is the result of bioenergetic compromise (4). Morphologic changes include swollen organelles and rupture of the cell membrane, leading to loss of osmoregulation and cellular fragmentation. **Necrosis is a less well regulated process that leads to spillage of protein contents, and this may incite a brisk immune response.** This is in contrast to the silent elimination of cells by apoptosis, which typically elicits a minimal immune response. There is evidence that some drugs may enhance necrotic death in tumors, and this may stimulate a beneficial antitumor immune response.

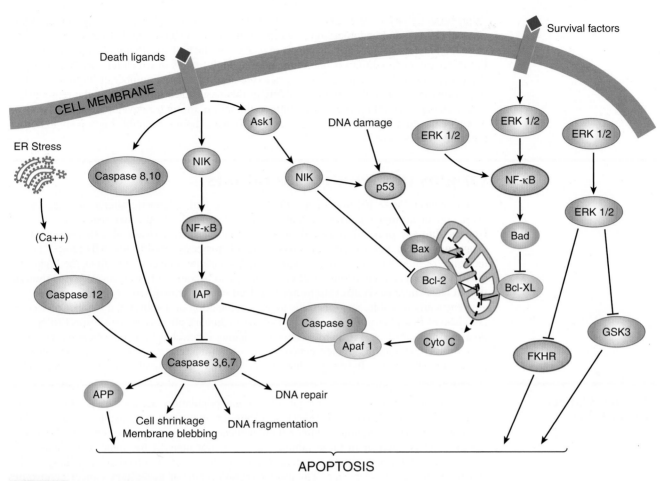

Figure 1.3 Apoptosis pathways.

Autophagy

Autophagy is a potentially reversible process in which a cell that is stressed "eats" itself (4). A wide range of stresses have been identified that may elicit autophagy (some of which may also elicit apoptosis), including growth factor deprivation and accumulation of reactive oxygen species. Unlike necrosis and apoptosis—in which loss of integrity of the cytoplasmic and nuclear membranes, respectively, are defining events—**autophagy is characterized by the formation of cytoplasmic autophagic vesicles into which cellular proteins and organelles are sequestered.** This may allow for cell survival if damaged organelles can be repaired. Conversely, the process may lead to cell death if these vesicles fuse with lysosomes with resultant degradation of their contents. Several cancer therapeutic agents have been shown to induce autophagy, while targeted disruption of genes such as *ATG5* that are involved in autophagy can inhibit cell death (4).

Cellular Senescence

Normal cells are only capable of undergoing division a finite number of times before becoming senescent. Cellular senescence is regulated by a biological clock related to progressive shortening of repetitive DNA sequences (TTAGGG) called **telomeres** that cap the ends of each chromosome. Telomeres are thought to be involved in chromosomal stabilization and in preventing recombination during mitosis. At birth, chromosomes have long telomeric sequences (150,000 bases) that become progressively shorter by 50 to 200 bases each time a cell divides. **Telomeric shortening is the molecular clock that triggers senescence** (Fig. 1.1). Malignant cells often avoid senescence by turning on expression of telomerase activity to prevent telomeric shortening (7). Telomerase is a ribonucleoprotein complex, and both the protein and RNA subunits have been identified. The RNA component serves as a template for telomeric extension, and the protein subunit catalyzes the synthesis of new telomeric repeats.

Telomerase activity is detectable in a high fraction of many cancers, including ovarian (8,9), cervical (10,11), and endometrial cancers (12). It has been suggested that detection of telomerase might be useful for early diagnosis of cancer, but lack of specificity is a significant issue. In this regard, endometrium is one of the normal adult tissues in which telomerase expression is most common (13). Perhaps this relates to the need for a large number of lifetime cell divisions because of rapid growth and shedding of this tissue each month during the reproductive years. Therapeutic approaches to inhibiting telomerase are under development that focus on reversing the immortalized state of cancer cells to make them susceptible once again to normal replicative senescence (7).

Origins of Genetic Alterations

Human cancers arise because of a series of genetic and epigenetic alterations that lead to disruption of normal mechanisms that govern cell growth, death, and senescence (14,15). **Genetic damage may be inherited or arise after birth as a result of either exposure to exogenous carcinogens or endogenous mutagenic processes within the cell** (Table 1.1). The incidence of most cancers increases with aging because the longer one is alive, the higher the likelihood that a cell will acquire sufficient damage to become fully transformed. **It is thought that at least three to six alterations are required to fully transform a cell.** Most cancer cells are genetically unstable, and this leads to an accumulation of a substantial number of secondary changes that play a role in evolution of the malignant phenotype with respect to growth, invasion, metastasis, and response to therapy, among other characteristics. Genetic instability also results in evolution of heterogeneous clones within a tumor. There is some evidence that progenitor cells (stem cells) exist within a tumor that may be relatively resistant to therapy (16).

Inherited Cancer Susceptibility

Although most cancers arise sporadically in the population because of acquired genetic damage, inherited mutations in cancer susceptibility genes are responsible for some cases. Families with these mutations exhibit a high incidence of specific types of cancers. The age of cancer onset is younger in these families, and it is not unusual for some individuals to be affected with multiple primary cancers. Many of the genes involved in hereditary cancer syndromes have been identified. **The most common forms of hereditary cancer syndromes predispose to breast or ovarian (*BRCA1, BRCA2*) and colon or endometrial (*HNPCC* genes) cancers** (Table 1.2). Examples of other hereditary cancer syndromes are also outlined in Table 1.2.

Tumor suppressor genes have been implicated most frequently in hereditary cancer syndromes, followed by DNA repair genes. In only a few instances are germ-line mutations in oncogenes responsible for hereditary cancers. Although affected individuals carry the germ-line alteration in every cell of their bodies, paradoxically, cancer susceptibility genes are characterized

Table 1.1 Origins of Genetic Damage in Human Cancers	
Type of Genetic Damage	*Examples*
Hereditary	
High-penetrance genes	*BRCA1, BRCA2, MLH1, MSH2*
Low-penetrance genes	*APC* I1307K in colorectal cancer
Exogenous Carcinogens	
Ultraviolet radiation	*TP53* and other genes in skin cancer
Tobacco	*K-ras* and *TP53* in lung cancer
Endogenous DNA Damage	
Cytosine methylation and deamination	*TP53* in ovarian and other cancers
Hydrolysis	Various genes
Spontaneous errors in DNA synthesis	Various genes
Oxidative stress with free radical damage	Various genes

Table 1.2 Hereditary Cancer Syndromes

Syndrome	Genes	Predominant Cancers
Cancer Types in Which Hereditary Syndromes Are Common		
Hereditary breast or ovarian cancer	*BRCA1, BRCA2*	Breast, ovary
Hereditary colorectal cancer	*HNPCC, MSH2, MLH1, PMS1, PMS2, MSH6*	Colon, endometrium, other GI tract, ovary
Familial adenomatous polyposis	*APC*	Colonic polyps and cancers
Familial melanoma	*CMM1, CMM2, CDK4, CDKN2 (p16)*	Melanoma
Rare Hereditary Cancer Syndromes		
Li-Fraumeni syndrome	*TP53*	Sarcomas, leukemias, breast, brain, and others
Wilm's tumor	*WT1*	Kidney
von Hippel-Lindau	*VHL*	Kidney and others
Neurofibromatosis	*NF1, NF2*	Neurofibromas
Retinoblastoma	*Rb*	Retinoblastoma, sarcomas
Multiple-endocrine neoplasia 1	*MEN1*	Thyroid, adrenal, pancreas, pituitary, parathyroid
Multiple-endocrine neoplasia 2	*ret**	Thyroid, adrenal, parathyroid
Hereditary papillary renal cancer	*met**	Papillary kidney

*Oncogenes

by a limited repertoire of cancers. In addition, there is no relationship between expression patterns of these genes in various organs and the development of specific types of cancers. For example, *BRCA1* expression is high in the testis, but men who inherit mutations in this gene are not predisposed to develop testicular cancer. The penetrance of cancer susceptibility genes is incomplete because all individuals who inherit a mutation do not develop cancer. The emergence of cancers in carriers depends on the occurrence of additional genetic alterations.

The familial cancer syndromes described above result from rare mutations that occur in less than 1% of the population. In addition, low-penetrance common genetic polymorphisms may also affect cancer susceptibility, albeit less dramatically (17). There are more than ten million polymorphic genetic loci in the human genome. Many of these polymorphisms are common, with the rarer allele occurring in more than 5% of individuals.

Although genetic polymorphisms would not be expected to increase risk sufficiently to produce familial cancer clustering, they could account for a significant fraction of cancers currently classified as sporadic because of their relatively high prevalence. For example, 6% of Ashkenazi Jews carry the rare allele of the I1307K polymorphism in the *APC* gene, which increases the risk of colorectal cancer by about 50% (18). The recent development of genomic technologies that can assess thousands of polymorphisms simultaneously in large numbers of individuals is fueling the search for additional genetic susceptibility polymorphisms. A more complete understanding of the genetic factors that affect cancer susceptibility could facilitate implementation of screening and prevention approaches in subsets of the population at increased risk.

Acquired Genetic Damage

The etiology of acquired genetic damage seen in cancers also has been elucidated to some extent. For example, a strong causal link exists between cigarette smoke and cancers of the aerodigestive tract and between ultraviolet radiation and skin cancer. **For many common forms of cancer** (colon, breast, endometrium, ovary) **a strong association with specific carcinogens does not exist.** It is thought that the genetic alterations responsible for these cancers may arise mainly because of endogenous mutagenic processes such as methylation, deamination, and hydrolysis of DNA. In addition, spontaneous errors in DNA synthesis may occur during the process of DNA replication associated with normal proliferation. Likewise, free radicals generated in response to inflammation and other cellular damage may cause DNA damage. These endogenous processes produce many mutations each day in every cell in the body. **Several families of highly effective DNA damage surveillance and repair genes exist, but some mutations may elude them.** The efficiency of these DNA damage-response systems varies between individuals because of genetic and other factors and may affect susceptibility to cancer.

Epigenetic Changes

Epigenetics changes are heritable changes that do not result from alterations in DNA sequence (15). Methylation of cytosine residues that reside next to guanine residues is the primary mechanism of epigenetic regulation, and this process is regulated by a family of DNA methyltransfereases. **Most cancers have globally reduced DNA methylation, which may contribute to genomic instability.** Conversely, selective hypermethylation of cytosines in the promoter regions of tumor suppressor genes may lead to their inactivation, and this may contribute to carcinogenesis.

There is a family of **imprinted genes** in which either the maternal or paternal copy is normally completely silenced because of methylation. Loss of imprinting in genes that stimulate proliferation, such as *insulin-like growth factor 2* (**IGF2**), may provide an oncogenic stimulus by increasing proliferation.

Acetylation and methylation of the histone proteins that coat DNA represent another level of epigenetic regulation that is altered in cancer. The underlying cause of these epigenetic alterations remains poorly understood, but they may represent appealing therapeutic targets.

Oncogenes

Alterations in genes that stimulate cellular growth (oncogenes) can cause malignant transformation (14,15). Oncogenes can be activated via several mechanisms. In some cancers, amplification of oncogenes with resultant overexpression of the corresponding protein has been noted. Instead of two copies of one of these genes, there may be many more copies. Some oncogenes may become overactive when affected by point mutations. Finally, oncogenes may be translocated from one chromosomal location to another and then come under the influence of promoter sequences that cause overexpression of the gene. This latter mechanism frequently occurs in leukemias and lymphomas but not in gynecologic cancers or other solid tumors.

In cell culture systems in the laboratory, **many genes that are involved in normal growth regulatory pathways can elicit transformation to overactive forms when altered to overactive forms via amplification, mutation, or translocation.** On this basis, a large number of genes have been classified as oncogenes. Studies in human cancers have suggested that the actual spectrum of genes altered in the development of human cancers is more limited. A number of genes that elicit transformation when activated *in vitro* have not been documented to undergo alterations in human cancers. In this section, the various classes of oncogenes will be summarized and particular attention paid to those that are altered in gynecologic cancers.

Cell Membrane Oncogenes: Peptide Growth Factors and Their Receptors

Peptide growth factors—such as those of the epidermal growth factor (EGF), platelet-derived growth factor (PDGF), and fibroblast growth factor (FGF) families—stimulate a cascade of molecular events that leads to proliferation by binding to cell membrane receptors (Fig. 1.4). Growth factors are involved in normal cellular processes such as development, stromal–epithelial communication, tissue regeneration, and wound healing. **Growth factors in the extracellular space can stimulate a cascade of molecular events that leads to proliferation by binding to cell membrane receptors.** Unlike endocrine hormones, which are secreted into the blood stream and act in distant target organs, peptide growth factors typically act in the local environment where they have been secreted.

The concept that autocrine growth stimulation may be a key strategy by which cancer cell proliferation becomes autonomous has received considerable attention. In this model, it is postulated that cancers secrete stimulatory growth factors that then interact with receptors on the same cell. Although peptide growth factors provide a growth stimulatory signal, **there is little evidence to suggest that overproduction of growth factors is a precipitating event in the development of most cancers.** Increased expression of peptide growth factors likely serves in most cases as a cofactor rather than as the driving force behind malignant transformation.

Cell membrane receptors that bind peptide growth factors are composed of an extracellular ligand-binding domain, a membrane spanning region, and a cytoplasmic tyrosine

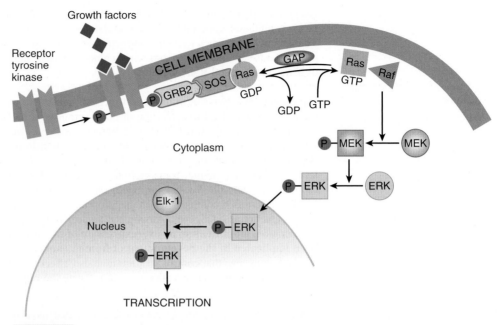

Figure 1.4   Mitogenic signal transduction pathways.

kinase domain (19). Binding of a growth factor to the extracellular domain results in aggregation and conformational shifts in the receptor and activation of the inner tyrosine kinase. This kinase phosphorylates tyrosine residues both on the growth factor receptor itself (**autophosphorylation**) and on molecular targets in the cell interior, leading to activation of secondary signals.

Growth of some cancers is driven by overexpression of receptor tyrosine kinases receptors. Therapeutic strategies that target receptor tyrosine kinases have been an active area of investigation. *Trastuzumab* is a monoclonal antibody that **blocks the HER-2/*neu* receptor,** and it is widely used in the treatment of breast cancers that overexpress this tyrosine kinase (20). *Cetuximab* is a monoclonal antibody that targets the epidermal growth factor receptor (EGFR), whereas *gefitinib* **is a direct inhibitor of the EGFR tyrosine kinase** (21). *Lapatinib* **is a dual EGFR/HER-2 kinase inhibitor.** *Imatinib* **antagonizes the activity of the BCR-ABL, c-kit, and PDGF receptor tyrosine kinases** and has proven effective in treatment of chronic myelogenous leukemias and gastrointestinal stromal tumors.

Intracellular Oncogenes

Following the interaction of peptide growth factors and their receptors, secondary molecular signals are generated to transmit the growth stimulus to the nucleus (Fig. 1.4). This function is served by a multitude of complex and overlapping signal transduction pathways that occur in the inner cell membrane and cytoplasm. Many of these signals involve phosphorylation of proteins by enzymes known as **nonreceptor kinases** (22). **These kinases transfer a phosphate group from ATP to specific amino acid residues of target proteins. The kinases that are involved in growth regulation are of two types: those that are phosphorylate tyrosine residues on proteins, including those of the SRC family (23); and others that are specific for serine or threonine residues such as AKT (24). The activity of kinases is regulated by phosphatases such as** *PTEN***,** which act in opposition to the kinases by removing phosphates from the target proteins.

Guanosine-triphosphate–binding proteins (G proteins) represent another class of molecules involved in transmission of growth signals (Fig 1.4). They are located on the inner aspect of the cell membrane and have intrinsic GTPase activity that catalyzes the exchange of guanine-triphosphate (GTP) for guanine-diphosphate (GDP). In their active GTP-bound form, G proteins interact with kinases that are involved in relaying the mitogenic signal, such as those of the MAP kinase family. Conversely, hydrolysis of GTP to GDP, which is stimulated by GTPase-activating proteins (GAPs), leads to inactivation of G proteins. **The *ras* family of G proteins is among the most frequently mutated oncogenes in human cancers** (e.g., gastrointestinal and endometrial cancers). Activation of *ras* genes usually involves point mutations in codons 12, 13, or 61 that result in constitutively activated molecules. The *BRAF* gene encodes a kinase that interacts with *ras* proteins in activating the MAP kinase pathway. *BRAF* mutations occur in many cancers that lack *ras* mutations, and most of these mutations involve codon 599 in the kinase domain (25). Therapeutic approaches to interfering with *ras* signaling are being developed, including farnesyltransferase inhibitors that block attachment of *ras* to the inner cell membrane, antisense oligonucleotides, and RNA interference (26).

Nuclear Oncogenes

If proliferation is to occur in response to signals generated in the cell membrane and cytoplasm, these events must lead to activation of nuclear transcription factors and other genetic products responsible for stimulating DNA replication and cell division. **Expression of several genes that encode nuclear proteins increases dramatically within minutes of treatment of cells with peptide growth factors.** Once induced, the products of these genes bind to specific DNA regulatory elements and induce transcription of genes involved in DNA synthesis and cell division. Examples include the *fos* and *jun* oncogenes, which dimerize to form the activator protein 1 (AP1) transcription complex. When inappropriately overexpressed, however, these transcription factors can act as oncogenes. Among the nuclear transcription factors involved in stimulating proliferation, **amplification or overexpression of members of the *myc* family has most often been implicated in the development of human cancers** (27). Many of the nuclear regulatory genes such as *myc* that control proliferation also affect the threshold for apoptosis. Thus, there is overlap in the molecular pathways that regulate the opposing processes of proliferation and apoptosis.

Genes involved in chromatin remodeling also that have been implicated as oncogenes, but primarily in hematologic malignancies rather than solid tumors. Finally, as discussed previously, genes encoding nuclear proteins that inhibit apoptosis (e.g., *bcl-2*) can act as oncogenes when altered to constituitively active forms.

Tumor Suppressor Genes

Loss of tumor suppressor gene function also plays a role in the development of most cancers. This usually involves a two-step process in which both copies of a tumor suppressor gene are inactivated. In most cases, there is mutation of one copy of a tumor suppressor gene and loss of the other copy because of deletion of a segment of the chromosome where the gene resides. There is also evidence that some tumor suppressor genes may be inactivated because of methylation of the promoter region of the gene (15). The promoter is an area proximal to the coding sequence that regulates whether the gene is transcribed from DNA into RNA. When the promoter is methylated, it is resistant to activation, and the gene is essentially silenced despite remaining structurally intact.

This two-hit paradigm is relevant to both hereditary cancer syndromes, in which one mutation is inherited and the second acquired, and sporadic cancers, in which both hits are acquired. Tumor suppressor gene products are found throughout the cell, reflecting their diverse functions. With the recognition that inactivation of tumor suppressor genes is a defining feature of cancers, genetic therapy strategies have been developed that aim to deliver functional copies of these lost genes to cancer cells.

Nuclear Tumor Suppressor Genes

The retinoblastoma gene was the first tumor suppressor gene discovered (28). It was found in the context of a rare hereditary cancer syndrome, as have many other tumor suppressor genes (Table 1.2). **The *Rb* gene plays a key role in the regulation of cell cycle progression** (Fig. 1.2). In the G_1 phase of the cell cycle, *Rb* protein binds to the E2F transcription factor and prevents it from activating transcription of other genes involved in cell cycle progression. G_1 arrest is maintained by cyclin-dependent kinase inhibitors that prevent phosphorylation of *Rb*, such as *p16*, *p21*, and *p27* (29). When *Rb* is phosphorylated by cyclin–cdk complexes, E2F is released and stimulates entry into the DNA synthesis phase of the cell cycle. Other cyclins and cdks are involved in progression from G_2 to mitosis. **Mutations in the *Rb* gene have been noted primarily in retinoblastomas and sarcomas** but rarely in other types of cancers. By maintaining G_1 arrest, the cdk inhibitors *p16*, *p21*, *p27*, and others act as tumor suppressor genes. Loss of *p16* tumor suppressor function as a result of genomic deletion or promoter methylation occurs in some cancers, including familial melanomas. Likewise, loss of *p21* and *p27* has been noted in some cancers.

Mutation of the *TP53* tumor suppressor gene is the most frequent genetic event described thus far in human cancers (Fig. 1.5) (30,31). The *TP53* gene encodes a 393 amino acid protein that plays a central role in the regulation of both proliferation and apoptosis. In normal cells, p53 protein resides in the nucleus and exerts its tumor suppressor activity by

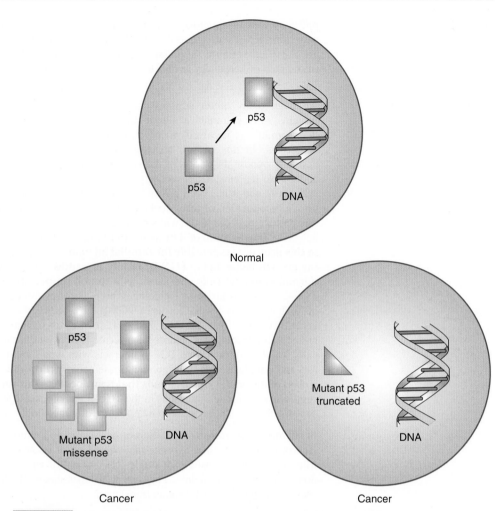

Normal

Mutant p53
missense

DNA

Cancer

Mutant p53
truncated

DNA

Cancer

Figure 1.5   Inactivation of the *p53* tumor suppressor gene by "dominant negative" missense mutation or by truncation mutation and deletion.

binding to transcriptional regulatory elements of genes, such as the cdk inhibitor *p21,* that act to arrest cells in G_1. The *MDM2* gene product degrades p53 protein when appropriate, whereas p14ARF down regulates *MDM2* when up regulation of p53 is needed to initiate cell cycle arrest.

Many cancers have missense mutations in one copy of the *TP53* gene that result in substitution of a single amino acid in exons 5 through 8, which encode the DNA binding domains (Fig 1.5). Although these mutant *TP53* genes encode full-length proteins, they are unable to bind to DNA and regulate transcription of other genes. Mutation of one copy of the *TP53* gene often is accompanied by deletion of the other copy, leaving the cancer cell with only mutant p53 protein. If the cancer cell retains one normal copy of the *TP53* gene, mutant p53 protein can complex with wild-type p53 protein and prevent it from oligimerizing and interacting with DNA. Because inactivation of both *TP53* alleles is not required for loss of p53 function, mutant p53 is said to act in a "dominant negative" fashion. Although normal cells have low levels of p53 protein because it is rapidly degraded, missense mutations encode protein products that are resistant to degradation. The resultant overaccumulation of mutant p53 protein in the nucleus can be detected immunohistochemically. A smaller fraction of cancers have mutations in the *TP53* gene that encode truncated protein products. In these cases, loss of the other allele occurs as the second event as is seen with other tumor suppressor genes.

Beyond simply inhibiting proliferation, normal p53 is thought to play a role in preventing cancer by stimulating apoptosis of cells that have undergone excessive genetic damage. In this regard, p53 has been described as the "guardian of the genome" because it delays entry into S phase until the genome has been cleansed of mutations. If DNA repair is inadequate, then p53 may initiate apoptosis, thereby eliminating cells with genetic damage. Likewise, other genes that repair damage to the DNA nucleotide sequence or strand breakage also sometimes are classified as tumor suppressors. These other genes will be discussed in the next sections in the context of hereditary gynecologic cancer syndromes.

Extranuclear Tumor Suppressor Genes

Although many tumor suppressor genes—including *TP53*, *Rb*, and *p16*—encode nuclear proteins, some extranuclear tumor suppressors have been identified. Theoretically, any protein that normally is involved in inhibition of proliferation has the potential to act as a tumor suppressor. In this regard, appealing candidates include phosphatases such as *PTEN* that normally oppose the action of the tyrosine kinases by dephosphorylating tyrosine residues. In addition to its phosphatase activity, *PTEN* is homologous to the cytoskeleton proteins tensin and auxin, and it has been postulated that *PTEN* might act to inhibit invasion and metastasis through modulation of the cytoskeleton. The *APC* tumor suppressor gene encodes a cytoplasmic protein involved in the wnt signaling pathway that regulates both cellular proliferation and adhesion. **Inactivation of *APC* leads to malignant transformation, and inherited mutations in this gene are responsible for familial adenomatous polyposis syndrome. The transforming growth factor-beta (TGF-β) family of peptide growth factors inhibit proliferation of normal epithelial cells and serve as a tumor suppressive pathway** (32). It is thought that TGF-β causes G_1 arrest by inducing expression of cyclin-dependent kinase inhibitors such as *p27*. Three closely related forms of TGF-β have been discovered that are encoded by separate genes (TGF-β1, TGF-β2, and TGF-β3). TGF-β is secreted from cells in an inactive form bound to a portion of its precursor molecule from which it must be cleaved to release biologically active TGF-β. Active TGF-β interacts with type I and type II cell surface TGF-β receptors and initiates serine or threonine kinase activity. **Prominent intracellular targets include a class of molecules called Smads that translocate to the nucleus and act as transcriptional regulators.** Although mutations in the TGF-β receptors and Smads have been reported in some cancers, this does not appear to be a feature of gynecologic cancers.

In addition to primary disregulation of oncogenes and tumor suppressor genes, altered expression of microRNAs that regulate the expression of these genes occurs in many cancers (33). MicroRNA genes consist of a single RNA strand of approximately 21 to 23 nucleotides that does not encode proteins. They bind to messenger RNAs that contain complementary sequences and can block protein translation.

Invasion and Metastasis

Metastasis is a process by which cancer cells spread from the primary tumor to distant sites (34). Cancer metastasis can proceed only if a series of sequential steps are completed, including proliferation, angiogenesis, invasion, embolism or circulation, transport, adherence in organs, adherence to vessel wall, and extravasation (Fig. 1.6) (34).

It has long been recognized that most types of cancer have an organ-specific pattern of metastasis. The propensity of various types of cancer to form metastases in specific organs was first proposed by Paget, who hypothesized that these patterns resulted from the "dependence of the seed (cancer cell) on the soil (the metastatic site)" (35). This hypothesis was suggested by the nonrandom pattern of metastasis. Paget concluded that metastases formed only when the seed and soil were compatible. **It is now appreciated at a molecular level that metastasis is dependent on a balance between stimulating factors from both the tumor and host cells *versus* inhibitory signals.** To produce metastasis, the balance must be weighted toward the stimulatory signals.

Cancer progression is a product of an evolving crosstalk between different cell types within the tumor and its surrounding supporting tissue, the tumor stroma (36). The tumor stroma contains a specific extracellular matrix as well as cellular components such as fibroblasts, immune and inflammatory cells, and blood-vessel cells. The interactive signaling between tumor and stroma contributes to the formation of a complex multicellular organ. The organ microenvironment can markedly change the gene-expression patterns of cancer cells and therefore their behavior and growth potential (36). Recent studies regarding chemokines and their receptors provide important clues regarding why some cancers metastasize to specific organs. For example, **breast cancer cells frequently express chemokine receptors CXCR4**

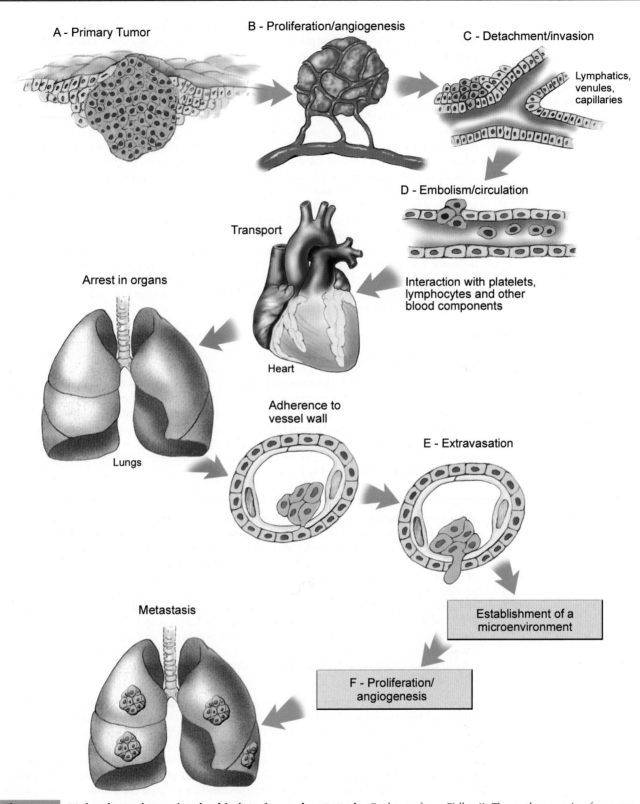

A - Primary Tumor

B - Proliferation/angiogenesis

C - Detachment/invasion

Lymphatics,
venules,
capillaries

D - Embolism/circulation

Transport

Interaction with platelets,
lymphocytes and other
blood components

Arrest in organs

Heart

Lungs

Adherence to
vessel wall

E - Extravasation

Establishment of a
microenvironment

Metastasis

F - Proliferation/
angiogenesis

Figure 1.6   **Molecular pathways involved in invasion and metastasis.** Redrawn from Fidler IJ. The pathogenesis of cancer metastasis: the "seed and soil" hypothesis revisited. *Nature Reviews Cancer* 2003;3:453–458.

and CCR7 at high levels. The specific ligands for these receptors, CXCL12 and CCL 21, are found at high levels in lymph nodes, lung, liver, and bone marrow, which are common sites for breast cancer metastasis.

Angiogenesis

All cells require oxygen and other nutrients for survival and growth, and cells must reside within 100 μm of a capillary in order to receive oxygen (37). Therefore, growth of new vessels, termed *angiogenesis,* is required for sustained malignant growth beyond approximately 1 mm in diameter. **Angiogenesis occurs as a result of a shift in balance toward proangiogenic factors within the tumor microenvironment** along with down regulation of antiangiogenic influences. **One of the primary mediators of angiogenesis is vascular endothelial growth factor A (VEGF-A)** (38), which increases vascular permeability, stimulates endothelial cell proliferation and migration, and promotes endothelial cell survival (39). **Other mediators of angiogenesis include tumor-derived factors and host stromal factors including interleukin-8, alpha v-beta 3 integrin, the tyrosine kinase receptor EphA2, and matrix metalloproteinases** (40). From a translational perspective, patient-specific tumor microenvironmental characteristics may influence the response to antiangiogenic therapy (41). **Antiangiogenesis therapies such as *Bevicizumab* that target the VEGF pathway are showing promise in ovarian cancer** and have already entered phase III clinical trials (40). Approaches targeting additional angiogenic pathways are also under clinical development.

Invasion

A critical first step in metastasis, and the primary feature that defines malignancy, **is invasion through the basement membrane.** This requires interplay between cancer cells and a permissive underlying stroma (42). Invasion of malignant cells through the basement membrane and endothelial cell migration for angiogenesis require degradation of the extracellular matrix. **This process is facilitated by a group of enzymes called matrix metalloproteinases (MMPs),** which are a family of zinc-dependent endopeptidases that digest collagen and other extracellular matrix components. They also stimulate proliferation and induce release of VEGF. **Ovarian tumors overexpress MMP-2 and MMP-9, and this increased expression correlates with aggressive clinical features** (43).

Adhesion

Tumor cell adhesion to the extracellular matrix within tissues greatly influences the ability of a malignant cell to invade and metastasize (44). **Given the shedding nature of ovarian cancer, adhesion molecules such as focal adhesion kinase, integrins, and E-cadherin have been evaluated for their role in peritoneal metastasis** (45). The proteins of the extracellular matrix consist of type I and IV collagens, laminins, heparin sulfate proteoglycan, fibronectin, and other noncollagenous glycoproteins (46). Cell adhesion to these proteins is mediated in part by a group of heterodimeric transmembrane proteins called *integrins,* which are composed of a noncovalently associated α and β subunit that define the integrin–ligand specificity (47). Approximately 18 β subunits and eight α subunits have been identified, and at least 24 receptor combinations exist (48). The intracellular domains of integrins interact with cytoskeletal components and are actively involved in generating intracellular signals.

Cadherins are another group of cell–cell adhesion molecules that are involved in development and maintenance of solid tissues. E-cadherins are the subgroup predominantly found in epithelial cells (49). These transmembrane proteins mediate cell–cell adhesion: Cadherins on neighboring cells preferentially bind to the same types of cadherins on adjacent cells. **E-cadherin is uniformly expressed in ovarian cancer, in low–malignant-potential tumors, in benign neoplasms, and—notably—in inclusion cysts of normal ovaries, but not in the normal surface epithelium** (50). Cadherin dysfunction is associated with loss of cell–cell cohesion, altered cellular motility, and increased invasiveness and metastatic potential. Changes in the composition of the cadherin–catenin complex, phosphorylation of components in the complex, and alterations in the interactions with the actin cytoskeleton have all been suggested as playing a role in regulating adhesion.

E-cadherin mutations occur only rarely (51), but cadherin expression may also be down regulated in the absence of mutations. **The cytoplasmic tails of cadherins exist as a macromolecular**

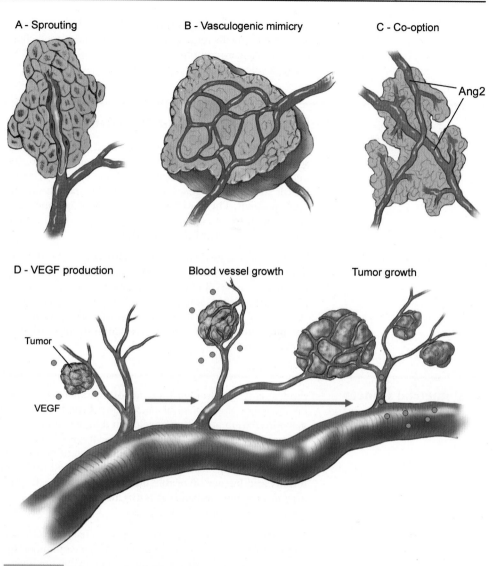

A - Sprouting

B - Vasculogenic mimicry

C - Co-option

Ang2

D - VEGF production

Blood vessel growth

Tumor growth

Tumor

VEGF

Figure 1.7   **The wnt signaling pathway.** Redrawn from Spannuth WA, Sood AK, Coleman RL. Angiogenesis as a strategic target for ovarian cancer therapy. *Nature Clinical Practice Oncology* 2008;5:194–204.

complex with β-catenin, which is involved in the wnt signaling pathways that regulate both adhesion and growth. Regulation of *β-catenin* activity also depends on the *APC* gene product and others in the wnt pathway (Fig. 1.7). Mutations in the *APC* gene that abrogate its ability to inhibit *β-catenin* activity are common in both the hereditary adenomatous polyposis coli syndrome and sporadic colon cancers (52). Likewise, mutations in the *β-catenin* gene that result in constitutively activated molecules also have been observed in some cancers, including endometrial cancers (53).

Tumor Microenvironment

Within the tumor microenvironment, other cell types also play a critical role in tumor growth and progression. For example, recent studies indicate that certain types of inflammatory cells, including macrophages and mast cells, and their associated cytokines confer an unfavorable prognosis and increased tumor growth. Conversely, the presence of an adaptive immune response characterized by cytotoxic T cells is associated with improved clinical outcome. In addition, cancer cells may evade immune recognition and destruction by various means, such as Fas ligand production to induce lymphocytice apoptosis and HLA-G secretion to inhibit natural-killer cell activity (54). Moreover, **cytokine production by cancer cells promotes**

growth and inhibits apoptosis. The mechanistic relationships between the microenvironment and tumor growth remain only partially understood, but immunomodulating strategies that target the cancer-promoting properties of both innate and adaptive immune cell populations are being developed.

Gynecologic Malignancies

Gynecologic cancers vary with respect to grade, histology, stage, response to treatment, and survival. It is now appreciated that this clinical heterogeneity is attributable to differences in underlying molecular pathogenesis. Some cancers arise in a setting of inherited mutations in cancer susceptibility genes, but most occur sporadically in the absence of a strong hereditary predisposition. **The spectrum of genes that are mutated varies between cancer types.** For each type of cancer, there are a few genes that are frequently mutated, while a wider spectrum are altered in a small fraction of cases (55).

There also is significant variety with respect to the spectrum of genetic changes within a given type of cancer. Cancers with a similar microscopic appearance may differ greatly at the molecular level. In some instances, molecular features may be predictive of clinical phenotypes such as stage, histologic type, and survival. As we gain a more complete understanding of the clinical implications of various genetic alterations in gynecologic cancers, **the molecular profile may prove valuable in predicting clinical behavior and response to treatment.**

Endometrial Cancer

Epidemiologic and clinical studies of endometrial cancer have suggested that there are two distinct types of endometrial cancer (56). **Type I cases are associated with unopposed estrogen stimulation and often develop in a background of endometrial hyperplasia.** Obesity is the most common cause of unopposed estrogen and is part of a metabolic syndrome that also includes insulin resistance and overexpression of insulin-like growth factors that may also play a role in carcinogenesis. **Type I cancers are well differentiated, endometrioid, early stage lesions and have a favorable outcome. In contrast, type II cancers are poorly differentiated or nonendometrioid (or both) and are more virulent.** They often present at an advanced stage, and survival is relatively poor.

In practice, not all cancers can be neatly characterized as either pure type I or II lesions, and endometrial cancers can also be viewed as a continuous spectrum with respect to etiology and clinical behavior. However, as the genetic events involved in the development of endometrial cancer have been elucidated, it has been found that specific alterations often, but not always, are seen primarily in either type I or II cases (Table 1.3).

Similar to other human cancers, endometrial cancers are believed to arise because of a series of genetic alterations. **A small minority of endometrial cancers occur in women with a strong hereditary predisposition because of germ-line mutations in DNA repair genes in the context of HNPCC syndrome.** A central unresolved issue in the understanding of endometrial carcinogenesis is the role of unopposed estrogenic stimulation. It has long been thought that estrogens may contribute to the development of endometrial cancer by virtue of their mitogenic effect on the endometrium. **A higher rate of proliferation in response to estrogens may lead to an increased frequency of spontaneous mutations.** In addition, when genetic damage occurs, regardless of the cause, the presence of estrogens may facilitate clonal expansion. It also has been postulated that estrogens may act as "complete carcinogens" that not only promote carcinogenesis by stimulating proliferation but also act as initiating agents by virtue of their carcinogenic metabolites. In contrast, **progestins oppose the action of estrogens by both down regulating estrogen receptor levels and decreasing proliferation and increasing apoptosis.**

Hereditary Endometrial Cancer

Approximately 3% to 5% of endometrial cancers arise because of inherited mutations in DNA repair genes in the context of hereditary nonpolyposis colon cancer (HNPCC) syndrome. HNPCC typically manifests as familial clustering of early onset colon cancer (57,58). There is also an increased incidence of several other types of cancers—most notably, endometrial cancer in women. The risk of ovarian, stomach, biliary tract, and other cancers also is

| Table 1.3 Characteristics of Type 1 versus Type 2 Endometrial Cancers |||
Clinical Features	Type 1	Type 2
BMI	Obese	Normal
Etiology	Unopposed estrogen	Sporadic
Precursor	Endometrial hyperplasia	None or *in situ* carcinoma
Histology	Endometrioid	Serous or clear cell
Grade	1, 2	2, 3
Stage	I, II	III, IV
Survival	Favorable	Poor
Molecular Features	Type 1	Type 2
TP53 mutation	Rare	>50%
HER-2/*neu*	Rare	>20%
PTEN mutation	>50%	Rare
β-catenin mutation	10–20%	Rare
PIK3CA mutation	>20%	Rare
K-ras mutation	10%	10%
MSI	20%	Rare
MLH1 methylation	20%	Rare

somewhat increased. The identification of the DNA mismatch repair genes responsible for HNPCC has facilitated the development of genetic testing (59). **Most HNPCC cases result from alterations in *MSH2* and *MLH1*. *MSH6*** mutations also are associated with an increased incidence of endometrial cancer (60). ***PMS1*** and ***PMS2*** have been implicated in a small number of these cancers as well. Loss of mismatch repair leads to a "mutator phenotype" in which genetic mutations accumulate throughout the genome, particularly in repetitive DNA sequences called **microsatellites.** Examples of microsatellite sequences include mono-, di-, and trinucleotide repeats (AAAA, CACACACA, and CAGCAGCAGCAG). **The propensity to accumulate mutations in microsatellite sequences is referred to as *microsatellite instability* (MSI).** Some microsatellite sequences are in noncoding areas of the genome, whereas others are within genes. It is thought that the accumulation of mutations in microsatellite sequences of tumor suppressor genes may inactivate them and accelerate the process of malignant transformation.

The Amsterdam and Bethesda criteria have been developed to provide clinical guidelines for the diagnosis of HNPCC based on the spectrum of cancers noted in a family. These criteria are inexact, and genetic testing should be considered in all families suspected of having HNPCC based on family history. Involvement of genetic counselors is useful in facilitating this process. **Analysis of cancers for microsatellite instability has been proposed as a genetic screening test for HNPCC. Among families with germ-line mutations in mismatch repair genes, MSI is seen in greater than 90% of colon cancers and approximately 75% of endometrial cancers** (61,62). However, MSI is found in 20% to 25% of endometrial cancers (63) and 15% to 20% of colorectal cancers overall (64), and most of these cases are attributable to silencing of the *MLH1* gene because of promoter methylation (65,66). **Another screening approach for HNPCC is immunohistochemical staining of tumors to determine where there has been a loss of MSH2 or MLH1 protein** (67). In cancers with MSI or loss of expression of one of the mismatch repair proteins, these genes can be sequenced to identify the disease-causing mutations, most of which cause truncated protein products. **Currently, mutational analysis of the responsible genes remains the gold standard for diagnosis of HNPCC** (59). Mutational analysis typically involves analysis of only *MSH2* and *MLH1,* which may overlook mutations in the other mismatch repair genes. Approximately half of families for which HNPCC is strongly suspected will be found to have a germ-line *MLH1* or *MSH2* mutation.

Endometrial cancer is the most common extracolonic malignancy is women with HNPCC. **The risk of a woman developing endometrial cancer has ranged from 20% to 60%** in various reports (68–70), and in some studies this exceeds the risk of colon cancer. In addition, **the risk of ovarian cancer is increased to approximately 5% to 12%.**

The most striking clinical feature of HNPCC-related cancers is early onset, typically at least ten years earlier than sporadic cases. The average age of women with sporadic endometrial cancers is in the early 60s, whereas cancers that arise in association with HNPCC are often diagnosed before the menopause (average age in the 40s) (68,71,72). The clinical features of HNPCC-associated endometrial cancers are similar to those of most sporadic cases (well differentiated, endometrioid, early stage), and survival is approximately 90% (71,73).

The mean age of onset of ovarian cancer in HNPCC families is in the early 40s, and the clinical features of these cancers generally are more favorable than sporadic cases (74). They are usually are early stage and well or moderately differentiated, and approximately 20% occur in the setting of synchronous endometrial cancers. However, **analysis of groups of patients with synchronous cancers of the ovary and endometrium has revealed that few of these exhibit microsatellite instability, and most probably are not attributable to HNPCC syndrome** (75).

The optimal strategy for prevention of HNPCC-associated mortality is unclear. Screening and surgical prophylaxis are both employed for colonic and extracolonic malignancies. Surveillance and prophylactic surgery should be considered early (between ages 25 and 35), generally ten years before the earliest onset of cancer in other relatives who had an HNPCC-related malignancy (72). **Transvaginal ultrasound has been proposed as a screening test for endometrial and ovarian cancer, but it appears to be relatively ineffective** (76). There is no evidence that CA125 or other blood markers facilitate early detection of endometrial cancer, but CA125 can be justified as a means of screening for HNPCC-associated ovarian cancer. **Endometrial biopsy may be the only screening test with sufficient sensitivity,** and it has been suggested that this should be employed periodically beginning around age 30 to 35. However, no data have been published demonstrating that this approach is superior with respect to decreasing mortality compared to simply performing biopsies in response to abnormal uterine bleeding.

The rationale for **prophylactic hysterectomy** in women with HNPCC is based on the high lifetime risk of endometrial cancer and the fact that the uterus does not serve a vital function once childbearing is complete. One study demonstrated that there were no cases of endometrial cancer in 61 HNPCC carriers who underwent prophylactic hysterectomy, whereas endometrial cancer developed in 69 of 210 (33%) who did not undergo surgery (77). On the other hand, because survival of women with HNPCC-associated endometrial cancers is approximately 90%, it is conceivable that prophylactic hysterectomy may not appreciably decrease mortality.

Some women in HNPCC families elect to undergo prophylactic colectomy. This provides an opportunity to remove the uterus as well. Hysterectomy in concert with colectomy, either via laparoscopy or laparotomy, should not greatly increase operative time or complications. If an endometrial biopsy has not been performed before prophylactic hysterectomy, the uterus should be opened intraoperatively and examined carefully. If a visual suspicion of cancer is confirmed by frozen section, then surgical staging can be performed. **In view of the increased risk of ovarian cancer in HNPCC syndrome, concomitant prophylactic salpingo-oophorectomy should be strongly considered.** Estrogen-replacement therapy following oophorectomy is not contraindicated in women with HNPCC because there is no evidence that this adversely affects the incidence of other cancers. In fact, **postmenopausal estrogen-replacement therapy in the general population substantially decreases colon cancer risk** (78).

Sporadic Endometrial Cancer

Cytogenetic studies have described gross chromosomal alterations in endometrial cancers, including changes in the number of copies of specific chromosomes (79). More recently, comparative genomic hybridization (CGH) studies have demonstrated areas of chromosomal loss and gain in both endometrial cancers and atypical hyperplasias (80,81). The most common sites of chromosomal gain are 1q, 8q, 10p, and 10q (82–84). Chromosomal losses also are frequently observed using CGH and in loss of heterozygosity studies (85). A correlation has been noted between higher numbers of chromosomal alterations on CGH and more virulent clinical features (86). The overall number of chromosomal alterations detected using CGH is lower in endometrial cancers relative to other cancer types.

Ploidy analysis simply measures total nuclear DNA content. **Approximately 80% of endometrial cancers have a normal diploid DNA content as measured by ploidy analysis.** Aneuploidy occurs in 20% and is associated with advanced stage, poor grade, nonendometrioid histology and poor survival (87). The frequency of aneuploidy (20%) is relatively low in endometrial cancers relative to ovarian cancers (80%). One might speculate that endometrial cancers more often present at an early stage than ovarian cancers because they usually have a lower level of genetic aberrations, as opposed to the conventional wisdom that attributes the favorable outcome of endometrial cancers to earlier diagnosis.

Finally, **patterns of genetic expression have been described using microarrays that distinguish between normal and malignant endometrium and between various histologic types of cancer** (85,88,89). Different types of microarrays have been employed by various groups, and study results often cannot be compared directly. In addition, selection of normal controls for comparison to cancers has not been uniform (90), and microdissection methods aimed at maximizing isolation of cancer have not always been employed (91). Global gene-expression profiles associated with both lymph node metastasis (92) and recurrence (93) have been identified in endometrial cancer. Studies to validate these biomarker panels and molecular-based prediction models are ongoing. This approach has the potential to dramatically increase our understanding of the molecular pathogenesis of endometrial cancer and to enhance prediction of clinical phenotypes.

Tumor Suppressor Genes

Inactivation of the *TP53* tumor suppressor gene is among the most frequent genetic events in endometrial cancers (30). **Overexpression of mutant p53 protein occurs in approximately 20% of endometrial adenocarcinomas and is associated with several known prognostic factors, including advanced stage,** poor grade, and nonendometrioid histology (87,94). Overexpression occurs in some 10% of stages I and II and 40% of stages III and IV cancers (94). Numerous studies have confirmed the strong association between *p53* overexpression and poor prognostic factors and decreased survival (95–101). In some of these studies, *p53* overexpression has been associated with worse survival even after controlling for stage (102,103). This suggests that loss of *p53* tumor suppressor function confers a particularly virulent phenotype. Although little is known regarding molecular alterations in uterine sarcomas, overexpression of mutant *p53* occurs in a majority of mixed mesodermal sarcomas of the uterus (74%) and in some leiomyosarcomas (104,105).

Endometrial cancers that overexpress p53 protein usually harbor missense mutations in exons 5 through 8 of the gene that result in amino acid substitutions in the protein (94,106–109). These mutations lead to loss of DNA binding activity. Because *TP53* mutations rarely, if ever, occur in endometrial hyplerplasias (106,110), this likely represents a late event in the development of type I endometrioid endometrial cancers. Alternatively, it is possible that acquisition of a *TP53* mutation leads to development of a virulent poorly differentiated or serous "type II" endometrial cancer that does not transition through a phase of hyperplasia, and it is associated with rapid spread of disease. In studies of papillary serous carcinoma, *TP53* mutation and p53 protein overexpression have been observed in the vast majority of cases, as well as in its putative dysplastic glandular precursor lesion (111,112).

Mutations in the *PTEN* tumor suppressor gene occur in approximately 30% to 50% of endometrial cancers (113–115), and this represents the most frequent genetic alteration described thus far in these cancers. Deletion of the second copy of the gene is also a frequent event, which results in complete loss of *PTEN* function. Most of these mutations are deletions, insertions, and nonsense mutations that lead to truncated protein products, whereas only about 15% are missense mutations that change a single amino acid in the critical phosphatase domain. The *PTEN* gene encodes a phosphatase that opposes the activity of cellular kinases. For example, it has been shown that loss of *PTEN* in endometrial cancers is associated with increased activity of the PI3 kinase with resultant phosphorylation of its downstream substrate Akt (116).

Mutations in the *PTEN* gene are associated with endometrioid histology, early stage and favorable clinical behavior (117). Well differentiated, noninvasive cases have the highest frequency of mutations. In addition, **PTEN mutations have been observed in 20% of endometrial hyperplasias,** suggesting that this is an early event in the development of some endometrioid type I endometrial cancers (118). It has been reported that loss of *PTEN* may occur in endometrial glands that appear normal, and it is proposed that this may represent the earliest event in endometrial carcinogenesis (119,120).

Synchronous endometrioid cancers are sometimes encountered in the endometrium and ovary that are indistinguishable microscopically. In some of these cases, identical *PTEN* mutations have been identified, suggesting that the ovarian tumor represents a metastasis from the endometrium (121). In other cases, the *PTEN* mutation seen in the endometrial cancer was not found in the ovarian tumor, suggesting that these represent two distinct primary cancers. *PTEN* mutations also have been observed in approximately 20% of endometrioid ovarian cancers that arise in the absence of endometrial cancers (122). As noted in the section on hereditary endometrial cancer, it has been shown that inherited mutations in DNA mismatch repair genes are responsible for the HNPCC syndrome. **Endometrial cancer is the second most common malignancy observed in women with HNPCC.**

Cancers that arise in these women with HNPCC syndrome are characterized by mutations in multiple microsatellite repeat sequences throughout the genome. **This microsatellite instability also has been seen in approximately 20% of sporadic endometrial cancers** (123,124). Endometrial cancers that exhibit microsatellite instability tend to be type I cancers. **Loss of mismatch repair in these cases usually results from silencing of the *MLH1* gene by promoter methylation** (65,66). Methylation of the *MLH1* promoter also has been noted in endometrial hyperplasias (124,125) and normal endometrium adjacent to cancers, suggesting that this is an early event in the development of some of these cancers (126). It is thought that global changes in methylation that result in decreased expression of a number of tumor suppressor and DNA repair genes may be a characteristic of some endometrial cancers, particularly type I cases (127,128). Loss of DNA mismatch repair may accelerate the process of malignant transformation by facilitating accumulation of mutations in microsatellite sequences present in genes involved in malignant transformation.

Several other tumor suppressor genes may play a role in the development of some endometrial cancers. The ***Par-4* gene** is a proapoptotic factor, and loss of expression of this gene occurs in some human cancers. Reduced expression occurs in approximately 40% of endometrial cancers and may be attributable to methylation of the promoter region of the gene (129). The ***Cables* gene** is a putative tumor suppressor involved in regulating phosphorylation of cyclin-dependent kinase 2 in a manner that restrains cell cycle progression. *Cables* mutant mice develop endometrial hyperplasia at an early age, and exposure to low levels of estrogen causes endometrial cancer (130). *Cables* expression is up regulated by estrogen and decreases following progestin treatment. Loss of *Cables* expression also occurs in human endometrial hyperplasias and cancers. Finally, mutations in the ***CDC4* gene,** which is involved in regulating cyclin E expression during cell cycle progression, have been noted in 16% of endometrial cancers (131). Mutations were accompanied by loss of the wild-type allele and were more common in cancers with poor prognostic factors such as high-grade and lymph node metastases. It is postulated that *CDC4* may act as a tumor suppressor by restraining the activity of cyclin E in promoting progression from G_1 to S phase.

Oncogenes

Alterations in oncogenes have been demonstrated in endometrial cancers, but these occur less frequently than inactivation of tumor suppressor genes (Table 1.3). Increased expression of the **HER-2/*neu*** receptor tyrosine kinase initially was noted in only 10% of endometrial cancers (99,132–135) and was associated with advanced stage and poor outcome. Recently, it has been suggested that **HER-2/*neu* overexpression may be more prevalent in patients with papillary serous endometrial cancers** (136–138). In a tissue microarray study of 483 endometrial cancers using immunohistochemical analysis and fluorescent *in situ*–hybridization (FISH), the highest rate of HER-2/*neu* overexpression and amplification was found in serous carcinomas (43% and 29%), whereas grade 1 endometrioid adenocarcinomas showed the lowest levels (3% and 1%) (138). These data also suggest that **therapies that target HER-2/*neu* may have a role in the treatment of papillary serous endometrial carcinomas.** The levels of HER-2/*neu* overexpression in endometrial cancers are much less striking than in breast cancers. With rare exception, *trastuzumab* (anti–HER-2/*neu* antibody) generally has not been a useful therapy in endometrial cancer.

The ***fms* oncogene** encodes a tyrosine kinase that serves as a receptor for macrophage-colony stimulating factor (M-CSF). Expression of *fms* in endometrial cancers was found to correlate with advanced stage, poor grade, and deep myometrial invasion (139,140). Subsequently, it was shown that *fms* and its ligand (M-CSF) usually were coexpressed in endometrial cancers, and it was proposed that this receptor–ligand pair might mediate an autocrine growth stimulatory pathway (141). In support of this hypothesis, M-CSF serum levels are increased in patients with endometrial cancer. In addition, M-CSF increases the invasiveness of cancer cell lines that express significant levels of *fms,* but it has no effect on cell lines with low levels of the receptor (142).

The *ras* oncogenes undergo point mutations in codons 12, 13, or 61 that result in constitutively activated molecules in many types of cancers. Initially, these codons of the K-*ras*, H-*ras*, and N-*ras* genes were examined in 11 immortalized endometrial cancer cell lines (143). Mutations in codon 12 of K-*ras* were seen in four cell lines, whereas three mutations were found in codon 61 of H-*ras*. Subsequent studies of primary endometrial adenocarcinomas have confirmed that codon 12 of K-*ras* is mutated in approximately 10% of U.S. cases and 20% of Japanese cases (106,144–150). These mutations occur more often, but not exclusively, in type I endometrial cancers. K-*ras* mutations also have been identified in some endometrial hyperplasias (145,150,151), which suggests that this may be a relatively early event in the development of some type I cancers.

As noted previously, the *PTEN* tumor suppressor gene, which normally acts to restrain *PI3K* activity, is frequently inactivated in type I endometrial cancers. Conversely, the **PIK3CA gene** is oncogenically activated in some cases. The catalytic subunit of *PI3K* (*PIK3CA*) is located on chromosome 3q26.3, and activating mutations in this gene have been described in several types of cancers. In an initial study, *PIK3CA* mutations were seen in 36% of endometrial cancers, and 24% of cases had mutations in both *PTEN* and *PIK3CA* (152). This suggested that there is an additive effect of two mutations in the same pathway. In a subsequent study, 39% of endometrial cancers and 7% of atypical endometrial hyperplasias were found to harbor mutations in *PIK3CA* (153). This study also implied that *PIK3CA* mutation occurred at the time of tumor invasion and could serve as a marker for invasion. As in the initial study, a high fraction of cases had mutations in both *PTEN* and *PIK3CA*. These and other studies confirm that *PIK3CA* activating mutations are common in endometrial cancers. Both inactivation of *PTEN* or unrestrained *PIK3CA* can lead to activation of AKT, which in turn leads to up regulation of the mammalian target of *rapamycin* (mTOR). Recent studies have suggested that mTOR inhibitors may have a role in the in the management of progesterone refractory hyperplasia and treatment of type I endometrial cancer (154,155).

Alterations in the wnt pathway involving E-cadherin, *APC*, and *β-catenin*, the product of the *CTNNB1* gene, have been noted in some endometrial cancers. E-cadherin is a transmembrane glycoprotein involved in cell–cell adhesion, and decreased expression in cancer cells is associated with increased invasiveness and metastatic potential (Fig. 1.7). E-cadherin mutations occur only rarely in endometrial cancers (51), but cadherin expression may also be down regulated in the absence of mutations (156,157). The cytoplasmic tail of E-cadherin exists as a macromolecular complex with the *β-catenin* and *APC* gene products, which link it to the cytoskeleton. It appears that a critical function of the *APC* tumor suppressor gene is to regulate phosphorylation of serine and threonine residues (codons 33, 37, 41, 45) in exon 3 of *β-catenin*, which results in degradation of *β-catenin*. Mutational inactivation of *APC* allows accumulation of *β-catenin*, which translocates to the nucleus and acts as a transcription factor to induce expression of cyclin D1 and perhaps other genes involved in cell cycle progression (157).

Germ-line *APC* mutations are responsible for the adenomatous polyposis coli syndrome, and somatic mutations are common in sporadic colon cancers, but ***APC* mutations have not been described in endometrial cancers** (52,158). The *APC* gene may be inactivated in some endometrial cancers because of promoter methylation. In addition, it has been shown that missense mutations in exon 3 of *β-catenin* lead to the same end result—namely, abrogation of the ability of *APC* to induce *β-catenin* degradation—which results in abnormal transcriptional activity. In view of this, **the *β-catenin* gene is considered an oncogene** (159). *β-catenin* mutations have been observed in several types of cancers, including hepatocellular, prostate, and endometrial cancers. **Mutation of *β-catenin* occurs in approximately 10% to 15% of endometrial cancers,** but abnormal accumulation of *β-catenin* protein occurs in approximately one-third of cases, suggesting that mechanisms other than mutation might be involved in some cases (53,158).

Mutations have also been observed in the fibroblast growth factor receptor 2 (*FGFR2*) gene in approximately 10% of endometrial cancers (160). *FGFR2* mutations were found almost exclusively in endometrioid cancers, and there was no association with clinical outcome. Further studies will be needed to evaluate the significance of the identified mutations and other mechanisms of increased *FGF* signaling in endometrial cancer as well as any potential clinical utility by drug targeting of the receptor.

Among nuclear transcription factors involved in stimulating proliferation, amplification of members of the *myc* family has most often been implicated in the development of human cancers. It has been shown that *c-myc* is expressed in normal endometrium (161) with higher expression in the proliferative phase. **Several studies have suggested that *myc* may be amplified in a fraction of endometrial cancers** (135,162,163).

Ovarian Cancer

Approximately 10% of ovarian cancers arise in women who carry germ-line mutations in cancer susceptibility genes—predominantly *BRCA1* or *BRCA2.* The vast majority of ovarian cancers are sporadic and arise because of accumulation of genetic damage.

The causes of acquired genetic alterations in the ovarian epithelium remain uncertain, but exogenous carcinogens, with the possible exception of talc, have not been strongly implicated. Some mutations may arise spontaneously because of increased epithelial proliferation required to repair ovulatory defects. Oxidative stress and free radical formation as a result of inflammation and repair at the ovulatory site may also contribute to accumulation of DNA damage. Regardless of the mechanisms involved, **reproductive events that decrease lifetime ovulatory cycles (e.g., pregnancy and birth control pills) are protective against ovarian cancer** (164). The protective effect of these factors is greater in magnitude than one would predict based on the extent that ovulation is interrupted, however. **Five years of oral contraceptive use provides a 50% risk reduction while only decreasing total years of ovulation by less than 20%.** There is evidence to suggest that the progestagenic milieu of pregnancy and the pill might also protect against ovarian cancer by increasing apoptosis of ovarian epithelial cells, thereby cleansing the ovary of cells that have acquired genetic damage (165). The action of other reproductive hormones such as estrogens, androgens, and gonadotropins also may contribute to the development of ovarian cancers.

Epithelial ovarian cancers are heterogeneous with respect to behavior (borderline versus invasive) and histologic type (serous, mucinous, endometrioid, clear cell). Although the strongest epidemiologic risk factors generally affect risk of all disease subsets, differences have been observed with respect to etiology and molecular alterations. For example, although it is thought that serous cancers arise from epithelial cells on the surface of the ovary or in underlying inclusion cysts or in the fallopian tube, **many endometrioid and clear cell cancers likely develop in deposits of endometriosis.**

Likewise, differences in the pattern of genetic alterations have been noted between histological types (Table 1.4). It has been proposed that ovarian tumors can be classified as low or high grade based on histology, clinical behavior, and molecular phenotypes (166). **Low-grade**

Table 1.4 Clinical and Molecular Characteristics of Histological Types of Ovarian Cancers	
Endometrioid and Clear Cell Cancers	Associated with endometriosis
	Usually early stage and favorable survival
	Frequent mutations in *PTEN, PIK3CA*
Mucinous Ovarian Cancers	Usually early stage
	Frequent mutations in K-*ras*
Low-Grade Serous Ovarian Cancer (Borderline, Well Differentiated)	Usually early stage and favorable survival
	Frequent mutations in K-*ras* and *BRAF*
High-Grade Serous Ovarian Cancer	Most common ovarian cancer histology in *BRCA1* and *BRCA2* mutation carriers
	Usually advanced stage and poor survival
	Frequent mutations in *TP53*
	Occasional overexpression of HER-2/*neu*, AKT2, *c-myc*

tumors are generally confined to the ovary at diagnosis and include low-grade serous carcinoma, mucinous, endometrioid, and clear cell carcinomas. They are genetically stable and characterized by mutations in a number of genes including K-*ras*, *BRAF*, *PTEN*, and *β-catenin*. High-grade cancers typically present at an advanced stage and are predominantly serous but also include carcinosarcoma and undifferentiated cancers. This group of tumors has a high level of genetic instability and is characterized by mutation of *TP53*.

As our understanding of the molecular pathogenesis of ovarian cancer continues to mature in the future, it is likely that the various disease subsets will be increasingly thought of as distinct entities that are defined by characteristic patterns of molecular signatures. Elucidation of the molecular basis for the clinical heterogeneity of ovarian cancer has the potential to facilitate future improvements in diagnosis, treatment, and prevention.

Hereditary Ovarian Cancer

It had long been suspected based on epidemiologic and family studies that approximately 10% of epithelial ovarian cancers are attributable to inheritance of mutations in high-penetrance cancer susceptibility genes. The *BRCA1* gene was identified on chromosome 17q in 1994, and *BRCA2* was identified on chromosome 13q in 1995. Inherited mutations in these two breast and ovarian cancer susceptibility genes are responsible for approximately 6% and 3% of ovarian cancers, respectively (167). Inherited mutations in the DNA mismatch repair genes involved in HNPCC that are described in the section on hereditary endometrial cancer are responsible for some 1% of ovarian cancer cases. The vast majority of *BRCA*-associated ovarian cancers are papillary serous (168), as are most peritoneal and fallopian tube cancers and some uterine cancers. Although there are conflicting reports regarding whether *BRCA* mutations increase the risk of serous cancers of the uterus (169,170), the evidence to support inclusion of serous fallopian tube cancers in this syndrome is stronger (171). In two studies, **BRCA mutations were found in 28%** (172) **and 17%** (173) **of women with fallopian tube cancer. Likewise, germ-line BRCA mutations have been reported in some studies in approximately one-third of those with primary peritoneal cancer** (173,174).

The *BRCA1* and *BRCA2* gene products complex with Rad51 and other proteins involved in repair of double-stranded DNA breaks (DSBs) by homologous recombination (175,176). *BRCA1* and *BRCA2* have been classified as tumor-suppressor genes because the nonmutated copy is invariably deleted in breast and ovarian cancers that arise in women who inherit a mutant gene. **In some studies, survival of BRCA carriers with ovarian cancer was better than that of sporadic cases** that were matched for age, stage, and other prognostic factors (177). It had been suggested that loss of DNA repair because of mutation of *BRCA1* or *BRCA2* might improve survival by rendering cancer cells more susceptible to chemotherapy. Poly(ADP-ribose) polymerase (PARP) is an enzyme involved in base excision repair, a key pathway in the repair of DNA single-strand breaks. Inhibition of PARP leads to the persistence of DNA lesions normally repaired by homologous recombination. Inhibitors of PARP recently have been shown to be highly selective for tumor cells with defects in the repair of DSBs by homologous recombination, particularly in the context of *BRCA1* or *BRCA2* mutation (178). Clinical trials are currently ongoing to determine the efficacy of PARP inhibitors in *BRCA* mutation carriers with recurrent ovarian cancer.

***BRCA1* and *BRCA2* mutations are associated with 60% to 90% lifetime risks of breast cancer, and this begins to manifest before age 30. *BRCA2* also increases the risk of breast cancer in men.** Screening, prophylactic mastectomy, and chemopreventives such as *tamoxifen* all play a role in decreasing breast cancer incidence and mortality. **The lifetime risk of ovarian cancer ranges from 20% to 40% in *BRCA1* carriers and 10% to 20% in *BRCA2* carriers,** but this increased risk is not manifest until the late 30s (179–183). **The median age of sporadic epithelial ovarian cancer is in the early to mid-60s, compared to the mid-40s and early 50s for *BRCA1*- and *BRCA2*-associated cases.**

It is unclear why only a fraction of women who carry *BRCA1* mutations develop ovarian cancer. It has been postulated that incomplete penetrance may result from the effect of modifying genes or gene–environment interactions (e.g., birth control pill use) (184). In some series, mutations in the carboxy terminus of *BRCA1* have been associated with a higher frequency of breast cancer relative to ovarian cancer (185). Conversely, mutations in the proximal amino end of the gene resulted in a higher likelihood of developing ovarian cancer. Likewise, some studies have suggested that ovarian cancer may occur more often in families with truncation mutations in exon 11 of *BRCA2* (186). Further studies are needed to examine whether a genotype–phenotype correlation exists.

23

BRCA1 and *2* mutations are rare and carried by fewer than one in 500 individuals in most populations, but there are some notable exceptions (187). Founder mutations that presumably arose thousands of years ago in a single ancestor have been identified in some ethnic groups. **The most common founder mutations described thus far are the *BRCA1* 185delAG and *BRCA2* 6174delT mutations that occur in approximately 1.0% and 1.4% of Ashkenazi Jews, respectively** (180,188). The high frequency of these mutations implies that they likely arose some 100 generations ago. A third less common founder mutation, *BRCA1* 5382insC, also has been noted in the Ashkenazi population. Because approximately one in 40 Ashkenazi individuals carries a *BRCA* founder mutation and testing for this panel of specific mutations is much less expensive, the threshold for genetic testing is much lower in this population.

Because mutations in *BRCA1* and *BRCA2* in the general population occur throughout the entire coding sequence, **the most reliable method of detecting mutations is complete gene sequencing.** The effort and cost involved in sequencing these large genes are relatively high, however, and currently it remains impractical to perform mutational analysis in low-risk individuals. The probability of finding a *BRCA1* or *BRCA2* mutation in a woman over age 50 who is the only individual in her family with ovarian or breast cancer is less than 3%. At the other extreme, in families with two cases of breast cancer and two cases of ovarian cancer, the probability of finding a mutation may be as high as 80% (186). **Testing generally has been advocated when the family history suggests at least a 5% probability of finding a mutation. In practical terms, this translates into two first- or second-degree relatives with either ovarian cancer at any age or breast cancer before age 50** (Fig. 1.8). However, some mutations are found in families with less impressive histories, particularly in families that contain few women.

It is preferable to begin by testing individuals in a high-risk family who already have been affected by cancer because a negative test in an unaffected individual may reflect failure to inherit the mutant allele even though others in the family carry a mutation. **When a specific mutation is identified in an affected individual, others in the family can be tested much more rapidly and inexpensively for that specific mutation.** Most deleterious *BRCA* mutations encode truncated protein products, but missense mutations that alter a single amino acid have been found to segregate with breast or ovarian cancer in some families (189). In a significant fraction of high-risk families, *BRCA* testing reveals sequence variants of uncertain significance or no detectable alterations, and these results represent a counseling dilemma. The search for *BRCA* genetic alterations may also involve sequencing of introns that lie between the coding exons. Intronic mutations may affect RNA splicing and can result in deletion of

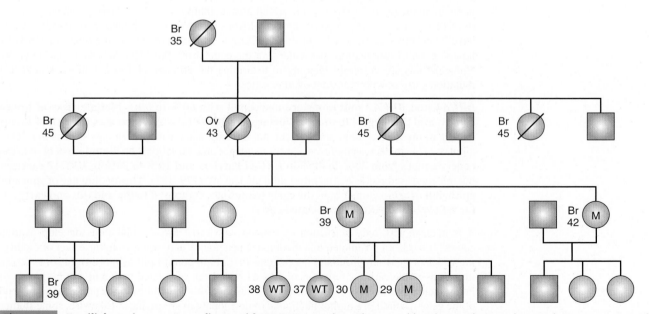

Figure 1.8   Familial ovarian cancer pedigree with *BRCA1* mutation. The age of family members and type of cancers are noted. Solid circles represent individuals affected with cancer, and slashes denote those who have died of cancer. Individuals denoted *M* have a mutation in *BRCA1*, whereas those denoted *WT* have normal *BRCA1* genes.

adjacent exons. In addition, genomic rearrangements may occur that inactivate *BRCA1* or *2* and identification of such alterations requires molecular testing beyond sequencing. **Failure to identify a *BRCA1* or *BRCA2* mutation in a family may be reassuring, but it must be tempered by the realization that *BRCA* mutational analysis may miss some mutations and that other undiscovered hereditary ovarian cancer genes may exist.**

Women should receive educational material and extensive counseling that explains the rationale and potential risks and benefits before they decide to undergo testing. Involvement of genetic counselors in this process is helpful because they have specialized training in nondirective counseling techniques that guide patients toward decisions that reflect their own beliefs and values. In addition, posttest counseling and follow-up are crucial to help women work through various issues, including decisions about prophylactic surgery and other interventions designed to decrease cancer mortality. Because it was feared that misuse of genetic information could have devastating consequences including difficulty in securing employment and life, health, or disability insurance, clinicians initially were hesitant to record genetic testing results in the medical record. **Because *BRCA* testing is now widely accepted and insurance companies generally cover the costs, results should be acknowledged in the medical record** chart because they form the basis for the decision to perform prophylactic surgery.

The value of screening for early stage ovarian cancer with CA125 or ultrasound is unproven but seems reasonable until controlled studies are available. Use of birth control pills as a chemopreventive also has been advocated because this is strongly protective against ovarian cancer in the general population. Oral contraceptives are a particularly attractive option for young women who have not yet completed childbearing, but the efficacy of this approach in *BRCA* carriers remains uncertain (184). **Because ovarian cancer has a 70% mortality rate, prophylactic bilateral salpinoophorectomy (BSO) should be discussed with all women who carry germ-line *BRCA1* or *BRCA2* mutations.** Fortunately, the incidence of ovarian cancer in mutation carriers does not begin to rise dramatically until the late 30s (190). This allows women time to bear children before considering BSO as they approach the end of their reproductive life span. The ovaries are internal organs, and most women experience only modest feelings of altered body image and self-esteem after they are removed. Insurance companies will almost always pay for prophylactic BSO in mutation carriers. High-risk women who lack *BRCA* mutations or those who have sequence alterations of uncertain significance may encounter greater reimbursement obstacles.

Prophylactic BSO is widely viewed as the most effective currently available means of decreasing ovarian cancer mortality in *BRCA* mutation carriers. There is strong evidence that this approach significantly decreases ovarian cancer mortality. In addition, prophylactic BSO can be performed laparoscopically in most women with an acceptably low incidence of serious complications. Discussion of the potential for adverse outcomes is particularly important in a setting in which a healthy disease-free individual is subjected to the risks inherent in abdominal surgery.

Patients who undergo prophylactic BSO may experience surgical menopause. In premenopausal women who do not have a personal history of breast cancer, estrogen replacement can be safely administered. Although historically there has been concern that estrogen replacement might increase the risk of breast cancer, this risk already is exceedingly high. In addition, systemic estrogen levels are lower in oophorectomized premenopausal women who are taking hormone replacement than if the ovaries had been left in place. **The therapeutic benefit of BSO in women with breast cancer has long been appreciated, and more recent studies support the contention that this intervention significantly reduces breast cancer risk in *BRCA* carriers** (191,192). Many *BRCA* carriers are identified after developing early onset breast cancer, and this group represents the most difficult in which to balance the risks and benefits of estrogen-replacement therapy.

Many patients elect to have the uterus removed as part of the surgical procedure because they have completed their family. Furthermore, **the likelihood of future exposure to *tamoxifen*,** which increases endometrial cancer risk two- to threefold, in the context of breast cancer prevention or treatment, also argues for concomitant hysterectomy. The more problematic issue in performing prophylactic BSO is whether the risk of malignant transformation is increased solely in the ovaries and fallopian tubes or in the entire field of mullerian-derived epithelia. **Peritoneal papillary serous carcinoma that is indistinguishable histologically or macroscopically from ovarian cancer has been described in rare instances following prophylactic**

salpingo-oophorectomy (193,194). These reports preceded the identification of *BRCA1* and *BRCA2*, however, and it is unclear what fraction of these women were mutation carriers. The origin of primary peritoneal cancers after prophylactic BSO is uncertain, and case reports have been published in which retrospective examination of the ovaries has revealed occult ovarian cancers that were not recognized by the pathologist (195). Thus, some cancers thought to originate in the peritoneal cavity may actually represent recurrences of occult ovarian cancer.

Some reports have noted an increased frequency of abnormalities in the ovarian epithelium (invaginations, inclusion cysts, stratification, and papillations) in *BRCA* carriers (196), but other studies have not confirmed the presence of a consistent pattern of premalignant histologic features (197,198). **Careful examination of prophylactic salpingo-oophorectomy specimens has led to the identification of occult cancers in as many as 12% of women in some series** (199,200). This adds support to the theory that primary peritoneal cancers that occur years after BSO may represent recurrences of ovarian cancer. Early stage fallopian tube cancers also have been found in *BRCA1* carriers undergoing prophylactic BSO (201). Thus, in view of these data, it seems reasonable to recommend that cytologic washings of the pelvis be obtained routinely in concert with prophylactic BSO and. Finally, the pathologist must be informed of the indication for prophylactic BSO and the surgery. Multiple sections of the fallopian tubes and ovaries should be examined to exclude the presence of an occult carcinoma. In this regard, **there is some evidence to suggest that the tubal fimbria rather than the ovarian epithelium may be the preferred site of cancer development in *BRCA1* and *BRCA2* mutation carriers** (202).

The efficacy of BSO in reducing breast and ovarian cancer in mutation carriers has been suggested by several retrospective studies. One study that examined the effect of prophylactic BSO revealed a 75% lower rate of breast and ovarian cancer (192). A separate study of 551 *BRCA1* and *BRCA2* carriers from various registries also found evidence of efficacy (191). **Among 259 women who had undergone prophylactic oophorectomy, 2.3% were found to have stage I ovarian cancer at the time of the procedure, and two women subsequently developed papillary serous peritoneal carcinoma.** Among controls, 58 women (19.9%) developed ovarian cancer after a mean follow-up of 8.8 years. With the exclusion of the six women whose cancer was diagnosed at surgery, prophylactic oophorectomy reduced the risk of coelomic epithelial cancer by 96%. Most recently, **an international registry study of more than 1,800 subjects with median follow-up of 3.5 years found that prophylactic BSO reduced ovarian, tubal, and peritoneal cancer risk by only 80%,** partly because of an estimated 6% residual lifetime risk of primary peritoneal cancer (203).

Sporadic Ovarian Cancer

Global Genomic Changes

Invasive epithelial ovarian carcinoma generally is a monoclonal disease that develops as a clonal expansion of a single transformed cell in the ovary (204). There is evidence, however, that some serous borderline tumors (134) as well as cancers that arise in the peritoneum of patients with *BRCA1* mutations may be polyclonal (205). Most ovarian cancers are characterized by a high degree of genetic damage that is manifest at the genomic and molecular levels. Gains and losses of various segments of the genome have been demonstrated using comparative genomic hybridization (206). Likewise, loss of heterozygosity (LOH), indicative of deletion of specific genetic loci, also has been demonstrated to occur at a high frequency on many chromosomal arms (207). It is unclear whether the wide range of genetic alterations in ovarian cancers reflects the need to alter several genes in the process of malignant transformation or results from generalized genomic instability. Both CGH and LOH studies have shown that **advanced stage, poorly differentiated cancers have a higher number of genetic changes than early stage, low-grade cases** (208–210).

It is estimated that the human genome contains some 25,000 genes. Microarray chips that contain sequences complementary to thousands of genes have been created that allow global assessment of the level of expression of each gene. Expression arrays have proven useful in predicting clinical phenotypes in several types of solid tumors. Many genes have been identified that appear to be up or down regulated in the process of malignant transformation (211,212). In addition, **microarrays have demonstrated patterns of gene expression that distinguish between histologic types** (213), **borderline and invasive cases** (214) **and between early and advanced stage disease** (212,215). Molecular signatures also have been identified that are predictive of response to therapy (216, 217) and survival (218). Further validation of genomic signatures is needed, but genomic approaches hold the exciting potential to guide selection of therapy in the future. Patients identified as having a "poor prognosis" molecular profile might be the best candidates for investigational trials of new therapies. Microarray analyses have also demonstrated that dysregulation of oncogenic molecular pathways varies considerably between ovarian cancers (219). This may provide the opportunity to incorporate biological therapies that target oncogenic pathways associated with src, *ras*, EGFR, and others based on an understanding of the underlying molecular alterations in a patient's cancer (216).

Tumor Suppressor Genes

Alteration of the *TP53* tumor suppressor gene is the most frequent genetic event described thus far in ovarian cancers (Table 1.4) (220–225). The frequency of overexpression of mutant *p53* is significantly higher in advanced stage (40% to 60%) relative to early stage cases (10% to 20%). The histologic distribution of early and advanced stage cases varies significantly, however, and may account for the difference in *TP53* mutation rate. In this regard, **approximately two-thirds of early stage serous ovarian cancers were found to have *TP53* mutations compared to only 21% of nonserous cases** (226). There is a suggestion that overexpression of mutant p53 protein may be associated with slightly worse survival in advanced stage ovarian cancers (220,222,224,225,227–230). Finally, although there is a high concordance between *TP53* missense mutations in exons 5 through 8 and protein overexpression, approximately 20% of advanced ovarian cancers contain mutations that result in truncated protein products, which usually are not overexpressed (221,230). Some of these mutations may lie outside of exons 5 to 8. **Overall, some 70% of advanced ovarian cancers have either missense or truncation mutations in the *TP53* gene.** Most *TP53* missense mutations are transitions rather than transversions or microdeletions (231,232), which suggests that these mutations occur spontaneously rather than resulting from exogenous carcinogens.

It has been suggested that loss of functional *p53* might confer a chemoresistant phenotype because of its role in chemotherapy-induced apoptosis. In this regard, several studies have examined the correlation between chemosensitivity and *TP53* mutation in ovarian cancers (233–236). Some have suggested a relationship between *p53* mutation and loss of chemosensitivity and resistance to therapy, but in other studies such a relationship has not been observed. It is likely that the status of the *TP53* gene is just one of a multitude of factors that determine chemosensitivity.

Overexpression of *p53* is rare in stage I serous borderline tumors and well-differentiated serous cancers, but it does occur in approximately 20% of advanced stage borderline cases (237,238). In a study of advanced serous borderline tumors, *p53* overexpression was associated with a sixfold higher risk of death (238). In some cases, invasive serous cancers may arise following an earlier diagnosis of borderline tumor. Ortiz et al. showed that ***TP53* mutational status was not concordant between the original borderline tumor and the subsequent invasive cancer** (239). This suggests that the invasive cancer either arises independently or as a clonal outgrowth within the original tumor.

Although mutations in the *Rb* tumor suppressor gene are not a common feature of ovarian cancers, recent evidence suggests that inactivation of *Rb* greatly enhances tumor formation in ovarian cells with *p53* mutations (240). In a mouse model in which these genes were inactivated in the ovarian epithelium, few cancers developed in response to loss of either *TP53* or *Rb* alone. When both genes were inactivated, epithelial ovarian cancers with serous features developed in almost all cases. Given that *Rb* mutations are rare in ovarian cancers, it is possible that inactivation of one of a number of genes in the *Rb* pathway can initiate transformation cooperatively with *TP53*. Inactivation of *Rb* itself may not be requisite. This mouse model of ovarian cancer has the potential to add greatly to our understanding of epithelial ovarian carcinogenesis.

The cyclin-dependent kinase (cdk) inhibitors act as tumor suppressors by virtue of their inhibition of cell cycle progression from G_1 to S phase. Expression of several cdk inhibitors appears to be decreased in some ovarian cancers. **In approximately 15% of ovarian cancers, *p16* undergoes homozygous deletions** (241). There is evidence to suggest that *p16* (242), CDKN2B (*p15*) (243), and some other tumor suppressor genes such as ***BRCA1*** (244,245) may be inactivated via transcriptional silencing because of promoter methylation rather than mutation or deletion. Likewise, decreased expression of the ***p21*** cdk inhibitor has been noted in a significant fraction of ovarian cancers despite the absence of inactivating mutations (246,247). Loss of CDKN1B (*p27*) also may occur and correlates with poor survival in some studies (248–251). It has been suggested that aberrant expression of *p27* in the cytoplasm may be most associated with poor outcome (252).

Normal ovarian epithelial cells are inhibited by the growth inhibitory peptide TGF-β, whereas most immortalized ovarian cancer cell lines are unresponsive (253,254). The effect of TGF-β on primary ovarian cancer cells obtained directly from patients is less straightforward. In studies conducted using ovarian cancer cells grown in monolayer culture, most remain sensitive to the growth inhibitory effect of TGF-β (254). In contrast, when ovarian cancer cells are grown in collagen matrix, they are unresponsive (255). There is some evidence that mutations may occur in cell surface TGF-β receptors or in the Smad family of genes that are involved in downstream signaling (256); in other studies, these signaling pathways were found to be intact (255). **Thus far, it has not been convincingly demonstrated that derangement of the TGF-β pathway plays a role in the development of ovarian cancers.**

Oncogenes

Ovarian cancers produce and are capable of responding to various peptide growth factors. For example, **epidermal growth factor** (257) **and transforming growth factor-alpha (TGF-α)** (258) are produced by some ovarian cancers that also express the receptor that binds these peptides (EGF receptor) (259,260). **Some cancers produce insulin-like growth factor-1 (IGF-1), IGF-1 binding protein, and express type 1 IGF receptor** (261). **Platelet-derived growth factor** also is expressed by many types of epithelial cells, including human ovarian cancer cell lines, but these cells usually are not responsive to PDGF (253,262,263). In addition, **ovarian cancers produce basic fibroblast growth factor** and its receptor, and basic FGF acts as a mitogen in some ovarian cancers (264). Ovarian cancers produce **macrophage-colony stimulating factor,** and serum levels of M-CSF are elevated in some patients (265). Because the **M-CSF receptor (*fms*)** is expressed by many ovarian cancers, this could constitute an autocrine growth stimulatory pathway in some cancers.(266). Ascites of patients with ovarian cancer also contains phospholipid factors such as LPA that stimulate proliferation and invasiveness of ovarian cancer cells (267). The edg-2 G-protein coupled receptors act as functional receptors for LPA. The finding that neutralization of LPA activity decreases growth and increases apoptosis of ovarian cancers suggests that manipulation of this pathway may be therapeutically beneficial (268).

Several groups also have demonstrated that normal ovarian epithelial cells produce, and are responsive to, many of the same peptide growth factors as malignant ovarian epithelial cells (260,269–271). Thus, despite cell culture data demonstrating autocrine and paracrine growth regulation of ovarian cancer cells by peptide growth factors, it remains unclear whether alterations in expression of growth factors are critical early events involved in the development of ovarian cancers. Alternatively, **it is possible that growth factors may primarily act as "necessary but not sufficient" cofactors that support growth and metastasis following malignant transformation.**

The HER-2/*neu* tyrosine kinase is a member of a family of related transmembrane receptors that includes the EGF receptor (272). Approximately 30% of breast cancers express increased levels of the HER-2/*neu* (273), often as a result of gene amplification. Overexpression of HER-2/*neu* in breast cancer has been associated with poor survival. **Expression of HER-2/*neu* is increased in a fraction of ovarian cancers and overexpression has been associated with poor survival in some studies** (273,274), **but not all** (275). Unlike breast cancers, ovarian cancers that exhibit HER-2/*neu* overexpression rarely have high-level gene amplification. Monoclonal antibodies that interact with HER-2/*neu* can decrease growth of breast and ovarian cancer cell lines that overexpress this receptor (276,277). Anti–HER-2/*neu* antibody therapy (*trastuzumab*) has demonstrated efficacy in the treatment of breast cancer and often is administered in concert with *paclitaxel*. A study performed by the Gynecologic Oncology Group found **only 11% of ovarian cancers exhibit significant HER-2/*neu* overexpression** (278). **The response rate to single-agent *trastuzumab* therapy was disappointingly low (7%),** but perhaps some benefit may be found in the future using combination regimens that also include *taxanes* or other *cytotoxics*.

Activating mutations in codons 12 and 13 the K-*ras* gene are rare in high-grade invasive serous ovarian cancers (279,280). Some types of cancers that lack K-*ras* mutations have activating mutations in codon 599 of the downstream *BRAF* gene, but this is not the case in high-grade serous ovarian cancers. In contrast, **K-*ras* mutations are common in borderline serous ovarian tumors, occurring in approximately 25% to 50% of cases** (281). In addition, **mutations in *BRAF* occur in some 20% of serous borderline cases lacking K-*ras* mutations** (282). Mutations in K-*ras* and *BRAF* have also been noted in cystadenoma epithelium adjacent to serous borderline tumors, suggesting that this is an early event in their development (25). **K-*ras* mutations have been noted in approximately 50% of mucinous ovarian cancers, but *BRAF* mutations have not been found** (283). These findings highlight the distinct differences in the molecular pathology between various histological types and between borderline tumors and invasive ovarian cancers (Table 1.4).

Similar to endometrial cancers, activation of the *PIK3CA* and *AKT2* oncogenes occurs in some ovarian cancers. The region of chromosome 3p26 that includes the phosphatidylinositol 3-kinase (*PIK3CA*) is amplified in some ovarian cancers (284). In addition, **activating mutations in *PIK3CA* occur in about 10% of ovarian cancers, and are much more common in endometrioid and clear cell cancers (20%) as compared to serous cancers (2%)** (285). Likewise, the *AKT2* serine/threonine kinase that is downstream of *PIK3CA* also has been shown to be amplified and overexpressed in some ovarian cancers (286). *PIK3CA* and *AKT2* kinase activity is opposed by the **PTEN phosphatase, and this tumor suppressor gene also is inactivated in about 20% of endometrioid ovarian cancers** (287).

Mutations in the β-*catenin* gene are a feature of some endometrial cancers. Similarly, β-*catenin* mutations are present in some 30% of endometrioid ovarian cancers (288) but not other histologic types. This provides further evidence of the molecular heterogeneity of the various histologic types of ovarian cancer (Table 1.4). In some endometrioid ovarian cancers with abnormal nuclear accumulation of β-*catenin* that lacked mutations, the *APC*, *AXIN1*, or *AXIN2* genes that regulate β-*catenin* activity were found to be mutated (288). This suggests that alterations in the wnt signaling pathway are a feature of endometrioid ovarian cancers. Mouse models in which the wnt and the PIK3/*PTEN* pathways are inactivated in the ovarian epithelium leads to the development of endometrioid cancer and endometriosis (289,290).

Increased activity of nuclear transcription factors and cyclins also may enhance malignant transformation. In this regard, amplification of the *c-myc* oncogene has been reported to occur in approximately 30% of ovarian cancers. Several studies have suggested that the *c-myc* gene is amplified in approximately 30% of cases (291–294). The overexpression of *c-myc* is observed most often in advanced stage serous cancers. Despite these reports of gene amplification, convincing evidence of *c-myc* protein overexpression has been less convincing. Some ovarian cancers have been reported to have increased expression of cyclin E, which is involved in cell cycle progression (295). In a study of advanced stage suboptimally debulked ovarian cancers, high cyclin E expression was associated with a six-month decrease in median survival (296). In some, but not all, cases, amplification of the cyclin E gene was found to be the underlying cause of overexpression. In a large study using a tissue array, **cyclin E overexpression has been was shown to be associated with serous and clear cell histology, advanced stage, and poor outcome** (297).

Cervical Cancer

Cervical cancer is the most common gynecologic malignancy worldwide and accounts for more than 400,000 cases annually. Molecular and epidemiologic studies have demonstrated that **sexually transmitted human papilloma virus (HPV) infections play a role in almost all cervical dysplasias and cancers** (298). HPV infection also is involved in the development of dysplasias and cancers of the vagina and vulva. The peak incidence of HPV infection is in the 20s and 30s, and the incidence of cervical cancer increases from the 20s to a plateau between ages 40 and 50. **Although HPV plays a major role in the development of most cervical cancers, only a small minority of women who are infected develop invasive cervical cancer.** This suggests that other genetic or environmental factors also are involved in cervical carcinogenesis. For example, **individuals who are immunosuppressed because of either HIV infection (299) or immunosuppressive drugs are more likely to develop dysplasia and invasive cervical cancer following HPV infection.**

Cervical screening programs in developed nations have dramatically reduced both the incidence of invasive cervical cancer and disease-related mortality. The recent development of vaccines against oncogenic HPV subtypes has the potential to further decrease the incidence of cervical dysplasia and cancer (300). Although cervical cancer mortality is low in the United States and Western Europe, it remains among the leading causes of cancer deaths in women in underdeveloped nations.

Human Papilloma Virus Infection

There are more than 100 HPV subtypes, but not all infect the lower genital tract. **HPV 16 and 18 are the most common types associated with cervical cancer** and are found in more than 80% of cases. **Types 31, 33, 35, 39, 45, 51, 52, 56, 58, 59, 68, 73, and 82 should be** considered high-risk types, and types 26, 53, and 66 should be considered probably carcinogenic (298). Low-risk types that may cause dysplasias or condyloma in the lower genital tract, but rarely cause cancers, include types 6, 11, 40, 42, 43, 44, 54, 61, 70, 72, and 81. The advent of HPV typing now allows assessment of whether patients carry high-risk or low-risk HPV types, and this has proven clinically useful in the management of patients with low-grade Pap smear abnormalities.

The HPV DNA sequence consists of 7,800 nucleotides divided into "early" and "late" open reading frames (ORFs). Early ORFs are within the first 4,200 nucleotides of the genome and encode proteins (E1–E8) that are important in viral replication and cellular transformation. Late ORFs (L1 and L2) are found within the latter half of the sequence and encode structural proteins of the virion. In oncogenic subtypes such as HPV 16 and 18, transformation may be accompanied by integration of episomal HPV DNA into the host genome. Opening of the episomal viral genome usually occurs in the E1–E2 region, resulting in a linear fragment for insertion. The location of the opening may be significant because E2 acts as a repressor of the *E6–E7 promoter,* and disruption of E2 can lead to unregulated expression of the *E6/E7 transforming genes.* HPV 16 DNA may be found in its episomal form in some cervical cancers, however, and unregulated E6–E7 transcription may occur independently of viral DNA integration into the cellular genome.

Examination of the biological effects of HPV-encoded proteins has shed light on the mechanisms of HPV-associated transformation. Expression of the E4 transcript results in the production of intermediate filaments that colocalize with cytokeratins. E4 proteins of oncogenic subtypes disrupt the cytoplasmic cytokeratin matrix, whereas those of nononcogenic strains do not. It has been suggested that this may facilitate the release of HPV particles in oncogenic subtypes such as HPV 16. The E5 oncogene encodes a 44–amino acid protein that usually forms dimers within the cellular membrane. The transforming properties of E5 appear to involve potentiation of membrane-bound epidermal growth factor receptors or platelet factor growth receptors. **The E6 and E7 oncoproteins are the main transforming genes of oncogenic strains of HPV** (Fig. 1.9) (301). Transfection of these genes *in vitro* results in immortalization and transformation of some cell lines. **The HPV E7 protein acts primarily by binding to and inactivating the Rb tumor suppressor gene product.** E7 contains two domains, one of which mediates binding to *Rb* while the other serves as a substrate for casein kinase II (CKII) phosphorylation. **Variations in oncogenic potential between HPV subtypes may be related to differences in the binding efficacy of E7 to Rb.** High-risk HPV types contain E7 oncoproteins that bind *Rb* with more affinity than E7 from low-risk types. The transforming activity of E7 may be increased by CKII mutation, implying a role for this binding site in the development of HPV-mediated neoplasias.

The E6 proteins of oncogenic HPV subtypes bind to and inactivate the TP53 tumor suppressor gene product (302,303). There also is a correlation between oncogenicity of

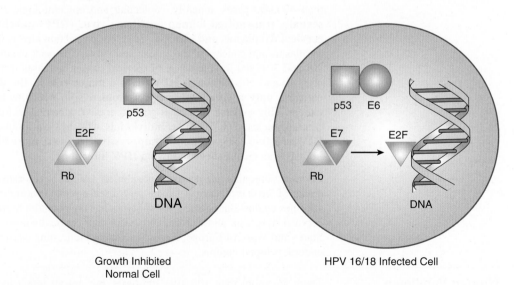

Growth Inhibited
Normal Cell

HPV 16/18 Infected Cell

Figure 1.9 Neutralization of *p53* and *Rb* by HPV 16/18 in cervical cancer.

various HPV strains and the ability of their E6 oncoproteins to inactivate *p53*. Inactivation of *Rb* and *p53* by E6 and E7 circumvents the need for mutational inactivation of these key growth regulatory genes.

HPV-negative cervical cancers are uncommon but have been reported to exhibit overexpression of mutant p53 protein (304). This suggests that inactivation of the *p53* tumor suppressor gene either by HPV E6 or by mutation is a requisite event in cervical carcinogenesis. In some studies, the levels of E6 and E7 in invasive cervical cancers have been found to predict outcome, whereas HPV viral load does not (305).

Genomic Changes

Comparative genomic hybridization techniques have been used to identify chromosomal loci that are either increased or decreased in copy number in cervical cancers. **A strikingly consistent finding of various studies is the high frequency of gains on chromosome 3q in both squamous cell cancers (306,307) and adenocarcinomas** (308). Other chromosomes that exhibit frequent gains include 1q and 11q. The most common areas of chromosomal loss include chromosomes 3p and 2q. For the most part, with the exception of the fragile histidine triad (*FHIT*) gene on chromosome 3p, it has not been proven that these genomic gains and losses result in the recruitment of specific oncogenes and tumor suppressor genes in the process of malignant transformation. It is conceivable that these chromosomal alterations may be frequent sequelae of infection with oncogenic HPVs while playing no significant role in the pathogenesis of cervical cancers. Abnormalities seen in invasive cancers using comparative genomic hybridization also have been identified in high-grade dysplasias, however, suggesting that these are early events in cervical carcinogenesis (307,309,310).

Oncogenes and Tumor Suppressor Genes

Only a small fraction of HPV-infected women develop cervical cancer. This suggests that additional genetic alterations are requisite for progression to high-grade dysplasia and cancer, but little is known regarding these events. Allele loss suggestive of involvement of tumor suppressor genes has been noted at loci on chromosomes 3p, 11p, and others. It is striking that **the cyclin-dependent kinase inhibitor *p16* is up regulated in almost all cervical dysplasias and cancers** (311). Clinical trials are ongoing to determine whether this will represent a useful adjunct to improve the positive predictive value of high-risk HPV testing for detection of cervical dysplasia.

The role of several oncogenes has been examined in cervical carcinomas, most prominently in the *ras* and *myc* genes. **Mutant *ras* genes are capable of cooperating with HPV in transforming cells *in vitro*.** There is some evidence that mutations in either K-*ras* or H-*ras* may play a role in a subset of cervical cancers (304,312–315). **Alterations in *ras* genes have not been seen in cervical intraepithelial neoplasia, suggesting that mutation of *ras* is a late event in the pathogenesis of some cervical cancers. In contrast, *c-myc* amplification and overexpression may be an early event in the development of some cervical cancers** (316). Overexpression of *c-myc* has been demonstrated in one-third of early invasive carcinomas and some CIN 3 lesions, but not in normal cervical epithelium or lower-grade dysplasia. Overexpression of *c-myc* gene may result from amplification of the gene (four- to 20-fold) in some cases. In some studies, amplification correlated with poor prognosis in early stage cases (317). Other studies have not confirmed the finding of amplification of *c-myc* in cervical cancers, however. Integration of the HPV genome near *c-myc* on chromosome 8q may lead to increased expression because of enhanced transcription of the gene rather than amplification. Further studies are needed to clarify the role of *ras* genes, *c-myc,* and other oncogenes in cervical carcinogenesis.

The fragile histidine triad gene localized within human chromosomal band 3p14.2 is frequently deleted in many different cancers, including cervical cancer (318–320). Decreased expression of this putative tumor suppressor gene is an early event in some cervical cancers (320,321). In one study, *FHIT* protein expression was markedly reduced or absent in 71% of invasive cancers, 52% of high-grade squamous intraepithelial lesions (HSILs) associated with invasive cancer, and 21% of HSILs without associated invasive cancer (320). In addition, reduced expression is associated with poor prognosis in advanced cervical cancers (322).

As is the case in endometrial and ovarian cancers, **it is thought that gene silencing resulting from promoter hypermethylation also may play a role in cervical carcinogenesis** (323,324). In this regard, the *RAS* association domain family 1A (*RASSF1A*) gene is located on chromosome 3p21.3 in an area that is frequently a site of deletions in cervical cancer. The function of this gene is not completely understood, but it is thought to be involved in *ras*-mediated signal transduction pathways. Although mutations in *RASSF1A* do not occur in cervical cancers, inactivation of the gene because of promoter methylation occurs in a fraction of cases, particularly adenocarcinomas (325,326).

Hypermethylation of genes associated with programmed cell death (apoptosis) or tumor suppressor genes have also been described in association with cervical cancer. Likewise, hypermethylation of HPV DNA that has been integrated into the host genome may also play a role in suppressing the transformation associated with viral oncogenes until other molecular alterations overcome this method of epigenetic silencing (327).

Gestational Trophoblastic Disease

The genetic alterations that underlie gestational trophoblastic disease have been elucidated to a great extent. **The most prominent feature of these tumors is an imbalance of parental chromosomes. In the case of partial moles, this involves an extra haploid copy of one set of paternal chromosomes, while complete moles generally are characterized by two complete haploid sets of paternal chromosomes and an absence of maternal chromosomes.** Although the risk of repeat molar pregnancy is only approximately 1%, women who have had two molar pregnancies have an approximate 25% risk of developing another mole. Although this suggests a hereditary defect that affects gametogenesis, this remains speculative. **Thus far, there is no convincing evidence that damage to specific tumor suppressor genes or oncogenes contributes to the development of gestational trophoblastic disease.** However, recent microarray studies have identified several genes that are differentially expressed compared to those found in normal villi, particularly genes associated with cellular apoptosis, immunosuppression, and cell invasion (328,329).

References

1. **Schwartz GK, Shah MA.** Targeting the cell cycle: a new approach to cancer therapy. *J Clin Oncol* 2005;23:9408–9421.
2. **Benz EJ, Jr., Nathan DG, Amaravadi RK, Danial NN.** Targeting the cell death-survival equation. *Clin Cancer Res* 2007;13:7250–7253.
3. **Danial NN.** bcl-2 family proteins: critical checkpoints of apoptotic cell death. *Clin Cancer Res* 2007;13:7254–7263.
4. **Amaravadi RK, Thompson CB.** The roles of therapy-induced autophagy and necrosis in cancer treatment. *Clin Cancer Res* 2007;13:7271–7279.
5. **Chao DT, Korsmeyer SJ.** bcl-2 family: regulators of cell death. *Annu Rev Immunology* 1998;16:395–419.
6. **Verdine GL, Walensky LD.** The challenge of drugging undruggable targets in cancer: lessons learned from targeting bcl-2 family members. *Clin Cancer Res* 2007;13:7264–7270.
7. **Shay JW, Keith WN.** Targeting telomerase for cancer therapeutics. *Br J Cancer* 2008;98:677–683.
8. **Kyo S, Takakura M, Tanaka M, Murakami K, Saitoh R, Hirano H, et al.** Quantitative differences in telomerase activity among malignant, premalignant, and benign ovarian lesions. *Clin Cancer Res* 1998;4:399–405.
9. **Wan M, Li WZ, Duggan BD, Felix JC, Zhao Y, Dubeau L, et al.** Telomerase activity in benign and malignant epithelial ovarian tumors. *J Natl Cancer Inst* 1997;89:437–441.
10. **Takakura M, Kyo S, Kanaya T, Tanaka M, Inoue M, et al.** Expression of human telomerase subunits and correlation with telomerase activity in cervical cancer. *Cancer Res* 1998;58:1558–1561.
11. **Kyo S, Takakura M, Tanaka M, Kanaya T, Inoue M, et al.** Telomerase activity in cervical cancer is quantitatively distinct from that in its precursor lesions. *Int J Cancer* 1998;79:66–70.
12. **Brien TP, Kallakury BV, Lowry CV, Ambros RA, Muraca PJ, Malfetano JH, et al.** Telomerase activity in benign endometrium and endometrial carcinoma. *Cancer Res* 1997;57:2760–2764.
13. **Kyo S, Takakura M, Kohama T, Inoue M.** Telomerase activity in human endometrium. *Cancer Res* 1997;57:610–614.
14. **Croce CM.** Oncogenes and cancer. *N Engl J Med* 2008;358:502–511.
15. **Esteller M.** Epigenetics in cancer. *N Engl J Med* 2008;358:1148–1159.
16. **Wicha MS, Liu S, Dontu G.** Cancer stem cells: an old idea—a paradigm shift. *Cancer Res* 2006;66:1883–1890.
17. **Stratton MR, Rahman N.** The emerging landscape of breast cancer susceptibility. *Nat Genet* 2008;40:17–22.
18. **Gryfe R, Di Nicola N, Lal G, Gallinger S, Redston M.** Inherited colorectal polyposis and cancer risk of the *APC* I1307K polymorphism. *Am J Hum Genet* 1999;64:378–384.
19. **Bublil EM, Yarden Y.** The EGF receptor family: spearheading a merger of signaling and therapeutics. *Curr Opin Cell Biol* 2007;19:124–134.
20. **Shepard HM, Jin P, Slamon DJ, Pirot Z, Maneval DC.** Herceptin. *Handb Exp Pharmacol* 2008;183–219.
21. **Kumar A, Petri ET, Halmos B, Boggon TJ.** Structure and clinical relevance of the epidermal growth factor receptor in human cancer. *J Clin Oncol* 2008;26:1742–1751.
22. **Schwartzberg PL.** The many faces of SRC: multiple functions of a prototypical tyrosine kinase. *Oncogene* 1998;17:1463–1468.
23. **Summy JM, Gallick GE.** Treatment for advanced tumors: SRC reclaims center stage. *Clin Cancer Res* 2006;12:1398–1401.
24. **Tokunaga E, Oki E, Egashira A, Sadanaga N, Morita M, Kakeji Y, et al.** Deregulation of the Akt pathway in human cancer. *Curr Cancer Drug Targets* 2008;8:27–36.
25. **Ho CL, Kurman RJ, Dehari R, Wang TL, Shih IeM.** Mutations of *BRAF* and *KRAS* precede the development of ovarian serous borderline tumors. *Cancer Res* 2004;64:6915–6918.
26. **Duursma AM, Agami R.** Ras interference as cancer therapy. *Semin Cancer Biol* 2003;13:267–273.
27. **Facchini LM, Penn LZ.** The molecular role of *myc* in growth and transformation: recent discoveries lead to new insights. *FASEB Journal* 1998;12:633–651.
28. **Leiderman YI, Kiss S, Mukai S.** Molecular genetics of *Rb1*—the retinoblastoma gene. *Semin Ophthalmol* 2007;22:247–254.
29. **Shapiro GI.** Cyclin-dependent kinase pathways as targets for cancer treatment. *J Clin Oncol* 2006;24:1770–1783.
30. **Berchuck A, Kohler MF, Marks JR, Wiseman R, Boyd J, Bast RC Jr., et al.** The *p53* tumor suppressor gene frequently is altered in gynecologic cancers. *Am J Obstet Gynecol* 1994;170:246–252.
31. **Soussi T.** *p53* alterations in human cancer: more questions than answers. *Oncogene* 2007;26:2145–2156.
32. **Elliott RL, Blobe GC.** Role of transforming growth factor Beta in human cancer. *J Clin Oncol* 2005;23:2078–2093.

33. **Calin GA, Croce CM.** MicroRNA-cancer connection: the beginning of a new tale. *Cancer Res* 2006;66:7390–7394.

34. **Fidler IJ.** The pathogenesis of cancer metastasis: the "seed and soil" hypothesis revisited. *Nat Rev Cancer* 2003;3:453–458.

35. **Paget S.** The distribution of secondary growths in cancer of the breast. *Cancer Metastasis Rev* 1989;8:98–101.

36. **Mueller MM, Fusenig NE.** Friends or foes—bipolar effects of the tumour stroma in cancer. *Nat Rev Cancer* 2004;4:839–849.

37. **Folkman J.** Angiogenesis in cancer, vascular, rheumatoid and other disease. *Nat Med* 1995;1:27–31.

38. **Frumovitz M, Sood AK.** Vascular endothelial growth factor (VEGF) pathway as a therapeutic target in gynecologic malignancies. *Gynecol Oncol* 2007;104:768–778.

39. **Senger DR, Galli SJ, Dvorak AM, Perruzzi CA, Harvey VS, Dvorak HF, et al.** Tumor cells secrete a vascular permeability factor that promotes accumulation of ascites fluid. *Science* 1983;219:983–985.

40. **Spannuth WA, Sood AK, Coleman RL.** Angiogenesis as a strategic target for ovarian cancer therapy. *Nat Clin Pract Oncol* 2008;5: 194–204.

41. **Jung YD, Ahmad SA, Akagi Y, Takahashi Y, Liu W, Reinmuth N, et al.** Role of the tumor microenvironment in mediating response to anti-angiogenic therapy. *Cancer Metastasis Rev* 2000;19:147–157.

42. **Liotta LA, Kohn EC.** The microenvironment of the tumour-host interface. *Nature* 2001;411:375–379.

43. **Kamat AA, Fletcher M, Gruman LM, Mueller P, Lopez A, Landen CN Jr, et al.** The clinical relevance of stromal matrix metalloproteinase expression in ovarian cancer. *Clin Cancer Res* 2006;12: 1707–1714.

44. **Boudreau N, Bissell MJ.** Extracellular matrix signaling: integration of form and function in normal and malignant cells. *Curr Opin Cell Biol* 1998;10:640–646.

45. **Hood JD, Cheresh DA.** Role of integrins in cell invasion and migration. *Nat Rev Cancer* 2002;2:91–100.

46. **Hay E.** *Biology of the extracellular matrix.* 1991; New York: Plenum Press.

47. **Hynes RO.** Integrins: versatility, modulation, and signaling in cell adhesion. *Cell* 1992;69:11–25.

48. **Morgan MR, Humphries MJ, Bass MD.** Synergistic control of cell adhesion by integrins and syndecans. *Nat Rev Mol Cell Biol* 2007;8:957–969.

49. **Hirohashi S.** Inactivation of the E-cadherin-mediated cell adhesion system in human cancers. *Am J Pathol* 1998;153:333–339.

50. **Sundfeldt K, Piontkewitz Y, Ivarsson K, Nilsson O, Hellberg P, Brännström M, et al.** E-cadherin expression in human epithelial ovarian cancer and normal ovary. *Int J Cancer* 1997;74:275–280.

51. **Risinger JI, Berchuck A, Kohler MF, Boyd J.** Mutations of the E-cadherin gene in human gynecologic cancers. *Nat Genet* 1994;7:98–102.

52. **O'Sullivan MJ, McCarthy TV, Doyle CT.** Familial adenomatous polyposis: from bedside to benchside. *Am J Clin Pathol* 1998;109: 521–526.

53. **Fukuchi T, Sakamoto M, Tsuda H, Maruyama K, Nozawa S, Hirohashi S, et al.** Beta-catenin mutation in carcinoma of the uterine endometrium. *Cancer Res* 1998;58:3526–3528.

54. **Paul P, Rouas-Freiss N, Khalil-Daher I, Moreau P, Riteau B, Le Gal FA, et al.** HLA-G expression in melanoma: a way for tumor cells to escape from immunosurveillance. *Proc Natl Acad Sci U S A* 1998;95:4510–4515.

55. **Wood LD, Parsons DW, Jones S, Lin J, Sjöblom T, Leary RJ, et al.** The genomic landscapes of human breast and colorectal cancers. *Science* 2007;318:1108–1113.

56. **Deligdisch L, Holinka CF.** Endometrial carcinoma: two diseases? *Cancer Detect Prev* 1987;10:237–246.

57. **Lynch HT, Lynch J.** Lynch syndrome: genetics, natural history, genetic counseling, and prevention. *J Clin Oncol* 2000;18:19S–31S.

58. **Annie Yu HJ, Lin KM, Ota DM, Lynch HT.** Hereditary nonpolyposis colorectal cancer: preventive management. *Cancer Treat Rev* 2003;29:461–470.

59. **Giardiello FM, Bresinger JD, Peterson GM.** *American Gastroenterological Association technical review: Hereditary colorectal cancer and genetic testing* 2001.

60. **Wijnen J, de Leeuw W, Vasen H, van der Klift H, Møller P, Stormorken A, et al.** Familial endometrial cancer in female carriers of *MSH6* germline mutations. *Nat Genet* 1999;23:142–144.

61. **Peltomäki P, Lothe RA, Aaltonen LA, Pylkkänen L, Nyström-Lahti M, Seruca R, et al.** Microsatellite instability is associated with tumors that characterize the hereditary non-polyposis colorectal carcinoma syndrome. *Cancer Res* 1993;53:5853–5855.

62. **Aaltonen LA, Peltomäki P, Leach FS, Sistonen P, Pylkkänen L, Mecklin JP, et al.** Clues to the pathogenesis of familial colorectal cancer. *Science* 1993;260:812–816.

63. **Kowalski LD, Mutch DG, Herzog TJ, et al.** Mutational analysis of *MLH1* and *MSH2* in 25 prospectively-acquired RER+ endometrial cancers. *Genes Chromosomes Cancer* 1997;18:219–227.

64. **Thibodeau SN, French AJ, Roche PC, Cunningham JM, Tester DJ, Lindor NM, et al.** Altered expression of *hMSH2* and *hMLH1* in tumors with microsatellite instability and genetic alterations in mismatch repair genes. *Cancer Res* 1996;56:4836–4840.

65. **Simpkins SB, Bocker T, Swisher EM, Mutch DG, Gersell DJ, Kovatich AJ, et al.** *MLH1* promoter methylation and gene silencing is the primary cause of microsatellite instability in sporadic endometrial cancers. *Hum Mol Genet* 1999;8:661–666.

66. **Salvesen HB, MacDonald N, Ryan A, Iversen OE, Jacobs IJ, Akslen LA, et al.** Methylation of *hMLH1* in a population-based series of endometrial carcinomas. *Clin Cancer Res* 2000;6: 3607–3613.

67. **Hampel H, Frankel W, Panescu J, Lockman J, Sotamaa K, Fix D, et al.** Screening for Lynch syndrome (hereditary nonpolyposis colorectal cancer) among endometrial cancer patients. *Cancer Res* 2006;66:7810–7817.

68. **Watson P, Vasen HF, Mecklin JP, Bernstein I, Aarnio M, Järvinen HJ, et al.** The risk of endometrial cancer in hereditary nonpolyposis colorectal cancer. *Am J Med* 1994;96:516–520.

69. **Dunlop MG, Farrington SM, Carothers AD, Wyllie AH, Sharp L, Burn J, et al.** Cancer risk associated with germline DNA mismatch repair gene mutations. *Hum Mol Genet* 1997;6:105–110.

70. **Aarnio M, Mecklin JP, Aaltonen LA, Nyström-Lahti M, Järvinen HJ.** Life-time risk of different cancers in hereditary non-polyposis colorectal cancer (HNPCC) syndrome. *Int J Cancer* 1995;64:430–433.

71. **Vasen HF, Watson P, Mecklin JP, Jass JR, Green JS, Nomizu T, et al.** The epidemiology of endometrial cancer in hereditary nonpolyposis colorectal cancer. *Anticancer Res* 1994;14:1675–1678.

72. **Brown GJ, St John DJ, Macrae FA, Aittomäki K.** Cancer risk in young women at risk of hereditary nonpolyposis colorectal cancer: implications for gynecologic surveillance. *Cancer Res* 2001;80: 346–349.

73. **Boks DE, Trujillo AP, Voogd AC, Morreau H, Kenter GG, Vasen HF.** Survival analysis of endometrial carcinoma associated with hereditary nonpolyposis colorectal cancer. *Int J Cancer* 2002;102: 198–200.

74. **Watson P, Bützow R, Lynch HT, Mecklin JP, Järvinen HJ, Vasen HF, et al.** The clinical features of ovarian cancer in hereditary nonpolyposis colorectal cancer. *Cancer Res* 2001;82:223–228.

75. **Shannon C, Kirk J, Barnetson R, Evans J, Schnitzler M, Quinn M, et al.** Incidence of microsatellite instability in synchronous tumors of the ovary and endometrium. *Clin Cancer Res* 2003;9:1387–1392.

76. **Dove-Edwin I, Boks D, Goff S, Kenter GG, Carpenter R, Vasen HF, Thomas HJ.** The outcome of endometrial carcinoma surveillance by ultrasound scan in women at risk of hereditary nonpolyposis colorectal carcinoma and familial colorectal carcinoma. *Cancer* 2002;94:1708–1712.

77. **Schmeler KM, Lynch HT, Chen LM, Munsell MF, Soliman PT, Clark MB, et al.** Prophylactic surgery to reduce the risk of gynecologic cancers in the Lynch syndrome. *N Engl J Med* 2006;354:261–269.

78. Writing group for the women's health initiative investigators. Risks and benefits of estrogen plus progestin in healthy postmenopausal women: principal results from the women's health initiative randomized controlled trial. *JAMA* 2003;288:321–333.

79. **Shah NK, Currie JL, Rosenshein N, Campbell J, Long P, Abbas F, et al.** Cytogenetic and FISH analysis of endometrial carcinoma. *Cancer Genet Cytogenet* 1994;73:142–146.

80. **Baloglu H, Cannizzaro LA, Jones J, Koss LG.** Atypical endometrial hyperplasia shares genomic abnormalities with endometrioid carcinoma by comparative genomic hybridization. *Hum Pathol* 2001;32:615–622.

81. **Kiechle M, Hinrichs M, Jacobsen A, Lüttges J, Pfisterer J, Kommoss F, et al.** Genetic imbalances in precursor lesions of

endometrial cancer detected by comparative genomic hybridization. *Am J Pathol* 2000;156:1827–1833.

82. **Suzuki A, Fukushige S, Nagase S, Ohuchi N, Satomi S, Horii A.** Frequent gains on chromosome arms 1q and/or 8q in human endometrial cancer. *Hum Genet* 1997;100:629–636.

83. **Sonoda G, du Manoir S, Godwin AK, Bell DW, Liu Z, Hogan M, et al.** Detection of DNA gains and losses in primary endometrial carcinomas by comparative genomic hybridization. *Genes Chromosomes Cancer* 1997;18:115–125.

84. **Hirasawa A, Aoki D, Inoue J, Imoto I, Susumu N, Sugano K, et al.** Unfavorable prognostic factors associated with high frequency of microsatellite instability and comparative genomic hybridization analysis in endometrial cancer. *Clin Cancer Res* 2003;9:5675–5682.

85. **Risinger JI, Maxwell GL, Chandramouli GV, Jazaeri A, Aprelikova O, Patterson T, et al.** Microarray analysis reveals distinct gene expression profiles among different histologic types of endometrial cancer. *Cancer Res* 2003;63:6–11.

86. **Suehiro Y, Umayahara K, Ogata H, Numa F, Yamashita Y, Oga A, et al.** Genetic aberrations detected by comparative genomic hybridization predict outcome in patients with endometrioid carcinoma. *Genes Chromosomes Cancer* 2000;29:75–82.

87. **Lukes AS, Kohler MF, Pieper CF, Kerns BJ, Bentley R, Rodriguez GC, et al.** Multivariable analysis of DNA ploidy, *p53*, and HER-2/*neu* as prognostic factors in endometrial cancer. *Cancer* 1994;73:2380–2385.

88. **Moreno-Bueno G, Sánchez-Estévez C, Cassia R, Rodríguez-Perales S, Díaz-Uriarte R, Domínguez O, et al.** Differential gene expression profile in endometrioid and nonendometrial carcinoma: *STK15* is frequently overexpressed and amplified in nonendometrioid carcinomas. *Cancer Res* 2003;63:5697–5702.

89. **Mutter GL, Baak JP, Fitzgerald JT, Gray R, Neuberg D, Kust GA, et al.** Global expression changes of constitutive and hormonally regulated genes during endometrial neoplastic transformation. *Gynecol Oncol* 2001;83:177–185.

90. **Maxwell GL, Chandramouli GV, Dainty L, Litzi TJ, Berchuck A, et al.** Microarray analysis of endometrial carcinomas and mixed mullerian tumors reveals distinct gene expression profiles associated with different histologic types of uterine cancer. *Clin Cancer Res* 2005;11:4056–4066.

91. **Wong YF, Cheung TH, Lo KW, Yim SF, Siu NS, Chan SC, et al.** Identification of molecular markers and signaling pathway in endometrial cancer in Hong Kong Chinese women by genome-wide gene expression profiling. *Oncogene* 2007;26:1971–82.

92. **Bidus MA, Risinger JI, Chandramouli GV, Dainty LA, Litzi TJ, Berchuck A, et al.** Prediction of lymph node metastasis in patients with endometrioid endometrial cancer using expression microarray. *Clin Cancer Res* 2006;12:83–88.

93. **Ferguson SE, Olshen AB, Viale A, Barakat RR, Boyd J.** Stratification of intermediate-risk endometrial cancer patients into groups at high risk or low risk for recurrence based on tumor gene expression profiles. *Clin Cancer Res* 2005;11:2252–2257.

94. **Kohler MF, Berchuck A, Davidoff AM, et al.** Overexpression and mutation of *p53* in endometrial carcinoma. *Cancer Res* 1992;52:1622–1627.

95. **Hachisuga T, Fukuda K, Uchiyama M, et al.** Immunohistochemical study of *p53* expression in endometrial carcinomas: correlation with markers of proliferating cells and clinicopathologic features. *Int J Gynecol Cancer* 1993;3:363–368.

96. **Hamel NW, Sebo TJ, Wilson TO, et al.** Prognostic value of *p53* and proliferating cell nuclear antigen expression in endometrial carcinoma. *Cancer Res* 1996;62:192–198.

97. **Inoue M, Okayama A, Fujita M, et al.** Clinicopathological characteristics of *p53* overexpression in endometrial cancers. *Int J Cancer* 1994;58:14–19.

98. **Ito K, Watanabe K, Nasim S, Sasano H, Sato S, Yajima A, et al.** Prognostic significance of *p53* overexpression in endometrial cancer. *Cancer Res* 1994;54:4667–4670.

99. **Khalifa MA, Mannel RS, Haraway SD, Walker J, Min KW.** Expression of EGFR, HER-2/*neu*, *p53*, and PCNA in endometrioid, serous papillary, and clear cell endometrial adenocarcinomas. *Cancer Res* 1994;53:84–92.

100. **Kohlberger P, Gitsch G, Loesch A, Tempfer C, Kaider A, Reinthaller A, et al.** p53 protein overexpression in early stage endometrial cancer. *Cancer Res* 1996;62:213–217.

101. **Service RF.** Research news: stalking the start of colon cancer. *Science* 1994;263:1559–1560.

102. **Clifford SL, Kaminetsky CP, Cirisano FD, Dodge R, Soper JT, Clarke-Pearson DL, et al.** Racial disparity in overexpression of the *p53* tumor suppressor gene in stage I endometrial cancer. *Am J Obstet Gynecol* 1997;176:S229–S232.

103. **Kohler MF, Carney P, Dodge R, Soper JT, Clarke-Pearson DL, Marks JR, et al.** *p53* overexpression in advanced-stage endometrial adenocarcinoma. *Am J Obstet Gynecol* 1996;175:1246–1252.

104. **Liu FS, Kohler MF, Marks JR, Bast RC Jr, Boyd J, Berchuck A.** Mutation and overexpression of the *p53* tumor suppressor gene frequently occurs in uterine and ovarian sarcomas. *Obstet Gynecol* 1994;83:118–124.

105. **Hall KL, Teneriello MG, Taylor RR, Lemon S, Ebina M, Linnoila RI, et al.** Analysis of Ki-*ras*, *p53*, and *MDM2* genes in uterine leiomyomas and leiomyosarcomas. *Cancer Res* 1997;65:330–335.

106. **Enomoto T, Fujita M, Inoue M, Rice JM, Nakajima R, Tanizawa O, et al.** Alterations of the *p53* tumor suppressor gene and its association with activation of the c-K-*ras*-2 protooncogene in premalignant and malignant lesions of the human uterine endometrium. *Cancer Res* 1993;53:1883–1888.

107. **Okamoto A, Sameshima Y, Yamada Y, Teshima S, Terashima Y, Terada M, et al.** Allelic loss on chromosome 17p and *p53* mutations in human endometrial carcinoma of the uterus. *Cancer Res* 1991;51:5632–5636.

108. **Ignar-Trowbridge D, Risinger JI, Dent GA, Kohler M, Berchuck A, McLachlan JA, et al.** Mutations of the *p53* gene in human endometrial carcinoma. *Molec Carcinog* 1992;5:250–253.

109. **Yaginuma Y, Westphal H.** Analysis of the *p53* gene in human uterine carcinoma cell lines. *Cancer Res* 1991;51:6506–6509.

110. **Kohler MF, Nishii H, Humphrey PA, Saski H, Marks J, Bast RC, et al.** Mutation of the *p53* tumor-suppressor gene is not a feature of endometrial hyperplasias. *Am J Obstet Gynecol* 1993;169:690–694.

111. **Tashiro H, Isacson C, Levine R, Kurman RJ, Cho KR, Hedrick L.** *p53* gene mutations are common in uterine serous carcinoma and occur early in their pathogenesis. *Am J Pathol* 1997;150:177–185.

112. **Jia L, Liu Y, Yi X, Miron A, Crum CP, Kong B, et al.** Endometrial glandular dysplasia with frequent *p53* gene mutation: a genetic evidence supporting its precancer nature for endometrial serous carcinoma. *Clin Cancer Res* 2008;14:2263–2269.

113. **Kong D, Suzuki A, Zou TT, Sakurada A, Kemp LW, Wakatsuki S, et al.** *PTEN*1 is frequently mutated in primary endometrial carcinomas. *Nat Genet* 1997;17:143–144.

114. **Risinger JI, Hayes AK, Berchuck A, Barrett JC.** *PTEN*/MMAC1 mutations in endometrial cancers. *Cancer Res* 1997;57:4736–4738.

115. **Tashiro H, Blazes MS, Wu R, Cho KR, Bose S, Wang SI, et al.** Mutations in *PTEN* are frequent in endometrial carcinoma but rare in other common gynecologic malignancies. *Cancer Res* 1997;57:3935–3940.

116. **Kanamori Y, Kigawa J, Itamochi H, Shimada M, Takahashi M, Kamazawa S, et al.** Correlation between loss of *PTEN* expression and Akt phosphorylation in endometrial carcinoma. *Clin Cancer Res* 2001;7:892–895.

117. **Risinger JI, Hayes K, Maxwell GL, Carney ME, Dodge RK, Barrett JC, et al.** *PTEN* mutation in endometrial cancers is associated with favorable clinical and pathologic characteristics. *Clin Cancer Res* 1998;4:3005–3010.

118. **Milner J, Ponder B, Hughes-Davies L, et al.** Transcriptional activation functions in *BRCA2*. *Nature* 1997;386:772–773.

119. **Mutter GL, Ince TA, Baak JP, Kust GA, Zhou XP, Eng C.** Molecular identification of latent precancers in histologically normal endometrium. *Cancer Res* 2001;61:4311–4314.

120. **Mutter GL, Lin MC, Fitzgerald JT, Kum JB, Baak JP, Lees JA, et al.** Altered *PTEN* expression as a diagnostic marker for the earliest endometrial precancers. *J Natl Cancer Inst* 2000;92:924–930.

121. **Lin WM, Forgacs E, Warshal DP, Yeh IT, Martin JS, Ashfaq R, et al.** Loss of heterozygosity and mutational analysis of the *PTEN/MMAC1* gene in synchronous endometrial and ovarian carcinomas. *Clin Cancer Res* 1998;4:2577–2583.

122. **Obata K, Morland SJ, Watson RH, Hitchcock A, Chenevix-Trench G, Thomas EJ, et al.** Frequent *PTEN/MMAC* mutations in endometrioid but not serous or mucinous epithelial ovarian tumors. *Cancer Res* 1998;58:2095–2097.

123. Risinger JI, Berchuck A, Kohler MF, Watson P, Lynch HT, Boyd J. Genetic instability of microsatellites in endometrial carcinoma. *Cancer Res* 1993;53:5100–5103.

124. Faquin WC, Fitzgerald JT, Lin MC, Boynton KA, Muto MG, Mutter GL. Sporadic microsatellite instability is specific to neoplastic and preneoplastic endometrial tissues. *Am J Clin Pathol* 2000;113: 576–582.

125. Esteller M, Catasus L, Matias-Guiu X, Mutter GL, Prat J, Baylin SB, et al. *hMLH1* promoter hypermethylation is an early event in human endometrial tumorigenesis. *Am J Pathol* 1999;155:1767–1772.

126. Kanaya T, Kyo S, Maida Y, Yatabe N, Tanaka M, Nakamura M, et al. Frequent hypermethylation of *MLH1* promoter in normal endometrium of patients with endometrial cancers. *Oncogene* 2003;22:2352–2360.

127. Risinger JI, Maxwell GL, Berchuck A, Barrett JC. Promoter hypermethylation as an epigenetic component in Type I and Type II endometrial cancers. *Ann N Y Acad Sci* 2003;983:208–212.

128. Momparler RL. Cancer epigenetics. *Oncogene* 2003;22:6479–6483.

129. Moreno-Bueno G, Fernandez-Marcos PJ, Collado M, Tendero MJ, Rodriguez-Pinilla SM, Garcia-Cao I, et al. Inactivation of the candidate tumor suppressor *par-4* in endometrial cancer. *Cancer Res* 2007;67:1927–1934.

130. Zukerberg LR, DeBernardo RL, Kirley SD, D'Apuzzo M, Lynch MP, Littell RD, et al. Loss of *cables,* a cyclin-dependent kinase regulatory protein, is associated with the development of endometrial hyperplasia and endometrial cancer. *Cancer Res* 2004;64:202–208.

131. Spruck CH, Strohmaier H, Sangfelt O, Müller HM, Hubalek M, Müller-Holzner, et al. *hCDC4* gene mutations in endometrial cancer. *Cancer Res* 2002;62:4535–4539.

132. Berchuck A, Rodriguez G, Kinney RB, Soper JT, Dodge RK, Clarke-Pearson DL, et al. Overexpression of HER-2/neu in endometrial cancer is associated with advanced stage disease. *Am J Obstet Gynecol* 1991;164:15–21.

133. Hetzel DJ, Wilson TO, Keeney GL, Roche PC, Cha SS, Podratz KC. HER-2/neu expression: a major prognostic factor in endometrial cancer. *Cancer Res* 1992;47:179–185.

134. Lu KH, Bell DA, Welch WR, Berkowitz RS, Mok SC. Evidence for the multifocal origin of bilateral and advanced human serous borderline ovarian tumors. *Cancer Res* 1998;58:2328–2330.

135. Monk BJ, Chapman JA, Johnson GA, Brightman BK, Wilczynski SP, Schell MJ, et al. Correlation of *c-myc* and HER-2/neu amplification and expression with histopathologic variables in uterine corpus cancer. *Am J Obstet Gynecol* 1994;171:1193–1198.

136. Slomovitz BM, Broaddus RR, Burke TW, Sneige N, Soliman PT, Wu W, et al. Her-2/neu overexpression and amplification in uterine papillary serous carcinoma. *J Clin Oncol* 2004;22:3126–3132.

137. Santin AD, Bellone S, Van Stedum S, Bushen W, De Las Casas LE, Korourian S, et al. Determination of HER2/neu status in uterine serous papillary carcinoma: comparative analysis of immunohistochemistry and fluorescence in situ hybridization. *Gynecol Oncol* 2005;98:24–30.

138. Morrison C, Zanagnolo V, Ramirez N, Cohn DE, Kelbick N, Copeland L, et al. HER-2 is an independent prognostic factor in endometrial cancer: association with outcome in a large cohort of surgically staged patients. *J Clin Oncol* 2006;24:2376–2385.

139. Kacinski BM, Carter D, Mittal K, Kohorn EI, Bloodgood RS, Donahue J, et al. High level expression of *fms* proto-oncogene mRNA is observed in clinically aggressive endometrial adenocarcinomas. *Int J Radiat Oncol Biol Phys* 1988;15:823–829.

140. Leiserowitz GS, Harris SA, Subramaniam M, Keeney GL, Podratz KC, Spelsberg TC. The proto-oncogene c-fms is overexpressed in endometrial cancer. *Cancer Res* 1993;49:190–196.

141. Kacinski BM, Chambers SK, Stanley ER, Carter D, Tseng P, Scata KA, et al. The cytokine CSF-1 (M-CSF), expressed by endometrial carcinomas *in vivo* and *in vitro,* may also be a circulating tumor marker of neoplastic disease activity in endometrial carcinoma patients. *Int J Radiat Oncol Biol Phys* 1990;19:619–626.

142. Filderman AE, Bruckner A, Kacinski BM, Deng N, Remold HG. Macrophage colony-stimulating factor (CSF-1) enhances invasiveness in CSF-1 receptor-positive carcinoma cell lines. *Cancer Res* 1992;52:3661–3666.

143. Boyd J, Risinger JI. Analysis of oncogene alterations in human endometrial carcinoma: prevalence of *ras* mutations. *Mol Carcinog* 1991;4:189–195.

144. Ignar-Trowbridge D, Risinger JI, Dent GA, Kohler M, Berchuck A, McLachlan JA, et al. Mutations of the Ki-*ras* oncogene in endometrial carcinoma. *Am J Obstet Gynecol* 1992;167:227–232.

145. Duggan BD, Felix JC, Muderspach LI, Tsao JL, Shibata DK. Early mutational activation of the c-Ki-*ras* oncogene in endometrial carcinoma. *Cancer Res* 1994;54:1604–1607.

146. Enomoto T, Inoue M, Perantoni AO, Terakawa N, Tanizawa O, Rice JM. K-*ras* activation in neoplasms of the human female reproductive tract. *Cancer Res* 1990;50:6139–6145.

147. Enomoto T, Inoue M, Perantoni AO, Buzard GS, Miki H, Tanizawa O, et al. K-*ras* activation in premalignant and malignant epithelial lesions of the human uterus. *Cancer Res* 1991;51:5308–5314.

148. Fujimoto I, Shimizu Y, Hirai Y, Chen JT, Teshima H, Hasumi K, et al. Studies on *ras* oncogene activation in endometrial carcinoma. *Cancer Res* 1993;48:196–202.

149. Mizuuchi H, Nasim S, Kudo R, Silverberg SG, Greenhouse S, Garrett CT. Clinical implications of K-*ras* mutations in malignant epithelial tumors of the endometrium. *Cancer Res* 1992;52: 2777–2781.

150. Sasaki H, Nishii H, Takahashi H, Tada A, Furusato M, Terashima Y, et al. Mutation of the Ki-*ras* protooncogene in human endometrial hyperplasia and carcinoma. *Cancer Res* 1993;53:1906–1910.

151. Mutter GL, Wada H, Faquin WC, Enomoto T. K-*ras* mutations appear in the premalignant phase of both microsatellite stable and unstable endometrial carcinogenesis. *Mol Pathol* 1999;52:257–262.

152. Oda K, Stokoe D, Taketani Y, McCormick F. High frequency of coexistent mutations of *PIK3CA* and *PTEN* genes in endometrial carcinoma. *Cancer Res* 2005;65:10669–10673.

153. Hayes MP, Wang H, Espinal-Witter R, Douglas W, et al. *PIK3CA* and *PTEN* mutations in uterine endometrioid carcinoma and complex atypical hyperplasia. *Clin Cancer Res* 2006;12:5932–5935.

154. Milam MR, Soliman PT, Chung LH, Schmeler KM, Bassett RL Jr, Broaddus RR, et al. Loss of phosphatase and tensin homologue deleted on chromosome 10 and phosphorylation of mammalian target of rapamycin are associated with progesterone refractory endometrial hyperplasia. *Int J Gynecol Cancer* 2008;18: 146–151.

155. Abraham RT, Gibbons JJ. The mammalian target of rapamycin signaling pathway: twists and turns in the road to cancer therapy. *Clin Cancer Res* 2007;13:3109–3114.

156. Fujimoto J, Ichigo S, Hori M, Tamaya T. Expressions of E-cadherin and alpha- and beta-catenin mRNAs in uterine endometrial cancers. *Eur J Gynaecol Oncol* 1998;19:78–81.

157. Hirohashi S. Inactivation of the E-cadherin-mediated cell adhesion system in human cancers. *Am J Pathol* 1998;153:333–339.

158. Moreno-Bueno G, Hardisson D, Sánchez C, Sarrió D, Cassia R, García-Rostán G, et al. Abnormalities of the APC/beta-catenin pathway in endometrial cancer. *Oncogene* 2002;21:7981–7990.

159. Mitra AB, Murty VV, Pratap M, Sodhani P, Chaganti RS. ERBB2 (HER2/neu) oncogene is frequently amplified in squamous cell carcinoma of the uterine cervix. *Cancer Res* 1994;54:637–639.

160. Pollock PM, Gartside MG, Dejeza LC, Powell MA, Mallon MA, Davies H, et al. Frequent activating FGFR2 mutations in endometrial carcinomas parallel germline mutations associated with craniosynostosis and skeletal dysplasia syndromes. *Oncogene* 2007.

161. Pollock PM, Gartside MG, Dejeza LC, Powell MA, Mallon MA, Davies H, et al. Immunocytochemical study of ras and myc proto-oncogene polypeptide expression in the human menstrual cycle. *Am J Obstet Gynecol* 1989;161:1663–1668.

162. Borst MP, Baker VV, Dixon D, Hatch KD, Shingleton HM, Miller DM. Oncogene alterations in endometrial carcinoma. *Cancer Res* 1990;38:364–366.

163. Williams JA Jr, Wang ZR, Parrish RS, Hazlett LJ, Smith ST, Young SR. Fluorescence in situ hybridization analysis of HER-2/neu, c-myc, and p53 in endometrial cancer. *Exp Mol Pathol* 1999;67:135–143.

164. Whittemore AS, Harris R, Itnyre J. Characteristics relating to ovarian cancer risk. Collaborative analysis of twelve US case-control studies: IV. the pathogenesis of epithelial ovarian cancer. *Am J Epidemiol* 1992;136:1212–1220.

165. Rodriguez GC, Walmer DK, Cline M, Krigman H, Lessey BA, Whitaker RS, et al. Effect of progestin on the ovarian epithelium of macaques: cancer prevention through apoptosis? *J Soc Gynecol Investig* 1998;5:271–276.

166. **Kurman RJ, Shih I.** Pathogenesis of ovarian cancer: lessons from morphology and molecular biology and their clinical implications. *Int J Gynecol Pathol* 2008;27:151–160.

167. **Narod SA, Boyd J.** Current understanding of the epidemiology and clinical implications of *BRCA1* and *BRCA2* mutations for ovarian cancer. *Curr Opin Obstet Gynecol* 2002;14:19–26.

168. **Stratton JF, Gayther SA, Russell P, Dearden J, Gore M, Blake P, et al.** Contribution of *BRCA1* mutations to ovarian cancer. *N Engl J Med* 1997;336:1125–1130.

169. **Levine DA, Lin O, Barakat RR, Robson ME, McDermott D, Cohen L, et al.** Risk of endometrial carcinoma associated with *BRCA* mutation. *Cancer Res* 2001;80:395–398.

170. **Lavie O, Hornreich G, Ben Arie A, Renbaum P, Levy-Lahad E, Beller U.** *BRCA1* germline mutations in women with uterine serous papillary carcinoma. *Obstet Gynecol* 2000;96:28–32.

171. **Brose MS, Rebbeck TR, Calzone KA, Stopfer JE, Nathanson KL, Weber BL.** Cancer risk estimates for *BRCA1* mutation carriers identified in a risk evaluation program. *J Natl Cancer Inst* 2002;94:1365–1372.

172. **Aziz S, Kuperstein G, Rosen B, Cole D, Nedelcu R, McLaughlin J, et al.** A genetic epidemiological study of carcinoma of the fallopian tube. *Gynecol Oncol* 2001;80:341–345.

173. **Levine DA, Argenta PA, Yee CJ, Marshall DS, Olvera N, Bogomolniy F, et al.** Fallopian tube and primary peritoneal carcinomas associated with *BRCA* mutations. *J Clin Oncol* 2003;21:4222–4227.

174. **Menczer J, Chetrit A, Barda G, Lubin F, Fishler Y, Altaras M, et al.** Frequency of *BRCA* mutations in primary peritoneal carcinoma in Israeli Jewish women. *Cancer Res* 2003;88:58–61.

175. **Powell SN, Kachnic LA.** Roles of *BRCA1* and *BRCA2* in homologous recombination, DNA replication fidelity and the cellular response to ionizing radiation. *Oncogene* 2003;22:5784–5791.

176. **Jasin M.** Homologous repair of DNA damage and tumorigenesis: the *BRCA* connection. *Oncogene* 2002;21:8981–8993.

177. **Rubin SC, Benjamin I, Behbakht K, Takahashi H, Morgan MA, LiVolsi VA, et al.** Clinical and pathological features of ovarian cancer in women with germ-line mutations of *BRCA1*. *N Engl J Med* 1996;335:1413–1416.

178. **Farmer H, McCabe N, Lord CJ, Tutt AN, Johnson DA, Richardson TB, et al.** Targeting the DNA repair defect in *BRCA* mutant cells as a therapeutic strategy. *Nature* 2005;434:917–921.

179. **Whittemore AS, Gong G, Itnyre J.** Prevalence and contribution of *BRCA1* mutations in breast cancer and ovarian cancer: results from three U.S. population-based case-control studies of ovarian cancer. *Am J Hum Genet* 1997;60:496–504.

180. **Struewing JP, Hartge P, Wacholder S, Baker SM, Berlin M, McAdams M, et al.** The risk of cancer associated with specific mutations of *BRCA1* and *BRCA2* among Ashkenazi Jews. *N Engl J Med* 1997;336:1401–1408.

181. **Risch HA, McLaughlin JR, Cole DE, Rosen B, Bradley L, Kwan E, et al.** Prevalence and penetrance of germline *BRCA1* and *BRCA2* mutations in a population series of 649 women with ovarian cancer. *Am J Hum Genet* 2001;68:700–710.

182. **Antoniou A, Pharoah PD, Narod S, Risch HA, Eyfjord JE, Hopper JL, et al.** Average risks of breast and ovarian cancer associated with *BRCA1* or *BRCA2* mutations detected in case series unselected for family history: a combined analysis of 22 studies. *Am J Hum Genet* 2003;72:1117–1130.

183. **Satagopan JM, Boyd J, Kauff ND, Robson M, Scheuer L, Narod S, et al.** Ovarian cancer risk in Ashkenazi Jewish carriers of *BRCA1* and *BRCA2* mutations. *Clin Cancer Res* 2002;8:3776–3781.

184. **Narod SA, Risch H, Moslehi R, Dørum A, Neuhausen S, Olsson H, et al.** Oral contraceptives and the risk of hereditary ovarian cancer. Hereditary Ovarian Cancer Clinical Study Group. *N Engl J Med* 1998;339:424–428.

185. **Gayther SA, Warren W, Mazoyer S, Russell PA, Harrington PA, Chiano M, et al.** Germline mutations of the *BRCA1* gene in breast and ovarian cancer families provide evidence for genotype-phenotype correlation. *Nat Genet* 1995;11:428–433.

186. **Shattuck-Eidens D, Oliphant A, McClure M, McBride C, Gupte J, Rubano T, et al.** *BRCA1* sequence analysis in women at high risk for susceptibility mutations. Risk factor analysis and implications for genetic testing. *JAMA* 1997;278:1242–1250.

187. **Szabo CI, King MC.** Population genetics of *BRCA1* and *BRCA2*. *Am J Hum Genet* 1997;60:1013–1020.

188. **Struewing JP, Abeliovich D, Peretz T, Avishai N, Kaback MM, Collins FS, et al.** The carrier frequency of the *BRCA1* 185delAG mutation is approximately 1 percent in Ashkenazi Jewish individuals. *Nat Genet* 1995;11:198–200.

189. **Deffenbaugh AM, Frank TS, Hoffman M, et al.** Characterization of common *BRCA1* and *BRCA2* variants. *Genet Test* 2002;6:119–121.

190. **Ford D, Easton DF, Bishop DT, et al.** Risks of cancer in *BRCA1*-mutation carriers. Breast Cancer Linkage Consortium. *Lancet* 1994;343:692–695.

191. **Rebbeck TR, Lynch HT, Neuhausen SL, Narod SA, Van't Veer L, Garber JE, et al.** Prevention and Observation of Surgical End Points Study Group., et al. Prophylactic oophorectomy in carriers of *BRCA1* or *BRCA2* mutations. *N Engl J Med* 2002;346:1616–1622.

192. **Kauff ND, Satagopan JM, Robson ME, Scheuer L, Hensley M, Hudis CA, et al.** Risk-reducing salpingo-oophorectomy in women with a *BRCA1* or *BRCA2* mutation. *N Engl J Med* 2002;346:1609–1615.

193. **Piver MS, Jishi MF, Tsukada Y, Nava G.** Primary peritoneal carcinoma after prophylactic oophorectomy in women with a family history of ovarian cancer. A report of the Gilda Radner Familial Ovarian Cancer Registry. *Cancer* 1993;71:2751–2755.

194. **Struewing JP, Watson P, Easton DF, Ponder BA, Lynch HT, Tucker MA.** Prophylactic oophorectomy in inherited breast/ovarian cancer families. *Monogr Natl Cancer Inst* 1995;33–35.

195. **Chen KT, Schooley JL, Flam MS.** Peritoneal carcinomatosis after prophylactic oophorectomy in familial ovarian cancer syndrome. *Obstet Gynecol* 1985;66:93S–94S.

196. **Salazar H, Godwin AK, Daly MB, Laub PB, Hogan WM, Rosenblum N, et al.** Microscopic benign and invasive malignant neoplasms and a cancer-prone phenotype in prophylactic oophorectomies. *J Natl Cancer Inst* 1996;88:1810–1820.

197. **Barakat RR, Federici MG, Saigo PE, Robson ME, Offit K, Boyd J.** Absence of premalignant histologic, molecular, or cell biologic alterations in prophylactic oophorectomy specimens from *BRCA1* heterozygotes. *Cancer* 2000;89:383–390.

198. **Stratton JF, Buckley CH, Lowe D, Ponder BA.** Comparison of prophylactic oophorectomy specimens from carriers and noncarriers of a *BRCA1* or *BRCA2* gene mutation. United Kingdom Coordinating Committee on Cancer Research (UKCCCR) Familial Ovarian Cancer Study Group. *J Natl Cancer Inst* 1999;91:626–628.

199. **Lu KH, Garber JE, Cramer DW, Welch WR, Niloff J, Schrag D, et al.** Occult ovarian tumors in women with *BRCA1* or *BRCA2* mutations undergoing prophylactic oophorectomy. *J Clin Oncol* 2000;18:2728–2732.

200. **Colgan TJ, Murphy J, Cole DE, Narod S, Rosen B.** Occult carcinoma in prophylactic oophorectomy specimens: prevalence and association with *BRCA* germline mutation status. *Am J Surg Pathol* 2001;25:1283–1289.

201. **Paley PJ, Swisher EM, Garcia RL, Agoff SN, Greer BE, Peters KL, et al.** Occult cancer of the fallopian tube in *BRCA-1* germline mutation carriers at prophylactic oophorectomy: a case for recommending hysterectomy at surgical prophylaxis. *Cancer Res* 2001;80:176–180.

202. **Medeiros F, Muto MG, Lee Y, Elvin JA, Callahan MJ, et al.** The tubal fimbria is a preferred site for early adenocarcinoma in women with familial ovarian cancer syndrome. *Am J Surg Pathol* 2006;30:230–236.

203. **Finch A, Beiner M, Lubinski J, Lynch HT, Moller P, Rosen B, et al.** Salpingo-oophorectomy and the risk of ovarian, fallopian tube, and peritoneal cancers in women with a *BRCA1* or *BRCA2* mutation. *JAMA* 2006;296:185–192.

204. **Jacobs IJ, Kohler MF, Wiseman RW, Marks JR, Whitaker R, et al.** Clonal origin of epithelial ovarian carcinoma: analysis by loss of heterozygosity, *p53* mutation, and X-chromosome inactivation. *J Natl Cancer Inst* 1992;84:1793–1798.

205. **Schorge JO, Muto MG, Welch WR, Bandera CA, Rubin SC, Bell DA, et al.** Molecular evidence for multifocal papillary serous carcinoma of the peritoneum in patients with germline *BRCA1* mutations. *J Natl Cancer Inst* 1998;90:841–845.

206. **Kallioniemi A, Kallioniemi OP, Sudar D, Rutovitz D, Gray JW, Waldman F, et al.** Comparative genomic hybridization for molecular cytogenetic analysis of solid tumors. *Science* 1992;258:818–821.

207. **Cliby W, Ritland S, Hartmann L, Dodson M, Halling KC, Keeney G, et al.** Human epithelial ovarian cancer allelotype. *Cancer Res* 1993;53:Suppl-8.

208. **Dodson MK, Hartmann LC, Cliby WA, DeLacey KA, Keeney GL, Ritland SR, et al.** Comparison of loss of heterozygosity patterns in invasive low-grade and high-grade epithelial ovarian carcinomas. *Cancer Res* 1993;53:4456–4460.

209. **Iwabuchi H, Sakamoto M, Sakunaga H, Ma YY, Carcangiu ML, Pinkel D, et al.** Genetic analysis of benign, low-grade, and high-grade ovarian tumors. *Cancer Res* 1995;55:6172–6180.

210. **Suzuki S, Moore DH 2nd, Ginzinger DG, Godfrey TE, Barclay J, Powell B, et al.** An approach to analysis of large-scale correlations between genome changes and clinical endpoints in ovarian cancer. *Cancer Res* 2000;60:5382–5385.

211. **Welsh JB, Zarrinkar PP, Sapinoso LM, Kern SG, Behling CA, Monk BJ, et al.** Analysis of gene expression profiles in normal and neoplastic ovarian tissue samples identifies candidate molecular markers of epithelial ovarian cancer. *Proc Natl Acad Sci U S A* 2001;98:1176–1181.

212. **Schummer M, Ng WV, Bumgarner RE, Nelson PS, Schummer B, Bednarski DW, et al.** Comparative hybridization of an array of 21,500 ovarian cDNAs for the discovery of genes overexpressed in ovarian carcinomas. *Gene* 1999;238:375–385.

213. **Schwartz DR, Kardia SL, Shedden KA, Kuick R, Michailidis G, Taylor JM, et al.** Gene expression in ovarian cancer reflects both morphology and biological behavior, distinguishing clear cell from other poor-prognosis ovarian carcinomas. *Cancer Res* 2002;62:4722–4729.

214. **Bonome T, Lee JY, Park DC, Radonovich M, Pise-Masison C, Brady J, et al.** Expression profiling of serous low malignant potential, low-grade, and high-grade tumors of the ovary. *Cancer Res* 2005;65:10602–10612.

215. **Shridhar V, Lee J, Pandita A, Iturria S, Avula R, Staub J, et al.** Genetic analysis of early- versus late-stage ovarian tumors. *Cancer Res* 2001;61:5895–5904.

216. **Dressman HK, Berchuck A, Chan G, Zhai J, Bild A, Sayer R, et al.** An integrated genomic-based approach to individualized treatment of patients with advanced-stage ovarian cancer. *J Clin Oncol* 2007;25:517–525.

217. **Spentzos D, Levine DA, Kolia S, Otu H, Boyd J, Libermann TA, et al.** Unique gene expression profile based on pathologic response in epithelial ovarian cancer. *J Clin Oncol* 2005;23:7911–7918.

218. **Berchuck A, Iversen ES, Lancaster JM, Pittman J, Luo J, Lee P, et al.** Patterns of gene expression that characterize long-term survival in advanced stage serous ovarian cancers. *Clin Cancer Res* 2005;11:3686–3696.

219. **Bild AH, Yao G, Chang JT, Wang Q, Potti A, Chasse D, et al.** Oncogenic pathway signatures in human cancers as a guide to targeted therapies. *Nature* 2006;439:353–357.

220. **Bennett M, Macdonald K, Chan SW, Luzio JP, Simari R, Weissberg P.** Cell surface trafficking of *Fas*: a rapid mechanism of *p53*-mediated apoptosis. *Science* 1998;282:290–293.

221. **Casey G, Lopez ME, Ramos JC, Plummer SJ, Arboleda MJ, Shaughnessy M, et al.** DNA sequence analysis of exons 2 through 11 and immunohistochemical staining are required to detect all known *p53* alterations in human malignancies. *Oncogene* 1996;13:1971–1981.

222. **Hartmann LC, Podratz KC, Keeney GL, Kamel NA, Edmonson JH, Grill JP, et al.** Prognostic significance of *p53* immunostaining in epithelial ovarian cancer. *J Clin Oncol* 1994;12:64–69.

223. **Kohler MF, Kerns BJ, Humphrey PA, Marks JR, Bast RC Jr, Berchuck A.** Mutation and overexpression of *p53* in early-stage epithelial ovarian cancer. *Obstet Gynecol* 1993;81:643–650.

224. **Marks JR, Davidoff AM, Kerns BJ, Humphrey PA, Pence JC, Dodge RK, et al.** Overexpression and mutation of *p53* in epithelial ovarian cancer. *Cancer Res* 1991;51:2979–2984.

225. **van der Zee AG, Hollema H, Suurmeijer AJ, Krans M, Sluiter WJ, Willemse PH, et al.** Value of P-glycoprotein, glutathione S-transferase pi, c-erbB-2, and *p53* as prognostic factors in ovarian carcinomas. *J Clin Oncol* 1995;13:70–78.

226. **Leitao MM, Soslow RA, Baergen RN, Olvera N, Arroyo C, Boyd J.** Mutation and expression of the *TP53* gene in early stage epithelial ovarian carcinoma. *Gynecol Oncol* 2004;93:301–306.

227. **Eltabbakh GH, Belinson JL, Kennedy AW, Biscotti CV, Casey G, Tubbs RR, et al.** *p53* overexpression is not an independent prognostic factor for patients with primary ovarian epithelial cancer. *Cancer* 1997;80:892–898.

228. **Henriksen R, Strang P, Backstrom T, Wilander E, Tribukait B, Oberg K.** Ki-67 immunostaining and DNA flow cytometry as prognostic factors in epithelial ovarian cancers. *Anticancer Res* 1994;14:603–608.

229. **Berns EM, Klijn JG, van Putten WL, de Witte HH, Look MP, Meijer-van Gelder ME, et al.** *p53* protein accumulation predicts poor response to *tamoxifen* therapy of patients with recurrent breast cancer. *J Clin Oncol* 1998;16:121–127.

230. **Havrilesky L, Darcy KM, Hamdan H, Priore RL, Leon J, Bell J, et al.** Relationship between *p53* mutation, *p53* overexpression and survival in advanced ovarian cancers treated on Gynecologic Oncology Group studies #114 and #132. *J Clin Oncol* 2003;21:3814–3825.

231. **Kohler MF, Marks JR, Wiseman RW, Jacobs IJ, Davidoff AM, Clarke-Pearson DL, et al.** Spectrum of mutation and frequency of allelic deletion of the *p53* gene in ovarian cancer. *J Natl Cancer Inst* 1993;85:1513–1519.

232. **Kupryjańczyk J, Thor AD, Beauchamp R, Merritt V, Edgerton SM, Bell DA, et al.** *p53* mutations and protein accumulation in human ovarian cancer. *Proc Natl Acad Sci U S A* 1993;90:4961–4965.

233. **Eliopoulos AG, Kerr DJ, Herod J, Hodgkins L, Krajewski S, Reed JC, et al.** The control of apoptosis and drug resistance in ovarian cancer: influence of *p53* and bcl-2. *Oncogene* 1995;11:1217–1228.

234. **Perego P, Giarola M, Righetti SC, Supino R, Caserini C, Delia D, et al.** Association between cisplatin resistance and mutation of *p53* gene and reduced bax expression in ovarian carcinoma cell systems. *Cancer Res* 1996;56:556–562.

235. **Righetti SC, Della Torre G, Pilotti S, Ménard S, Ottone F, Colnaghi MI, et al.** A comparative study of *p53* gene mutations, protein accumulation, and response to cisplatin-based chemotherapy in advanced ovarian carcinoma. *Cancer Res* 1996;56:689–693.

236. **Havrilesky LJ, Elbendary A, Hurteau JA, Whitaker RS, Rodriguez GC, Berchuck A.** Chemotherapy-induced apoptosis in epithelial ovarian cancers. *Obstet Gynecol* 1995;85:1007–1010.

237. **Berchuck A, Kohler MF, Hopkins MP, Humphrey PA, Robboy SJ, Rodriguez GC, et al.** Overexpression of *p53* is not a feature of benign and early-stage borderline epithelial ovarian tumors. *Cancer Res* 1994;52:232–236.

238. **Gershenson DM, Deavers M, Diaz S, Tortolero-Luna G, Miller BE, Bast RC Jr, et al.** Prognostic significance of *p53* expression in advanced-stage ovarian serous borderline tumors. *Clin Cancer Res* 1999;5:4053–4058.

239. **Ortiz BH, Ailawadi M, Colitti C, Muto MG, Deavers M, Silva EG, et al.** Second primary or recurrence? Comparative patterns of *p53* and K-*ras* mutations suggest that serous borderline ovarian tumors and subsequent serous carcinomas are unrelated tumors. *Cancer Res* 2001;61:7264–7267.

240. **Flesken-Nikitin A, Choi KC, Eng JP, Shmidt EN, Nikitin AY.** Induction of carcinogenesis by concurrent inactivation of *p53* and *Rb1* in the mouse ovarian surface epithelium. *Cancer Res* 2003;63:3459–3463.

241. **Schultz DC, Vanderveer L, Buetow KH, Boente MP, Ozols RF, Hamilton TC, et al.** Characterization of chromosome 9 in human ovarian neoplasia identifies frequent genetic imbalance on 9q and rare alterations involving 9p, including *CDKN2*. *Cancer Res* 1995;55:2150–2157.

242. **McCluskey LL, Chen C, Delgadillo E, Felix JC, Muderspach LI, Dubeau L.** Differences in *p16* gene methylation and expression in benign and malignant ovarian tumors. *Cancer Res* 1999;72:87–92.

243. **Liu Z, Wang LE, Wang L, Lu KH, Mills GB, Bondy ML, et al.** Methylation and messenger RNA expression of p15INK4b but not p16INK4a are independent risk factors for ovarian cancer. *Clin Cancer Res* 2005;11:4968–4976.

244. **Esteller M, Silva JM, Dominguez G, Bonilla F, Matias-Guiu X, Lerma E, et al.** Promoter hypermethylation and *BRCA1* inactivation in sporadic breast and ovarian tumors. *J Natl Cancer Inst* 2000;92:564–569.

245. Baldwin RL, Nemeth E, Tran H, Shvartsman H, Cass I, Narod S, et al. *BRCA1* promoter region hypermethylation in ovarian carcinoma: a population-based study. *Cancer Res* 2000;60:5329–5333.

246. Schmider A, Gee C, Friedmann W, Lukas JJ, Press MF, Lichtenegger W, et al. *p21* (WAF1/CIP1) protein expression is associated with prolonged survival but not with *p53* expression in epithelial ovarian carcinoma. *Cancer Res* 2000;77:237–242.

247. Levesque MA, Katsaros D, Massobrio M, Genta F, Yu H, Richiardi G, et al. Evidence for a dose-response effect between *p53* (but not p21WAF1/Cip1) protein concentrations, survival, and responsiveness in patients with epithelial ovarian cancer treated with platinum-based chemotherapy. *Clin Cancer Res* 2000;6:3260–3270.

248. Masciullo V, Ferrandina G, Pucci B, Fanfani F, Lovergine S, Palazzo J, et al. p27Kip1 expression is associated with clinical outcome in advanced epithelial ovarian cancer: multivariate analysis. *Clin Cancer Res* 2000;6:4816–4822.

249. Sui L, Dong Y, Ohno M, Sugimoto K, Tai Y, Hando T, et al. Implication of malignancy and prognosis of p27(kip1), Cyclin E, and Cdk2 expression in epithelial ovarian tumors. *Cancer Res* 2001;83:56–63.

250. Hurteau JA, Allison BM, Brutkiewicz SA. Expression and subcellular localization of the cyclin-dependent kinase inhibitor p27(Kip1) in epithelial ovarian cancer. *Cancer Res* 2001;83:292–298.

251. Korkolopoulou P, Vassilopoulos I, Konstantinidou AE, Zorzos H, Patsouris E, Agapitos E, et al. The combined evaluation of p27Kip1 and Ki-67 expression provides independent information on overall survival of ovarian carcinoma patients. *Cancer Res* 2002; 85:404–414.

252. Rosen DG, Yang G, Cai KQ, Bast RC Jr, Gershenson DM, Silva EG, et al. Subcellular localization of p27kip1 expression predicts poor prognosis in human ovarian cancer. *Clin Cancer Res* 2005; 11:632–637.

253. Berchuck A, Olt GJ, Everitt L, Soisson AP, Bast RC Jr, Boyer CM, et al. The role of peptide growth factors in epithelial ovarian cancer. *Obstet Gynecol* 1990;75:255–262.

254. Hurteau J, Rodriguez GC, Whitaker RS, Shah S, Mills G, Bast RC, Berchuck A. Transforming growth factor-beta inhibits proliferation of human ovarian cancer cells obtained from ascites. *Cancer* 1994;74:93–99.

255. Baldwin RL, Tran H, Karlan BY. Loss of *c-myc* repression coincides with ovarian cancer resistance to transforming growth factor beta growth arrest independent of transforming growth factor beta/Smad signaling. *Cancer Res* 2003;63:1413–1419.

256. Wang D, Kanuma T, Mizunuma H, Takama F, Ibuki Y, Wake N, et al. Analysis of specific gene mutations in the transforming growth factor-beta signal transduction pathway in human ovarian cancer. *Cancer Res* 2000;60:4507–4512.

257. Bauknecht T, Kiechle M, Bauer G, Siebers JW. Characterization of growth factors in human ovarian carcinomas. *Cancer Res* 1986;46:2614–2618.

258. Kommoss F, Wintzer HO, Von Kleist S, Kohler M, Walker R, Langton B, et al. In situ distribution of transforming growth factor-a in normal human tissues and in malignant tumours of the ovary. *J Pathol* 1990;162:223–230.

259. Morishige K, Kurachi H, Amemiya K, Fujita Y, Yamamoto T, Miyake A, et al. Evidence for the involvement of transforming growth factor-a and epidermal growth factor receptor autocrine growth mechanism in primary human ovarian cancers *in vitro*. *Cancer Res* 1991;51:5322–5328.

260. Rodriguez GC, Berchuck A, Whitaker RS, Schlossman D, Clarke-Pearson DL, Bast RC Jr. Epidermal growth factor receptor expression in normal ovarian epithelium and ovarian cancer. II. Relationship between receptor expression and response to epidermal growth factor. *Am J Obstet Gynecol* 1991;164:745–750.

261. Yee D, Morales FR, Hamilton TC, Von Hoff DD. Expression of insulin-like growth factor I, its binding proteins, and its receptor in ovarian cancer. *Cancer Res* 1991;51:5107–5112.

262. Henriksen R, Funa K, Wilander E, Bäckström T, Ridderheim M, Oberg K. Expression and prognostic significance of platelet-derived growth factor and its receptors in epithelial ovarian neoplasms. *Cancer Res* 1993;53:4550–4554.

263. Sariban E, Sitaras NM, Antoniades HN, Kufe DW, Pantazis P. Expression of platelet-derived growth factor (PDGF)-related transcripts and synthesis of biologically active PDGF-like proteins by human malignant epithelial cell lines. *J Clin Invest* 1988;82:1157–1164.

264. Di Blasio AM, Cremonesi L, Viganó P, Ferrari M, Gospodarowicz D, Vignali M, et al. Basic fibroblast growth factor and its receptor messenger ribonucleic acids are expressed in human ovarian epithelial neoplasms. *Am J Obstet Gynecol* 1993;169:1517–1523.

265. Kacinski BM, Stanley ER, Carter D, Chambers JT, Chambers SK, Kohorn EI, et al. Circulating levels of CSF-1 (M-CSF) a lymphohematopoietic cytokine may be a useful marker of disease status in patients with malignant ovarian neoplasms. *Int J Radiat Oncol Biol Phys* 1989;17:159–164.

266. Toy EP, Chambers JT, Kacinski BM, Flick MB, Chambers SK. The activated macrophage colony-stimulating factor (CSF-1) receptor as a predictor of poor outcome in advanced epithelial ovarian carcinoma. *Cancer Res* 2001;80:194–200.

267. Furui T, LaPushin R, Mao M, Khan H, Watt SR, Watt MA, et al. Overexpression of edg-2/vzg-1 induces apoptosis and anoikis in ovarian cancer cells in a lysophosphatidic acid-independent manner. *Clin Cancer Res* 1999;5:4308–4318.

268. Tanyi JL, Morris AJ, Wolf JK, Fang X, Hasegawa Y, Lapushin R, et al. The human lipid phosphate phosphatase-3 decreases the growth, survival, and tumorigenesis of ovarian cancer cells: validation of the lysophosphatidic acid signaling cascade as a target for therapy in ovarian cancer. *Cancer Res* 2003;63:1073–1082.

269. Lidor YJ, Xu FJ, Martínez-Maza O, Olt GJ, Marks JR, Berchuck A, et al. Constitutive production of macrophage colony stimulating factor and interleukin-6 by human ovarian surface epithelial cells. *Exp Cell Res* 1993;207:332–339.

270. Siemans CH, Auersperg N. Serial propagation of human ovarian surface epithelium in culture. *J Cell Physiol* 1991;134:347–356.

271. Ziltener HJ, Maines-Bandiera S, Schrader JW, Auersperg N. Secretion of bioactive interleukin-1, interleukin-6 and colony-stimulating factors by human ovarian surface epithelium. *Biol Reprod* 1993;49:635–641.

272. Tzahar E, Yarden Y. The ErbB-2/HER2 oncogenic receptor of adenocarcinomas: from orphanhood to multiple stromal ligands. *Biochem Biophys Acta* 1998;1377:M25–M37.

273. Slamon DJ, Godolphin W, Jones LA, Holt JA, Wong SG, Keith DE, et al. Studies of HER-2/*neu* proto-oncogene in human breast and ovarian cancer. *Science* 1989;244:707–712.

274. Berchuck A, Kamel A, Whitaker R, Kerns B, Olt G, Kinney R, et al. Overexpression of HER-2/*neu* is associated with poor survival in advanced epithelial ovarian cancer. *Cancer Res* 1990;50: 4087–4091.

275. Rubin SC, Finstad CL, Wong GY, Almadrones L, Plante M, Lloyd KO. Prognostic significance of HER-2/*neu* expression in advanced ovarian cancer. *Am J Obstet Gynecol* 1993;168:162–169.

276. Rodríguez GC, Boente MP, Berchuck A, Whitaker RS, O'Briant KC, Xu F, et al. The effect of antibodies and immunotoxins reactive with HER-2/*neu* on growth of ovarian and breast cancer cell lines. *Am J Obstet Gynecol* 1993;168:228–232.

277. Pietras RJ, Pegram MD, Finn RS, Maneval DA, Slamon DJ. Remission of human breast cancer xenografts on therapy with humanized monoclonal antibody to HER-2 receptor and DNA-reactive drugs. *Oncogene* 1998;17:2235–2249.

278. Bookman MA, Darcy KM, Clarke-Pearson D, Boothby RA, Horowitz IR. Evaluation of monoclonal humanized anti-HER2 antibody, *trastuzumab,* in patients with recurrent or refractory ovarian or primary peritoneal carcinoma with overexpression of HER2: a phase II trial of the Gynecologic Oncology Group. *J Clin Oncol* 2003;21: 283–290.

279. Haas M, Isakov J, Howell SB. Evidence against ras activation in human ovarian carcinomas. *Mol Biol Med* 1987;4:265–275.

280. Feig LA, Bast RC Jr, Knapp RC, Cooper GM. Somatic activation of *rasK* gene in a human ovarian carcinoma. *Science* 1984;223: 698–701.

281. Mok SC, Bell DA, Knapp RC, Fishbaugh PM, Welch WR, Muto MG, et al. Mutation of K-*ras* protooncogene in human ovarian epithelial tumors of borderline malignancy. *Cancer Res* 1993;53: 1489–1492.

282. Singer G, Oldt R III, Cohen Y, Wang BG, Sidransky D, Kurman RJ, et al. Mutations in *BRAF* and *KRAS* characterize the development of low-grade ovarian serous carcinoma. *J Natl Cancer Inst* 2003;95:484–486.

283. **Gemignani ML, Schlaerth AC, Bogomolniy F, Barakat RR, Lin O, Soslow R, et al.** Role of *KRAS* and *BRAF* gene mutations in mucinous ovarian carcinoma. *Cancer Res* 2003;90:378–381.

284. **Shayesteh L, Lu Y, Kuo WL, Baldocchi R, Godfrey T, et al.** *PIK3CA* is implicated as an oncogene in ovarian cancer. *Nat Genet* 1999;21:99–102.

285. **Campbell IG, Russell SE, Choong DY, Montgomery KG, Ciavarella ML, Hooi CS, et al.** Mutation of the *PIK3CA* gene in ovarian and breast cancer. *Cancer Res* 2004;64:7678–7681.

286. **Cheng JQ, Godwin AK, Bellacosa A, Taguchi T, Franke TF, et al.** *AKT2*, a putative oncogene encoding a member of a subfamily of protein-serine/threonine kinases, is amplified in human ovarian carcinomas. *Proc Natl Acad Sci U S A* 1992;89:9267–9271.

287. **Obata K, Morland SJ, Watson RH, Hitchcock A, Chenevix-Trench G, Thomas EJ, et al.** Frequent *PTEN*/MMAC mutations in endometrioid but not serous or mucinous epithelial ovarian tumors. *Cancer Res* 1998;58:2095–2097.

288. **Wu R, Zhai Y, Fearon ER, Cho KR.** Diverse mechanisms of beta-catenin deregulation in ovarian endometrioid adenocarcinomas. *Cancer Res* 2001;61:8247–8255.

289. **Wu R, Hendrix-Lucas N, Kuick R, Zhai Y, Schwartz DR, Akyol A, et al.** Mouse model of human ovarian endometrioid adenocarcinoma based on somatic defects in the Wnt/beta-catenin and *PI3K/PTEN* signaling pathways. *Cancer Cell* 2007;11:321–333.

290. **Dinulescu DM, Ince TA, Quade BJ, Shafer SA, Crowley D, Jacks T.** Role of K-*ras* and *PTEN* in the development of mouse models of endometriosis and endometrioid ovarian cancer. *Nat Med* 2005; 11:63–70.

291. **Berns EM, Klijn JG, Henzen-Logmans SC, Rodenburg CJ, van der Burg ME, Foekens JA.** Receptors for hormones and growth factors (onco)-gene amplification in human ovarian cancer. *Int J Cancer* 1992;52:218–224.

292. **Sasano H, Garrett CT, Wilkinson DS, Silverberg S, Comerford J, Hyde J.** Protooncogene amplification and tumor ploidy in human ovarian neoplasms. *Hum Pathol* 1990;21:4:382–391.

293. **Serova DM.** Amplification of *c-myc* proto-oncogene in primary tumors, metastases and blood leukocytes of patients with ovarian cancer. *Eksp Onkol* 1987;9:25–27.

294. **Tashiro H, Miyazaki K, Okamura H, Iwai A, Fukumoto M.** *c-myc* overexpression in human primary ovarian tumors: Its relevance to tumor progression. *Int J Cancer* 1992;50:828–833.

295. **Marx J.** Research news: How cells cycle towards cancer. *Science* 1994;263:319–321.

296. **Farley J, Smith LM, Darcy KM, Sobel E, O'Connor D, Henderson B, et al.** Cyclin E expression is a significant predictor of survival in advanced, suboptimally debulked ovarian epithelial cancers: a Gynecologic Oncology Group study. *Cancer Res* 2003; 63:1235–1241.

297. **Rosen DG, Yang G, Deavers MT, Malpica A, Kavanagh JJ, Mills GB, Liu J.** Cyclin E expression is correlated with tumor progression and predicts a poor prognosis in patients with ovarian carcinoma. *Cancer* 2006;106:1925–1932.

298. **Muñoz N, Bosch FX, de Sanjosé S, Herrero R, Castellsagué X, International Agency for Research on Cancer Multicenter Cervical Cancer Study Group, et al.** Epidemiologic classification of human papillomavirus types associated with cervical cancer. *N Engl J Med* 2003;348:518–527.

299. **Sun XW, Kuhn L, Ellerbrock TV, Chiasson MA, Bush TJ, Wright TC Jr., et al.** Human papillomavirus infection in women infected with the human immunodeficiency virus. *N Engl J Med* 1997;337:1343–1349.

300. **Koutsky LA, Ault KA, Wheeler CM, Brown DR, Barr E, Alvarez FB, et al.** A controlled trial of a human papillomavirus type 16 vaccine. *N Engl J Med* 2002;347:1645–1651.

301. **Scheffner M, Werness BA, Huibregtse JM, Levine AJ, Howley PM.** The E6 oncoprotein encoded by human papillomavirus types 16 and 18 promotes the degradation of *p53*. *Cell* 1990;63: 1129–1136.

302. **Scheffner M, Münger K, Byrne JC, Howley PM.** The state of the *p53* and retinoblastoma gene in human cervical carcinoma cell lines. *Proc Natl Acad Sci U S A* 1991;88:5523–5527.

303. **Werness BA, Levine AJ, Howley PM.** Association of human papillomavirus types 16 and 18 E6 proteins with *p53*. *Science* 1990; 248:76–79.

304. **Parker MF, Arroyo GF, Geradts J, Sabichi AL, Park RC, Taylor RR, et al.** Molecular characterization of adenocarcinoma of the cervix. *Cancer Res* 1997;64:242–251.

305. **de Boer MA, Jordanova ES, Kenter GG, Peters AA, Corver WE, Trimbos JB, et al.** High human papillomavirus oncogene mRNA expression and not viral DNA load is associated with poor prognosis in cervical cancer patients. *Clin Cancer Res* 2007;13:132–138.

306. **Narayan G, Pulido HA, Koul S, Lu XY, Harris CP, Yeh YA, et al.** Genetic analysis identifies putative tumor suppressor sites at 2q35-q36.1 and 2q36.3-q37.1 involved in cervical cancer progression. *Oncogene* 2003;22:3489–3499.

307. **Umayahara K, Numa F, Suehiro Y, Sakata A, Nawata S, Ogata H, et al.** Comparative genomic hybridization detects genetic alterations during early stages of cervical cancer progression. *Genes Chromosomes Cancer* 2002;33:98–102.

308. **Yang YC, Shyong WY, Chang MS, Chen YJ, Lin CH, Huang ZD, et al.** Frequent gain of copy number on the long arm of chromosome 3 in human cervical adenocarcinoma. *Cancer Genet Cytogenet* 2001;131:48–53.

309. **Lin WM, Michalopulos EA, Dhurander N, Cheng PC, Robinson W, Ashfaq R, et al.** Allelic loss and microsatellite alterations of chromosome 3p14.2 are more frequent in recurrent cervical dysplasias. *Clin Cancer Res* 2000;6:1410–1414.

310. **Kirchhoff M, Rose H, Petersen BL, Maahr J, Gerdes T, Lundsteen C, et al.** Comparative genomic hybridization reveals a recurrent pattern of chromosomal aberrations in severe dysplasia/carcinoma in situ of the cervix and in advanced-stage cervical carcinoma. *Genes Chromosomes Cancer* 1999;24:144–150.

311. **Wang SS, Trunk M, Schiffman M, Herrero R, Sherman ME, Burk RD, et al.** Validation of p16INK4a as a marker of oncogenic human papillomavirus infection in cervical biopsies from a population-based cohort in Costa Rica. *Cancer Epidemiol Biomarkers Prev* 2004;13:1355–1360.

312. **Grendys EC Jr, Barnes WA, Weitzel J, Sparkowski J, Schlegel R.** Identification of H, K, and N-*ras* point mutations in stage IB cervical carcinoma. *Cancer Res* 1997;65:343–347.

313. **Koulos JP, Wright TC, Mitchell MF, Silva E, Atkinson EN, Richart RM.** Relationships between c-Ki-*ras* mutations, HPV types, and prognostic indicators in invasive endocervical adenocarcinomas. *Cancer Res* 1993;48:364–369.

314. **Riou G, Barrois M, Sheng ZM, Duvillard P, Lhomme C.** Somatic deletions and mutations of c-Ha-*ras* gene in human cervical cancers. *Oncogene* 1988;3:329–333.

315. **Van Le L, Stoerker J, Rinehart CA, Fowler WC.** H-*ras* condon 12 mutation in cervical dysplasia. *Cancer Res* 1993;49:181–184.

316. **Riou G, Lê MG, Favre M, Jeannel D, Bourhis J, Orth G.** Human papillomavirus-negative status and *c-myc* gene overexpression: independent prognostic indicators of distant metastasis for early-stage invasive cervical cancers. *J Natl Cancer Inst* 1992;84: 1525–1526.

317. **Bourhis J, Lê MG, Barrois M, Gerbaulet A, Jeannel D, Duvillard P, et al.** Prognostic value of *c-myc* proto-oncogene overexpression in early invasive carcinoma of the cervix. *J Clin Oncol* 1990;8: 1789–1796.

318. **Birrer MJ, Hendricks D, Farley J, Sundborg MJ, Bonome T, Walts MJ, et al.** Abnormal FHIT expression in malignant and premalignant lesions of the cervix. *Cancer Res* 1999;59:5270–5274.

319. **Huang LW, Chao SL, Chen TJ.** Reduced FHIT expression in cervical carcinoma: correlation with tumor progression and poor prognosis. *Cancer Res* 2003;90:331–337.

320. **Connolly DC, Greenspan DL, Wu R, Ren X, Dunn RL, Shah KV, et al.** Loss of FHIT expression in invasive cervical carcinomas and intraepithelial lesions associated with invasive disease. *Clin Cancer Res* 2000;6:3505–3510.

321. **Liu FS, Hsieh YT, Chen JT, Ho ES, Hung MJ, Lin AJ.** FHIT (fragile histidine triad) gene analysis in cervical intraepithelial neoplasia. *Cancer Res* 2001;82:283–290.

322. **Krivak TC, McBroom JW, Seidman J, Venzon D, Crothers B, MacKoul PJ, et al.** Abnormal fragile histidine triad (FHIT) expression in advanced cervical carcinoma: a poor prognostic factor. *Cancer Res* 2001;61:4382–4385.

323. **Dong SM, Kim HS, Rha SH, Sidransky D.** Promoter hypermethylation of multiple genes in carcinoma of the uterine cervix. *Clin Cancer Res* 2001;7:1982–1986.

324. **Virmani AK, Muller C, Rathi A, Zoechbauer-Mueller S, Mathis M, Gazdar AF.** Aberrant methylation during cervical carcinogenesis. *Clin Cancer Res* 2001;7:584–589.

325. **Wong YF, Selvanayagam ZE, Wei N, Porter J, Vittal R, Hu R, et al.** Expression genomics of cervical cancer: molecular classification and prediction of radiotherapy response by DNA microarray. *Clin Cancer Res* 2003;9:5486–5492.

326. **Kuzmin I, Liu L, Dammann R, Geil L, Stanbridge EJ, Wilczynski SP, et al.** Inactivation of *RAS* association domain family 1A gene in cervical carcinomas and the role of human papillomavirus infection. *Cancer Res* 2003;63:1888–1893.

327. **Dueñas-González A, Lizano M, Candelaria M, Cetina L, Arce C, Cervera E.** Epigenetics of cervical cancer. An overview and therapeutic perspectives. *Mol Cancer* 2005;4:38.

328. **Kim SJ, Lee SY, Lee C, Kim I, An HJ, Kim JY, et al.** Differential expression profiling of genes in a complete hydatidiform mole using cDNA microarray analysis. *Gynecol Oncol* 2006;103:654–660.

329. **Feng HC, Tsao SW, Ngan HY, Xue WC, Chiu PM, Cheung AN.** Differential expression of insulin-like growth factor binding protein 1 and ferritin light polypeptide in gestational trophoblastic neoplasia: combined cDNA suppression subtractive hybridization and microarray study. *Cancer* 2005;104:2409–2416.

2 Biologic, Targeted, and Immune Therapies

Oliver Dorigo
Otoniel Martínez-Maza
Jonathan S. Berek

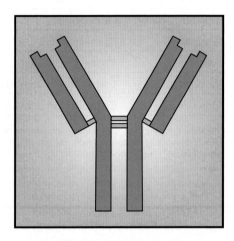

Cancer is caused by a series of events that include the accumulation of successive molecular lesions and alterations in the tumor microenvironment (1). Molecular lesions include overexpression, amplification, or mutations of oncogenes; deletion of tumor suppressor genes; and the inappropriate expression of growth factors and their cellular receptors. In addition to these molecular changes, the formation of new blood vessels **(angiogenesis)** and the lack of effective host antitumor immune responses create a microenvironment that supports the growth of cancer (2). Our improved understanding of these mechanisms presents an opportunity for the development of novel therapeutic approaches (3). This chapter provides an overview of biologic, targeted, and immunotherapeutic strategies for gynecologic cancers.

Biologic and Targeted Therapies

The growth of cancer cells is crucially dependent on oncogenic signal transduction pathways. Extracellular signals are transmitted to the cancer cell via transmembrane receptors. Activation of the **epidermal growth factor receptors (EGFR, HER2, HER3, and HER4),** for example, stimulates a cascade of intracellular proteins that ultimately lead to changes in gene expression. **Novel therapeutics are targeted to modulate these signal transduction pathways by blocking the extracellular transmembrane receptors or interfering with intracellular proteins such as tyrosine kinases further downstream. This novel therapeutic approach is also termed** *molecular targeting* (4). It is accomplished by either monoclonal antibodies that bind to transmembrane receptors and serum proteins such as **vascular endothelial growth factor (VEGF)** or chemical, small-molecule inhibitors that prevent activation of signal transduction proteins. **Targeting the signaling cascade inhibits the proliferation of cancer cells, induces apoptosis, and blocks metastasis. The specificity of these molecules is based on the assumption that cancer cells are overexpressing various proteins in the signal transduction pathways, therefore presenting a preferred target compared to normal cells.** Conceptually, this should result in more cancer cell–specific therapy and less clinical side effects because of sparing of normal tissue (5). At this time, a large variety of molecular-targeting strategies are being tested for efficacy in clinical trials (Table 2.1).

Table 2.1 Targeted Therapies in Cancer Disease			
Targeted Pathway	Drug	Chemistry	Main Molecular Targets
Angiogenesis	Bevacizumab	Humanized monoclonal antibody	VEGF-A
	VEGF-Trap	Fusion protein	VEGF-A (-B,C,D,E)
Epidermal Growth Factor Receptors	Trastuzumab	Humanized monoclonal antibody	HER2
	Pertuzumab	Humanized monoclonal antibody	HER2
	Cetuximab	Chimerized monoclonal antibody	EGFR
	Gefitinib	Quinazoline	EGFR ATP binding domain
	Erlotinib	Quinazoline	EGFR ATP binding domain
	Lapatinib	Quinazoline	EGFR, HER2, ERK1 and 2, Akt
Tyrosine Kinases	Temsirolimus	Rapamycin analog	mTOR
Multiple Kinases	Sorafenib	Carboxamide derivative	raf, c-kit, VEGFR-2,–3, FLT-3, PDGFR-β
	Sunitinib	Carboxamide derivative	PDGFR, VEGFR-1,–2,–3, c-kit, FLT-3

Abbreviations: VEGF, vascular endothelial growth factor; VEGFR, vascular endothelial growth factor receptor; PDGFR, platelet-derived endothelial cell growth factor receptor; HER2, human epidermal growth factor; EGFR, epidermal growth factor receptor; mTOR, mammalian target of rapamycin; FLT3, fms-like tyrosine kinase 3, raf, raf oncogene.

Angiogenesis

The formation of new blood vessels (neoangiogenesis) is a normal process during embryonic development, tissue remodeling, and wound healing (6). Malignant tumors are able to induce angiogenesis by secreting paracrine factors that promote the formation of new blood vessels. **Angiogenesis is a complex process that is influenced by various pro- and antiangiogenic factors, including VEGF, interleukin 8, platelet-derived endothelial cell growth factor, and angiopoietins. Overexpression of these angiogenic factors leads to neovascularization and increased supply of nutrients and oxygen to the tumor.**

Three main therapeutic strategies that target angiogenesis are currently being explored for the treatment of cancer patients (7). One group of agents targets VEGF (e.g., *bevacizumab*, VEGF-Trap), the second group prevents VEGF from binding to its receptor (*pertuzumab*), and a third group of agents inhibits tyrosine kinase activation and downstream signaling in the angiogenesis signaling cascade (*valatanib, sunitenib*) (8).

Vascular Endothelial Growth Factor

VEGF is overexpressed in gynecologic malignancies, therefore presenting an excellent target for therapy (9). Inhibition of VEGF-induced angiogenic signaling decreases tumor microvascular density and causes death of solid tumors in various preclinical models. Several agents are now available for clinical use; all target the VEGF signaling pathway. The most widely used agent at this time is *bevacizumab,* a humanized, recombinant monoclonal antibody that binds to all isoforms of VEGF-A. *Bevacizumab* has been approved for the treatment of colorectal carcinoma based on improved overall survival in combination with chemotherapy in patients with metastatic colorectal cancer in (10,11). In addition, *bevacizumab* has shown promising effects in metastatic non-small cell lung cancer and recurrent or metastatic breast carcinoma in (12).

In ovarian carcinoma, various clinical trials have demonstrated the efficacy of *bevacizumab* treatment. In a study by the Gynecologic Oncology Group, 62 patients received single agent *bevacizumab* 15 mg/kg intravenously every 21 days (13). Thirteen patients (21%) showed clinical responses with two complete and 11 partial responses. The median response duration was 10 months, and 25 patients (41.3%) survived progression free for at least 6 months. In a second trial, *bevacizumab* treatment of 44 patients with recurrent, platinum-resistant ovarian carcinoma resulted in partial responses in seven patients (15.9%) and stable disease in 27 (61.4%) (14). Median progression-free survival was 4.4 months with a median survival of 10.7 months.

Bevacizumab **has also been used in combination with other agents.** In a phase II study of 13 patients with recurrent ovarian or primary peritoneal carcinoma, combination treatment with *bevacizumab* (15 mg/kg i.v. every 21 days) and *erlotinib* (150 mg/day orally) resulted in one complete response and one partial response for a total response rate of 15% (12). Seven patients had stable disease. Another trial investigated the combination of *bevacizumab* (10 mg/kg every 14 days) and oral *cyclophosphamide* (50 mg/day orally) in 70 patients with recurrent ovarian cancer (15). Partial responses were observed in 17 patients (24%), with a median time to progression and survival of 7.2 and 16.9 months, respectively. The probability of being alive and progression free at 6 months was 56%. Serum levels of VEGF and thrombospondin-1 were determined in four patients and showed a decrease over time but did not correlate with clinical outcome. The combination of *bevacizumab* and weekly *taxane* therapy was evaluated in a small series of patients (16). All nine evaluable patients had a decrease of serum CA125 and a significant improvement of their disease-related symptoms.

Bevacizumab-**related side effects include venous and arterial thrombosis, hemorrhage, nephrotic syndrome with proteinuria, hypertension, rare leukoencephalopathy, and bowel perforation.** The risk factors in particular for bowel perforation under *bevacizumab* treatment are not well identified but include tumor involving the intestines and bowel resection. The incidence of bowel perforation in ovarian cancer patient during *bevacizumab* treatment is reported in several clinical trials. In one trial, five of 44 patients (11.4%) experienced treatment related gastrointestinal perforation (14), while others have not reported any such complication (13). Recent reviews have suggested that the incidence of bowel perforation for ovarian cancer patients receiving *bevacizumab* is approximately 5% to 7% (17,18).

The Gynecologic Oncology Group has initiated a clinical trial that will evaluate the addition of *bevacizumab* to first-line chemotherapy after primary tumor debulking (19). Patients receive *bevacizumab* in combination with *carboplatin* and *paclitaxel* followed by *bevacizumab* alone for consolidation. **A similar trial by the Gynecologic Cancer InterGroup is designed to evaluate the safety and efficacy of adding *bevacizumab* to standard chemotherapy (*carboplatin* and *paclitaxel*) in patients with advanced epithelial ovarian or primary peritoneal cancer (ICON7) (19).**

Various other targeting strategies of angiogenic pathways are currently being investigated (7). **VEGF-Trap** (AVE 0005) is a recombinant fusion protein that consists of the extracellular domain of VEGF receptors VEGFR1 and VEGFR2 fused to the FC portion of immunoglobulin G1 (20). VEGF is inactivated by binding to the ligand-binding domain of this fusion protein followed by destruction of this complex via immune system–mediated mechanisms. **Small-molecule tyrosine kinase inhibitors that target the VEGF pathway include *pazopanib*, *vatalanib*, and *sunitinib*. *Pazopanib* is a multitarget receptor tyrosine kinase inhibitor against VEGFR1, VEGFR2, VEGFR3, platelet-derived growth factor receptor (PDGFR), and c-kit (3).** Similarly, *vatalanib* (PTK787) targets multiple VEGF-receptor tyrosine kinases. *Sunitinib* (SU11248) inhibits PDGR, VEGFR, c-kit, and SLT3 and has shown promising results in renal cell cancer and gastrointestinal stromal tumors. Trials in gynecologic malignancies are ongoing to test the efficacy of these agents in patients.

Epidermal Growth Factor Receptor Inhibitors

The epidermal growth factor receptor pathway plays an important role in regulation of growth and differentiation of epithelial cells through regulation of cell division, migration, adhesion, differentiation, and apoptosis (21). **The epidermal growth factor receptor family consists of four members including EGFR (HER1), HER2, HER3, and HER4 (22). EGFR overexpression has been reported in 35% to 70% of patients with epithelial ovarian cancer (23,24). In endometrial cancer, EGFR is overexpressed in 43% to 67% of tumors and is associated with shortened disease-free and overall survival (25–27). In addition, amplification of the HER2 gene is commonly found in endometrial carcinoma.** Overexpression of the HER2 receptor is more prevalent in nonendometrial cancer and is associated with an aggressive form of the disease. In uterine serous papillary carcinoma, HER2 gene amplification can be demonstrated in as many as 42% of cases (28).

Various agents directed against epidermal growth factor receptors are available (29). *Trastuzumab* is a humanized monoclonal antibody that binds to the extracellular domain of HER2 (30). Blockade of HER2 affects various molecules that ultimately decreases cell proliferation. *Pertuzumab* is another humanized monoclonal antibody that binds to a different epitope of HER2 compared to *trastuzumab*. Binding to HER2 prevents dimerization of the receptor,

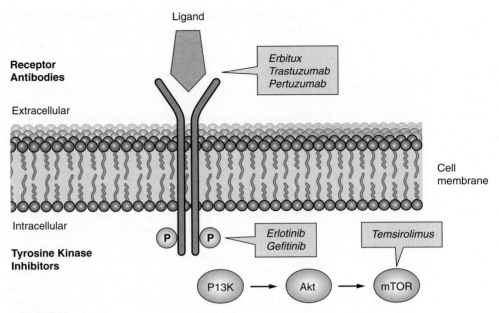

Figure 2.1   Inhibition of epidermal growth factor receptor signaling.

which is required for its function (31). *Cetuximab* is a chimeric monoclonal antibody that binds to EGFR, thereby preventing dimerization and activation (32). *Gefitinib* is a small-molecule tyrosine kinase inhibitor of EGFR that prevents phosphorylation of the receptor by binding to the intracellular ATP-binding domain of the receptor (33). *Erlotinib* is a small-molecule tyrosine kinase inhibitor of EGRF that prevents phosphorylation of the intracellular domain of the EGFR receptor. *Lapatinib* (GW572016) inhibits both EGFR and HER2 (Fig. 2.1).

Epidermal Growth Factor Receptor

Inhibition of EGFR signaling is accomplished by using either monoclonal antibodies against the extracellular receptor or small-molecule inhibitors against the intracellular kinase domain. Both strategies results in inhibition of phosphorylation or receptor activation.

Erlotinib is a potent reversible inhibitor of EGFR tyrosine kinase that blocks receptor *autophosphorylation* and has been used for the treatment of ovarian carcinoma. In one study, 34 patients were treated with single-agent *erlotinib* (150 mg/day orally) for as long as 48 weeks (34). Two patients showed a partial response lasting 8 and 17 weeks. Fifteen patients (44%) had stable disease, and 17 patients (50%) progressed under treatment. The side effects of *erlotinib* were mainly confined to tissues with strong expression of EGFR: Skin rashes and diarrhea were observed in 68% and 38% of patients, respectively.

Erlotinib has been used in combination with *docetaxel* and *carboplatin* as first-line treatment after surgical cytoreduction in patients with ovarian, fallopian tube, and primary peritoneal cancers (35). In this study, 23 evaluable patients showed five complete and seven partial responses. The treatment was well tolerated; main side effects were neutropenia and skin rashes. The study demonstrated the feasibility and tolerability of *erlotinib* in conjunction with chemotherapy.

Cetuximab (C225, *Erbitux*) is a chimerized monoclonal antibody against EGFR. Treatment of patients with primary ovarian or peritoneal cancer using *cetuximab* has shown only modest activity in screened patients with EGFR-positive tumors. *Cetuximab* in combination with *carboplatin* resulted in three complete (10.7%) and six partial (21.4%) responses in 28 patients with recurrent ovarian cancer (36). Twenty-six of these 28 patients (92.8%) had EGFR-positive tumors. **The combination of *paclitaxel*, *carboplatin*, and *cetuximab* for first-line chemotherapy of stage III ovarian cancer patients resulted in progression-free survival of 14.4 months and was therefore not significantly prolonged compared to historical data (37).**

Gefitinib (ZD1839 *Iressa*) is a low molecular weight *quinazoline* derivative that inhibits the activation of EGFR tyrosine kinase via competitive binding of the ATP-binding domain of the receptor. In a clinical trial by the Gynecologic Oncology Group, 27 patients with recurrent or persistent epithelial ovarian cancer were treated with 500 mg *gefitinib* daily (38). Four patients (14.8%) survived progression free for more than 6 months with one objective response (3.6%). Commonly observed toxicity included skin rash and diarrhea. Interestingly, EGFR expression was associated with longer progression-free survival and possibly longer survival. The patient with the only objective antitumor response had a tumor with a mutation in the catalytic domain of the tumor's EGFR (2235dEL15). This patient received 29 cycles of *gefitinib* and had a progression-free survival of approximately 27 months.

In a separate trial, 24 patients with recurrent epithelial ovarian cancer were treated with *gefitinib* 500 mg daily (39). All tumor samples had detectable levels of EGFR and PGFR. Of 16 patients who completed more than two cycles of therapy, no complete or partial responses were observed. However, analysis of clinical samples showed that *gefitinib* inhibited phosphorylation of EGFR, thereby providing a conceptual proof of targeted therapy.

Treatment of patients with recurrent ovarian cancer using the combination of *gefitinib*, *carboplatin*, and *paxitaxel* resulted in a high overall response rate of 63% (40). Interestingly, antitumor responses were observed in 35% of patients with platinum-resistant disease compared to a 73% response rate in patients with platinum-sensitive disease. Based on the preliminary data, none of the 18 patients treated showed EGFR receptor mutations.

***Gefitinib* has also been used in combination with *tamoxifen*.** In 56 patients with primary ovarian or fallopian tube cancer, treatment with *tamoxifen* (40 mg/day) and *gefitinib* (500 mg/day) did not result in objective antitumor responses, but 16 patients had stable disease (41). In squamous and adenocarcinoma of the cervix, *gefitinib* (500 mg/day) treatment resulted in disease stabilization in six of 28 patients (20%) but no clinical responses (42). The median duration of stable disease was 111.5 days with a median overall survival of 107 days.

Lapatinib is a small-molecule inhibitor of both the HER2 and EGFR tyrosine kinase receptor.

The rationale for using *lapatinib* in endometrial carcinoma is supported mainly by studies in human cancer cell lines. Its efficacy in endometrial cancer is being investigated currently in clinical trials (28).

HER-2/*neu*

The HER-2/*neu* receptor is activated by homo- or heterodimerization, resulting in tyrosine phosphorylation and subsequent activation of various downstream signals that among other functions control cellular proliferation, migration, and invasion. ***Trastuzumab* is a recombinant, humanized IgG1 monoclonal antibody that is specific for the extracellular domain of HER-2/*neu*. Binding of the antibody to HER-2/*neu* prevents activation of the receptor with a subsequent increase of apoptosis *in vitro* and *in vivo*, impaired DNA damage repair, and inhibition of tumor neovascularization** (30). Preclinical models have suggested that the therapeutic activity may also depend on innate immune effector cells that mediate antibody-dependent cellular cytotoxicity. In addition, *trastuzumab* influences the adaptive immune response and augments antigen processing and presentation (43). In breast cancer, the addition of *trastuzumab* to adjuvant chemotherapy for patients with HER-2/*neu*–positive tumors significantly decreases the hazard ratio for recurrence and subsequently improves survival (44).

The HER-2/*neu* oncogene is overexpressed in several gynecologic malignancies, including 20% to 30% of ovarian cancers (45). The largest clinical trial evaluating HER2/*neu* as a target in ovarian or primary peritoneal carcinoma was conducted by the Gynecologic Oncology Group (46). **Of 837 tumor samples screened for HER2/*neu* expression, 95 patients (11.4%) were found to have tumors with HER/*neu* overexpression.** Forty-one patients with HER2/*neu*-positive tumors received *trastuzumab* weekly. Single-agent treatment resulted in one complete (2.4%) and two partial (4.9%) responses, with a median duration of response of 8 weeks (range 2 to 104 weeks). The authors concluded that **single-agent *trastuzumab* in recurrent ovarian cancer was of limited value because of the low frequency of HER-2/*neu* overexpression and the low rate of clinical antitumor response.**

HER2/*neu* overexpression is infrequent in cervical cancer. In one study, only one of 35 (2.9%) cervical carcinomas showed strong expression of HER2/*neu* (47).

In uterine papillary serous carcinoma, 12 of 68 (18%) tumors showed HER2/*neu* overexpression; this was associated with a worse overall prognosis (48). In a separate study, five of 19 specimens (26%) stained strongly for HER2/*neu* protein receptor (49).

Mitogen-Activated Protein Kinase Pathways	**The mitogen-activated protein (MAP) kinase cascades are activated by various cofactors, inflammatory cytokines, and stress** (50). The signaling cascades include various molecules, including RAS, MEK1/2, ERK1/2, and p38 MAPK. Various molecules have been developed that target this pathway but are mostly still under investigation. *Sorafenib* is among the first of the agents with clinically proven efficacy. *Sorafenib* is a competitive inhibitor of *raf* that has been approved for treatment of renal cell carcinoma and hepatocellular carcinoma (51). Besides targeting *raf, sorafenib* also inhibits VEGFR2 and VEGFR3, FT3, c-kit, and PDGFR-β.
The PI3-kinase/Akt/ mTOR Pathway	**The phosphoinositide3-kinase (PI3-kinase)/Akt/mTOR pathway is a major oncogenic signaling pathway in various cancers** (52). **Activation of this pathway can be demonstrated in more than 80% of endometrial cancers, 50% to 70% of epithelial ovarian cancers, and approximately 50% of cervical cancers** (53–55). Activation of PI3-kinase by various growth factors such as platelet-derived growth factor (PDGF) or insulin growth factor results in phosphorylation and therefore activation of the central oncogenic protein Akt. Activated Akt is released from the membrane and elicits downstream effects mainly by phosphorylating signal transduction proteins such as *BAD,* FKHR, Caspase 9, and mammalian target of rapamycin (mTOR). Activation of these downstream signals leads to an increase in cellular proliferation, invasiveness, drug resistance, and neoangiogenesis. The *PTEN* (phosphatase and tensin homologue deleted on chromosome 10) gene is a tumor suppressor gene that is located on chromosome 10q23 and encodes a dual-specificity phosphatase for both lipid and protein substrates (56). *PTEN* decreases the activation of Akt in the *PTEN*/PI3-kinase/Akt pathway.
	Several inhibitors of PI3-kinase/Akt/mTOR signaling are currently in clinical trials (57,58). **Rapamycin** or **rapamycin** analogues, for example, **block the activity of mTOR,** a protein complex responsible for increasing protein synthesis and cellular proliferation (59). Several mTOR inhibitors, including RAD001 and CCI779, and specific PI3-kinase inhibitors are currently under development in preclinical models and clinical trials. PI3-kinase/Akt/mTOR inhibitors have been used in endometrial cancer with limited benefit (60). However, the results from clinical trials using mTOR inhibitors in renal cell carcinomas and glioblastomas are very encouraging (61).

Immunotherapy

Failure of functional immunity contributes to the genesis of virus-associated cancers, such as those caused by human papilloma virus (HPV) or Epstein-Barr virus. The greatest success story involving the enhancement of immunity to combat gynecologic cancer is the development of vaccines against HPV, which are highly effective for the prevention of cervical dysplasia and cancer (62). Although many effective induced antitumor immune responses have been described, **the relative role of natural antitumor immune responses in the detection and destruction of cancer cells,** at least as was envisioned originally when the concept of immune surveillance was first defined (63), **is still unclear.** Some researchers suggest that immune responses are mainly involved in protection from virus-associated cancers but not other forms of cancer (64).

Cancer is a common disease, and overt immune deficiency certainly is not necessary for its development. However, recent studies have shown that many cancers, including those that are not known to have a viral etiology, are seen with increased frequency in patients who have dysfunctional immunity. In a recent metaanalysis of cancer incidence in populations known to be immune deficient (e.g., organ-transplant recipients, patients with HIV infection), Grulich and co-workers (65) found an increased incidence of several common cancers, suggesting that impaired immunity can contribute to the development of cancer.

Components of the Immune System Involved in Antitumor Responses	**Various types of human immune responses can target tumor cells. Immune responses can be categorized as humoral or cellular, a distinction based on the observation in experimental systems that some immune responses could be transferred by serum (humoral) and others by cells (cellular). In general, humoral responses refer to antibody responses;** antibodies are antigen-reactive, soluble, bifunctional molecules composed of specific antigen-binding

sites associated with a constant region that directs the biologic activities of the antibody molecule, such as binding to effector cells or complement activation (Fig. 2.2). Cellular immune responses generally refer to cytotoxic responses mediated directly by activated immune cells rather than by the production of antibodies (Fig. 2.3).

Nearly all immune responses involve both humoral and cellular components and require the coordinated activities of populations of lymphocytes operating in concert with each other and with antigen-presenting cells. These activities result in various effector functions such as antibody production, cytokine secretion, and the stimulation and expansion of cytotoxic T cells. Cellular interactions involved in immune responses include direct cell–cell contact, as well as cellular interactions mediated by the secretion of, and response to, cytokines. The latter are biologic messenger molecules that play important roles in the genesis, amplification, and effector functions of immune responses.

T lymphocytes play a pivotal role by acting as helper cells in the generation of humoral and cellular immune responses and by acting as effector cells in cellular responses. Cytotoxic T cells are effector T cells that can directly interact with, and kill, target cells by

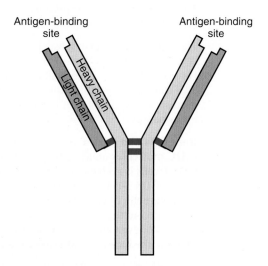

Figure 2.2   The basic immunoglobulin structure.

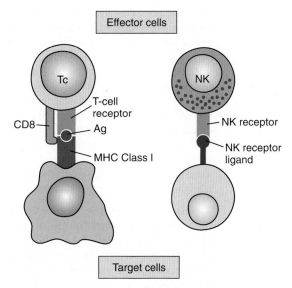

Figure 2.3   Cell-mediated cytotoxicity: two different types of cell-mediated cytotoxicity.

the release of cytotoxic molecules and the induction of target cell apoptosis. T-lymphocyte precursors mature into functional T lymphocytes in the thymus, where they learn to recognize antigen in the context of the major histocompatibility complex (MHC) molecules of the individual. Most T lymphocytes with the capability of responding to self-antigens are removed during thymic development. T lymphocytes are distinguished from other types of lymphocytes by their biologic activities and by the expression of distinctive cell surface molecules, including the T-cell antigen receptor and the CD3 molecular complex. T lymphocytes recognize specific antigens by interactions that involve the T-cell antigen receptor (Fig. 2.2) (66).

There are two major subsets of T lymphocytes: T helper/inducer cells, which express the CD4 cell surface marker; and T suppressor/cytotoxic cells, which express the CD8 marker. CD4 T lymphocytes can provide help to B lymphocytes, resulting in antibody production, and also can act as helper cells for other T lymphocytes. Much of the helper activity of T lymphocytes is mediated by the production of cytokines. CD4 T cells have been further subdivided into TH1 (cellular immunity/proinflammatory) and TH2 (antibody response–promoting) subsets, based on the pattern of cytokine production and the biological properties of these cells. Recent studies have identified a subset of T cells that inhibit autoreactive cells, perhaps acting to prevent autoimmune responses (67). This subset of T cells has been called *regulatory T cells.* Other recently described T-cell subsets include TH17 cells, which are important in driving immune responses to bacteria and fungi (68,69).

The CD8 T-lymphocyte subset includes cells that are cytotoxic and can directly kill target cells. A major biologic role of such cytotoxic T lymphocytes is the lysis of virus-infected cells. However, cytotoxic T lymphocytes can directly mediate the lysis of tumor cells. Effector T cells also can contribute to antitumor immune responses by producing cytokines, such as tumor necrosis factor (TNF), that induce tumor cell lysis and can enhance other antitumor cell effector responses.

Both CD4 and CD8 T cells respond to antigen only when it is presented in the context of MHC molecules on antigen-presenting cells or target cells or both. The T-cell receptor on CD4 T cells is restricted to responding to antigen plus MHC class II molecules; the receptor on CD8 T-cells is restricted to responding to antigen plus MHC class I molecules. In addition, both T-cell subsets require a second simultaneous costimulatory signal for optimal stimulation in the absence of which the T cells may be induced to enter a state of unresponsiveness or even apoptosis. **Therefore, provision of effective costimulatory signals is necessary for the induction of effective antitumor responses by activated T cells.**

B lymphocytes are the cells that produce and secrete antibodies, which are antigen-binding molecules (Fig. 2.2). B lymphocytes develop from pre-B cells and, after exposure to antigen and appropriate activation signals, differentiate to become plasma cells—cells that produce large quantities of antibodies. Mature B lymphocytes use cell-surface immunoglobulin molecules as antigen receptors. **In addition to producing antibodies, B lymphocytes play another important role: They can serve as efficient antigen-presenting cells for T lymphocytes.** Although the production of antitumor antibodies does not appear to play a central role in host antitumor immune responses, **monoclonal antibodies reactive with tumor-associated antigens have proved to be very useful in antitumor therapy, as well as in the detection of tumors or of tumor-associated molecules.** Unfortunately, no truly unique tumor-specific antigens have been identified, and most tumor-related antigens are expressed to some extent on nonmalignant tissues. Also, because some monoclonal antibodies are of murine and not human origin, the host's immune system can recognize and respond to murine monoclonal antibodies. This has led to the development of **"humanized"** monoclonal antibodies (genetically engineered monoclonal antibodies composed of human constant regions with specific antigen-reactive murine variable regions), with the aim of avoiding many of the problems associated with the administration of murine monoclonal antibodies.

Macrophages and dendritic cells also play key roles in the generation of adaptive, lymphocyte-mediated immune responses by acting as antigen-presenting cells. Helper/inducer (CD4) T lymphocytes, bearing a T-cell receptor of appropriate antigen and self-specificity, are activated by antigen-presenting cells that display processed antigen combined with self-MHC molecules (Fig. 2.2). Antigen-presenting cells also provide costimulatory signals that are important for the induction of T-lymphocyte activation. In addition to serving as antigen-presenting cells, macrophages can ingest and kill microorganisms and act as cytotoxic antitumor killer cells. These cells also produce various cytokines, including IL-1,

IL-6, chemokines, IL-10, and TNF, which are involved in many immune responses. These monocyte-produced cytokines can have direct effects on tumor cell growth and development, both as growth-inducing and growth-inhibiting factors.

Natural killer (NK) cells are cells that have large granular lymphocytic morphology, do not express the CD3 T-cell receptor complex, and do not respond to specific antigens. NK cells can lyse target cells, including tumor cells, unrestricted by the expression of antigen or self-MHC molecules on the target cell. Therefore, NK cells are effector cells in an innate (non–antigen-restricted) immune response and may play a vital role in immune responses to tumor cells. The cells that can effect antibody-dependent cellular cytotoxicity (ADCC) are NK-like cells.

Cytokines are soluble mediator molecules that induce, enhance, or effect immune responses. Cytokines are produced by various types of cells and play critical roles not only in immune responses but also in biologic responses outside of the immune response, such as hematopoiesis or the acute-phase response. T helper 1(TH1) and TH2 cells, which control the nature of an immune response by secreting characteristic and mutually antagonistic sets of cytokines (9–11), are defined by the cytokines they produce. TH1 clones produce IL-2 and IFN-, whereas TH2 clones produce IL-4, IL-5, IL-6, and IL-10. TH1 cytokines promote cell-mediated and inflammatory responses, whereas TH2 cytokines enhance antibody production. Most immune responses involve both TH1 and TH2 components.

Research has identified CD4-positive T cells that participate in the maintenance of immuno-logic self-tolerance by actively suppressing the activation and expansion of self-reactive lymphocytes. These cells are called regulatory T cells, or Treg cells. Treg cells are characterized by the expression of CD25 (the IL-2 receptor-chain) and the transcription factor FoxP3 (70,71). Treg cell activity is thought to be important in preventing the development of autoimmune diseases. Removal of Treg also may enhance immune responses against infectious agents or cancer. Although much remains to be learned about the role of Treg activity in anti-tumor immunity, it is clear that such cells may play a role in modulating host responses to cancer.

Therapeutic Strategies

There is great interest in developing effective biologic and immune therapies for gynecologic malignancies. For example, patients with small-volume or microscopic residual peritoneal ovarian cancer are attractive candidates for immunotherapy or biologic therapy, especially approaches based on regional peritoneal immunotherapy or biotherapy (72,73). Also, many patients with advanced disease are immunocompromised, suggesting a role for immune-enhancing therapeutic approaches. Dysplastic and cancerous cervical epithelial cells infected with HPV, an oncogenic virus, also present an attractive target for immune enhancement-based therapeutic strategies, including the development of therapeutic vaccines for HPV. Advances in molecular biology, biotechnology, immunology, and cytokine biology have resulted in the availability of many new, promising immunotherapeutic approaches for gynecologic cancers.

The state of the art in immunotherapy for ovarian cancer and other gynecologic malignancies has been considered and described in detail in several recent excellent reviews (74–77), and the reader is referred to these publications for more detailed information on immunotherapy for gynecologic cancers. Examples of the current use of immunotherapy in clinical trials, both monoclonal antibody-based and therapies-based on enhanced cellular immune responses, are provided below.

Monoclonal Antibodies and Antibody-Based Immunotherapy

Monoclonal antibodies have played an important role in both the development of immunotherapeutic agents and tumor markers. Monoclonal antibodies also have been used for radioimmunodetection (78,79) **and are being used for treatment.** Monoclonal antibodies can potentially induce antitumor responses in various ways: (i) by complement activation and subsequent tumor cell lysis; (ii) by directly inducing antiproliferative effects, perhaps by interaction with tumor cell surface signaling molecules; (iii) by enhancing the activity of phagocytic cells, which can interact with immune complexes containing monoclonal antibodies; and (iv) by mediating ADCC via interactions of the Fc portion of monoclonal antibodies with Fc receptors on cells that mediate ADCC (80). In addition, monoclonal antibodies can be labeled with either radioactive particles or antitumor drugs and used to focus these agents onto tumor cells (81). In fact, some monoclonal antibody-based drugs are currently approved and being used for the treatment of cancer with great success. These FDA-approved monoclonal antibody-based anticancer drugs include: *bevacizumab* (*Avastin*) for treatment of colon and lung cancer, *cetuximab* (*Erbitux*) for the treatment of colon and head and neck cancer, *gemtuzumab* (*Mylotarg*) for the treatment of acute myelogenous leukemia, *rituximab* (*Rituxan*) for the treatment of non-Hodgkin's lymphoma, and *trastuzumab* (*Herceptin*) for the treatment of breast cancer.

Several clinical trials have utilized monoclonal antibodies directed against ovarian cancer antigens, including CA125, folate receptor, MUC1 antigen, and tumor-associated glyco-protein 72 (76). Evidence that CA125 can act as a tumor antigen that stimulates humoral and cellular immune responses is derived from various *in vitro* studies and clinical trials. *Oregovomab* (B43.13) is a murine monoclonal antibody to CA125 that has been used for the treatment of ovarian cancer. The antibody binds to circulating CA125, resulting in the formation of immune complexes (antibody–antigen complexes). These immune complexes are recognized as foreign, mainly because of the murine component. They are taken up by antigen-presenting cells, allowing the processing of the autologous CA125 antigen, ultimately leading to induction of CA125-specific antibodies, helper T cells, and cytolytic T cells.

In 2004, Berek et al. reported on the use of *oregovomab* for maintenance therapy in patients with ovarian cancer after first-line treatment. A subgroup of patients with favorable prognostic factors had a significantly longer time to relapse compared to patients in the placebo group (82). A five-year follow-up report in 2008 documented a median survival of 57.5 months for the *oregovomab* group and 48.6 months for the placebo group (83). These differences were not statistically significant. However, **the velocity of the rise in CA125 levels at relapse was found to be a highly significant predictor of postrelapse outcome.**

Another antibody network–based strategy has employed anti-idiotype vaccines in patients with relapsed ovarian cancer. ACA125 is a murine anti-idiotypic antibody that mimics an antigenic epitope on CA125 (75,76,84,85). Therefore, antibodies generated to ACA125 have the potential to react with antigenic epitopes on CA125, with ACA125 serving as an antiidio-type vaccine that would enhance immune responses to CA125 (75). Treatment with ACA125 resulted in both humoral and cellular responses, and those patients who had detectable anti-ACA125 responses showed a longer mean survival time than those who did not develop responses (86,87).

Abagovomab is an anti-idiotypic antibody that mimics the CA125 antigen. The initial results of *abagovomab* treatment in patients with ovarian cancer were reported by Sabbatini et al. and showed that all patients developed an anti-idiotypic antibody response (Ab3) (88). In addition, the generation of T-cell immunity to CA125 was demonstrated in five patients. While patients had measurable serum CA125 levels in both trials, neither trial analyzed CA125 expression in tumor tissue. A large international, multicenter trial is underway to investigate the effect of *abagovomab* as consolidation treatment in patients with ovarian cancer.

Adoptive Immunotherapy

Adoptive immunotherapy involves the *ex vivo* expansion of antitumor immune cells followed by the administration of such effector cells. It has provided another immune system–based approach for antitumor therapy (74,75,89–92). **Adoptive immunotherapy, involving the infusion of large numbers of autologous *ex vivo*–activated immune effector cells, has been shown to produce tumor regression in various animal and human tumors** (90), and it has been seen to produce the best results seen to date in tumor immunotherapy (74). This approach can provide large numbers of tumor-specific T cells with the capacity to specifically kill tumor cells and can potentially lead to the complete elimination of residual tumor cells (74).

Early approaches used peripheral blood mononuclear cells exposed to IL-2 *ex vivo* to lead to the generation of lymphokine-activated killer (LAK) cells that are cytotoxic for a variety of tumor cells (93,94). Although experimental treatment of human subjects with LAK cells and IL-2 yielded some responses, considerable toxicity was seen (72,89–92,94–98). Given that (1) the overall response rate to LAK treatment is low, (2) this type of adoptive immunother-apy can result in high morbidity, and (3) it is impractical in most medical settings, **adoptive immunotherapy with LAK cells does not appear to be a practical option for the treatment of ovarian cancer.** The use of immunotherapy based on *ex vivo*–stimulated tumor-infiltrating lymphocytes or tumor-associated lymphocytes from ascites, with or without added IL-2, also has been examined in ovarian cancer (74,92,97,98).

It is clear that optimization of such adoptive immunotherapies is needed in terms of the cell source, the forms of stimulation, the methods for *ex vivo* expansion, and the cytokines that are given during such treatment (74). Potentially important refinements of these approaches include (i) the use of dendritic cells (DCs) as antigen-presenting cells (APCs) to stimulate T cells, (ii) the provision of effective costimulatory signals to the responding T cells by *APC,* and (iii) host conditioning with immunosuppressive chemotherapy before the adoptive transfer of cells (74,99).

Dendritic Cell and Tumor Vaccine Therapy

Cancers may develop or progress because immune system cells are not given a strong enough signal to become activated to destroy the tumor cells. In some cases, cancers are able to down regulate immune responses as cytokines or other molecules produced by tumor cells, such as IL-10 (100), can inhibit antitumor immune responses. It may be possible to counter this lack of antitumor immune responsiveness by enhancing *APC* activity, providing tumor-associated antigens in a manner that can better induce the generation of anti-tumor effector T cells (tumor vaccine therapy), or both.

A thorough overview of the rationale and design of potential tumor vaccines for ovarian cancer can be found in recent review papers (74,75). At this time, tumor vaccine approaches include (i) vaccination with defined tumor-associated antigens, or DNA vaccines that encode for tumor-associated antigens; and (ii) vaccination with whole tumor cell preparations with and without the coadministration of antigen-presenting cells such as dendritic cells. Adjuvants have been used to enhance the immunogenicity of tumor vaccines (74).

Various tumor-associated antigens are potential immunogens for tumor vaccines, including (i) differentiation antigens, (ii) new antigens created by mutation of genes encoding host cell proteins, (iii) molecules that are overexpressed on tumor cells (i.e., HER2, NY-ESO-1, CA125), and (iv) viral antigens from oncogenic viruses (i.e., HPV-encoded antigens) (75). **Experimental tumor vaccine therapy in ovarian cancer has been carried out using the NY-ESO-1 antigen.** Nearly half of epithelial ovarian cancers are NY-ESO-1 positive (101). Vaccination with a peptide from NY-ESO-1 resulted in the generation of both cellular and humoral immunity to this antigen, in most vaccinated patients (102). **Vaccines based on HER2 also have been tested in ovarian cancer patients, with such treatment resulting in the induction of specific T-cell responses in most patients** (103).

Human papilloma virus—specifically, HPV subtypes 16, 18, 31, and 45—has been implicated as the major etiologic agent in cervical cancer. HPV-infected dysplastic and cancerous cervical epithelial cells consistently retain and express two of the viral genes, *E6* and *E7,* that respectively interact with and disrupt the function of the *p53* and retinoblastoma tumor-suppressor gene products. **Factors other than infection with HPV, such as cellular immune function, play an important role in determining whether the infection of cervical epithelial cells regresses or progresses to cancer.** This has led to the development of prophylactic and therapeutic vaccines to HPV, as well as treatment approaches based on the enhancement of host immune function.

Human papilloma virus vaccines have been shown to have an exceptional level of efficacy (62), clearly reducing the incidence of both HPV-16 and -18 infections and HPV-16 and -18–related cervical intraepithelial neoplasia. The HPV vaccines *Gardasil* and *Cerverix* use HPV-like particles as immunogens to generate neutralizing antibodies for HPV. These findings suggest that HPV-based therapeutic cancer vaccines may also be effective for the control of cervical cancer (77).

The choice of target antigens for therapeutic vaccines to HPV positive cancers is of great importance and requires careful consideration of the expression of virus-encoded antigens in tumor cells (77). **HPV *E6* and *E7* are attractive antigens for use in therapeutic vaccines** because these HPV-encoded proteins are involved in cellular transformation and therefore are consistently expressed in HPV-positive tumor cells. Candidate therapeutic HPV vaccines include DNA vaccines, with recent research aimed at enhancing the potency and delivery of such vaccines by linking vaccine DNA to MHC class II–associated invariant chain (77,104) or by fusion of HPV DNA to the sorting signal of lysosomal-associated membrane protein type 1 to enhance MHC class II–mediated antigen presentation (77,105,106). Clinical trails with such DNA-based vaccines are currently being planned (77).

Dendritic cells are highly effective antigen-presenting cells and play a central role in the induction of both CD4 and CD8 T-cell responses. Dendritic cells can be pulsed with tumor

antigen peptides or bioengineered to express tumor antigens, allowing them to be used in experimental therapies that aim to enhance antitumor immunity. Exposure of T cells to dendritic cells pulsed with ovarian cancer–derived antigenic preparations resulted in the generation of cytolytic effector T cells that could kill autologous tumor cells *in vitro* (107–109). In a phase I clinical trial, Hernando and co-workers (110) showed that patients with advanced gynecological malignancies could be effectively vaccinated with dendritic cells pulsed with a nontumor test antigen, keyhole limpet hemocyanin (KLH), and autologous tumor antigens. Lymphoproliferative responses to KLH and to tumor lysate stimulation were noted. The treatment was safe, well tolerated, immunologically active, and generally devoid of significant adverse effects.

Given the exceptional ability of dendritic cells to serve as potent antigen-presenting cells in the induction of T-cell responses, an attractive approach would be to combine tumor vaccines with *ex vivo*–generated dendritic cell preparations. Dendritic cells can be generated *ex vivo* from peripheral blood mononuclear cells using various strategies (74,111–114). Such *ex vivo*–generated dendritic cells can be pulsed with tumor antigens or vaccines or with DNA- or RNA-encoding tumor antigens, before administration, and have resulted in the induction of antitumor responses in preclinical studies (74,115–117).

Several major challenges need to be overcome for the successful development of effective DC-based therapies for ovarian cancer: (i) the identification of tumor-associated or tumor-specific antigens, (ii) the development of means to induce optimal DC maturation after antigen uptake, (iii) the development of schemes for generation of DCs that maintain optimal antigen-presenting cell activity and do not produce immunosuppressive factors, and (iv) the development of *ex vivo* expansion techniques that provide sufficient numbers of DCs for effective immunotherapy (74,118–120). **As more is learned about the immunogenicity of current tumor-associated antigens, novel cancer-associated antigens are identified, and the techniques of DC activation and antigen expression are better developed, DC-based immunotherapy may provide a therapeutic alternative for the treatment of these cancers.**

Biologic Response Modifier and Cytokine Therapy: Modulation of Host Immunity

Most early experimental biologic therapies for metastatic ovarian cancer involved biologic response modifiers such as ***Corynebacterium parvum*** (a heat-killed, gram-negative anaerobic bacillus), ***bacillus Calmette-Guérin*** (BCG), or modifications of these agents (121–123). Exposure to *C. parvum* resulted in the nonspecific enhancement of host immune responses, including the induction of an acute inflammatory response (123). Biologic response modifier therapy for ovarian cancer, including treatment with *C. parvum* and BCG, was examined in several studies (121,123–125). However, intraperitoneal (IP) treatment with *C. parvum* induced a profound local reaction, including peritoneal fibrosis, and its toxicity precluded more widespread testing.

Malignancies that tend predominantly to grow in the peritoneal cavity, such as residual ovarian cancer, have been treated in many experimental trials with IP drugs, most frequently with cytotoxic chemotherapeutic agents (126). IP biologic response modifier therapy, immunotherapy with cytokines, and gene therapy have been proposed and used for similar reasons. These approaches have the additional advantage of potentially inducing the activation of regional immune effector mechanisms in the peritoneal cavity (73). This might be particularly true for cytokine-based treatment strategies or for adoptive immunotherapies because activated immune effector cells may require direct contact with the malignant target cells for most effective antitumor activity.

Various cytokines have been tested in clinical trials, to date producing mixed results (74). This includes trials of IFN-α and IFN-γ, TNF-α, and IL-2. In recent studies, treatment of patients with refractory ovarian cancer with intravenous recombinant human IL-12, a TH1-inducing cytokine, resulted in disease stabilization in about half of the treated patients (127). **IP treatment with IL-12 in patients with carcinomatosis from mesotheliomas, müllerian or gastrointestinal carcinomas, showed a 10% complete response rate and disease stabilization in nearly half of the treated patients** (128). In a recent phase II trial, treatment with subcutaneously administered **IL-2 and oral retinoic acid** was reported to improve survival in patients who had ovarian cancer responding to chemotherapy (129).

The recent identification of T-cell subpopulations that have potent immunoregulatory properties, such as Treg cells and TH17 cells, provides new opportunities for the design of

host immune system–modulating therapies with the aim of enhancing immune responses to cancer. Treg cells, which are immunoinhibitory regulatory T cells, can inhibit the induction of cytotoxic T cells and may thereby inhibit host antitumor immune responses. Increased levels of Treg cells in ascites, blood and tumor, have been seen in patients with advanced ovarian cancer (130). These Treg cells can inhibit antitumor immunity and promote tumor cell growth in ovarian cancer (131). Therefore, blocking the action of these Treg cells is clearly an important target in the development of new immunotherapeutic approaches to combat cancer. Studies aimed at blocking Treg activity in patients with cancer have been initiated using monoclonal antibodies targeting CD25, a cell-surface molecule commonly expressed on these cells. To date, these studies have not resulted in enhanced anticancer immune responses (132), and more refined approaches to target Treg need to be developed.

TH17 cells are another recently identified regulatory T-cell subpopulation, characterized by the secretion of IL-17. They have the ability to modulate Treg activity (68,69,133). The role of TH17 cells in cancer has not been clearly defined. In a recent animal study, it was reported that provision of IL-2 in the tumor microenvironment was associated with decreased TH17 activity and increased Treg activity (133). Although much more work needs to be done to define the role of TH17 cells in down regulating Treg activity, and perhaps in enhancing antitumor responses, future experimental treatment strategies aimed at enhancing TH17 activity may be of value in enhancing antitumor immune responses.

References

1. **Hanahan D, Weinberg RA.** The hallmarks of cancer. *Cell* 2000;100:57–70.
2. **Collinson FJ, Hall GD, Perren TJ, Jayson GC.** Development of antiangiogenic agents for ovarian cancer. *Expert Rev Anticancer Ther* 2008;8:21–32.
3. **Ashouri S, Garcia AA.** Current status of signal transduction modulators in the treatment of gynecologic malignancies. *Curr Treat Options Oncol* 2007;8:383–392.
4. **Markman M.** The promise and perils of "targeted therapy" of advanced ovarian cancer. *Oncology* 2008;74:1–6.
5. **Murdoch D, Sager J.** Will targeted therapy hold its promise? An evidence-based review. *Curr Opin Oncol* 2008;20:104–111.
6. **Goede V, Schmidt T, Kimmina S, Kozian D, Augustin HG.** Analysis of blood vessel maturation processes during cyclic ovarian angiogenesis. *Lab Invest* 1998;78:1385–1394.
7. **Martin L, Schilder R.** Novel approaches in advancing the treatment of epithelial ovarian cancer: the role of angiogenesis inhibition. *J Clin Oncol* 2007;25:2894–2901.
8. **Grothey A, Ellis LM.** Targeting angiogenesis driven by vascular endothelial growth factors using antibody-based therapies. *Cancer J* 2008;14:170–177.
9. **Alvarez AA, Krigman HR, Whitaker RS, Dodge RK, Rodriguez GC.** The prognostic significance of angiogenesis in epithelial ovarian carcinoma. *Clin Cancer Res* 1999;5:587–591.
10. **Cohen MH, Gootenberg J, Keegan P, Pazdur R.** FDA drug approval summary: *bevacizumab* plus FOLFOX4 as second-line treatment of colorectal cancer. *Oncologist* 2007;12:356–361.
11. **Hurwitz H, Fehrenbacher L, Novotny W, Cartwright T, Hainsworth J, Heim W, et al.** Bevacizumab plus *irinotecan, fluorouracil,* and *leucovorin* for metastatic colorectal cancer. *N Engl J Med* 2004;350:2335–2342.
12. **Sandler AB, Johnson DH, Herbst RS.** Anti-vascular endothelial growth factor monoclonals in non-small cell lung cancer. *Clin Cancer Res* 2004;10:4258s–4262s.
13. **Burger RA, Sill MW, Monk BJ, Greer BE, Sorosky JI.** Phase II trial of *bevacizumab* in persistent or recurrent epithelial ovarian cancer or primary peritoneal cancer: a Gynecologic Oncology Group Study. *J Clin Oncol* 2007;25:5165–5171.
14. **Cannistra SA, Matulonis UA, Penson RT, Hambleton J, Dupont J, Mackey H, et al.** Phase II study of *bevacizumab* in patients with platinum-resistant ovarian cancer or peritoneal serous cancer. *J Clin Oncol* 2007;25:5180–5186.
15. **Garcia AA, Hirte H, Fleming G, Yang D, Tsao-Wei DD, Roman L, et al.** Phase II clinical trial of *bevacizumab* and low-dose metronomic oral *cyclophosphamide* in recurrent ovarian cancer: a trial of the California, Chicago, and Princess Margaret Hospital phase II consortia. *J Clin Oncol* 2008;26:76–82.
16. **Cohn DE, Valmadre S, Resnick KE, Eaton LA, Copeland LJ, Fowler JM.** *Bevacizumab* and weekly *taxane* chemotherapy demonstrates activity in refractory ovarian cancer. *Gynecol Oncol* 2006;102:134–139.
17. **Wright JD, Secord AA, Numnum TM, Rocconi RP, Powell MA, Berchuck A, et al.** A multi-institutional evaluation of factors predictive of toxicity and efficacy of *bevacizumab* for recurrent ovarian cancer. *Int J Gynecol Cancer* 2008;18:400–406.
18. **Badgwell BD, Camp ER, Feig B, Wolff RA, Eng C, Ellis LM, Cormier JN.** Management of *bevacizumab*-associated bowel perforation: a case series and review of the literature. *Ann Oncol* 2008;19:577–582.
19. **Auranen A, Grénman S.** Radiation therapy and biological compounds for consolidation therapy in advanced ovarian cancer. *Int J Gynecol Cancer* 2008;18 Suppl 1:44–46.
20. **Lu C, Thaker PH, Lin YG, Spannuth W, Landen CN, Merritt WM, et al.** Impact of vessel maturation on antiangiogenic therapy in ovarian cancer. *Am J Obstet Gynecol* 2008;198:477.e1–e9; discussion 477.e9–10.
21. **Kumar A, Petri ET, Halmos B, Boggon TJ.** Structure and clinical relevance of the epidermal growth factor receptor in human cancer. *J Clin Oncol* 2008;26:1742–1751.
22. **Wieduwilt MJ, Moasser MM.** The epidermal growth factor receptor family: biology driving targeted therapeutics. *Cell Mol Life Sci* 2008;65:1566–1584.
23. **Psyrri A, Kassar M, Yu Z, Bamias A, Weinberger PM, Markakis S, et al.** Effect of epidermal growth factor receptor expression level on survival in patients with epithelial ovarian cancer. *Clin Cancer Res* 2005;11:8637–8643.
24. **de Graeff P, Crijns AP, Ten Hoor KA, Klip HG, Hollema H, Oien K, et al.** The ErbB signalling pathway: protein expression and prognostic value in epithelial ovarian cancer. *Br J Cancer* 2008;99:341–349.
25. **Khalifa MA, Abdoh AA, Mannel RS, Haraway SD, Walker JL, Min KW.** Prognostic utility of epidermal growth factor receptor overexpression in endometrial adenocarcinoma. *Cancer* 1994;73:370–376.
26. **Scambia G, Benedetti Panici P, Ferrandina G, Battaglia F, Distefano M, D'Andrea G, et al.** Significance of epidermal growth factor receptor expression in primary human endometrial cancer. *Int J Cancer* 1994;56:26–30.

27. **Wang D, Konishi I, Koshiyama M, Mandai M, Nanbu Y, Ishikawa Y, et al.** Expression of c-erbB-2 protein and epidermal growth receptor in endometrial carcinomas. Correlation with clinicopathologic and sex steroid receptor status. *Cancer* 1993;72:2628–2637.

28. **Konecny GE, Venkatesan N, Yang G, Dering J, Ginther C, Finn R, et al.** Activity of *lapatinib*, a novel HER2 and EGFR dual kinase inhibitor in human endometrial cancer cells. *Br J Cancer* 2008;98:1076–1084.

29. **Vaidya AP, Parnes AD, Seiden MV.** Rationale and clinical experience with epidermal growth factor receptor inhibitors in gynecologic malignancies. *Curr Treat Options Oncol* 2005;6:103–114.

30. **Hudis CA.** *Trastuzumab*—mechanism of action and use in clinical practice. *N Engl J Med* 2007;357:39–51.

31. **Attard G, Kitzen J, Blagden SP, Fong PC, Pronk LC, Zhi J, et al.** A phase Ib study of *pertuzumab*, a recombinant humanised antibody to HER2, and *docetaxel* in patients with advanced solid tumours. *Br J Cancer* 2007;97:1338–1343.

32. **Galizia G, Lieto E, De Vita F, Orditura M, Castellano P, Troiani T, et al.** *Cetuximab*, a chimeric human mouse anti-epidermal growth factor receptor monoclonal antibody, in the treatment of human colorectal cancer. *Oncogene* 2007;26:3654–3660.

33. **Wang S, Guo P, Wang X, Zhou Q, Gallo JM.** Preclinical pharmacokinetic/pharmacodynamic models of *gefitinib* and the design of equivalent dosing regimens in EGFR wild-type and mutant tumor models. *Mol Cancer Ther* 2008;7:407–417.

34. **Gordon AN, Finkler N, Edwards RP, Garcia AA, Crozier M, Irwin DH, et al.** Efficacy and safety of *erlotinib* HCl, an epidermal growth factor receptor (HER1/EGFR) tyrosine kinase inhibitor, in patients with advanced ovarian carcinoma: results from a phase II multicenter study. *Int J Gynecol Cancer* 2005;15:785–792.

35. **Vasey PA, Gore M, Wilson R, Rustin G, Gabra H, Guastalla JP, et al.** A phase Ib trial of *docetaxel, carboplatin,* and *erlotinib* in ovarian, fallopian tube, and primary peritoneal cancers. *Br J Cancer* 2008;98:1774–1780.

36. **Secord AA, Blessing JA, Armstrong DK, Rodgers WH, Miner Z, Barnes MN, et al.** Phase II trial of *cetuximab* and *carboplatin* in relapsed platinum-sensitive ovarian cancer and evaluation of epidermal growth factor receptor expression: a Gynecologic Oncology Group study. *Gynecol Oncol* 2008;108:493–499.

37. **Konner J, Schilder RJ, DeRosa FA, Gerst SR, Tew WP, Sabbatini PJ, et al.** A phase II study of *cetuximab/paclitaxel/carboplatin* for the initial treatment of advanced-stage ovarian, primary peritoneal, or fallopian tube cancer. *Gynecol Oncol* 2008;110:140–145.

38. **Schilder RJ, Sill MW, Chen X, Darcy KM, Decesare SL, Lewandowski G, et al.** Phase II study of *gefitinib* in patients with relapsed or persistent ovarian or primary peritoneal carcinoma and evaluation of epidermal growth factor receptor mutations and immunohistochemical expression: a Gynecologic Oncology Group Study. *Clin Cancer Res* 2005;11:5539–5548.

39. **Posadas EM, Liel MS, Kwitkowski V, Minasian L, Godwin AK, Hussain MM, et al.** A phase II and pharmacodynamic study of *gefitinib* in patients with refractory or recurrent epithelial ovarian cancer. *Cancer* 2007;109:1323–1330.

40. **Lacroix L, Pautier P, Duvillard P, Motte N, Saulnier P, Bidart JM, et al.** Response of ovarian carcinomas to *gefitinib-carboplatin-paclitaxel* combination is not associated with EGFR kinase domain somatic mutations. *Int J Cancer* 2006;118:1068–1069.

41. **Wagner U, du Bois A, Pfisterer J, Huober J, Loibl S, Lück HJ, et al.** *Gefitinib* in combination with tamoxifen in patients with ovarian cancer refractory or resistant to platinum-*taxane* based therapy—a phase II trial of the AGO Ovarian Cancer Study Group (AGO-OVAR 2.6). *Gynecol Oncol* 2007;105:132–137.

42. **Goncalves A, Fabbro M, Lhomme C, Gladieff L, Extra JM, Floquet A, et al.** A phase II trial to evaluate *gefitinib* as second- or third-line treatment in patients with recurring locoregionally advanced or metastatic cervical cancer. *Gynecol Oncol* 2008;108:42–46.

43. **Reich O, Liegl B, Tamussino K, Regauer S.** p185HER2 overexpression and HER2 oncogene amplification in recurrent vulvar Paget's disease. *Mod Pathol* 2005;18:354–357.

44. **De Laurentiis M, Cancello G, Zinno L, Montagna E, Malorni L, Esposito A, et al.** Targeting HER2 as a therapeutic strategy for breast cancer: a paradigmatic shift of drug development in oncology. *Ann Oncol* 2005;16(suppl 4):iv7–13.

45. **Tuefferd M, Couturier J, Penault-Llorca F, Vincent-Salomon A, Broet P, Guastalla JP, et al.** HER2 status in ovarian carcinomas: a multicenter GINECO study of 320 patients. *PLoS ONE* 2007;2:e1138.

46. **Bookman MA, Darcy KM, Clarke-Pearson D, Boothby RA, Horowitz IR.** Evaluation of monoclonal humanized anti-HER2 antibody, *trastuzumab*, in patients with recurrent or refractory ovarian or primary peritoneal carcinoma with overexpression of HER2: a phase II trial of the Gynecologic Oncology Group. *J Clin Oncol* 2003;21:283–290.

47. **Chavez-Blanco A, Perez-Sanchez V, Gonzalez-Fierro A, Vela-Chavez T, Candelaria M, Cetina L, et al.** HER2 expression in cervical cancer as a potential therapeutic target. *BMC Cancer* 2004;4:59.

48. **Slomovitz BM, Broaddus RR, Burke TW, Sneige N, Soliman PT, Wu W, et al.** Her-2/*neu* overexpression and amplification in uterine papillary serous carcinoma. *J Clin Oncol* 2004;22:3126–3132.

49. **Villella JA, Cohen S, Smith DH, Hibshoosh H, Hershman D.** HER-2/*neu* overexpression in uterine papillary serous cancers and its possible therapeutic implications. *Int J Gynecol Cancer* 2006;16:1897–1902.

50. **McCubrey JA, Milella M, Tafuri A, Martelli AM, Lunghi P, Bonati A, et al.** Targeting the *Raf*/MEK/ERK pathway with small-molecule inhibitors. *Curr Opin Investig Drugs* 2008;9:614–630.

51. **Adnane L, Trail PA, Taylor I, Wilhelm SM.** *Sorafenib* (BAY 43-9006, *Nexavar*), a dual-action inhibitor that targets *RAF*/MEK/ERK pathway in tumor cells and tyrosine kinases VEGFR/PDGFR in tumor vasculature. *Methods Enzymol* 2006;407:597–612.

52. **Jiang BH, Liu LZ.** PI3K/*PTEN* signaling in tumorigenesis and angiogenesis. *Biochem Biophys Acta* 2008;1784:150–158.

53. **Mutter GL, Lin MC, Fitzgerald JT, Kum JB, Baak JP, Lees JA, et al.** Altered *PTEN* expression as a diagnostic marker for the earliest endometrial precancers. *J Natl Cancer Inst* 2000;92:924–930.

54. **Cully M, You H, Levine AJ, Mak TW.** Beyond *PTEN* mutations: the PI3K pathway as an integrator of multiple inputs during tumorigenesis. *Nat Rev Cancer* 2006;6:184–192.

55. **Castellvi J, Garcia A, Rojo F, Ruiz-Marcellan C, Gil A, Baselga J, et al.** Phosphorylated 4E binding protein 1: a hallmark of cell signaling that correlates with survival in ovarian cancer. *Cancer* 2006;107:1801–1811.

56. **Salmena L, Carracedo A, Pandolfi PP.** Tenets of *PTEN* tumor suppression. *Cell* 2008;133:403–414.

57. **LoPiccolo J, Blumenthal GM, Bernstein WB, Dennis PA.** Targeting the PI3K/Akt/mTOR pathway: effective combinations and clinical considerations. *Drug Resist Updat* 2008;11:32–50.

58. **Marone R, Cmiljanovic V, Giese B, Wymann MP.** Targeting phosphoinositide 3-kinase: moving towards therapy. *Biochim Biophys Acta* 2008;1784:159–185.

59. **Wullschleger S, Loewith R, Hall MN.** TOR signaling in growth and metabolism. *Cell* 2006;124:471–484.

60. **Gadducci A, Tana R, Cosio S, Fanucchi A, Genazzani AR.** Molecular target therapies in endometrial cancer: from the basic research to the clinic. *Gynecol Endocrinol* 2008;24:239–249.

61. **Motzer RJ, Escudier B, Oudard S, Hutson TE, Porta C, Bracarda S, et al.** Efficacy of *everolimus* in advanced renal cell carcinoma: a double-blind, randomised, placebo-controlled phase III trial. *Lancet* 2008;372:449–456.

62. **FUTURE II Study Group.** Quadrivalent vaccine against human papillomavirus to prevent high-grade cervical lesions. *N Engl J Med* 2007;356:1915–1927.

63. **Burnet FM.** The concept of immunological surveillance. *Prog Exp Tumor Res* 1970;13:1–27.

64. **Klein G, Klein E.** Surveillance against tumors—is it mainly immunological? *Immunol Lett* 2005;100:29–33.

65. **Grulich AE, van Leeuwen MT, Falster MO, Vajdic CM.** Incidence of cancers in people with HIV/AIDS compared with immunosuppressed transplant recipients: a meta-analysis. *Lancet* 2007;370:59–67.

66. **Owen M.** T-cell receptors and MHC molecules. In: **Roitt I, Borstoff J, Male D, eds.** *Immunology*, 5th ed. St. Louis: Mosby-Year Book, 1998.

67. **Zou W.** Regulatory T cells, tumour immunity and immunotherapy. *Nat Rev Immunol* 2006;6:295–307.

68. **Bettelli E, Carrier Y, Gao W, Korn T, Strom TB, Oukka M, et al.** Reciprocal developmental pathways for the generation of pathogenic effector TH17 and regulatory T cells. *Nature* 2006;441:235–238.
69. **Bronte V.** TH17 and cancer: friends or foes? *Blood* 2008;112:214.
70. **Sakaguchi S, Sakaguchi N, Shimizu J, Yamazaki S, Sakihama T, Itoh M, et al.** Immunologic tolerance maintained by CD25+ CD4+ regulatory T cells: their common role in controlling autoimmunity, tumor immunity, and transplantation tolerance. *Immunol Rev* 2001;182:18–32.
71. **Shevach EM.** CD4+ CD25+ suppressor T cells: more questions than answers. *Nat Rev Immunol* 2002;2:389–400.
72. **Bookman MA, Bast RC Jr.** The immunobiology and immunotherapy of ovarian cancer. *Semin Oncol* 1991;18:270–291.
73. **Bookman MA.** Biological therapy of ovarian cancer: current directions. *Semin Oncol* 1998;25:381–396.
74. **Chu CS, Kim SH, June CH, Coukos G.** Immunotherapy opportunities in ovarian cancer. *Expert Rev Anticancer Ther* 2008;8:243–257.
75. **Odunsi K, Sabbatini P.** Harnessing the immune system for ovarian cancer therapy. *Am J Reprod Immunol* 2008;59:62–74.
76. **Oei AL, Sweep FC, Thomas CM, Boerman OC, Massuger LF.** The use of monoclonal antibodies for the treatment of epithelial ovarian cancer (review). *Int J Oncol* 2008;32:1145–1157.
77. **Wu TC.** Therapeutic human papillomavirus DNA vaccination strategies to control cervical cancer. *Eur J Immunol* 2007;37:310–314.
78. **Epenetos AA, Shepherd J, Britton KE, Mather S, Taylor-Papadimitriou J, Granowska M, et al.** 123I radioiodinated antibody imaging of occult ovarian cancer. *Cancer* 1985;55:984–987.
79. **Epenetos AA, Hooker G, Krausz T, Snook D, Bodmer WF, Taylor-Papadimitriou J.** Antibody-guided irradiation of malignant ascites in ovarian cancer: a new therapeutic method possessing specificity against cancer cells. *Obstet Gynecol* 1986;68:71S–74S.
80. **Berek JS, Martinez-Maza O, Montz FJ.** The immune system and gynecologic cancer. In: **Coppelson MT, Morrow CP, eds.** *Gynecologic oncology.* Edinburgh: Churchill-Livingstone;1992: 119–151.
81. **Ortiz-Sanchez E, Helguera G, Daniels TR, Penichet ML.** Antibody-cytokine fusion proteins: applications in cancer therapy. *Expert Opin Biol Ther* 2008;8:609–632.
82. **Berek JS, Taylor PT, Gordon A, Cunningham MJ, Finkler N, Orr J Jr, et al.** Randomized, placebo-controlled study of *oregovomab* for consolidation of clinical remission in patients with advanced ovarian cancer. *J Clin Oncol* 2004;22:3507–3516.
83. **Berek JS, Taylor PT, Nicodemus CF.** CA125 velocity at relapse is a highly significant predictor of survival post relapse: results of a 5-year follow-up survey to a randomized placebo-controlled study of maintenance *oregovomab* immunotherapy in advanced ovarian cancer. *J Immunother* 2008;31:207–214.
84. **Schlebusch H, Wagner U, Grunn U, Schultes B.** A monoclonal anti-idiotypic antibody ACA125 mimicking the tumor-associated antigen CA125 for immunotherapy of ovarian cancer. *Hybridoma* 1995;14:167–174.
85. **Wagner U.** Antitumor antibodies for immunotherapy of ovarian carcinomas. *Hybridoma* 1993;12:521–528.
86. **Reinartz S, Köhler S, Schlebusch H, Krista K, Giffels P, Renke K, et al.** Vaccination of patients with advanced ovarian carcinoma with the anti-idiotype ACA125: immunological response and survival (phase Ib/II). *Clin Cancer Res* 2004;10:1580–1587.
87. **Wagner U, Köhler S, Reinartz S, et al.** Immunological consolidation of ovarian carcinoma recurrences with monoclonal anti-itiotype antibody ACA125: Immune responses and survival in palliative treatment. *Clin Cancer Res* 2001;7:1154–1162. Commentary by **Foon, K, Bhattacharya-Chatterjee, M.** Are solid tumor anti-idiotype vaccines ready for prime time? *Clin Cancer Res* 2001;7: 1112–1115.
88. **Sabbatini P, Dupont J, Aghajanian C, Derosa F, Poynor E, Anderson S, et al.** Phase I study of *abagovomab* in patients with epithelial ovarian, fallopian tube, or primary peritoneal cancer. *Clin Cancer Res* 2006;12:5503–5510.
89. **Rosenberg SA.** Immunotherapy of cancer by systemic administration of lymphoid cells plus interleukin-2. *J Biol Response Mod* 1984;3:501–511.
90. **Rosenberg SA, Lotze MT.** Cancer immunotherapy using interleukin-2 and interleukin-2-activated lymphocytes. *Annu Rev Immunol* 1986;4:681–709.

91. **Rosenberg SA, Lotze MT, Muul LM, Leitman S, Chang AE, Ettinghausen SE, et al.** Observations on the systemic administration of autologous lymphokine-activated killer cells and recombinant interleukin-2 to patients with metastatic cancer. *N Engl J Med* 1985;313:1485–1492.
92. **Lotzova E.** Role of human circulating and tumor-infiltrating lymphocytes in cancer defense and treatment. *Nat Immun Cell Growth Regul* 1990;9:253–264.
93. **Urba WJ, Clark JW, Steis RG, Bookman MA, Smith JW 2nd, Beckner S, et al.** Intraperitoneal lymphokine-activated killer cell/interleukin-2 therapy in patients with intra-abdominal cancer: immunologic considerations. *J Natl Cancer Inst* 1989;81:602–611.
94. **Steis RG, Urba WJ, VanderMolen LA, Bookman MA, Smith JW 2nd, Clark JW, et al.** Intraperitoneal lymphokine-activated killer-cell and interleukin-2 therapy for malignancies limited to the peritoneal cavity. *J Clin Oncol* 1990;8:1618–1629.
95. **Berek JS, Lichtenstein AK, Knox RM, Jung TS, Rose TP, Cantrell JL, et al.** Synergistic effects of combination sequential immunotherapies in a murine ovarian cancer model. *Cancer Res* 1985;45:4215–4218.
96. **West WH, Tauer KW, Yannelli JR, Marshall GD, Orr DW, Thurman GB, et al.** Constant-infusion recombinant interleukin-2 in adoptive immunotherapy of advanced cancer. *N Engl J Med* 1987;316:898–905.
97. **Topalian SL, Solomon D, Avis FP, Chang AE, Freerksen DL, Linehan WM, et al.** Immunotherapy of patients with advanced cancer using tumor-infiltrating lymphocytes and recombinant interleukin-2: a pilot study. *J Clin Oncol* 1988;6:839–853.
98. **Aoki Y, Takakuwa K, Kodama S, Tanaka K, Takahashi M, Tokunaga A, et al.** Use of adoptive transfer of tumor-infiltrating lymphocytes alone or in combination with *cisplatin*-containing chemotherapy in patients with epithelial ovarian cancer. *Cancer Res* 1991;51:1934–1939.
99. **Dudley ME, Wunderlich JR, Yang JC, Sherry RM, Topalian SL, Restifo NP, et al.** Adoptive cell transfer therapy following non-myeloablative but lymphodepleting chemotherapy for the treatment of patients with refractory metastatic melanoma. *J Clin Oncol* 2005;23:2346–2357.
100. **Gotlieb WH, Abrams JS, Watson JM, Velu TJ, Berek JS, Martinez-Maza O.** Presence of interleukin 10 (IL-10) in the ascites of patients with ovarian and other intra-abdominal cancers. *Cytokine* 1992;4:385–390.
101. **Odunsi K, Jungbluth AA, Stockert E, Qian F, Gnjatic S, Tammela J, et al.** NY-ESO-1 and LAGE-1 cancer-testis antigens are potential targets for immunotherapy in epithelial ovarian cancer. *Cancer Res* 2003;63:6076–6083.
102. **Odunsi K, Qian F, Matsuzaki J, Mhawech-Fauceglia P, Andrews C, Hoffman EW, et al.** Vaccination with an NY-ESO-1 peptide of HLA class I/II specificities induces integrated humoral and T cell responses in ovarian cancer. *Proc Natl Acad Sci U S A* 2007;104:12837–12842.
103. **Disis ML, Schiffman K, Guthrie K, Salazar LG, Knutson KL, Goodell V, et al.** Effect of dose on immune response in patients vaccinated with an HER-2/*neu* intracellular domain protein–based vaccine. *J Clin Oncol* 2004;22:1916–1925.
104. **Brulet JM, Maudoux F, Thomas S, Thielemans K, Burny A, Leo O, et al.** DNA vaccine encoding endosome-targeted human papillomavirus type 16 *E7* protein generates CD4+ T cell-dependent protection. *Eur J Immunol* 2007;37:376–384.
105. **Wu TC, Guarnieri FG, Staveley-O'Carroll KF, Viscidi RP, Levitsky HI, Hedrick L, et al.** Engineering an intracellular pathway for major histocompatibility complex class II presentation of antigens. *Proc Natl Acad Sci U S A* 1995;92:11671–11675.
106. **Ji H, Wang TL, Chen CH, Pai SI, Hung CF, Lin KY, et al.** Targeting human papillomavirus type 16 *E7* to the endosomal/lysosomal compartment enhances the antitumor immunity of DNA vaccines against murine human papillomavirus type 16 *E7*-expressing tumors. *Hum Gene Ther* 1999;10:2727–2740.
107. **Santin AD, Hermonat PL, Ravaggi A, Bellone S, Pecorelli S, Cannon MJ, et al.** *In vitro* induction of tumor-specific human lymphocyte antigen class I-restricted CD8 cytotoxic T lymphocytes by ovarian tumor antigen-pulsed autologous dendritic cells from patients with advanced ovarian cancer. *Am J Obstet Gynecol* 2000;183:601–609.

108. **Santin AD, Hermonat PL, Ravaggi A, Bellone S, Cowan C, Korourian S, et al.** Development, characterization and distribution of adoptively transferred peripheral blood lymphocytes primed by human papillomavirus 18 *E7*–pulsed autologous dendritic cells in a patient with metastatic adenocarcinoma of the uterine cervix. *Eur J Gynaecol Oncol* 2000;21:17–23.

109. **Zhao X, Wei YQ, Peng ZL.** Induction of T cell responses against autologous ovarian tumors with whole tumor cell lysate-pulsed dendritic cells. *Immunol Invest* 2001;30:33–45.

110. **Hernando JJ, Park TW, Kubler K, Offergeld R, Schlebusch H, Bauknecht T.** Vaccination with autologous tumour antigen-pulsed dendritic cells in advanced gynaecological malignancies: clinical and immunological evaluation of a phase I trial. *Cancer Immunol Immunother* 2002;51:45–52.

111. **Inaba K, Turley S, Yamaide F, Iyoda T, Mahnke K, Inaba M, et al.** Efficient presentation of phagocytosed cellular fragments on the major histocompatibility complex class II products of dendritic cells. *J Exp Med* 1998;188:2163–2173.

112. **Mackensen A, Herbst B, Chen JL, Kohler G, Noppen C, Herr W, et al.** Phase I study in melanoma patients of a vaccine with peptide-pulsed dendritic cells generated *in vitro* from CD34(+) hematopoietic progenitor cells. *Int J Cancer* 2000;86:385–392.

113. **Thurner B, Roder C, Dieckmann D, Heuer M, Kruse M, Glaser A, et al.** Generation of large numbers of fully mature and stable dendritic cells from leukapheresis products for clinical application. *J Immunol Methods* 1999;223:1–15.

114. **Thurner B, Haendle I, Roder C, Dieckmann D, Keikavoussi P, Jonuleit H, et al.** Vaccination with mage-3A1 peptide-pulsed mature, monocyte-derived dendritic cells expands specific cytotoxic T cells and induces regression of some metastases in advanced stage IV melanoma. *J Exp Med* 1999;190:1669–1678.

115. **Finn OJ.** Cancer vaccines: between the idea and the reality. *Nat Rev Immunol* 2003;3:630–641.

116. **Paul S, Acres B, Limacher JM, Bonnefoy JY.** Cancer vaccines: challenges and outlook in the field. *IDrugs* 2007;10:324–328.

117. **Tabi Z, Man S.** Challenges for cancer vaccine development. *Adv Drug Deliv Rev* 2006;58:902–915.

118. **Cannon MJ, O'Brien TJ, Underwood LJ, Crew MD, Bondurant KL, Santin AD.** Novel target antigens for dendritic cell-based immunotherapy against ovarian cancer. *Exp Rev Anticancer Ther* 2002;2:97–105.

119. **McIlroy D, Gregoire M.** Optimizing dendritic cell-based anticancer immunotherapy: maturation state does have clinical impact. *Cancer Immunol Immunother* 2003;52:583–591.

120. **McIlroy D, Tanguy-Royer S, Le Meur N, Guisle I, Royer PJ, Leger J, et al.** Profiling dendritic cell maturation with dedicated microarrays. *J Leukoc Biol* 2005;78:794–803.

121. **Berek JS, Knapp RC, Hacker NF, Lichtenstein A, Jung T, Spina C, et al.** Intraperitoneal immunotherapy of epithelial ovarian carcinoma with *Corynebacterium parvum*. *Am J Obstet Gynecol* 1985;152:1003–1010.

122. **Lichtenstein A, Berek J, Bast R, Spina C, Hacker N, Knapp RC, et al.** Activation of peritoneal lymphocyte cytotoxicity in patients with ovarian cancer by intraperitoneal treatment with *Corynebacterium parvum*. *J Biol Response Mod* 1984;3:371–378.

123. **Bast RC Jr, Berek JS, Obrist R, Griffiths CT, Berkowitz RS, Hacker NF, et al.** Intraperitoneal immunotherapy of human ovarian carcinoma with *Corynebacterium parvum*. *Cancer Res* 1983;43:1395–1401.

124. **Mantovani A, Sessa C, Peri G, Allavena P, Introna M, Polentarutti N, et al.** Intraperitoneal administration of *Corynebacterium parvum* in patients with ascitic ovarian tumors resistant to chemotherapy: effects on cytotoxicity of tumor-associated macrophages and NK cells. *Int J Cancer* 1981;27:437–446.

125. **Gusdon JP Jr, Homesley HD, Jobson VW, Muss HB.** Treatment of advanced ovarian malignancy with chemoimmunotherapy using autologous tumor and *Corynebacterium parvum*. *Obstet Gynecol* 1983;62:728–735.

126. **Howell SB, Kirmani S, Lucas WE, Zimm S, Goel R, Kim S, et al.** A phase II trial of intraperitoneal *cisplatin* and *etoposide* for primary treatment of ovarian epithelial cancer. *J Clin Oncol* 1990;8:137–145.

127. **Hurteau JA, Blessing JA, DeCesare SL, Creasman WT.** Evaluation of recombinant human interleukin-12 in patients with recurrent or refractory ovarian cancer: a gynecologic oncology group study. *Gynecol Oncol* 2001;82:7–10.

128. **Lenzi R, Rosenblum M, Verschraegen C, Kudelka AP, Kavanagh JJ, Hicks ME, et al.** Phase I study of intraperitoneal recombinant human interleukin 12 in patients with Müllerian carcinoma, gastrointestinal primary malignancies, and mesothelioma. *Clin Cancer Res* 2002;8:3686–3695.

129. **Recchia F, Saggio G, Cesta A, Candeloro G, Nuzzo A, Lombardo M, et al.** Interleukin-2 and 13-cis retinoic acid as maintenance therapy in advanced ovarian cancer. *Int J Oncol* 2005;27:1039–1046.

130. **Woo EY, Chu CS, Goletz TJ, Schlienger K, Yeh H, Coukos G, et al.** Regulatory CD4(+)CD25(+) T cells in tumors from patients with early-stage non-small cell lung cancer and late-stage ovarian cancer. *Cancer Res* 2001;61:4766–4772.

131. **Curiel TJ, Coukos G, Zou L, Alvarez X, Cheng P, Mottram P, et al.** Specific recruitment of regulatory T cells in ovarian carcinoma fosters immune privilege and predicts reduced survival. *Nat Med* 2004;10:942–949.

132. **Powell DJ Jr, Felipe-Silva A, Merino MJ, Ahmadzadeh M, Allen T, Levy C, et al.** Administration of a CD25-directed immunotoxin, LMB-2, to patients with metastatic melanoma induces a selective partial reduction in regulatory T cells *in vivo*. *J Immunol* 2007;179:4919–4928.

133. **Kryczek I, Wei S, Zou L, Altuwaijri S, Szeliga W, Kolls J, et al.** Cutting edge: TH17 and regulatory T cell dynamics and the regulation by IL-2 in the tumor microenvironment. *J Immunol* 2007;178:6730–6733.

3

Chemotherapy

Maurie Markman

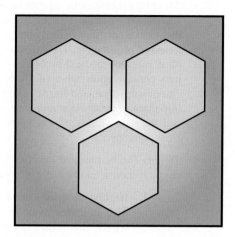

General Principles

Tumor Growth and Chemotherapy

A wide variety of chemotherapeutic agents is available, and the selection and dose of drugs is determined by the relative benefits of individual agents, as well as combinations, based on the results of phase II and phase III trials. Most antineoplastic agents have a narrow therapeutic index, and the choice of treatment is based on several factors, including age, performance status, comorbidities, organ function, tumor type, and whether or not a patient has had previous chemotherapy (Table 3.1).

Table 3.1 Issues to Be Considered before Using Antineoplastic Drugs
1. Natural History of the Particular Malignancy
a. Diagnosis of a malignancy made by biopsy
b. Rate of disease progression
c. Extent of disease spread
2. Patient's Circumstances and Tolerance
a. Age, general health, underlying diseases
b. Extent of previous treatment
c. Adequate facilities to evaluate, monitor, and treat potential drug toxicities
d. The patient's emotional, social, and financial situation
3. Likelihood of Achieving a Beneficial Response
a. Cancers in which chemotherapy is curative in some patients (e.g., ovarian germ cell tumors)
b. Cancers in which chemotherapy has demonstrated improvement in survival (e.g., epithelial ovarian cancer)
c. Cancers that respond to treatment but in which improved survival has not been clearly demonstrated (e.g., metastatic cervical cancer)
d. Cancers with marginal or no response to chemotherapy (e.g., melanoma)

It is important to have a good understanding of the likely natural history of each patient's malignancy. This may influence decisions regarding when to initiate treatment, particularly when chemotherapy is being administered with palliative intent, and it also may be appropriate to withhold chemotherapy in asymptomatic patients with indolent metastatic disease. **Chemotherapy should be restricted to patients in whom the diagnosis of cancer has been confirmed by either biopsy or cytology.**

All chemotherapeutic agents have potential side effects, and it is important to ascertain whether the patient has measurable disease or elevated tumor markers before commencing treatment, particularly in patients with metastatic disease, so that response can be assessed objectively. The extent of previous therapy and the patient's age, general health, and other relevant medical problems (e.g., neuropathy from long-standing diabetes) are all taken into consideration when deciding on the choice of treatment. In addition, the patient's emotional, social, and financial status must be respected and taken into consideration. It is also important to clearly communicate the aims and objectives of therapy, the likelihood of benefit, and the side effects of treatment so the patient can make an informed decision regarding chemotherapy.

Tumors can be grouped into the following four categories by their likelihood of chemotherapeutic response and benefit from treatment:

1. **Highly chemosensitive tumors—treatment administered with curative intent. This includes ovarian germ cell tumors and gestational trophoblastic tumors where chemotherapy is curative for most patients.** Toxicity is acceptable if the probability of cure is high, but every effort must be made to limit toxicity and reduce side effects without compromising the chance of cure such as by inappropriate dose reductions or prolonged delay between cycles.

2. **Chemosensitive, but cure is uncommon. This includes advanced epithelial ovarian cancer, where response rates are in excess of 70% to 89%, but most patients will eventually relapse. Chemotherapy improves survival but does not restore a normal life expectancy in the majority of patients.** Individuals with these tumors usually benefit from chemotherapy, and it should be offered unless there are exceptional circumstances.

3. **In the third group (e.g., uterine leiomyosarcoma), responses to chemotherapy are relatively low, and the impact of treatment on overall survival is unclear.** In this setting, it is not unreasonable to consider a patient's overall medical condition in the determination of the relative risks versus benefits of cytotoxic drug therapy.

4. **Relatively chemoresistant tumors (e.g., metastatic melanoma) where responses to chemotherapy are low and very unpredictable.** If treatment is considered, every effort should be made to include these patients in well-designed, prospective clinical trials testing new treatment approaches.

Differential Sensitivity

Chemotherapeutic agents must have greater activity against tumors than against normal tissues. The therapeutic window between antitumor effect and normal tissue toxicity may be small because most chemotherapeutic agents work by disrupting DNA or RNA synthesis, affecting crucial cellular enzymes, or altering protein synthesis.

Normal cells also use these vital cellular processes in ways similar to those of malignant cells, particularly fetal or regenerating tissue or normal cell populations in which constant cell proliferation is required (e.g., bone marrow, gastrointestinal epithelium, and hair follicles). As a result, the differential effect of antineoplastic drugs on tumors compared with normal tissues is quantitative rather than qualitative, and some degree of injury to normal tissue is produced by every chemotherapeutic agent. The normal tissue toxicity produced by most chemotherapeutic agents correlates with the intrinsic cellular proliferation of the target tissue. Hence, blood count suppression, mucosal injury, and alopecia are commonly seen with most chemotherapeutic regimens.

Therapeutic Index

For any particular chemotherapeutic agent, the net effect on the patient is often referred to as the drug's *therapeutic index* **(i.e., a ratio of the doses at which therapeutic effect and toxicity occur).** Cancer chemotherapy requires a balance of therapeutic effect and toxicity to optimize the therapeutic index. Because the window of toxicity is often narrow for available chemotherapeutic agents, successful chemotherapy depends on pharmacologic and biologic factors.

Biologic Factors Influencing Treatment

Cell Kinetic Concepts

Both normal and tumorous tissues have a certain growth capacity and are influenced and regulated by various internal and external forces. The differential growth and regulatory influences occurring in both normal and tumorous tissues form the basis of effective cancer treatment. The exploitation of these differences forms the basis for the effective use of both radiation and chemotherapy in cancer management.

Patterns of Normal Growth

All normal tissues have the capacity for cellular division and growth. However, normal tissues grow in substantially different patterns. There are three general types of normal tissue growth: static, expanding, and renewing.

1. The **static** population comprises relatively well-differentiated cells that, after initial proliferative activity in the embryonic and neonatal period, rarely undergo cell division. Typical examples are striated muscle and neurons.

2. The **expanding** population of cells is characterized by the capacity to proliferate under special stimuli (e.g., tissue injury). Under those circumstances, the normally quiescent tissue (e.g., liver or kidney) undergoes a surge of proliferation with regrowth.

3. The **renewing** population of cells is constantly in a proliferative state. There is constant cell division, a high degree of cell turnover, and constant cell loss. This occurs in bone marrow, epidermis, and gastrointestinal mucosa.

Normal tissues with a static pattern of growth are rarely seriously injured by drug therapy, whereas renewing cell populations such as bone marrow, gastrointestinal mucosa, and spermatozoa are commonly injured.

Cancer Cell Growth

Tumor cell growth represents a disruption in the normal cellular brake mechanisms, resulting in continued proliferation and eventual death of the host. It is not the speed of cell proliferation but the failure of the regulated balance between cell loss and cell proliferation that differentiates malignant cells from normal cells.

Gompertzian Growth

The characteristics of cancer growth have been assessed by multiple studies in animals and more limited studies in humans. When tumors are extremely small, growth follows an exponential pattern but later seems to slow. Such a growth pattern is known as **Gompertzian growth**. Strictly speaking, this means exponential growth with exponential growth retardation over the entire duration of tumor growth. More simply, **Gompertzian growth means that, as a tumor mass increases in size, the time required to double the tumor's volume also increases.**

Doubling Time

The doubling time of a human tumor is the time it takes for the mass to double its size. There is considerable variation in doubling times of human tumors. For example, embryonal tumors, lymphomas, and some malignant mesenchymal tumors have relatively fast doubling times (20 to 40 days), whereas adenocarcinomas and squamous cell carcinomas have relatively slow doubling times (50 to 150 days). **In general, metastases have faster doubling times than primary tumors.**

If it is assumed that exponential growth occurs early in a tumor's history and that a tumor starts from a single malignant stem cell, then

1. a 1-mm mass will have undergone approximately 20 tumor doublings

2. a 5-mm mass (a size that might be first visualized on a radiograph) will have undergone 27 doublings

3. a 1-cm mass will have undergone 30 doublings

Were such a lesion discovered clinically, the physician would assume that the tumor had been detected early. The reality is that it would have already undergone 30 doublings or been present approximately 60% of its life span.

Unfortunately, our current diagnostic methods detect tumors only relatively late in their growth, and metastases may well have occurred long before there is obvious evidence of the primary lesion. The second implication of tumor kinetics is that, in late stages of tumor growth, a very few doublings in tumor mass have a dramatic impact on the size of the tumor. Once a tumor becomes palpable (1 cm in diameter), only three more doublings would produce an enormous tumor mass (8 cm in diameter).

Cell Cycle

Information on growth patterns and doubling times relates to the growth of the tumor mass as a whole. The kinetic behavior of individual tumor cells has been well described, and a classic cell cycle model has been produced (Fig. 3.1).

1. **M phase (mitotic phase)** of the cell cycle is the phase of cell division.
2. **G_1 phase (postmitotic phase)** is a period of variable duration when cellular activities and protein and RNA synthesis continue. These G_1 cells can differentiate or continue in the proliferative cycle.
3. **S phase (DNA synthetic phase)** is the period in which new DNA replication occurs.
4. **G_2 phase (postsynthetic phase)** is the period in which the cell has a diploid number of chromosomes and twice the DNA content of the normal cell. The cell remains in this phase for a relatively short time and then enters the mitotic phase again.
5. **G_0 phase (the resting phase)** is the time during which cells do not divide. Cells may move in and out of the G_0 phase.

The generation time is the duration of the cycle from M phase to M phase. Variation occurs in all phases of the cell cycle, but the variation is greatest during the G_1 period. The reasons for this variation are complex and not completely understood.

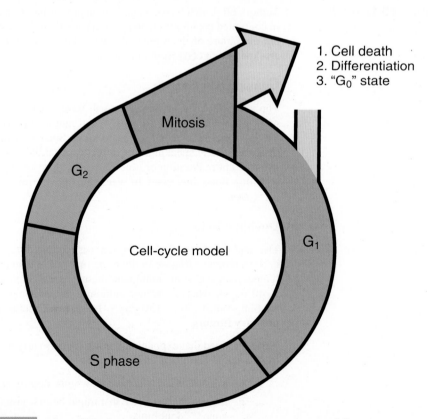

Figure 3.1   **The cell cycle.** After cell division, a cell can (1) die, (2) differentiate, or (3) enter resting (G_0) phase. Cells in the latter two phases can reenter the cycle at G_1.

These cell cycle events have important implications for the cancer therapist. Differential sensitivities to chemotherapy and radiation therapy are associated with different proliferative states. **Dividing cancer cells that are actively traversing the cell cycle are very sensitive to chemotherapeutic agents.** Cells in a resting state (G_0) are relatively insensitive to chemotherapeutic agents, although they occupy space and contribute to the bulk of the tumor.

Cell Kinetics

In cell kinetic studies performed on human tumors, the duration of the S phase (DNA synthesis phase) is relatively similar for most human tumors, ranging from a low of 10 hours to a high of approximately 31 hours. The length of the cell cycle in human tumors varies from slightly more than half a day to perhaps 5 days. **With cell cycle times in the range of 24 hours and doubling times in the range of 10 to 1,000 days, it is clear that only a small proportion of tumor cells are in active cell division at any one time.**

Two major factors that affect the rate at which tumors grow are the **growth fraction** and **cell death. The growth fraction is the number of cells in the tumor mass that are actively undergoing cell division.** There is a marked variation in the growth fraction of tumors in human beings, ranging from 25% to almost 95%. In the past, it was thought that human tumors contained billions of cells, all growing slowly. In actuality, only a small fraction of cells in a tumor mass are rapidly proliferating; the remainder are out of the cell cycle and quiescent. **Cancer "stem cells" are a very small population of cells that appear to be relatively chemoresistant; these play a major role in the development and progression of cancers.**

Tumor growth may be altered by the following:

1. **cytotoxic chemotherapy,** which alters both the generation time and the growth fraction of a tumor
2. **hormones,** which appear to alter the growth fraction without changing the generation time
3. **radiation therapy,** which alters both the generation time and the growth fraction
4. **alterations in oxygen tension and vascular supply,** which alter the growth fraction without altering generation time
5. **immunologic therapies,** which seem to alter both generation time and growth fraction

Cell Cycle–Specific versus Cell Cycle–Nonspecific Drugs

Antineoplastic agents have complex mechanisms of action and alter cells in a wide variety of ways. Different drugs have different sites of action in the cell cycle, and their effectiveness is also a function of the proliferative capacity of the tissue involved. With the use of some of these kinetic concepts, it is possible to classify chemotherapeutic agents on the basis of their cell cycle specificity and their site of maximal drug action within the cell cycle (Table 3.2).

Cell Cycle–Nonspecific   Cell cycle–nonspecific agents kill in all phases of the cell cycle and are not too dependent on proliferative activity.

Cell Cycle–Specific   Cell cycle–specific agents, such as *hydroxyurea*, depend on the proliferative activity and on the phase of the cell cycle for their action. The agents kill in only one

Table 3.2 Cell Cycle Specificity of Chemotherapeutic Agents	
Classification	**Examples**
Cell cycle–specific, proliferation dependent	*hydroxyurea, cytosine arabinoside*
Cell cycle–specific, less proliferation dependent	*5-fluorouracil, methotrexate*
Cell cycle–nonspecific, proliferation dependent	*cyclophosphamide, actinomycin D, carboplatin, cisplatin*
Cell cycle–nonspecific, less proliferation dependent	*paclitaxel, topotecan*

Table 3.3 Site of Action in the Cell Cycle	
Portion of Cell Cycle	*Drugs*
G$_1$	*actinomycin D*
Early S	*hydroxyurea, cytosine arabinoside, 5-fluorouracil, methotrexate*
Late S	*doxorubicin*
G$_2$	*bleomycin, etoposide, teniposide, carboplatin, cisplatin, topotecan*, radiation
M	*paclitaxel, vincristine, vinblastine*

phase of the cell cycle, and cells not in that phase are not injured. They tend to be most effective against tumors with relatively long S phases and against those tumors in which there is a relatively high growth fraction and a rapid rate of proliferation. Between these two broad classifications, there is a spectrum of drugs with variable degrees of cell cycle and proliferation dependence.

In addition to cell cycle and proliferative sensitivity, chemotherapeutic agents may exert a greater effect in a particular phase of the cell cycle. Thus, chemotherapeutic agents can be grouped according to their site of action in the cell cycle and the extent of their dependence on proliferative activity (Table 3.3).

Log Kill Hypothesis

From knowledge of basic cellular kinetics, there have emerged certain concepts of chemotherapy that have proven useful in the design of chemotherapeutic regimens. In experimental tumor systems in animals, survival of the animal is inversely proportional to the number of cells implanted or to the size of the tumor at the time treatment is initiated (1). Treatment immediately after tumor implantation or when the tumor is subclinical in size results in more cures than when the tumor is clinically obvious and large.

Chemotherapeutic agents appear to work by first-order kinetics; that is, they kill a constant fraction of cells rather than a constant number. This concept has important conceptual implications in cancer treatment. For instance, a single exposure of tumor cells to an antineoplastic drug might be capable of producing 2- to 5-logs of cell kill. With typical body tumor burdens of 10^{12} cells (1 kg), a single dose of chemotherapy is unlikely to be curative. This explains the need for intermittent courses of chemotherapy to achieve the magnitude of cell kill necessary to produce tumor regression and cure. It also provides a rationale for multiple-drug or combination chemotherapy.

The cure rate would be significantly improved if small tumors were present, but cell masses of 10^1 to 10^4 cells are too small for clinical detection. **This is the basis for using adjuvant chemotherapy in early stages of disease** when subclinical metastases are likely to be present in many patients.

Drug Resistance and Tumor Cell Heterogeneity

Chemotherapeutic agents often are active when initially used in cancer treatment, but tumors commonly become resistant during chemotherapy. Hence, patients often have an initial remission followed by a recurrence that is no longer responsive to the drugs that were initially effective.

Various cellular mechanisms are involved in drug resistance. Resistant tumor cells may display increased deactivation or decreased activation of drugs, allow increased drug efflux, or resist normal drug uptake. In some instances, altered specificity to an inhibiting enzyme or increased production of the target enzyme occurs to explain drug resistance on a pharmacologic basis.

Theories for Overcoming Drug Resistance

It has been suggested that spontaneous mutation to phenotypic drug resistance occurs in rapidly growing malignant tumors: This is the somatic mutation theory (2). **The theory suggests that most mammalian cells start with intrinsic sensitivity to antineoplastic drugs but develop spontaneous resistance at variable rates.** This concept—the Goldie-Coldman hypothesis—has been applied to the growth of malignant tumors and has important clinical implications.

Goldie and Coldman developed a mathematical model that relates curability to the time of appearance of singly or doubly resistant cells. Assuming a natural mutation rate, the model predicts a variation in size of the resistant fraction in tumors of the same size and type, depending on the mutation rate and the point at which the first mutation develops. Given such assumptions, **the proportion of resistant cells in any untreated tumor is likely to be small,** and the initial response to treatment would not be influenced by the number of resistant cells. In clinical practice, this means that **a complete remission could be obtained even if resistant cells were present.** The failure to cure such a patient, however, would be directly dependent on the presence of resistant cells.

This model of spontaneous drug resistance implies that:

1. Tumors are curable with chemotherapy if no permanently resistant cells are present and if chemotherapy is begun before resistance develops.

2. If only one antineoplastic agent is used, then the probability of cure diminishes rapidly with the development of a single resistant line.

3. Minimizing the emergence of drug-resistant clones requires multiple effective drugs and that they be applied as early as possible in the course of the patient's disease.

4. The rate of spontaneous mutation to resistance occurs at approximately the natural frequency of 1 in 10,000 to 1 in 1,000,000 cell divisions.

This model predicts that alternating cycles of treatment should be superior to the sequential use of particular agents because sequential use of antineoplastic drugs would allow for the development and regrowth of a doubly resistant line. The intrinsic frequency of spontaneous mutation to drug resistance is also likely to be influenced by etiological factors responsible for tumor development. Lung or bladder cancers, for instance, result from exposure to multiple carcinogenic chemicals and may have a higher spontaneous mutation rate than is seen in other tumors. Under these circumstances, numerous drug-resistant clones may be present even before the tumors are clinically evident. This would explain the inability of antineoplastic therapy to cure a number of the common malignancies.

An alternative hypothesis, developed by Norton and Simon, focuses on the Gompertzian growth rates exhibited by malignant tumors (3,4). This mathematical model suggests that the efficacy of treatment of tumors exhibiting sensitivity to particular chemotherapeutic agents will be enhanced if single agents, or combination regimens, are delivered at their optimal dose levels in a so-called dose-dense manner rather than as alternating regimens.

The fundamental difference between the Norton-Simon and Goldie-Coldman models is that in the former approach, the individual drugs are given in sequence at their optimal levels to produce a cytotoxic effect, whereas in the later strategy, which focuses on the rapid administration of as many active agents as possible, dose levels of individual drugs will frequently need to be modified because of overlapping toxic effects (e.g., bone marrow suppression).

Randomized trials in breast cancer have provided important evidence in support of the Norton-Simon hypothesis, with novel strategies being designed to deliver active drugs in the dose-dense manner. High-risk gestational trophoblastic tumors are very chemosensitive, and treatment with EMA-CO every 6 to 7 days is an example of a dose-dense regimen.

Pleiotropic Drug Resistance

If the failure of drug treatment depends on the spontaneous appearance of resistant cells, an understanding of drug resistance is crucial to therapeutic success. A wide variety of mechanisms for drug resistance has been described, although these mechanisms usually confer resistance to a particular drug or drug family. **The phenomenon of pleiotropic drug resistance occurs when certain drug-resistance mechanisms confer crossresistance to structurally dissimilar drugs with different mechanisms of action** (5).

Some pleiotropic resistant cells contain a cell surface P glycoprotein with a molecular weight of 170 kilodaltons. In general, the appearance of pleiotropic drug resistance is associated with the cell's impaired ability to accumulate and retain antineoplastic drugs. It has been further demonstrated that this P glycoprotein is directly related to the expression of resistance, and cells that revert to sensitive ones lose this membrane glycoprotein.

Dose Intensity and High-Dose Chemotherapy

Studies in human solid tumors *in vitro* frequently demonstrate steep dose-response curves, suggesting the importance of full drug dosage.

Although retrospective data suggested that dose intensity may be important, **several prospective randomized trials in epithelial ovarian cancer have failed to demonstrate an improved outcome by either increasing the dose of *cisplatin* or *carboplatin* per cycle or extending the duration of treatment beyond 5 to 6 cycles** (6–8). In addition, two recent randomized studies of high-dose chemotherapy (with bone marrow or peripheral progenitor stem cell support) for advanced ovarian cancer failed to demonstrate superior survival compared to standard dose regimens (9,10).

Although evidence does not suggest dose-intensive approaches improve outcome, there is certainly a minimum dose below which survival will be compromised. Unfortunately, this dose is difficult to determine. **In general, the goal should be to maintain dose intensity consistent with an acceptable toxicity profile in each individual patient.** The severity of neutropenia can frequently be reduced through the administration of a bone marrow stimulatory agent (e.g., granulocyte colony stimulating factor). These drugs can be either administered at the time of documented severe bone marrow suppression or given prophylactically with chemotherapeutic regimens known to have a high risk of grade 3 or 4 myelosuppression.

Even though **a commercially available agent has been shown to increase platelet counts** and decrease the need for platelet transfusions, its role in the treatment of gynecologic cancers remains to be defined.

Pharmacologic Factors Influencing Treatment

Pharmacologically, it is useful to describe effective chemotherapy as concentration over time of the active agent or its metabolite at the primary site of antitumor action. Although it is not possible to determine exact pericellular pharmacokinetics, substantial information on important pharmacokinetic factors is available (11).

$$\textbf{Drug effect} = \textbf{Drug concentration} \times \textbf{Duration of exposure} = \textbf{C} \times \textbf{T}$$

Because direct measurements often are not possible, considerable focus is given to plasma concentration $\times$ time (C $\times$ T) analyses. Many important factors influence this pharmacokinetic result, including route of administration and drug absorption, transportation, distribution, biotransformation, inactivation, excretion, and interactions with other drugs.

Route of Administration and Absorption

Traditionally, drugs have been given orally, intravenously, or intramuscularly. Over the past decade, considerable attention has been given to the **regional** administration of chemotherapeutic agents, particularly in ovarian cancer (12–15). **The intraperitoneal approach is based on the concept that the peritoneal clearance of the agent is slower than its plasma clearance** and, as a result, an increased concentration of the drug in the peritoneal cavity is maintained while plasma concentrations are low.

Studies of a wide variety of chemotherapeutic agents have demonstrated a differential concentration of 30- to 1,000-fold, depending on the molecular weight, charge, and lipid solubility of the particular drug. Clinical trials in ovarian cancer have been performed with *cisplatin, carboplatin, paclitaxel,* and drug combinations (12). A number of reports have noted that approximately 30% of patients with ovarian cancer who have small volume residual disease after initial systemic platinum-based chemotherapy can achieve a surgically defined complete response following second-line treatment with intraperitoneal *cisplatin.*

Several randomized trials have now revealed that the intraperitoneal administration of *cisplatin* as primary therapy of small volume advanced ovarian cancer (largest tumor nodule within the peritoneal cavity ≤ 1 cm in maximal diameter) **results in an improvement in both the time to subsequent disease progression and overall survival compared with intravenous delivery of this agent, but toxicity may be increased** (13–15). It is anticipated that ongoing research with intraperitoneal therapy will define strategies that will reduce the side effects associated with regional drug delivery (16).

Drug Distribution

Antineoplastic agents usually produce their antitumor effect by interacting with intracellular target molecules. As a result, it is critically important that a particular drug or active metabolite be able to arrive at the cancer cell in sufficient concentration for lethal effect. After absorption, drugs may be bound to serum albumin or other blood components; their ability to penetrate various body compartments, vascular spaces, and extracellular sites is highly influenced by plasma protein binding, relative ionization at physiologic pH, molecular size, and lipid solubility.

Sanctuary Sites Unique circumstances may produce sanctuary sites, which are areas where the tumor is inaccessible to anticancer drugs and the drug concentration over time is insufficient for cell kill. Examples of such sanctuary sites include the cerebrospinal fluid and areas of large tumor masses with central tumor necrosis and low oxygen tension.

Cell Penetration Although some drugs enter the target cell by simple diffusion, in some instances cellular penetration is an active process. As an example, many of the *alkylating agents* depend on a carrier transport system for cellular penetration. For large macromolecules, it may be necessary for pinocytosis to accomplish cellular entry.

Drug Metabolism

Many antineoplastic agents are active as intact molecules, but some require metabolism to an active form. Many of the antimetabolites require phosphorylation for cell entry. The alkylating agent *cyclophosphamide* requires absorption and liver metabolism to be activated. Attention to these unique metabolic requirements is needed for appropriate drug selection. For example, if direct installation of an alkylating agent is required, an agent that is active as an intact drug should be selected (e.g., *Thiotepa* or *nitrogen mustard*), rather than *cyclophosphamide,* because the latter drug requires hepatic biotransformation and would not be active locally. Not only is initial activation important but also the rate of metabolic degradation of the active drug or metabolite is important in determining antitumor activity. As an example, a major mechanism of drug resistance in ovarian cancer is increased metabolism of *alkylating agents* because of increased intracellular enzymes (e.g., glutathione-S-transferase).

Excretion

Most chemotherapeutic agents are excreted through the kidney or liver. Because overall kidney or liver function is critical to normal drug excretion, it is necessary to modify the dosage of certain agents when either of these organs is functionally impaired.

Certain drugs (e.g., *vincristine, doxorubicin, paclitaxel*) are excreted primarily through the liver, and others (e.g., *methotrexate*) are excreted almost entirely by the kidney. Most experimental protocols and cooperative group trials contain formulas for dose modification for specific organ impairments that influence drug excretion.

Drug Interactions

There are multiple opportunities for clinically important drug interactions to occur during cancer treatment. These interactions may increase or decrease the antitumor activity of a particular agent, or they may increase or modify its toxicity. Types of drug interaction of potential importance include those listed in Table 3.4.

Important drug interactions with antineoplastic drugs include the following.

1. The *alkylating agents* are highly reactive compounds and may produce direct chemical or physical inactivation when multiple drugs are mixed.

2. Intestinal absorption of certain chemotherapeutic agents is altered by antibiotics that suppress bowel flora (e.g., reduced absorption of oral *methotrexate*), resulting in its decreased circulating level.

3. Drugs such as *cisplatin* or *methotrexate* bind to albumin or plasma proteins and may be displaced from that binding by drugs that bind to similar sites, such as *aspirin*

				Bioavailable
Effect	**Caused by**	**Interaction**	**Resulting in**	**Drug**
↓ **Renal function/excretion**	nephrotoxic antibiotics	*methotrexate; cisplatin*	↓ Excretion	↑
↓ **Hepatic metabolism/biliary excretion**	*vincristine*	*doxorubicin*	↓ Excretion	↑
↑ **Displacement from albumin or plasma proteins**	sulfonamides; salicylates	*methotrexate; cisplatin*	↓ Binding	↑
↑ **Intestinal absorption**	*neomycin*	*methotrexate*	↓ Absorption	↓
↑ **Direct chemical interaction**	*mannitol*	*cisplatin*	↑ Excretion	↓
↑ **Direct effect on metabolism**	*phenobarbitol* *methotrexate* *5-fluorouracil*	*cyclophosphamide* *5-fluorouracil* *methotrexate*	↑ Metabolism ↑ Activation ↓ Metabolism	↑ ↓

Table 3.4 Drug Interactions in Cancer Chemotherapy

or *sulfa,* thereby increasing the circulating level of bioavailable *cisplatin* or *methotrexate.*

4. Alterations in drug activation may occur, as when *methotrexate* increases *5-fluorouracil* activation; conversely, drug interaction may antagonize antitumor effect, as when *5-fluorouracil* impairs the antifolate action of *methotrexate.*

5. Nephrotoxic antibiotics frequently alter *methotrexate* excretion and may increase the renal toxicity of *cisplatin.*

Principles of Combination Chemotherapy

Combination chemotherapy has become the standard approach to the management of many adult solid tumors, including breast cancer and female pelvic malignancies. The enthusiasm for combinations results from several significant limitations inherent in single-agent chemotherapy. In addition, **there is a solid theoretic basis for combination chemotherapy from a knowledge of cellular kinetics, drug metabolism, drug resistance, and tumor heterogeneity.**

Limitations of Single-Drug Therapy

The major limitations of single-agent chemotherapy are the following.

1. Toxicity limits the dose and duration of drug administration and thus restricts the tumor cell kill achievable.

2. Adaptive mechanisms allow cell survival and eventual regrowth of resistant tumor cells in spite of lethal effects produced in the bulk of the tumor.

3. Drug resistance may spontaneously develop.

4. Multidrug or pleiotropic drug resistance may develop.

Several different mechanisms of resistance are seen with antineoplastic agents, and some of these are listed in Table 3.5. Most problems inherent in single-drug therapy cannot be corrected by simply altering the dose or schedule of that single drug. As a result, increasing use has been made of multidrug combination chemotherapy.

Combination Chemotherapy Mechanisms

Different chemotherapeutic agents may act in different phases of the tumor cell cycle. Use of multiple drugs with different cellular kinetic characteristics reduces the tumor mass more completely than any individual chemotherapeutic agent while minimizing the impact of single-drug resistance. For instance, if a cell cycle–nonspecific agent is administered, producing a 2-log cell kill in a tumor mass with 10^9 cells, and no further therapy is given, then a minor tumor response will occur, followed by tumor regrowth and no impact on survival. If a cell cycle–specific agent produces a similar degree of cell kill, only the cells coming into cell cycle

Table 3.5 Mechanisms of Resistance to Anticancer Drugs	
Mechanism	*Example Drug*
Insufficient activation of drug	*intraperitoneal cyclophosphamide, 5-fluorouracil*
Insufficient drug intake or defective drug transport	*methotrexate, daunomycin, paclitaxel*
Increased activation	*cytosine arabinoside*
Increased utilization of an alternative biochemical pathway (salvage)	*cytosine arabinoside, 5-fluorouracil*
Increased concentration of the target enzyme	*methotrexate*
Rapid DNA repair of a drug-related lesion	*alkylating agents, cisplatin, carboplatin*
Gene amplification	*methotrexate*
Altered enzyme expression	*topotecan*

will be affected by such an agent. Simply by using combinations or sequences of cell cycle–specific and –nonspecific agents, log kill can be enhanced in tumors. With identification of appropriate combinations and proper sequencing, sufficient log kill may be achieved to produce a cure.

Drug Resistance

Combination chemotherapy can help to circumvent spontaneous mutations to drug resistance. After initial cell kill, the residual tumor may contain drug-resistant cells. **The probability of the emergence of drug-resistant cells in any given population is reduced if two or more agents with different mechanisms of action can be used in a tightly sequenced treatment scheme.**

Drug Interaction

Drug interactions may be additive, synergistic, or antagonistic. Combinations that result in improved therapy because of increased antitumor activity or decreased toxicity are said to be **synergistic. Additive** therapies produce enhanced antitumor activity equivalent to the sum of both agents acting singly. Finally, antitumor agents may actually **antagonize** the effect of each other, producing a lesser therapeutic effect than when used singly. For example, *5-fluorouracil* prevents the antifolate action of *methotrexate* when used before *methotrexate* administration.

Schedule Dependency

In some instances, the same drugs used in different sequences may produce a widely varied effect, suggesting the importance of schedule dependency. An example is the reduced cardiac toxicity demonstrated for weekly low-dose *doxorubicin* compared with high-dose bolus *doxorubicin*. Although schedule dependency has been an important, well-documented phenomenon in experimental tumors, its importance is less well defined for human cancer chemotherapy.

The general principles that allowed the development of successful combinations are shown in Table 3.6. Although these cannot be used in every regimen and some overlap in toxicities is common, these concepts are a central feature of most of the regimens now being used successfully in cancer treatment.

Remission

Once a treatment regimen has been selected, it is necessary to have some standardized way to evaluate the response to drug treatment. The terms *complete remission* (or *response*) and *partial remission* (or *response*) are used frequently and provide a convenient way to describe responses and compare various published regimens.

Complete Remission (Response)   **Complete remission (response) is the complete disappearance of all objective evidence of tumor as well as the resolution of all signs and symptoms referable to the tumor.** Complete regressions of cancer are those associated in general with significant prolongation of survival.

Partial Remission (Response)   **A partial remission (response) has been variously defined as a 30% to 50% reduction in the size of all measurable lesions along with some degree of**

Table 3.6 Important Factors in the Design of Drug Combinations
1. The drugs used must be active as single agents against the particular tumor.
2. The drugs should have different mechanisms of action to minimize emergence of drug resistance.
3. The drugs should have a biochemical basis of additive and preferably synergistic effects.
4. The drugs chosen should have a different spectrum of toxicity so they can be used for maximum cell kill at (or near) full doses.
5. The drugs chosen should be administered intermittently so that cell kill is enhanced and prolonged immunosuppression is minimized.

subjective improvement and the absence of any new lesions during therapy. Partial remissions translate in general into improved well-being for the patient but only occasionally are associated with longer overall survival.

Finally, various terms indicate lesser responses, such as objective response or minor response, but such responses rarely result in any significant improvement in survival.

RECIST Criteria

The Response Evaluation Criteria in Solid Tumors (RECIST) have been used to measure the effect of chemotherapy in an individual patient and are now used in all clinical trials (Table 3.7).

Baseline documentation of "target" and "nontarget" lesions before treatment in clinical trials is essential. All measurable lesions up to a maximum of 5 lesions per organ and 10 lesions in total, representative of all involved organs, should be identified as target lesions and recorded and measured at baseline. Target lesions should be selected on the basis of their size (lesions with the longest diameter) and their suitability for accurate repeated measurements (either clinically or by imaging techniques).

A sum of the longest diameter (LD) for all target lesions should be calculated and reported as the baseline sum LD. The baseline sum LD should be used as the reference by which to characterize the objective tumor response. All other lesions (or sites of disease) should be identified as nontarget lesions and should also be recorded at baseline. Measurements of these lesions are not required, but the presence or absence of each should be noted throughout follow-up.

Dose Adjustment

Patients vary in their tolerance to chemotherapy, and tailoring the treatment to a particular patient is often necessary, particularly when treatment is administered with palliative intent. One convenient method involves the use of a "sliding scale." A typical scheme for adjusting chemotherapy based on myelosuppression is presented in Table 3.8. Doses of myelosuppressive agents are reduced if the patient proves very sensitive to the regimen but can be returned to full levels if tolerance improves in subsequent courses.

Table 3.7 RECIST Definitions of Response	
Complete response (CR)	Disappearance of all target lesions
Partial response (PR)	At least a 30% decrease in the sum of the longest diameter (LD) of target lesions, taking as reference the baseline sum LD
Progressive disease (PD)	At least a 20% increase in the sum of the LD of target lesions, taking as reference the smallest sum LD recorded since the treatment started or the appearance of one or more new lesions
Stable disease (SD)	Neither sufficient shrinkage to qualify for PR nor sufficient increase to qualify for PD, taking as reference the smallest sum LD since the treatment started

Table 3.8 Drug Dose Adjustments for Combination Chemotherapy (Sliding Scale Based on Bone Marrow Toxicity)

If White Blood Count before Starting the Next Course Is	Then Dosage Is
>4,000/mm³	100% of all drugs
3,999–3,000/mm³	100% of nonmyelotoxic agents and 50% of each myelotoxic agent
2,999–2,000/mm³	100% of nonmyelotoxic agents and 25% of each myelotoxic agent
1,999–1,000/mm³	50% of nonmyelotoxic agents and 25% of myelotoxic agents
999–0/mm³	No drug until blood counts recover

If the Platelet Count before Starting Next Course Is	Then Dosage Is
>100,000/mm³	100% of all drugs
50,000–100,000/mm³	100% of nonmyelotoxic drugs and 50% of myelotoxic drugs
<50,000/mm³	No drug until blood counts recover

Many experimental protocols provide for an escalation of drug dose if no significant toxicity is experienced with initial courses of therapy. A sliding scale offers the best opportunity to give the maximum amount of therapy possible. The sliding scale presented is based only on bone marrow toxicity. If the drugs used in any particular combination have other serious toxicities, such as renal or hepatic toxicity, then sliding scales based on the other toxicities are used to minimize toxicity but maximize therapeutic effect.

Because *carboplatin* is cleared renally and severe marrow toxicity occasionally occurs, dose-adjustment scales based on renal function have been developed (Table 3.9). Dose adjustments are based on the *glomerular filtration rate* (GFR) or creatinine clearance and the target serum concentration multiplied by the *area under curve (AUC)* or platelet nadir for the drug's antitumor activity (17). The formula is:

$$\text{Dose (mg)} = \text{Target AUC} \times (\text{GFR} + 25)$$

The desired target AUC is 4 to 5 mg/mL for previously treated patients and 5 to 7 mg/mL for those previously untreated. The use of these dose-adjustment schemes tailored to the particular toxicity allows for safer administration of chemotherapeutic agents.

Drug Toxicity

Antineoplastic drugs are among the most toxic agents used in modern medicine. Many of the toxic side effects, particularly those to organ systems with a rapidly proliferating cell population, are dose related and predictable. Usually, the mechanism of toxicity is similar to the mechanism that produces the desired cytocidal effect on tumors. Even organs with limited cell proliferation can be damaged by chemotherapeutic agents in either a dose-related or an idiosyncratic fashion. In almost all instances, chemotherapeutic agents are used in doses that produce some degree of toxicity to normal tissues.

Severe systemic debility, advanced age, poor nutritional status, or direct organ involvement by primary or metastatic tumor can result in unexpectedly severe side effects of chemotherapy. Idiosyncratic drug reactions also can have severe and unexpected consequences. As a result, careful monitoring of patients receiving cancer chemotherapy is a major responsibility of the treating physician.

Hematologic Toxicity

The proliferating cells of the erythroid, myeloid, and megakaryocytic series of the bone marrow are highly susceptible to damage by many of the commonly used antineoplastic agents. **Granulocytopenia and thrombocytopenia are predictable side effects** of most of the

Table 3.9 *Carboplatin* Dosing

Area under the Curve (AUC) Method: Calvert Formula

Dose (mg) = target AUC (mg/mL × min) × [CrCl (mL/min) + 25]

CrCl = creatinine clearance

Guidelines

Untreated adults target AUC for *carboplatin* alone	= 5 − 7
Previously treated adults target AUC for *carboplatin* alone	= 4 − 5
Target AUC for *carboplatin* in combination	= 5 − 6

Platelet Nadir Method: Egorin Formula

Untreated patients

Dose (mg/M^2) = 0.091 × (CrCl/BSA) × (PreRx Plt − Desired nadir Plt/PreRx Plt × 100) + 86

Previously treated patients

Dose (mg/M^2) = 0.091 × (CrCl/BSA) × [(PreRx Plt − Desired nadir Plt/PreRx Plt × 100) − 17] + 86

M^2 = meters squared; BSA = body surface area; PreRx Plt = pretreatment platelet count

Creatinine Clearance (CrCl)

Based on a timed urine collection

$$\frac{\text{urine creatinine}}{\text{serum creatinine}} \times \frac{\text{urine volume}}{\text{time}}$$

Based on age, weight, and serum creatinine

Method of Cockcroft and Gault

$$\text{CrCl men} = \frac{(140 - \text{age}) \times (\text{lean body weight})}{(\text{serum creatinine}) \times 72}$$

CrCl women = CrCl men × 0.85

Method of Jeliffe

$$\frac{\text{CrCl}}{1.73} = \frac{100}{\text{serum creatinine}} - 2$$

CrCl = mL/min; time = duration of collection in minutes; age = years; weight = kg; Urine Volume = mL; urine creatinine = mg/dL; serum creatinine = mg/dL

Modified from **Calvert AH, Newell DR, Gumbrell, et al.** *Carboplatin* dosage: prospective evaluation of a simple formula based on renal function. *J Clin Oncol* 1989;7:1748–1756; and **Egorin MJ, Van Echo DA, Olman EA, et al.** Prospective validation of a pharmacologically based dosing scheme for the cisdiamminedichloroplatinum (II) analogue diamminecyclobutanedicarboxylatoplatinum. *Cancer Res* 1985;45:6502–6506; and modified and reproduced with permission from **Rubin SC.** *Chemotherapy of gynecologic cancers: Society of Gynecologic Oncologists handbook,* 2nd ed. Philadelphia: Lippincott Williams and Wilkins, 2004.

commonly used antitumor agents and are seen with all effective regimens of combination chemotherapy. The severity and duration of these side effects are variable and depend on the drugs, the dose, the schedule, and the patient's previous exposure to radiation or chemotherapy.

In general, acute granulocytopenia occurs 6 to 12 days after administration of most myelosuppressive chemotherapeutic agents, and recovery occurs in 21 to 24 days; platelet suppression occurs 4 to 5 days later, with recovery after white cell count recovery. Several agents are unique in producing delayed bone marrow suppression, among them *mitomycin C* and the nitrosoureas. Marrow suppression from these drugs commonly occurs at 28 to 42 days, with recovery 40 to 60 days after treatment.

Granulocytopenia   **Patients with an absolute granulocyte count of less than 500/mm^3 for 5 days or longer are at high risk of rapidly fatal sepsis.** The wide use of empiric, broad-spectrum antibiotics in febrile granulocytopenic patients with cancer has significantly decreased the likelihood of life-threatening toxicity. **The importance of quickly initiating broad-spectrum antibiotics in the presence of fever in a neutropenic patient, even in the absence of localizing signs of infection, cannot be overemphasized.** Granulocytopenic patients should have their temperature checked every 4 hours and must be examined frequently for evidence of infection. The availability of hematopoietic growth factors has enabled physicians to reduce the duration of granulocytopenia in certain patients.

Before the initiation of antibiotics in a febrile granulocytopenic patient, cultures of possible sites of infection (e.g., blood, urine, sputum, recent surgical wound, indwelling intravenous delivery device) should be obtained. In addition, a detailed physical examination (including the throat, perianal region, and skin) should be performed, looking for a specific site of infection, which may influence the choice of antibiotic therapy (e.g., catheter infection).

Thrombocytopenia   **Patients with sustained thrombocytopenia who have platelet counts of less than 20,000/mm³ are at risk of spontaneous hemorrhage, particularly gastrointestinal or acute intracranial hemorrhage.** Routine platelet transfusions for platelet counts below 10,000 to 20,000/mm³ have significantly reduced the risk of spontaneous hemorrhage. It is common to transfuse 6 to 10 units of donor platelets to the patient with a platelet count of less than 20,000/mm³. Repeat transfusions at intervals of 2 to 3 days for the duration of the severe thrombocytopenia are indicated. Although patients with platelet counts exceeding 50,000/mm³ do not commonly experience severe bleeding, transfusion at this level is indicated:

1. if the patient manifests active bleeding
2. if the patient has active peptic ulcer disease
3. before and during surgical procedures

A posttransfusion platelet count performed one hour after platelet administration should show an appropriate incremental increase. If no posttransfusion platelet increase occurs, it is likely that there has been previous sensitization to random donor platelets, and the patient requires single-donor human leukocyte antigen-matched platelets for future transfusions.

***Recombinant interleukin-11* can be considered for use in patients with, or anticipated to develop, severe thrombocytopenia.** The drug is administered subcutaneously beginning 6 to 24 hours after chemotherapy (50 μg/kg once daily) and continued until the platelet count exceeds 50,000/mm³. Treatment with this agent should be discontinued at least 2 days before the next chemotherapy.

Gastrointestinal Toxicity

The gastrointestinal tract is a frequent site of serious antineoplastic drug treatment toxicity. **Mucositis** caused by a direct effect on the rapidly dividing epithelial mucosal cells is common; concomitant granulocytopenia allows the injured mucosa to become infected and serve as a portal of entry for bacteria and fungi into the bloodstream. Impaired cellular immunity because of underlying disease or corticosteroid therapy also can contribute to extensive infection of the gastrointestinal tract. Other side effects related to the gastrointestinal tract include **impaired intestinal motility,** resulting from the autonomic neuropathic effect of vinca alkaloids (*vincristine* and *vinblastine*), and **nausea and vomiting,** induced by many anticancer drugs.

Upper Gastrointestinal   The onset of mucositis is frequently 3 to 5 days earlier than that of myelosuppression. Lesions of the mouth and pharynx are difficult to distinguish from candidiasis and herpes simplex infection. **Esophagitis** resulting from direct drug toxicity can be confused with radiation esophagitis or infections with bacteria, fungi, or herpes simplex because they all produce dysphagia and retrosternal burning pain. Mild oral candidiasis (thrush) responds to several oral agents. More intensive therapy will be required for esophageal or severe oral candidiasis or herpes simplex infections. Symptomatic management of painful upper gastrointestinal inflammation includes warm saline mouth rinses and topical anesthetics such as viscous lidocaine. Intravenous fluids or hyperalimentation may be required.

Lower Gastrointestinal   Mucositis in the lower gastrointestinal tract is invariably associated with diarrhea. Serious complications include bowel perforation, hemorrhage, and necrotizing enterocolitis.

Necrotizing enterocolitis includes a spectrum of severe diarrheal illnesses that can be fatal in a granulocytopenic patient. Broad-spectrum antibiotic therapy may predispose the patient to necrotizing enterocolitis, as does cytotoxic chemotherapy, which can interfere with the integrity of the bowel wall. This condition is more common in patients receiving intensive chemotherapy (e.g., patients with leukemia), but it can be observed with treatment of solid tumors (e.g., gynecological malignancies). The most common organism associated with this extremely serious condition is *Pseudomonas aeruginosa*. Symptoms of necrotizing enterocolitis include watery or bloody diarrhea, abdominal pain, sore throat, nausea, vomiting, and fever. Physical examination usually reveals abdominal tenderness and distention. The performance of an abdominal or pelvic computed tomographic scan or ultrasound will be helpful in the evaluation of this constellation of signs and symptoms. Treatment includes the administration of broad-spectrum antibiotics with specific activity against aerobic gram-negative rods and anaerobes. Nasogastric decompression, intravenous fluids, and bowel rest may also be required. In the neutropenic patient, recovery of normal blood counts is essential for improvement of the condition. Surgical intervention is occasionally necessary.

Immunosuppression

Most anticancer drugs are capable of producing suppression of cellular and, to a lesser extent, humoral immunity. The magnitude and duration of the immunosuppression vary with the dose and schedule of drug administration and have been inadequately characterized for most chemotherapeutic agents. However, **most of the acute immunosuppressive side effects do not persist after completion of drug treatment.** Laboratory studies suggest a decrease in host defenses during treatment associated with a rebound to complete or nearly complete restoration 2 to 3 days after treatment is completed. This short-term immunosuppressive effect has led to increased use of intermittent chemotherapy regimens to allow immunologic recovery during courses of treatment.

Dermatologic Reactions

Several important drug toxicities involve skin reactions. **Skin necrosis and sloughing may result from extravasation of certain irritating chemotherapeutic agents such as *doxorubicin, actinomycin D, mitomycin C, vinblastine, vincristine,* and *nitrogen mustard.*** The extent of necrosis depends on the quantity of drug extravasated and can vary from local erythema to chronic ulcerative necrosis. Management often includes immediate removal of the intravenous line, local infiltration of corticosteroids, ice pack therapy four times a day for 3 days, and elevation of the affected limb. Long-term monitoring of the affected area is required, and surgical debridement and full-thickness skin grafting are often necessary for severe lesions.

Alopecia is a very most common side effect. Although not intrinsically injurious, it has major emotional consequences for patients. Agents commonly associated with severe hair loss include the anthracycline antibiotics, taxanes such as *paclitaxel or docetaxel,* and *alkylating agents* such as *cyclophosphamide.* Most commonly used drug combinations, however, produce variable degrees of alopecia. Alopecia is reversible, and regrowth usually begins several weeks after treatment is completed. Attempts to minimize alopecia by using a variety of methods such a scalp cooling have been tried with varying degrees of success, depending on the drugs used.

Generalized allergic skin reactions can occur with chemotherapeutic agents, as they do with other drugs, and can sometimes be severe. Other skin reactions occasionally seen with chemotherapeutic agents include increased skin pigmentation (*bleomycin*), photosensitivity reactions, transverse banding or nail loss, folliculitis (*actinomycin D, methotrexate*), and radiation recall reactions (*doxorubicin*).

Liposomal doxorubicin, an agent demonstrated to be active in platinum-refractory ovarian cancer, can produce a painful dermatologic syndrome characterized by desquamation of the skin, most often involving **the hands and feet** (18). Blistering, focal or disseminated, can also be observed.

Hepatic Toxicity

Modest elevations in aminotransferase, alkaline phosphatase, and bilirubin levels are frequently seen with many anticancer agents, but they resolve soon after treatment is completed. Nevertheless, more severe reactions do occur. **Long-term administration of *methotrexate* induces hepatic fibrosis that can progress to cirrhosis.** The cirrhosis and drug-induced hepatitis should be managed by withdrawal of the toxic agent, with the same supportive measures that are used for hepatitis or cirrhosis of any cause.

Preexisting liver disease or exposure to other hepatotoxins may increase the risk. Antimetabolites, such **as *6-mercaptopurine* and *6-thioguanine,*** can produce reversible cholestatic jaundice. Transient liver enzyme abnormalities are seen with *cytosine arabinoside,* the nitrosoureas, and **L-asparaginase.** *Mithramycin,* an agent occasionally used to control hypercalcemia, frequently causes marked elevations in liver enzyme levels associated with clotting disorders and renal insufficiency.

Pulmonary Complications

Patients with cancer have a wide variety of problems that can manifest as pulmonary complications. Respiratory compromise resulting from lung metastases, pulmonary emboli, radiation pneumonitis, tumor-induced neuromuscular dysfunction, and pneumonia all may be significant complications. In addition, direct pulmonary toxicity from commonly used anticancer drugs is sometimes seen.

Interstitial Pneumonitis   Interstitial pneumonitis with pulmonary fibrosis is the usual pattern of lung damage associated with cytotoxic drugs. Agents likely to cause such an effect are **bleomycin, alkylating agents, gemcitabine,** and **the nitrosoureas.** The physical and chest radiologic findings are not easily distinguishable from those of interstitial pneumonitis resulting from infectious agents, viruses, or lymphangitic spread of cancer.

Management of drug-induced interstitial pneumonitis includes discontinuation of the suspected agent and supportive care. Steroids may be of symptomatic benefit in some patients.

Cardiac Toxicity

Cardiac toxicity is seen with several important cancer chemotherapeutic agents. Although the myocardium consists of largely nondividing cells, drugs of the anthracycline antibiotic class—specifically, *doxorubicin* and *daunomycin*—can cause severe cardiomyopathy.

The risk of cardiac toxicity increases with the total cumulative dose of *doxorubicin*. For this reason, a cumulative dose of 500 mg/m^2 of ideal body surface area is now widely used as the maximum tolerable dose of *doxorubicin*. With careful and frequent monitoring of left ventricular function by means of ejection fraction studies, therapy can be continued to higher doses if no satisfactory alternative exists. **More infrequently, anthracyclines and *paclitaxel* can cause acute arrhythmias** that usually disappear within a few days of drug treatment. They appear not to be related to total drug dose. Anthracycline cardiac toxicity is potentiated by radiation.

The medical management of cardiomyopathy induced by anthracyclines is supportive but usually unsatisfactory. **Early detection of cardiac compromise with radionuclide cardiac scintigraphy before the clinical manifestations of congestive heart failure appear is important.** Discontinuation of the drug at the first indication of decreasing left ventricular function minimizes the risk of cardiovascular decompensation.

Rarely, *cyclophosphamide* has been reported to produce cardiotoxicity, particularly in the massive doses used in conjunction with bone marrow transplantation. With conventional doses of *cyclophosphamide*, this complication is unlikely. *Busulfan* and *mitomycin C* have been reported to cause endocardial fibrosis and myocardial fibrosis, respectively. In some patients, *5-fluorouracil* has been reported to be a rare cause of angina pectoris.

Cardiac toxicity has also been recognized as an important side effect of *trastuzumab*, a novel targeted therapy (HER-2/*neu* receptor) commonly used in the management of breast cancer, especially when the agent is delivered with *doxorubicin* or *paclitaxel* (19).

A major toxicity of the antiangiogenic agent *bevacizumab* is the development of hypertension (20). In a patient with preexisting cardiac abnormalities, this effect has the potential to result in deterioration of heart function. This concern is likely to increase as this class of agents is increasingly used in routine clinical practice in the management of gynecologic malignancies.

Genitourinary Toxicity

In addition to chemotherapeutic agents, various other cancer-related complications may produce chronic azotemia or acute renal failure, including fluid depletion, infection, tumor infiltration of the kidney, ureteral obstruction by tumor, radiation damage, and tumor lysis syndrome.

Drugs that cause kidney damage include:

1. *cisplatin,* which produces renal tubular toxicity associated with azotemia and magnesium wasting

2. *methotrexate,* which can precipitate in the renal tubules, causing oliguric renal failure (*methotrexate* toxicity can be prevented by maintenance of a high urine volume and alkalinization of the urine)

3. **nitrosoureas,** which cause a chronic interstitial nephritis with chronic renal failure

4. **mitomycin C,** which causes a systemic microangiopathic hemolysis and acute renal failure

Metabolites of cyclophosphamide are irritants to the bladder mucosa and **cause a chronic hemorrhagic cystitis,** particularly during high-dose or prolonged treatment. Vigorous hydration and diuresis can reduce the risk of this complication.

Treatment of drug-related genitourinary toxicity requires discontinuation of the possibly nephrotoxic drugs and volume expansion to increase glomerular filtration. Specific metabolic abnormalities, such as hyperuricemia and hypomagnesemia, should be corrected. If oliguria develops or if medical management is unsuccessful in restoring acceptable kidney function, then short-term peritoneal dialysis or hemodialysis may be required. Daily administration of 3 L of fluid containing 100 to 150 mEq of sodium bicarbonate per liter maintains the urinary pH above 7. Because *methotrexate* is poorly dialyzed, prolonged toxic levels can result if *leucovorin* rescue therapy is not continued until the *methotrexate* concentration is less than $5 \times 10^{-8}\ M$.

N-acetylcysteine or **mesna** (*sodium mercaptoethanesulfonate*) **has been used in conjunction with very high doses of cyclophosphamide or ifosfamide to prevent bladder toxicity** by inactivating the toxic metabolite (*acrolein*). Persistent hemorrhagic cystitis that does not respond to conservative management may be treated with ε-*aminocaproic acid.*

Neurotoxicity

Many antineoplastic drugs are associated with some central or peripheral neurotoxicity. These neurologic side effects usually are mild, but occasionally they can be severe.

Vinca Alkaloids   The vinca alkaloids (**vincristine, vinblastine,** and **vindesine**) are commonly associated with peripheral motor, sensory, and autonomic neuropathies, which are the major side effects of *vincristine.* Toxicity first appears as loss of deep tendon reflexes with distal paresthesias. Cranial nerves can be affected, and the autonomic neuropathy can appear as adynamic ileus, urinary bladder atony with retention, or hypotension. All of these neurologic toxicities from the vinca alkaloids are slowly reversible after cessation of the offending drug.

Cisplatin   Cisplatin produces ototoxicity, peripheral neuropathy, and, rarely, retrobulbar neuritis and blindness. High doses of *cisplatin,* which may be used in ovarian cancer therapy, are particularly likely to produce a progressive and somewhat delayed peripheral neuropathy. This defect is characterized by sensory impairment and loss of proprioception, whereas motor strength usually is preserved. Progression of this neuropathy 1 to 2 months after cessation of high-dose *cisplatin* has been reported.

Paclitaxel   Paclitaxel is associated with the development of a peripheral sensory neuropathy. The incidence and severity of symptoms relate to the peak levels of the agent reached in the plasma. In addition, the combination of *paclitaxel* and *cisplatin* (or *carboplatin*) has the potential to be more neurotoxic than either agent used alone (21).

Other Drugs   Rarely, *5-fluorouracil* can be associated with **an acute cerebellar toxicity,** apparently related to its metabolism to fluorocitrate, a neurotoxic metabolite of the parent compound. **Hexamethylmelamine** has been reported to produce **peripheral neuropathy and encephalopathy.** Some improvement in the peripheral neuropathy has been reported with administration of B vitamin supplements, but therapeutic effectiveness may be reduced.

Vascular and Hypersensitivity Reactions

Occasionally, severe hypersensitivity reactions in the form of anaphylaxis develop with chemotherapeutic agents. In rare cases, this has been associated with **cyclophosphamide, doxorubicin, cisplatin,** intravenous **melphalan, and high-dose methotrexate. Bleomycin** administration may be associated with marked fever reactions, anaphylaxis, Raynaud's phenomenon, and a chronic scleroderma-like reaction. The same reactions have been reported with *procarbazine, etoposide,* and *teniposide.*

Hypersensitivity reactions have been seen with **paclitaxel** and are believed to result from hypersensitivity to the *cremophor* vehicle. They can be ameliorated with intravenous infusions of *dexamethasone* (20 mg), *diphenhydramine* (50 mg), and *cimetidine* (300 mg) 30 minutes before *paclitaxel* is administered. A similar incidence of hypersensitivity reactions is observed with **docetaxel,** a closely related antineoplastic agent to *paclitaxel.*

Carboplatin and *cisplatin* may be associated with a significant risk of hypersensitivity reactions in patients who have been treated with more than six total courses of a platinum agent (22).

Second Malignancies

Many antineoplastic agents are mutagenic and teratogenic. The potential of these agents to induce second malignancies appears to vary with the class of agent (23). ***Alkylating agents*** (especially *melphalan*), *procarbazine,* and the nitrosoureas **seem to be the major offenders. Prolonged use of *etoposide* has also been associated with the development of leukemia.**

The cumulative 7-year risk of acute nonlymphocytic leukemia developing in patients treated primarily with oral *melphalan* for ovarian cancer is as high as 9.6% in patients receiving therapy for more than 1 year (24). Although *cisplatin* has also been suggested to be associated with the development of acute leukemia, the risk is lower than with the *alkylating agents* (25).

Evidence from long-term studies of Hodgkin's disease suggests a major risk with combined chemotherapy and radiation therapy. In such patients, there is a risk of acute leukemia as well as an increase in solid tumors, seen particularly in the radiation ports. An increase in the frequency of acute leukemia has been reported in patients treated for Hodgkin's disease, multiple myeloma, and ovarian cancer. The second malignancy commonly occurs 4 to 7 years after successful therapy. Encouragingly, evidence suggests that after 11 years, the risk of acute leukemia in patients treated for Hodgkin's disease decreases to that of the normal population.

The long-term follow-up of women cured of choriocarcinoma, primarily with antimetabolite therapy, reveals no evidence of an increased risk of second malignancy. Radiation alone also appears to produce a relatively low risk of late leukemia, as do chemotherapeutic regimens alone, particularly those without *alkylating agents* or *procarbazine.* Combination chemotherapy (including *cisplatin*-based treatment of ovarian cancer) and limited-field radiation therapy increase the risk only slightly.

Particularly high risks are associated with:

1. **extensive radiation therapy plus combination chemotherapy**
2. **prolonged *alkylating agent* therapy (longer than 1 year)**
3. **age older than 40 years at initial treatment**

Gonadal Dysfunction

Many cancer chemotherapeutic agents have profound and lasting effects on testicular and ovarian function. **Chemotherapeutic agents, particularly *alkylating agents*, can cause azoospermia and amenorrhea.** Secondary sexual characteristics related to hormonal function usually are less disturbed. Prolonged intensive combination chemotherapy commonly produces azoospermia in men, and recovery is uncommon.

The onset of amenorrhea and ovarian failure is accompanied by an elevation of the serum follicle-stimulating hormone and luteinizing hormone and a decrease in the serum estradiol level. Occasionally, this hormonal pattern can be seen before the onset of amenorrhea. If the characteristic pattern is seen, patients should be advised to consider conception because these findings predict premature ovarian failure and early menopause.

When short-term intensive chemotherapy is used, particularly with antimetabolites, vinca alkaloids, or antitumor antibiotics, injury to the reproductive system is less common. For example, men treated for testicular cancer, children with acute leukemia, and women cured of gestational trophoblastic disease or ovarian germ cell malignancies usually have recovered reproductive capacity after therapy (26–29).

Chemotherapy in Pregnancy

Risk of congenital abnormalities from chemotherapeutic agents is highest during the first trimester, especially when antimetabolites (e.g., *cytosine arabinoside* or *methotrexate*) and *alkylating agents* are used. **Chemotherapy administered during the second or third trimesters usually is not associated with an increase in fetal abnormalities,** although the number of patients studied is relatively small (see Chapter 17).

Metabolic Abnormalities

Inappropriate Antidiuretic Hormone Secretion   Inappropriate antidiuretic hormone secretion is characterized by hyponatremia, high urine osmolality, and high urinary sodium values, and it is associated with several malignancies, most commonly small cell carcinoma of the lung. It can also be seen as a complication of vinca alkaloids. Symptoms are primarily neurologic and include altered mental status, confusion, lethargy, seizures, and coma. The severity of symptoms is related to the rapidity of development of hyponatremia. The diagnosis rests on:

1. the documentation of hyponatremia
2. the presence of a urine that is hypertonic to plasma
3. the exclusion of hypothyroidism or adrenal insufficiency

Hyperuricemia   Hyperuricemia may be a complication of effective cancer chemotherapy in certain tumors, particularly hematologic malignancies in which rapid tumor lysis is seen in response to initial treatment. Rapid tumor lysis releases predominant intracellular ions and uric acid and can result in life-threatening hyperkalemia, hyperphosphatemia, hypocalcemia, and hyperuricemia. Renal failure associated with hyperuricemia can be severe. **Prevention of the *tumor lysis syndrome* requires maintenance of a high urinary output, maintenance of high urinary pH (above 7.0), and prophylactic use of the xanthine oxidase inhibitor *allopurinol*.**

Antineoplastic Drugs

Alkylating Agents

This class of antineoplastic agent acts primarily by chemically interacting with DNA. These drugs form extremely unstable alkyl groups that react with nucleophilic (electron-rich) sites on many important organic compounds such as nucleic acids, proteins, and amino acids. These interactions produce the primary cytotoxic effects.

Mechanism

Alkylating agents commonly bind to the N-7 position of guanine and to other key DNA sites. In doing so, they interfere with accurate base pairing, crosslink DNA, and produce single- and double-stranded breaks. This results in the inhibition of DNA, RNA, and protein synthesis.

Table 3.10 *Alkylating Agents* Used for Gynecologic Cancer

Drug	Route of Administration	Common Treatment Schedules	Common Toxicities	Diseases Treated
Cyclophosphamide (Cytoxan)	PO, IV	1.5–3.0 mg/kg/day orally 10–50 mg/kg IV every 1–4 weeks 600–1,000 mg/m² every 3–4 weeks	Myelosuppression, cystitis ± bladder fibrosis, alopecia, hepatitis, amenorrhea, azoospermia	Breast, ovarian cancer, soft tissue sarcomas
Chlorambucil (Leukeran)	PO	0.03–0.1 mg/kg/day	Myelosuppression, gastrointestinal distress, dermatitis, hepatotoxicity	Ovarian cancer
Melphalan (Alkeran, L-PAM)	PO	0.2 mg/kg/day × 5 days every 4–6 weeks	Myelosuppression, nausea and vomiting (rare), mucosal ulceration (rare), second malignancies	Ovarian, breast cancer
Triethylenethiophosphoramide (TSPA, Thiotepa)	IV / Intracavitary	IV: 0.8 mg/kg every 4–6 weeks / Intracavitary: 45–60 mg	Myelosuppression, nausea and vomiting, headaches, fever (rare)	Ovarian, breast cancer; intracavitary for malignant effusions
Ifosphamide (Ifex)	IV	1.0 or 1.2 g/m²/day × 5 days with *mesna*: 200 mg/m² immediately before and 4 and 8 h after *ifosphamide*	Myelosuppression, bladder toxicity, central nervous system dysfunction, renal toxicity	Cervical, ovarian cancer

PO, oral; IV intravenous.

Because some effects of *alkylating agents* are similar to those of irradiation, these drugs are often called **radiomimetic.** Most of the effective *alkylating agents* are bifunctional or polyfunctional, and have two or more potentially unstable alkyl groups per molecule. These bifunctional *alkylating agents* allow crosslinkage of DNA that results in cellular disruption.

Because all *alkylating agents* have similar mechanisms of action, there tends to be crossresistance to other agents of the same class.

Drugs

Although several hundred *alkylating agents* exist, those most commonly in use include **cyclophosphamide, melphalan, Thiotepa, chlorambucil**, and **ifosfamide**.

In addition to the more common *alkylating agents*, several antineoplastic agents of different types are usually classified as alkylating-like agents, although their precise mechanism of action is less well understood and is probably not exclusively alkylation. These include the nitrosoureas, *DTIC* (*dacarbazine*), and the platinum analogs *cisplatin* and *carboplatin*.

The characteristics of the commonly used *alkylating agents* are listed in Table 3.10, and the alkylating-like agents are listed in Table 3.11.

Antitumor Antibiotics

The antitumor antibiotics are antineoplastic drugs that, in general, have been isolated as natural products from fungi found in the soil. These natural products usually have extremely complex and different chemical structures, although they function in general by forming complexes with DNA.

Mechanism

The interaction between these drugs and DNA often involves intercalation: The compound is inserted between DNA base pairs. A second mechanism thought to be important in their antitumor action is the formation of free radicals capable of damaging DNA, RNA, and vital proteins. Other effects include metal ion chelation and alteration of tumor cell membranes. This class of antineoplastic agents is thought to be *cell cycle–nonspecific.*

Drugs

Major drugs in this family include the anthracycline antibiotics *doxorubicin, liposomal doxorubicin*, and *daunorubicin*, as well as *actinomycin D, bleomycin, mitomycin C*, and *mithramycin*.

Anthracyclines   **The anthracyclines are antibiotics isolated from the fungi *Streptomyces*.** These pigmented compounds have an anthraquinone nucleus attached to an amino sugar and have multiple mechanisms of action. Because of the planar structure of the anthraquinone moiety, these agents act as intercalators in the DNA double helix. In addition, they are known

Table 3.11 Alkylating-Like Agents Used for Gynecologic Cancer				
Drug	*Route of Administration*	*Common Treatment Schedules*	*Common Toxicities*	*Diseases Treated*
Cisplatin	IV	10–20 mg/m²/day × 5 every 3 weeks 40–75 mg/m² every 1–3 weeks	Nephrotoxicity, tinnitus and hearing loss, nausea or and vomiting, myelosuppression, peripheral neuropathy	Ovarian and germ cell carcinomas, cervical, endometrial cancer
Carboplatin	IV	300–400 mg/m² × 6 every 3–4 weeks AUC 4–7.5	Less neuropathy, ototoxicity, and nephrotoxicity than *cisplatin*; more hematopoietic toxicity, especially thrombocytopenia, than *cisplatin*	Ovarian and germ cell carcinomas, endometrial cancer
Dacarbazine (DTIC)	IV	2–4.5 mg/kg/day × 10 days every 4 weeks	Myelosuppression, nausea and vomiting, flu-like syndrome, hepatotoxicity	Uterine sarcomas, soft tissue sarcomas

IV, intravenous; AUC, area under "concentration versus time" curve.

to chelate divalent cations and are avid calcium binders. These agents cause single-stranded DNA breaks, inhibit DNA repair, and actively generate free radicals that are capable of producing DNA damage. Anthracyclines are capable of reacting directly with cell membranes, disrupting membrane structure, and altering membrane function.

Bleomycin   *Bleomycin* was also **isolated from the *Streptomyces* fungus.** Its structure contains a DNA-binding fragment and an ion-binding unit. It appears to produce its antitumor action primarily by producing single- and double-stranded breaks in DNA, mainly at sites of guanine bases. The drug is primarily excreted in the urine, and increased toxicity may be seen in patients with impaired renal function.

Mitomycin C   *Mitomycin C* is another antibiotic that was **isolated from the *Streptomyces* fungus.** It is activated *in vivo* into an alkylating agent that can bind DNA, producing crosslinks and inhibiting DNA synthesis. In addition, it has a quinone moiety that can generate free radical reactions similar to those seen with the anthracycline antibiotics. It is administered intravenously and is degraded primarily by metabolism. Renal clearance is not a major mechanism of excretion.

Mithramycin   *Mithramycin* is an antitumor antibiotic **isolated from another *Streptomyces* species.** It has intrinsic antitumor properties and is also effective in the management of **hypercalcemia.** Its primary mechanism of action seems to be the inhibition of RNA synthesis, although it binds to DNA and inhibits DNA and protein synthesis.

Some of the important characteristics of the antitumor antibiotics are listed in Table 3.12.

Table 3.12 Antitumor Antibiotics Used for Gynecologic Cancer

Drug	Route of Administration	Common Treatment Schedules	Common Toxicities	Diseases Treated
Actinomycin D (dactinomycin, Cosmegen)	IV	0.3–0.5 mg/m² IV × 5 days every 3–4 weeks	Nausea and vomiting, skin necrosis, mucosal ulceration, myelosuppression	Germ cell ovarian tumors, choriocarcinoma, soft tissue sarcoma
Bleomycin (Blenoxane)	IV, SC, IM, IP	10–20 units/m² 1–2 times/week to total dose of 400 units; for effusions, 60–120 units	Fever, dermatologic reactions, pulmonary toxicity, anaphylactic reactions	Cervical, germ cell ovarian tumors, malignant effusions
Mitomycin-C (Mutamycin)	IV	10–20 mg/m² every 6–8 weeks	Myelosuppression, local vesicant, nausea and vomiting, mucosal ulcerations, nephrotoxicity	Breast, cervical, ovarian cancer
Doxorubicin (Adriamycin)	IV	60–90 mg/m² every 3 weeks or 20–35 mg/m² every day × 3 every 3 weeks	Myelosuppression, alopecia, cardiotoxicity, local vesicant, nausea and vomiting, mucosal ulcerations	Ovarian, breast, endometrial cancer
Mithramycin (Mithracin)	IV	20–50 mg/kg/day every 4–6 weeks; hypercalcemia: 25 mg/kg every 3–4 days	Nausea and vomiting, hemorrhagic diathesis, hepatotoxicity, renal toxicity, fever, myelosuppression, facial flushing	Hypercalcemia of malignancy
Liposomal doxorubicin (Doxil)	IV	40–50 mg/m² every 4 weeks	Palmar-plantar erythrodysesthesia, myelosuppression, stomatitis	Ovarian and endometrial cancers

IV, intravenous; SC, subcutaneous; IM, intramuscular; IP, intraperitoneal.

Antimetabolites

The antimetabolite family of antineoplastic agents interacts with vital intracellular enzymes, leading to their inactivation or to the production of fraudulent products incapable of normal intracellular function. In general, their structures resemble analogs of normal purines and pyrimidines, or they resemble normal substances that are vital for cell function. Some antimetabolites are active as intact drugs, and others require biotransformation to active agents.

Mechanism

Although many of these agents act at different sites in biosynthetic pathways, they appear to exert their antitumor activity by disrupting functions crucial to the viability of the cell. These effects are usually more disruptive to actively proliferating cells; thus, the antimetabolites are classed in general as **cell cycle–specific** agents.

Drugs

Although hundreds of antimetabolites have been investigated in cancer treatment, only a few are commonly used. They include:

1. the folate antagonist *methotrexate*, which inhibits the enzyme dihydrofolate reductase
2. the purine antagonists *6-mercaptopurine* and *6-thioguanine*
3. the pyrimidine antagonists *5-fluorouracil (5-FU)* and *cytosine arabinoside*
4. the ribonucleotide reductase inhibitor *hydroxyurea*
5. the nucleoside analog *gemcitabine*

In most instances, the antimetabolites are used not as single drugs but in combinations because of their cell cycle specificity and their capacity for complementary inhibition. Antimetabolites commonly used in the treatment of gynecologic malignancies are summarized in Table 3.13.

Plant Alkaloids

The most common plant alkaloids in use are the vinca alkaloids, natural products derived from the common periwinkle plant (*Vinca rosea*), although the *epipodophyllotoxins* and *paclitaxel* are used frequently in gynecologic malignancies (Table 3.14). Like most natural products, these compounds are large and complex molecules, but *vincristine* and *vinblastine* differ only by a single methyl group on one side chain.

Mechanism

Vincristine and *vinblastine* act primarily by binding to vital intracellular microtubular proteins, particularly tubulin. Tubulin binding produces inhibition of microtubule assembly and destruction of the mitotic spindle, and cells are arrested in mitosis. In general, this class of antineoplastic

Table 3.13 Antimetabolites Used for Gynecologic Cancer

Drug	Route of Administration	Common Treatment Schedules	Common Toxicities	Diseases Treated
5-Fluorouracil (fluorouracil, 5-FU)	IV	10–15 mg/kg/week	Myelosuppression, nausea and vomiting, anorexia, alopecia	Breast, ovarian cancer
Methotrexate (MTX, amethopterin)	PO, IV, intrathecal	PO: 15–40 mg/day × 5 days; IV: 240 mg/m² with leucovorin rescue; intrathecal: 12–15 mg/m²/week	Mucosal ulceration, myelosuppression, hepatotoxicity, allergic pneumonitis; with intrathecal: meningeal irritation	Choriocarcinoma, breast, ovarian cancer
Hydroxyurea (Hydrea)	PO, IV	1–2 g/m²/day for 2–6 weeks	Myelosuppression, nausea and vomiting, anorexia	Cervical cancer
Gemcitabine (Gemzar)	IV	800–1000 mg/m²/ week × 3 weeks, followed by 1 week rest, then repeated	Myelosuppression, fever	Ovarian, breast Cancer, Leiomyosarcoma

IV, intravenous; PO, oral.

Table 3.14 Plant Alkaloids				
Drug	Route of Administration	Common Treatment Schedules	Common Toxicities	Diseases Treated
Vincristine (Oncovin)	IV	0.01–0.03 mg/kg/week	Neurotoxicity, alopecia, myelosuppression, cranial nerve palsies, gastrointestinal	Ovarian germ cell, sarcomas, cervical cancer
Vinblastine (Velban)	IV	5–6 mg/m² every 1–2 weeks	Myelosuppression, alopecia, nausea and vomiting, neurotoxicity	Ovarian germ cell, choriocarcinoma
Epipodophyllotoxin (etoposide, VP-16)	IV	300–600 mg/m² divided over 3–4 days every 3–4 weeks	Myelosuppression, alopecia, hypotension	Ovarian germ cell, choriocarcinoma
	PO	50 mg/m²/day × 21 days, then 1 week rest, then repeat		Ovarian cancer
Paclitaxel (Taxol)	IV	135–250 mg/m² as a 3- to 24-hour infusion every 3 weeks	Myelosuppression, alopecia, allergic reactions, cardiac arrhythmias	Ovarian, breast cancer
Vinorelbine (Navelbine)	IV	20–25 mg/m² weekly	Myelosuppression, constipation, peripheral neuropathy	Ovarian, breast cancer
Docetaxel (Taxotere)	IV	60–100 mg/m² every 3–4 weeks	Myelosuppression, alopecia, hypersensitivity reactions, peripheral edema	Breast, ovarian cancer

IV, intravenous; PO, oral.

agent is believed to be **cell cycle–specific.** At high concentrations, these drugs also have effects on nucleic acid and protein synthesis.

Paclitaxel has a unique mechanism of action. It binds preferentially to microtubules and results in their polymerization and stabilization. *Paclitaxel*-treated cells contain large numbers of microtubules, free and in bundles that result in disruption of microtubular function and, ultimately, cell death. Renal clearance is minimal (5%).

Drugs

Vinblastine is used primarily in the treatment of ovarian germ cell tumors. Its **primary toxicity is myelosuppression.** In contrast, *vincristine* causes little myelosuppression. Its primary **dose-limiting toxicity is peripheral neuropathy.** *Vincristine* has been used in the treatment of cervical carcinoma.

A second family of plant alkaloids has been documented to have significant antitumor properties. Members of this family, known as **the *epipodophyllotoxins,* are extracts from the mandrake plant.** Although the primary plant extracts had tubulin-binding properties similar to those of the vinca alkaloids, the active derivative, *etoposide,* does not seem to function either by inhibiting mitotic spindle formation or by tubulin binding. Rather, the drug appears to function by causing single-stranded DNA breaks. Unlike many of the other compounds that act primarily by DNA interactions, the agent appears to be **cell cycle–specific** and **schedule-dependent.** The dose-limiting toxicity is myelosuppression. Other toxicities include an infusion rate–limited hypotension, nausea, vomiting, anorexia, and alopecia.

Paclitaxel is a complex agent in the class of drugs known as *taxanes.* Its major toxic effects include bone marrow suppression, alopecia, myalgias, arthralgias, and hypersensitivity reactions (29). **The most common dose-limiting toxicity is granulocytopenia,** although with

Table 3.15 Topoisomerase-1 Inhibitors				
Drug	*Route of Administration*	*Common Treatment Schedules*	*Common Toxicity*	*Disease Treated*
Topetecan (Hycamtin)	IV	1.25–1.5 mg/m²/day × 5 days, every 3–4 weeks	Myelosuppression	Ovarian cancer
Irinotecan (Camptosar)	IV	250–300 mg/m² every 3–4 weeks or 125 mg/m²/wk × 4, followed by 2 weeks rest	Myelosuppression, diarrhea	Cervix, ovarian cancer

certain schedules the limiting toxicity is **peripheral sensory neuropathy.** The drug is active in cancers of the ovary, endometrium, cervix, and breast.

A second taxane, ***docetaxel,*** is also active in cancers of the ovary, endometrium, and breast (30). The dose-limiting toxicity of *docetaxel* is bone marrow suppression, principally neutropenia. Hypersensitivity reactions are also observed.

Topoisomerase-1 Inhibitors

This class of antineoplastic agent exerts its cytotoxic effect through inhibition of the enzyme topoisomerase-1 (Table 3.15) (31). This is a critically important enzyme in DNA replication, repair, and transcription. Topoisomerase-1 inhibitors bind to the enzyme–DNA complex, leading to permanent strand breaks and cell death.

Topotecan, the first topoisomerase-1 inhibitor approved for clinical use in the United States, is active in platinum-refractory ovarian cancer and cervical cancer. The major toxicity of the agent is bone marrow suppression. The drug was developed for administration on a 5-day schedule but is frequently utilized on an more convenient weekly schedule. An oral formulation of the drug is currently undergoing investigation.

Irinotecan, a second topoisomerase-1 inhibitor, has revealed activity in both cancers of the ovary and cervix (31). The major side effects of the agent are bone marrow suppression and diarrhea.

Other Agents

There are additional agents that are employed in the management of gynecologic malignancies (Table 3.16).

Of particular interest are a group of agents currently classified as being **antiangiogenic drugs** (e.g., *bevacizumab*) that appear to exert their biological effects on either the normal or abnormal blood vessels delivering nutrients to the malignancy (20,32). To date, experience with this class of drugs in the management of gynecologic malignancies is limited, but existing data suggest these agents may ultimately play an important role in routine disease management.

New Drug Trials

A number of chemotherapeutic agents have been studied experimentally but are not commercially available. Many of these agents have already demonstrated activity against human tumors, but sufficient evidence to allow human experimentation has not yet been acquired. In addition, many investigational agents are being studied in phase I and phase II trials.

Table 3.16 Miscellaneous Agent				
Drug	*Route of Administration*	*Common Treatment Schedules*	*Common Toxicities*	*Disease Treated*
Hexamethylmelamine (altretamine) (Hexalen)	PO	120 mg/m²/day × 14 days every 4 weeks	Nausea and vomiting, myelosuppression, neurotoxicity, skin rashes	Ovarian, breast cancer
Bevacizumab (Avastin)	IV	15 mg/kg every 21 days	Hypertension, proteinuria, bowel perforation	Breast, colon, lung, ovarian cancer

Phase I Trials   These studies define the spectrum of toxicity of a new chemotherapeutic agent and are complete when the dose-limiting toxicity of any particular dose and schedule has been defined.

Phase II Trials   These studies usually use the dose established from phase I trials and apply this dose and schedule to selected tumor types of importance.

Phase III Trials   These studies compare one effective treatment with another in a randomized fashion.

References

1. **Skipper HE, Schabel FM Jr, Mullett LB.** Implications of biochemical, cytokinetic, pharmacologic, and toxicologic relationships in the design of optimal therapeutic schedules. *Cancer Chemother Rep* 1950;54:431–450.

2. **Goldie JH, Coldman AJ.** A mathematical model for relating the drug sensitivity of tumors to their spontaneous mutation rate. *Cancer Treat Rep* 1979;63:1727–1733.

3. **Norton L, Simon R.** Predicting the course of Gompertzian growth. *Nature* 1976;264:542–544.

4. **Norton L, Simon R.** The Norton-Simon hypothesis revisited. *Cancer Treat Rep* 1986;70:163–169.

5. **Ling V.** Drug resistance and membrane alteration in mutants of mammalian cells. *Can J Genet Cytol* 1975;17:503–515.

6. **Hakes TB, Chalas E, Hoskins WJ, et al.** Randomized prospective trial of 5 versus 10 cycles of *cyclophosphamide, doxorubicin,* and *cisplatin* in advanced ovarian carcinoma. *Gynecol Oncol* 1992; 45:284–289.

7. **McGuire WP, Hoskins WJ, Brady MS, Homesley HD, Creasman WT, Berman LM, et al.** Assessment of dose-intensive therapy in suboptimally debulked ovarian cancer: a Gynecologic Oncology Group study. *J Clin Oncol* 1995;13:1589–1599.

8. **Gore M, Mainwaring P, A'Hern R, MacFarlane V, Slevin M, Harper P, et al.** Randomized trial of dose-intensity with single-agent *carboplatin* in patients with epithelial ovarian cancer. *J Clin Oncol* 1998;16:2426–2434.

9. **Mobus V, Wandt H, Frickhofen N, et al.** Phase III trial of high-dose sequential chemotherapy with peripheral blood stem cell support compared with standard dose chemotherapy for first-line treatment of advanced ovarian cancer: Intergroup trial of the AGO-Ovar-AIO and EBMT. *J Clin Oncol* 2007;25:4187–4193.

10. **Grenman S, Wiklund T, Jalkanen J, et al.** A randomized phase III study comparing high-dose chemotherapy to conventionally dosed chemotherapy for stage III ovarian cancer: the Finnish Ovarian Cancer (FINOVA) study. *Eur J Cancer* 2006;42:2196–2199.

11. **Chu E, DeVita VT Jr.** Principles of Medical Oncology. In: **DeVita VT Jr, Hellman S, Rosenberg SA, eds.** *Cancer: principles and practice of oncology,* 7th ed. Philadelphia: Lippincott–Raven Publishers, 2005:295–306.

12. **Markman M.** Intraperitoneal antineoplastic drug delivery: rationale and results. *Lancet Oncol* 2003;4:277–283.

13. **Alberts DS, Liu PY, Hannigan EV, O'Toole R, Williams SD, Young JA, et al.** Intraperitoneal *cisplatin* plus intravenous *cyclophosphamide* versus intravenous *cisplatin* plus intravenous *cyclophosphamide* for stage III ovarian cancer. *N Engl J Med* 1996;335:1950–1955.

14. **Markman M, Bundy BN, Alberts DS, Fowler JM, Clark-Pearson DL, Carson LF, et al.** Phase III trial of standard-dose intravenous *cisplatin* plus *paclitaxel* versus moderately high-dose *carboplatin* followed by intravenous *paclitaxel* and intraperitoneal *cisplatin* in small-volume stage III ovarian carcinoma: an intergroup study of the Gynecologic Oncology Group, Southwestern Oncology Group, and Eastern Cooperative Oncology Group. *J Clin Oncol* 2001;19: 1001–1007.

15. **Armstrong DK, Bundy B, Wenzel L, et al.** Intraperitoneal *cisplatin* and *paclitaxel* in ovarian cancer. *N Engl J Med* 2006;354:34–43.

16. **Markman M, Walker JL.** Intraperitoneal chemotherapy of ovarian cancer: a review, with a focus on practical aspects of treatment. *J Clin Oncol* 2006;24:988–994.

17. **Calvert AH, Newell DR, Gumbrell LA, O'Reilly S, Burnell M, Boxall FE, et al.** *Carboplatin* dosage: prospective evaluation of a simple formula based on renal function. *J Clin Oncol* 1989;7: 1748–1756.

18. **Muggia FM, Hainsworth JD, Jeffers S, Miller P, Groshen S, Tan M, et al.** Phase II study of *liposomal doxorubicin* in refractory ovarian cancer: antitumor activity and toxicity modification by liposomal encapsulation. *J Clin Oncol* 1997;15:987–993.

19. **Perez EA, Rodeheffer R.** Clinical cardiac tolerability of *trastuzumab*. *J Clin Oncol* 2004;22:322–329.

20. **Burger RA, Sill MW, Monk BJ, Greer BE. Sorosky JI.** Phase II trial of *bevicizumab* in persistent or recurrent epithelial ovarian cancer or primary peritoneal cancer: A Gynecologic Oncology Group study. *J Clin Oncol* 2007;25:515–5171.

21. **Connelly E, Markman M, Kennedy A, Webster K, Kulp B, Peterson G, et al.** *Paclitaxel* delivered as a 3-hr infusion with *cisplatin* in patients with gynecologic cancers: unexpected incidence of neurotoxicity. *Gynecol Oncol* 1996;62:166–168.

22. **Markman M, Kennedy A, Webster K, Elson P, Peterson G, Kulp B, et al.** Clinical features of hypersensitivity reactions to *carboplatin*. *J Clin Oncol* 1999;17:1141–1145.

23. **Van Leeuwen FE, Travis LB.** Second cancers. In: **DeVita VT Jr, Hellman S, Rosenberg SA, eds.** *Cancer: principles and practice of oncology,* 7th ed. Philadelphia: Lippincott–Raven Publishers, 2005:2575–2601.

24. **Greene MH, Boice JD Jr, Greer BE, Blessing JA, Dembo AJ.** Acute nonlymphocytic leukemia after therapy with *alkylating agents* for ovarian cancer: a study of five randomized clinical trials. *N Engl J Med* 1982;307:1416–1421.

25. **Travis LB, Holowaty EJ, Bergfeldt K, Lynch CF, Kohler BA, Wiklund T, et al.** Risk of leukemia after platinum-based chemotherapy for ovarian cancer. *N Engl J Med* 1999;340:351–357.

26. **Bower M, Newlands ES, Holden L, Short D, Brock C, Rustin GJS, et al.** EMA/CO for high-risk gestational trophoblastic tumors: results from a cohort of 272 patients. *J Clin Oncol* 1997;15: 2636–2643.

27. **Brewer M, Gershenson DM, Herzog CE, Mitchell MF, Silva EG, Wharton JT.** Outcome and reproductive function after chemotherapy for ovarian dysgerminoma. *J Clin Oncol* 1999;17:2670–2675.

28. **Tangir J, Zelterman D, Ma W, Schwartz PE.** Reproductive function after conservative surgery and chemotherapy for malignant germ cell tumors of the ovary. *Obstet Gynecol* 2003;101:251–257.

29. **Low JJ, Perrin LC, Crandon AJ, Hacker NF.** Conservative surgery to preserve ovarian function in patients with malignant ovarian germ cell tumors: a review of 74 cases. *Cancer* 2000;89:391–398.

30. **Gelmon K.** The taxoids: *paclitaxel* and *docetaxel*. *Lancet* 1994; 344:1267–1272.

31. **Pizzolato JF, Saltz LB.** The *camptothecins*. *Lancet* 2003;361: 2235–2242.

32. **Cannistra SA, Matulonis UA, Person RT, et al.** Phase II study of *bevicizumab* in patients with platinum-resistant ovarian caner or peritoneal serous cancer. *J Clin Oncol* 25:5180–5186.

4 Radiation Therapy

Patricia J. Eifel

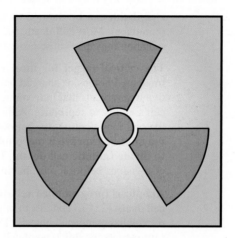

Radiation therapy plays a major role in the treatment of patients with gynecologic malignancies. For women with cervical cancer, radiation therapy is the primary treatment for patients with advanced disease (1,2), yields cure rates equal to those seen after radical surgery for patients with early tumors (3–5), and reduces the risk of local recurrence after surgery for patients with high-risk features (6,7). For women with endometrial cancer, radiation therapy reduces the risk of local recurrence after hysterectomy for patients with high-risk features (8) and is a potentially curative primary treatment for patients with inoperable cancers (9,10). In selected women with ovarian cancer, postoperative, adjuvant, whole-abdominal radiation therapy improves long-term survival (11,12). Radiation therapy is also the primary curative treatment for most patients with invasive vaginal cancer (13,14), and it has an expanding role in the management of carcinomas of the vulva (15–17).

Computer technology and information systems have transformed many aspects of radiation-therapy practice in the past two decades, making possible three-dimensional treatment planning based on computed tomography (CT) and magnetic resonance imaging (MRI), optimized inverse planning, computer-controlled treatment delivery, and remote afterloading brachytherapy. These techniques enable radiation oncologists to restrict radiation-dose distributions to specified target volumes, thereby delivering the maximal dose to the tumor, while sparing normal tissues as much as possible.

Radiation biologists and clinicians have also continued to advance our understanding of the molecular mechanisms involved in radiation-induced cell death, the nature of drug–radiation interactions, and the importance of radiation dose, and the time over which it is given, and the dose per fraction. **In 1999 and 2000, the results of randomized clinical trials demonstrated a significant improvement in pelvic disease control and survival when concurrent chemotherapy was added to radiation therapy for patients with locally advanced cervical cancer** (18–21). These results led to one of the most significant changes in the standard treatment of gynecologic cancers in decades.

In this chapter, the basic principles of radiation therapy, radiation biology, and radiation physics are reviewed and an overview of the indications for and techniques of radiation therapy in the treatment of gynecologic malignancies is presented.

Radiation Biology

Radiation Damage and Repair

Cellular Effects of Ionizing Radiation

Cell death can be defined as the loss of clonogenic capacity (i.e., the ability of the cell to reproduce). Most cell death due to ionizing radiation is mitotic cell death. However, ionizing radiation may also cause programmed cell death (apoptosis).

The critical target for most radiation-induced cell death is the DNA within the cell's nucleus. Photons or charged particles interact with intracellular water to produce highly reactive free radicals that in turn interact with DNA to produce strand breaks that interfere with the cell's ability to reproduce. Although this interaction may cause a cell's "reproductive death," the cell may continue to be metabolically alive for some time. **Radiation-induced damage may not be expressed morphologically until days or months later when the cell attempts to divide (mitotic cell death).** In some cases, a damaged cell may undergo a limited number of divisions before it dies, having lost the ability to reproduce indefinitely.

Apoptosis (programmed cell death) may also play an important role in radiation-induced cell death (22). In contrast to mitotic cell death apoptosis may occur before cell division or after the cell has completed mitosis. **The plasma membrane and nuclear DNA may both be important targets for this type of cell death.** Apoptosis appears to be a particularly important mechanism of radiation-induced cell death in certain postmitotic normal tissues, including human salivary glands and lymphocytes. Radiation-induced apoptosis has also been observed in some proliferating normal tissues and tumors. Biologists are actively studying the pathways that regulate the expression of radiation-induced apoptosis in the hope that they can be exploited to improve local tumor control.

Cell-Survival Curves

The effects of ionizing radiation on the survival of mammalian cell populations *in vitro* are typically expressed graphically as dose-response or *"cell-survival"* curves (23). The surviving fraction of cells is plotted (on an exponential scale) against the dose of radiation (on a linear scale). Experimental data using single doses of sparsely ionizing radiation (e.g., x-rays, gamma rays, electrons, or protons) typically produce cell-survival curves with two components (Fig. 4.1): a shoulder region and an exponential region.

Several mathematical models, based on different hypothetical mechanisms of cell killing, have been devised to describe radiation dose–response relationships. These include:

1. the multitarget model (also referred to as the N-D_0 model)
2. the linear-quadratic model (also referred to as the α/β model)

The multitarget model (Fig. 4.1A) is described by the expression $\log_e N = D_q/D_0$, where N and D_q measure the width of the shoulder and D_0 is the slope of the final exponential portion of the survival curve. This model derives from the classic target theory, which holds that each cell contains multiple sensitive targets, all of which must be hit to kill the cell. The presence of a shoulder region is believed to reflect accumulation of **sublethal injury** in some of the irradiated cells (24). Although the multitarget model accurately describes the exponential portion of the dose–response curve, it is a poor fit to experimental data in the shoulder region. In particular, it fails to predict the approximately linear slope (D_1) of the initial portion of the shoulder (Fig. 4.1B).

The linear-quadratic model describes the dose–response relationship according to the equation $S = e - \alpha + \beta D^2$, where S is the surviving fraction, D is the dose of radiation, and α and β are constants (Fig. 4.1B). This model presupposes two components to cell death: one that is proportional to the dose (αD) and one that is proportional to the square of the dose (βD^2). The dose at which the linear and quadratic components are equal is α/β (Fig. 4.1A). This model fits experimental data particularly well for the first few logs of cell death, which are most relevant to fractionated and low-dose-rate (LDR) irradiation, but it is continuously bending on a log-linear plot. This bend is inconsistent with experimental data that demonstrate a straight line on a log-linear plot for the distal portion of the cell-survival curve.

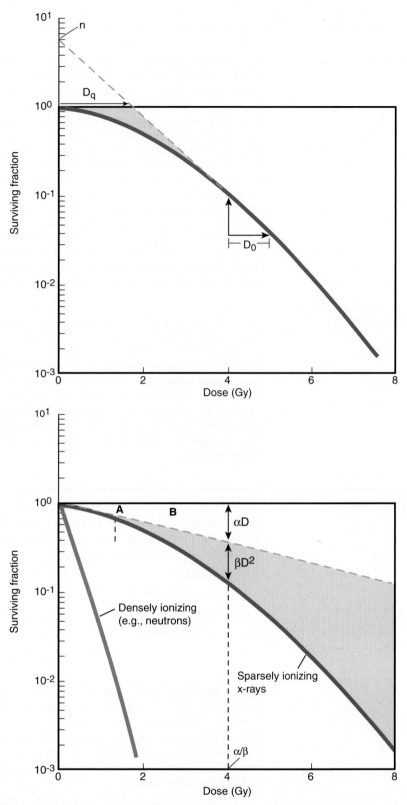

Figure 4.1 **Parameters commonly used to characterize the relationship between radiation dose and cell survival in mammalian culture.** In the multitarget, or N-D_0, model **(A)**, N is the extrapolation number, N and D_q measure the width of the shoulder, and D_0 represents the slope of the final exponential portion of the survival curve. The multitarget model provides an accurate description of experimental data in the exponential portion of the survival curve. The linear-quadratic model **(B)** more accurately describes the shape of the initial shoulder portion of the curve. Because the shoulder has more influence on fractionated radiation therapy, the linear-quadratic model is more often used to predict the results of fractionated clinical radiation therapy. Modified from **Hall EJ.** *Radiobiology for the radiologist,* 5th ed. Philadelphia: Lippincott Williams & Wilkins, 2000, with permission.

Fractionation

Conventional radiation therapy usually is given in a fractionated course with daily doses of 180 to 200 cGy (centiGray) per fraction. Hypothetical cell-survival curves for normal tissue and tumor cells illustrate the advantage of fractionation (Fig. 4.2). When a dose of radiation is divided into multiple smaller doses separated by an interval sufficient to allow maximum repair of sublethal injury, a relatively shallow dose–response curve is achieved, reflecting a repetition of the shoulder of the single-dose cell-survival curve. The slope of the fractionated-dose cell-survival curve depends on the character of the shoulder (N and D_q). The sparing effect of fractionation is greatest for cells with a response to radiation characterized by a relatively broad shoulder, reflecting the cells' greater ability to accumulate and repair sublethal damage during the interfraction interval. Many normal tissues and some poorly responsive tumors exhibit this type of response to fractionated irradiation *in vivo* and *in vitro*. In contrast, most tumors and some acutely responding normal tissues (e.g., bone marrow and intestinal crypt cells) have a dose–response curve with a relatively narrow shoulder, implying relatively little sparing effect of fractionation. **The difference between the *fractionation sensitivity* of tumors and normal tissues is an important determinant of the *therapeutic ratio* (the difference between tumor control and normal tissue complications) of fractionated irradiation.**

Dose-Rate Effect

So far, this discussion of cell-survival curves and fractionation has referred to radiation given in acute exposures—that is, at a rate of 100 cGy per minute or greater. At these dose rates, the shoulder of the survival curve is pronounced. However, **as the dose rate is decreased, cells have a greater opportunity to repair sublethal injury during the exposure. This is called the *dose-rate effect*.** The slope of the survival curve becomes increasingly shallow and the shoulder less apparent (Fig. 4.3) until a dose rate is reached at which all sublethal injury is repaired. **In experimental systems, the dose-rate effect appears to be much more pronounced for normal cells than for tumor cells. This differential effect implies a favorable therapeutic ratio that is exploited with LDR intracavitary and interstitial brachytherapy.**

The Four Rs

The biological effect of a given dose of radiation is influenced by the dose, fraction size, interfraction interval, and time over which the dose is given. Four factors, classically referred to as "the four Rs of radiobiology," govern the influence of dose, time, and fractionation on the cellular response to radiation. These are:

1. repair
2. repopulation
3. redistribution
4. reoxygenation

Repair

As previously discussed, **because fractionated irradiation permits greater recovery of sublethal injury during treatment, a higher total dose of radiation is required to achieve a given biological effect when the total dose is divided into smaller fractions.** The broader the shoulder of the survival curve, the greater the increase in dose required to achieve the same level of cell death achieved by a single dose. Two-dose experiments with varying interfraction intervals indicate that a space of at least 4 hours, and probably more than 6 hours, is necessary to complete repair of accumulated sublethal injury. Clinical studies tend to confirm these findings; for this reason, altered-fractionation protocols usually require a minimum interval of 4 to 6 hours between treatments.

Repopulation

Repopulation **refers to the cell proliferation that occurs during the delivery of radiation.** The magnitude of the effect of repopulation on the dose required to produce a given level of cell death depends on the doubling time of the cells involved. For cells with a relatively short doubling time, a significant increase in dose may be required to compensate for a protraction in the delivery time. This phenomenon may be of considerable practical importance. The speed of repopulation of normal tissues that manifest radiation injury soon after exposure (skin, mucosal surfaces, etc.) limits contraction of a course of fractionated irradiation. However,

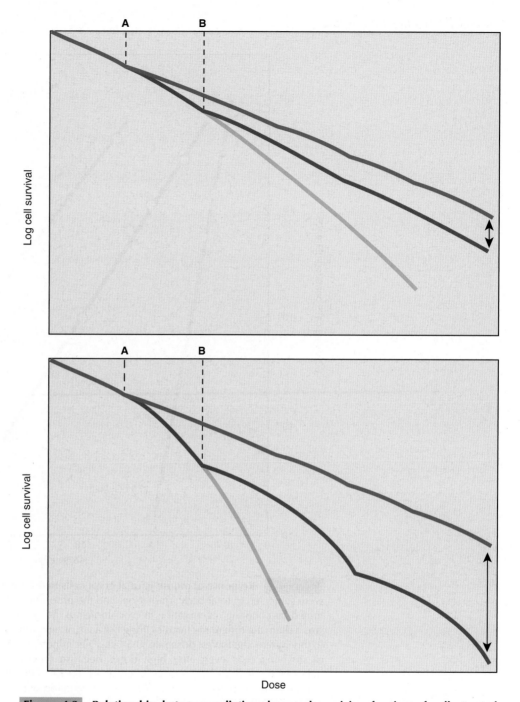

Figure 4.2 Relationship between radiation dose and surviving fraction of cells treated *in vitro* with radiation delivered in a single dose or in fractions. **Top = Most tumors and acutely responding normal tissues. Bottom = Late-responding normal tissues.** For most tumors and acutely responding normal tissues, the cellular response to single doses of radiation is described by a curve with a relatively shallow initial shoulder (Top, yellow line). Cellular survival curves for late-responding normal tissues (Bottom, yellow line) have a more pronounced shoulder, suggesting that these cells have a greater capacity to accumulate and repair sublethal radiation injury. When the total dose of radiation is delivered in several smaller fractions (Dose A [dose/fraction] = blue line, or a larger fraction Dose B [dose/fraction] = red line), the response to each fraction is similar and the overall radiation survival curve reflects multiple repetitions of the initial portion of the single-dose survival curve. Note that the total dose required to kill a specific proportion of the cells decreases as the dose per fraction increases (red line). Arrows indicate the differential effects of relatively large versus small fractions of radiation. The greater differential effects of fractionated irradiation on normal tissues (Bottom) than on tumor (Top) reflect the greater capacity of late-responding normal tissues to accumulate and repair sublethal radiation injury. (From **Karcher KH, Kogelnik HD, Reinartz G [eds]:** *Progress in Radio-Oncology II.* New York, Raven Press, 1982, pp. 287–296).

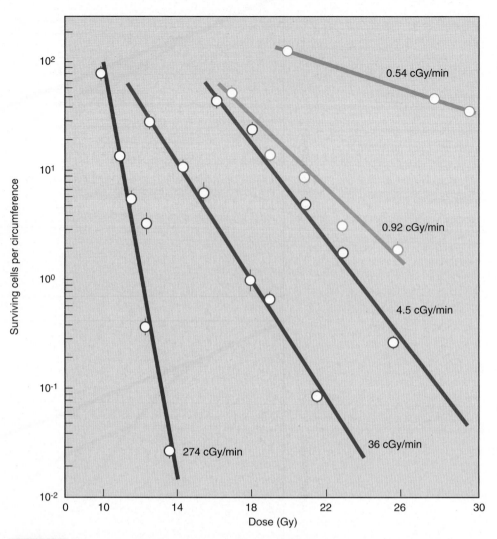

Figure 4.3   **Response of mouse jejunal crypt cells to different dose rates of γ rays.** The mice were subjected to total body irradiation, and the proportion of surviving crypt cells was determined by counting regenerating microcolonies in the crypts 3.5 days after irradiation. There was a dramatic difference in cell killing because of repair of sublethal injury at low dose rates. In this system, the lowest dose rate (0.54 cGy per minute) causes little reduction in the number of surviving cells even after high doses because repopulation during the long exposure balances the cell killing from radiation. From **Fu KK, Phillips TL, Kane LJ, et al.** Tumor and normal tissue response to irradiation *in vivo*: variation with decreasing dose rates. *Radiology* 1975;114:709–716, with permission.

unnecessary protraction probably reduces the effectiveness of a dose of radiation by permitting time for repopulation of malignant clonogens during treatment (25,26). In addition, **cytotoxic treatments—including chemotherapy, radiation therapy, and possibly surgical resection—may actually trigger an increase in the proliferation rate of surviving clonogens. This** *accelerated repopulation* **may increase the detrimental effect of treatment delays and may influence the effectiveness of sequential multimodality treatments (27,28).**

Redistribution

Studies of synchronized cell populations have shown significant differences in the radiosensitivity of cells in different phases of the cell cycle (29). Cells are usually most sensitive to radiation in the late G$_2$ phase and during mitosis and are most resistant in the mid- to late S and early G$_1$ phases. When asynchronous dividing cells receive a fractionated dose of radiation, the first fraction tends to synchronize the cells by killing off those in sensitive phases of the cell cycle. Cells remaining in the S phase then begin to progress to a more sensitive phase of the cell cycle during the interval before the next fraction is given. This redistribution of cells to a more sensitive phase of the cell cycle tends to increase the overall cell death achieved from a fractionated dose of ionizing radiation, particularly if the cells have a relatively short cell cycle time.

Reoxygenation

The sensitivity of fully oxygenated cells to sparsely ionizing radiation is approximately three times that of cells irradiated under anoxic conditions. This makes oxygen the most effective known radiation sensitizer. The molecular interactions responsible for the oxygen effect are not completely understood, but it is believed that oxygen stabilizes the reactive free radicals produced by the ionizing events. The ratio between the dose needed to achieve a given level of cell death under oxygenated versus hypoxic conditions is referred to as the **oxygen enhancement ratio** (Fig. 4.4).

Most normal tissues are fully oxygenated, but significant hypoxia occurs in at least some solid tumors, rendering the resulting hypoxic cells relatively resistant to the effects of radiation. However, **the clinical importance of tumor hypoxia is uncertain because hypoxic cells initially tend to become better oxygenated during a course of fractionated irradiation** (30). This phenomenon, called **reoxygenation,** tends to increase the response of tumors to a dose of fractionated radiation.

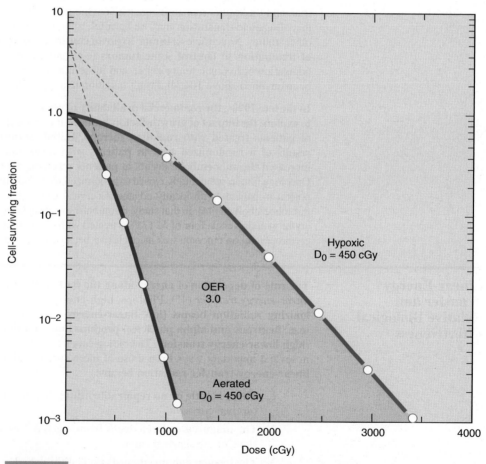

Figure 4.4 **Survival curves for mammalian cells irradiated under aerated and hypoxic conditions.** The dose required to produce a given level of damage is approximately three times greater under hypoxic or anoxic conditions than under fully oxygenated conditions. The ratio of doses is the oxygen enhancement ratio (OER). Sometimes the shoulder also is reduced under hypoxic conditions. Modified from **Hall EJ.** *Radiobiology for the radiologist,* 5th ed. Philadelphia: Lippincott Williams & Wilkins, 2000, with permission.

Treatment Strategies for Overcoming Radioresistance of Hypoxic Cells

Many treatment strategies have been explored to overcome the relative radioresistance of hypoxic cells in human solid tumors (31–35). These include:

1. **hyperbaric oxygen or carbogen breathing**
2. **red cell transfusion or growth factors**
3. **pharmacologic agents** (e.g., *misonidazole*) that act as hypoxic cell sensitizers
4. **high-linear-energy-transfer radiation**

None of these approaches has clearly demonstrated an improvement in outcome; however, most of the studies have been severely compromised by technical or logistical problems.

Numerous retrospective studies have found correlations between the minimum hemoglobin level during treatment and outcome, but all of them have been compromised by possible confounding risk factors (36–38). Even with multivariate analysis, investigators cannot rule out the possibility that patients whose hemoglobin levels fell despite transfusion also had tumors that were more aggressive or less responsive to treatment. Studies of intratumoral oxygen tension also suggest that hypoxic tumors tend to have a poor prognosis; however, this correlation appears to be present even in surgically treated patients and may in part reflect a tendency for biologically aggressive tumors to be hypoxic (39).

An early randomized study of transfusion in anemic patients with locally advanced cervical cancer (40) hinted at improved local control when oxygen-carrying capacity was increased. However, the findings of this small study have not yet been confirmed in a larger prospective trial, and the results remain inconclusive. One group of investigators (41) has even suggested that allogeneic transfusion may be harmful, although their results conflict with those of most other studies. Nevertheless, **tumor hypoxia continues to be one probable cause of the failure of irradiation to control some tumors** (e.g., advanced cervical cancers with a significant population of hypoxic tumor cells), and most clinicians recommend that the hemoglobin level be maintained above 10 g/dl during radiation therapy (42).

In the late 1990s, the commercial availability of recombinant erythropoietin led investigators to explore the impact of growth-factor–induced increases in hemoglobin level on the outcome of patients treated with radiation therapy. Initial enthusiasm was tempered by negative results of a randomized trial in patients with head and neck cancer and by reports of increased thromboembolic events in patients receiving erythropoietin (43). The Gynecologic Oncology Group prematurely closed a randomized trial of chemoradiation with or without erythropoietin in patients with locally advanced cervical cancer because of concerns about the risk of thromboembolism (44). In that study, thrombotic events occurred in 11 of 57 (19.3%) who received erythropoietin versus four of 52 (7.7%) treated with chemoradiation alone ($p = NS$); the impact of erythropoietin on outcome was inconclusive because of the small number of patients in the study.

Linear-Energy Transfer and Relative Biological Effectiveness

The rate of deposition of energy along the path of the radiation beam is referred to as its *linear-energy transfer* (45). **Photons, high-energy electrons, and protons produce sparsely ionizing radiation beams (low linear-energy-transfer), whereas larger atomic particles (e.g., neutrons and alpha particles) produce much more densely ionizing radiation beams (high linear-energy transfer).** The biological effects of densely ionizing radiation beams differ in several important ways from those of more sparsely ionizing radiation beams. **With high-linear-energy-transfer radiation beams:**

1. **There is little or no repairable injury** and therefore no shoulder on the tumor cell-survival curve.
2. **The magnitude of cell death from a given dose is greater,** increasing the terminal slope of the survival curve.
3. **The oxygen enhancement ratio is diminished.**

The unit of *relative biological effectiveness* **is used to compare the effects of different radiation beams. Relative biological effectiveness is defined as the ratio between a test radiation dose and that of 250-kV x-rays needed to produce a specific biological effect.** The relative biological effectiveness may differ somewhat according to the tissue and biological end point being studied.

In practice, few facilities exist for the production of high-linear-energy-transfer beams, and their use has had no major impact on the results of treatment for gynecologic malignancies.

Hyperthermia

Temperature is another factor that can modify the effect of ionizing radiation (46). Supraphysiological temperatures alone can be toxic to cells because heat is preferentially toxic to cells in a low-pH environment (frequent in areas of hypoxia) and to cells in the relatively radioresistant S phase of the cell cycle. **Temperatures in the range of 42° to 43°C sensitize cells to radiation both by reducing the shoulder and by increasing the slope of the cell-survival curve.** Because of the different vascular supplies of tumors and normal tissues, hyperthermia may produce greater temperature elevations in tumors, increasing the possible therapeutic advantage when heat is combined with irradiation. Biologists and clinicians have been trying to find ways to exploit this effect for many years but have been hampered by technological limitations on the ability to selectively heat deep-seated tumors (47). A trial from Amsterdam (48) reported that survival was improved when hyperthermia was used with irradiation in patients with locally advanced cervical cancer. The patients in this study received relatively low doses of radiation, did not receive concurrent chemotherapy, and had poorer than expected pelvic disease control in the control arm, but the findings suggest that the approach may still deserve further study.

Interactions between Radiation and Drugs

Drugs and radiation interact in a number of ways to modify cellular responses. Steel and Peckham (49) categorized these interactions into four groups: spatial cooperation (independent action), additivity, supraadditivity, and subadditivity.

Spatial Cooperation (Independent Action)

Spatial cooperation is the situation in which drugs and radiation act independently with different targets and mechanisms of action so that the total effect of the combination is equal to that of each agent separately. For example, a site that is protected from chemotherapy (e.g., the brain) may be treated with radiation to prevent recurrence. Alternatively, a drug may be used to destroy microscopic distant disease while radiation is used to sterilize local tumor.

Additivity

Additivity is the situation in which two agents act on the same target to cause damage that is equal to the sum of their individual toxic effects.

Supraadditivity

When there is supraadditivity, a drug potentiates the effect of radiation, causing a greater response than would be expected from simple additivity.

Subadditivity

With subadditivity, the amount of cell death that results from the use of two agents is less than that expected from simple additivity (the amount may still be greater than expected from either treatment alone).

Clinically, it is difficult to determine which mode of interaction occurs when two agents are used concurrently. When a greater response is observed than would be expected from radiation alone, the interaction is often described as synergistic but may be only additive or even subadditive.

Therapeutic Ratio

Ionizing radiation interacts with all the tissues in its path, not just tumor tissue. Radiation can be considered an effective cancer treatment only if there is a differential biological effect on tumor and normal tissues. **The difference between tumor control and normal tissue complications is referred to as the therapeutic gain or therapeutic ratio.**

In general, the relationship between the probability of tumor cure or the probability of normal tissue injury and the dose of radiation can be described by a sigmoid curve (Fig. 4.5). At relatively low radiation doses, there is an insufficient amount of cell death to produce any likelihood of tumor cure. As the dose is increased, a threshold is reached at which some cures begin to be observed. For most tumor systems, the likelihood of cure rises rapidly as the radiation dose is increased beyond this threshold and then reaches a plateau. The shape

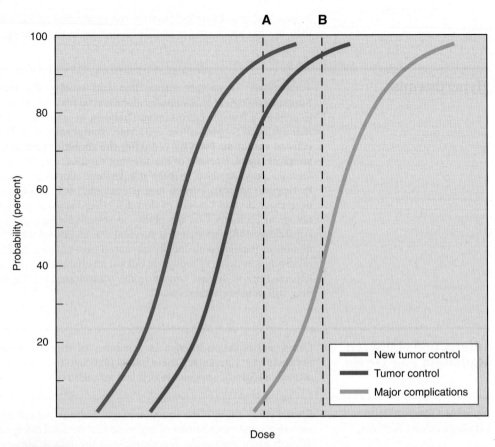

Figure 4.5   Theoretical sigmoid dose–response curves for tumor control and severe complications. The therapeutic ratio is related to the distance between the two curves. Dose A controls tumor in 80% of cases with a 5% incidence of complications. Dose B yields a 10% to 15% increase in the tumor control probability but a much greater risk of complications, narrowing the therapeutic ratio. A leftward shift of the tumor control probability curve (e.g., by the addition of sensitizing drugs) broadens the window for complication-free cure.

and slope of the dose–response curve vary according to the tumor type and size (50, 51). A similar sigmoid relationship is seen when the likelihood of complications is plotted against the radiation dose. If the sigmoid curve for normal tissue complications is to the right of the sigmoid curve for tumor control, then treatment with doses that fall between the two curves may achieve tumor control without causing complications. The difference between these curves represents the **therapeutic ratio.** The primary goal of radiation research efforts is to improve the therapeutic ratio by increasing the separation between these dose–response curves, maximizing the probability of complication-free tumor control.

Effects of Radiation on Normal Tissues

The extent of radiation damage to normal tissues depends on a number of factors, including the radiation dose, the organ, the volume of tissue irradiated, and the division rate of the irradiated cells. **Tissues that have rapid cell turnover (i.e., tissues whose functional activity requires constant cell renewal) tend to manifest radiation injury soon after exposure,** often during a fractionated course of radiation therapy. **Examples of acutely reacting tissues include most epithelia (e.g., skin, hair, gastrointestinal mucosa, bone marrow, and reproductive tissues).** In contrast, **tissues that have slower cell turnover (i.e., tissues whose functional activity does not require constant cell renewal) tend to manifest radiation injury months or years after exposure to radiation. Examples of late-reacting tissues are the connective tissues, muscle, and neural tissues.** In some normal tissues, cell death may occur through the mechanism of apoptosis. Although apoptosis is not the primary mechanism of damage in most normal tissue injury, it is important in the response of lymphocytes, salivary gland cells, and a small proportion of intestinal crypt cells (22).

Acute Reactions

Acute reactions to pelvic irradiation, such as diarrhea, are usually associated with mucosal denudation, which in turn stimulates an increase in cell proliferation (52). This regenerative response is usually sufficient to prevent serious side effects with weekly doses of 900 to 1,000 cGy given in five fractions. This empirically derived schedule is the most commonly used for clinical radiation therapy. If treatment is accelerated to deliver the dose over much shorter periods, then the regenerative capacity of the epithelium may be over-whelmed and the acute reaction so severe that a break in treatment is needed to allow for epithelial regeneration. The severity of acute reactions also depends on the volume of the normal tissues irradiated and the specific nature of the tissues.

Late Reactions

The pathogenesis of late radiation complications (i.e., those that occur months to years after radiation therapy) differs from that of acute reactions and is still incompletely understood. **It has been hypothesized that late effects of radiation result from:**

1. **damage to vascular stroma** that causes an epithelial proliferation with decreased blood supply and subsequent fibrosis

2. **damage to slowly or infrequently proliferating parenchymal stem cells** that eventually results in loss of tissue or organ function (52)

Because late-reacting tissues are not proliferating rapidly, the duration of a course of radiation treatment does not alter their tolerance. However, late-responding normal tissues tend to be quite sensitive to changes in the dose per fraction so that a strong correlation is seen between the radiation fraction size and the risk of late complications. Thus, **for a given dose of radiation administered over a given period, the risk of late effects will be greater with larger fractions.** This fractionation effect is responsible for the advantage of altered fractionation schedules in clinical settings in which late normal tissue reactions are severely dose limiting (53–55) (Fig. 4.2). This fractionation effect also has important implications for treatments such as high-dose-rate (HDR) brachytherapy and intensity-modulated radiation therapy (IMRT), where a portion of the target (and possibly adjacent normal tissues) frequently receives doses of more than 2 Gy per fraction.

The likelihood of developing serious late effects from radiation depends on many factors, including but not limited to the dose of radiation, the radiation dose per fraction, the volume of tissue irradiated, the radiation-dose rate, patient characteristics, other treatments (such as surgery or chemotherapy), and the end point being measured. Some tissues—such as the liver, kidney, and lung—consist of functional subunits that are arranged more or less in parallel; these tissues can tolerate a high dose of radiation given to a small portion of the organ without serious late effects but tend to be relatively sensitive to moderate whole-organ doses. Other organs, such as bowel or ureter, are organized in a serial fashion—delivery of a damaging dose to even a small portion of the organ can cause total organ failure. For all of the reasons discussed previously, normal tissue tolerances cannot be described in terms of simple dose limits. However, some generalizations can be made about the tolerance of individual tissues (doses refer to external radiation given in daily fractions of 1.8 to 2 Gy or with LDR brachytherapy).

Uterus   **The uterus and cervix are typically described as resistant to radiation;** however, what is really meant by this is that the uterus can be treated to very high doses (more than 100 Gy in some cases) without the patient developing serious complications in adjacent critical structures (e.g., bowel and bladder). The uterus probably cannot sustain pregnancy after such doses. Even moderate doses of 40 to 50 Gy probably cause enough smooth muscle atrophy to prohibit successful term pregnancy, but this has rarely been tested. Women who received 20 to 30 Gy or more to the uterus during the perimenarchal period have become pregnant but tend to have spontaneous second-trimester abortions, probably because of underdevelopment of the uterus. Patches of endometrium frequently continue to function after doses of 50 Gy or more.

Ovary   **The radiation dose required to cause ovarian failure is highly dependent on the patient's age.** Perimenarchal girls may continue to menstruate and can even become pregnant after receiving as much as 30 Gy to the ovaries; however, they usually experience premature menopause 10 to 20 years later. **Most adult women have ovarian failure after 20 Gy;** as little as 5 to 10 Gy can induce menopause in older premenopausal women.

Vagina   The radiation tolerance of the vagina depends on the region (upper, mid-, lower, anterior, posterior, or lateral) and length of vagina treated as well as radiation dose, fraction size, dose rate, hormonal support, and other factors. **Small portions of the surface of the lateral apical vagina can be treated to a very high dose ($\geq$140 Gy) without causing major complications in adjacent structures.** However, these high doses do cause atrophy and shortening of the apical vagina. The vaginal tolerance dose is less if treatment includes more than the apical vagina or if the dose includes the posterior, or distal vagina. Even moderate doses (40 to 50 Gy) may decrease the elasticity of the vagina, although it is sometimes difficult to distinguish the direct effects of radiation from those of tumor, altered hormonal environment, aging, and other factors.

Small Intestine   The risk of small intestinal side effects is highly dependent on the radiation dose and volume irradiated and on the patient's history. **In the absence of complicating factors, the entire small intestine can tolerate doses of as much as 30 Gy without major late effects.** Smaller volumes can tolerate 45 to 50 Gy with a low risk of complications; the risk of chronic diarrhea and bowel obstruction increases rapidly with doses greater than 60 Gy and approaches 100% if a significant volume of small bowel receives 70 Gy or more. The risk of bowel obstruction is significantly increased in patients who have a history of major transperitoneal surgery, pelvic infection, or heavy smoking (56).

Rectum   **In most cases, the entire rectum can tolerate 45 to 50 Gy with a low risk of major sequelae. Small portions of the anterior rectal wall can tolerate doses of at least 70 to 75 Gy.** However, the risk of serious late effects (severe bleeding, obstruction, fistula) increases steeply as the volume of rectum treated to high dose is increased.

Bladder   **The entire bladder can be treated to 45 to 50 Gy with a very low rate of serious morbidity.** This dose may have subtle effects on bladder contractility, particularly in patients who have also undergone radical hysterectomy. **Small portions of the bladder tolerate doses of 80 Gy or more with a low risk of major morbidity (severe bleeding, contracture, fistula).** However, the dose–response relationship is poorly defined in this range because it is difficult to accurately determine the maximum dose given to the bladder during intracavitary treatments.

Ureter   **Surgically undisturbed ureters appear to tolerate 85 to 90 Gy** of combined external-beam and LDR intracavitary treatment with a low risk of stricture.

Kidneys   **Most patients can tolerate as much as 18 to 22 Gy to both kidneys** with very little risk of long-term damage. Higher doses cause permanent damage to renal parenchyma. If the patient has normal renal function, then 50% or more of the renal parenchyma can be treated to a high dose without causing renal failure; however, renal hypertension may occur if an entire kidney is obliterated with radiation. Underlying renal disease or concurrent use of chemotherapy can decrease renal tolerance.

Liver   **In most cases, the liver can tolerate as much as 30 Gy** (at 1.5 Gy per fraction) to the entire organ, although this dose will cause transient elevation of alkaline phosphatase levels and can cause dysfunction in a small proportion of patients. Higher doses cause serious damage to liver parenchyma but can be tolerated if delivered to a portion of the liver only. Tolerance is highly dependent on underlying hepatic function and can be markedly decreased with concurrent delivery of some chemotherapeutic agents and during periods of hepatocyte regeneration (for example, after partial hepatectomy).

Spinal Cord and Nerves   Transverse myelitis and paralysis can occur in a small proportion of patients who receive doses as low as 50 Gy to the spinal cord, and the risk increases rapidly as the dose approaches 60 Gy at 2 Gy per fraction. However, **peripheral nerves, including the cauda equina,** are rarely affected after 50 Gy and **usually tolerate doses as high as 60 Gy without serious sequelae.**

Bone   As little as 10 to 15 Gy of radiation causes transient depletion of bone marrow elements. **With doses of more than 30 to 40 Gy, permanent damage is done to supporting elements, and bone marrow within the irradiated area will not repopulate normally.** This damage can be seen as fatty replacement of the marrow cavity on MRI. The risk of fracture after radiation therapy depends on the bone irradiated, the volume of bone in the high-dose region, bone density, coexistent steroid use, and other factors. **Symptomatic fracture is rare**

after treatment with 40 to 45 Gy of pelvic radiation. However, routine MRI sometimes detects small, usually asymptomatic insufficiency fractures of the pelvis after this dose (57). Hip fracture may be seen after doses as low as 40 Gy to the entire femoral head and neck, and the risk probably increases rapidly as the dose approaches 60 Gy.

Treatment Strategies to Exploit Differences between Tumor and Normal Tissue in the Response to Fractionated Radiation Therapy

A variety of altered fractionation schemes have been devised to exploit the different sensitivities of tumor and normal tissues to fractionation and the possible effects of tumor cell repopulation. These include **hyperfractionation,** in which the dose per fraction is reduced, the number of fractions and total dose are increased, and the overall treatment time is relatively unchanged; **accelerated fractionation,** in which the dose per fraction is unchanged, the overall treatment duration is reduced, and the total dose is unchanged or decreased; and **hypofractionation,** in which the dose per fraction is increased, the number of fractions and total dose are reduced, and the overall treatment time is decreased.

With hyperfractionation, treatment is usually given two or more times daily with at least 4 to 6 hours between fractions to allow repair of sublethal injury. This scheme should permit delivery of a higher dose of radiation without increasing the risk of late complications or the overall duration of treatment. Hyperfractionation schemes may have an advantage if the increased dose delivered per day does not cause unacceptable acute effects and if patients are willing to accept the added inconvenience of two or three treatments daily.

Accelerated fractionation schemes do not reduce the risk of late effects and tend to increase the acute effects of treatment but may be advantageous because treatment is completed over a shorter time, reducing tumor cell repopulation during treatment (55). However, such schemes are likely to be of limited value in the management of gynecologic malignancies because acute side effects tend to limit the rate of treatment delivery.

Hypofractionation schedules are usually avoided when treatment is likely to cure the patient because the α/β of late-responding normal tissues is less than the α/β of most tumors, meaning that large fractions have a therapeutic disadvantage. Malignant melanoma, which appears to have a relatively low α/β, may be a rare exception to this pattern. Hypofractionated schedules are frequently used for palliative treatment because they are convenient and produce rapid symptom relief. However, **the necessary reduction in dose reduces the likelihood of complete eradication of tumor within the treatment field. Hypofractionation may be particularly beneficial if the tumor target is some distance from critical structures and if the radiation treatment plan is characterized by a rapid dose gradient** such that the target receives a relatively high dose per fraction while normal tissue structures receive no more than approximately 2 Gy per fraction. Under ideal circumstances, HDR brachytherapy plans and some highly conformal external-beam plans achieve this favorable geometry.

Combinations of Surgery and Radiation Therapy

Because surgery and radiation therapy are both effective treatments, clinicians have tried to improve locoregional control or reduce treatment morbidity by combining the two modalities. **Theoretically, surgery may remove bulky tumor that may be difficult to control with tolerable doses of radiation, and radiation may sterilize microscopic disease at the periphery of the surgical bed.** The two modalities have been combined in a number of ways:

1. **preoperative irradiation**
2. **diagnostic surgery (surgical staging) followed by definitive irradiation**
3. **intraoperative irradiation**
4. **surgical resection followed by postoperative irradiation**
5. **combinations of these approaches**

Preoperative Irradiation

Preoperative irradiation is sometimes used to sterilize possible microscopic disease at the margins of a planned operative site. This is potentially most useful when the surgeon anticipates close margins adjacent to a critical structure—for example, the urethra or anus in a patient with locally advanced vulvar cancer.

Preoperative irradiation has largely been abandoned in favor of postoperative irradiation, which can be planned when information from the surgical specimen is available and which avoids unnecessarily treating patients with very-early-stage disease. Preoperative irradiation is still sometimes used to treat patients with stage II endometrial cancer that grossly involves the cervix and is also used in some patients with bulky cervical cancers. This is because the dose deliverable to paravaginal tissues is much greater when the uterus is still in place to hold an intrauterine applicator than after surgery, when only an intravaginal applicator can be used.

Some studies have suggested that lower doses of radiation may be required to sterilize microscopic disease in a tumor bed undisturbed by surgery because an intact vascular supply is better able to deliver oxygen. Because the risk of operative complications is increased after high-dose radiation, doses given when surgical resection is anticipated are usually lower than doses given when a tumor is irradiated definitively. **The greatest risk of preoperative radiation therapy is that if the tumor remains unresectable, the effectiveness of additional irradiation will be markedly decreased by the long interval between treatments.**

Intraoperative Irradiation

In some cases, intraoperative irradiation can be delivered with a permanent implant (using ^{125}I or ^{198}Au), with afterloading catheters in the operative bed (using ^{192}Ir), or with a special electron beam or orthovoltage unit in the operating room. These approaches deliver radiation directly to the site of maximum risk when the target can be visualized directly and normal tissues nearest the treatment area can be removed from the radiation field. **Removal of normal tissues from the treatment field is an important physical advantage of intraoperative external-beam techniques** that must counterbalance the biological disadvantage to any normal tissues remaining in the field when an entire dose is delivered in a single large fraction.

Postoperative Irradiation

Postoperative irradiation has been demonstrated to improve locoregional control and even survival in several settings important to gynecologic oncologists. **In vulvar cancer,** postoperative pelvic and groin irradiation reduces the risk of groin recurrence and improves the survival rate of patients with multiple positive inguinal nodes (16). **In endometrial cancer,** postoperative pelvic irradiation reduces the incidence of pelvic recurrences in patients with high-risk disease (8,58,59). **In cervical cancer,** postoperative pelvic irradiation reduces pelvic recurrence in patients with lymph node involvement and in those with high-risk features in the primary tumor (6,7).

Combination Approaches

Combined therapy is optimized when the treatment plan exploits the complementary advantages of the two treatments. This requires close cooperation between specialists at the time of the patient's initial evaluation. Because the morbidity of combined therapy is often greater than that of single-modality therapy, combined treatment should usually be limited to situations in which a combined approach is likely to improve survival, permit organ preservation, or significantly reduce the risk of local recurrence compared with the expected results from treatment with either modality alone (60).

Physical Principles

Ionizing Radiations Used in Therapy

Ionizing radiations lie on the high-energy portion of the electromagnetic spectrum and are characterized by their ability to excite, or ionize, atoms in an absorbing material. The nuclear decay of radioactive nuclei can produce several types of radiation, including uncharged gamma (γ) rays, negatively charged beta (β) rays (electrons), positively charged alpha (α) particles (helium ions), and neutrons. The resulting ionizing radiations are exploited therapeutically in brachytherapy treatments (using ^{226}Ra, ^{137}Cs, ^{186}Ir, and other isotopes) or to produce teletherapy beams (e.g., ^{60}Co). The average energy of the photons produced by the decay of radioactive cobalt is 1.2 million eV (MeV).

Most external-beam therapy is delivered via linear accelerators that produce photon beams (x-rays) by bombarding a target such as tungsten with accelerated electrons. Varying the energy of the accelerated electrons produces therapeutic x-rays of different energies. X-rays and γ-rays are both composed of photons and differ only in that x-rays are produced by extranuclear forces and γ-rays are produced by intranuclear forces.

Interactions of Radiation with Matter

X-Rays and γ-Rays

Photons interact with matter by means of three distinct mechanisms: the photoelectric effect, Compton scatter, and pair production.

The photoelectric effect is most important at energies used for diagnostic purposes. Absorption by the photoelectric effect is proportional to Z^3, where Z is the atomic number of the absorbing material. This effect is responsible for the increased absorption of bone that provides contrast between bone and soft tissue with diagnostic x-ray beams of 250 kV or less. However, the increased bone absorption, high skin dose, and poor penetration with such beams make these beams unsuitable for most modern therapeutic applications. Superficial kilovoltage radiation beams, delivered using a transvaginal cone, are occasionally used for patients with large bleeding exophytic tumors to achieve hemostasis before definitive treatment (61).

Modern therapeutic beams of 1 to 20 megavolts (MV) produce photons that interact with tissues primarily by Compton scatter. In this process, incident photons interact with loosely bound outer-shell electrons, ejecting them from the atom. Both the photon and the electron go on to interact with other atoms, causing additional ionizations. Compton-scatter absorption is independent of Z but varies according to the density of the absorbing material. This accounts for the poor contrast of radiation portal verification films.

Photons that are absorbed by Compton scatter produce an increasing number of scattered electrons and ionizations as they penetrate beneath the surface of an absorbing material. This creates a buildup region just below the surface that is responsible for the **skin-sparing** characteristic of modern high-energy therapy beams (Fig. 4.6). **The maximum dose from a megavoltage beam is reached at 0.5 to 3.0 cm below the skin surface, depending on the photon energy.** At greater depths, the dose decreases at a fairly constant rate that is related to the beam energy. The greater skin-sparing effects and penetration of energy beams of 15 MV or greater make them particularly useful for pelvic treatment.

Pair production absorption is related to Z^2. In soft tissue, this type of absorption begins to dominate only at photon energies of more than approximately 30 MeV, so pair production is of limited importance in current radiation therapy planning.

Electrons and Other Particles

Several types of particle beams are used in radiation therapy: electron beams, proton beams, and neutron beams.

Electrons are very light particles. When they interact with matter, they tend to lose most of their energy in a single interaction. The dose from an electron beam is relatively homogenous up to a depth that is related to the beam's energy (Fig. 4.6). Beyond this depth, the dose decreases very rapidly to nearly zero. Electrons are used to treat relatively superficial targets without delivering a significant dose to underlying tissues. The approximate depth (in centimeters) at which the rapid falloff in dose occurs can be estimated by dividing the electron energy by 3.

Protons are positively charged particles that are much heavier than electrons. Protons scatter minimally as they interact with matter, deposit increasing amounts of energy as they slow down, and then stop at a depth related to their initial energy. This results in rapid deposition of most of their energy at depth (called the **Bragg peak**), with a steep falloff in dose to near zero shortly after the peak. Modulating the energy can spread this peak out. **The absence of an exit dose makes proton beams ideal for conformal therapy, and interest in their use has increased as the cost of producing proton generators has become somewhat more reasonable.** The physics support, quality assurance, and clinical requirements needed to safely treat patients with protons are complex, highly specialized, and time consuming. Although in some difficult clinical situations, protons clearly provide at least a theoretical dosimetric advantage over photons, there are as yet no randomized comparisons. Also, because the depth of penetration of protons is highly dependent on the density of intervening tissue, the presence of variable gas-filled structures (e.g., bowel) in the midpelvis may limit applications in gynecologic oncology.

97

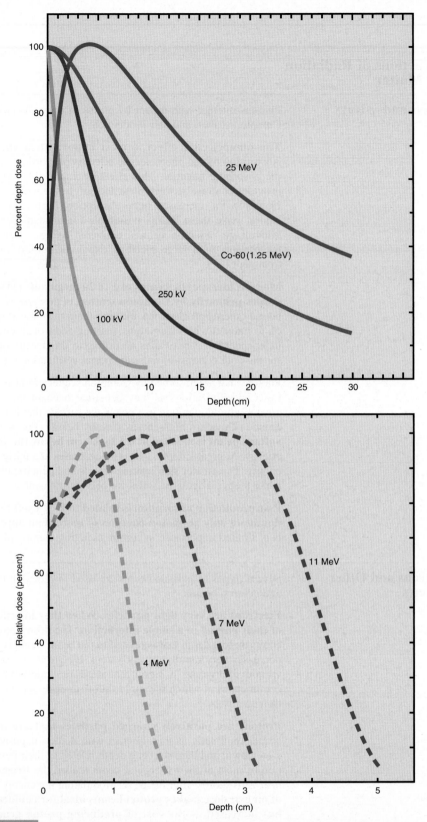

Figure 4.6 **Depth dose curves for selected x-ray and γ-ray beams (top).** As the energy increases, the depth of maximum dose (D_{max} or D_{100}) increases. For kilovoltage beams, the dose is maximum at the skin surface. With appositionally directed megavoltage beams (e.g., ^{60}Co or 25-MeV photon beams), the maximum dose is reached at a depth beyond the skin surface, producing skin sparing. High-energy beams also penetrate more deeply, making them more useful for treatment of deep-seated pelvic tumors.
Depth dose curves for electron beam fields of selected energies (bottom). The depth of maximum dose increases with increasing energy. At depths just below the maximum, the dose falls off rapidly, sparing deeper tissues.

Neutrons are neutral particles that tend to deposit most of their energy in a single intranuclear event. For this reason, there is little or no repairable injury and therefore no shoulder on the tumor cell-survival curve. The falloff of a neutron dose is similar to that of a photon beam of 4 to 6 MV, but the high relative biological effectiveness of densely ionizing neutron beams has been of interest to clinical investigators. However, **clinical studies of neutron treatments in cervical cancer patients were plagued by high complication rates** (62), and neutrons are rarely if ever used to treat gynecologic tumors today.

Measurement of Absorbed Dose

Absorbed dose is a measure of the energy deposited by the radiation source in the target material. **The unit currently used to measure radiation dose is the Gray (Gy), equal to 1 joule per kilogram of absorbing material.** Before the early 1980s, absorbed doses of radiation were measured in radians (rads), where 1 rad = 1 cGy and 1 Gy = 100 rad.

The rate of decay of a sample of radioactive material (such as radium or cesium) is referred to as the activity of the sample and is measured in curies (Ci), where 1 Ci = 3.7×10^{10} disintegrations per second, and 1 mCi = 10^{-3} Ci.

Safe delivery of radiation depends on precise calibration of radiation source activities and machine output. These are measured using sensitive ionization chambers in *phantoms* that simulate tissue density. Periodic calibrations of equipment and sources are a vital part of quality assurance in any radiation oncology department.

Inverse Square Law

The dose of radiation from a source to any point in space varies according to the inverse of the square of the distance from the source to the point (63). This relationship is particularly important for brachytherapy applications because it results in a rapid falloff of dose as distance from an intracavitary or interstitial source is increased.

Radiation Techniques

Radiation therapy is delivered in three ways.

1. **Teletherapy:** X-rays are delivered from a source at a distance from the body (external-beam therapy).
2. **Brachytherapy:** Radiation sources are placed within or adjacent to a target volume (intracavitary or interstitial therapy).
3. **Radioactive solutions:** Solutions that contain isotopes (e.g., radioactive colloidal gold or ^{32}P) are introduced into a cavity (e.g., the peritoneum) to treat the walls of the cavity.

Teletherapy

Several terms are commonly used to describe the dose distributions produced by external-beam irradiation of tissues.

Percentage depth dose is the change in dose with depth along the central axis of a radiation beam (Fig. 4.6).

$D_{\mathbf{max}}$ is the maximum dose delivered to the treated tissue. With a single appositional photon beam, the D_{max} is located at a distance below the tissue surface that increases with the energy of the photon beam (Fig. 4.6).

Source to skin distance is the distance between the source of x-rays (e.g., a cobalt source or the target in a linear accelerator) and the skin surface.

Isocenter is a point within the patient that remains a fixed distance from the radiation source as the treatment source (gantry) is rotated around the patient (Fig. 4.7).

Source to axis distance is the distance from the source of x-rays to the isocenter.

Isodose curve is a line or surface that connects points of equal radiation dose (Fig. 4.8).

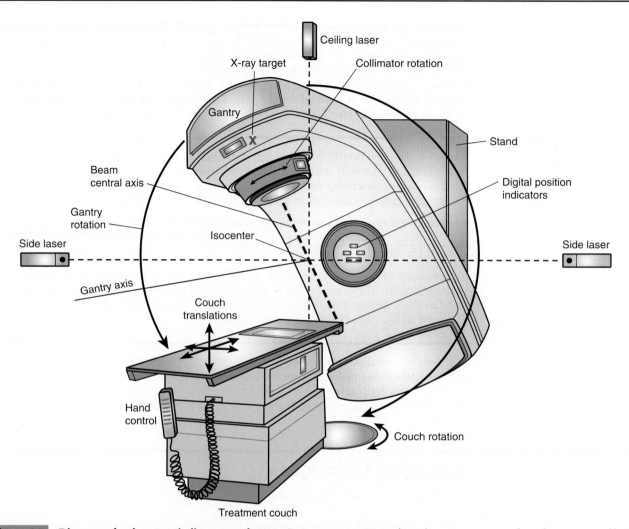

Figure 4.7   Diagram of a therapeutic linear accelerator. Patients are positioned on the treatment couch with a system of lasers that are aligned precisely with the center of the radiation beam. Collimators in the treatment head, located on a rotating gantry, define the size and rotation of the radiation field. The treatment couch can also be rotated around the central axis of the radiation beam. Beam-modifying devices such as shielding blocks and wedges can be attached to a tray beneath the collimator (not shown). From **Karzmark CJ, Nunan CS, Tanabe E.** *Medical electron accelerators.* New York: McGraw-Hill, 1993, with permission.

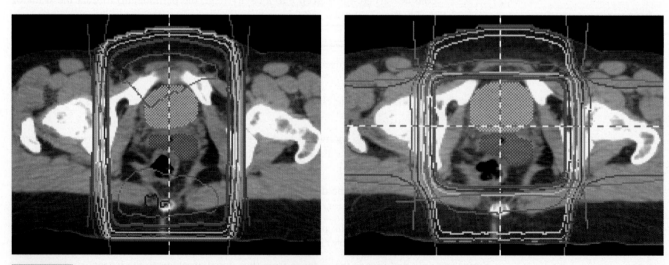

Figure 4.8   Isodose distribution for external-beam irradiation of the pelvis using an 18-MV beam. (A) A pair of parallel opposed anterior and posterior fields. **(B)** Anterior, posterior, and two lateral fields (four-field box technique). The heavy red isodose line represents the region of tissue treated to ≥45 Gy.

Many factors influence the dose distribution in tissue from a single external beam of photons. These include:

1. **The energy of the beam** (determined by its voltage). Higher-energy photon beams are more penetrating than lower-energy beams. In other words, the dose of radiation delivered to deep tissues relative to more superficial tissues is greater with higher-energy beams. Higher-energy beams also have a larger **buildup region** than lower-energy beams; this results in a relative sparing of the skin surface, facilitating irradiation of deep tissues (Fig. 4.6).

2. **The distance from the source to the patient.** As the source to skin distance increases, the percentage depth dose increases.

3. **The size of the radiation field.** The percentage depth dose increases with increasing field size because of the increasing contribution of internal scatter to the radiation dose. This effect is greatest with relatively low-energy radiation beams.

4. **The patient's contour and the angle of the beam's incidence.**

5. **The density of tissues in the target volume** (particularly air versus soft tissue).

6. **A variety of beam-shaping devices placed between the radiation source and the patient** that alter the shape or distribution of the radiation dose.

Modern linear accelerators permit many variations in these factors (Fig. 4.7). A rotational gantry permits *isocentric* beam arrangements that maintain a fixed distance between the beam's source and a point within the patient. This facilitates accurate patient setup and treatment planning.

Most radiation therapy treatment plans combine two or more beams to create a dose distribution designed to accomplish three aims: (i) **to maximize the dose of radiation delivered to the target;** (ii) **to produce a relatively homogeneous dose within the volume of interest** to minimize hot or cold spots that would increase the risks of complications or recurrence, respectively; and (iii) **to minimize the dose delivered to uninvolved tissues,** taking into account the different tolerances of various normal tissues.

The treatment plan must include the primary target volume (gross tumor or tumor bed), any areas at risk for microscopic spread of disease, and a margin of tissue to account for uncertainties in the location of the target, reproducibility of the setup, and organ motion. The overall plan is often designed to deliver different doses to areas of greater or lesser risk (e.g., gross versus microscopic residual disease) by boosting areas at greater risk with smaller treatment fields after initial treatment to a relatively large volume. Two opposing beams (e.g., anterior–posterior and posterior–anterior) usually produce a relatively homogeneous distribution of dose within the intervening tissue with some sparing of the skin surface. In many cases, **multiple fields may be used to "focus" the high-dose region to conform more closely to a deep target volume** (Fig. 4.8).

Modern technology has made it possible to use computers to optimize the beam arrangements required in treatment plans that incorporate many fields and beam-shaping devices. These conformal treatment plans may provide a very tight distribution of dose around the target volume. The simplest form of conformal therapy uses fairly conventional beam arrangements but exploits modern CT-based treatment-planning techniques to more accurately define the target volume and to design blocks that conform closely to that volume. CT reconstructions permit more accurate shaping of fields that enter the patient from oblique angles. **Multileaf collimators** have computer-controlled leaves that can form irregularly shaped fields, replacing hand-loaded beam-shaping devices. Because the therapist no longer needs to enter the room to replace blocks on each field, it is possible to treat patients with more fields and more complex beam arrangements in a treatment visit of acceptable duration.

More recently, attention has been focused on IMRT (Fig. 4.9). This form of highly conformal radiation therapy uses complex computer algorithms to optimize delivery of radiation from multiple beam angles. The physician must carefully contour target volumes and all critical normal tissue structures on each slice of a CT scan that has been obtained in the treatment position. The minimum and maximum acceptable doses of radiation to be delivered to each area are specified. Inverse planning techniques (based on the physician's designation of targets and avoidance structures rather than specific radiation fields) are used to design an optimized plan, which usually includes multiple irregularly shaped fields from each of several (usually six to nine) beam angles.

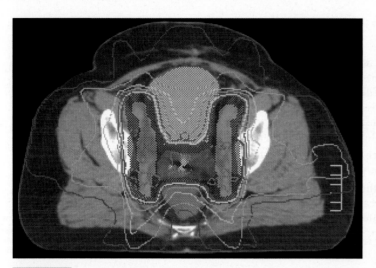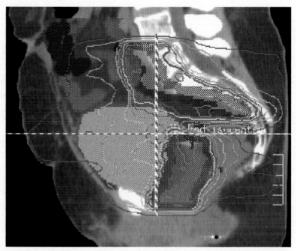

Figure 4.9   **Dose distribution obtained using intensity-modulated radiation therapy (IMRT) to treat the pelvic lymph nodes after hysterectomy.** In this case, each of seven fields was modulated to obtain a distribution that covered the iliac and presacral lymph nodes while sparing bowel in the central pelvis from high dose. A somewhat larger volume receives low-dose radiation than with standard techniques, and the very tight dose distribution requires an accurate understanding of anatomy, tissues at risk, and internal organ motion.

The leaves of multileaf collimators enter the field or retract dynamically to deliver the desired amount of radiation to tissues within the target. Very tightly conforming radiation distributions can be obtained with this approach. However, the time required to plan treatments is lengthened, as is the duration of daily treatments. Quality assurance is also very demanding for this type of treatment because the fields are less readily visualized than static radiation fields. **In the past 5 years, the use of IMRT and other highly conformal radiation techniques has increased exponentially.** In many cases, **these techniques clearly can be used to reduce the dose delivered to normal tissues** during a course of radiation therapy. However, the opportunities for error also are increased; unlike traditional treatments that were based on relatively simple, empirically tested field shapes and distributions, **IMRT plans are entirely dependent on the clinician's understanding of the target volume and tissues at risk.** If the clinician misses or fails to correctly designate tissues at risk for disease, the computerized inverse planning process will tend to result in exclusion of areas of possible tumor involvement or overtreatment of critical structures. **Because the dose of radiation falls off rapidly outside the designated target volume, IMRT plans require a high degree of confidence in the distribution of disease, a clear understanding of internal organ motion, and meticulous patient immobilization. Because there are as yet no level-1 data confirming the benefit of IMRT in treatment of gynecologic neoplasms,** payers may consider the treatment experimental and decline payment.

Brachytherapy

Intracavitary Treatment

Any treatment that involves placement of radioactive sources within an existing body cavity is termed *intracavitary* treatment. The most common gynecologic applications of intracavitary therapy involve placement of intrauterine or intravaginal applicators that are subsequently loaded with encapsulated radioactive sources (e.g., ^{137}Cs or ^{192}Ir) (Table 4.1). Applicator systems vary in their appearance and configuration, but those used for radical treatment of cervical or uterine cancer tend to have several features in common. These applicators usually consist of a hollow tube, or **tandem,** and some form of intravaginal receptacle for additional sources. The greatest variation between systems is in the vaginal applicators, which differ in their shape, the orientation of sources, and the presence or absence of shielding (64,65). One applicator that is commonly used to treat intact carcinomas of the cervix is the Fletcher-Suit-Delclos system. Important characteristics of this system are the arrangement of vaginal sources perpendicular to the tandem and the presence of internal shielding that reduces the dose to the rectum from the vaginal sources by as much as 25%. The Fletcher-Williamson applicator (Fig. 4.10) is similar to the Fletcher-Suit-Delclos applicator but is adapted for use with an iridium stepping source (66).

Table 4.1 Isotopes Used in Gynecologic Oncology				
Element	Isotope	Half-Life	E_γ (MeV)	E_β (MeV)
Phosphorus	^{32}P	14.3 days	None	1.7 (max)
Iodine	^{125}I	60.2 days	0.028_{avg}	None
	^{131}I	8.06 days	0.08–0.63	0.61 (max)
Cesium	^{137}Cs	30 years	0.662	0.514, 1.17
Iridium	^{192}Ir	74 days	0.32–0.61	0.24, 0.67
Gold	^{198}Au	2.7 days	0.41–1.1	0.96 (max)
Radium	^{226}Ra	1,620 years	0.19–0.6	3.26 (max)
Cobalt	^{60}Co	5.26 years	1.17–1.33	0.313 (max)

E_γ, gamma-ray energy; E_β, beta-ray energy; MeV, million electron volts.

The vaginal ring applicator is commonly used with high dose rate HDR systems and has geometry similar to that of the unshielded Delclos miniovoids used with Fletcher-type applicator systems. Other applicator systems, such as the Delclos dome cylinder, have been designed specifically for treatment of the vaginal apex after hysterectomy (67).

Figure 4.11 illustrates a typical pear-shaped isodose distribution produced by a line of intrauterine sources and Fletcher-Suit-Delclos vaginal colpostats loaded with ^{137}Cs. **Intracavitary brachytherapy has proven very useful in the treatment of cervical cancer because it allows a very high dose of radiation to be delivered to a small volume surrounding the applicator** (i.e., the cervix and paracervical tissues) without excessive treatment of normal tissues that are

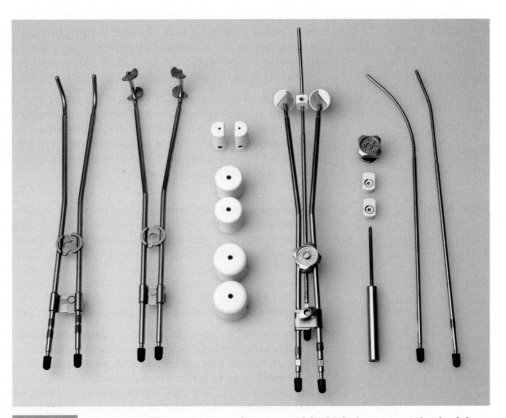

Figure 4.10   Fletcher-Williamson type applicators used for high-dose-rate and pulsed dose-rate intracavitary applications. Note the tungsten shields located in the inferior-medial position anteriorly and posteriorly in the small (2 cm) ovoid inserts.

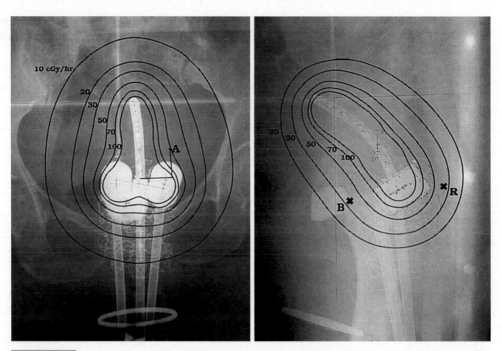

Figure 4.11 **Posterior–anterior and lateral views of a Fletcher-Suit–Delclos applicator system loaded with** ^{137}**Cs sources for treatment of invasive cervical cancer.** Units on the isodose contours are cGy per hour. Point A *(A)*, bladder *(B)*, and rectal *(R)* reference points are indicated on the figure. From **Eifel PJ, Berek JS, Thigpen JT.** Cancer of the cervix, vagina, and vulva. In **DeVita V, Hellman S, Rosenberg S, eds.** *Cancer: principles and practice of oncology.* Philadelphia: JB Lippincott Co., 2001;1526–1556, with permission.

more distant from the sources. Because of the rapid change in dose over short distances, accurate positioning of the intracavitary applicator and sources is very important. Packing or retraction of the bladder and rectum can significantly reduce the dose to portions of these organs by distancing them from the vaginal sources.

To minimize the exposure of medical personnel to radiation, most modern applicator systems are loaded with radioactive sources after adequate positioning has been confirmed with anterior–posterior and lateral x-rays of the pelvis. In many cases, **remote afterloading devices are used to automatically retract sources from the applicator to a lead-lined safe when someone enters the patient's room,** further reducing the radiation exposure to visitors and medical personnel.

Dose Rate

Historically, most brachytherapy was delivered at a low dose rate, most commonly 40 to 60 cGy per hour. These dose rates take maximum advantage of the dose-rate effect described above, differentially sparing late-responding normal tissues as compared with acutely responding tissues and tumor cells. The dose of LDR intracavitary therapy needed to radically treat cervical cancer is usually delivered in 72 to 96 hours during one or two hospital admissions. Although some investigators have tried to reduce the duration of these treatments by doubling the dose rate (from 40 cGy per hour to 80 cGy per hour), the limited clinical data on this approach suggest that doubling the dose rate results in a less favorable therapeutic ratio (68).

In the past two decades, the advent of computer-controlled remote afterloading has made it possible to deliver brachytherapy treatments at high dose rates (in minutes rather than hours). **HDR treatment may offer practical advantages for the patient because it is typically performed on an outpatient basis,** although more applications are usually required. **With this technique, a single very high activity source of** ^{192}**Ir is remotely inserted into the intracavitary applicator.** Based on the treatment plan, during each treatment the source is advanced in individual "steps" to deliver radiation throughout the treatment volume. Because of the high activity of the source (usually about 10 Ci), treatment must be delivered in a heavily shielded room, and strict safety and quality assurance standards must be met. **HDR therapy has become**

more popular in the past 15 years, particularly for intracavitary gynecologic applications. This is partly because of the practical advantages for physicians who center most of their practice in an outpatient clinical setting, but another factor is the recent interruption in the supply of cesium sources suitable for LDR gynecologic brachytherapy. Many clinicians remain reluctant to change to HDR therapy because of the **theoretical radiobiological disadvantages of large-fraction irradiation and the absence of well-controlled randomized clinical trials comparing HDR and LDR regimens** (69).

An alternative to HDR therapy that is commonly used in Europe but only recently introduced in the United States is pulsed dose-rate (PDR) brachytherapy. With this approach, treatment is given in intermittent pulses, using a single stepping source of ^{192}Ir, similar to but lower in activity than the source used for HDR brachytherapy. If treatment is delivered in hourly pulses of 40 to 50 cGy, the tissue sparing should be nearly identical to that achieved with LDR brachytherapy. PDR holds several advantages over true LDR brachytherapy. The sources are readily obtainable, patients are able to receive nursing care and have visitors as they wish during the intervals between pulses, and the stepping source method permits somewhat more flexibility in treatment planning. The equipment can be used for either interstitial or intracavitary brachytherapy, and because the applicators are identical to those used for HDR, clinicians who choose to have both options available to their patients require only one set of applicators.

The total brachytherapy dose to point A must be reduced when converting from LDR to HDR regimens. The appropriate dose and dose per fraction is based on calculations of the estimated biologically effective dose (BED) on tumor and normal tissues. BED is derived from the linear-quadratic formula described earlier in this chapter and is equal to the total nominal dose (nd) times the relative effectiveness: **BED = (nd) × (1 + $d/(\alpha/\beta)$)**, where d is the dose per fraction. For example: Assuming α/β values of 10 and 3 for tumor and for normal tissues, respectively, a fractionation scheme in which a total dose of 30 Gy is given in five fractions of 6 Gy each would result in:

$$\text{Tumor BED} = (30) \times (1 + 6/10) = 48 \text{ Gy}_{10}$$

$$\text{Normal tissue BED} = (30) \times (1 + 6/3) = 90 \text{ Gy}_3$$

Clinicians often express these doses in the more familiar terms of the equivalent dose at 2 Gy per fraction, which is equal to $\text{BED}/[1 + 2/(\alpha/\beta)]$. Using this calculation, the above example would yield equivalent doses of 40 and 54 Gy, respectively, for tumor and normal tissues. In other words, the effect on normal tissues is about 35% greater than would be expected from the same tumor-effective dose given at 2 Gy per fraction or with LDR brachytherapy (which, at 40 to 45 cGy per hour, has an effect similar to that of a dose divided in 2-Gy fractions).

Obviously, this differential effect would make HDR unacceptable if the normal tissues received the same dose as tumor. Fortunately, with good applicator positioning, effective packing of the bladder and rectum, and optimal source positioning, the total dose and dose per fraction delivered to normal tissues are usually considerably lower than those delivered to tumor, making it possible to achieve a ratio of tumor to normal tissue effect that is similar to what is achieved with LDR. **If the tumor is very large or the vaginal anatomy is unfavorable, the nominal doses to tumor and normal tissues may be similar;** in these cases, patients may be more effectively treated with LDR, PDR, or a larger than usual number of HDR fractions (69–72).

It is important that dose fractionation schemes used for HDR therapy produce tumor control and complication rates approximately equivalent to those seen with LDR therapy. The optimal dose per fraction of HDR therapy is unknown and is probably patient specific, but, in general, **increasing the number of fractions and concomitantly decreasing the dose per fraction appears to reduce the rate of moderate and severe complications** (71,73).

The most common HDR regimen used in the United States is probably five fractions of 5.5 to 6 Gy each to point A after 45 Gy to the pelvis, although there is wide variation in the number of fractions (2 to 13) and the dose per fraction (3 to 9 Gy) (74,75). Because large single fractions of radiation permit less recovery of sublethal injury than LDR irradiation, HDR therapy doses that yield a rate of tumor control equivalent to that seen with LDR therapy might result in an increased risk of late complications. However, with intracavitary treatment of the cervix, vulnerable normal tissues (primarily the rectum and bladder) are often some distance from the tumor site and therefore may receive a significantly lower dose and dose per fraction than the prescription point (usually point A).

Interstitial Implants

Interstitial brachytherapy refers to the placement of radioactive sources within tissues. Various sources of radiation—such as ^{192}Ir, ^{198}Au, ^{103}Pd, and ^{125}I—may be obtained as radioactive wires or seeds. ^{192}Ir may be obtained as separate sources that are usually distributed at regular intervals (usually 1 cm) in Teflon tubes or as wires with activity specified in terms of the mCi per cm. Sources may be positioned in the tumor or tumor bed in a variety of ways:

1. **Permanent seed implants (usually ^{125}I, ^{103}Pd, or ^{198}Au)** can be inserted using a specialized seed inserter. These implants are most commonly used to treat prostate cancer but have sometimes been used to treat pelvic or aortic lymph nodes, particularly in the case of nodal recurrence after irradiation.

2. **Temporary Teflon catheter implants** can be placed intraoperatively and subsequently loaded with radioactive sources (usually ^{192}Ir). These are sometimes used to treat tumor beds (76).

3. **Temporary transperineal template-guided interstitial needle implants** can be placed using a Lucite template with regularly spaced holes and a central obturator that can hold a tandem or additional needles. Needles are afterloaded, usually with ^{192}Ir. These implants are used to treat vaginal and some cervical tumors. In some cases, particularly for treatment of apical vaginal lesions, guidance by laparoscopy or laparotomy may facilitate needle placement (77–79).

4. **Temporary transperineal implants can also be placed freehand,** an approach that may allow better control of needle placement in selected cases. Freehand implants are particularly useful for treating urethral and vaginal tumors (Fig. 4.12) (80).

Most gynecologic interstitial implants are temporary LDR implants. Like intracavitary therapy, interstitial therapy delivers a relatively high dose of radiation to a small volume, sparing the surrounding normal tissues. However, **the risk to normal tissues adjacent to the**

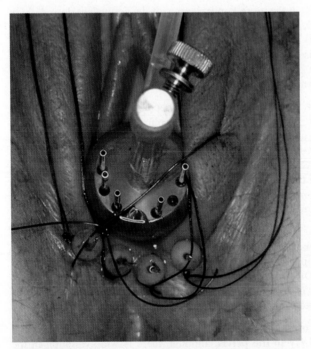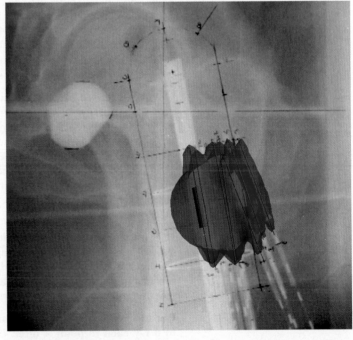

Figure 4.12 **Interstitial implant for a stage II distal vaginal cancer.** Needles are individually inserted transperineally; a finger is placed in the vagina while the needles are inserted to monitor the position of each needle relative to the tumor and mucosal surface. *Left:* A Lucite cylinder in the vagina displaces uninvolved vagina from the needles and has channels for additional sources at the periphery of the cylinder. *Right:* Postoperative radiographs show placement of the needles with a superimposed dose cloud that encloses the volume treated to 30 Gy.

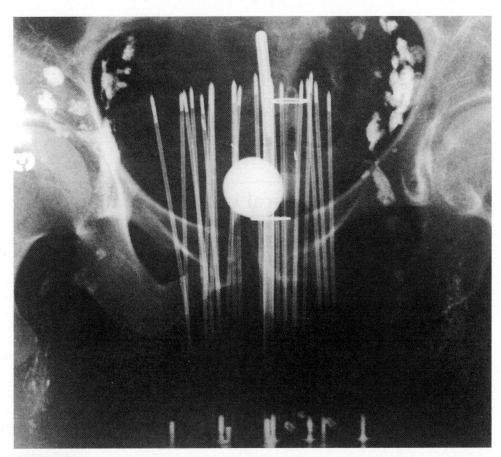

Figure 4.13 **Interstitial implant for an advanced cervical cancer.** Reproduced from Dr. Mark Schray, Division of Radiation Oncology, Mayo Clinic, with permission.

tumor or in the tumor bed may still be significant, particularly if the needle placement is inaccurate.

Some investigators have advocated the use of template-guided interstitial brachytherapy to treat difficult cases of locally advanced cervical cancer (81,82) (Fig. 4.13). The ability to place sources in the lateral parametrium with this technique suggests a theoretical advantage over intracavitary treatment for patients with pelvic wall involvement. Some investigators have claimed high local control rates with this approach (81,82). However, survival rates are not clearly superior to those achieved with combined external-beam and intracavitary therapy, and the risk of major complications also may be greater (78,79).

The radiation oncology community remains polarized as to the appropriateness of interstitial therapy for patients with intact cervical carcinomas, and as yet no randomized trials have been conducted to compare the therapeutic ratio of conventional intracavitary irradiation with that of interstitial treatment. Interstitial implants may also be used in a variety of other gynecologic applications, including vaginal cancer, vaginal recurrence of cervical or endometrial cancer, and urethral cancer.

Intraperitoneal Radioisotopes

Intraperitoneal radioisotopes have been used to treat epithelial ovarian cancer in an effort to address the transperitoneal spread of the disease (83). **Radioactive chromic phosphate (^{32}P) has largely replaced colloidal gold (^{198}Au) for peritoneal treatment.** The longer half-life (14.3 days), pure β decay, and higher mean energy (0.698 MeV) of ^{32}P yield slightly longer exposures, fewer radiation protection problems, and deeper tissue penetration than what is observed with ^{198}Au.

If a radioisotope is evenly distributed within the peritoneum, it is theoretically possible to irradiate the entire peritoneal surface. However, the pattern of energy deposition within the abdomen and the dose delivered beneath the peritoneal surfaces depend on many factors, including the physical characteristics of the isotope used, the energies of its decay products, and the distribution of the isotope within the peritoneal cavity. **In practice, isotope is seldom distributed uniformly to the peritoneal and omental surfaces** (84). Postsurgical adhesions may limit the free flow of fluid, and this nonuniform distribution may result in underdosage of some peritoneal sites and overdosage of some normal tissues. This may result in unacceptable complications, particularly if intraperitoneal and external-beam irradiation are combined (85). Although randomized studies have demonstrated similar survival rates for patients with early ovarian cancer treated with ^{32}P or single-agent chemotherapy, the role of intraperitoneal treatment still has not been clearly established (86), and this approach is rarely used today.

Clinical Uses of Radiation

Cervical Cancer

Although specific radiation-therapy techniques may vary, the curative treatment of cervical cancer usually includes a combination of external pelvic irradiation and brachytherapy, often with concurrent chemotherapy. The goal of radiation therapy is to eliminate cancer in the cervix, paracervical tissues, and regional lymph nodes (64). All of these regions can be encompassed in a pelvic radiation field. However, the dose that can be delivered to the pelvis is limited by the tolerance of intrapelvic normal tissues, most importantly the rectosigmoid, bladder, and small bowel. Because the bulkiest tumor is usually in the cervix, this region typically requires higher doses than the rest of the pelvis to achieve locoregional control. Fortunately, it is usually possible to deliver these high doses with intracavitary therapy.

Treatment Volume

Typical external-beam fields are designed to include the primary tumor, paracervical tissues, and iliac and presacral lymph nodes, all with 1.5- to 2-cm margins. If the common iliac or aortic nodes are involved, then the treatment fields are usually extended to include at least the lower paraaortic region.

The borders of the typical anterior–posterior and posterior–anterior pelvic fields are as follows:

1. **Inferior**—at the midpubis or 3 to 4 cm below the most distal disease in the cervix or vagina (usually demonstrated using a radioopaque vaginal marker).

2. **Superior**—at the L4–L5 interface or at the bifurcation of the aorta so that the common iliac nodes are encompassed. For patients with very small tumors that are at least risk for extensive nodal spread, the upper border may be placed at the L5–S1 interface. For patients who have lymph node involvement, the field may be extended to include paraaortic nodes.

3. **Lateral**—1 to 2 cm lateral to the pelvic lymph nodes as visualized on a lymphangiogram or at least 1 cm lateral to the margins of the bony pelvis. Appropriate shielding along the common iliac nodes decreases the amount of sigmoid and small bowel in the field.

Every effort should be made to minimize the high-dose treatment volume while adequately encompassing the tumor and its regional lymph nodes. **Using four beams (anterior, posterior, and right and left lateral) rather than an opposed pair of anterior and posterior beams** (Fig. 4.8) **can sometimes reduce the volume of tissue irradiated to a high dose.** However, great care must be taken not to shield the primary tumor, uterosacral disease, or external iliac nodes when lateral fields are used (87,88). For some patients with locally advanced tumors, the amount of tissue spared with lateral fields may be relatively small after these areas are included. The additional bone marrow treated with lateral fields may also be a consideration if chemotherapy is part of the treatment plan. However, when the pelvis is treated after hysterectomy, four or more fields usually produce a more favorable dose distribution than two opposed fields. Some clinicians have advocated the use of highly conformal radiation-therapy techniques such as IMRT to treat the whole pelvis (89,90). When these highly conformal techniques are used, particular care must be taken to adequately cover the target volume and account for tumor response and internal organ motion.

For most patients with locally advanced disease, an initial course of treatment is given with external-beam irradiation and concurrent chemotherapy. **Four to five weeks (40 to 45 Gy) of** chemoradiation usually decreases endocervical disease and shrinks exophytic tumor, facilitating optimal intracavitary therapy. The dose to the central tumor is then supplemented with one or two LDR intracavitary treatments or with a variable number of HDR treatments. If the initial tumor volume is small or there is an excellent tumor response to external-beam irradiation and concurrent chemotherapy, then brachytherapy may be given earlier in the patient's treatment. Because the number of brachytherapy treatments is greater with HDR therapy than with LDR therapy, practitioners who use the HDR approach often begin brachytherapy before external-beam therapy has been completed, if the initial tumor response has been adequate. The balance between external-beam and intracavitary therapy may vary somewhat according to the tumor extent (64). However, several studies have suggested that intracavitary therapy is critically important to successful treatment, even for patients with very bulky stage IIIB tumors (1,91).

Patients with International Federation of Gynecology and Obstetrics (FIGO) stage IA disease can often be treated with intracavitary irradiation alone. Most patients with stage IB1 disease have a sufficiently high risk of metastasis to the pelvic lymph nodes to justify at least a moderate dose of pelvic radiation (e.g., 39.6 Gy) to sterilize possible microscopic regional disease.

For patients with carcinoma of the cervix who have vaginal hemorrhage, hemostasis can usually be achieved with vaginal packing, application of Monsel's solution, and rapid initiation of external-beam irradiation. For patients with excessive bleeding, transvaginal irradiation (if available) or several days of accelerated pelvic radiation therapy (e.g., 1.8 Gy twice daily) may be helpful.

Radiation Dose

The total doses of radiation to the central tumor and regional nodes are tailored according to the amount of disease in those sites (92). A number of methods have been used to prescribe and specify the doses delivered with intracavitary therapy. Most radiation oncologists specify treatment using some variation of the Manchester system, which uses two primary reference points (Fig. 4.11):

1. Point A—a point 2 cm lateral and 2 cm superior to the external cervical os in the plane of the implant.
2. Point B—a point 3 cm lateral to point A.

Although the cGy doses from intracavitary and external-beam radiation therapy may not be biologically equivalent (particularly with HDR therapy), these doses are frequently summed to determine the total doses to points A and B. The total dose to point A (from external-beam and LDR intracavitary therapy) believed to be adequate to achieve central disease control is usually between 75 Gy (for small stage IB1 cancers) and 90 Gy (for bulky or locally advanced disease). The prescribed dose to point B is 45 to 65 Gy, depending on the extent of parametrial and sidewall disease.

Prescription and treatment planning cannot be limited to specification of the dose to these reference points. Other factors that should be considered include the following:

1. the position and length of the intrauterine tandem, which influence the loading of the tandem.
2. the type and position of vaginal applicators, which influence the loading of the vaginal applicators.
3. the quality of the vaginal packing.
4. the size of the central tumor before and after external-beam treatment.
5. the vaginal surface dose (usually limited to 120 to 140 Gy).
6. the proximity of the system to the bladder and rectum.
7. the dose rate (or fraction size).

A number of methods and reference doses have been described to estimate the maximum dose to the bladder and rectum on the basis of orthogonal reference films of the implants. The most common method for specifying normal tissue doses is to calculate the doses to reference points defined by the International Commission on Radiation Units and Measurements (Figure 4.11) (93). Using this method, the bladder reference point is placed at the posterior edge of a Foley bulb filled with 7 cc of contrast material; the rectal point is located 5 mm posterior to the vaginal applicator or packing (whichever is most posterior) at the level of the vaginal sources. Three-dimensional reconstructions of intracavitary placements suggest that most methods that use orthogonal x-rays to estimate the dose to normal structures tend to underestimate the true maximum dose (94). For this reason, it is important to qualitatively examine each intracavitary system rather than to depend solely on normal-tissue reference points.

Some centers also document the total **milligram-Radium-equivalent hours** (mgRaEq-hr) of each intracavitary system. This number, obtained by multiplying the mgRaEq of cesium or radium in the system by the number of hours the radioactive sources are left in place, cannot be used as the sole measure of any treatment but is sometimes used to limit the total integral dose to the pelvis. The doses to points at a substantial distance from the system are roughly proportional to the total mgRaEq-hr because, as the distance increases, the dose rate approaches that from a single point source of similar activity. In general, after 40 to 45 Gy of external-beam irradiation, the total mgRaEq-hr (from intracavitary radiation therapy given at 40 to 60 cGy/hr) should not exceed 6,000 to 6,500. An alternative measure is the **reference air kerma, defined as the total dose delivered at 1 meter from the center of the activity and measured in μGy.m^2**; this unit serves the same purpose but can more easily be used with isotopes other than radium or cesium.

There is a growing movement toward use of image-guided brachytherapy (IGBT) with treatment planning based on CT or MRI images obtained with the implant in place. Ideally, IGBT would include true three-dimensional imaging and calculations of the distribution of dose to tumor and normal tissues with accompanying dose limits derived from clinically derived dose-effect data. There currently are very few clinical data derived from patients treated with IGBT; logistical problems also create significant impediments to true IGBT. As a first step, many clinicians are obtaining at least ultrasonic or CT images of intracavitary systems to rule out unsuspected uterine perforation (a potential source of serious complications) and to provide closer estimates of relationships between critical structures and radiation sources.

Results of Treatment

Radiation therapy is extremely effective in the treatment of stage IB1 cervical cancer, producing central and pelvic disease control rates of greater than 98% and greater than 95%, respectively, and disease-specific survival rates of approximately 90% (2,4). **Pelvic control rates decrease as tumor size and FIGO stage increase,** although large single-institution experiences report 5-year pelvic control rates of 60% to 70% and disease-specific survival rates of 40% to 50% even for bulky stage IIIB cancers treated with radiation alone (e.g., before routine use of concurrent chemotherapy) (1,2). Although these control rates clearly indicated a need for more effective treatment of these advanced lesions, it is remarkable that such massive carcinomas, usually more than 7 cm in diameter, can be controlled even half the time with radiation therapy alone. This undoubtedly reflects the remarkable effectiveness of carefully planned combinations of external-beam and intracavitary radiation therapy.

During the past decade, studies have demonstrated a significant improvement in pelvic disease control and survival when *cisplatin*-containing chemotherapy is delivered concurrently with radiation for patients with locoregionally advanced cervical cancer (19–21,95–97). Several of the regimens tested in these studies also included **5-*fluorouracil.*** This drug is known to be a potent radiation sensitizer, particularly effective in the treatment of gastrointestinal malignancies, but its contribution to chemoradiation in patients with carcinoma of the cervix is still uncertain. Other randomized trials suggest that ***mitomycin C*** (98, 99) and ***epirubicin*** (100) also may improve outcome when they are delivered concurrently with radiation to patients with locally advanced cervical cancer.

Adjuvant Pelvic Radiation Therapy after Radical Hysterectomy

For patients with stage IB and IIA cervical cancer treated with radical hysterectomy and pelvic lymphadenectomy, lymph node involvement is probably the strongest predictor of local recurrence and death: Patients with nodal involvement have survival rates of only 50% to 60% of those of patients with negative nodes (101,102). **Parametrial involvement and involvement of surgical margins also predict a high rate of pelvic recurrence and are**

considered to be indications for postoperative irradiation. In 2000, the Southwest Oncology Group published results of a study comparing postoperative radiation with combined chemoradiation in patients who had positive lymph nodes, parametrium, or surgical margins; the study demonstrated a 50% reduction in the risk of recurrence when *cisplatin* and *fluorouracil* were added to pelvic irradiation (96).

For patients with negative nodes but high-risk primary tumor features (i.e., tumor size >4 cm, deep stromal invasion, or vascular space involvement), **postoperative irradiation has also been demonstrated to produce a significant reduction in the risk of recurrence** (7,103). This is discussed further in Chapter 9.

The drawback of adjuvant pelvic radiation therapy is a somewhat greater risk of major complications than with surgery alone or radiation alone (5,7). For this reason, a National Cancer Institute Consensus Conference (60) concluded that "primary therapy should avoid the routine use of both radical surgery and radiation therapy," suggesting that patients who are known to have high-risk factors at initial evaluation may be better treated with radical radiation therapy.

Recurrent Cervical Cancer

Patients who have an isolated pelvic recurrence after radical hysterectomy can sometimes be treated successfully with aggressive radiation therapy. The prognosis is best for patients with isolated central recurrences that are not fixed to the pelvic wall and do not involve pelvic nodes. These patients have 5-year survival rates as high as 60% to 70% (104). For patients whose tumors involve the pelvic wall or lymphnodes; a few groups report better than a 20% 5-year survival rate for radiation alone. Some groups have reported encouraging results with combined chemoradiation (105). It probably is reasonable to extrapolate from recent randomized trials that demonstrate improved survival with concurrent chemoradiation for locally advanced cervical cancer to justify a similar approach in patients with pelvic recurrences.

Complications

Late complications of radical irradiation for cervical cancer occur in 5% to 15% of patients and are related to the dose per fraction, the total dose administered, and the volume irradiated (106). Patient factors such as a history of pelvic infection, heavy smoking, previous abdominal surgery, and diabetes mellitus may increase the risk of complications (56,107). The positioning of the intracavitary system also may influence the risk of complications. **Late effects may be seen in the bladder** (hematuria, fibrosis and contraction, or fistulas) **and in the rectosigmoid or terminal ileum** (bleeding, stricture, obstruction, or perforation). **Agglutination of the apex of the vagina is common.** Severe vaginal shortening is less common and is probably correlated with the patient's age, menopausal status, and sexual activity and with the initial extent of disease (108,109). Unfortunately, our understanding of the factors influencing sexual dysfunction in patients treated for cervical cancer is still incomplete. Most gastrointestinal complications occur within 30 months of radiation therapy, although late effects may occur many years after treatment (109).

In the United States, late complications of radiation therapy (occurring more than 90 days after treatment) are usually scored according to the Radiation Therapy Oncology Group/European Organization for Research and Treatment of Cancer Late Radiation Morbidity Scheme, which is part of the National Cancer Institute system for reporting of adverse events (Table 4.2). However, it is important to recognize that with today's multimodality treatments, several factors may contribute to adverse events. In Europe, many groups use the Franco-Italian Glossary, a scoring system that incorporates early and late surgical and radiation-related side effects (110).

Palliation

Radiation therapy plays an important role in the palliation of metastatic cervical cancer. **Short courses of palliative irradiation, such as 2,000 cGy in five fractions or 3,000 cGy in 10 fractions, usually will alleviate symptoms related to bony metastases or paraaortic nodal disease.** Such treatment also may relieve symptoms related to pressure from enlarging mediastinal or supraclavicular nodal disease.

Table 4.2 RTOG and EORTC Late Radiation Morbidity Scoring Scheme[a]

Adverse Event[b]	Grade				
	0	1	2	3	4
Bladder	No change from baseline	Slight epithelial atrophy; minor telangiectasia (microscopic hematuria)	Moderate frequency; generalized telangiectasia; intermittent macroscopic hematuria	Severe frequency and dysuria; severe generalized telangiectasia (often with petechiae); frequent hematuria; reduction in bladder capacity (<150 mL)	Necrosis; contracted bladder (capacity <100 mL), severe hemorrhagic cystitis, fistula
Bone	No change from baseline	Asymptomatic; reduced bone density	Moderate pain or tenderness; irregular bone sclerosis	Severe pain or tenderness; dense bone sclerosis	Necrosis; spontaneous fracture
Joint	No change from baseline	Mild joint stiffness; slight limitation of movement	Moderate stiffness; intermittent or moderate joint pain; moderate limitation of movement	Severe joint stiffness; pain with severe limitation of movement	Necrosis; complete fixation
Kidney	No change from baseline	Transient albuminuria; no hypertension; mild impairment of renal function; urea 25–35 mg %; creatinine 1.5–2.0 mg %; creatinine clearance >75%	Persistent moderate albuminuria (2+); mild hypertension; no related anemia; moderate impairment of renal function; urea >36–60 mg %; creatinine clearance >50%–74%	Severe albuminuria; severe hypertension; persistent anemia (<10 g %; severe renal failure; urea >60 mg %; creatinine clearance <50%)	Malignant hypertension; uremic coma; urea >100 mg %
Liver	No change from baseline	Mild lassitude; nausea; dyspepsia; slightly abnormal liver function	Moderate symptoms; some abnormal liver function tests; serum albumin normal	Disabling hepatic insufficiency; liver function tests grossly abnormal; low albumin; edema or ascites	Necrosis; hepatic coma or encephalopathy
Vagina	No change from baseline	Partial stenosis or shortening but less than complete occlusion	Complete occlusion; telangiectasis with frequent bleeding	Radionecrotic ulcer	Fistula to bladder, bowel, or peritoneal cavity
Small, large intestine	No change from baseline	Mild diarrhea; mild cramping; bowel movement ≥5× daily; slight rectal discharge or bleeding	Moderate diarrhea and colic; bowel movement >5× daily; excessive rectal mucus or intermittent bleeding	Obstruction or bleeding, requiring surgery	Necrosis; perforation fistula
Spinal cord	No change from baseline	Mild Lhermitte's syndrome	Severe Lhermitte's syndrome	Objective neurologic findings at or below cord level treatment	Mono-, para-, quadriplegia
Subcutaneous tissue	No change from baseline	Slight induration (fibrosis) and loss of subcutaneous fat	Moderate fibrosis but asymptomatic; slight field contracture; <10% linear reduction	Severe induration and loss of subcutaneous tissue; field contracture; >10% linear reduction	Necrosis

RTOG, Radiation Therapy Oncology Group; EORTC, European Organization for Research and Treatment of Cancer

[a]Used for adverse events occurring more than 90 days after radiation therapy.

[b]Includes sites most pertinent to treatment of gynecologic malignancies.

Endometrial Cancer

The role of radiation therapy in the treatment of endometrial carcinoma is discussed in greater detail in Chapter 10. **Indications for radiation therapy in the treatment of endometrial cancer are as follows:**

1. **adjuvant treatment to prevent locoregional recurrence** after hysterectomy and bilateral salpingo-oophorectomy.

2. **preoperative treatment for patients with very extensive cervical stromal involvement.**

3. **curative treatment for some patients with medical problems that preclude surgery** and for occasional patients with stage III disease involving the vagina.

4. **curative treatment for patients with isolated vaginal or pelvic recurrence,** usually using a combination of external-beam and intracavitary or interstitial radiation therapy.

5. **palliative treatment of massive pelvic or metastatic disease.**

In the past, disease confined to the uterus was often treated with preoperative intracavitary radiation therapy. An intracavitary line source was placed in the uterus, or the uterus was packed with multiple radium (Heyman's) capsules or cesium (Simon's) capsules (111). Preoperative irradiation reduces the risk of vaginal apex recurrence but has never been proven to improve survival, although no randomized studies have been done to compare preoperative and postoperative irradiation (112,113). Because tailored postoperative irradiation appears to achieve similar pelvic control rates and avoids unnecessary over-treatment of patients whose hysterectomy findings predict a negligible risk of recurrence, preoperative irradiation has been abandoned for most patients (112,114,115).

Most patients with stage I endometrial cancer have minimally invasive grade 1–2 tumors, which rarely recur after hysterectomy alone and usually need no additional treatment. The use of adjuvant pelvic radiation therapy is usually confined to patients with deeply invasive lesions or other high-risk findings at surgery (e.g., lymph node involvement or cervical stromal involvement) (112,114,115). Adjuvant pelvic radiation therapy reduces the risk of pelvic recurrence but has never been proven to improve survival. In 2004, the Gynecologic Oncology Group reported results of a randomized trial addressing this question in patients with intermediate-risk FIGO stage I cancers. This study demonstrated a reduction in the overall risk of pelvic (particularly vaginal) recurrence without a significant difference in overall survival for patients who received postoperative pelvic radiation therapy (116). However, using subset analysis, the authors identified a subset of patients with high-intermediate-risk disease who may benefit from adjuvant radiation therapy. In another randomized trial, Creutzberg et al. (58) found that postoperative radiation therapy reduced the risk of pelvic recurrence but had no significant impact on survival. Unfortunately, both of these trials included a large number of patients who had relatively favorable findings (grade 1 disease or <50% invasion); neither trial included a sufficient number of patients who had grade 3 tumors or deep myometrial invasion to rule out clinically important differences in these subgroups.

Uterine papillary serous cancers have a particularly poor prognosis and an inclination to spread intraperitoneally in a manner similar to that seen with ovarian cancers. Whole-abdominal irradiation appears to be valuable treatment for some patients with minimal residual disease after hysterectomy (117,118), although many groups favor the use of adjuvant chemotherapy with or without local radiation therapy for this group of patients.

For patients with endometrial cancer, the potential benefit of adjuvant treatment must be balanced against the risk of complications for each patient. Extensive staging lymphadenectomy appears to increase the risk of serious bowel complications after radiation therapy (119,120).

Ovarian Cancer

Several independent investigators have established a curative role for whole-abdominal and pelvic irradiation for some subsets of patients with epithelial ovarian cancer (121–124). Survival rates are strongly correlated with initial disease stage and volume of residual disease. The best survival rates are for patients with stage II disease and for those whose macroscopic residual disease was confined to the pelvis—a situation in which a relatively high dose of radiation can be given.

Because transperitoneal spread is the most common route of dissemination of ovarian cancer, radiation fields that encompass the whole peritoneal cavity are more likely to be curative than those that treat only the pelvis or lower abdomen. **However, normal tissues in the upper abdomen (e.g., kidney, liver, bowel, and spinal cord) limit the dose of radiation that can be delivered to the whole abdomen to approximately 22 Gy.** Somewhat higher doses can be delivered to portions of the upper abdomen that do not include the most sensitive normal structures. Because 22 Gy is insufficient to control macroscopic disease, patients with gross upper abdominal disease cannot be expected to benefit from whole-abdominal irradiation. **Although a curative benefit has been established for whole-abdominal radiation therapy, randomized studies have never determined the relative benefits of abdominopelvic radiation therapy and combination platinum-based chemotherapy in appropriately selected patients with minimal residual disease.**

Radiation therapy may also be helpful in the palliation of pain, bleeding, or other symptoms from ovarian cancer. **Occasionally, patients who have localized recurrences may experience prolonged disease-free survival after localized radical radiation therapy, particularly if all macroscopic disease can be surgically resected initially.**

The high response rates but frequent relapses observed after treatment of ovarian cancer with chemotherapy have encouraged investigators to add whole-abdominal irradiation either as a salvage treatment for incomplete responses or as part of an up-front multimodality treatment program. Many small single-arm studies of sequential treatments have been reported, and they show varied results. A retrospective analysis of the Toronto data suggested an improved outcome for high-risk patients treated with sequential chemotherapy and whole-abdominal irradiation compared with historical controls treated with radiation alone (125). However, three randomized studies have compared chemotherapy alone with multimodality treatment (126–128) with disappointing results. Although some patients with minimal residual disease may benefit, **in general the data do not support routine use of sequential chemotherapy and abdominopelvic irradiation.** Poor tolerance after extensive chemotherapy and the possible induction of accelerated repopulation of resistant clonogens during treatment are among the reasons suggested for the failure of this approach in most hands (121,129,130).

Technique

Early studies of whole-abdominal radiation therapy used a **"moving-strip" technique** in which a 10-cm-high field (usually ^{60}Co) was moved by 2.5-cm increments so that each "strip" received 8 or 10 fractions, usually of 2.25 Gy each (131,132). With the advent of high-energy linear accelerators, this approach was replaced by an **open-field technique** (Fig. 4.14). These two techniques have been compared in randomized trials that demonstrated no significant difference in survival and a lower rate of bowel complications (1% versus 6%) with the open-field technique (132,133). **Most abdominopelvic irradiation techniques include a boost to**

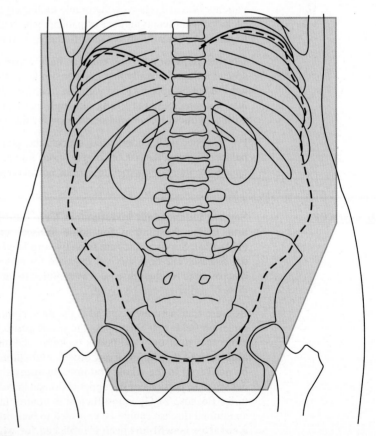

Figure 4.14   **Treatment portals for carcinoma of the ovary or for uterine papillary serous carcinoma.** The field must encompass the entire peritoneal cavity. Shielding is usually added to limit the dose to the kidneys to less than 18 to 20 Gy. The liver dose is usually limited to 25 Gy.

the pelvis, and some investigators boost the paraaortic nodes and medial diaphragms ("T boost") to 40 to 45 Gy after initial whole-abdominal treatment (123). The design of abdominopelvic fields requires careful simulation using fluoroscopy and CT-based planning to confirm adequate coverage of the peritoneal surfaces and diaphragms and proper shielding of sensitive structures.

Toxicity

Acute side effects of abdominopelvic irradiation include nausea, anorexia, general fatigue, and diarrhea in most patients (134). These symptoms are usually fairly well controlled with appropriate medications. Approximately 10% of patients develop significant myelotoxicity (platelet count <100,000 or neutrophil count <1,500). The risk of significant toxicity is much higher in patients who undergo abdominopelvic irradiation after chemotherapy, and the risk depends on the drugs and the duration of previous chemotherapy. As many as 40% of patients treated with abdominopelvic irradiation have transiently elevated levels of alkaline phosphatase, but symptomatic hepatitis is rare if the dose of radiation to the liver does not exceed 27 Gy. In the absence of tumor recurrence, late bowel complications are rare, but the risk tends to increase with the extent and number of previous abdominal operations (particularly lymphadenectomy) (135).

Vulvar Cancer

The role of radiation therapy in the treatment of vulvar cancer has increased dramatically during the past 25 years. Improved radiation-therapy equipment and techniques have reduced the toxicity that discouraged early attempts to treat the vulva with radiation, and prospective studies have increased interest in this effective modality. In particular, the landmark randomized study published by Homesley and colleagues in 1986 demonstrated a marked improvement in survival when patients with positive lymph nodes were treated with pelvic and inguinal irradiation after vulvectomy and lymphadenectomy (16). The role of radiation for treatment of vulvar cancer is explored in more detail in Chapter 13.

In brief, **the possible benefits of radiation therapy in the treatment of vulvar cancer** include: (i) reduced risk of regional recurrence and improved survival in patients with **inguinal node metastases** (16); (ii) reduced risk of vulvar recurrence in patients with **positive surgical margins, multiple local recurrences,** or other high-risk features (136,137); and (iii) **avoidance of exenterative surgery in patients whose disease involves the anus or urethra** (138). Radiation therapy may also be an alternative to inguinal lymphadenectomy in selected patients with clinically negative groins (17,139).

Several reports have emphasized the critical importance of careful radiation-therapy technique in treating patients with vulvar cancer (17,139,140). A number of approaches have been developed to decrease the dose to the femoral heads from groin irradiation. In most cases, adequate coverage of the volume at risk is readily achieved without risking serious femoral morbidity. However, this can only be accomplished with detailed CT-based treatment planning.

In general, the total dose of radiation should be tailored to the amount of residual disease, with doses of approximately 45 to 50 Gy for microscopic disease and 60 Gy or higher for positive margins, extracapsular nodal extension, or macroscopic residual disease.

When necessary, the dose to portions of the vulva at high risk for recurrence can be "boosted" with an *en face* electron field. This approach minimizes the amount of tissue exposed to high doses and thereby reduces acute skin reactions. **Carefully designed IMRT may be useful in selected cases.** Bolus may be needed to increase the dose to superficial tissues in the "buildup region" of photon and low-energy electron beams. Treatment interruptions should be minimized to avoid possible tumor proliferation during breaks in radiation therapy.

The use of concurrent "sensitizing" chemotherapy (e.g., continuous-infusion *fluorouracil* or *cisplatin*) to improve control rates has been explored in a number of uncontrolled studies (141–147). The encouraging response rates and long-term control of gross disease reported in these trials and the successful use of chemoradiation in cervical and anal cancer are bound to increase interest in this approach in the future.

Acute moist desquamation of the skin of the inguinal creases and vulva is expected. Symptoms may be reduced with careful local care, sitz baths, avoidance of tight clothing, and immediate treatment of superimposed fungal or bacterial infections. Superinfection with *Candida* species is particularly frequent during treatment. **Late complications may include lymphedema, particularly after radical groin dissection. Atrophy, telangiectasia, and fibrosis of the skin or subcutaneous tissues can occur** and may be related to the daily fraction size and total dose, tissue destruction from tumor, and the extent of local surgery.

Vaginal Cancer

Although small apical vaginal lesions can sometimes be resected, the intimate relationship of the vagina to the bladder and rectum usually makes it impossible to perform curative surgical resection without sacrificing those organs. **For this reason, most patients who have invasive vaginal cancers are treated with radiation therapy, which achieves cure rates that are, stage for stage, similar to those achieved with radiation therapy for patients with cervical cancer** (13,14,148). Treatment usually consists of a combination of external-beam irradiation and brachytherapy. Interstitial or intracavitary techniques may be used, depending on the size and site of the primary lesion and its response to external-beam therapy (Fig. 4.12). Because the dose gradient from intracavitary therapy is very steep, interstitial techniques are usually used to treat tumors that are more than 3 to 5 mm thick. Tumors that are very advanced, diffuse, or fixed or that extensively involve the rectovaginal septum may be boosted to a high dose using conformal external-beam therapy or IMRT. The vaginal apex can move 2 to 3 cm with bladder filling and emptying; this internal organ motion should be carefully considered during treatment planning.

Concurrent chemoradiation may have a role in the treatment of vaginal cancers, although there are no large trials in this group of patients. Many clinicians believe that similarities in histology and behavior justify the use of regimens that have been proven beneficial for cervical cancer to treat locally advanced vaginal cancers. Also, because vaginal cancer is very rare and the radiation-therapy techniques are specialized, patients with this disease may benefit from referral to centers with relatively large gynecologic radiation oncology practices.

References

1. **Logsdon MD, Eifel PJ.** FIGO IIIB squamous cell carcinoma of the cervix: an analysis of prognostic factors emphasizing the balance between external beam and intracavitary radiation therapy. *Int J Radiat Oncol Biol Phys* 1999;43:763–775.
2. **Stehman FB, Perez CA, Kurman RJ, Thigpen JT.** Uterine cervix. In: **Hoskins W, Perez C, Young R, eds.** *Principles and practice of gynecologic oncology.* Philadelphia: JB Lippincott Co., 2000:591–662.
3. **Eifel PJ.** Radiotherapy versus radical surgery for gynecologic neoplasms: carcinomas of the cervix and vulva. *Front Radiat Ther Oncol* 1993;27:130–142.
4. **Eifel PJ, Morris M, Wharton JT, Oswald MJ.** The influence of tumor size and morphology on the outcome of patients with FIGO stage IB squamous cell carcinoma of the uterine cervix. *Int J Radiat Oncol Biol Phys* 1994;29:9–16.
5. **Landoni F, Maneo A, Colombo A, Placa F, Milani R, Perego P, et al.** Randomised study of radical surgery versus radiotherapy for stage IB–IIA cervical cancer. *Lancet* 1997;350:535–540.
6. **Morrow CP.** Is pelvic radiation beneficial in the postoperative management of Stage IB squamous cell carcinoma of the cervix with pelvic node metastases treated by radical hysterectomy and pelvic lymphadenectomy? *Gynecol Oncol* 1980;10:105–110.
7. **Sedlis A, Bundy BN, Rotman MZ, Lentz SS, Muderspach LI, Zaino RJ.** A randomized trial of pelvic radiation therapy versus no further therapy in selected patients with stage IB carcinoma of the cervix after radical hysterectomy and pelvic lymphadenectomy: a Gynecologic Oncology Group study. *Gynecol Oncol* 1999;73: 177–183.
8. **Aalders J, Abeler V, Kolstad P, Onsrud M.** Postoperative external irradiation and prognostic parameters in stage I endometrial carcinoma: clinical and histopathologic study of 540 patients. *Obstet Gynecol* 1980;56:419–427.
9. **Grigsby PW, Perez CA.** Radiotherapy alone for medically inoperable carcinoma of the cervix: stage IA and carcinoma *in situ. Int J Radiat Oncol Biol Phys* 1991;21:375–378.
10. **Kupelian PA, Eifel PJ, Tornos C, Burke TW, Delclos L, Oswald MJ.** Treatment of endometrial carcinoma with radiation therapy alone. *Int J Radiat Oncol Biol Phys* 1993;27:817–824.
11. **Dembo A, Bush R, Beale F, Bean HA, Pringle JF, Sturgeon J, et al.** Ovarian carcinoma: improved survival following abdominopelvic irradiation in patients with a completed pelvic operation. *Am J Obstet Gynecol* 1979;134:793–800.
12. **Dembo AJ.** Radiotherapeutic management of ovarian cancer. *Semin Oncol* 1984;11:238–250.
13. **Frank SJ, Jhingran A, Levenback C, Eifel PJ.** Definitive treatment of vaginal cancer with radiation therapy. *Int J Radiat Oncol Biol Phys* 2003;57:S194.
14. **Kirkbride P, Fyles A, Rawlings GA, Manchul L, Levin W, Murphy KJ, et al.** Carcinoma of the vagina—experience at the Princess Margaret Hospital (1974–1989). *Gynecol Oncol* 1995;56: 435–443.
15. **Boronow RC.** Combined therapy as an alternative to exenteration for locally advanced vulvo-vaginal cancer: rationale and results. *Cancer* 1982;49:1085–1091.
16. **Homesley HD, Bundy BN, Sedlis A, Adcock L.** Radiation therapy versus pelvic node resection for carcinoma of the vulva with positive groin nodes. *Obstet Gynecol* 1986;68:733–740.
17. **Katz A, Eifel PJ, Jhingran A, Levenback CF.** The role of radiation therapy in preventing regional recurrences of invasive squamous cell carcinoma of the vulva. *Int J Radiat Oncol Biol Phys* 2003;57: 409–418.
18. **Keys HM, Bundy BN, Stehman FB, Muderspach LI, Chafe WE, Suggs CL 3rd, et al.** *Cisplatin,* radiation, and adjuvant hysterectomy compared with radiation and adjuvant hysterectomy for bulky stage IB cervical carcinoma. *N Engl J Med* 1999;340:1154–1161.
19. **Morris M, Eifel PJ, Lu J, Grigsby PW, Levenback C, Stevens RE, et al.** Pelvic radiation with concurrent chemotherapy compared with pelvic and para-aortic radiation for high-risk cervical cancer. *N Engl J Med* 1999;340:1137–1143.

20. Rose PG, Bundy BN, Watkins EB, Thigpen JT, Deppe G, Maiman MA, et al. Concurrent *cisplatin*-based chemotherapy and radiotherapy for locally advanced cervical cancer. *N Engl J Med* 1999;340:1144–1153.

21. Eifel PJ, Winter K, Morris M, Levenback C, Grigsby PW, Cooper J, et al. Pelvic irradiation with concurrent chemotherapy versus pelvic and para-aortic irradiation for high-risk cervical cancer: an update of Radiation Therapy Oncology Group trial (RTOG) 90-01. *J Clin Oncol* 2004;22:872–880.

22. Dewey WC, Ling CC, Meyn RE. Radiation-induced apoptosis: relevance to radiotherapy. *Int J Radiat Oncol Biol Phys* 1995; 33:781–796.

23. Hall EJ, Giaccia AJ. *Radiobiology for the radiologist*, 6th ed. Philadelphia: Lippincott Williams & Wilkins, 2006.

24. Elkind MM, Sutton H. Radiation response of mammalian cells grown in culture: 1. repair of x-ray damage in surviving Chinese hamster cells. *Radiat Res* 1960;13:556.

25. Fyles A, Keane TJ, Barton M, Simm J. The effect of treatment duration in the local control of cervix cancer. *Radiother Oncol* 1992;25:273–279.

26. Lanciano RM, Pajak TF, Martz K, Hanks GE. The influence of treatment time on outcome for squamous cell cancer of the uterine cervix treated with radiation: a patterns-of-care study. *Int J Radiat Oncol Biol Phys* 1993;25:391–397.

27. Parsons JT, Bova FJ, Million RR. A re-evaluation of split-course technique for squamous cell carcinoma of the head and neck. *Int J Radiat Oncol Biol Phys* 1980;6:1645–1652.

28. Tannock IF, Browman G. Lack of evidence for a role of chemotherapy in the routine management of locally advanced head and neck cancer. *J Clin Oncol* 1986;4:1121–1126.

29. Terasima R, Tolmach LJ. X-ray sensitivity and DNA synthesis in synchronous populations of HeLa cells. *Science* 1963;140:490.

30. Kallman RF. The phenomenon of reoxygenation and its implications for fractionated radiotherapy. *Radiology* 1972;105:135–142.

31. Dische S, Anderson PJ, Sealy R, Watson ER. Carcinoma of the cervix—anaemia, radiotherapy and hyperbaric oxygen. *Br J Radiol* 1983;56:251–255.

32. Sundfør K, Tropé C, Suo Z, Bergsjø P. Normobaric oxygen treatment during radiotherapy for carcinoma of the uterine cervix. Results from a prospective controlled randomized trial. *Radiother Oncol* 1999;50:157–165.

33. Leibel S, Bauer M, Wasserman T, Marcial V, Rotman M, Hornback N, et al. Radiotherapy with or without *misonidazole* for patients with stage IIIB or IVA squamous cell carcinoma of the uterine cervix: preliminary report of a Radiation Therapy Oncology Group randomized trial. *Int J Radiat Oncol Biol Phys* 1987;13:541–549.

34. Overgaard J, Bentzen SM, Kolstad P, Kjoerstad K, Davy M, Bertelsen K, et al. *Misonidazole* combined with radiotherapy in the treatment of carcinoma of the uterine cervix. *Int J Radiat Oncol Biol Phys* 1989;16:1069–1072.

35. Thomas G. The effect of hemoglobin level on radiotherapy outcomes: the Canadian experience. *Semin Oncol* 2001;28:60–65.

36. Girinski T, Pejovic-Lenfant M, Bourhis J, Campana F, Cosset JM, Petit C, et al. Prognostic value of hemoglobin concentrations and blood transfusions in advanced carcinoma of the cervix treated by radiation therapy: results of a retrospective study of 386 patients. *Int J Radiat Oncol Biol Phys* 1989;16:37–42.

37. Grogan M, Thomas GM, Melamed I, Wong FL, Pearcey RG, Joseph PK, et al. The importance of hemoglobin levels during radiotherapy for carcinoma of the cervix. *Cancer* 1999;86:1528–1536.

38. Kapp KS, Poschauko J, Geyer E, Berghold A, Oechs AC, Petru E, et al. Evaluation of the effect of routine packed red blood cell transfusion in anemic cervix cancer patients treated with radical radiotherapy. *Int J Radiat Oncol Biol Phys* 2002;54:58–66.

39. Sundfør K, Lyng H, Rofstad EK. Tumour hypoxia and vascular density as predictors of metastasis in squamous cell carcinoma of the uterine cervix. *Br J Cancer* 1998;78:822–827.

40. Bush R. The significance of anemia in clinical radiation therapy. *Int J Radiat Oncol Biol Phys* 1986;12:2047–2050.

41. Santin AD, Bellone S, Parrish RS, Coke C, Dunn D, Roman J, et al. Influence of allogeneic blood transfusion on clinical outcome during radiotherapy for cancer of the uterine cervix. *Gynecol Obstet Invest* 2003;56:28–34.

42. Höckel M, Knoop C, Schlenger K, Vorndran B, Baussmann E, Mitze M, et al. Intratumoral pO2 predicts survival in advanced cancer of the uterine cervix. *Radiother Oncol* 1993;26:45–50.

43. Henke M, Laszig R, Rübe C, Schäfer U, Haase KD, Schilcher B, et al. Erythropoietin to treat head and neck cancer patients with anaemia undergoing radiotherapy: randomised, double-blind, placebo-controlled trial. *Lancet* 2003;362:1255–1260.

44. Thomas G, Ali S, Hoebers FJ, Darcy KM, Rodgers WH, Patel M, et al. Phase III trial to evaluate the efficacy of maintaining hemoglobin levels above 12.0 g/dl with erythropoietin vs above 10.0 g/dl without erythropoietin in anemic patients receiving concurrent radiation and *cisplatin* for cervical cancer. *Gynecol Oncol* 2008;108:317–325.

45. Fowler JF. Rationales for high linear energy transfer radiotherapy. In: Steel G, Adams GE, Peckham MJ, eds. *The biological basis for radiotherapy*. New York: Elsevier, 1983:261.

46. Hall EJ. *Radiobiology for the radiologist*, 5th ed. Philadelphia: Lippincott Williams & Wilkins, 2000.

47. Perez CA, Gillespie B, Pajak T, Hornback NB, Emami B, Rubin P. Quality assurance problems in clinical hyperthermia and their impact on therapeutic outcome: a report by the Radiation Therapy Oncology Group. *Int J Radiat Oncol Biol Phys* 1989;16:551–558.

48. Franckena M, Stalpers LJ, Koper PC, Wiggenraad RG, Hoogenraad WJ, van Dijk JD, et al. Long-term improvement in treatment outcome after radiotherapy and hyperthermia in locoregionally advanced cervix cancer: an update of the Dutch Deep Hyperthermia Trial. *Int J Radiat Oncol Biol Phys* 2008;70:1176–1182.

49. Steel GG, Peckham M. Exploitable mechanisms in combined radiotherapy-chemotherapy: the concept of additivity. *Int J Radiat Oncol Biol Phys* 1979;5:317–322.

50. Fletcher GH. Clinical dose response curves of human malignant epithelial tumours. *Br J Radiol* 1973;46:1–12.

51. Shukovsky LJ. Dose, time volume relationships in squamous cell carcinoma of the supraglottic larynx. *Am J Roentgenol Radiat Ther Nucl Med* 1970;108:27.

52. Withers HR, Mason KA. The kinetics of recovery in irradiated colonic mucosa of the mouse. *Cancer* 1974;34 (suppl):896–903.

53. Peters LJ, Ang KK. Unconventional fractionation schemes in radiotherapy. In: *Important advances in oncology*. Philadelphia: J. B. Lippincott, 1986;269–285.

54. Thames HD Jr, Withers HR, Peters LJ, Fletcher GH. Changes in early and late radiation responses with altered dose fractionation: implications for dose-survival relationships. *Int J Radiat Oncol Biol Phys* 1982;8:219–226.

55. Thames HD Jr, Peters LJ, Withers HR, Fletcher GH. Accelerated fractionation vs hyperfractionation: rationales for several treatments per day. *Int J Radiat Oncol Biol Phys* 1983;9:127–138.

56. Eifel PJ, Jhingran A, Bodurka DC, Levenback C, Thames H. Correlation of smoking history and other patient characteristics with major complications of pelvic radiation therapy for cervical cancer. *J Clin Oncol* 2002;20:3651–3657.

57. Konski A, Sowers M. Pelvic fractures following irradiation for endometrial carcinoma. [see comments]. *Int J Radiat Oncol Biol Phys* 1996;35:361–367.

58. Creutzberg CL, van Putten WL, Koper PC, Lybeert ML, Jobsen JJ, Wárlám-Rodenhuis CC, et al. Surgery and postoperative radiotherapy versus surgery alone for patients with stage-1 endometrial carcinoma: multicentre randomised trial. PORTEC Study Group. Post Operative Radiation Therapy in Endometrial Carcinoma. *Lancet* 2000;355:1404–1411.

59. Roberts JA, Brunetto VI, Keys HM, Zaino R, Spirtos NM, Bloss JD. A phase III randomized study of surgery vs surgery plus adjunctive radiation therapy in intermediate-risk endometrial adenocarcinoma (GOG No. 99). *Gynecol Oncol* 1998;68:135(abst).

60. National Institutes of Health. National Institutes of Health Consensus Development Conference Statement on Cervical Cancer. *Gynecol Oncol* 1997;66:351–361.

61. Seider MJ, Peters LJ, Wharton JT, Oswald MJ. Safety of adjunctive transvaginal beam therapy in the treatment of squamous cell carcinoma of the uterine cervix. *Int J Radiat Oncol Biol Phys* 1988;14:729–735.

62. Maor MH, Gillespie BW, Peters LJ, Wambersie A, Griffin TW, Thomas FJ, et al. Neutron therapy in cervical cancer: results of a phase III RTOG study. *Int J Radiat Oncol Biol Phys* 1988;14:885–891.

63. **Kahn F.** *The physics of radiation therapy.* 3rd ed. Philadelphia: Lipincott Williams & Wilkins, 2003.

64. **Fletcher GH.** Female pelvis. In: **Fletcher GH, ed.** *Textbook of radiotherapy.* Philadelphia: Lea & Febiger, 1980.

65. **Delclos L, Fletcher GH, Sampiere V, Grant WH 3rd.** Can the Fletcher gamma ray colpostat system be extrapolated to other systems? *Cancer* 1978;41:970–979.

66. **Viswanathan AN, Petereit DG.** Gynecologic Brachytherapy. In: **Devlin P, ed.** *Brachytherapy: techniques and applications.* Philadelphia: Lippincott Williams & Wilkins; 2006. pp. 223–268.

67. **Delclos L, Fletcher GH, Moore EB, Sampiere V.** Minicolpostats, dome cylinders, other additions and improvements of the Fletcher-suit afterloadable system: indications and limitations of their use. *Int J Radiat Oncol Biol Phys* 1980;6:1195–1206.

68. **Haie-Meder C, Kramar A, Lambin P, Lancar R, Scalliet P, Bouzy J, et al.** Analysis of complications in a prospective randomized trial comparing two brachytherapy low dose rates in cervical carcinoma. *Int J Radiat Oncol Biol Phys* 1994;29:953–960.

69. **Eifel PJ.** High dose-rate brachytherapy for carcinoma of the cervix: high tech or high risk? *Int J Radiat Oncol Biol Phys* 1992;24:383–386.

70. **Kapp KS, Stuecklschweiger GF, Kapp DS, Hackl AG.** Dosimetry of intracavitary placements for uterine and cervical carcinoma: results of orthogonal film, TLD, and CT-assisted techniques. *Radiother Oncol* 1992;24:137–146.

71. **Petereit DG, Pearcey R.** Literature analysis of high dose rate brachytherapy fractionation schedules in the treatment of cervical cancer: is there an optimal fractionation schedule? *Int J Radiat Oncol Biol Phys* 1999;43:359–366.

72. **Petereit DG, Sarkaria JN, Potter DM, Schink JC.** High-dose-rate versus low-dose-rate brachytherapy in the treatment of cervical cancer: analysis of tumor recurrence—the University of Wisconsin experience. *Int J Radiat Oncol Biol Phys* 1999;45:1267–1274.

73. **Lancker M, Storme G.** Prediction of severe late complications in fractionated, high-dose-rate brachytherapy in gynecological applications. *Int J Radiat Oncol Biol Phys* 1991;20:1125–1129.

74. **Nag S, Orton C, Young D, Erickson B.** The American Brachytherapy Society survey of brachytherapy practice for carcinoma of the cervix in the United States. *Gynecol Oncol* 1999;73:111–118.

75. **Eifel PJ, Moughan J, Owen JB, Katz A, Mahon I, Hanks GE.** Patterns of radiotherapy practice for patients with squamous carcinoma of the uterine cervix. A Patterns of Care study. *Int J Radiat Oncol Biol Phys* 1999;43:351–358.

76. **Höckel M, Baußmann E, Mitze M, Knapstein PG.** Are pelvic side-wall recurrences of cervical cancer biologically different from central relapses? *Cancer* 1994;74:648–655.

77. **Erickson B, Gillin MT.** Interstitial implantation of gynecologic malignancies. *J Surg Oncol* 1997;66:285–295.

78. **Hughes-Davies L, Silver B, Kapp D.** Parametrial interstitial brachytherapy for advanced or recurrent pelvic malignancy: The Harvard/Stanford experience. *Gynecol Oncol* 1995;58:24–27.

79. **Monk BJ, Tewari K, Burger RA, Johnson MT, Montz FJ, Berman ML.** A comparison of intracavitary versus interstitial irradiation in the treatment of cervical cancer. *Gynecol Oncol* 1997;67:241–247.

80. **Delclos L, Fletcher GH.** Gynecologic cancers. In: **Levitt SH, Kahn FM, Potish RA, ed.** *Technological basis of radiation therapy: practical clinical applications.* Philadelphia: Lea & Febiger, 1992;193–227.

81. **Martinez A, Edmundson GK, Cox RS, Gunderson LL, Howes AE.** Combination of external beam irradiation and multiple-site perineal applicator (MUPIT) for treatment of locally advanced or recurrent prostatic, anorectal, and gynecologic malignancies. *Int J Radiat Oncol Biol Phys* 1985;11:391–398.

82. **Syed AMN, Puthwala AA, Neblett D.** Transperineal interstitial-intracavitary "Syed-Neblett" applicator in the treatment of carcinoma of the uterine cervix. *Endocuriether Hyperther Oncol* 1986;2:1–13.

83. **Rosenshein NB.** Radioisotopes in the treatment of ovarian cancer. *Clin Obstet Gynaecol* 1983;10:279–295.

84. **Reed GW, Watson ER, Chesters MS.** A note on the distribution of radioactive colloidal gold following *intraperitoneal* injection. *Br J Radiol* 1961;34:323.

85. **Klaassen D, Starreveld A, Shelly W, Miller A, Boyes D, Gerulath A, et al.** External beam pelvic radiotherapy plus intraperitoneal radioactive chromic phosphate in early stage ovarian cancer: a toxic combination. *Int J Radiat Oncol Biol Phys* 1985;11:1801–1804.

86. **Young RC, Walton LA, Ellenberg SS, Homesley HD, Wilbanks GD, Decker DG, et al.** Adjuvant therapy in stage I and stage II epithelial ovarian cancer. Results of two prospective randomized trials. *N Engl J Med* 1990;322:1021–1027.

87. **Chao C, Williamson JF, Grigsby PW, Perez CA.** Uterosacral space involvement in locally advanced carcinoma of the uterine cervix. *Int J Radiat Oncol Biol Phys* 1998;40:397–403.

88. **Kim RY, McGinnis LS, Spencer SA, Meredith RF, Jennelle RL, Salter MM.** Conventional four-field pelvic radiotherapy technique without CT treatment planning in cancer of the cervix: potential geographic miss. *Radiother Oncol* 1994;30:140–145.

89. **Ahmed RS, Kim RY, Duan J, Meleth S, De Los Santos JF, Fiveash JB.** IMRT dose escalation for positive para-aortic lymph nodes in patients with locally advanced cervical cancer while reducing dose to bone marrow and other organs at risk. *Int J Radiat Oncol Biol Phys* 2004;60:505–512.

90. **Mundt AJ, Roeske JC, Lujan AE.** Intensity-modulated radiation therapy in gynecologic malignancies. *Med Dosim* 2002;27:131–136.

91. **Lanciano RM, Martz K, Coia LR, Hanks GE.** Tumor and treatment factors improving outcome in stage III-B cervix cancer. *Int J Radiat Oncol Biol Phys* 1991;20:95–100.

92. **Fletcher GH, Hamberger AD.** Squamous cell carcinoma of the uterine cervix. Treatment technique according to size of the cervical lesion and extension. In: **Fletcher GH, ed.** *Textbook of radiotherapy.* 3rd ed. Philadelphia: Lea & Febiger, 1980;720–778.

93. **International Commission on Radiation Units and Measurements.** *Dose and volume specification for reporting intracavitary therapy in gynecology.* Vol 38. Bethesda, MD: International Commission on Radiation Units and Measurements, 1985.

94. **Pelloski CE, Palmer M, Chronowski GM, Jhingran A, Horton J, Eifel PJ.** Comparison between CT-based volumetric calculations and ICRU reference-point estimates of radiation doses delivered to bladder and rectum during intracavitary radiotherapy for cervical cancer. *Int J Radiat Oncol Biol Phys* 2005;62:131–137.

95. **Keys HM, Bundy BN, Stehman FB, et al.** Weekly *cisplatin* chemotherapy during irradiation improves survival and reduces relapses for patients with bulky stage IB cervical cancer treated with irradiation and adjuvant hysterectomy: results of a randomized GOG trial. *Gynecol Oncol* 1998;68:100.

96. **Peters WA 3rd, Liu PY, Barrett RJ 2nd, Stock RJ, Monk BJ, Berek JS, et al.** Concurrent chemotherapy and pelvic radiation therapy compared with pelvic radiation therapy alone as adjuvant therapy after radical surgery in high-risk early-stage cancer of the cervix. *J Clin Oncol* 2000;18:1606–1613.

97. **Whitney CW, Sause W, Bundy BN, Malfetano JH, Hannigan EV, Fowler WC Jr, et al.** A randomized comparison of *fluorouracil* plus *cisplatin* versus *hydroxyurea* as an adjunct to radiation therapy in stages IIB–IVA carcinoma of the cervix with negative para-aortic lymph nodes: a Gynecologic Oncology Group and Southwest Oncology Group study. *J Clin Oncol* 1999;17:1339–1348.

98. **Roberts KB, Urdaneta N, Vera R, Vera A, Gutierrez E, Aguilar Y, et al.** Interim results of a randomized trial of *mitomycin C* as an adjunct to radical radiotherapy in the treatment of locally advanced squamous-cell carcinoma of the cervix. *Int J Cancer* 2000;90:206–223.

99. **Lorvidhaya V, Chitapanarux I, Sangruchi S, Lertsanguansinchai P, Kongthanarat Y, Tangkaratt S, et al.** Concurrent *mitomycin C, 5-fluorouracil,* and radiotherapy in the treatment of locally advanced carcinoma of the cervix: a randomized trial. *Int J Radiat Oncol Biol Phys* 2003;55:1226–1232.

100. **Wong LC, Ngan HY, Cheung AN, Cheng DK, Ng TY, Choy DT.** Chemoradiation and adjuvant chemotherapy in cervical cancer. *J Clin Oncol* 1999;17:2055–2060.

101. **Alvarez RD, Potter ME, Soong SJ, Gay FL, Hatch KD, Partridge EE, et al.** Rationale for using pathologic tumor dimensions and nodal status to subclassify surgically treated stage IB cervical cancer patients. *Gynecol Oncol* 1991;43:108–112.

102. **van Bommel PF, van Lindert AC, Kock HC, Leers WH, Neijt JP.** A review of prognostic factors in early-stage carcinoma of the cervix

(FIGO I B and II A) and implications for treatment strategy. *Eur J Obstet Gynecol Reprod Biol* 1987;26:69–84.

103. **Rotman M, Sedlis A, Piedmonte MR, Bundy B, Lentz SS, Muderspach LI, et al.** A phase III randomized trial of postoperative pelvic irradiation in stage IB cervical carcinoma with poor prognostic features: follow-up of a Gynecologic Oncology Group study. *Int J Radiat Oncol Biol Phys* 2006;65:169–176.

104. **Ijaz T, Eifel PJ, Burke T, Oswald MJ.** Radiation therapy of pelvic recurrence after radical hysterectomy for cervical carcinoma. *Gynecol Oncol* 1998;70:241–246.

105. **Thomas G, Dembo A, Beale F, Bean H, Bush R, Herman J, et al.** Concurrent radiation, *mitomycin C,* and 5-*fluorouracil* in poor prognosis carcinoma of the cervix: preliminary results of a phase I-II study. *Int J Radiat Oncol Biol Phys* 1984;10:1785–1790.

106. **Hamberger AD, Unal A, Gershenson DM, Fletcher GH.** Analysis of the severe complications of irradiation of carcinoma of the cervix: whole pelvis irradiation and intracavitary radium. *Int J Radiat Oncol Biol Phys* 1983;9:367–371.

107. **Kucera H, Enzelsberger H, Eppel W, Weghaupt K.** The influence of nicotine abuse and diabetes mellitus on the results of primary irradiation in the treatment of carcinoma of the cervix. *Cancer* 1987;60:1–4.

108. **Bruner DW, Lanciano R, Keegan M, Corn B, Martin E, Hanks GE.** Vaginal stenosis and sexual function following intracavitary radiation for the treatment of cervical and endometrial carcinoma. *Int J Radiat Oncol Biol Phys* 1993;27:825–830.

109. **Eifel PJ, Levenback C, Wharton JT, Oswald MJ.** Time course and incidence of late complications in patients treated with radiation therapy for FIGO stage IB carcinoma of the uterine cervix. *Int J Radiat Oncol Biol Phys* 1995;32:1289–1300.

110. **Chassagne D, Sismondi P, Horiot JC, Sinistrero G, Bey P, Zola P, et al.** A glossary for reporting complications of treatment in gynecological cancers. *Radiother Oncol* 1993;26:195–202.

111. **Heyman J.** The so-called Stockholm method and the results of treatment of uterine cancer at the Radiumhemmet. *Acta Radiol* 1935;22:129.

112. **Eifel PJ, Ross J, Hendrickson M, Cox RS, Kempson R, Martinez A.** Adenocarcinoma of the endometrium. Analysis of 256 cases with disease limited to the uterine corpus: treatment options. *Cancer* 1983;52:1026–1031.

113. **Jones HW.** Treatment of adenocarcinoma of the endometrium. *Obstet Gynecol Surv* 1975;30:147–169.

114. **Calais G, Vitu L, Descamps P, Body G, Reynaud-Bougnoux A, Lansac J, et al.** Preoperative or postoperative brachytherapy for patients with endometrial carcinoma stage I and II. *Int J Radiat Oncol Biol Phys* 1990;19:523–527.

115. **Piver MS, Yazigi R, Blumenson L, Tsukada Y.** A prospective trial comparing hysterectomy, hysterectomy plus vaginal radium, and uterine radium plus hysterectomy in stage I endometrial carcinoma. *Obstet Gynecol* 1979;54:85–89.

116. **Keys HM, Roberts JA, Brunetto VL, Zaino RJ, Spirtos NM, Bloss JD, et al., for the Gynecologic Oncology Group.** A phase III trial of surgery with or without adjunctive external pelvic radiation therapy in intermediate risk endometrial adenocarcinoma: a Gynecologic Oncology Group study. *Gynecol Oncol* 2004;92:744–751.

117. **Hendrickson M, Ross M, Eifel P, Martinez A, Kempson R.** Uterine papillary serous carcinoma: a highly malignant form of endometrial adenocarcinoma. *Am J Surg Pathol* 1982;6:93–108.

118. **Mallipeddi P, Kapp DS, Teng NNH.** Long-term survival with adjuvant whole abdominopelvic irradiation for uterine papillary serous carcinoma. *Cancer* 1993;71:3076–3081.

119. **Corn BW, Lanciano RM, Greven KM, Noumoff J, Schultz D, Hanks GE, et al.** Impact of improved irradiation technique, age and lymph node sampling on the severe complication rate of surgically staged endometrial cancer patients: a multivariate analysis. *J Clin Oncol* 1994;12:510–515.

120. **Greven KM, Lanciano RM, Herbert SH, Hogan PE.** Analysis of complications in patients with endometrial carcinoma receiving adjuvant irradiation. *Int J Radiat Oncol Biol Phys* 1991;21:919–923.

121. **Dembo A.** The sequential multiple modality treatment of ovarian cancer. *Radiother Oncol* 1985;3:187–192.

122. **Fuller DB, Sause WT, Plenk HP, Menlove RL.** Analysis of postoperative radiation therapy in Stage I through III epithelial ovarian carcinoma. *J Clin Oncol* 1987;5:897–905.

123. **Martinez A, Schray MF, Howes AE, Bagshaw MA.** Postoperative radiation therapy for epithelial ovarian cancer: the curative role based on a 24-year experience. *J Clin Oncol* 1985;3:901–911.

124. **Weiser EB, Burke TW, Heller PB, Woodward J, Hoskins WJ, Park RC.** Determinants of survival of patients with epithelial ovarian carcinoma following whole abdomen irradiation (WAR). *Gynecol Oncol* 1988;30:201–208.

125. **Ledermann JA, Dembo AJ, Sturgeon JFG, Fine S, Bush RS, Fyles AW, et al.** Outcome of patients with unfavorable optimally cytoreduced ovarian cancer treated with chemotherapy and whole abdominal irradiation. *Gynecol Oncol* 1991;41:30–35.

126. **Bruzzone M, Repetto L, Chiara S, Campora E, Conte PF, Orsatti M, et al.** Chemotherapy versus radiotherapy in the management of ovarian cancer patients with pathological complete response or minimal residual disease at second look. *Gynecol Oncol* 1990;38:392–395.

127. **Lambert HE, Rustin GJS, Gregory WM, Nelstrop AE.** A randomized trial comparing single-agent *carboplatin* with *carboplatin* followed by radiotherapy for advanced ovarian cancer: a North Thames Ovary Group study. *J Clin Oncol* 1993;11:440–448.

128. **Lawton F, Luesley D, Blackledge G, Hilton C, Kelly K, Latief T, et al.** A randomized trial comparing whole abdominal radiotherapy with chemotherapy following *cisplatinum* cytoreduction in epithelial ovarian cancer. West Midlands Ovarian Cancer Group Trial II. *Clin Oncol* (R Coll Radiol) 1990;2:4–9.

129. **Eifel PJ, Gershenson DM, Delclos L, Wharton JT, Peters LJ.** Twice-daily, split-course abdominopelvic radiation therapy after chemotherapy and positive second-look laparotomy for epithelial ovarian carcinoma. *Int J Radiat Oncol Biol Phys* 1991;21: 1013–1018.

130. **Hacker N, Berek J, Burnison C, Heintz PM, Juillard GJ, Lagasse LD.** Whole abdominal radiation as salvage therapy for epithelial ovarian cancer. *Obstet Gynecol* 1985;65:60–66.

131. **Delclos L, Murphy M.** Evaluation of tolerance during treatment, late tolerance, and better evaluation of clinical effectiveness of the cobalt 60 moving strip technique. *Am J Roentgenol Radiat Ther Nucl Med* 1966;96:75–80.

132. **Dembo AJ, Bush RS, Beale FA, et al.** A randomized clinical trial of moving strip versus open field whole abdominal irradiation in patients with invasive epithelial cancer of ovary. *Int J Radiat Oncol Biol Phys* 1983;9:97.

133. **Fazekas JT, Maier JG.** Irradiation of ovarian carcinomas: a prospective comparison of the open-field and moving-strip techniques. *Am J Roentgenol Radium Ther Nucl Med* 1974;120:118–123.

134. **Dembo AJ.** Abdominopelvic radiotherapy in ovarian cancer. *Cancer* 1985;55:2285–2290.

135. **van Bunningen B, Bouma J, Kooijman C, Wárlám-Rodenhuis CC, Heintz AP, van Lindert A.** Total abdominal irradiation in stage I and II carcinoma of the ovary. *Radiother Oncol* 1988;11:305–310.

136. **Faul C, Miramow D, Gerszten K, Huang C, Edwards R.** Isolated local recurrence in carcinoma of the vulva: prognosis and implications for treatment. *Int J Gynecol Cancer* 1998;8:409–414.

137. **Faul CM, Mirmow D, Huang Q, Gerszten K, Day R, Jones MW.** Adjuvant radiation for vulvar carcinoma: improved local control. *Int J Radiat Oncol Biol Phys* 1997;38:381–389.

138. **Thomas GM, Dembo AJ, Bryson SC, Osborne R, DePetrillo AD.** Changing concepts in the management of vulvar cancer. *Gynecol Oncol* 1991;42:9–21.

139. **Petereit DG, Mehta MP, Buchler DA, Kinsella TJ.** A retrospective review of nodal treatment for vulvar cancer. *Am J Clin Oncol* 1993;16:38–42.

140. **Koh WJ, Chiu M, Stelzer KJ, Greer BE, Mastras D, Comsia N, et al.** Femoral vessel depth and the implications for groin node radiation. *Int J Radiat Oncol Biol Phys* 1993;27:969–974.

141. **Eifel PJ, Morris M, Burke TW, Levenback C, Gershenson DM.** Preoperative continuous infusion *cisplatinum* and 5-*fluorouracil* with radiation for locally advanced or recurrent carcinoma of the vulva. *Gynecol Oncol* 1995;59:51–56.

142. **Koh WJ, Wallace HJ 3rd, Greer BE, Cain J, Stelzer KJ, Russell KJ, et al.** Combined radiotherapy and chemotherapy in the management of local-regionally advanced vulvar cancer. *Int J Radiat Oncol Biol Phys* 1993;26:809–816.

143. **Moore DH, Thomas GM, Montana GS, Saxer A, Gallup DG, Olt G.** Preoperative chemoradiation for advanced vulvar cancer: a

phase II study of the Gynecologic Oncology Group. *Int J Radiat Oncol Biol Phys* 1998;42:79–85.

144. **Berek JS, Heaps JM, Fu YS, Juillard GJ, Hacker NF.** Concurrent *cisplatin* and *5-fluorouracil* chemotherapy and radiation therapy for advanced-stage squamous carcinoma of the vulva. *Gynecol Oncol* 1991;42:197–201.

145. **Levin W, Goldberg G, Altaras M, Bloch B, Shelton MG.** The use of concomitant chemotherapy and radiotherapy prior to surgery in advanced stage carcinoma of the vulva. *Gynecol Oncol* 1986;25:20–25.

146. **Thomas G, Dembo A, DePetrillo A, Pringle J, Ackerman I, Bryson P, et al.** Concurrent radiation and chemotherapy in vulvar carcinoma. *Gynecol Oncol* 1989;34:263–267.

147. **Wahlen SA, Slater JD, Wagner RJ, Wang WA, Keeney ED, Hocko JM, et al.** Concurrent radiation therapy and chemotherapy in the treatment of primary squamous cell carcinoma of the vulva. *Cancer* 1995;75:2289–2294.

148. **Frank SJ, Deavers MT, Jhingran A, Bodurka DC, Eifel PJ.** Primary adenocarcinoma of the vagina not associated with diethylstilbestrol (DES) exposure. *Gynecol Oncol* 2007;105:470–474.

5

Pathology

Christina S. Kong
Teri A. Longacre
Michael R. Hendrickson

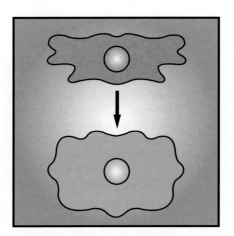

The individual organs within the genital tract make up an extended müllerian system that can give rise to a wide variety of histologically similar tumors. Because of this extended müllerian system, tumor classification and assignment of primary site can be problematic. This chapter provides an overview of the main tumors that are encountered in the female genital tract, emphasizing key histopathologic features and pertinent ancillary diagnostic studies.

To maximize the information provided by pathologic examination, it is important that the treating clinician understand basic concepts of gynecologic oncologic pathology. It is similarly important for the pathologist to understand basic clinical, radiologic, and serologic data. **The integration of clinical, radiologic, and pathologic information is central to intraoperative evaluation and ultimately to treatment planning, and it occurs best within the framework of the multidisciplinary tumor board** seen in most major cancer centers.

Cervix

Squamous Lesions of the Cervix

Terminology

There are several systems for classifying preneoplastic lesions of the cervix, so it is useful to be familiar with all the systems because the terms can be used interchangeably (Table 5.1). Over the years, the classification systems have moved toward fewer, more clinically relevant categories. The most recent is the **Bethesda system,** which was developed for providing uniform diagnostic terminology for cervical cytologic specimens but is now also used for histologic diagnoses. **It has two categories: low-grade squamous intraepithelial lesion (LSIL) and high-grade squamous intraepithelial lesion (HSIL).** The LSIL category encompasses condyloma and cervical intraepithelial neoplasia (CIN) grade 1, whereas the HSIL category encompasses CIN 2 and CIN 3. CIN 1 is equivalent to mild dysplasia, CIN 2 to moderate dysplasia, and CIN 3 to severe dysplasia and carcinoma *in situ*. The Bethesda system and CIN terminology are the most widely used.

Low-Grade Squamous Intraepithelial Lesion

There are three main subtypes of LSIL. **Flat condylomas** lack the exophytic growth pattern and are more frequently associated with intermediate and high-risk HPV types. These are the most common in the cervix. **Condyloma acuminatum** is the classic genital wart with an exophytic

Table 5.1 Terminology for Cervicovaginal Squamous Intraepithelial Lesions			
Low-Grade Squamous Intraepithelial Lesion		*High-Grade Squamous Intraepithelial Lesion*	
Cervical Intraepithelial Neoplasia (CIN)			
Condyloma	CIN 1	CIN 2	CIN 3
	Mild dysplasia	Moderate dysplasia	Severe dysplasia

growth pattern. It is typically associated with low-risk HPV types 6 and 11. **Immature condylomas** are the least common and exhibit a filiform, papillary growth pattern; they are associated with low-risk HPV types.

LSIL is characterized by thickened mucosa with enlarged, dark cells that have low nuclear-to-cytoplasmic ratios in the upper layers (Fig. 5.1). Binucleation can be seen in 90% of LSIL, and when the nuclei are surrounded by an irregularly shaped and sharply punched out halo, they are known as *koilocytes*. However, binucleation and halos both can be seen as part of a reactive process. With reactive change, the nucleus is minimally enlarged and not hyperchromatic, and the halo is less distinct, round, and uniform. Glycogen vacuoles can also appear as round, uniform halos. In addition, LSIL can be mimicked by a squamous papilloma (also known as an *ectocervical* or *fibroepithelial polyp*). **Squamous papillomas lack koilocytes and have central fibrovascular cores that are not typical of condylomas.**

The ASCUS-LSIL Triage Study studied interobserver variability in the diagnosis of squamous intraepithelial lesion (SIL) on biopsy (1). More than 2,700 cervical biopsies and loop electrosurgical excision procedure (LEEP) specimens were examined by one to two staff pathologists at one of four centers across the United States and then reviewed by one of four quality control (QC) pathologists. **There was agreement on the diagnosis of LSIL in 43% of cases, but 41% of the cases diagnosed by the staff pathologists as LSIL were downgraded by the QC pathologists to negative.** Of note, most of the downgraded cases were positive for high-risk HPV, raising the question of which diagnosis was correct. The significance of this finding was not addressed by the study.

High-Grade Squamous Intraepithelial Lesion

HSIL are characterized by atypical, dark cells with high nuclear-to-cytoplasmic ratios that involve one-third to two-thirds of the epithelium in cases of CIN 2 (Fig. 5.2) or more than two-thirds in cases of CIN 3 (Fig. 5.3). The involved mucosa is notable for disorderly arrangement

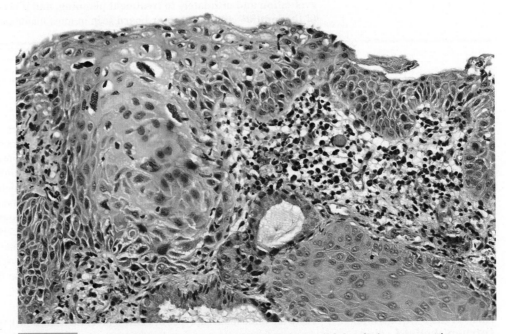

Figure 5.1   Low-grade squamous intraepithelial lesion (mild dysplasia, CIN 1). The mucosa is thickened with dysplastic cells and koilocytes in the upper layers.

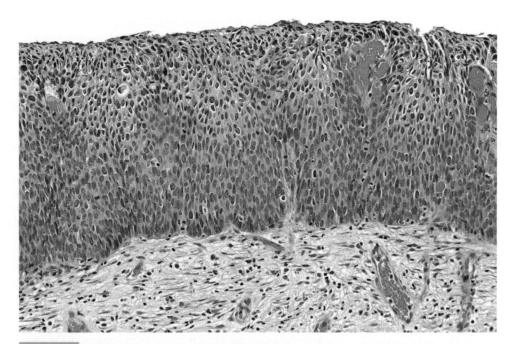

Figure 5.2   **High-grade squamous intraepithelial lesion (moderate dysplasia, CIN 2).** Dysplastic cells with high nuclear-to-cytoplasmic ratios involve less than two-thirds of the mucosa.

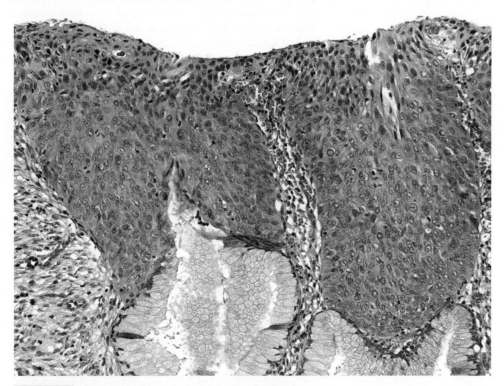

Figure 5.3   **High-grade squamous intraepithelial lesion (severe dysplasia, CIN 3).** The squamous mucosa is notable for full thickness atypia and extension of the dysplastic cells down into endocervical glands.

of cells with loss of polarity and crowding. Mitotic figures in the upper half of the mucosa are commonly identified.

Immature squamous metaplasia and atrophy can be difficult to distinguish from HSIL because they are also characterized by cells with high nuclear-to-cytoplasmic ratios. However, the nuclei in squamous metaplasia and atrophy should lack crowding and appear uniform with smooth nuclear membranes. Mitotic figures can be seen near the basal layer but not in the upper half of the mucosa. In indeterminate cases, immunohistochemical stain for p16^{INK4a}, a surrogate marker for high-risk HPV, can be helpful (2). In some cases, for various reasons (e.g., tangential sectioning, small dissociated fragment, cautery artifact), a distinction cannot be made between LSIL and HSIL. These are best characterized as SIL of indeterminate grade.

The ALT study found good reproducibility for the histologic diagnosis of HSIL with concordance in 76.9% of cervical biopsies and 80.2% of LEEP specimens (1).

Squamous Cell Carcinoma

Cervical squamous cell carcinomas (SCCs) can be subdivided into two main groups: microinvasive carcinomas and invasive carcinomas. *Microinvasive carcinoma* **(FIGO* stage IA1) is defined as microscopic disease with ≤3.0 mm stromal invasion and ≤7.0 mm horizontal extent. For accurate measurements, the entire lesion needs to be visible with requires negative surgical margins. Although lymphatic-vascular invasion (LVI) is acknowledged as a poor prognostic factor, the presence or absence of LVI does not change the FIGO stage. The depth of invasion is measured from the basement membrane at the point of invasion to the deepest invasive focus** (Fig. 5.4). Morphologically, microinvasive carcinoma is characterized by jagged fingers extending from the base of HSIL into the submucosa and surrounded by chronic inflammation and loose, fibroblastic stroma (i.e., desmoplasia). Often at the point of invasion, the neoplastic cells become more differentiated and have abundant eosinophilic cytoplasm that may be keratinizing. Microinvasive carcinoma can be difficult to distinguish from HSIL, especially when HSIL involves endocervical glands or is associated with previous biopsy site changes. Examining multiple-level sections of the same focus can be helpful.

Squamous cell carcinomas that are clearly invasive can be keratinizing or nonkeratinizing and range from well differentiated to poorly differentiated. Well- to moderately differentiated invasive SCC is characterized by cohesive nests and sheets of neoplastic cells with abundant eosinophilic cytoplasm and distinct cell borders (Fig. 5.5). Keratin pearl formation, central keratinization, and necrosis within nests may also be identified. With poorly differentiated carcinomas, keratinization may be minimal or absent, and they may be difficult to

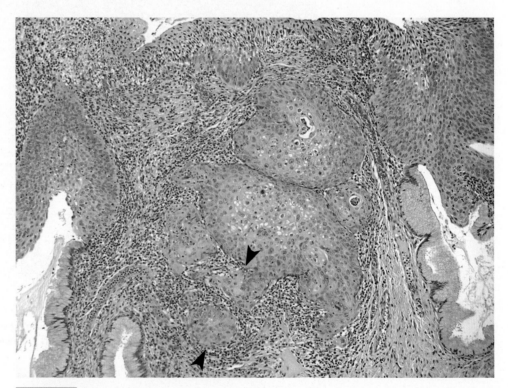

Figure 5.4   **Microinvasive squamous cell carcinoma of the cervix.** Invasion is measured from the basement membrane at the point of invasion (upper arrow) to the deepest invasive focus (lower arrow). FIGO* Stage IA1 cervical cancer is defined by a depth of invasion ≤3 mm and horizontal extent ≤7 mm in a specimen with negative margins.

*International Federation of Gynecology and Obstetrics

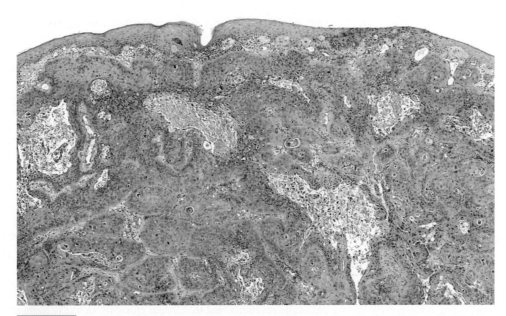

Figure 5.5   **Invasive squamous cell carcinoma of the cervix, moderately differentiated keratinizing.** Keratinization and necrosis within nests of malignant squamous cells are present.

distinguish from other types of poorly differentiated carcinomas (e.g., adenocarcinoma). **Grade and type have not been found to be prognostically significant.** Instead, depth of invasion, lymphatic or vascular invasion, and size are important prognostic variables.

Human Papilloma Virus

Human papilloma virus (HPV) DNA has been detected in virtually all cases of cervical dysplasia and carcinoma, and it is considered to be a necessary but not sufficient cause for the development of the vast majority of invasive cervical carcinomas. Although a variety of HPV types may infect epithelial cells, the risk of oncogenic transformation is most strongly linked to several specific high-risk types. **In 2003, a large epidemiologic study by the International Agency for Research on Cancer (IARC) pooled data from nine countries and identified 15 high-risk HPV types** (16, 18, 31, 33, 35, 39, 45, 51, 52, 56, 58, 59, 68, 73, and 82), three probable high-risk types (26, 53, and 66), and 12 low-risk types (6, 11, 40, 42, 43, 44, 54, 61, 70, 72, 81, and CP6108). **The IARC met again in 2005 to reassess the carcinogenicity of HPV and revised the original list of high-risk types to include 13 types: 16, 18, 31, 33, 35, 39, 45, 51, 52, 56, 58, 59, and 66** (3). Most investigators now believe that persistent infection with high-risk HPV types is associated with the subsequent development of high-grade dysplasia and invasive carcinoma (4). A substantial proportion of LSIL are also associated with infection by high-risk HPV types, but many infections are transitory (4,5).

Cervicovaginal Cytology (Pap Testing)

Specimen Preparation Methods

There are two main specimen types for cervicovaginal cytology: conventional smear and liquid-based preparation. Conventional smears involve directly smearing material onto a glass slide and then immediately fixing the specimen with ethanol. The advantages of conventional smears are their low cost and the lack of need for specialized equipment to process specimens. The disadvantages are lack of uniformity in specimen preparation and unsatisfactory smears because of obscuring inflammation, obscuring blood, or thick areas in the smear.

Liquid-based preparations involve placing the cytologic material in a liquid fixative instead of directly smearing it on a glass slide. The two most commonly used are **ThinPrep** (Hologic, Bedford, MA) and **SurePath** (BD Diagnostics, Burlington, NC). ThinPrep uses a methanol-based fixative and a filter preparation for making the slide. SurePath uses an ethanol-based fixative and a Ficoll gradient. SurePath also employs a detachable head for the collection device so the entire specimen is submitted for processing. **The advantages of liquid-based preparations are uniformity in slide preparation and fewer unsatisfactory specimens.** The disadvantages are significantly higher cost and the necessity for specialized processing equipment for each liquid-based method.

Who Signs Out Pap Tests?

Cervicovaginal cytologic specimens are predominantly screened by board-certified cytotechnologists. In some small laboratories, the primary screening of the slides is performed by a pathologist. If the Pap test is negative for intraepithelial lesion or malignancy and lacks reactive or reparative changes, then the final report can be issued by the cytotechnologist. **Quality control review by a second senior cytotechnologist or a pathologist is performed on at least 10% of all negative cases and on all cases for patients with a history of an abnormal Pap test.** If any reactive, reparative, or epithelial abnormalities are found, then the slide is reviewed by a pathologist who will issue the final report.

The Clinical Laboratory Improvement Act of 1988 set limits on the number of Pap tests that can be reviewed by a cytotechnologist in a 24-hour period. The nationwide limit is 100 nonimaged or 200 imaged slides per day, but individual states can set lower limits (e.g., 80 nonimaged or 160 imaged slides in California). Currently, there is a requirement that all pathologists and cytotechnologists who interpret Pap tests pass an annual proficiency test.

The Bethesda System

In 1988, the National Cancer Institute sponsored a workshop in Bethesda, Maryland, to develop uniform diagnostic terminology for Pap tests. The resulting classification system has undergone multiple revisions, and the system currently in use is Bethesda 2001 (6) (Table 5.2).

According to the Bethesda system, the Pap test report should include the following categories: specimen type (e.g., conventional, liquid based), specimen adequacy, and interpretation or result. A general categorization category and educational notes and suggestions are optional. If

Table 5.2 2001 Bethesda System	
	Bethesda 2001
Specimen Type	Conventional Liquid-based (specify type: e.g., ThinPrep, SurePath) Other
Specimen Adequacy	Satisfactory for evaluation Unsatisfactory for evaluation
General Categorization (Optional)	Negative for intraepithelial lesion or malignancy Epithelial cell abnormality Other: Endometrial cells in a woman >40 years of age
Interpretation or Result	Negative for intraepithelial lesion or malignancy (specify organisms, other nonneoplastic findings)
Squamous	Atypical squamous cells of undetermined significance (ASC-US) *or* cannot exclude HSIL (ASC-H) Low-grade squamous intraepithelial lesion (LSIL) High-grade squamous intraepithelial lesion (HSIL) Squamous cell carcinoma
Glandular	Atypical endocervical, endometrial *or* glandular cells (NOS or favor neoplastic) Endocervical adenocarcinoma *in situ* Adenocarcinoma
Other	Endometrial cells in a woman >40 years of age Other malignant neoplasms
Ancillary Testing	HPV, GC, *Chlamydia*: Include description of test method(s) and results
Automated Review	Specify device and result if slide is examined by an imaging system
Educational Notes and Suggestions (Optional)	Based on ASCCP management guidelines

Table 5.3 Lubricants Less Likely to Interfere with ThinPrep Samples	
Brand	*Company*
KY Jelly	Johnson & Johnson
Surgilube	E. Fougera & Co.
Astroglide	Biofilm, Inc.
Crystelle	Deltex Pharmaceuticals

automated screening is performed (e.g., ThinPrep Imager or BD FocalPoint), then the device and result are also reported. If ancillary testing is performed, then the results may be indicated in the Pap test report or reported separately.

Specimen adequacy is divided into "**satisfactory for evaluation**" and "**unsatisfactory for evaluation.**" The presence or absence of transformation zone cells (i.e., endocervical cells or squamous metaplastic cells) and quality indicators (e.g., obscuring blood or inflammation, scant cellularity) are indicated under the umbrella of "satisfactory for evaluation." Specimens can be unsatisfactory for a variety of reasons, and this will be indicated on the report. Some specimens are rejected and not processed; these are usually the result of a broken slide or empty collection vial. Others are found to be unsatisfactory after processing and examination of the slide. A common cause of unsatisfactory ThinPrep specimens is the use of lubricants containing carbomers or carbopol polymers when obtaining the sample. Cytyc has distributed a nonexhaustive list of lubricants that are less likely to interfere with processing (Table 5.3). Another common cause of unsatisfactory specimens is obscuring blood. Although liquid-based systems can remove blood from the sample, the ThinPrep system is able to handle less blood than the SurePath Ficoll gradient.

Squamous Cell Abnormalities

LSIL in cervical cytology specimens is characterized by enlarged (more than three times the size of an intermediate cell nucleus), dark nuclei with irregular, thickened nuclear membranes. When the cells are binucleated and surrounded by a sharply defined, irregularly shaped halo with a peripheral rim of thickened cytoplasm, then the cell is known as a *koilocyte* (Fig. 5.6). **Although koilocytes are pathognomonic for a diagnosis of LSIL, they are not required.** LSIL can be diagnosed based on cells with enlarged, dark, irregular nuclei and no cytoplasmic halo. Koilocytes can be mimicked by prominent glycogen vacuoles or inflammatory halos (Fig. 5.7). In these cases, the area of perinuclear clearing is not sharply demarcated and tends to be round and regular with the nucleus centrally located. **When the findings fall short of LSIL, the diagnosis of** *atypical squamous cells of undetermined significance* **(ASC-US) is used** (Fig. 5.8). Usually, this is because one of the nuclear features is lacking: The nuclei are not quite large enough (2.5 to 3 times the size of an intermediate cell nucleus), dark enough, or irregular enough.

HSIL is characterized by cells with dark nuclei, irregular nuclear membranes and high nuclear-to-cytoplasmic ratios (Fig. 5.9). The dysplastic cells can occur singly, in sheets, or as syncytial aggregates. The chromatin ranges from coarse to bland, and the cytoplasm from delicate to dense. The nuclei vary in size and are frequently smaller than those seen with LSIL. With liquid-based preparations, dispersed abnormal single cells are more common than aggregates. In addition, with ThinPrep, the nuclei may not be dark; the diagnosis relies on finding single cells with irregular nuclear membranes and high nuclear-to-cytoplasmic ratios.

Mimics of HSIL include squamous metaplasia, atrophy, repair, endometrial cells, histiocytes, and endocervical cells. Atrophy and squamous metaplasia can be especially difficult to distinguish from HSIL. With **atrophic changes,** the basal and parabasal cells have high nuclear-to-cytoplasmic ratios with enlarged, dark nuclei, and the background can resemble tumor diathesis (Fig. 5.10). The distinction from HSIL relies on finding smooth nuclear membranes, flat monolayer sheets, and lack of variability in nuclear size and shape. **Squamous metaplastic cells** have high nuclear-to-cytoplasmic ratios and dense cytoplasm but smooth nuclear membranes. **If the cytologic features fall short of a diagnosis of HSIL, then the diagnosis of** *atypical squamous cells–cannot exclude HSIL* **(ASC-H) is used.** If dysplastic cells are clearly present but do not quite meet criteria for HSIL, then the changes are characterized as *LSIL cannot exclude HSIL.*

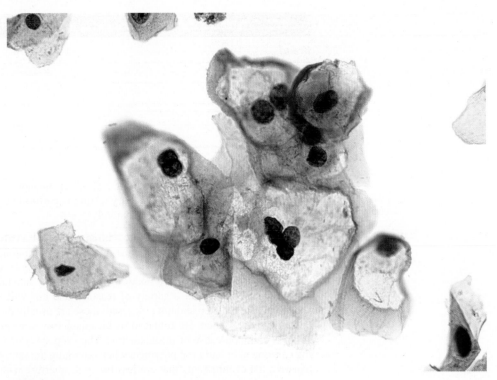

Figure 5.6 **Low-grade squamous intraepithelial lesion.** Koilocytes have sharply delineated, irregular halos and multiple, dark nuclei with irregular nuclear borders. (Papanicolaou stain)

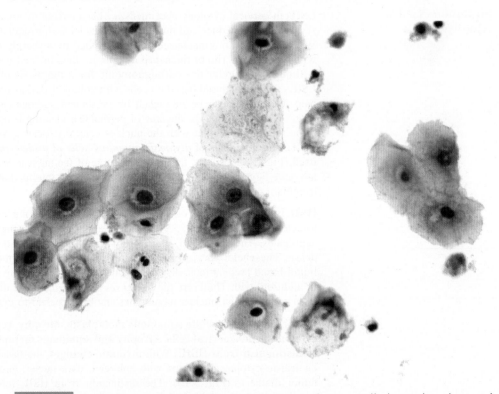

Figure 5.7 **Inflammatory halos.** Perinuclear clearing with a centrally located nucleus and hazy edges can be seen with infections (e.g., trichomonas) and can be mistaken for koilocytes. (Papanicolaou stain)

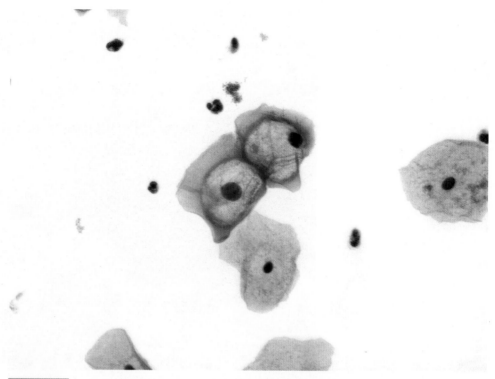

Figure 5.8 **Atypical squamous cells of undetermined significance (ASC-US).** The nucleus is 2.5 times the size of the intermediate cell nucleus, and the nuclear membranes are smooth. (Papanicolaou stain)

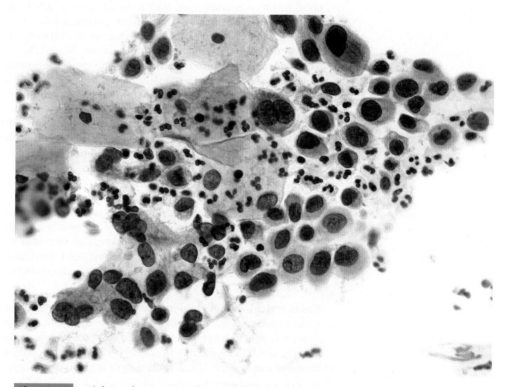

Figure 5.9 **High-grade squamous intraepithelial lesion.** The dysplastic cells have dark nuclei with focal nuclear membrane irregularities and high nuclear-to-cytoplasmic ratios. (Papanicolaou stain)

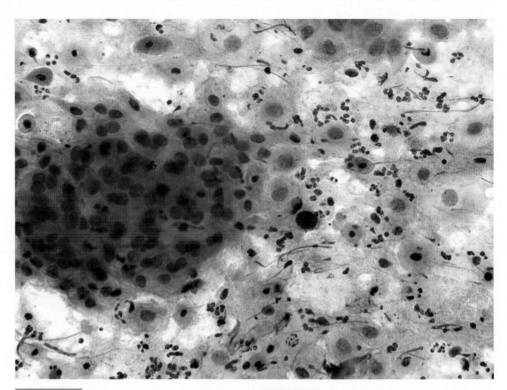

Figure 5.10 **Atrophy.** Atrophic vaginitis is characterized by sheets of parabasal cells and an inflammatory background that can mimic squamous cell carcinoma. (Papanicolaou stain)

The cytologic diagnosis of squamous cell carcinoma implies invasive carcinoma because carcinoma *in situ* is encompassed within the category of HSIL. Keratinizing SCC has single cells with dense, dark nuclei and dense, orangeophilic (i.e., orange-colored) cytoplasm. Nonkeratinizing SCC has syncytial aggregates as well as single cells with coarse chromatin and poorly defined cell borders with delicate basophilic (i.e., blue-colored) cytoplasm. **Macronucleoli and tumor diathesis** (i.e., necrosis, degenerating blood, inflammation) can be seen with both but more frequently with nonkeratinizing SCC. **With liquid-based preparations, tumor diathesis is seen as necrotic material clinging to the edges of cell groups and is less apparent than on conventional smears where it is spread across the background** (Fig. 5.11). **SCC can be difficult to distinguish from HSIL** because there is significant morphologic overlap between these two entities. Because keratinization can be seen with both, the findings of macronucleoli and tumor diathesis are more reliable indicators of SCC but are not always present. However, for both HSIL and SCC, the next step is colposcopy with biopsy, which will provide material for more definitive assessment for invasive carcinoma.

Glandular Cell Abnormalities

The diagnosis of "atypical glandular cells" accounts for less than 1% of all Pap tests. However, significant disease is present in 9% to 38% of cases with HSIL as the most common abnormal finding (7). Other findings include endocervical adenocarcinoma *in situ*, cervical carcinoma, endometrial pathology including carcinoma, and extrauterine carcinoma. Postmenopausal women have a higher rate of abnormality with a significant cervical or endometrial abnormality found in more than 30% of cases.

Endocervical adenocarcinoma *in situ* (AIS) is characterized by enlarged, elongated nuclei with irregular nuclear membranes and coarse chromatin arranged radially as rosettes or in strips as crowded palisades (Fig. 5.12). When the cytoplasm is partially stripped away, the palisading nuclei can resemble an array of feathers. This feature is referred to as *feathering* and is considered characteristic of AIS. Mitotic figures are also commonly present.

Endocervical AIS can be closely mimicked by tubal metaplasia, direct sampling of the endometrium, and HSIL involving endocervical glands. Tubal metaplasia is distinguished by the lack of nuclear crowding and smooth nuclear membranes. The presence of cilia is characteristic but not always seen. **Direct sampling of endometrium** can yield strips and sheets of atypical glandular cells with feathering, rosette formation, and frequent mitotic figures.

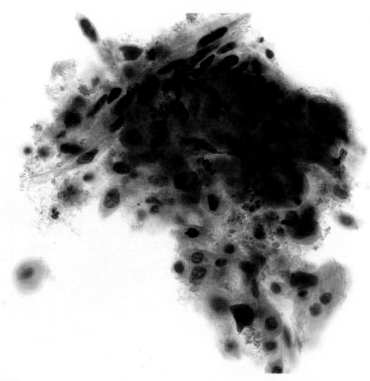

Figure 5.11   **Squamous cell carcinoma.** Necrosis in liquid-based preparations is characterized by granular debris that clings to the edges of tumor cell clusters. (Papanicolaou stain)

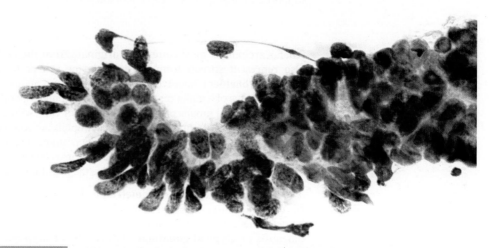

Figure 5.12   **Endocervical adenocarcinoma *in situ*.** Palisading nuclei stripped of cytoplasm ("feathering") is a characteristic feature. The nuclei are enlarged and elongated with coarse chromatin. (Papanicolaou stain)

Identifying small, tightly cohesive endometrial stromal cells can help in the distinction from AIS. Sampling of endometrial tissue can occur as the result of cervical endometriosis or inadvertent sampling of the lower uterine segment or endometrial cavity (Fig. 5.13). The latter occurs more frequently in patients who have a shortened cervix resulting from previous LEEP or cone biopsy. The presence of glands embedded in stroma should raise the possibility of direct endometrial sampling. **HSIL involving endocervical glands** can be distinguished from AIS by the lack of palisading, presence of single cells with high nuclear-to-cytoplasmic ratios and irregular nuclear membranes, or evidence of keratinization. AIS and HSIL can coexist. If the features fall short of a diagnosis of AIS, depending on the degree of atypia present, the following Bethesda diagnoses may be used: "Atypical endocervical cells, not otherwise specified (NOS)" or "Atypical endocervical cells, favor neoplastic." The latter diagnosis is associated with a higher likelihood of finding a clinically significant lesion on biopsy.

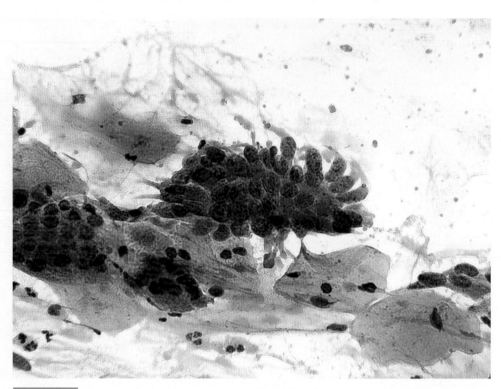

Figure 5.13 **Endometriosis.** Direct sampling of endometrial glands can mimic endocervical adenocarcinoma *in situ*. The smooth nuclear membranes and lack of nuclear crowding support a benign process. (Papanicolaou stain)

Adenocarcinomas most commonly originate from the endocervix or endometrium but can also represent spread from an extrauterine source (e.g., ovary, breast, stomach, colon, kidney, or bladder). Invasive endocervical adenocarcinomas resemble AIS but are distinguished by the presence of a tumor diathesis in the background. Endometrial carcinoma is characterized by three-dimensional groups or papillary clusters of cells with enlarged nuclei and often vacuolated cytoplasm (Fig. 5.14). Intracytoplasmic neutrophils are common. When the tumor cells have large cytoplasmic vacuoles and are associated with psammoma bodies, then the findings are suggestive of a **serous carcinoma.** Adenocarcinoma cells in a clean background or with unusual morphology that is not typical of a uterine primary raise the possibility of metastatic disease (Fig. 5.15).

The diagnosis of **atypical endometrial cells** is used when endometrial cell clusters are noted for mild nuclear enlargement, vacuolated cytoplasm, or cytoplasmic neutrophils. If it cannot be determined whether the atypical cells are endocervical or endometrial in origin, then the diagnosis of **atypical glandular cells (NOS) or atypical glandular cells, favor neoplastic** can be used.

Other

The diagnosis of "**endometrial cells in a woman 40 years of age and older**" is used when benign-appearing exfoliated endometrial stromal or glandular cells are identified in a cervical cytology specimen from a woman aged 40 or older. The age cutoff was set by the Bethesda system 2001 because menstrual data, menopausal status, hormonal therapy, and clinical risk factors are frequently unknown to the laboratory. For asymptomatic, premenopausal women, no further studies are recommended. However, endometrial sampling is recommended for symptomatic premenopausal women and all postmenopausal women (7).

Ancillary Testing

HPV testing has become routine since the ASCUS LSIL Triage (ALT) Study (8) and the publication of the American Society for Colposcopy and Cervical Pathology (ASCCP) *Consensus Guidelines for the Management of Women with Cervical Cytological Abnormalities*. Initially, **Digene Hybrid Capture II** was the only commercially available HPV test and had the additional distinction of being the assay used in the ALT study. In the intervening time, several different assays that use multiple different methodologies have become commercially available.

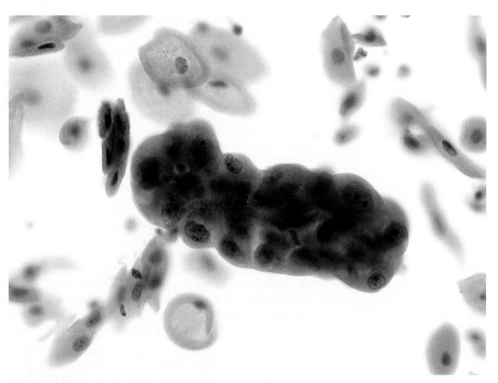

Figure 5.14 Endometrial carcinoma. Three-dimensional papillary clusters of cells with enlarged nuclei. (Papanicolaou stain)

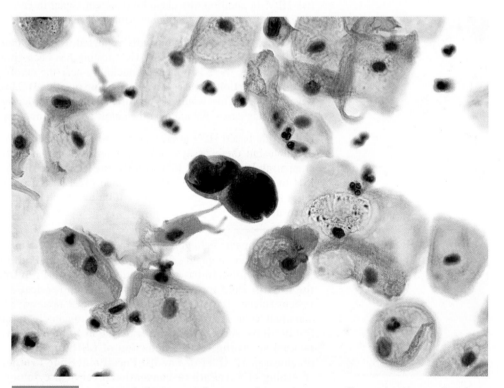

Figure 5.15 Metastatic breast carcinoma. Adenocarcinoma cells in a background without inflammation and necrosis raise the possibility of spread from an extrauterine source. (Papanicolaou stain)

Some are **direct tests for HPV such as *in situ* hybridization (ISH)**, whereas others are **surrogate markers such as p16^{INK4A} and ProEx C. Polymerase chain reaction (PCR) is the traditional gold standard for HPV detection,** and two assays by Roche, currently available in Europe, are undergoing FDA approval in the United States.

Digene Hybrid Capture II (HC2) has been approved by the FDA for use in triaging patients with a cervical cytology diagnosis of ASC-US and for triaging patients over age 30 with negative cervical cytology (8). It can be performed on cervical swabs or liquid-based cervical cytology samples. The method involves hybridization of the full genomic HPV RNA probe with the target DNA, followed by capture onto a solid phase and chemiluminescent detection. **The FDA-approved threshold for a positive result is** 1.0 RLU/PC (relative light unit to positive control specimen ratio), which corresponds to approximately ~1 pg/mL **or 5,000 HPV DNA copies per test well** (9).

HC2 utilizes two RNA probes, one directed at low-risk HPV types (6, 11, 42, 43, 44) and another at high-risk HPV types (16, 18, 31, 33, 35, 39, 45, 51, 52, 56, 58, 59, 68). Only the high-risk HPV assay has clinical utility because low-risk HPV has no oncogenic potential. Since HC2 was developed, HPV 68 has been reclassified out of the high-risk category, whereas HPV 66 is now considered high risk. Although the high-risk probe does not directly target HPV 66, studies have shown that HPV 66 is detected through cross-reactivity. **One of the main criticisms of HC2 is decreased specificity because of cross-reactivity, but the benefit of cross-reactivity is increased clinical sensitivity**. As exemplified by HPV 66, cross-reactivity can allow for the detection of HPV types not currently classified as high risk.

Positive results with HC2 testing for high-risk HPV have been reported in many patients who have no cytologic or histologic evidence of dysplasia. False positive results with HC2 can occur as the result of cross-reactivity or signal leak. De Cremoux et al. reported a false positive rate of 6.2% with 1.9% because of cross-reactivity and 4.3% because of signal leak (10). **Cross-reactivity with high-risk HPV DNA occurred in cases that had very high loads of low-risk HPV;** similar cross-reactivity with low-risk types occurred with high loads of high-risk HPV. In addition, the chemiluminescent signal in cases with high viral loads also led to false positive results in contiguous samples because of leaking of the signal.

Currently, HC2 results are usually reported as positive or negative based on the assigned cutoff of 1.0 RLU/PC. Although HC2 testing has been shown to have good interlaboratory reproducibility, there is poor reproducibility near the cutoff point of 1.0 RLU/PC (11). **In a significant portion of cases with borderline positive HC2 results, PCR analysis for HPV is negative** (12). This would argue for including a borderline category when reporting HC2 results to flag cases that are near the cutoff point and may represent a false positive result.

Other slide-based HPV assays such as *in situ* hybridization, p16^{INK4A} and ProEx C are also available but these assays lack the extensive validation of Digene HC2. Limited studies comparing Ventana HPV ISH with Digene HC2 have shown insufficient sensitivity for HPV ISH to replace HC2 for ASC-US triage (13,14). Assays intended for triage or screening purposes should be very sensitive with a low false negative rate and high negative predictive value.

Automated Screening

The main impetus behind developing automated screening systems was to increase productivity and improve quality. Both **ThinPrep** and **SurePath** have imaging systems that can be used with their liquid-based preparations. **The ThinPrep Imaging System was approved by the FDA in 2003** for dual review of ThinPrep cervical cytology slides. After the imaging system screens the slide, the cytotechnologist reviews 22 selected fields of view. If any abnormal cells are seen, then the slide is manually rescreened by the cytotechnologist. **Studies have shown the ThinPrep system to have equivalent or better sensitivity than manual screening for the detection of LSIL and HSIL, and higher specificity for the diagnosis of HSIL** (15). **The BD FocalPoint Slide Profiler is FDA approved for primary screening of SurePath or conventional cervical cytology slides. It functions as a triage device,** allowing a portion of slides to be archived with no further review by a cytotechnologist and identifying cases that are more likely to contain significant abnormalities, requiring further review. The BD FocalPoint GS Imaging System is a new location-guided screening system that can be used in conjunction with the Slide Profiler. The guided screener will direct the cytotechnologist to the fields of view containing the abnormal areas detected by image analysis.

Glandular Lesions of the Cervix

Terminology

A variety of terms have been used to describe preinvasive glandular lesions of the cervix, including *atypia*, *dysplasia*, and *adenocarcinoma in situ*. Unlike cervical squamous lesions, cervical glandular dysplasia is a poorly defined and controversial entity. Glandular lesions that exhibit some but not all the features of adenocarcinoma *in situ* have been associated with *in situ* and invasive adenocarcinoma, but the diagnostic criteria, clinical implications, prevalence, and progression rate of these lesions are not uniformly agreed upon (16).

Adenocarcinoma *In Situ*

The histological diagnosis of adenocarcinoma *in situ* (ACIS) requires unequivocal dysplastic changes, which are typically manifested by low-power basophilia, nuclear hyperchromasia with either fine or coarsely granular chromatin, nuclear apoptotic or karyorrhectic debris, apical mitotic figures, and loss of polarity (which may be subtle) (Fig. 5.16). The involved glands exhibit a lobular architecture that may appear more pronounced than adjacent uninvolved endocervical glands, but irregular infiltration into stroma is absent. Partial gland involvement is common. Recently, a superficial form of ACIS has been described in the superficial columnar mucosa featuring similar cytologic alterations but less pronounced atypia. This lesion is thought to occur more commonly in a younger age group (mean, 26 years) and so has been interpreted as an "early" form of ACIS (17).

A variety of processes mimic ACIS, including tubal or tuboendometrial metaplasia, endometriosis, and reactive endocervical cells, as well as several endocervical cell alterations that do not necessarily appear to represent a reactive process (18). These latter alterations often pose the most diagnostic difficulty and are classified on the basis of the abnormality present: endocervical glandular hyperplasia, mitotically active endocervical mucosa, stratified endocervical mucosa, and atypical oxyphilic metaplasia.

In recent years, the use of biomarkers, particularly a combination of Ki-67 and p16, has been used in the differential diagnosis of ACIS. In general, strong, diffuse expression of

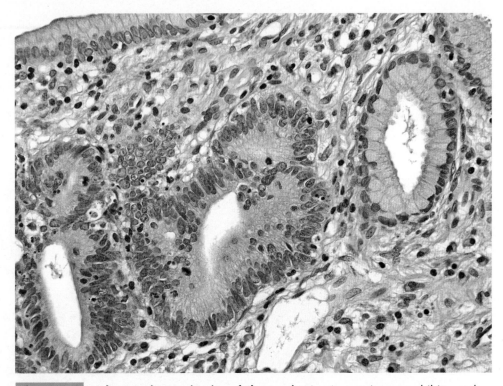

Figure 5.16 **Adenocarcinoma *in situ* of the cervix.** *In situ* carcinoma exhibits nuclear hyperchromasia, stratification, irregular chromatin, and apical mitotic figures. A normal endocervical gland is present on the right.

p16 in conjunction with increased Ki-67 is more commonly associated with ACIS, whereas weak or focal p16 expression with or without increased Ki-67 is more supportive of an ACIS mimic (19). Exceptions occur, so it is important to be thoroughly aware of the variant expression patterns of these markers in the individual lesions in order to prevent over-interpretation on the basis of staining patterns alone (20).

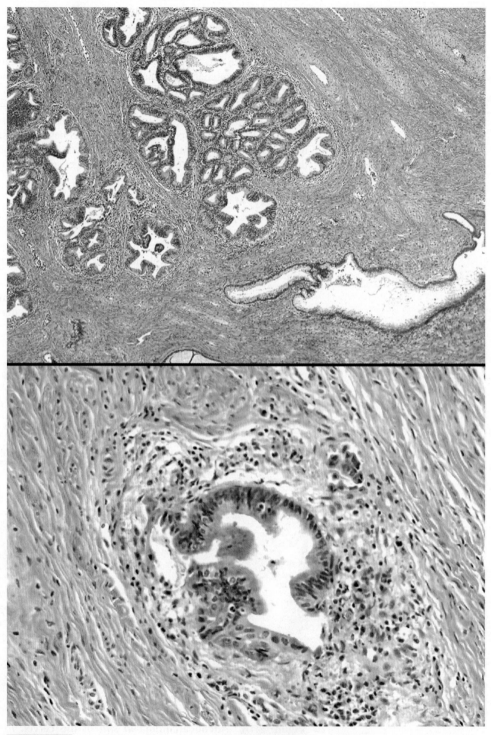

Figure 5.17 **Invasive adenocarcinoma of the cervix.** Deeply infiltrative glands are irregular in contour and surrounded by edematous stroma. (top, low power; bottom, high power)

Invasive Adenocarcinoma

The diagnosis of invasive cervical adenocarcinoma can be very difficult in early or superficially invasive lesions as well as in limited (superficial) biopsy specimens. Unlike squamous carcinoma of the cervix, invasion may not be associated with a significant stromal reaction; in these instances, identification of invasion is based on the presence of significant glandular irregularity, an infiltrative gland pattern, and the presence of enlarged, complex neoplastic glandular structures deep to the normal endocervical crypts (Fig. 5.17).

Because of the difficulties in diagnosing early invasive lesions, the concept of "microinvasive adenocarcinoma" is not as well accepted as it is for microinvasive squamous cell carcinoma; nevertheless, a maximum depth of invasion of 3 mm with negative margins and no lymphovascular invasion is considered by most clinicians as the upper limit for consideration for conservative management. Measurements are made from the surface and expressed in millimeters.

Invasive adenocarcinoma of the usual or endocervical type accounts for 60% to 70% of cervical adenocarcinomas. Two variants—adenoma malignum (minimal deviation adenocarcinoma) and **villoglandular adenocarcinoma**—are very uncommon but the source of frequent diagnostic problems. **Other histologic subtypes include serous, clear cell, endometrioid, mesonephric, intestinal type, adenoid basal, adenoid cystic, and neuroendocrine carcinoma** (18,21). Only those with distinctive clinical or differential diagnostic problems that affect prognosis or treatment are discussed.

Minimal Deviation Carcinoma (Adenoma Malignum)

This tumor, which is characterized by a deceptively benign histologic appearance, accounts for <10% of all cervical adenocarcinomas. Patients present with irregular bleeding, diffuse cervical enlargement, or vaginal mucus discharge. **An association with Peutz-Jeghers syndrome has been reported** (21). A wide age range has been reported, but virtually all patients are older than 20 years of age.

Microscopically, the tumor features cystically dilated, irregular (claw-shaped) glands with minimal cytologic atypia and minimal stromal reaction (Fig. 5.18). The diagnosis is most easily established by careful search for foci of cytologic atypia, stromal reaction, or conventional-type adenocarcinoma. This tumor can replace normal endocervical and endometrial glandular tissue, mimicking mucinous metaplasia in uterine curettings and biopsy. Intracytoplasmic carcinoembryonic antigen (CEA) staining may he helpful is some cases, but not all adenoma malignum carcinomas are CEA positive and normal endocervical glands may express CEA on occasion, although usually only along the surface (glycocalyx). These carcinomas do not stain for p16.

Villoglandular Carcinoma

This tumor occurs predominantly in young women and is characterized by villoglandular architectural growth pattern and low nuclear grade. These tumors have a good prognosis but only if they are exophytic with minimal or no invasion (Fig. 5.19). **An association with HPV has been reported,** and these tumors may be p16 positive.

Clear Cell Carcinoma

Clear cell carcinoma may occur in young (diethystilbestrol exposure *in utero*) or older women and may arise in the ectocervix (typically, associated with diethystilbestrol exposure) or endocervix. A variety of patterns—including tubulocystic, glandular, solid, and papillary—may be seen (21).

Mesonephric Carcinoma

Mesonephric remnants may develop hyperplasia and carcinoma; often a spectrum of these changes is seen in the carcinomas (21). The carcinomas often pose significant diagnostic difficulty because of their lateral and deep location within the cervix. **There may be no surface component.** Ductal, retiform, tubular, solid, and spindle patterns may be seen in the carcinomas. Most are low to moderate nuclear grade, so some cases may be difficult to distinguish from florid mesonephric hyperplasia. The distinction is often based on loss of lobular architecture and infiltrative pattern. Diagnosis of higher-grade mesonephric adenocarcinoma is based on identification of residual normal or hyperplastic mesonephric tubules with their characteristic eosinophilic luminal material. Prognosis is uncertain because of the limited numbers of cases but probably similar to usual endocervical adenocarcinoma. These tumors are not known to be associated with HPV, and most are p16 negative.

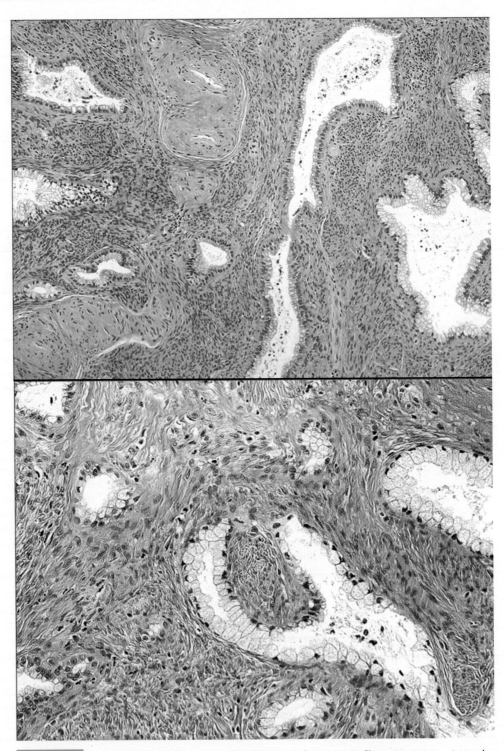

Figure 5.18 **Minimal deviation adenocarcinoma (adenoma malignum).** Large, irregular mucinous glands typically show bland or minimally atypical cytological features. (top, low power; bottom, high power)

Neuroendocrine Carcinoma

Neuroendocrine carcinoma, small- and large-cell variants, account for less than 5% of all cervical carcinomas. These highly aggressive tumors may present as small lesions, but most are deeply invasive. They exhibit the usual features of a neuroendocrine carcinoma; high mitotic rates and necrosis are common (Fig. 5.20). **Neuroendocrine carcinoma is often associated with ACIS, HSIL, and conventional invasive cervical adenocarcinoma.** Most harbor HPV-18 and are p16-positive. **Rarely, well-differentiated neuroendocrine carcinoma (carcinoid)**

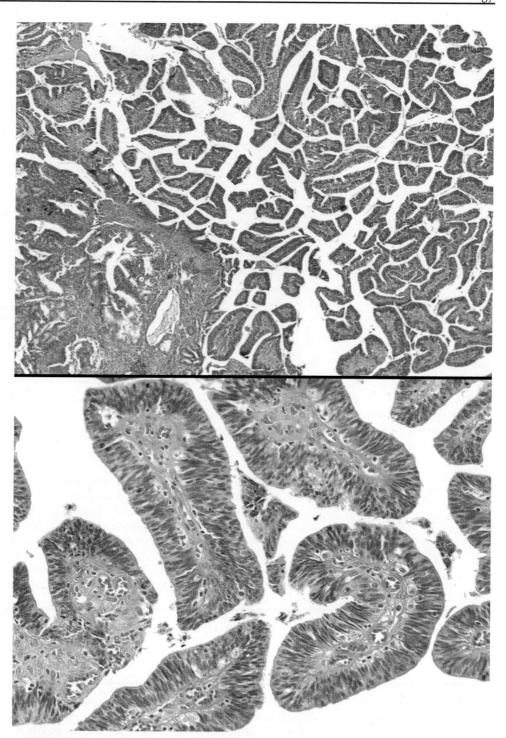

Figure 5.19   Villoglandular adenocarcinoma of cervix. Slender, elongate villi are lined by well-differentiated epithelium with an exophytic growth pattern. This tumor is associated with a good prognosis, provided there is minimal or no cervical stromal invasion. (top, low power; bottom, high power)

may occur in the cervix, and the prognosis for this tumor may be better. Metastasis should always be excluded.

Adenoid Basal Carcinoma (Adenoid Basal Epithelioma)

Adenoid basal cell carcinoma (epithelioma) occurs in postmenopausal, elderly women (mean age 65 years). Most are asymptomatic, and the tumor is discovered during evaluation of an atypical Pap smear. Indeed, it is often associated with HSIL. The cervix is often normal on

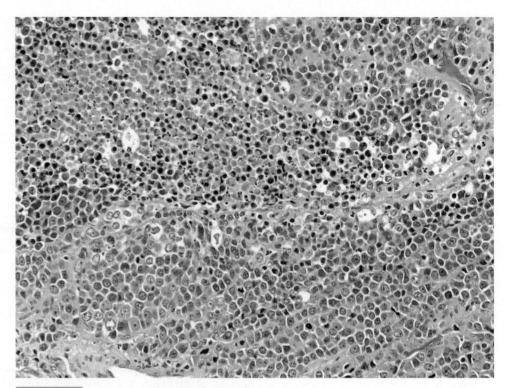

Figure 5.20 **Neuroendocrine carcinoma of cervix.** Malignant cells with high mitotic index are arranged in a sheetlike growth pattern. Necrosis is often present in these clinically aggressive tumors.

colposcopic and physical examination. The tumor is cytologically bland (often looks like "bland squamous cell carcinoma") and features basaloid, adenoid, and squamoid differentiation. The adenoid areas consist of small, closely packed tubules, occasionally with intraluminal secretions reminiscent of mesonephric tubules (Fig. 5.21). There is typically no stromal response. Mitotic figures are rare or absent. The tumor has a favorable prognosis and needs to be distinguished from the adenoid cystic pattern of cervical adenocarcinoma, which does not have a favorable prognosis (21). **Because of the extremely favorable prognosis associated with adenoid basal carcinoma, the diagnostic term** *adenoid basal epithelioma* **is preferred.**

Adenoid Cystic Carcinoma	Unlike adenoid basal carcinoma (epithelioma), **adenoid cystic carcinoma is a clinically aggressive neoplasm.** It is composed of cribriform nests containing eosinophilic hyaline material within the gland lumens, resembling adenoid cystic carcinoma of the salivary gland
Localization of Adenocarcinoma: Primary versus Metastasis	Distinction between primary endometrial and primary endocervical adenocarcinoma may be difficult in biopsy and curettage specimens, especially when no precursor lesion is present. When clinical and histologic evaluation fails to clearly identify a carcinoma as cervical or endometrial in origin, an immunohistochemical panel that includes several markers, such as estrogen receptor (ER), progesterone receptor (PgR), vimentin, CEA, and p16 is often useful (19,22,23). Using this particular panel (Table 5.4), **glandular proliferations that are ER/ PgR-positive, vimentin-positive, CEA-negative, and p16-negative are almost always endometrial origin** (Fig. 5.22), whereas those that are ER and PgR negative, vimentin negative, CEA positive, and p16 positive are very likely to be endocervical in origin (Fig. 5.23). However, overexpression of p16 can occur in a variety of other carcinomas independent of HPV status, including uterine (as well as cervical) serous carcinoma. Because the distinction between these two sites of origin may be based on whether a strong staining pattern with p16 is focal or diffuse in an individual case, this pattern of reactivity is most useful in whole tissue sections. In limited samplings, such as are encountered in routine biopsy and curettage specimens, these patterns may be misleading.

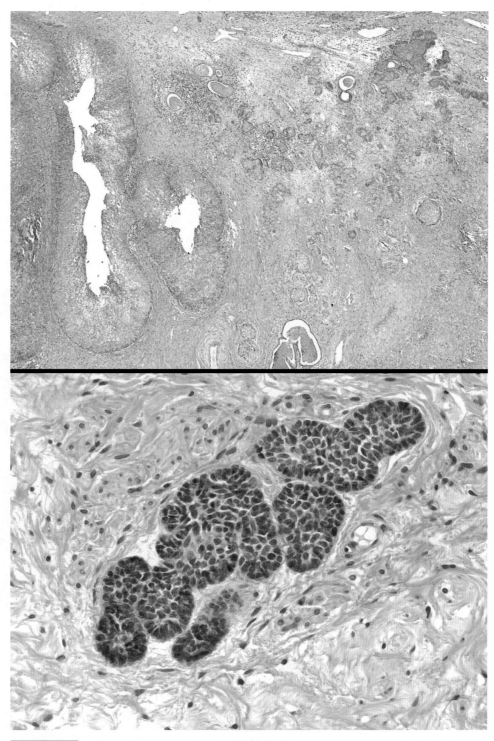

Figure 5.21   **Adenoid basal carcinoma (epithelioma).** This variant of cervical adenocarcinoma is characterized by nests of bland basaloid and squamoid cells in the cervical stroma. A squamous intraepithelial lesion is typically present in the overlying mucosa. This neoplasm is often referred to as *adenoid basal epithelioma* because it has a very favorable prognosis. (top, low power; bottom, high power)

Metastatic Carcinoma

The most common sites of origin for metastatic carcinomas presenting in uterine curettings are breast, stomach, ovary, and colon. Most patients have a previous history of carcinoma, and the metastasis is not the first presentation of disease. Lymphoma and melanoma, although rare, also continue to pose diagnostic problems when encountered in this location

Table 5.4 Distinguishing Endometrial from Endocervical Adenocarcinoma		
	Endocervical	*Endometrial*
Clinical or Radiologic	Dominant mass in cervix	Dominant mass in uterine fundus
H&E	Cancer containing fragments differ from endometrial functionalis fragments (dimorphic pattern) Adenocarcinoma *in situ* in associated endocervical glands Associated squamous intraepithelial lesion	Mergence of malignant fragments with less atypical patterns in other fragments (endometrial hyperplasia/metaplasia) Stromal foam cells No adenocarcinoma *in situ* in associated cervical fragments
Immunohistochemistry	CEA positive ER- and PgR-negative Vimentin-negative p16-positive	CEA negative ER- and PgR-positive Vimentin-positive p16-negative
HPV *in situ*	Positive	Negative

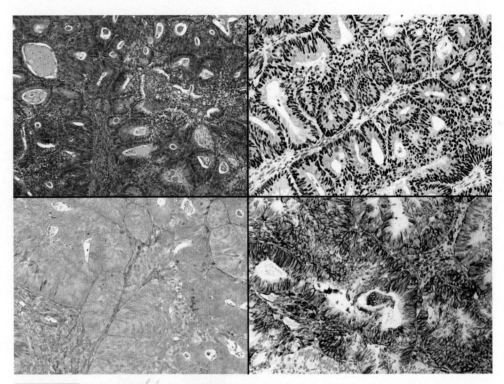

Figure 5.22 **Endometrial adenocarcinoma** (upper left). Endometrial adenocarcinoma is typically ER/PgR-positive (upper right), vimentin-positive (lower right), and p16-negative (lower left).

because of their mimicry of undifferentiated carcinoma or sarcoma. Use of a basic panel for undifferentiated tumors and a low threshold for suspecting metastasis will prevent most misclassifications.

Mesenchymal Tumors

Stromal and smooth muscle tumors may occur in the cervix; they resemble their more common uterine counterparts. Although the vagina is the more common site, embryonal rhabdomyosarcoma may also occur in the cervix; in contrast to vaginal rhabdomyosarcoma, which is more common in children, **cervical rhabdomyosarcoma tends to occur in young adults.** Most are embryonal, but spindle and alveolar variants may also be seen.

Mixed Epithelial and Mesenchymal Tumors

The same mixed epithelial and mesenchymal tumors that occur in the uterine corpus may occur in the cervix. They tend to exhibit the same patient demographics as their uterine counterparts, but cervical adenosarcomas tend to occur at a younger age (24). Most present during the

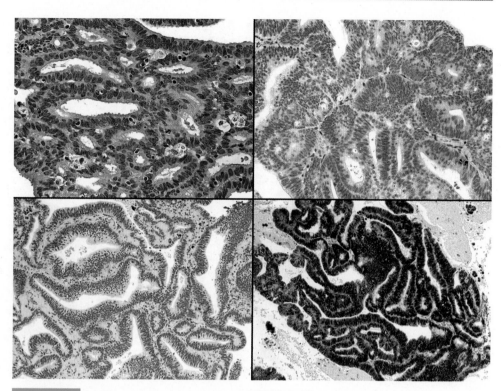

Figure 5.23 **Endocervical adenocarcinoma** (upper left). In contrast to endometrial adeno-carcinoma (see Figure 5.22), endocervical adenocarcinoma is typically Er/PgR negative (upper right), vimentin negative (lower left), and p16 positive (lower right).

reproductive years with abnormal bleeding and recurrent polyps. Data are limited, but most appear to have a more favorable prognosis, possibly because of the early detection of low-stage disease in the majority of patients. As in uterine corpus tumors, depth of invasion and sarcomatous overgrowth are adverse prognostic indicators.

Other Tumors

A variety of other neoplasms may arise in the uterine cervix. **These include alveolar soft part sarcoma, rhabdomyoma, and nerve sheath tumors.** Alveolar soft part sarcomas of the female genital tract appear to have a better prognosis than their counterparts in other sites. **Yolk sac tumors** may also occur in the cervicovaginal region. **Melanoma, lymphoma, and leukemia** usually involve the cervix secondarily either as metastases or in the setting of widespread disease (18).

Vagina

Squamous Lesions of the Vagina

Squamous Intraepithelial Lesion

Preneoplastic lesions of the vagina are termed *vaginal intraepithelial neoplasia* (VAIN) and graded from 1 to 3. Similar to the cervix, condyloma and **VAIN 1** correlate with LSIL and **VAIN 2 and VAIN 3** correlate with HSIL. LSIL and HSIL in the vagina have the same morphologic features as those in the cervix. LSIL can be mimicked by vaginal papillomatosis, which exhibits papillary architecture, parakeratosis, and cytoplasmic halos. However, papillomatosis lacks significant acanthosis and nuclear atypia. HSIL can be mimicked by atrophy and immature squamous metaplasia, but can be distinguished by a lack of nuclear atypia in the latter two entities.

Squamous Cell Carcinoma

Primary squamous cell carcinoma of the vagina is uncommon. Vaginal SCC more frequently occurs as a result of secondary involvement by extension from the cervix or vulva. The morphologic features are the same as for the cervix. In patients with vaginal adenosis, immature

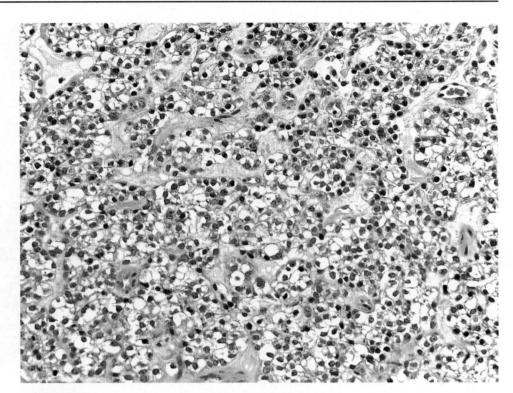

Figure 5.24 **Clear cell adenocarcinoma of vagina.** In this solid pattern of clear cell carcinoma, sheets of malignant cells with clear cytoplasm extensively replace normal tissue.

squamous metaplasia involving areas of adenosis can be mistaken for invasive SCC, but the two entities can be readily distinguished by the lack of cytologic atypia and lack of desmoplastic response with the benign process.

Glandular Lesions of the Vagina	Clear cell adenocarcinoma is the most common malignant glandular lesion in the vagina, followed by endometrioid, mucinous, and mesonephric subtypes. The latter histologic subtypes occur predominantly in perimenopausal women.
Clear Cell Adenocarcinoma	**Clear cell carcinoma of the cervicovaginal region is strongly linked to *in utero* exposure to diethylstilbestrol (DES)** and has decreased in incidence with decreased use of this teratogen. It typically **occurs in association with adenosis.** Although the upper vagina is the most common site of involvement in DES-exposed women, the cervix is the most commonly affected site in non–DES-exposed women. The appearance is the same as the ovarian counterpart (Fig. 5.24). Prognosis is determined by tumor size, depth of invasion, and lymph node involvement.
Adenosis	The presence of glandular epithelium in the vagina is termed *adenosis*. Adenosis may exhibit mucinous endocervical-like epithelium or tuboendometrioid epithelium. It is often asymptomatic but may be detected by colposcopic examination. Atypical adenosis, which exhibits architectural and cytological atypia, is often seen in association with clear cell adenocarcinoma.
Fibroepithelial Stromal Polyp	Fibroepithelial stromal polyp is a common, typically small, exophytic polypoid lesion occurring in reproductive-aged women, most commonly in the vagina, but also in the vulva and cervix. Almost one-third occur during pregnancy. The polyps often occur in the anterior wall and range in size from 0.5 cm to 4.0 cm. Histologically, they are characterized by small spindle cells and enlarged, stellate multinucleated cells in a myxoid stroma (Fig. 5.25). Mitotic figures can be prominent and may raise the suspicion for a malignant process. However, fibroepithelial stromal polyps are distinguished from sarcoma botryoides by the absence of a cambium layer.

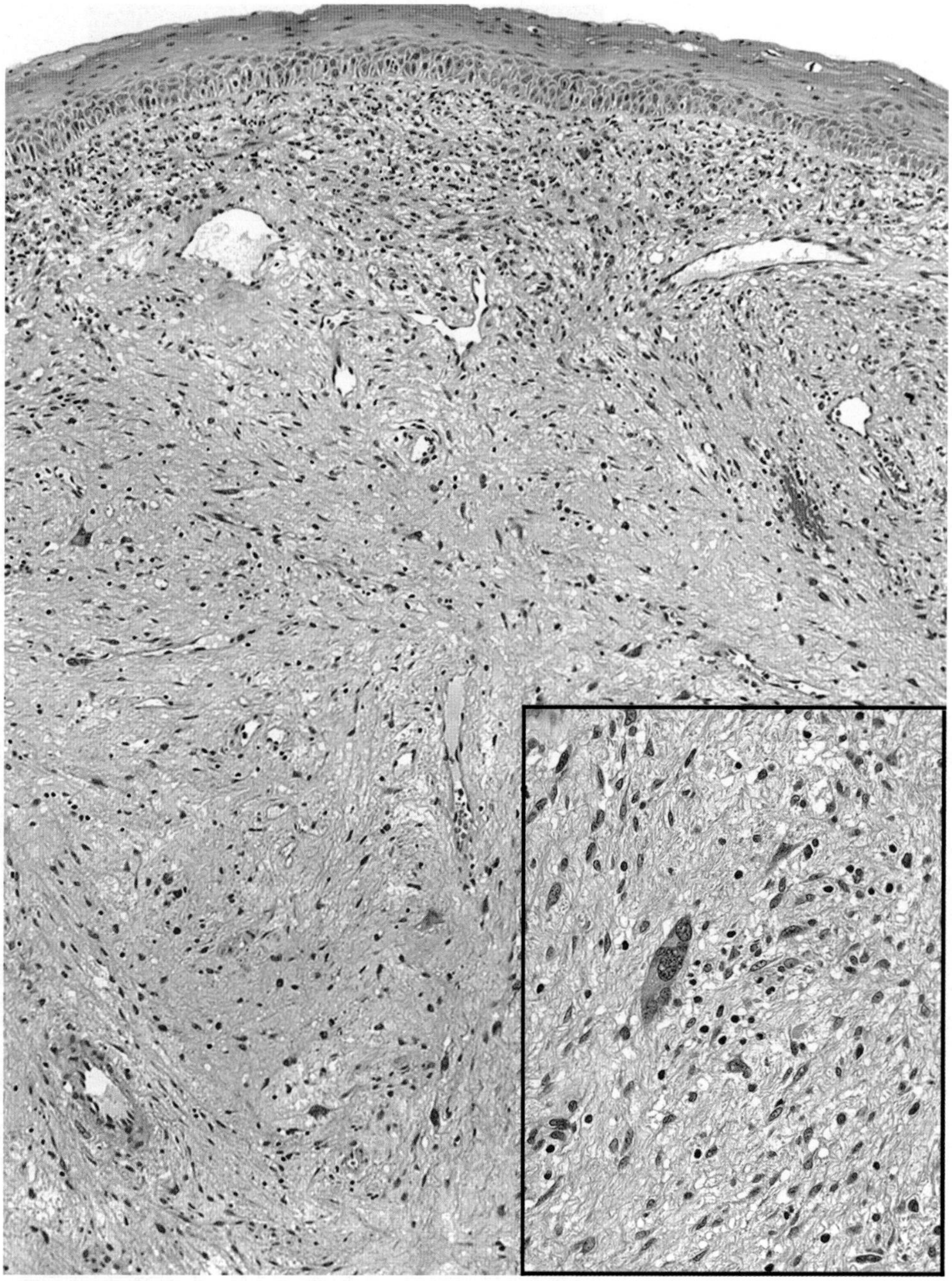

Figure 5.25   **Fibroepithelial stromal polyp.** Atypical stromal cells (inset) may simulate a malignancy, but this is a benign, probably reactive process. Although the lesion extends to the surface epithelium, there is no cellular condensation (forming a so-called cambium layer) at the surface; the absence of a cambium layer helps to distinguish this lesion from sarcoma botyroides on a limited sampling (see Figure 5.26). This polyp occurs most commonly in the vagina but can also be seen in the vulva and cervix.

Sarcoma Botyroides

Embryonal rhabdomyosarcoma is the most common vaginal sarcoma; it occurs almost always in infants and children, but rare cases have been reported in young adults and post-menopausal women. The tumors present as polypoid vaginal masses, often protruding through the introitus, that may vary in size from 0.2 cm to 12 cm. Microscopically, the tumor is composed of small, round to oval or spindle cells surrounded by an edematous, myxoid stroma (Fig. 5.26). **A characteristically dense, cellular cambium layer can be seen in the**

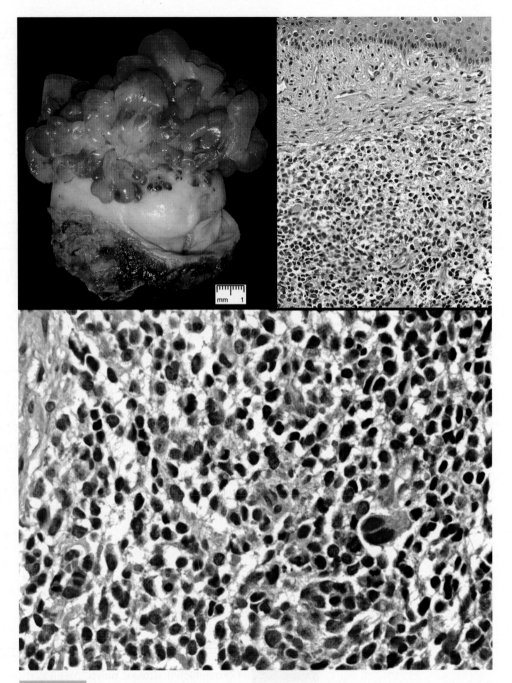

Figure 5.26   Sarcoma botyroides (embryonal rhabdomyosarcoma). *Top left:* Botyroid growth pattern of cervical embryonal rhabdomyosarcoma. Courtesy of Dr. Matthew Quick. *Top right:* Stellate cells set in myxoid stroma are more condensed beneath the surface epithelium, forming a distinct cambium layer. *Bottom:* Small cells with hyperchromatic nuclei are punctuated by larger cells with more abundant eosinophilic cytoplasm.

subepithelial zone. Rhabdomyoblasts (strap cells) are present but may be sparse or ill defined. Identification of rhabdomyoblasts can be facilitated by immunostaining for myogenin or Myo-D1.

Wide local excision and combination chemotherapy is the preferred treatment for sarcoma botyroides. Staging in children is based on the Intergroup Rhabdomyosarcoma Study group classification; adults are staged according to the TNM and FIGO system. Most rhabdomyosarcomas in the vulvovaginal region are of the embryonal type, but rare tumors are of the alveolar type, which has a worse prognosis.

Melanoma

Melanoma is the second most common malignancy to occur in the vagina (after squamous cell carcinoma). Affected patients are typically 60 years of age and present with vaginal bleeding. Most, but not all lesions are pigmented, nodular or flat, and measure 2 cm to 3 cm in size at diagnosis; ulceration may be present. **The anterior wall of the lower third of the vagina is the most common site.** The diagnosis may be difficult on small biopsies because an *in situ* component or pagetoid spread is often absent. Epithelioid cell lesions may resemble carcinoma, whereas spindle cell lesions may create confusion for sarcoma. Immuno-histochemical stains for melanoma markers are often required to establish a diagnosis. The prognosis is poor.

Postoperative Spindle Cell Nodule

A variety of reactive processes may occur within the vagina, particularly following surgical procedures. One such lesion is composed of a cellular, spindle cell proliferation that may simulate a neoplastic process. This lesion has been designated as postoperative spindle cell nodule.

Vulva

Squamous Cell Lesions of the Vulva

Terminology

Similar to the cervix, different terminology systems are in use to describe preneoplastic lesions of the vulva (25) (Table 5.5). These systems resemble the ones used for the cervix. Low-grade vulvar intraepithelial lesion (LVIL) encompasses condyloma acuminatum and VIN 1, whereas high-grade vulvar intraepithelial lesion (HVIL) encompasses VIN 2, VIN 3, and carcinoma *in situ*. The main difference lies in whether VIN is graded. **The latest 2003 World Health Organization (WHO) classification grades VIN on a scale of 1 to 3, with VIN 3 further subdivided into classic type and simplex type.** In contrast, **the International Society for the Study of Vulvovaginal Disease (ISSVD) decided in 2004 to eliminate the category of VIN 1 and to abolish grading of VIN.** This decision was based on the lack of evidence that condylomas, which account for the majority of VIN 1 lesions, progress to carcinoma and the lack of interobserver reproducibility for diagnosing VIN 1 or for distinguishing between VIN 2 and VIN 3 (26). The ISSVD retained the distinction between classic VIN and simplex (differentiated) VIN. Given the variability in terminology, it is best to determine what terminology system the pathologist is using, especially if the diagnosis is "vulvar intraepithelial neoplasia (VIN)" with no further specification.

Vulvar Intraepithelial Neoplasia

The two-tiered Bethesda-like system is a simple way to view precursor lesions of the vulva. LVIL consists predominantly of condyloma acuminata, which are associated with low-risk HPV types 6 and 11 (Fig. 5.27) Flat condylomas are uncommon in the vulva but may be

Table 5.5 Terminology for Precursor Lesions of Vulvar Squamous Cell Carcinoma

WHO 2003	ISSVD 2004	Synonyms
Condyloma acuminatum	Condyloma acuminatum	n/a
VIN 1	n/a	Flat condyloma, mild dysplasia
VIN 2	VIN, usual type	Moderate dysplasia
VIN 3		Severe dysplasia, carcinoma *in situ*, Bowen's disease, bowenoid papulosis, bowenoid dysplasia
Carcinoma *in situ* (simplex type) VIN 3	VIN, differentiated type	n/a

WHO, World Health Organization; ISSVD, International Society for the Study of Vulvar Disease; SIL, squamous intraepithelial lesion; VIN, vulvar intraepithelial neoplasia.

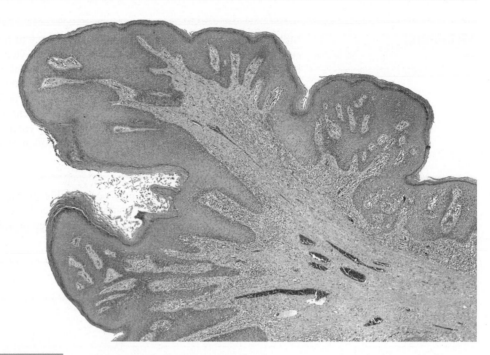

Figure 5.27   Condyloma. Exophytic condylomas are common in the vulva and are associated with low-risk HPV types 6 and 11.

associated with high-risk HPV. Fibroepithelial polyps (skin tags) and hymenal mucosa can be mistaken for exophytic condylomas. Nonspecific inflammatory atypia or psoriasis can be misdiagnosed as flat condylomas.

HVIL can be subdivided into two main types of VIN 3: classic (Bowenoid) VIN and simplex (differentiated) VIN. These two types of VIN 3 underscore the two different pathways—HPV related and HPV unrelated—that lead to the development of vulvar squamous cell carcinoma. **High-risk HPV is identified in 53% to 90% of cases of classic VIN 3, with HPV 16 as the most common type** (27). However, HPV 18, 31, 33, 35, 51, 52, and 68 have also been isolated from cases of classic VIN (28). In contrast, **HPV is rarely identified in simplex VIN** (28).

Classic VIN is commonly multicentric with extension to the perineum and involvement of the cervix and vagina. There are three patterns or subtypes of classic VIN: warty, basaloid, and pagetoid. The **warty pattern** is characterized by prominent koilocytosis or warty architecture (Fig. 5.28), whereas the **basaloid** is more poorly differentiated (Fig. 5.29). The atypia involves two-thirds or more of the epithelium and is notable for disorganization, cells with high nuclear-to-cytoplasmic ratios, dark irregular nuclei, and numerous mitotic figures, including abnormal forms. Dyskeratotic cells are often present, and the dysplastic cells frequently extend down pilosebaceous units, which can mimic invasive carcinoma. The **pagetoid subtype** is rare but important to recognize because it can closely mimic extramammary Paget's disease. The distinction between these two entities requires special stains because histologically they are both characterized by single cells and clusters of cells with pale cytoplasm involving the squamous epithelium of the vulva.

Simplex VIN is localized to the vulva and usually identified adjacent to areas of invasive carcinoma in elderly patients. It is rarely identified prospectively (29). The morphologic changes of simplex VIN are subtle and characterized by nuclear atypia of the basal cell layer and expansion of the basal layer into elongated, narrow, branching rete ridges (Fig. 5.30) The nuclei can range from relatively small, dark and irregular to enlarged and pleomorphic. Maturation is also abnormal as exhibited by the presence of enlarged keratinocytes with large, pleomorphic nuclei and abundant, markedly eosinophilic cytoplasm in the mid- to superficial layers. These abnormal keratinocytes can also extend into the basal layer and involve the rete ridges (29). The thickness of the epithelium is variable and can be atrophic or acanthotic (i.e., thickened). The differential diagnosis for simplex VIN includes lichen sclerosus with squamous hyperplasia and other benign dermatologic conditions such as lichen simplex chronicus, psoriasis, spongiotic dermatitis, and candida vulvitis.

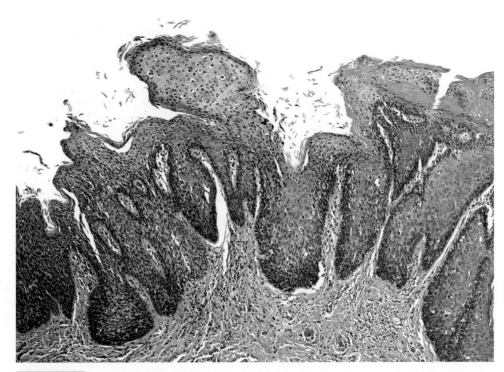

Figure 5.28   **Classic VIN, warty.** Prominent koilocytosis is present on the surface and overlies severe atypia involving two-thirds of the underlying epithelium.

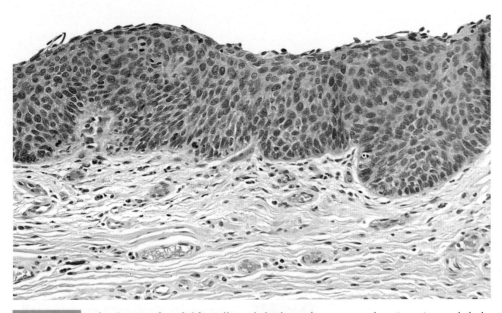

Figure 5.29   **Classic VIN, basaloid.** Cells with high nuclear-to-cytoplasmic ratios and dark, irregular nuclei involve the full thickness of the squamous epithelium.

Lichen sclerosus is considered a risk factor for the development of vulvar squamous cell carcinoma. It appears to play a role in the HPV-independent pathway. Lichen sclerosus is negative for HPV and is more frequently identified in association with simplex VIN than with classic VIN (27,28).

Squamous Cell Carcinoma   **Primary invasive squamous cell carcinomas of the vulva can be subdivided into two main types: conventional squamous cell carcinoma and verrucous carcinoma.** Conventional squamous cell carcinomas can exhibit different growth patterns, including

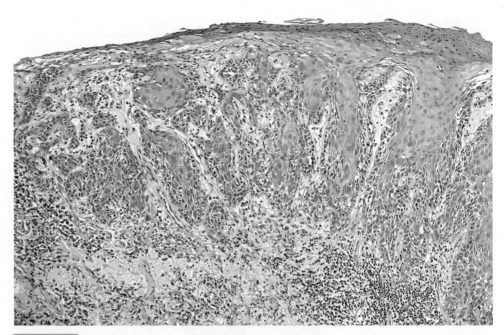

Figure 5.30   Simplex VIN. Abnormal keratinocytes with abundant, markedly eosinophilic cytoplasm involve the mid- to superficial layers and extend into the elongated, branching rete ridges.

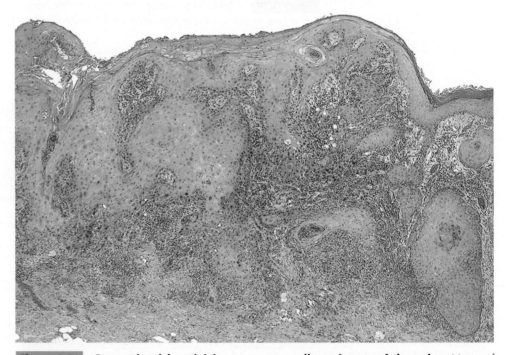

Figure 5.31   Conventional keratinizing squamous cell carcinoma of the vulva. Nests of well-differentiated tumor cells jaggedly invade into the stroma on microscopic examination.

warty, basaloid, and keratinizing (Fig. 5.31). Invasive squamous cell carcinomas that have warty or basaloid features are typically associated with classic VIN and high-risk HPV, whereas well-differentiated keratinizing squamous cell carcinomas are more commonly associated with simplex VIN (27).

Verrucous carcinoma is a rare special variant of squamous cell carcinoma that is slow growing and has minimal metastatic potential. It is typically exophytic, well circumscribed, and composed of hyperkeratotic fronds of cytologically bland squamous epithelium. The interface with the underlying stroma characteristically consists of a pushing border with associated chronic inflammation (Fig. 5.32).

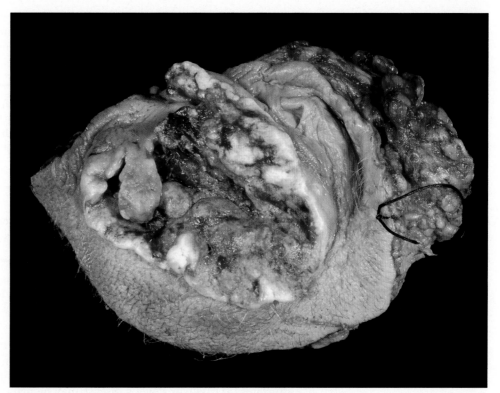

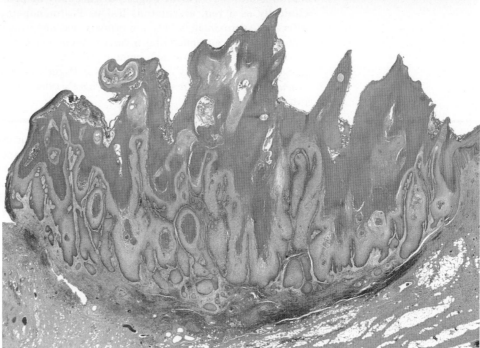

Figure 5.32   **Verrucous carcinoma of the vulva.** *Top:* Vulvectomy specimen shows exophytic verrucous tumor. *Bottom:* The tumor is exophytic with hyperkeratotic fronds of bland squamous epithelium and well circumscribed with a pushing border with the underlying stroma.

Bartholin Cyst

Bartholin duct cyst is the most common cystic growth in the vulva. It occurs posteriorly in the vulvar vestibule. Excision is usually reserved for those lesions that fail to respond to conservative management. However, some investigators recommend excision of Bartholin gland cysts to exclude adenocarcinoma when cysts or abscesses occur in patients more than 40 years of age. The cyst lining is often variable: Endocervical-like mucinous, squamous, and transitional epithelium is often present. The presence of atypia, cellular stratification, or mitotic figures are concerning features and should warrant full pathologic examination of the entire cyst wall to exclude carcinoma.

Bartholin Gland Adenocarcinoma

An uncommon tumor, this neoplasm affects women 50 years of age and older. The clinical impression is usually that of a Bartholin duct cyst. **Histologic types include adenocarcinoma, squamous cell carcinoma, adenoid cystic carcinoma, and hybrid types.** A transition zone to adjacent Bartholin gland confirms the diagnosis. Approximately 20% of patients have ipsilateral groin lymph node metastases at initial diagnosis.

Fibroepithelial Stromal Polyp

Fibroepithelial stromal polyps also occur on the vulva but are most commonly seen in the vagina. They may be single or multiple. **Fibroepithelial stromal polyps probably represent a reactive lesion rather than a true neoplasm.**

Hidradenoma Papilliferum

A rare benign glandular neoplasm, papillary hidradenoma usually occurs in the region of the intralabial sulcus in adult women. The tumor is well circumscribed and composed of complex, branching papillae lined by a double layer of outer myoepithelial and inner epithelial cells (31).

Extramammary Paget's Disease

Paget's disease of the vulva is an intraepithelial neoplasm characterized by large, round cells with abundant, pale cytoplasm, often forming small intracytoplasmic lumina or gland-like structures (31). **Vulvar Paget's disease may be primary or secondary and presents clinically as a red, eczematous lesion. Postmenopausal women are most commonly affected.** Approximately 90% are primary and noninvasive (cutaneous), whereas 10% are associated with an underlying invasive carcinoma (cutaneous, anorectal, urothelial). All forms of Paget's disease are immunoreactive for cytokeratin and epithelial membrane antigen. Classic primary cutaneous vulvar Paget's disease also expresses CK7 and HER-2/*neu* (Fig. 5.33), whereas secondary Paget's often exhibits an immunophenotype of the primary site of origin.

Mesenchymal Tumors

A variety of specialized genital stromal neoplasms occur in the vulvovaginal region of reproductive-aged women (32). Most are small, hormonally responsive, and clinically indolent. The most common specialized genital stromal tumors are **angiomyofibroblastoma, cellular angiofibroma, and superficial angiomyxoma** (33). Often mistaken clinically for a Bartholin gland cyst, these specialized genital stromal lesions may recur locally if incompletely excised, but they are not associated with aggressive clinical behavior.

Prepubertal vulval fibroma is unlikely to be confused with any of the typical vulvar mesenchymal lesions because of its predilection for prepubertal females. This lesion, which most commonly involves the labia majora, presents as a unilateral or, rarely, bilateral, ill-defined, and painless subcutaneous vulvar mass with microscopic features that suggest a hamartomatous process.

Other mesenchymal neoplasms that behave in a clinically benign fashion include lipoma, neurofibroma, schwannoma, granular cell tumor, glomus tumor, and hemangioma.

Dermatofibrosarcoma protuberans is a low-grade cutaneous tumor with a high risk for recurrence if incompletely excised. High-grade sarcomas that most commonly occur in the vulva include **rhabdomyosarcoma, proximal epithelioid sarcoma, alveolar soft part sarcoma, Ewing's sarcoma and peripheral primitive neuroectodermal tumor, and postradiation angiosarcoma.**

Rarely, smooth muscle tumors may involve the vulvar region. Criteria for malignancy differ from those for uterine smooth muscle tumors and are based on size (>5 cm), mitotic index (>5 mitotic figures per 10 high-power fields), infiltrative margins, and cellular atypia.

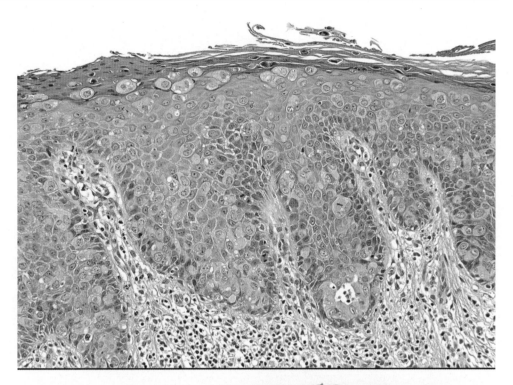

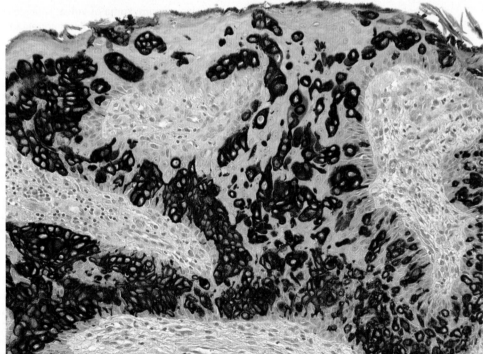

Figure 5.33   Paget's disease of vulva. *Top:* Paget cells are confined to the intraepidermal compartment, forming small glandlike structures. *Bottom:* The Paget cells express cytokeratin 7.

Aggressive Angiomyxoma

Aggressive angiomyxoma occurs in the deep vulvar and inguinal soft tissue and is characterized by a paucicellular spindle cell proliferation separated by loose myxoid stroma (Fig. 5.34). Mitotic activity is low. Despite the bland histologic appearance, it is an infiltrative

Figure 5.34   Aggressive angiomyxoma of vulva. Paucicellular spindle cell proliferation separated by loose myxoid stroma. Despite the bland appearance, this is an infiltrative tumor with a propensity for recurrence if incompletely excised.

tumor that may locally invade deep pelvic structures if incompletely excised (31). Aggressive angiomyxoma occurs most commonly during the third to fifth decades. The clinical impression frequently includes Bartholin's gland cyst or hernia; the extent of disease is often underestimated.

Melanocytic Tumors

Malignant melanoma accounts for less than 10% of all vulvar malignancies and consists of three types: mucosal or acral lentiginous, nodular, and superficial spreading. As many as 25% are unclassified. Vulvar melanoma occurs more commonly in elderly, white women and typically presents as a nodular mass that may be pigmented; satellite lesions are common. Melanomas express S-100 protein, HMB-45, and Melan A (Fig. 5.35). Clark levels and Breslow thickness should be reported for all vulvar melanomas.

Benign, atypical, and dysplastic nevi occur in the vulva. **Benign nevi** may be congenital or acquired. **Atypical vulvar nevi** (atypical melanocytic nevi of the genital type) occur primarily in young, reproductive-aged women and are characterized by atypical superficial melanocytes and variably sized junctional melanocytic nests. They are distinguished from melanoma on the basis of small size, circumscription, absence of pagetoid spread, significant cytological atypia and mitotic activity in the deeper dermal melanocytes. **Atyical vulvar nevi** may appear more atypical during pregnancy. They are not associated with dysplastic nevi elsewhere. **Dysplastic** nevi also occur predominantly in younger women but exhibit an irregular border; microscopically, clusters of atypical spindled and epithelioid nevus cells with prominent nucleoli and nuclear pleomorphism are seen. Unlike atypical vulvar nevi, dysplastic vulvar nevi may be associated with dysplastic nevi elsewhere on the trunk and extremities.

Other Neoplasms

Other tumors that occur in the vulva include cutaneous adnexal tumors, tumors that arise from specialized anogenital mammary-like glands, and tumors of minor vestibulary gland and Skene gland origin (31).

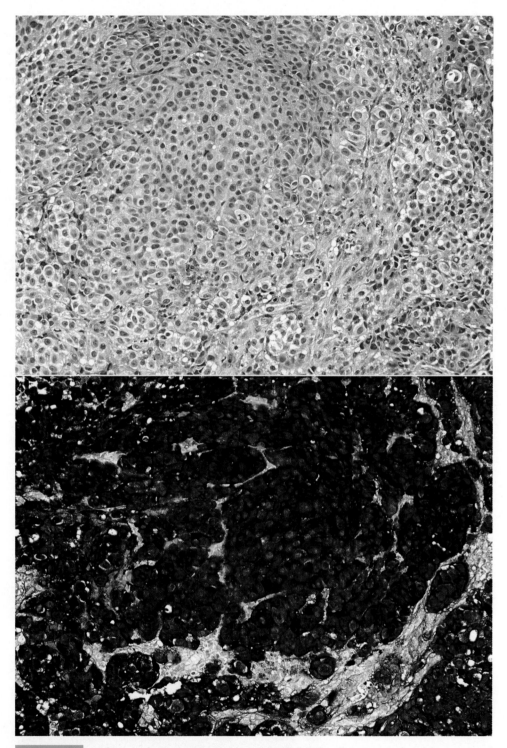

Figure 5.35   Vulvar melanoma. *Top:* Nests of epithelioid cells extensively replace normal vulvar tissue. *Bottom:* Strong expression of S100 protein.

Uterine Corpus

Endometrial Neoplasms   The endometrial morphologic changes with which the gynecologic oncologist is concerned are limited and chiefly involve endometrial carcinoma and its precursors. This section focuses on these proliferations and those that figure in their differential diagnosis.

In discussing endometrial nonsecretory proliferations it is helpful to realize that **the endometrium can give rise to a variety of epithelial phenotypes that are more commonly encountered in other parts of the müllerian-derived system: the ovary, the fallopian tubes and the endocervix. The term *metaplasia* is used for benign epithelial proliferations of this type, and *special variant carcinomas* is used for the malignant patterns.** Endometrial epithelial proliferations, whether benign or malignant, typically feature mixtures of these differentiated epithelial types. The carcinoma precursors feature this mixed epithelial phenotype in varying degrees, hence the full designation *hyperplasia/metaplasia*, which is to be understood when *hyperplasia* is used unmodified.

Endometrial Hyperplasia/Metaplasia

The term *endometrial hyperplasia* denotes a proliferating endometrium featuring glandular architectural abnormalities that result in glandular crowding and take the form of either **cystic dilatation of glands (simple hyperplasia)** or **glandular budding (complex hyperplasia).** Current taxonomy further stratifies hyperplastic endometria on the basis of their

Table 5.6 Features of Endometrial Hyperplasias

	Simple (without Atypia)	Complex (without Atypia)	Atypical (Simple or Complex)*
Histology	Increased number of round glands, which may be cystically dilated ("Swiss cheese"). The stroma participates in the process so the glands are not markedly crowded. No cytologic atypia.	The glands are closely packed and have irregular contours; little stroma remains between glands. No cytologic atypia.	Cytologic atypia (nuclear pleomorphism, loss of polarity, prominent nucleoli). Architecture may be either simple or (more commonly) complex.
Clinical	Premenopausal women; anovulatory bleeding	Perimenopausal and postmenopausal women	Postmenopausal
Premalignant potential[a]	Slight (<5%)	5%–15%	≥30%

*Most atypical hyperplasia are complex

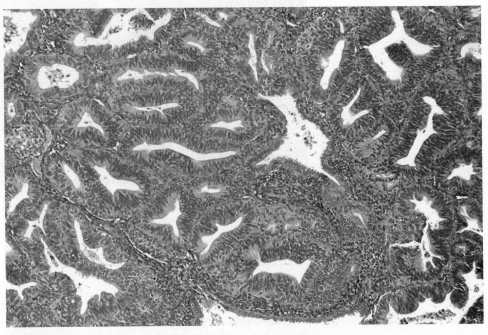

Figure 5.36   **Simple endometrial hyperplasia without atypia.** An increased number of round glands is seen, some of which are cystically dilated. There is no cytologic atypia.

cytologic features into **atypical endometrial hyperplasia** and **nonatypical endometrial hyperplasia**, the latter term implying that significant cytologic atypia is absent. The risk posed by hyperplasia for the subsequent development of endometrial carcinoma is roughly correlated with the degree of cytologic atypia present. The assessment of atypia is subject to observer disagreement. The WHO classification is simplified to *simple without atypia, complex without atypia,* and *atypical hyperplasia* (simple or complex) (Table 5.6) (Figs. 5.36 and 5.37).

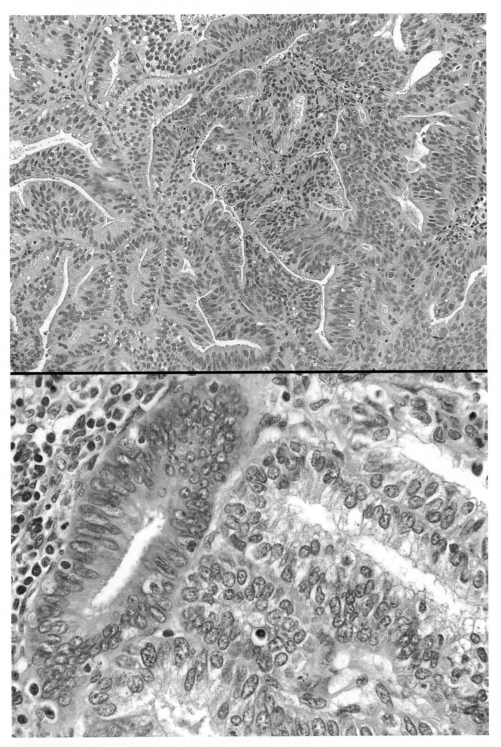

Figure 5.37   Complex atypical hyperplasia. Crowded, irregular glands show little intervening stroma. The glands show rounded, pleomorphic nuclei with prominent nucleoli. (top, low power; bottom, high power)

Differential Diagnosis

Atrophic or Weakly Proliferative Endometrium with the Architecture of Hyperplasia
When a complex hyperplasia is the last unshed endometrium of a postmenopausal woman and the epithelium subsequently becomes atrophic in the wake of estrogen withdrawal, then the pattern often mimics hyperplasia. Confusion is avoided when it is noted that the epithelium is atrophic and not proliferating.

Well-Differentiated Adenocarcinoma (Usual or Special Variant)   This is the chief differential diagnostic consideration and, unfortunately, the one that exhibits among the highest levels of expert disagreement in gynecologic pathology. The reasons for this are set out elsewhere, (41) and the differential diagnosis is discussed below.

Endometrial Carcinoma

Histologic Types

First, carcinomas may be classified in terms of their differentiated histopathologic features (Table 5.7). The endometrium gives rise to a variety of differentiated carcinomas, but more than 80% are glandular neoplasms that resemble the epithelium found in endometrial hyperplasia. **Squamous or squamoid (*morular*) differentiation is commonly encountered in this endometrioid or usual adenocarcinoma.** The term *endometrioid* is used to denote this histologic pattern and to distinguish it from *endometrial,* which is the generic term for carcinomas that originated anatomically in the endometrium. Other müllerian-differentiated types (e.g., serous, clear cell, mucinous) make up the remainder of endometrial carcinomas, the so-called special variants.

Endometrial carcinomas may also be grouped with an eye to the hormonal (and associated epidemiologic) background in which they arise: **hyperestrogenic settings (type I) or hypoestrogenic settings (type II).**

Patients in the first group **(type I)** tend to be between 40 and 60 years of age (although carcinoma can develop in younger women, including, in rare instances, those in their 20s). **They may have a history of chronic anovulation or estrogen hormone-replacement therapy,** and the carcinomas are usually well differentiated, stage I, nonmyoinvasive tumors associated with endometrial hyperplasia/metaplasia (found either concurrently or in previous endometrial samplings). **Most of the tumors are estrogen and progesterone receptor (ER and PgR) positive and *p53* negative** and express low levels of the proliferation antigen Ki-67. Patients in this first group have a very favorable prognosis after hysterectomy.

In contrast, patients in the second group **(type II)** tend to be elderly and typically have no history of hyperestrogenism. In these cases, the surrounding nonneoplastic endometrium is almost always atrophic or only weakly estrogen supported, but there may be an *in situ* component with high-grade cytologic features. **The carcinomas that develop in this group of patients are usually of the special variant type with a poor prognosis or are high-grade**

Table 5.7 Classification of Endometrial Carcinoma
Endometrioid (Usual) Carcinoma (includes glandular and villoglandular patterns)
(a) Secretory
(b) Ciliated cell
(c) With squamous differentiation (includes adenoacanthoma and adenosquamous carcinomas—see text)
Special Variant Carcinomas
(a) Serous
(b) Clear cell
(c) Mucinous
(d) Pure squamous cell
(e) Mixed
(f) Undifferentiated

endometrioid neoplasms that are high stage with deep myoinvasion. They tend to be ER and PgR negative, strongly express p53, and show high Ki-67 labeling.

Most endometrial adenocarcinomas are of endometrioid type. In these tumors, malignant glands are lined by stratified, often elongated, nuclei, reminiscent of benign endometrial epithelium. A distinct subtype of endometrioid carcinoma is **villoglandular carcinoma,** in which there are long, slender papillae lined by relatively bland cells with cigar-shaped nuclei (Fig. 5.38).

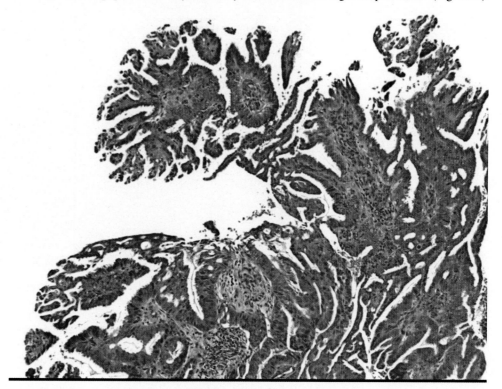

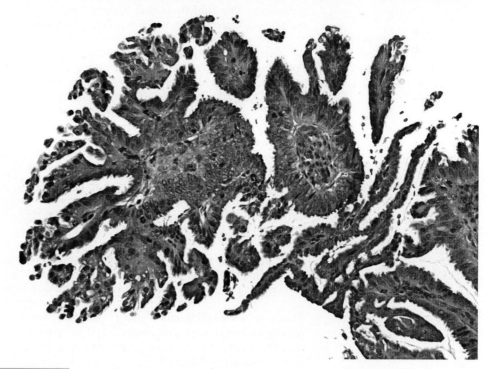

Figure 5.38   **Villoglandular carcinoma.** Delicate, elongated papillae (analogous to villous structures in villous adenomas of the large bowel) are lined by small, complex, epithelial buds. (top, low power; bottom, high power)

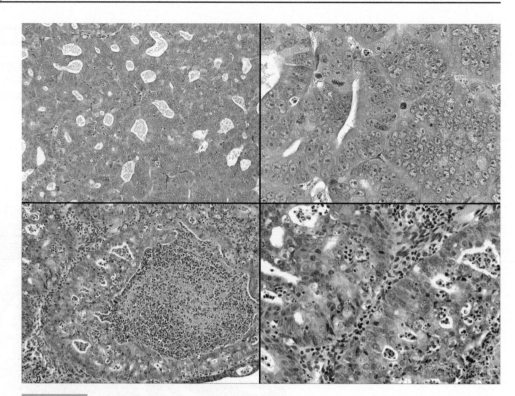

Figure 5.39   **Well-differentiated endometrioid adenocarcinoma.** Back-to-back glands with minimal or no intervening stroma (upper left) and cytologic atypia (note prominent nucleoli, upper right) are features of usual endometrial carcinoma. Glandular nests with extensive cribriforming is another common pattern seen in endometrioid adenocarcinoma (lower left and lower right). Note that in this example, the cytologic atypia is not significantly different from that seen in endometrial hyperplasia (lower right) and the diagnosis of carcinoma is based on complex architecture.

Villoglandular carcinoma is a low-grade tumor with an excellent prognosis; the main reason for recognizing this subtype is that it should not be confused with serous carcinoma of the endometrium (see below), which is also papillary but has a much worse prognosis.

Well-Differentiated Adenocarcinoma versus Atypical Hyperplasia or Metaplasia	A variety of morphologic definitions of well-differentiated adenocarcinoma have been published over the years and differ in various respects (34,35). Most require a certain level of cytologic atypia or architectural complexity. Architectural complexity usually takes the form of one or more of the following: extensive budding and branching of glands and papillary structures with superimposed secondary structures (buds or secondary papillae) and a cribriform pattern (Fig. 5.39). Expert disagreement over cases in this gray zone is common. Fortunately, this disagreement impedes clinical decision making in only a small subset of patients, including those with comorbidities or those for whom uterine conservation is important.
Adenocarcinoma with Squamous Elements	Squamous elements are very common in endometrioid adenocarcinoma of all grades (Fig. 5.40). The presence of squamous differentiation does not affect the prognosis. Of importance, the squamous areas (benign or malignant), which typically form sheets, are excluded when determining architectural grade (see below).
Secretory and Ciliary Carcinomas	Other subtypes of endometrioid adenocarcinoma include the rare secretory carcinoma and ciliated carcinomas. These are well differentiated and have a favorable prognosis. These morphologic patterns can also be seen focally in an otherwise ordinary endometrioid carcinoma.
Mucinous Adenocarcinoma	**Mucinous adenocarcinoma** (Fig. 5.41) **is usually low-grade and low-stage and is frequently seen in women treated with *tamoxifen*.** If this pattern is seen in an endometrial sampling, the anatomic origin—cervix or endometrium—may be in doubt. Strategies for illuminating this issue are set out in Table 5.5.

Serous Carcinoma   **This tumor makes up between 5% and 10% of all endometrial carcinomas and is known for its aggressive behavior** (36–38). It typically affects

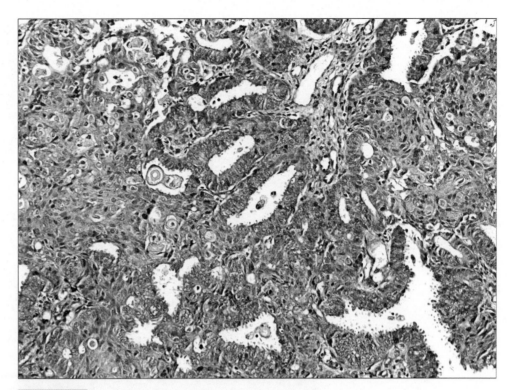

Figure 5.40   Endometrioid adenocarcinoma with squamous elements. A solid area of benign-appearing squamous cells is seen in the right half of the field.

postmenopausal women and arises in the setting of endometrial atrophy. The hallmarks of this carcinoma are a **tendency for myometrial invasion, extensive lymphatic space invasion, and early (and clinically inapparent) dissemination** beyond the uterus (most often in the form of diffuse peritoneal involvement). Microscopically, the tumor is composed of complex papillary fronds lined by highly malignant cells possessing prominent, eosinophilic nucleoli (Fig. 5.42). Uterine serous carcinoma generally lacks ER and PgR and is strongly immunoreactive for *p53*. **Serous carcinoma of endometrium is not graded; it is regarded as a high-grade tumor by definition.**

Only a minority of papillary proliferations of the endometrium are serous carcinomas; more frequent are papillary hyperplasia/metaplasias and villoglandular endometrioid carcinomas. All of these are benign or low-grade proliferations and must be distinguished from serous carcinoma (Table 5.8). Metastatic serous carcinoma to the endometrium must also be excluded.

In Situ **Serous Carcinoma (Endometrial Intraepithelial Carcinoma)**	This lesion is characterized by replacement of benign (often atrophic) endometrial epithelium by highly malignant cells resembling serous carcinoma (Fig. 5.43) (38). It is regarded as a precursor of serous carcinoma and is sometimes seen adjacent to it (39).
Clear Cell Carcinoma	Primary clear cell carcinoma of the endometrium is histologically indistinguishable from clear cell carcinoma in the ovary. This neoplasm combines high-grade cytologic features characterized by enlarged, angulated nuclei and large, irregular nucleoli with cytoplasmic clearing (at least in focal areas). The architecture may be papillary, glandular, or sheetlike. When it is glandular, the tumor cell nuclei often protrude into the luminal space, giving rise to a **hobnail or tombstone appearance** (Fig. 5.44). **The differential diagnosis includes** first, the hypersecretory change (**Arias-Stella reaction**) (Fig. 5.45) seen both in pregnancy and with the use of progestational medication; and, second, the clinically nonaggressive **secretory variant of endometrioid carcinoma.**
Squamous Cell Carcinoma	Primary squamous cell carcinoma of the endometrium is very rare and is much less common than extension of a primary uterine cervical carcinoma to the endometrium. Primary squamous cell carcinoma of the endometrium may be associated with cervical stenosis and pyometra.

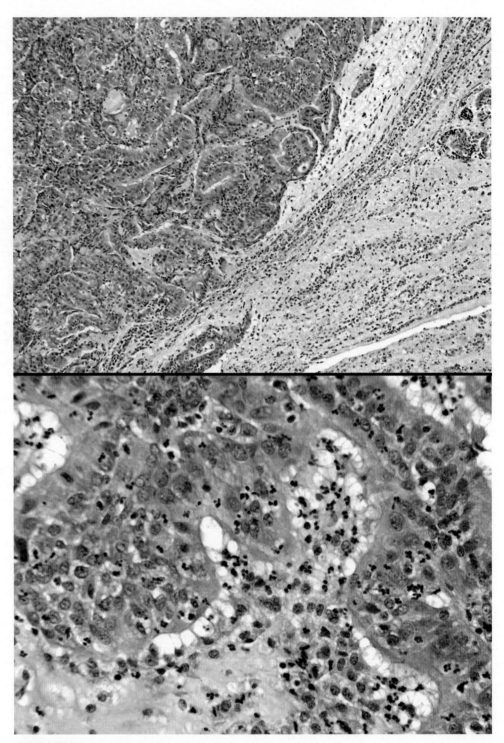

Figure 5.41 **Mucinous adenocarcinoma.** Confluent and cribriform glands are lined by mucinous epithelium. (top, low power; bottom, high power)

Undifferentiated Carcinoma

This is a tumor that shows no glandular or squamous differentiation. It represents 1% to 2% of all endometrial carcinomas and has epidemiologic features similar to those of endometrioid carcinoma.

Mixed Carcinoma

Tumor heterogeneity is, of course, ubiquitous and a well-established consequence of tumor progression; endometrial carcinomas are no exception. When differences between components become sufficiently striking, the term *mixed* is employed. To qualify for this diagnosis, the minor component(s) should compose 10% or more of the tumor.

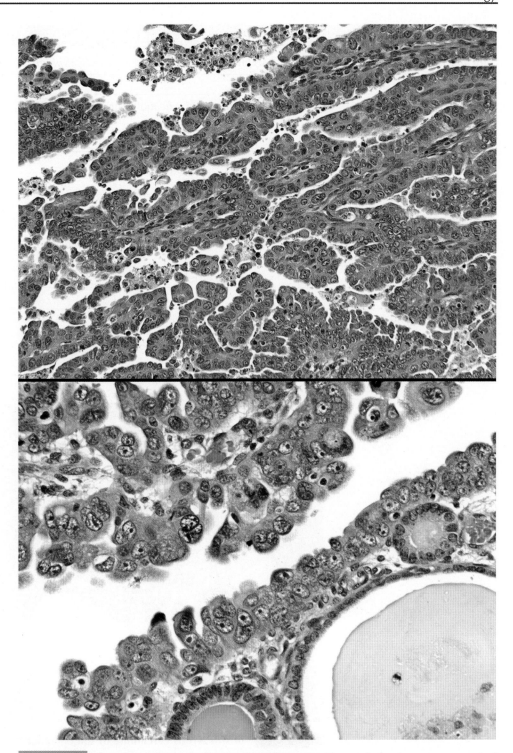

Figure 5.42   **Serous carcinoma of the endometrium.** Papillae and glands are composed of malignant cells with marked nuclear atypia. (top, low power; bottom, high power)

Histologic Grading of Endometrioid Carcinoma

The histologic grade is assigned according to the percentage of solid epithelial growth (not including areas of squamous differentiation).

1. **FIGO grade 1: The tumor exhibits well-formed glands and has 5% or less of solid growth pattern.**

Table 5.8 Papillary Proliferations of the Endometrium

Anticipated Clinical Behavior	Architecture of Connective Tissue Scaffolding	Cytologic Atypia
Benign		
Papillary syncytial metaplasia	Epithelial stratification with a papillary configuration	Minimal
Papillary change	Three-dimensional papillae	Minimal
Villoglandular hyperplasia	Sheets or folia	Minimal to moderate
Type I carcinomas		
Villoglandular endometrioid carcinoma	Sheets or folia	Moderate to severe
Endometrioid carcinomas with small nonvillous papillae	Epithelial stratification with a papillary configuration	Minimal to moderate
Mucinous carcinoma	Sheets or folia	Moderate to severe
Type II carcinomas		
Uterine (papillary) serous carcinoma	Three-dimensional papillae	Markedly atypical

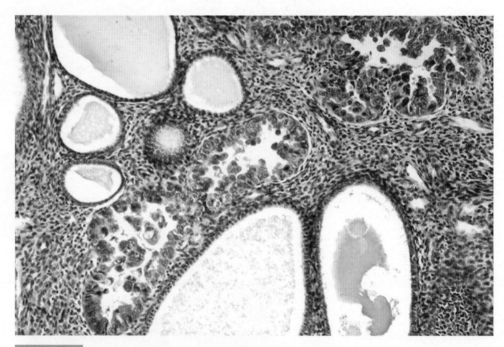

Figure 5.43   *In situ* **serous carcinoma of the endometrium.** High-grade nuclear atypia of serous carcinoma contrasts with benign, inactive glandular epithelium of the adjacent, nonhyperplastic endometrium.

2. **FIGO grade 2: The solid growth pattern occupies between 6% and 50% of the tumor.**

3. **FIGO grade 3: Tumors display more than 50% solid epithelial growth.**

Severe nuclear atypia raises the grade by one, but the possibility of a nonendometrioid (serous or clear cell) carcinoma should always be excluded in this situation.

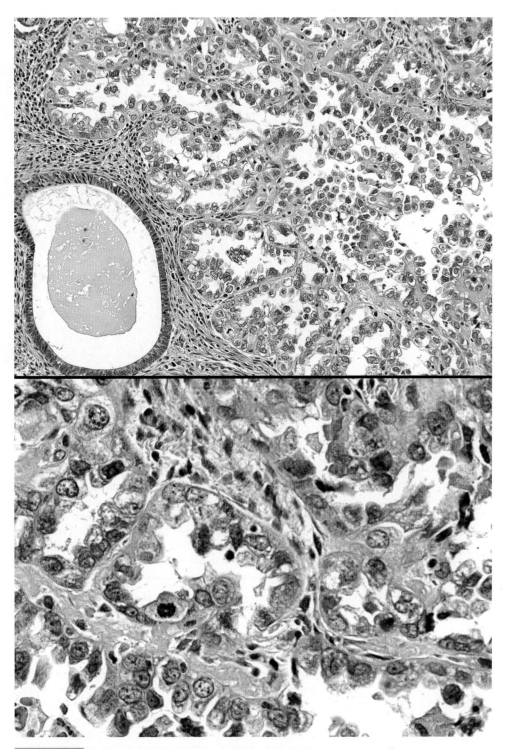

Figure 5.44 **Clear cell carcinoma of the endometrium.** Malignant glands are lined by anaplastic hobnail cells with clear cytoplasm. (top, low power; bottom, high power)

Pathologic Staging of Endometrial Carcinoma

Endocervical Involvement   Endocervical involvement is usually diagnosed on the hysterectomy specimen. Infrequently, it may be diagnosed from an endocervical curettage, but the cancer present in the endocervical curettage is usually a contamination from the uterine cavity.

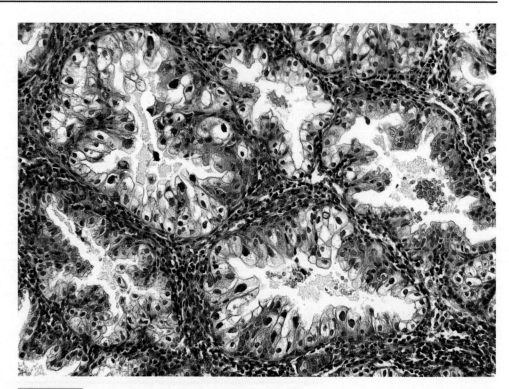

Figure 5.45   Arias-Stella reaction of the endometrium. The glandular lining shows enlarged hobnail cells with clear cytoplasm and "smudged" nuclei, a pattern that may mimic clear cell carcinoma.

Myometrial Invasion

The depth of myometrial invasion is expressed as a proportion of the myometrium invaded by carcinoma; in the FIGO staging system, this is reported as inner or outer half. The presence of lymphatic or vascular space invasion is not used to determine the depth of invasion. Involvement of adenomyosis by adenocarcinoma may resemble myometrial invasion on intra-operative visual examination; the presence of residual endometrial stroma or benign basalis glands between the tumor and myometrium is a helpful microscopic differentiating feature.

Ovarian Involvement

Simultaneous primary involvement should be considered before diagnosing ovarian metastases with well differentiated uterine endometrioid carcinoma. In most such cases, the uterine tumor shows minimal or no myometrial invasion and there is no lymphovascular or cervical stromal invasion.

Mesenchymal Neoplasms

Endometrial stromal tumors and smooth muscle tumors account for the majority of mesenchymal neoplasms in the uterine corpus. Although most endometrial stromal neoplasms are easily separated from smooth muscle neoplasms, there is a range over which clear distinction is not possible using conventional light microscopy and immunohistochemistry. These "mixed" tumors are occasionally referred to as stromomyomas; however, when such lesions remain ambiguous despite immunohistochemical analysis and the probability of an endometrial stromal proliferation is high on other grounds, they should be assigned to the endometrial stromal group for management purposes (40).

Smooth Muscle Tumors

Smooth muscle tumors are the most common mesenchymal neoplasm in the uterus. Most are composed of interlacing fascicles of spindle-shaped smooth muscle fibers (Fig. 5.46), but **epithelioid** (Fig. 5.47) and **myxoid** (Fig. 5.48) **variants** are also seen.

Leiomyoma

Leiomyomas represent the most common tumor of the uterus. They present during reproductive years and are often multiple. The typical gross appearance is that of a well circumscribed, solid, white to tan myometrial nodule with a trabeculated surface on cut sections.

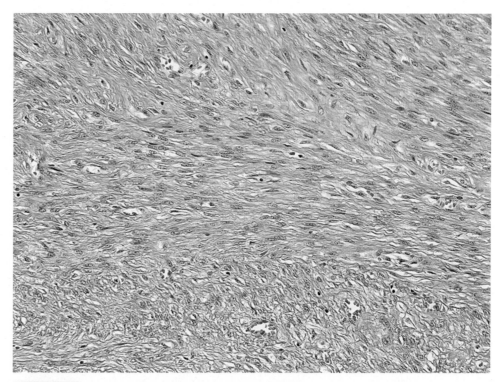

Figure 5.46 **Uterine smooth muscle tumor (leiomyoma), standard morphology.** The usual smooth muscle tumor forms a discrete intramyometrial fibrous mass. Bland spindle cell histology features ovoid, blunt-ended nuclei with no atypia.

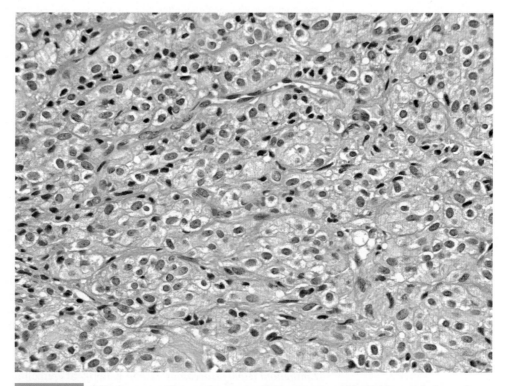

Figure 5.47 **Uterine smooth muscle tumor (leiomyoma), epithelioid morphology.** Some smooth muscle tumors exhibit pronounced epithelioid histology, mimicking epithelial processes.

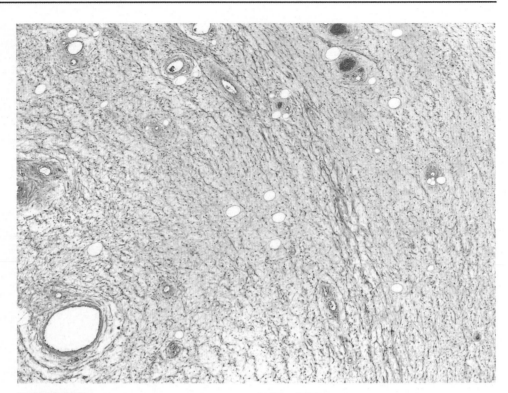

Figure 5.48   **Uterine smooth muscle tumor (leiomyoma), myxoid morphology.** Rarely, smooth muscle tumors undergo extensive myxoid change. In these cases, a myxoid leiomyosarcoma must be excluded.

Degenerative changes may alter this appearance, and edema, hemorrhage, fibrosis, and hyaline (infarction-type) necrosis are commonly seen. **Occasionally, mitotically active leiomyomas containing 15 or more mitotic figures per 10 high-power fields may be encountered; in the absence of other atypical features** (i.e., coagulative tumor cell necrosis or significant cytologic atypia), **these neoplasms are clinically benign (41).**

Cellular Leiomyoma

Leiomyomas exhibiting dense cellularity without tumor cell necrosis or significant cytologic atypia are designated cellular leiomyomas; these cellular neoplasms are clinically benign but may be confused with endometrial stromal neoplasms (Fig. 5.49). They are distinguished from stromal tumors by the presence of diffuse expression of the smooth muscle markers desmin and caldesmon with minimal or absent expression of CD10 (41).

Atypical Leiomyoma

Leiomyomas that exhibit diffuse or multifocal moderate to severe cytologic atypia, but no tumor cell necrosis or increased mitotic index (>10 mitotic figures per 10 high-power fields) are designated atypical leiomyomas with low potential for recurrence (Fig. 5.50). Most such tumors are clinically benign, although local recurrence may rarely occur (42).

Leiomyosarcoma

Leiomyosarcomas are uncommon uterine tumors but are the most common sarcoma in the uterus. They typically affect adult women in the perimenopausal years. Leiomyosarcomas are typically solitary, fleshy, and necrotic intramural tumors. **The presence of coagulative tumor cell necrosis, moderate to severe cytologic atypia, and numerous mitotic figures distinguish leiomyosarcoma from leiomyoma** (Fig. 5.51). Leiomyosarcoma is a highly malignant neoplasm, and the prognosis is poor.

Epithelioid leiomyosarcomas exhibit patterns of epithelioid differentiation in addition to the usual features of malignancy seen in the more conventional leiomyosarcoma: cytologic atypia, tumor cell necrosis, and increased mitotic index (5 mitotic figures per 10 high-power fields) (41).

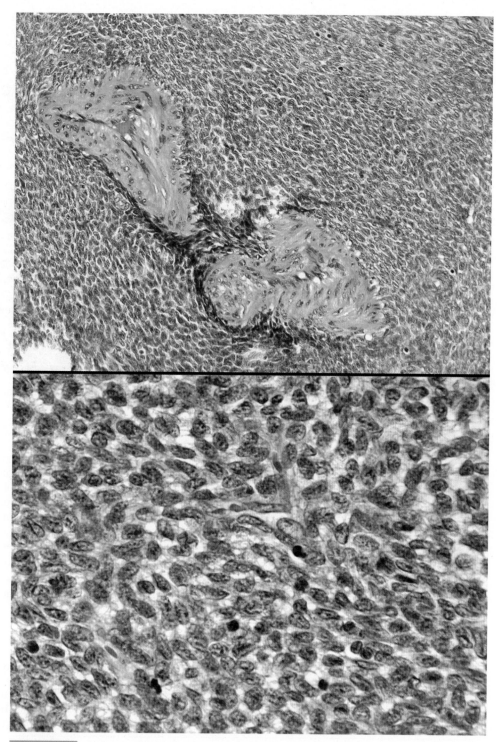

Figure 5.49   **Cellular leiomyoma.** Leiomyomas with marked cellularity may mimic endometrial stromal differentiation (see Figures 5.53 and 5.54). (top, low power; bottom, high power)

Myxoid leiomyosarcoma is a large, gelatinous neoplasm that usually appears to be circumscribed on gross examination. Microscopically, the smooth muscle cells are usually widely separated by myxoid material (Fig. 5.52). The characteristic low cellularity partly accounts for the presence of only a few mitotic figures per 10 high-power fields in most myxoid leiomyosarcomas. Despite the low mitotic counts, myxoid leiomyosarcoma has the same unfavorable prognosis as typical leiomyosarcoma (41).

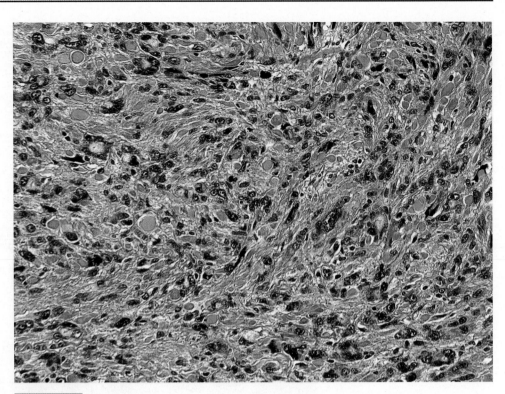

Figure 5.50 **Atypical leiomyoma.** Diffuse, marked nuclear atypia in the absence of tumor cell necrosis and increased mitotic index is classified as atypical leiomyoma, which has a low risk of recurrence.

Smooth Muscle Tumor of Uncertain Malignant Potential	Uterine smooth muscle tumors that cannot be reliably diagnosed as benign or malignant are designated as tumors of uncertain malignant potential. This diagnosis is used when there is uncertainty concerning the type of necrosis (hyaline versus coagulative), the subtype of smooth muscle differentiation (standard versus epithelioid versus myxoid), the degree of cytologic atypia or the mitotic index (41).
Smooth Muscle Neoplasms with Unusual Growth Patterns	Uterine smooth muscle tumors may demonstrate unusual patterns of distribution. As in other uterine smooth muscle neoplasms, the tumors showing these unusual patterns of distribution may exhibit standard spindle, epithelioid, or myxoid histology (41).
Diffuse Leiomyomatosis	Diffuse leiomyomatosis refers to the presence of numerous, histologically benign small smooth muscle nodules diffusely distributed throughout the uterus. The nodules range up to 3 cm in diameter, but most are less than 1 cm. This condition is benign.
Intravenous Leiomyomatosis	This condition is characterized by the presence of cords of histologically benign smooth muscle growing within venous channels beyond the confines of a leiomyoma. Extension into pelvic veins and, on occasion, the inferior vena cava and right heart may be seen.
Benign Metastasizing Leiomyoma	This clinicopathologic condition consists of the presence of histologically benign smooth muscle tumors in the lung, pelvic lymph nodes, or abdomen in association with a histologically benign uterine smooth muscle tumor. Typically, the uterine tumor is removed years before the extrauterine tumors are detected.
Disseminated Peritoneal Leiomyomatosis	Disseminated peritoneal leiomyomatosis is a rare condition characterized by widespread nodules of histologically benign smooth muscle in the omentum and peritoneum, often numbering in the tens to hundreds. The nodules are usually small, firm, gray to white, and cover the peritoneal surfaces, clinically simulating a disseminated malignancy. This condition typically occurs during the reproductive years and many patients are pregnant at the time of diagnosis. Despite the alarming appearance, disseminated peritoneal leiomyomatosis is usually

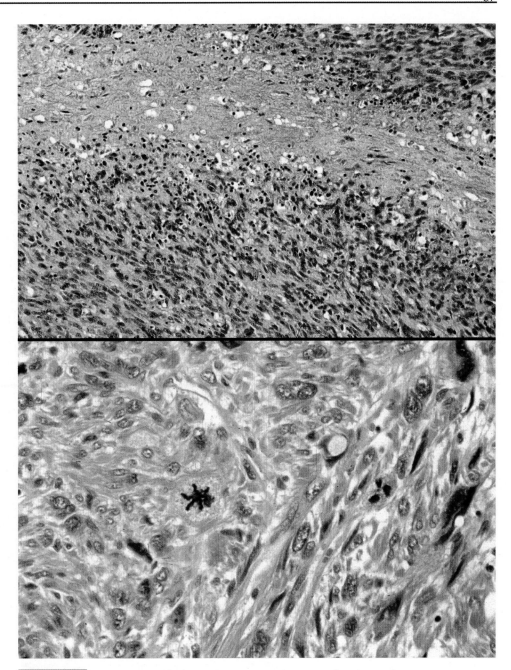

Figure 5.51   **Uterine leiomyosarcoma.** Diagnostic criteria for uterine leiomyosarcoma are diffuse atypia, tumor cell necrosis, and increased mitotic index. (top, low power; bottom, high power)

associated with an indolent clinical course and can be treated conservatively with long-term follow-up.

Endometrial Stromal Tumors

Neoplasms in the endometrial stromal group resemble the stroma of normal proliferative phase endometrium. In the uterus, they are divided into two main categories: **endometrial stromal nodule** and **endometrial stromal sarcoma.** Both are composed of a monomorphous population of ovoid to spindled cells possessing scanty cytoplasm and small, bland, uniform nuclei with evenly distributed chromatin. These cells are embedded in an abundant reticulin framework that contains a highly characteristic, delicate, arborizing vasculature. Focal hyaline thickening of the vessel walls and collagen bands may be present. Endometrial stromal nodule is clinically benign, whereas endometrial stromal sarcoma may recur, sometimes many years after the primary tumor has been removed.

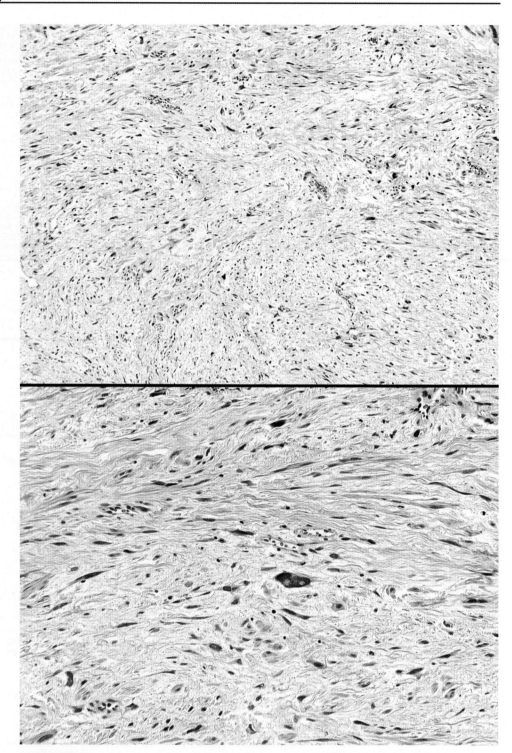

Figure 5.52   Uterine myxoid leiomyosarcoma. This rare variant of uterine leiomyosarcoma may exhibit clinically aggressive behavior in the absence of significant mitotic activity (>2 mitotic figures per 50 high-power fields). The presence of cytologic atypia and tumor cell necrosis distinguishes this infiltrative lesion from myxoid leiomyoma. (top, low power; bottom, high power)

Endometrial Stromal Nodule

Endometrial stromal nodule is well circumscribed, usually small, and intramural (Fig. 5.53). Infiltration of the myometrium or uterine vasculature is absent. Because diagnosis is based on complete circumscription and absence of lymphovascular invasion, the distinction between stromal nodule and stromal sarcoma can usually be made only at the time of hysterectomy.

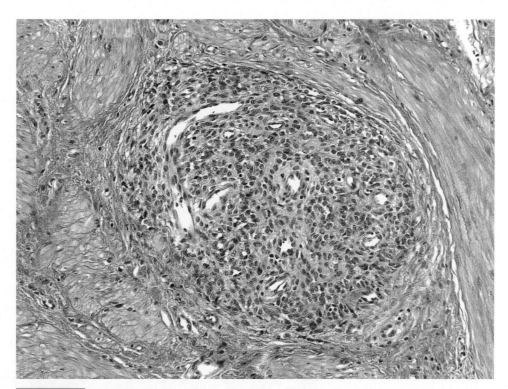

Figure 5.53   **Endometrial stromal nodule.** Endometrial stromal tumors are composed of small, uniform cells with scant cytoplasm similar to stromal cells in normal proliferative phase endometrium. When an endometrial stromal tumor is well circumscribed and there is no lymphovascular invasion, it is clinically benign and classified as an endometrial stromal nodule.

Endometrial Stromal Sarcoma (Low Grade)

Endometrial stromal sarcoma accounts for less than 20% of all uterine sarcomas, occurs almost exclusively in adults, and has a peak incidence in the fifth decade; more than **three-quarters of women are premenopausal.** There is no association with previous irradiation nor do patients share the risk profile of patients with endometrial carcinoma. Endometrial stromal sarcoma is **an indolent neoplasm with a protracted clinical course.** At the time of clinical presentation, most tumors are confined to the uterus. Extrauterine disease is associated with a higher risk for recurrence but is still compatible with long-term survival. Patients come to clinical attention because of a mass that may be associated with abdominal pain or uterine bleeding. When advanced, the uterus is asymmetrically enlarged by a typically yellow or tan tumor mass that infiltrates the surrounding normal myometrium, often extending into the endometrial cavity as a polypoid growth. **The neoplasm is distinguished from endometrial stromal nodule by (i) the presence of infiltrating margins or (ii) vascular invasion** (Fig. 5.54). In most cases, mitotic figures are difficult to find, but occasional tumors have in excess of 10 mitotic figures per 10 high-power fields. Although it was traditional to grade endometrial stromal sarcoma based on mitotic index, this classification currently has relatively little utility in diagnostic practice and patient management (43). **Endometrial stromal sarcoma should be distinguished from "undifferentiated sarcoma,"** a clinically highly aggressive neoplasm, which shares with endometrial stromal sarcoma a generally undifferentiated appearance but has a greater degree of cytologic atypia.

Undifferentiated Uterine Sarcoma

Undifferentiated uterine sarcoma is much less common than low-grade endometrial stromal sarcoma (44). Undifferentiated uterine sarcomas are easily recognized as cytologically malignant and are composed of highly cellular, often pleomorphic, undifferentiated rounded to spindled cells with a high mitotic index (Fig. 5.55). Most resemble the undifferentiated malignant stroma often encountered in carcinosarcomas. Undifferentiated uterine sarcomas, in sharp contrast to endometrial stromal sarcomas, are aggressive neoplasms with a high incidence of metastases.

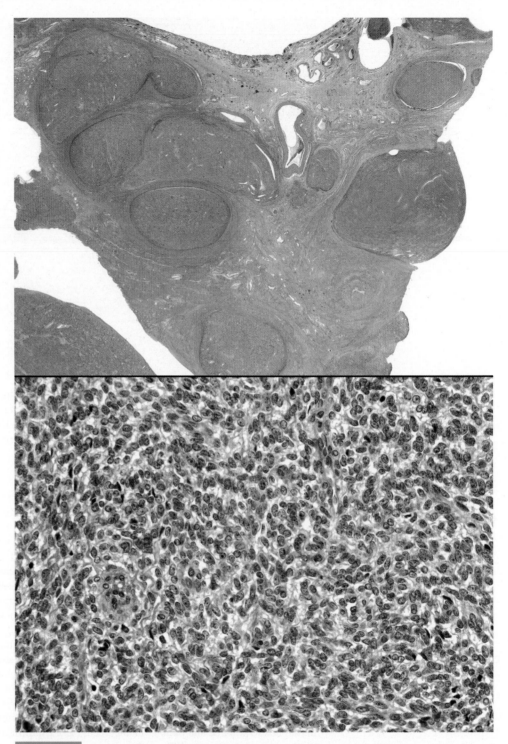

Figure 5.54 **Endometrial stromal sarcoma.** The presence of infiltrative margins and lymphovascular invasion distinguish low-grade endometrial stromal sarcoma from benign stromal nodule. (top, low power; bottom, high power)

Mixed Müllerian Neoplasms

Mixed müllerian neoplasms are biphasic epithelial–mesenchymal proliferations that exhibit a range of clinical behaviors from benign to highly malignant. **Adenofibroma, adenomyoma**, and **atypical polypoid adenomyoma** are the common biphasic epithelial–mesenchymal lesions at the benign end of the spectrum, whereas **adenosarcoma** and **carcinosarcoma** represent the malignant end of the spectrum (Table 5.9).

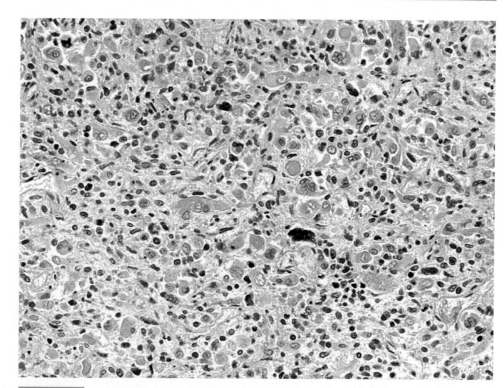

Figure 5.55 **Undifferentiated uterine sarcoma.** Mesenchymal tumors showing marked cellularity, cytologic atypia, and high mitotic index are classified as undifferentiated uterine sarcomas. Heterologous elements may also be present.

Table 5.9 Mixed Müllerian Neoplasms

Mesenchymal Elements		Epithelial Elements	
		Benign	Malignant
	Benign	Adenomyoma Adenomyosis Atypical polypoid adenomyoma	[Carcinofibroma]
	Malignant	Adenosarcoma Endometrial stromal sarcoma 　with glandular elements	Carcinosarcoma • Homologous • Heterologous

Adenofibroma

Adenofibromas are considered to be clinically benign with little risk for recurrence once they are completely excised. They typically have broad, fibrotic to mildly cellular stroma with intervening cleftlike epithelial-lined surfaces morphologically similar to phyllodes tumor of the breast (Fig. 5.56). Authorities differ on the appropriate mitotic index for distinguishing adenofibroma from adenosarcoma. Zaloudek and Norris advocate a threshold of 4 mitotic figures per 10 high-power fields (45), whereas Clement and Scully suggest a threshold of 2 mitotic figures per 10 high-power fields (46). In most instances, the 4 mitotic figures per 10 high-power fields criterion is sufficient to diagnose adenosarcoma, but tumors with particularly cellular stroma or borderline mitotic counts are best regarded as being of uncertain malignant potential, particularly if subepithelial condensation is present (see **Adenosarcoma** below).

Atypical Polypoid Adenomyoma

Atypical polypoid adenomyoma is a polypoid endometrial proliferation composed of irregular glands set in a stroma composed of smooth muscle or, more commonly, smooth muscle and fibrous tissue (Fig. 5.57). Morular or squamous metaplasia is present in most cases and is often florid. The endometrial samplings typically consist of large fragments or chunks of tissue

175

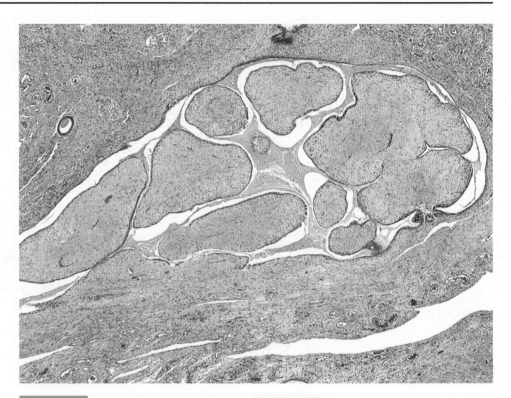

Figure 5.56 **Adenofibroma of uterus.** Irregular, clefted glands are surrounded by prominent paucicellular and mitotically inactive stroma.

simulating carcinoma. The condition occurs in premenopausal or perimenopausal women; a clinical history of infertility is not uncommon. These lesions can recur locally but do not have metastatic potential. Reproductive conservation utilizing procedures short of hysterectomy is warranted for the conventional APA, provided there is continual follow-up (47).

Adenosarcoma

Adenosarcoma is an uncommon, predominantly low-grade malignant biphasic tumor that is composed of benign epithelial elements and sarcomatous stroma. Most patients with uterine corpus adenosarcoma are postmenopausal. **An association with unopposed estrogen and *tamoxifen* therapy has been reported.**

Uterine corpus adenosarcoma typically presents as a polypoid growth that protrudes through the cervical os or appears to arise from the cervix or lower uterine segment; often there is a history of recurrent polyps, which in retrospect may represent early or subtle forms of adenosarcoma. Microscopically, the tumor consists of uniformly distributed, often cystic, and irregularly contoured glandular elements, often with internal papillations scattered throughout a variably cellular stroma. The stroma forms a characteristic hypercellular collar or cuff (so-called cambium layer) around the glands, often producing irregular, stellate glandular configurations (Fig. 5.58).

Approximately 25% of adenosarcomas are myoinvasive. Most patients with uterine adenosarcoma are cured by hysterectomy. However, deep myoinvasion, lymphovascular invasion, high-grade heterologous stroma, stromal overgrowth, and extrauterine spread are associated with disease recurrence. Stromal overgrowth is defined as pure stromal proliferation constituting greater than 25% of the tumor. Approximately 10% to 25% of patients with uterine adenosarcoma die of their disease. This figure rises to 50% for those whose tumors contain stromal overgrowth.

Adenosarcoma often represents a challenge for the pathologist because of significant overlap with adenofibroma and other forms of benign polyp. Most adenosarcomas arise in the uterine corpus, but cervical, vaginal, tubal, ovarian, and primary peritoneal adenosarcomas also occur. Involvement of additional extragenital sites in women has been linked to endometriosis.

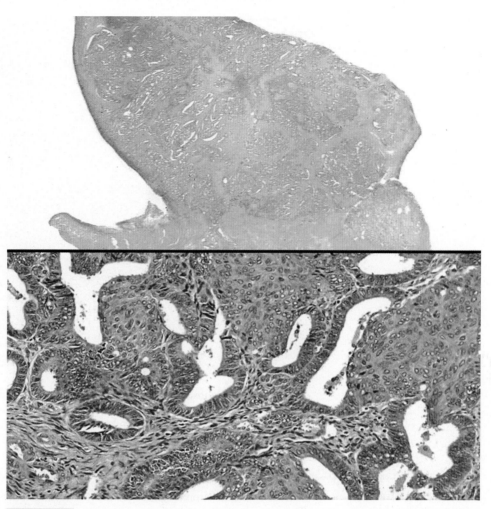

Figure 5.57 **Atypical polypoid adenomyoma.** This polyp typically occurs in the lower uterine segment and is composed of complex endometrioid glands with squamous metaplasia set in a fibromuscular stroma. (top, low power; bottom, high power)

Carcinosarcoma

Despite the long entrenched terminology of "malignant mixed müllerian tumor," carcinosarcoma is the current preferred designation for mixed neoplasms composed of carcinoma and sarcoma. **With rare exceptions, carcinosarcoma is a disease of elderly menopausal women; there is an association with prior pelvic radiation.** Most patients present with uterine bleeding; the typical appearance is that of a fleshy, necrotic and hemorrhagic, polypoid mass that fills the uterine cavity and extends through the cervical os. The cardinal rule for diagnosing carcinosarcoma requires the presence of a distinct biphasic neoplasm, composed of separate but admixed malignant-appearing epithelial and mesenchymal elements (Fig. 5.59). The mesenchymal and epithelial elements should not merge with one another. Both the high-grade nuclear features and the biphasic pattern of this neoplasm are obvious in the typical case. **The stromal components may be *homologous*** (leiomyosarcoma, stromal sarcoma, fibrosarcoma) **or *heterologous*** (chondrosarcoma, rhabdomyosarcoma, osteosarcoma, liposarcoma). Although tradition holds that heterologous elements do not bear on prognosis, a recent study from Memorial Sloan-Kettering suggests that surgical stage I uterine carcinosarcoma with heterologous elements may be more aggressive than carcinosarcoma without heterologous elements (48). Prognosis is also dependent on stage, the size of the tumor, and the depth of myometrial invasion.

Ovary

Four broad histogenetic categories of ovarian tumors are observed: surface epithelial–stromal tumors (65% to 70%), sex cord-stromal tumors (15% to 20%), germ cell tumors (5% to 10%), and metastases (5%).

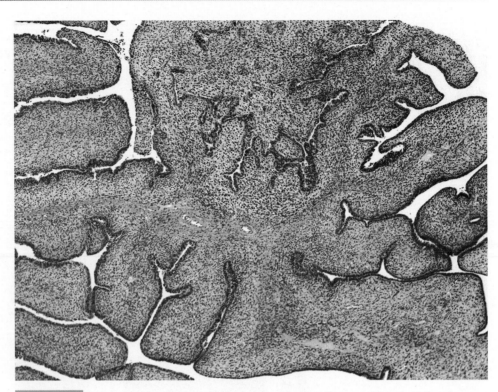

Figure 5.58 **Adenosarcoma of uterus.** In contrast to adenofibroma, the stroma in adenosarcoma is cellular and mitotically active. Stromal condensation around the glandular component forms a characteristic cambium layer.

Surface Epithelial–Stromal Tumors

Surface epithelial–stromal tumors are the most common neoplasms of the ovary (Table 5.10). They consist of six types: serous, mucinous, endometrioid, clear cell, transitional, and undifferentiated (49,50). Tumors with squamous differentiation have also historically been included among the surface epithelial–stromal tumors, but pure squamous tumors are rare; most arise in teratomas.

Serous Tumors

Tumors with serous differentiation represent 45% of surface epithelial–stromal ovarian neoplasms; they are characterized by epithelial cells resembling those of the fallopian tube and encompass a group of three biologically distinct entities: benign serous cystadenofibroma, serous tumor of low malignant potential (serous borderline tumor), and serous carcinoma.

Benign Serous Tumors

Benign serous cystadenomas or cystadenofibromas constitute almost one-half of all serous ovarian neoplasms. Benign serous tumors occur over a wide age range but are most common in the reproductive age group. They are often bilateral and composed of varying amounts of fibrous stroma and cysts. They range in size from 1 cm to 10 cm (rarely as large as 30 cm). The cysts are unilocular or multilocular and may contain papillary projections. Surface papillomas may also be present. Microscopically, the cysts are lined by a simple layer of epithelium that recapitulates the ciliated epithelial cells of the fallopian tube.

Serous Tumors of Low Malignant Potential (Serous Borderline Tumors)

Serous tumors of low malignant potential constitute approximately 15% of all ovarian serous neoplasms and account for the vast majority of all borderline surface epithelial–stromal neoplasms. They occur at a slightly younger age than serous carcinoma (mean 45 years versus 60 years). They are more often bilateral and larger than benign serous tumors and may present with disease beyond the confines of the ovary. Serous neoplasms in the low malignant potential group are predominately cystic with variable amounts of papillary epithelial projections, although solid tumors with surface papillary excrescences may also occur. Microscopically, serous tumors of low malignant potential are composed of architecturally complex branching

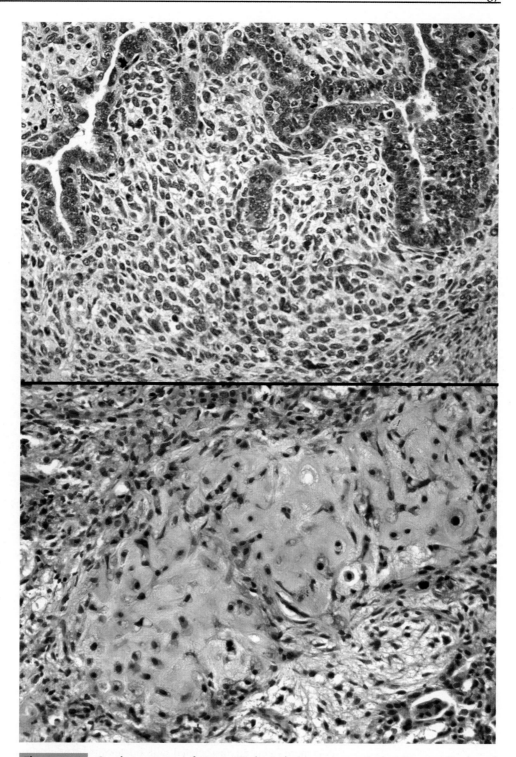

Figure 5.59   Carcinosarcoma of uterus. Biphasic lesion composed of malignant glands and stroma (top). Heterologous elements, such as cartilage depicted here, may be present in carcinosarcoma (bottom).

papillary and micropapillary structures not unlike that of low-grade serous carcinomas, but they do not feature destructive invasion of the ovarian stroma. The nuclei are uniform or mildly atypical (Fig. 5.60). Mitotic activity is low. Psammoma bodies are often present but are not diagnostic.

Micropapillary Pattern   Approximately 10% of serous tumors of low malignant potential contain foci of significant micropapillary architecture, defined as nonhierarchical branching of

179

Table 5.10 Histologic Classification of Surface-Epithelial Stromal Tumors	
Histologic Type*	*Total (%)*
Serous	46
Mucinous	36
Endometrioid	8
Clear	3
Transitional	2
Undifferentiated	2
Mixed	3

*Tumors with squamous differentiation have also been included among the surface epithelial–stromal tumors, but pure squamous tumors are rare. Most arise in an epidermoid or dermoid cyst.

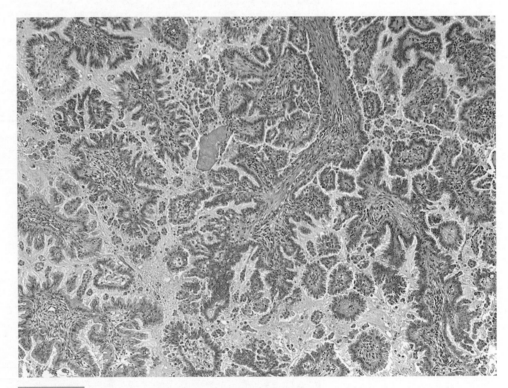

Figure 5.60   Serous borderline tumor (low malignant potential). Papillae are lined by stratified tubal type epithelium with tufting. Mitotic activity is minimal, and cytologic atypia is mild to moderate. There is no stromal invasion.

slender, elongated papillae that are at least five times as long as they are wide (Fig. 5.61) *or* a sievelike cribriform pattern occupying a continuous 5-mm extent. The micropapillary variant is more frequently associated with bilaterality, ovarian surface involvement, and the presence of extraovarian disease (51). When the extraovarian disease is invasive, serous tumors of low malignant potential with micropapillary architecture have a poorer prognosis.

Stromal Microinvasion   Stromal microinvasion, defined as 5 mm in linear extent or 10 mm^2 in area, may be found in 10% to 15% of serous tumors of low malignant potential. Stromal microinvasion is characterized by eosinophilic cells or small micropapillae lying within stromal spaces beneath larger papillae (Fig. 5.62). It is seen more frequently during pregnancy. Although it may be associated with a small, long-term risk of disease recurrence when occurring in patients who are not pregnant, the overall prognosis is favorable. Stromal microinvasion appears to represent a histologic link between serous tumors of low malignant potential and low-grade serous carcinoma and is likely a bona fide form of early invasion (52).

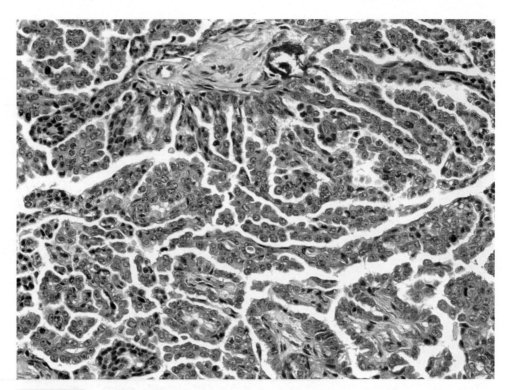

Figure 5.61   Serous borderline tumor with micropapillary pattern. In this variant, the papillae are elongated and at least fivefold longer than their width. Ovarian surface involvement, bilaterality, and extraovarian implants are more common in this variant than in the usual serous borderline tumor.

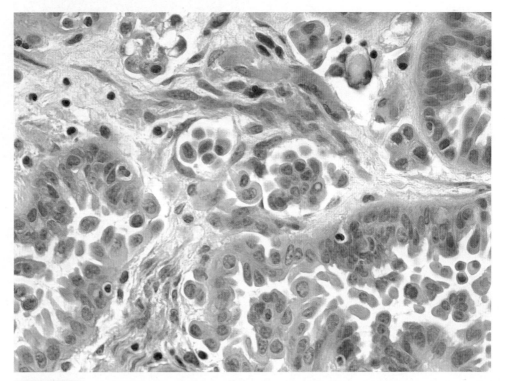

Figure 5.62   Stromal microinvasion in serous borderline tumor. Small foci of intrastromal single cells and small, nonbranching papillae may be seen in 10% to 15% of serous borderline tumors. Although such foci likely represent early stromal invasion, their presence does not warrant a diagnosis of carcinoma, provided they are small (<5 mm) and show no significant cytologic atypia.

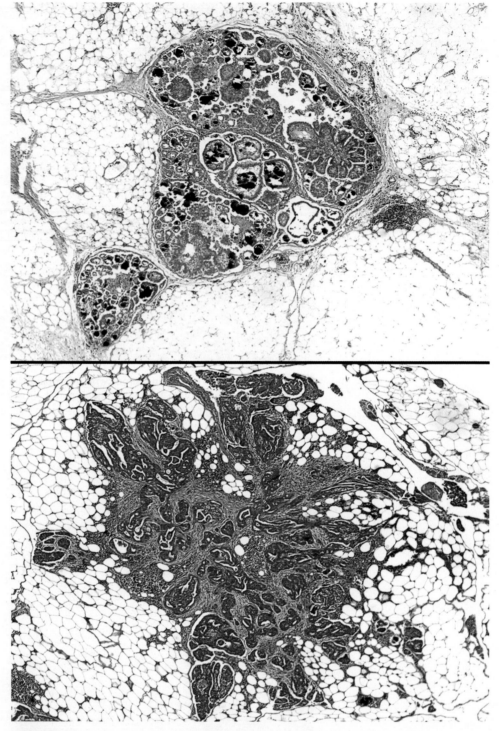

Figure 5.63 *Top:* **Noninvasive implant of serous borderline tumor.** *Bottom:* **Invasive implant of serous borderline tumor.** Unlike noninvasive implants, invasive implants have an irregular stromal interface.

Extraovarian Disease   Approximately 30% to 40% of serous tumors of low malignant potential are associated with similar-appearing lesions in the pelvis and intraabdominal sites, including lymph nodes. These lesions, termed *implants*, may be microscopic or macroscopic and are subclassified as noninvasive or invasive types, based on the presence of destructive infiltration into underlying normal tissue structures (Fig. 5.63). **Noninvasive implants are divided into**

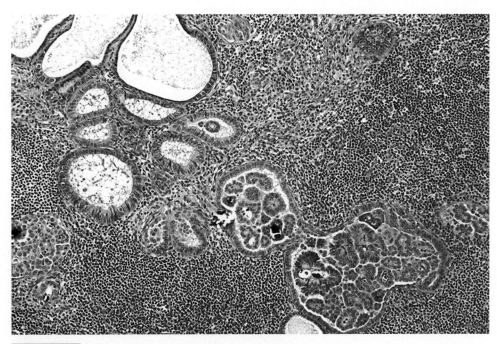

Figure 5.64 **Lymph node involvement by serous borderline tumor.** Lymph node involvement by serous borderline tumor can be florid but does not confer a poorer prognosis.

epithelial and desmoplastic types, depending on whether or not there is an associated stromal response. The distinction between noninvasive and invasive implants is important because **extraovarian invasive disease is associated with a significantly poorer prognosis** (53). At times it is difficult to determine whether an implant is invasive or not; in these instances, the implants may be classified as indeterminate. Implants that are indeterminate for invasion appear to have a prognosis that is intermediate to that of noninvasive and invasive implants (54).

Lymph node involvement (Fig. 5.64) occurs in 20% to 30% of cases of ovarian serous tumor of low malignant potential (55), but the presence of lymph node involvement does not confer a worse prognosis unless it exhibits an invasive pattern.

Endosalpingiosis frequently coexists with serous low malignant potential (borderline) lesions in the peritoneum and lymph nodes, but the presence of endosalpingiosis alone does not upstage disease. The frequent coexistence of endosalpingiosis with "implants" of ovarian serous tumor of low malignant potential would seem to support the concept that serous tumors may arise in endosalpingiosis in at least a subset of cases.

Serous Carcinoma   Serous carcinoma accounts for 35% to 40% of all serous ovarian neoplasms and approximately 75% of ovarian surface epithelial–stromal carcinomas. Ovarian serous carcinoma tends to occur in the sixth to seventh decades (mean 56 years). **Grossly, serous carcinoma is bilateral in 60% of cases** and is solid and cystic or mostly solid. Microscopically, serous carcinomas exhibit fine papillae (low-grade carcinoma) that can become fused and form solid sheets of cells with slitlike spaces (high-grade carcinoma). Marked nuclear atypia and numerous mitotic figures, which may be atypical, are characteristic in the high-grade tumors (Fig. 5.65). **Psammoma bodies are often present** but are not specific.

Ovarian serous carcinoma is graded using either a three-tiered system based on architecture and cytology or a two-tiered system based on the degree of nuclear atypia and the mitotic index (56,57). **The high-grade (grades 2 and 3) serous carcinomas are the most common surface epithelial carcinomas and are associated with *p53* mutations and somatic or germ-line abnormalities of *BRCA1* or *BRCA2*.** Low-grade (grade 1) serous carcinomas (Fig. 5.66) are much less common than high-grade serous carcinomas, accounting for less than 10% of serous carcinomas. The low-grade (grade 1) serous carcinomas exhibit mutations in *B-RAF* and *K-RAS,* similar to those seen in serous tumors of low malignant potential (58).

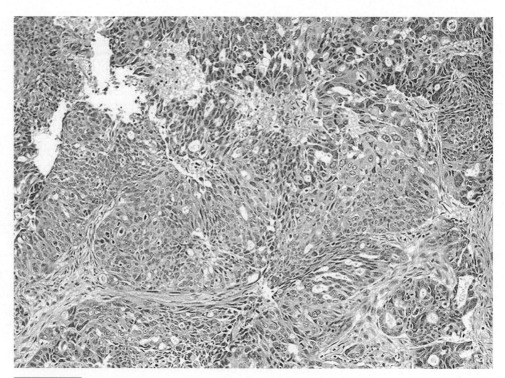

Figure 5.65   High-grade serous carcinoma of ovary. Sheets and papillae show marked nuclear pleomorphism and frequent mitotic figures.

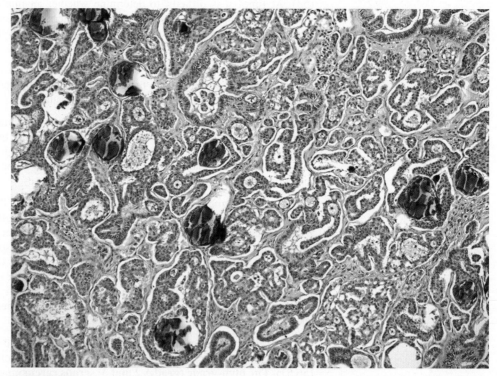

Figure 5.66   Low-grade serous carcinoma of ovary. Simple and branching papillae invade stroma but show moderate cytologic atypia and low mitotic activity.

High-grade serous carcinoma is the most common gynecologic tumor to occur in women with germ-line *BRCA1* and *BRCA2* mutations; **serous carcinoma may also develop in the fallopian tubes and on the surface of the peritoneum.**

Serous psammocarcinoma, a very rare variant of low-grade serous carcinoma, is defined by the presence of massive psammomatous calcification (at least 75% of the tumor cell nests contain a psammoma body), predominant extraovarian disease distribution, and low-grade cytologic atypia. The prognosis for serous psammocarcinoma is favorable (59).

Mucinous Tumors

Surface epithelial tumors with mucinous differentiation account for 15% of all ovarian neoplasms in the United States and Europe. These tumors are characterized by epithelial cells resembling those of the endocervix (endocervical-like) or gastrointestinal tract (intestinal type). Like the serous tumors, they encompass a group of three distinct entities: benign mucinous cystadenoma or adenofibroma, mucinous borderline tumor (tumor of low malignant potential), and mucinous carcinoma (50,60).

Benign Mucinous Tumors

Almost 80% of all mucinous ovarian neoplasms are benign unilocular or multilocular cystadenomas. They occur in a wide age range but are most commonly diagnosed in the reproductive age group. Benign mucinous tumors are typically unilateral and can reach a very large size, extending to 30 cm or more in diameter. Microscopically, the tumors are composed of a columnar epithelial lining with abundant, pale-staining intracellular mucin that resembles endocervical or gastric-type epithelium. Goblet cells may be present but are uncommon in benign mucinous tumors (in contrast to intestinal-type mucinous tumors of low malignant potential or mucinous carcinomas).

Mucinous Tumors of Low Malignant Potential (Mucinous Borderline Tumors), Intestinal Type

Mucinous borderline tumors account for 10% to 15% of all mucinous ovarian tumors; the intestinal type is most common. **Mucinous borderline tumors of intestinal type are unilateral and often larger than benign mucinous tumors.** They occur most commonly during the late reproductive years (mean 45 years). Microscopically, the multilocular cysts are lined by variably stratified mucinous epithelium forming complex papillary folds. The individual cells show mild to moderate cytological atypia with increased mitotic figures (Fig. 5.67). Goblet cells are present. The presence of marked or severe nuclear atypia involving the full thickness of stratified epithelium (i.e., not limited to the crypts) is classified as *intraepithelial carcinoma*.

Two patterns of microinvasion are recognized in mucinous borderline tumors of intestinal type. **The first pattern consists of infiltration of stroma by individual cells or small nests of cells that are cytologically similar to the cells elsewhere in the borderline tumor.** Such foci must not exceed 5 mm in linear extent or 10 mm^2 in area. This is an uncommon finding in mucinous borderline tumors (in comparison to the frequency of microinvasion in serous borderline tumors). **The second, more common pattern of microinvasion consists of one or more small foci (≤5 mm in linear extent or ≤10 mm^2 in area) of nests, individual cells, and glands exhibiting cytological features of high-grade carcinoma cells; this latter pattern is classified as** *microinvasive* **carcinoma.** Foci of microinvasive carcinoma are of uncertain prognostic significance, but their presence should prompt a search by the pathologist for larger foci of invasive carcinoma (49).

Mucinous Tumors of Low Malignant Potential (Mucinous Borderline Tumors), Endocervical-Like

Mucinous borderline tumors of müllerian (endocervical) type are bilateral in as much as 40% of cases and have a strong association with endometriosis, which is present in as much as 50% of cases. The mean age of patients with endocervical-like mucinous borderline tumors is mid-30s. These tumors are composed of complex papillae, architecturally similar to those of serous borderline tumors, lined by columnar mucin-secreting epithelium and ciliated eosinophilic epithelium. Nuclear atypia is mild to moderate, and mitotic figures may be present. Typically, there is a prominent neutrophilic infiltrate in the stroma of the papillae. Stromal microinvasion, similar to that in serous borderline tumors may be present. Extraovarian implants may also be present in as much as 20% of cases, but their presence has not been associated with a poorer prognosis.

Mucinous Carcinoma, Intestinal Type

Mucinous carcinomas account for less than 10% of all mucinous ovarian neoplasms. Two different patterns of invasion are recognized, both of which may coexist in a single tumor. The confluent glandular or expansile invasive pattern is recognized by marked glandular crowding

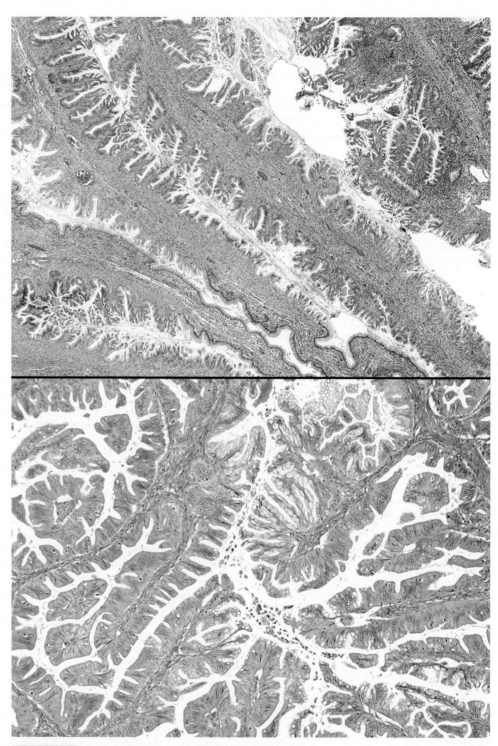

Figure 5.67   Mucinous borderline tumor, intestinal type. Papillary growth pattern, stratification, and nuclear atypia distinguish these tumors from cystadenoma. Intestinal differentiation is exemplified by goblet cells and, in some cases, Paneth cells. There is no stromal invasion. (top, low power; bottom, high power)

with little intervening stroma (Fig. 5.68). The destructive stromal invasive pattern, which is less common, is recognized by irregular nests and single cells with malignant cytological features infiltrating stroma (Fig. 5.69). The presence of stromal invasion, whether of destructive or confluent type, must exceed 5 mm in linear extent or 10 mm^2 in area in order to be classified as carcinoma; otherwise a diagnosis of microinvasive carcinoma is warranted.

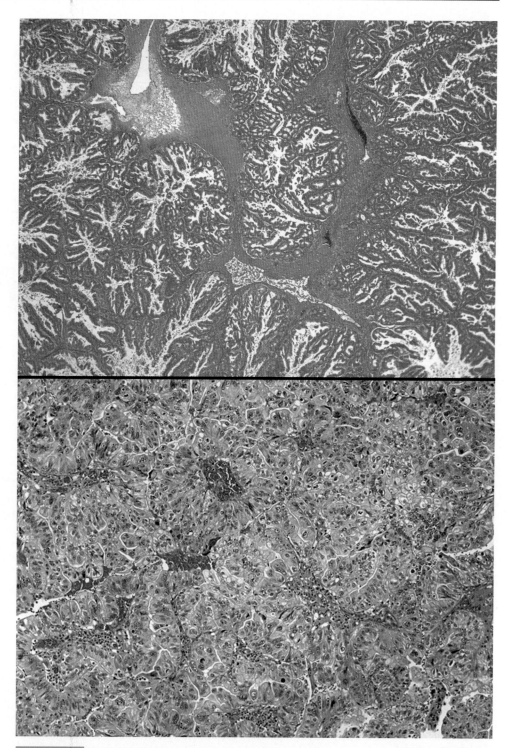

Figure 5.68   Mucinous adenocarcinoma of ovary. Expansile stromal invasion in a mucinous ovarian tumor is classified as mucinous carcinoma, but it does not appear to confer the same ominous prognosis as mucinous ovarian tumors with destructive stromal invasion (see Figure 5.69). (top, low power; bottom, high power)

Most primary mucinous carcinomas of the ovary are confined to the ovary at the time of diagnosis; an advanced stage mucinous carcinoma involving the ovary at first diagnosis should be evaluated as a possible metastasis from other sites, particularly the gastrointestinal tract (49).

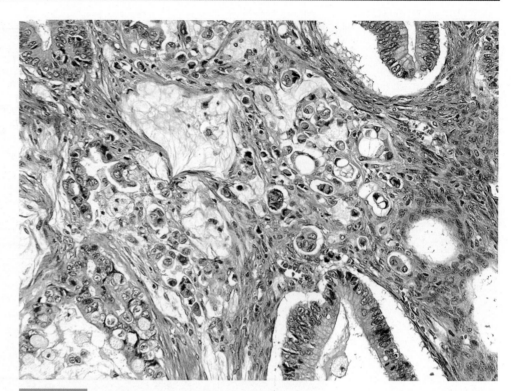

Figure 5.69 **Mucinous adenocarcinoma of ovary.** Destructive stromal invasion in a mucinous ovarian tumor is classified as mucinous carcinoma. Metastasis—for example, from the gastrointestinal tract—should always be considered, especially in the presence of high-stage disease or bilateral ovarian involvement.

Mucinous Tumor with Pseudomyxoma Peritonei

Although ovarian mucinous tumors associated with pseudomyxoma peritonei are listed as a distinct category by the WHO, **most of these tumors are metastases from primary mucinous tumors of the vermiform appendix** (Fig. 5.70). Rarely, primary ovarian mucinous tumors of the intestinal type are associated with pseudomyxoma peritonei; these tumors typically have an associated teratomatous component in the ovary (61,62). The natural history of these tumors is not well understood.

Endometrioid Tumors

Surface epithelial tumors with endometrioid differentiation exhibit the glandular or stromal histologic features of endometrial glands and stroma. Ovarian tumors showing endometrioid differentiation account for **less than 10% of all surface epithelial–stromal tumors.**

Benign Endometrioid Tumors and Endometrioid Tumors of Low Malignant Potential (Endometrioid Borderline Tumors)

Benign endometrioid tumors are rare and, when present, typically unilateral. Borderline endometrioid tumors may be bilateral (30%). Both are clinically benign. The tumors resemble their uterine counterparts and are composed of glandular or villoglandular proliferations, which may show cytoplasmic clearing or secretory-type changes with sub- or supranuclear vacuolization. Squamous metaplasia is common. The changes in borderline endometrioid tumors are analogous to those seen in complex atypical hyperplasia of the endometrium, in that there is both cytological and architectural atypia but no stromal invasion.

Endometrioid Carcinoma

The typical ovarian endometrioid carcinoma is comparable to FIGO grade 1 or 2 endometrioid adenocarcinoma of the uterus, although occasional tumors have a higher-grade, more solid growth pattern. Squamous metaplasia is common, as are other metaplastic changes (secretory, ciliated cell, oxyphilic, mucinous). Endometrioid carcinomas of the ovary exhibit a wide array of patterns that may pose differential diagnostic problems for the pathologist; these include spindled, tubular, insular, trabecular, microglandular, adenoid basal, and adenoid cystic. When prominent, these patterns may mimic Sertoli cell or Sertoli-Leydig cell tumors, carcinoid tumors, or granulosa cell tumors (Fig. 5.71). Metastases from the gastrointestinal tract may also

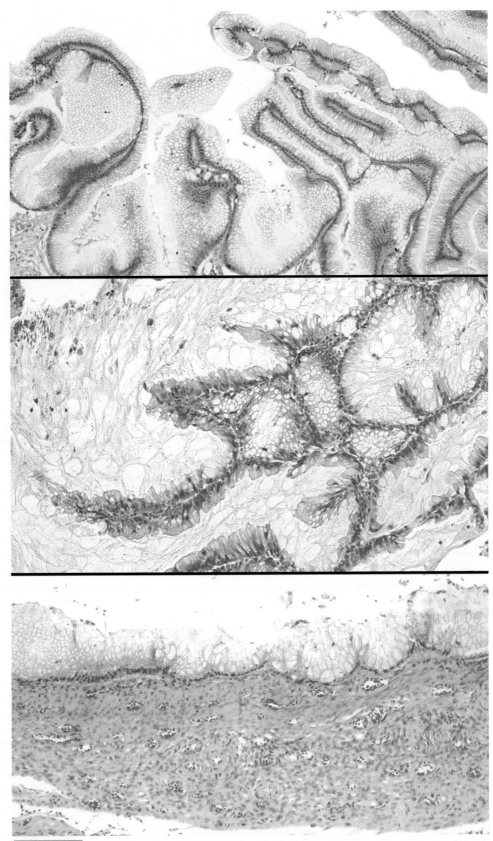

Figure 5.70   Pseudomyxoma peritonei. Cytologically low-grade mucinous epithelium is present within pools of mucin in the ovarian stroma (top), peritoneum (middle), and within the appendix (bottom) in this condition. Most cases are associated with an appendiceal mucinous neoplasm; rarely, this condition is encountered in mucinous ovarian tumors arising in a mature teratoma.

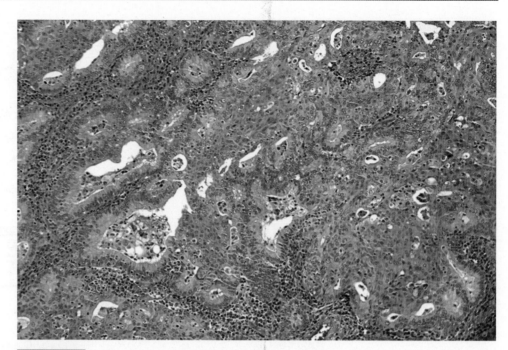

Figure 5.71   **Endometrioid adenocarcinoma of ovary.** Ovarian endometrioid carcinoma has similar morphology to endometrial endometrioid carcinoma, including squamous cell differentiation.

simulate a primary endometrioid carcinoma. **An association with endometriosis, either ovarian or elsewhere in the pelvis, is observed in as much as 40% of cases. Simultaneous primary endometrioid carcinomas in the uterus are present in 20% of cases** (49).

Clear Cell Tumors

Surface epithelial stromal tumors with clear cell differentiation are characterized by epithelial cells containing glycogen-rich clear cytoplasm and hobnail cells with varying degrees of fibrous stroma. Once considered to be of mesonephric origin, clear cell surface epithelial tumors are now recognized as derivatives of the müllerian tract. **Clear cell tumors account for 3% of all surface epithelial stromal tumors. Almost all are malignant.**

Benign Clear Cell Tumors and Clear Cell Tumors of Low Malignant Potential (Borderline Clear Cell Tumors)

The benign and borderline clear cell adenofibromatous tumors are extremely rare (<1% of clear cell tumors) and present in the second to seventh decade of life.

Clear Cell Carcinoma

Clear cell carcinomas tend to occur in the fifth to seventh decade (10% in the fourth decade). There is an unexplained increased prevalence of clear cell carcinoma in Japan relative to Western countries. Two-thirds of women with clear cell carcinoma are nulliparous. **More than one-half have associated endometriosis** involving the ovary or other pelvic sites. **When associated with endometriosis, mixed clear cell and endometrioid carcinoma may occur.** Patients with clear cell carcinoma are at risk for developing **paraneoplastic hypercalcemia or pelvic venous thromboses.** Most clear cell carcinomas, even when advanced stage, are unilateral (49). The tumors are composed of glands, tubules, cysts, or solid sheets of polyhedral cells with optically clear or eosinophilic granular cytoplasm (Fig. 5.72). Hobnail cells are characteristic. Psammoma bodies may be present, and as much as 25% of cases contain eosinophilic hyaline bodies. Clear cell carcinomas of the ovary are not graded (49).

Transitional Cell (Brenner) Tumors

Transitional cell tumors are thought to arise through metaplasia of the ovarian surface epithelium and are analogous to Walthard nests, which are transitional-type epithelial inclusions occurring beneath the serosa of the fallopian tubes and in the hilar regions of the ovaries. They are uncommon (3% of all surface epithelial–stromal tumors). Most are clinically benign.

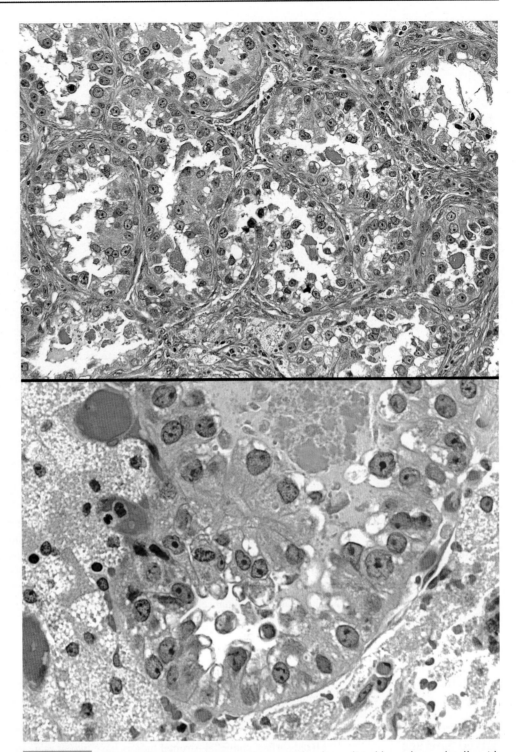

Figure 5.72   Clear cell adenocarcinoma of ovary. Glands are lined by polygonal cells with clear cytoplasm and enlarged, hyperchromatic, and pleomorphic nuclei. (top, low power; bottom, high power)

Benign Transitional Cell (Brenner) Tumor

Brenner tumors are the most common type of ovarian transitional cell tumor. They are often microscopic or incidental findings discovered at laparotomy for unrelated pelvic conditions. They affect patients during the fourth to eighth decades (mean 50 years). They are typically solid, unilateral tumors with small cysts on cut section; most are less than 2 cm. A gritty consistency may be present because of flecks of calcification (Fig. 5.73). They may be associated with a mucinous cystic tumor. Microscopically, they contain nests of cytologically bland cells with urothelial appearance surrounded by a prominent fibromatous stroma. The individual nests may be solid or microcystic with an inner mucinous epithelial lining.

191

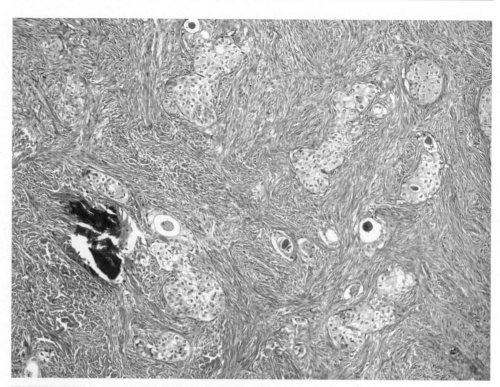

Figure 5.73 **Brenner tumor of ovary.** Nests of transitional epithelium are set in fibrous stroma. Stromal calcifications may impart a gritty texture.

Transitional Cell (Brenner) Tumor of Low Malignant Potential (Borderline)	Borderline tumors are typically unilateral, solid and cystic, and usually larger (10 cm to 25 cm) than benign Brenner tumors. Microscopically, they feature coarse papillary fronds lined by multilayered uroepithelium that resembles low-grade papillary urothelial carcinoma of the urinary tract. Despite their epithelial proliferation, these tumors are clinically benign.
Malignant Brenner Tumor	Malignant transitional cell tumors *with* benign or atypical proliferating transitional elements are designated as malignant Brenner tumors. These tumors show nuclear pleomorphism, hyperchromasia, and numerous mitotic figures, as well as destructive stromal invasion.
Transitional Cell Carcinoma	Malignant transitional cell tumors *without* benign or atypical proliferating transitional elements are designated as transitional cell carcinomas. The diagnosis of transitional cell carcinoma is highly subjective.
Undifferentiated Epithelial Tumors	Undifferentiated carcinomas lack histological features of a specific müllerian cell type. They are invariably high grade. Because undifferentiated areas are common in high-grade ovarian carcinomas that contain specific features of serous, clear cell, or other differentiation elsewhere, pure undifferentiated carcinomas are infrequent (49).
Mixed Surface Epithelial–Stromal Tumors	Mixed surface epithelial–stromal tumors have two or more differentiated histologic cell types, each of which account for at least 10% of the tumor.
Sex Cord–Stromal Tumors	Sex cord–stromal tumors demonstrate ovarian, testicular, or a mixture of ovarian and testicular cell differentiation (63). **Many of the tumors of this subtype variably express inhibin,** a feature that is often used in confirming the presence of sex cord–stromal differentiation.
Adult Granulosa Cell Tumors	Adult granulosa cell tumor is the most common sex cord–stromal tumor in the ovary. This tumor **occurs in females over a wide age range** (mean 52 years) but is more common in late reproductive years than in the pediatric age group. Patients often present with estrogenic symptoms (50).

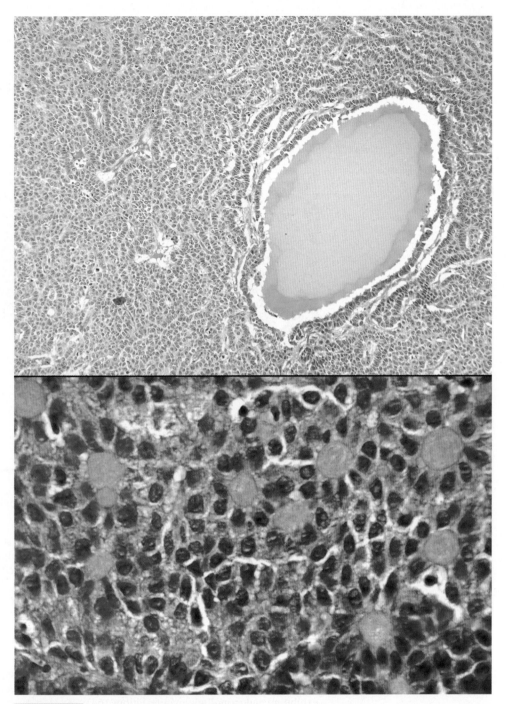

Figure 5.74   **Adult granulosa cell tumor.** *Top:* Ribbons of cells with coffee-bean nuclei surround a macrofollicle. The mitotic index is usually low in these tumors. *Bottom:* Microfollicular pattern with Call-Exner bodies.

Adult granulosa cell tumors are unilateral and solid, solid and cystic, or predominantly cystic. Microscopically, they are characterized by a proliferation of ovoid, predominantly uniform cells with an open chromatin pattern and nuclear grooves (Fig. 5.74). Mitotic figures are present but typically few in number. A variety of patterns can be observed, including trabecular, insular, diffuse (*sarcomatoid*), and **microfollicular,** featuring characteristic **Call-Exner bodies** (small round spaces filled with eosinophilic material formed by the surrounding granulosa cells). Macrofollicles are also present in most adult granulosa cell tumors. Adult granulosa cell tumor is **a neoplasm of low malignant potential;** recurrences may occur many years after initial diagnosis. The most important prognostic feature is stage of disease.

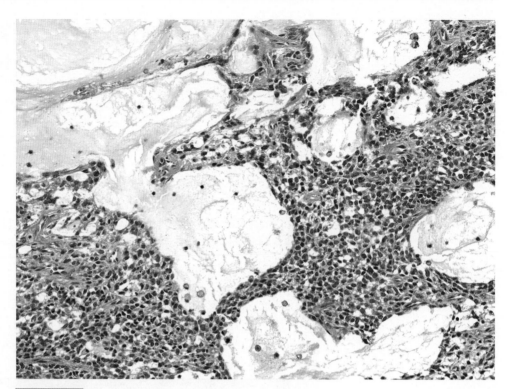

Figure 5.75 **Juvenile granulosa cell tumor.** Macrofollicles in this tumor are surrounded by cells with more hyperchromatic and often more mitotically active nuclei than those in the adult type.

Juvenile Granulosa Cell Tumors

Juvenile granulosa cell tumors tend to occur in younger women (97% occur in females younger than age 30). Patients often present with isosexual pseudoprecocity or menstrual irregularities.

Most juvenile granulosa cell tumors are unilateral and low stage with a macroscopic appearance similar to the adult granulosa cell tumor. They are distinguished from the adult variant by the presence of larger, more irregular follicles and rounded, more atypical nuclei that are euchromatic or hyperchromatic and nongrooved (Fig. 5.75). Mitotic figures are often numerous. **Most juvenile granulosa cell tumors are clinically benign;** approximately 10% of patients develop recurrences, typically within the first 5 years of initial diagnosis (63).

Sertoli-Leydig Cell Tumors

Sertoli-Leydig cell tumors occur most commonly in women in their mid-20s but can occur in females as young as 2 and as old as 75 years. **Approximately one-third of patients present with virilization;** estrogenic manifestations are less frequent. Almost one-half of patients exhibit no endocrinologic manifestations (64).

Sertoli-Leydig cell tumors are typically unilateral and low stage, but 10% may have ovarian surface involvement. Less than 5% exhibit extraovarian spread at diagnosis. Most are solid or solid and cystic, and pale yellow or tan in color. The characteristic features are tubules or cords of Sertoli cells with interspersed nests of Leydig cells enmeshed in primitive gonadal stroma (Fig. 5.76). **Rarely, a Sertoli-only cell tumor can be seen.** Approximately 20% have heterologous elements, which may be epithelial or mesenchymal and include mucinous, cartilaginous, neuroendocrinological (carcinoid tumor), or skeletal muscular (rhabdomyosarcoma) differentiation. Retiform elements resembling rete testis are seen in 15% of cases. The tumors are graded on the basis of the degree of Sertoli tubule formation and the extent of primitive stroma. Well-differentiated tumors have a mitotic index of less than 5 mitotic figures per 10 high-power fields, whereas poorly differentiated tumors have a mitotic index greater than 10 mitoses per 10 high-power fields, and intermediate tumors have an intermediate mitotic index.

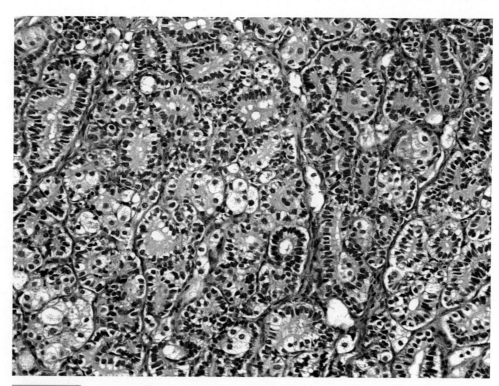

Figure 5.76   **Sertoli-Leydig cell tumor.** Sertoli tubules with interspersed Leydig cells form this well-differentiated tumor.

Sex-Cord Tumor with Annular Tubules	A rare variant of Sertoli cell tumor, the sex-cord tumor with annular tubules is distinguished by the presence of simple or complex annular tubules composed of Sertoli cells arranged antipodally around hyaline material (Fig. 5.77). Tumors are unilateral and often associated with hormonal manifestations. As much as 25% are clinically malignant (50). **One-third occur in patients with Peutz-Jeghers syndrome;** when they occur in this setting, sex-cord tumor with annular tubules are clinically benign, bilateral, and small, often incidental findings.
Gynandroblastoma	When sex cord–stromal tumors contain minor components of other types of sex cord–stromal tumor, the tumor is usually designated by the major component. However, when a tumor is composed of an admixture of well differentiated Sertoli cell tubules and granulosa cell elements, and the second cell population makes up at least 10% of the tumor, the tumor is classified as gynandroblastoma, and the relative contribution and subtypes are reported. Most such tumors are benign.
Fibroma–Thecoma	This group of stromal tumors is composed of spindle or oval cells with scant (**fibroma**) or more abundant, pale, lipid-rich cytoplasm (**thecoma**) associated with varying degrees of collagen. **Estrogenic manifestations are generally absent in fibromas but occur in as many as 60% of patients with thecomas.** Tumors in this group tend to occur in middle age (fibroma) or after menopause (thecoma). Most are unilateral, solid, or solid and microcystic, and they vary from gray or white (fibroma) to bright yellow (thecoma). Microscopically, the tumors are composed of cells arranged in fascicles or a storiform pattern; calcification and hyaline plaques may be seen (Fig. 5.78). Patients with nevoid basal cell carcinoma syndrome develop ovarian fibromas at a younger age; in this setting, the fibromas are bilateral, multinodular, and calcified. **Almost all fibromas and thecomas are clinically benign. Some fibromas present with ascites and pleural effusion (Meigs syndrome),** which resolves on removal of the tumor.
Sclerosing Stromal Cell Tumors	These stromal tumors occur in young women and are rarely associated with endocrine manifestations. They are unilateral and clinically benign. Sclerosing stromal tumors are distinguished by the presence of alternating, relatively hypercellular and hypocellular areas of

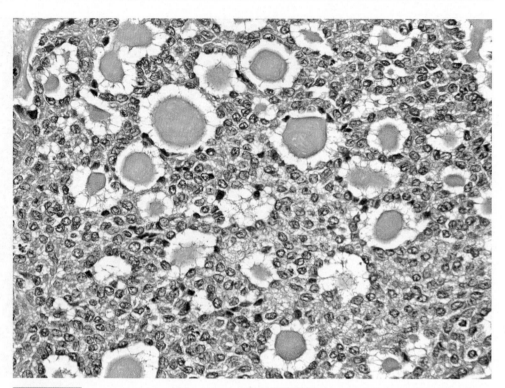

Figure 5.77   **Sex-cord tumor with annular tubules.** Prominent hyaline bodies are surrounded by a proliferation of complex annular tubules. This tumor may be associated with Peutz-Jeghers syndrome and is typically incidental and clinically benign in that setting. Those tumors that are not associated with the syndrome may recur and demonstrate clinically aggressive behavior.

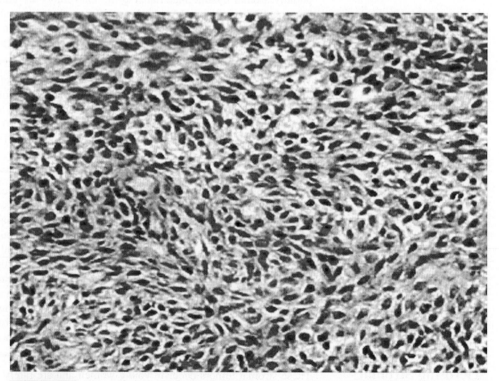

Figure 5.78   **Fibroma–thecoma of ovary.** Spindle-shaped cells are dispersed in a variably fibrous stroma.

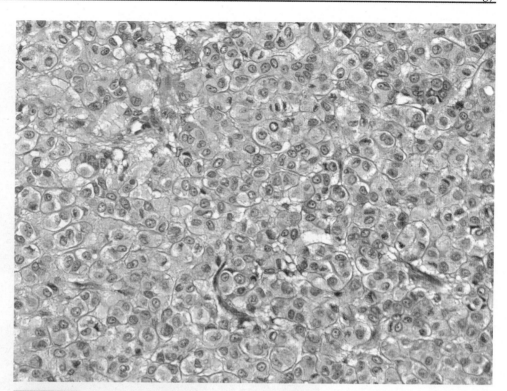

Figure 5.79   Steroid cell tumor of ovary. Nests of polygonal cells with central rounded nuclei may exhibit finely vacuolated, eosinophilic, or, less commonly, optically clear cytoplasm.

stromal proliferation arranged in a pseudolobular pattern. An extensive, thin-walled vascular pattern is often present.

Steroid Cell Tumors, Not Otherwise Specified

Steroid cell tumors tend to occur in young, reproductive-aged women (25% younger than 30 years of age). These tumors are unilateral. Most are confined to the ovary at diagnosis, but as many as 20% have extraovarian spread at diagnosis and 30% are clinically malignant. Endocrine manifestations, when present, tend to be androgenic, although estrogenic, progestogenic, and Cushingoid manifestations may also be seen (63). Most are solid and pale yellow or orange, with the color depending on the steroid content. Microscopically, the tumors are composed of solid nests of uniform, round, or polygonal cells with distinct cell borders and central nuclei that contain small but distinct nucleoli (Fig. 5.79). The cytoplasm may be finely vacuolated or eosinophilic and granular. Most tumors are mitotically inactive with fewer than 2 mitotic figures per 10 high-power fields; tumors with a high mitotic index may be more aggressive.

Leydig Cell Tumors and Stromal Luteomas

Steroid cell tumors, not otherwise specified, must be distinguished from Leydig cell tumors and stromal luteomas, both of which tend to exhibit a benign clinical course. **Leydig cell tumors are recognized by the presence of Reinke crystals.** They are either small and typically hilar in location or large and replacing most of the ovarian parenchyma. **Stromal luteomas** are typically small (less than 3 cm), well-circumscribed tumors that occur within (and are circumscribed by) the ovarian stroma. **A size criterion of 1 cm has been imposed to distinguish Leydig cell tumors and stromal luteomas from benign, nonneoplastic ovarian steroid cell proliferations** (see below).

Germ Cell Tumors

These tumors are derived from the primordial germ cells of the ovary. Most are mature cystic teratomas and are clinically benign. The remaining germ cell tumors are malignant; most occur in children or adolescent females (63).

Mature Cystic Teratoma

Mature teratomas are typically cystic, although solid variants do occur. They have a wide age range, occurring in females from 2 to 80 years (mean 32 years). As many as 15% are bilateral at presentation. **Mature teratomas are one of the most common ovarian neoplasms,**

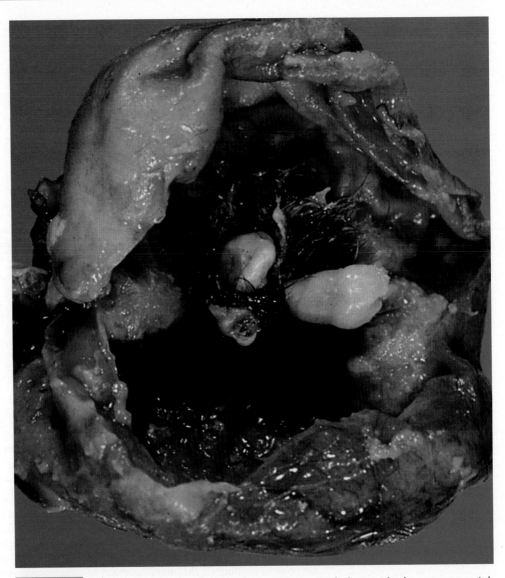

Figure 5.80 **Mature teratoma.** Cystic neoplasm contains teeth, hair and sebaceous material.

accounting for 30% to 45% of all ovarian tumors and as much as 60% of all benign ovarian tumors. Recurrences may occur in the residual ipsilateral ovary following cystectomy, particularly when the tumors are multiple or ruptured. **The presence of *mature glial implants* in the peritoneum (grade 0 implants) does not adversely affect prognosis** (50) (Fig. 5.80).

Monodermal mature teratomas are not uncommon in the ovary and include struma **ovarii** (thyroid), **carcinoid, strumal carcinoid, ependymoma**, and **primitive neuroectodermal tumor.**

The development of a **secondary somatic carcinoma may rarely occur** in mature teratomas in postmenopausal women. **Squamous carcinoma and adenocarcinoma,** usually of intestinal type, account for most cases of secondary carcinoma. **Secondary sarcomas** are less common and tend to occur in younger patients.

Immature Teratoma

Immature teratomas are distinguished from mature teratomas by the presence of variable amounts of immature embryonal tissue, typically in the form of immature neuroectodermal tissue (Fig. 5.81). Prognosis is dependant on grade and stage of disease. Tumors are graded on the basis of the amount of immature tissue present. Grading is traditionally based on a three-tiered system, although a two-tiered system may be more reproducible. Treatment of immature teratomas has evolved in recent years. Surgery alone is considered curative in children and

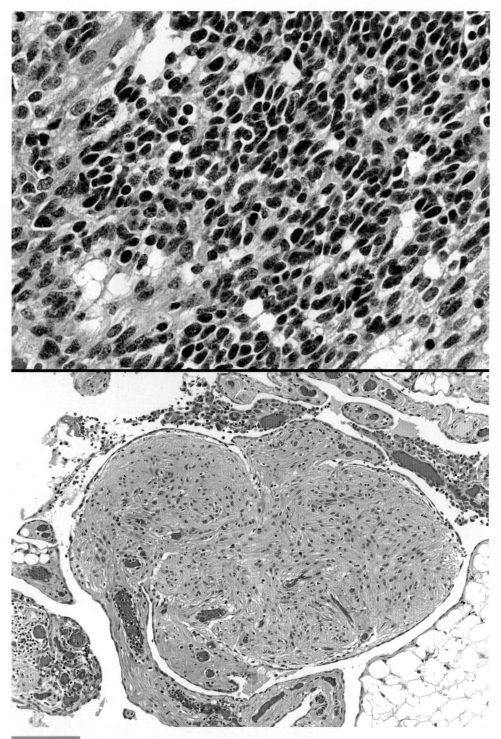

Figure 5.81   Immature teratoma. *Top:* Teratomas are graded on the amount of immature tissue, most commonly manifested by immature neural tissue, that is present. *Bottom:* In contrast, the presence of mature glial tissue does not affect prognosis, even when it forms nodular deposits throughout the peritoneum (gliomatosis).

adolescent patients with immature teratomas regardless of the grade. Chemotherapy is used for patients who relapse.

Dysgerminoma

Dysgerminoma is identical to its testicular counterpart, the seminoma. The ovarian tumors are unilateral in 80% of patients, large (mean 15 cm), solid, and tan in appearance; cyst formation is seen in areas of infarction. Most occur in the second and third decade, although 5% present

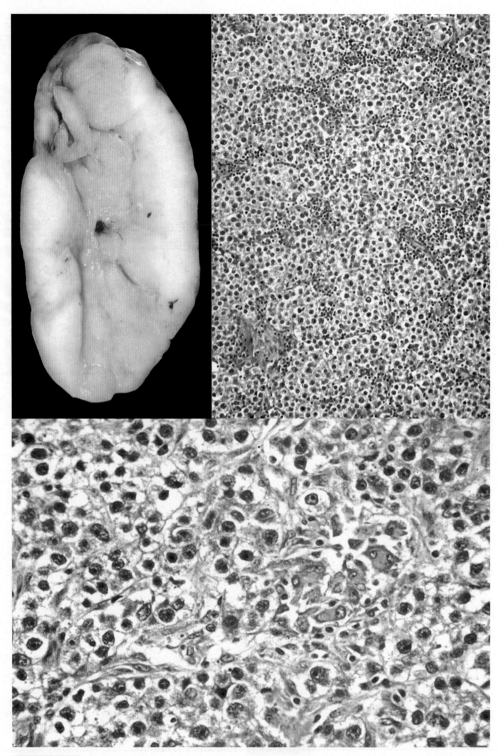

Figure 5.82 **Dysgerminoma.** *Top left:* Solid, pale tan lobulated growth pattern is characteristic of dysgerminoma. *Top right and bottom:* The tumor is composed of sheets of ovoid to polygonal cells with clear cytoplasm, prominent cell borders and central nuclei with multiple small nucleoli. Interspersed mature lymphocytes are characteristic.

in children less than 5 years of age. The tumors are composed of a diffuse proliferation of rounded cells with discrete cell membranes and central nuclei with one to four prominent nucleoli (Fig. 5.82). Lymphocytes and granulomas are often present. Some tumors contain syncytiotrophoblastic cells, which may be associated with elevated serum beta-human chorionic gonadotropin. The neoplastic cells express placental alkaline phosphatase, CD117, and

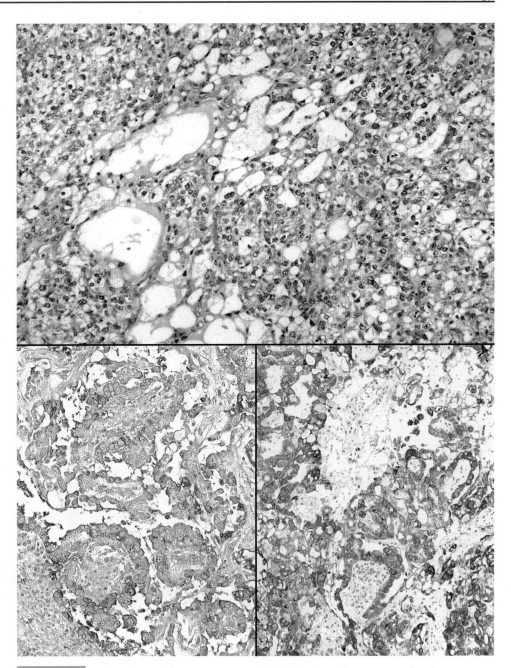

Figure 5.83 **Yolk sac tumor of ovary.** *Top:* Microcystic reticular pattern of yolk sac tumor. *Bottom:* These tumors express AFP (left) and glypican-3, as well as SALL4 (right).

OCT 3/4. Calcifications should prompt consideration for the presence of concomitant gonadoblastoma (50).

Yolk Sac Tumor

Yolk sac tumor (endodermal sinus tumor) occurs in females from as young as 17 months to 43 years (mean 20 years). The tumor is usually unilateral, solid, and cystic with areas of hemorrhage and necrosis. A reticular or tubulocystic pattern with **Schiller-Duval bodies** is characteristic, but microcystic, macrocystic, solid, and glandular patterns are also seen (Fig. 5.83). Yolk sac tumors are associated with elevated serum alpha fetoprotein (AFP). The tumors express AFP, cytokeratin, and glypigan-3, and SALL4 (65).

Gonadoblastoma

This tumor is composed of dysgerminoma cells admixed with sex-cord derivatives resembling Sertoli or granulosa cells. Gonadoblastoma is typically diagnosed in children or young adults. **Most are bilateral,** but this may not be macroscopically apparent. Calcifications within hyalinized bodies of the sex-cord component are seen in more than 80% of cases. **Almost all gonadoblastomas are associated with an underlying gonadal disorder, either pure or mixed dysgenesis, with a Y chromosome being detected.**

Embryonal Carcinoma

Pure embryonal carcinoma is rare in the ovary but may be admixed with other germ cell tumors; this appears to be particularly common in gonadoblastomas. Embryonal carcinoma expresses cytokeratin, CD117, OCT 3/4, and CD30.

Miscellaneous Ovarian Tumors

The ovary gives rise to a variety of other benign and malignant tumors that do not easily sort into one or another of the major ovarian tumor categories. Most of these tumors are extremely rare and include such diverse entities as **paraganglioma; myxoma; small cell carcinoma, hypercalcemic type; small cell carcinoma, pulmonary type; and large-cell neuroendocrine carcinoma,** among others (66). Only small cell carcinoma, hypercalcemic type occurs with sufficient frequency to warrant discussion in this chapter.

Small Cell Carcinoma, Hypercalcemic Type

This is an uncommon, highly malignant tumor presenting in young women, often in association with paraneoplastic hypercalcemia. The tumors are usually large and unilateral, even in the presence of advanced stage disease. Approximately 50% of tumors are confined to the ovary at presentation, and these tumors appear to have a better prognosis than tumors with extraovarian spread. Small cell carcinoma, hypercalcemic type is typically composed of small, undifferentiated and mitotically active cells (Fig. 5.84), although large cells may be present and, in some cases, form the predominant cell type. The tumor cells grow in solid sheets punctuated by variably sized follicle-like spaces. Mucinous epithelium may be seen in as many as 15% of tumors (66).

Small cell carcinoma, hypercalcemic type should not be confused with small cell carcinoma, pulmonary type. The latter tumor occurs in postmenopausal women and is histologically and immunohistologically similar to small cell neuroendocrine carcinoma of the lung.

Secondary Tumors of the Ovary (Metastases)

Tumors secondarily involving the ovary include **carcinoma, lymphoma or leukemia, melanoma, and sarcoma.** The tubular gastrointestinal tract, particularly **the colon, is the most common source of metastatic carcinoma** (Fig. 5.85), followed by the breast and pancreatobiliary tract. However, tumors arising in any site may secondarily spread to the ovary; the relative

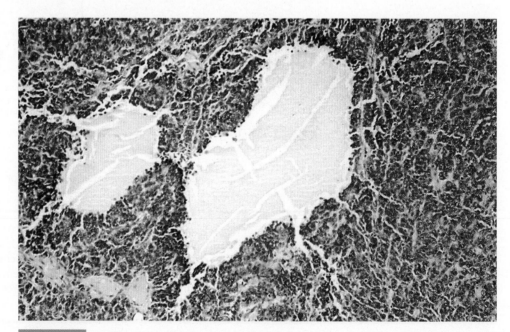

Figure 5.84 **Small cell carcinoma, hypercalcemic type of ovary.** Sheets of immature small cells with high mitotic index are punctuated by follicle-like spaces containing eosinophilic material.

frequency of the primary site varies in different countries, depending on the relative incidence of various types of cancer and on changing patterns in the treatment of these cancers. The classic **Kruckenberg tumor** refers to **metastatic signet-ring carcinoma** involving the ovaries (Fig. 5.86), which typically arises in the stomach, appendix, or large bowel. A variety of features may suggest an ovarian metastasis; these include bilateral disease, surface nodules, extensive lymphatic involvement, and diameter smaller than 10 cm.

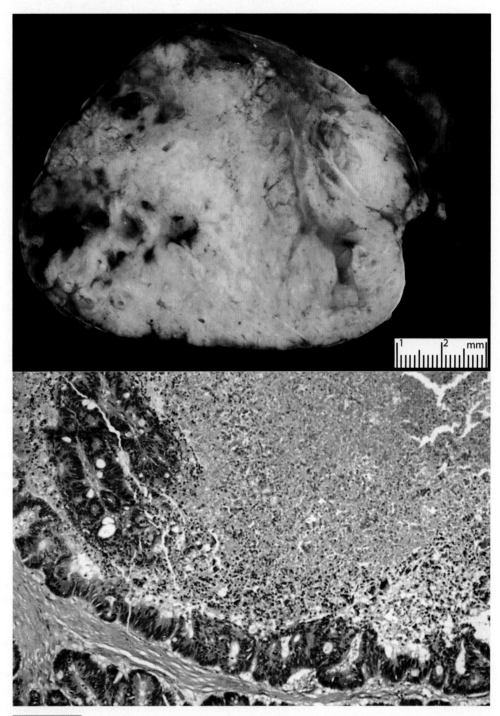

Figure 5.85   **Metastatic colorectal adenocarcinoma.** *Top:* Metastatic colorectal carcinoma often simulates a primary ovarian tumor. Note the smooth external capsule. *Bottom:* A garland gland pattern and the presence of extensive "dirty cell" necrosis secondary to the presence of necrotic cellular debris within gland lumens are characteristic of metastatic colorectal carcinoma.

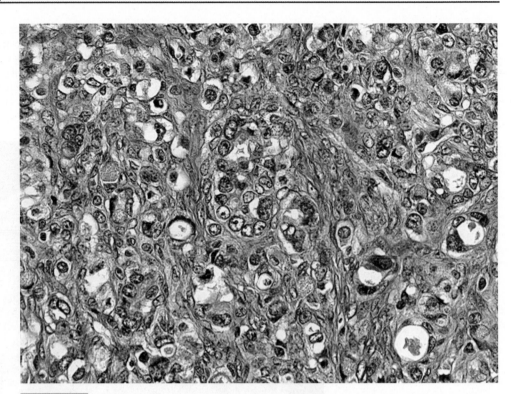

Figure 5.86 **Metastatic gastric signet-ring adenocarcinoma (Kruckenberg tumor).** Metastatic signet-ring carcinomas are often associated with ovarian stromal hyperplasia, which may mimic a stromal process.

Nonneoplastic Lesions of the Ovary

Many nonneoplastic lesions of the ovary may mimic an ovarian neoplasm. Most occur during the reproductive years. Some are associated with infertility. These include **cysts of follicular origin, massive ovarian edema, stromal hyperplasia and hyperthecosis, endometriosis,** and a variety of **pregnancy-associated changes** (67).

Cysts of Follicular Origin

Cysts of follicular origin are classified as **follicular or luteal,** depending on whether the cyst lining is composed of nonluteinized or luteinized granulosa and theca cells. By definition larger than 3 cm, most cysts of follicular origin do not exceed 8 cm in diameter. Rupture of a follicular or corpus luteal cyst may cause abrupt abdominal pain or hemoperitoneum.

Polycystic Ovarian Disease (Sclerocystic Ovaries)

Sclerocystic ovaries show bilateral ovarian enlargement with numerous cortical cysts, most measuring less than 3 cm, underlying a white fibrous band of cortical tissue. The etiology of this relatively common condition is heterogeneous, but in many cases the underlying defect has been attributed to insulin resistance of peripheral tissue or an abnormality of the hypothalamic-pituitary-ovarian axis. Patients present with anovulation, menstrual dysfunction, and hyperandrogenemia (**Polycystic Ovarian Syndrome, Stein-Leventhal syndrome**).

Massive Ovarian Edema

Massive ovarian edema occurs predominantly in children, adolescents, and young women. The etiology is uncertain but is thought to be the result of partial lymphatic or venous obstruction leading to accumulation of edema fluid and ovarian enlargement. Patients present with abdominal pain, abdominal distention, or menstrual irregularities. Affected patients may show features of virilism, hirsutism, and, rarely, precocious pseudopuberty. The affected ovary is gelatinous because of fluid accumulation within the interstitium of the ovary, separating and sometimes involving preexisting follicular structures (67).

Stromal Hyperplasia

Stromal hyperplasia is found predominantly in the postmenopausal age group. The ovaries are enlarged bilaterally by hyperplastic stroma, which may contain luteinized cells. **The condition is benign and generally asymptomatic,** often discovered incidentally during surgery for other causes.

Stromal Hyperthecosis

Stromal hyperthecosis may be seen in association with stromal hyperplasia in postmenopausal women but can also occur in reproductive-age women. Virilization, acne, obesity, hypertension, and glucose intolerance may be seen in association with stromal hyperthecosis in premenopausal women. **A small percentage of patients have HAIR-AN (hyperandrogenism, insulin resistance, and acanthosis nigricans) syndrome.** The ovaries are bilaterally enlarged by a proliferation of theca cells similar to those of the theca interna.

Endometriois

Endometriois commonly presents during the reproductive years and ranges from single or multiple microscopic deposits of ectopic endometrial glands and stroma to large hemorrhagic cysts (endometriomas) simulating a tumor mass. The larger cysts should be carefully examined to exclude the presence of an occult clear cell or endometrioid carcinoma.

Polypoid Endometriosis

Rarely, foci of endometriois may form large, polypoid masses on the ovary, fallopian tube, bowel, or peritoneum (Fig. 5.87). Most of the reported lesions have followed a benign clinical course (68), but complete excision and thorough microscopic examination should be performed to exclude adenosarcoma, stromal sarcoma, or adenocarcinoma arising in the setting of endometriosis.

Pregnancy Luteoma

Pregnancy luteoma is a benign condition that occurs in the second half of pregnancy and regresses after delivery. One or both ovaries are enlarged by single or multiple nodules of steroid cells with abundant, eosinophilic cytoplasm. Necrosis and degenerative changes may be present. Most are discovered during cesarean section.

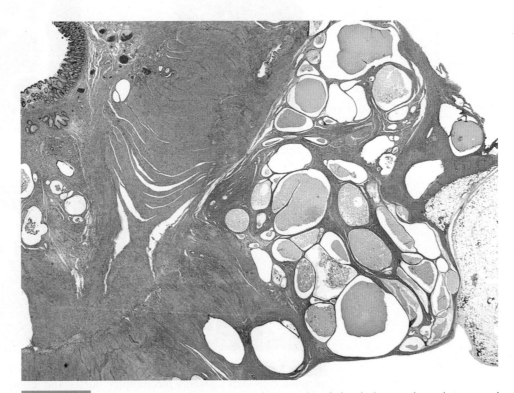

Figure 5.87   Polypoid endometriosis. When large and multifocal, these polypoid masses of ectopic endometrial tissue may simulate a neoplasm.

Large Solitary Luteinized Cyst of Pregnancy and the Puerperium

Large solitary luteinized follicular cyst of pregnancy and the puerperium is a rare, unilateral, thin-walled cyst lined by large cells with abundant cytoplasm with focal pleomorphic and hyperchromatic nuclei. These atypical cells are thought to be degenerative. A distinct theca layer is absent.

Hyperreactio Luteinalis

Hyperreactio luteinalis is characterized by bilateral ovarian enlargement secondary to the development of multiple luteinized cysts. This condition is rare in normal pregnancy but may occur in 10% to 40% of women with gestational trophoblastic disease and in women undergoing ovulation induction (especially those with preexisting polycystic ovaries).

Fallopian Tube

The traditional, admittedly arbitrary criteria to distinguish serous carcinoma of the ovary from serous carcinoma of the peritoneum are based on the presence of at least 5 mm of ovarian parenchymal involvement or, in the case of low-stage disease, by the exclusive presence of ovarian (surface or parenchymal) involvement. Primary serous carcinoma of the fallopian tube, once considered to be very rare, has been based on the exclusion of primary ovarian and uterine disease. The historical basis for these distinctions rests largely on the hypothesis that most serous carcinomas arise either from the surface epithelium of the ovary or from inclusion glands within the ovarian parenchyma.

This hypothesis has been challenged in the last several years by the revival of the **alternative theory that serous carcinoma arises from the epithelium of the fimbria of the fallopian tube.** The detection of tubal intraepithelial carcinoma (Fig. 5.88) in women undergoing risk-reducing salpingo-oophorectomy, in women with ovarian serous carcinoma, and in women with peritoneal serous carcinoma has buffeted this claim and generated renewed interest in the tubal fimbria as a candidate source of serous carcinoma. Whether all such examples reflect primary tubal epithelium as the source of carcinoma or secondary involvement by carcinoma arising elsewhere is currently unanswerable, except in those cases in which the fallopian tube is the only site of involvement. **A p53 signature has been identified in the fimbriated tubal**

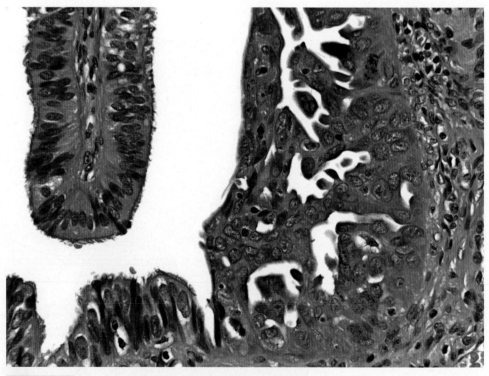

Figure 5.88   Serous tubal intraepithelial carcinoma. Tubal mucosa is focally replaced by stratified cells with markedly pleomorphic nuclei. The lesion is confined to the mucosa and typically occurs in the fimbria and distal fallopian tube in women with *BRCA* germ-line mutations.

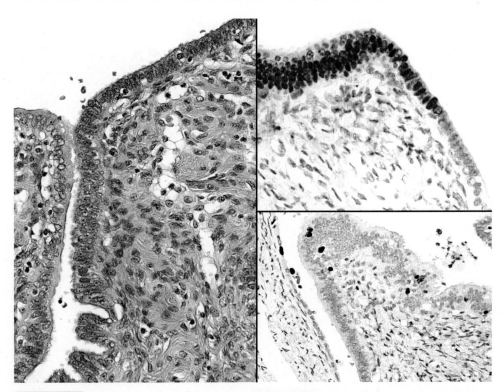

Figure 5.89 **Fallopian tube with "p53 signature."** Histologically normal tubal mucosa (left) may exhibit nuclear over-expression of p53 (top right), but low Ki-67 proliferation rate (bottom right). Although it has been proposed that this lesion may be a precursor to serous tubal carcinoma, it is not known to be associated with an adverse prognosis in the absence of morphological carcinoma.

epithelium that may represent a precursor lesion of tubal intraepithelial carcinoma (Fig. 5.89), but this requires further study (69). Metastases not uncommonly involve the fallopian tube mucosa and serosa.

The fallopian tubes from all risk-reducing salpingo-oophorectomy specimens should be serially sectioned and completely examined microscopically in order to exclude occult tubal intraepithelial carcinoma (70).

Primary Tubal Carcinoma

Serous carcinoma is the most common histologic subtype of carcinoma to occur in the fallopian tube (Fig. 5.90), but **endometrioid neoplasms** (adenofibroma, borderline, and carcinoma) **may also occur.** The distinction among the three types of endometrioid tumor and serous tumors is based on the criteria for these distinctions that are used elsewhere in the female genital tract.

Adenomatoid Tumor

Adenomatoid tumors are common, benign mesothelial neoplasms arising in the subserosa of the paratubal region, but they may also be seen in the uterus and, rarely, in the ovary. When occurring in the fallopian tube, they are small, firm tan white nodules, often measuring less than 1 cm in diameter. The uterine tumors are usually larger and arise in the myometrium. The presence of tubular and signet-ring–like cells may simulate a metastatic carcinoma (Fig. 5.91).

Gestational Trophoblastic Disease

Gestatational trophoblastic disease arises as a result of abnormal placental development with a resultant proliferation of syncytiotrophoblastic, cytotrophoblastic, or intermediate trophoblastic tissue (71).

Hydatidiform Mole

Hydatidiform mole is the most common form of gestatational trophoblastic disease and is divided into complete or partial moles. **The complete mole is diploid (46XX or 46XY)** and derived entirely from paternal chromosomes because of fertilization of an empty ovum by a

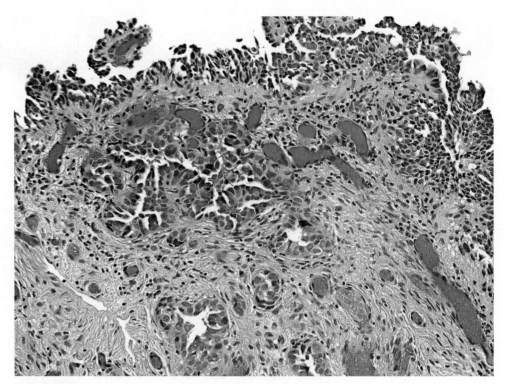

Figure 5.90   **Invasive serous carcinoma, fallopian tube.** Superficial invasion into the tubal stroma is seen in this early invasive serous tubal carcinoma.

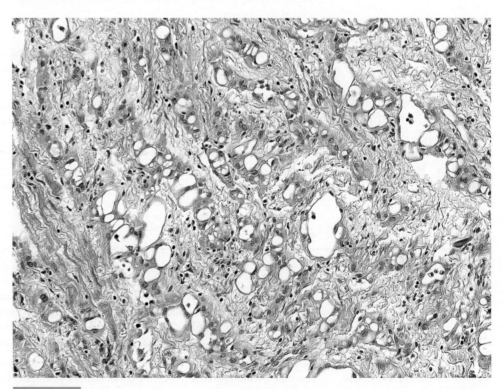

Figure 5.91   **Adenomatoid tumor, fallopian tube.** Signet-ring appearance may simulate metastatic carcinoma.

single spermatozum, whereas **partial mole is triploid (69XXX, 69XXY, or 69XYY)** and derived from fertilization of a normal egg by two spermatozoa.

Complete Hydatidiform Mole

Complete moles exhibit uniformly enlarged, hydropic villi with variable degrees of circumferential trophoblastic proliferation. The well-developed, second-trimester complete moles are visualized as transparent, grapelike vesicles on macroscopic examination, but complete moles in early trimester abortuses may be difficult to detect even on microscopic examination. Because complete moles are paternally derived, proteins encoded by paternally imprinted genes are not expressed in the villous stromal tissue or cytotrophoblast of complete moles. One of these proteins, p57, may be used to establish the diagnosis of complete moles in diagnostically more difficult cases (Fig. 5.92).

Complete moles may progress to invasive mole or choriocarcinoma. Progression is associated with progressively rising serum beta human chorionic gonadotropin levels.

Partial Hydatidiform Mole

Partial moles exhibit a dimorphic population of small and larger villi with lesser degrees of trophoblastic proliferation. **Most are associated with a fetus.** Progression of partial mole to invasive mole or choriocarcinoma is rare or nonexistent.

Invasive Mole

Invasive mole is diagnosed on the basis of invasion into myometrium or its blood vessels (Fig. 5.93). Common sites of extrauterine spread include the vagina, vulva, and lung.

Choriocarcinoma

Choriocarcinoma is a highly malignant tumor composed of syncytiotrophoblastic and cytotrophoblastic cells arranged in a bilaminar configuration (Fig. 5.94). Chorionic villi are almost always absent. Hemorrhage and necrosis are common. Patients often present with profuse vaginal bleeding. Distant lung, brain, or liver metastases may also be present.

Placental Site Trophoblastic Tumor

This very uncommon form of gestational trophoblastic disease is composed of intermediate trophoblastic cells (Fig. 5.95). The tumor may form a discrete mass or irregularly infiltrate the myometrium, causing uterine enlargement. Although most placental site trophoblastic tumors follow a benign clinical course, the behavior is unpredictable, and occasional tumors spread throughout the uterus and metastasize to distant sites.

An epithelioid variant, composed of smaller, more epithelioid cells resembling squamous cell carcinoma, appears to be more aggressive (71).

Exaggerated Placental Site

Exaggerated placental site is a benign condition marked by an exuberance of intermediate trophoblastic cells that may simulate placental site trophoblastic tumor. The lesion is no different from the usual implantation site, but the individual intermediate trophoblastic cells are larger and more numerous; nuclear hyperchromasia may also be present. Unlike placental site trophoblastic tumor, chorionic villi and syncytiotrophoblastic giant cells are typically present, mitotic figures are rare or absent, and there is no necrosis.

Placental Site Nodule and Plaque

Placental site nodules are **essentially hyalinized implantation sites.** They occur during the reproductive years and may be a cause of uterine bleeding or an incidental finding. They are discrete lesions, forming nodules or plaques, but occasionally they may present as multiple fragments or lesions in a uterine sampling (Fig. 5.96). A history of pregnancy may be remote or even absent. Placental site nodule or plaque is **a benign process** and not to be confused with placental site trophoblastic tumor.

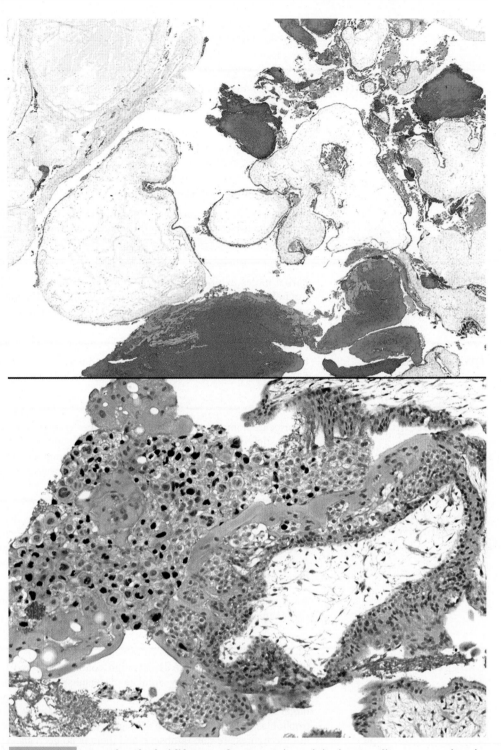

Figure 5.92   Complete hydatidiform mole. *Top:* Enlarged, hydropic villi correspond to the grapelike vesicles seen in curettage specimens. *Bottom:* Villous stromal cells and cytotrophoblast cells do not express paternally imprinted nuclear p57 in complete hydatidiform mole.

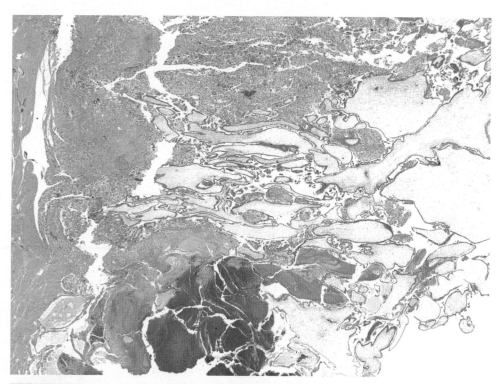

Figure 5.93   Invasive mole. Complete hydatidiform mole with exuberant trophoblastic proliferation invades the myometrium in this hysterectomy specimen.

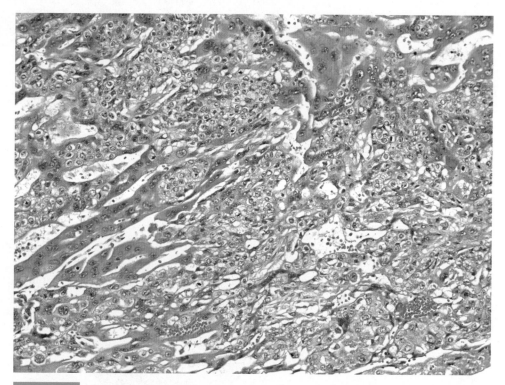

Figure 5.94   Choriocarcinoma. Bilaminar pattern of syncytiotrophoblastic and cytotrophoblastic cells is diagnostic of this tumor.

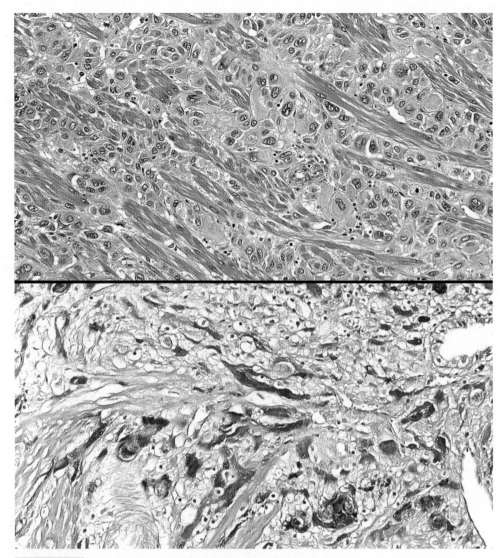

Figure 5.95 **Placental site trophoblastic tumor.** *Top:* Large, atypical eosinophilic and polygonal cells diffusely infiltrate the deep myometrium. *Bottom:* Human placental lactogen is expressed by the neoplastic intermediate trophoblastic cells.

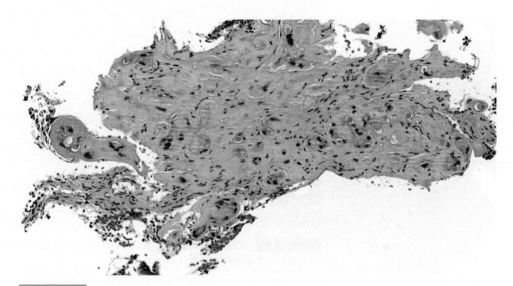

Figure 5.96 **Placental site nodule.** Discrete nodules or plaques of hyalinized intermediate trophoblastic tissue may be seen in curettage specimens.

References

1. **Stoler MH, Schiffman M.** Interobserver reproducibility of cervical cytologic and histologic interpretations: realistic estimates from the ASCUS-LSIL Triage Study. *JAMA* 2001;285:1500–1505.

2. **Kong CS, Balzer BL, Troxell ML, Patterson BK, Longacre TA.** p16INK4A immunohistochemistry is superior to HPV *in situ* hybridization for the detection of high-risk HPV in atypical squamous metaplasia. *Am J Surg Pathol* 2007;31:33–43.

3. **Cogliano V, Baan R, Straif K, Grosse Y, Secretan B, El Ghissassi F.** Carcinogenicity of human papillomaviruses. *Lancet Oncol* 2005;6:204.

4. **Ho GY, Bierman R, Beardsley L, Chang CJ, Burk RD.** Natural history of cervicovaginal papillomavirus infection in young women. *N Engl J Med* 1998;338:423–428.

5. Human papillomavirus testing for triage of women with cytologic evidence of low-grade squamous intraepithelial lesions: baseline data from a randomized trial. The Atypical Squamous Cells of Undetermined Significance/Low-Grade Squamous Intraepithelial Lesions Triage Study (ALTS) Group. *J Natl Cancer Inst* 2000;92: 397–402.

6. **Solomon D, Nayar R, eds.** *The Bethesda system for reporting cervical cytology.* New York: Springer, 2004.

7. **Wright TC Jr., Massad LS, Dunton CJ, Spitzer M, Wilkinson EJ, Solomon D.** 2006 consensus guidelines for the management of women with abnormal cervical cancer screening tests. *Am J Obstet Gynecol* 2007;197:346–355.

8. **Solomon D, Schiffman M, Tarone R.** Comparison of three management strategies for patients with atypical squamous cells of undetermined significance: baseline results from a randomized trial. *J Natl Cancer Inst* 2001;93:293–299.

9. **Sherman ME, Schiffman M, Cox JT.** Effects of age and human papilloma viral load on colposcopy triage: data from the randomized Atypical Squamous Cells of Undetermined Significance/Low-Grade Squamous Intraepithelial Lesion Triage Study (ALTS). *J Natl Cancer Inst* 2002;94:102–107.

10. **De Cremoux P, Coste J, Sastre-Garau X, Thioux M, Bouillac C, Labbe S, et al.** Efficiency of the hybrid capture 2 HPV DNA test in cervical cancer screening. A study by the French Society of Clinical Cytology. *Am J Clin Pathol* 2003;120:492–499.

11. **Carozzi FM, Del Mistro A, Confortini M, Sani C, Puliti D, Trevisan R, et al.** Reproducibility of HPV DNA testing by hybrid capture 2 in a screening setting. *Am J Clin Pathol* 2005;124: 716–721.

12. **Castle PE, Lorincz AT, Mielzynska-Lohnas I, Scott DR, Glass AG, Sherman ME, et al.** Results of human papillomavirus DNA testing with the hybrid capture 2 assay are reproducible. *J Clin Microbiol* 2002;40:1088–1090.

13. **Davis-Devine S, Day SJ, Freund GG.** Test performance comparison of inform HPV and hybrid capture 2 high-risk HPV DNA tests using the SurePath liquid-based Pap test as the collection method. *Am J Clin Pathol* 2005;124:24–30.

14. **Hesselink AT, van den Brule AJ, Brink AA, Berkhof J, van Kemenade FJ, Verheijen RH, et al.** Comparison of hybrid capture 2 with *in situ* hybridization for the detection of high-risk human papillomavirus in liquid-based cervical samples. *Cancer* 2004;102: 11–18.

15. **Biscotti CV, Dawson AE, Dziura B, Galup L, Darragh T, Rahemtulla A, et al.** Assisted primary screening using the automated ThinPrep Imaging System. *Am J Clin Pathol* 2005;123: 281–287.

16. **Ioffe OB, Sagae S, Moritani S, Dahmoush L, Chen TT, Silverberg SG.** Proposal of a new scoring scheme for the diagnosis of noninvasive endocervical glandular lesions. *Am J Surg Pathol* 2003;27:452–460.

17. **Witkiewicz A, Lee KR, Brodsky G, Cviko A, Brodsky J, Crum CP.** Superficial (early) endocervical adenocarcinoma *in situ*: a study of 12 cases and comparison to conventional AIS. *Am J Surg Pathol* 2005;29:1609–1614.

18. **Crum CP, Nucci MR, Lee KR.** The cervix. In: **Mills SE, ed.** *Sternberg's diagnostic surgical pathology.* New York: Lippincott Williams & Wilkins, 2009.

19. **Ansari-Lari MA, Staebler A, Zaino RJ, Shah KV, Ronnett BM.** Distinction of endocervical and endometrial adenocarcinomas: immunohistochemical p16 expression correlated with human papillomavirus (HPV) DNA detection. *Am J Surg Pathol* 2004;28: 160–167.

20. **Kong CS, Gilks CB, Longacre TA.** Immunohistochemical stain for p16 can be misleading in distinguishing endometrial from endocervical adenocarcinoma in small tissue samples. *Mod Pathol* 2005;18.

21. **Young RH, Clement PB.** Endocervical adenocarcinoma and its variants: their morphology and differential diagnosis. *Histopathology* 2002;41:185–207.

22. **Staebler A, Sherman ME, Zaino RJ, Ronnett BM.** Hormone receptor immunohistochemistry and human papillomavirus *in situ* hybridization are useful for distinguishing endocervical and endometrial adenocarcinomas. *Am J Surg Pathol* 2002;26:998–1006.

23. **Alkushi A, Irving J, Hsu F, Dupuis B, Liu CL, Van De Rijn M, et al.** Immunoprofile of cervical and endometrial adenocarcinomas using a tissue microarray. *Virchows Arch* 2003;442:271–277.

24. **Park HM, Park MH, Kim YJ, Chun SH, Ahn JJ, Kim CI, et al.** Müllerian adenosarcoma with sarcomatous overgrowth of the cervix presenting as cervical polyp: a case report and review of the literature. *Int J Gynecol Cancer* 2004;14:1024–1029.

25. **Scurry J, Wilkinson EJ.** Review of terminology of precursors of vulvar squamous cell carcinoma. *J Low Genit Tract Dis* 2006;10: 161–169.

26. **Sideri M, Jones RW, Wilkinson EJ, Preti M, Heller DS, Scurry J, et al.** Squamous vulvar intraepithelial neoplasia: 2004 modified terminology, ISSVD Vulvar Oncology Subcommittee. *J Reprod Med* 2005;50:807–810.

27. **Hart WR.** Vulvar intraepithelial neoplasia: historical aspects and current status. *Int J Gynecol Pathol* 2001;20:16–30.

28. **van der Avoort IA, Shirango H, Hoevenaars BM, Grefte JM, de Hullu JA, de Wilde PC, et al.** Vulvar squamous cell carcinoma is a multifactorial disease following two separate and independent pathways. *Int J Gynecol Pathol* 2006;25:22–29.

29. **Medeiros F, Nascimento AF, Crum CP.** Early vulvar squamous neoplasia: advances in classification, diagnosis, and differential diagnosis. *Adv Anat Pathol* 2005;12:20–26.

30. **Nucci MR, Young RH, Fletcher CD.** Cellular pseudosarcomatous fibroepithelial stromal polyps of the lower female genital tract: an underrecognized lesion often misdiagnosed as sarcoma. *Am J Surg Pathol* 2000;24:231–240.

31. **Stoler MH, Mills SE, Frierson HFJ.** The vulva and vagina. In: **Mills SE, ed.** *Sternberg's diagnostic surgical pathology.* New York: Lippincott Williams & Wilkins, 2009.

32. **Nielsen GP, Young RH.** Mesenchymal tumors and tumor-like lesions of the female genital tract: a selective review with emphasis on recently described entities. *Int J Gynecol Pathol* 2001;20:105–127.

33. **Nucci MR, Fletcher CD.** Vulvovaginal soft tissue tumours: update and review. *Histopathology* 2000;36:97–108.

34. **Longacre TA, Chung MH, Jensen DN, Hendrickson MR.** Proposed criteria for the diagnosis of well-differentiated endometrial carcinoma. A diagnostic test for myoinvasion. *Am J Surg Pathol* 1995;19:371–406.

35. **Kurman R, Norris H.** Evaluation of criteria for distinguishing atypical endometrial hyperplasia from well-differentiated carcinoma. *Cancer* 1982;49:2547–2559.

36. **Hendrickson M, Ross J, Eifel P, Martinez A, Kempson R.** Uterine papillary serous carcinoma: a highly malignant form of endometrial adenocarcinoma. *Am J Surg Pathol* 1982;6:93–108.

37. **Hendrickson MR, Longacre TA, Kempson RL.** Uterine papillary serous carcinoma revisited. *Gynecol Oncol* 1994;54:261–263.

38. **Sherman ME, Bitterman P, Rosenshein NB, Delgado G, Kurman RJ.** Uterine serous carcinoma. A morphologically diverse neoplasm with unifying clinicopathologic features. *Am J Surg Pathol* 1992;16: 600–610.

39. **Soslow RA, Pirog E, Isacson C.** Endometrial intraepithelial carcinoma with associated peritoneal carcinomatosis. *Am J Surg Pathol* 2000;24:726–732.

40. **Kempson RL, Hendrickson MR.** Smooth muscle, endometrial stromal, and mixed müllerian tumors of the uterus. *Mod Pathol* 2000;13:328–342.

41. **Longacre TA, Atkins KA, Kempson RL, Hendrickson MR.** The uterine corpus. In: **Mills S, ed.** *Sternberg's diagnostic surgical patholology.* Philadelphia: Lippincott Williams & Wilkins, 2009.

42. **Bell SW, Kempson RL, Hendrickson MR.** Problematic uterine smooth muscle neoplasms. A clinicopathologic study of 213 cases. *Am J Surg Pathol* 1994;18:535–558.

43. **Chang K, Crabtree G, Lim-Tan S, Kempson R, Hendrickson M.** Primary uterine endometrial stromal neoplasms. A clinicopathologic study of 117 cases. *Am J Surg Pathol* 1990;14:415–438.

44. **Hendrickson MR, Longacre TA, Kempson RL.** Pathology of uterine sarcomas. In: **Coukos G, Rubin, SC, eds.** *Cancer of the uterus.* New York: Marcel Dekker, 2005;149–194.

45. **Zaloudek C, Norris H.** Adenofibroma and adenosarcoma of the uterus: a clinicopathologic study of 35 cases. *Cancer* 1981;48:354–366.

46. **Clement P, Scully R.** Müllerian adenosarcoma of the uterus: a clinicopathologic analysis of 100 cases with a review of the literature. *Hum Pathol* 1990;21:363–381.

47. **Longacre TA, Chung MH, Rouse RV, Hendrickson MR.** Atypical polypoid adenomyofibromas (atypical polypoid adenomyomas) of the uterus. A clinicopathologic study of 55 cases. *Am J Surg Pathol* 1996;20:1–20.

48. **Ferguson SE, Tornos C, Hummer A, Barakat RR, Soslow RA.** Prognostic features of surgical stage I uterine carcinosarcoma. *Am J Surg Pathol* 2007;31:1653–1661.

49. **Longacre TA, Gilks CB.** Surface epithelial stromal tumors. In: **Nucci M, Oliva E, eds.** *Gynecologic pathology.* Philadelphia: Elsevier, 2008.

50. **Lee KR, Tavassoli FA, Prat J, Dietel M, Gersell DJ, Karseladze AI, et al.** Tumours of the ovary and peritoneum. In: **Tavassoli FA, Devillee, P, eds.** *Tumours of the breast and female genital organs.* Lyon: IARC Press, 2003;119–124.

51. **Bell DA, Longacre TA, Prat J, Kohn EC, Soslow RA, Ellenson LH, et al.** Serous borderline (low malignant potential, atypical proliferative) ovarian tumors: workshop perspectives. *Hum Pathol* 2004;35:934–948.

52. **McKenney JK, Balzer BL, Longacre TA.** Patterns of stromal invasion in ovarian serous tumors of low malignant potential (borderline tumors): A re-evaluation of the concept of stromal microinvasion. *Am J Surg Pathol* 2006;30:1209–1221.

53. **Bell DA, Longacre TA, Prat J, Kohn EC, Soslow RA, Ellenson LH, et al.** Serous borderline (low malignant potential, atypical proliferative) ovarian tumors: workshop perspectives. *Hum Pathol* 2004;35:934–948.

54. **Longacre TA, McKenney JK, Tazelaar HD, Kempson RL, Hendrickson MR.** Ovarian serous tumors of low malignant potential (borderline tumors): outcome-based study of 276 patients with long-term (> or =5-year) follow-up. *Am J Surg Pathol* 2005;29:707–723.

55. **McKenney JK, Balzer BL, Longacre TA.** Lymph node involvement in ovarian serous tumors of low malignant potential (borderline tumors): pathology, prognosis, and proposed classification. *Am J Surg Pathol* 2006;30:614–624.

56. **Malpica A, Deavers MT, Lu K, Bodurka DC, Atkinson EN, Gershenson DM, et al.** Grading ovarian serous carcinoma using a two-tier system. *Am J Surg Pathol* 2004;28:496–504.

57. **Shimizu Y, Kamoi S, Amada S, Hasumi K, Akiyama F, Silverberg SG.** Toward the development of a universal grading system for ovarian epithelial carcinoma. I. Prognostic significance of histopathologic features—problems involved in the architectural grading system. *Gynecol Oncol* 1998;70:2–12.

58. **Shih Ie M, Kurman RJ.** Ovarian tumorigenesis: a proposed model based on morphological and molecular genetic analysis. *Am J Pathol* 2004;164:1511–1518.

59. **Gilks CB, Bell DA, Scully RE.** Serous psammocarcinoma of the ovary and peritoneum. *Int J Gynecol Pathol* 1990;9:110–121.

60. **Ronnett BM, Kajdacsy-Balla A, Gilks CB, Merino MJ, Silva E, Werness BA, et al.** Mucinous borderline ovarian tumors: points of general agreement and persistent controversies regarding nomenclature, diagnostic criteria, and behavior. *Hum Pathol* 2004;35:949–960.

61. **McKenney JK, Soslow RA, Longacre TA.** Ovarian mature teratomas with mucinous epithelial neoplasms: morphologic heterogeneity and association with pseudomyxoma peritonei. *Am J Surg Pathol* 2008;32:645–655.

62. **Vang R, Gown AM, Zhao C, Barry TS, Isacson C, Richardson MS, et al.** Ovarian mucinous tumors associated with mature cystic teratomas: morphologic and immunohistochemical analysis identifies a subset of potential teratomatous origin that shares features of lower gastrointestinal tract mucinous tumors more commonly encountered as secondary tumors in the ovary. *Am J Surg Pathol* 2007;31:854–869.

63. **Young RH, Clement PB, Scully RE.** Sex cord-stromal, steroid cell, and germ cell tumors of the ovary. In: **Mills SE, ed.** *Sternberg's diagnostic surgical pathology.* Philadelphia: Lippincott Williams & Wilkins, 2009.

64. **Scully RE, Clement PB, Young RH.** Ovarian surface epithelial-stromal tumors. In: **Mills SE, ed.** *Sternberg's diagnostic surgical pathology.* Philadelphia: Lippincott Williams & Wilkins, 2009.

65. **Esheba GE, Pate LL, Longacre TA.** Oncofetal protein glypican-3 distinguishes yolk sac tumor from clear cell carcinoma of the ovary. *Am J Surg Pathol* 2008;32:600–607.

66. **Clement PB, Young RH, Scully RE.** Miscellaneous primary tumors, secondary tumors, and non-neoplastic lesions of the ovary. In: **Mills SE, ed.** *Sternberg's diagnostic surgical pathology.* Philadelphia: Lippincott Williams & Wilkins, 2009.

67. **Longacre TA, Gilks CB.** Nonneoplastic lesions of the ovary. In: **Nucci M, Oliva E, eds.** *Gynecologic pathology.* Philadelphia: Elsevier, 2008.

68. **Parker RL, Clement PB, Chercover DJ, Sornarajah T, Gilks CB.** Early recurrence of ovarian serous borderline tumor as high-grade carcinoma: a report of two cases. *Int J Gynecol Pathol* 2004;23:265–272.

69. **Folkins AK, Jarboe EA, Saleemuddin A, Lee Y, Callahan MJ, Drapkin R, et al.** A candidate precursor to pelvic serous cancer (p53 signature) and its prevalence in ovaries and fallopian tubes from women with *BRCA* mutations. *Gynecol Oncol* 2008;109:168–173. Epub 2008 Mar 14.

70. **Longacre TA, Oliva E, Soslow RA.** Recommendations for the reporting of fallopian tube neoplasms. *Virchows Arch* 2007;450:25–29.

71. **Shih IE, Mazur MT, Kurman RJ.** Gestational trophoblastic disease. In: **Mills SE, ed.** *Sternberg's diagnostic surgical pathology.* Philadelphia: Lippincott Williams & Wilkins, 2009.

6

Epidemiology and Biostatistics

Daniel W. Cramer

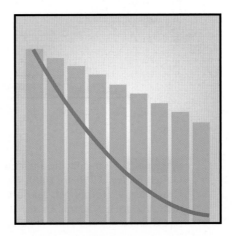

The disciplines of epidemiology and biostatistics apply to gynecologic oncology in defining cancer occurrence and survival, identifying risk factors, and implementing strategies for treatment or prevention, including the proper design of clinical trials. As such, epidemiology and biostatistics are essential to the practice of evidence-based medicine. In this chapter, some key principles of epidemiology and biostatistics are considered under the headings of descriptive statistics, etiologic studies, statistical inference and validity, and cancer risk and prevention. Readers should refer to standard statistical and epidemiologic texts for more detailed discussion and computational formulas (1,2).

Descriptive Statistics

Cancer is described in populations by statistics related to its occurrence and survival afterward. How cancer varies by age, ethnicity, and geography are of particular interest. Descriptive statistics about cancer in the United States can be obtained from the National Cancer Institute through its Web site: http://www.seer.cancer.gov/. Descriptive statistics about cancer in the world can be obtained from the International Agency for Research on Cancer through its Web site: http://www-dep.iarc.fr/.

Incidence

The incidence rate (IR) is defined as the number of new cases of disease in a population within a specified time period:

$$\text{IR} = \text{New cases/Person-time}$$

The fact that time is a component of the denominator should help clinicians avoid the misapplication of this term to **prevalence,** another measure of disease occurrence that includes both old and new cases.

Cancer Incidence and Mortality **Cancer incidence or mortality is usually stated as cases (or deaths) per 100,000 people per year, or as cases per 100,000 person-years.** Incidence or mortality is measured in a specific population over a specific period. For example, country or state cancer registries count the number of new cancer cases diagnosed or cases of dying among residents over a year and divide that figure by census estimates of the total population in the region.

Crude Incidence or Mortality Crude incidence or mortality is the total number of new cancers (or deaths) that occur over a specified time in the entire population.

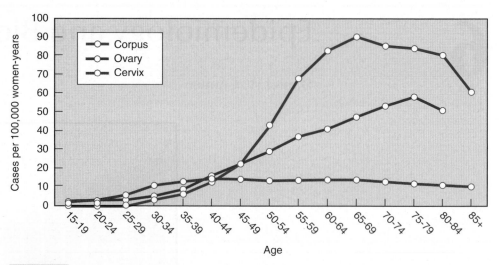

Figure 6.1   **Age-specific incidence curves for the gynecologic cancers in women in the United States, 1996 to 2000.** Modified from **Ries LAG MD, Krapcho M, Stinchcomb DG, Howlader N, Horner MJ, Mariotto A, et al., eds.** *SEER Cancer Statistics Review, 1975–2005.* Bethesda, MD: National Cancer Institute. Available at: http://seer.cancer.gov/csr/1975_2005/. Based on November 2007 SEER data submission posted to the SEER Web site 2008.

Age-Specific Incidence or Mortality   **Age-specific incidence (or mortality) is the number of new cancers (or deaths) that occur over a specified time among individuals of a particular age group divided by the total population in that same age group.** Age-specific incidence or mortality rates are the best way to describe the occurrence of cancer in a population and are commonly graphed in 5- or 10-year groups. Annual age-specific incidence and mortality curves for the common malignant gynecologic cancers in the United States based on all women in the Surveillance, Epidemiology, and End Results (SEER) survey area for 1996 to 2000 (3) are shown in Figures 6.1 and 6.2.

Invasive cervical cancer shows a gradual rise and plateau after 50 years of age at approximately 16 cases per 100,000 women-years. Cancer of the corpus (largely endometrium) rises during the perimenopause and peaks at approximately 90 cases per 100,000 women-years after 60 years of age. Cancer of the ovary also displays an increase during the perimenopause and peaks after age 70 years at approximately 60 cases per 100,000 women-years. Cancer mortality curves display similar age patterns, but ovarian cancer is revealed as the most lethal of the

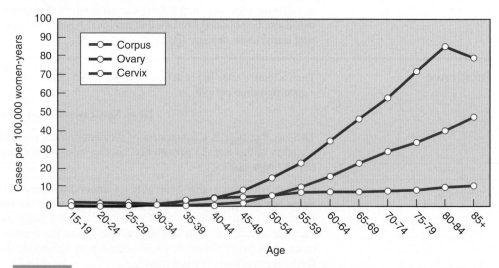

Figure 6.2   **Age-specific mortality curves for the gynecologic cancers in women in the United States, 1996 to 2000.** Modified from **Ries LAG MD, Krapcho M, Stinchcomb DG, Howlader N, Horner MJ, Mariotto A, et al., eds.** *SEER Cancer Statistics Review, 1975–2005.* Bethesda, MD: National Cancer Institute. Available at: http://seer.cancer.gov/csr/1975_2005/. Based on November 2007 SEER data submission posted to the SEER Web site 2008.

Table 6.1 Lifetime Risk of Acquiring or Dying from Gynecologic Cancers in White and Black U.S. Women*

	Risk of Acquiring (%)			Risk of Dying (%)		
	All	**White**	**Black**	**All**	**White**	**Black**
Cervix	0.7	0.7	1.0	0.2	0.2	0.4
Corpus	2.5	2.6	2.0	0.5	0.5	0.8
Ovary	1.4	1.5	1.0	1.0	1.1	0.8

*Data from 1975–2000. **Ries LAG, Melbert D, Krapcho M, Stinchcomb DG, Howlader N, Horner MJ, et al., eds.** *SEER Cancer Statistics Review, 1975–2005.*

gynecologic cancers. *In situ* cervical cancers are no longer being tabulated by the SEER registries. The vast majority of these cases are seen between ages 20 and 50, with a peak occurrence of approximately 200 cases per 100,000 women per year at ages 25 to 29. In addition, SEER is no longer counting ovarian tumors of borderline malignancy, accounting for a decline of 21% in incidence and 6% in mortality between 2004 and 2006.

Cumulative Incidence or Mortality **Cumulative incidence (or mortality) may be thought of as the proportion of people who develop disease (or die from it) during some period of observation.** Cumulative "incidence" is technically a misnomer because it does not contain time in the denominator but, rather, is expressed as a percentage. The cumulative IR (CIR) may be crudely approximated from age-specific IRs by the following formula:

$$\mathbf{CIR = \Sigma IR_i(\Delta T_i)}$$

where IR_i is the age-specific rate for the i age stratum and ΔT_i is the size of the age interval of the i stratum (usually 5 years). Cumulative incidence, summed over the age range 0 to 85 years, yields the "lifetime risk" for cancer occurrence or death. Lifetime risks that a woman in the United States will have or die from cancer of the cervix, corpus, or ovary are shown in Table 6.1 and confirm that a U.S. woman has a greater risk of acquiring cancer of the corpus than cervical or ovarian cancer but a higher risk of dying from ovarian cancer than cervical or endometrial cancer combined.

Age-Adjusted Incidence or Mortality **Age-adjusted incidence (AAI) or mortality is obtained by summing weighted averages of the incidence or mortality rates for each age stratum.** The weight is derived from the age distribution of a standard population:

$$\mathbf{AAI = \frac{\Sigma IR_i(W_i)}{\Sigma W_i}}$$

where IR_i is the IR in the i age stratum, and W_i is the number of people in the i stratum in the standard population. Age-adjusted rates are better than crude rates for summarizing incidence or mortality when comparing cancer occurrence among populations that may differ in their age structure. An "old" population would have a higher crude incidence of ovarian cancer and a lower crude incidence of carcinoma *in situ* of the cervix than a "young" population, even though both populations might have identical age-specific incidences for each disease. Cancer rates adjusted to the "world population standard" are shown in Table 6.2.

Worldwide, cervical cancer is the most important of the gynecologic cancers and is second only to breast cancer in overall occurrence. Cervical cancer is most frequent in southern Africa and Central America and least frequent in North America and parts of Asia. Cancer of the corpus is least frequent in Africa and Asia and most frequent in North America. Ovarian cancer is least frequent in Africa and Asia and most frequent in northern Europe.

Prevalence

Prevalence (P) is the proportion of people who have a particular disease or condition at a specified time. Prevalence can be calculated by multiplying incidence times the average duration of disease:

$$\mathbf{Prevalence = Incidence \times Average\ duration\ of\ disease}$$

Table 6.2 Age-Adjusted Incidence Rate* for the Gynecologic Cancers in Comparison with Other Major Cancers in Women							
Region	Breast	Colon	Lung	Stomach	Cervix	Corpus	Ovary
World	37.4	14.6	12.1	10.4	16.2	6.5	6.6
Northern Africa	23.2	4.0	2.2	2.5	12.1	2.4	2.6
Southern Africa	33.4	9.0	6.9	3.7	38.2	3.5	5.2
Eastern Africa	19.5	4.1	1.2	5.5	42.7	3.2	5.8
Western Africa	18.2	3.5	0.6	3.6	29.3	2.2	4.6
Northern America	99.4	32.9	35.6	3.4	7.7	22.0	10.7
Central America	25.9	7.4	6.5	10.8	30.6	4.5	7.2
South America	46.0	14.8	7.6	12.2	28.6	6.7	7.7
Eastern Asia	22.9	12.5	17.7	20.6	7.4	2.5	3.7
Southeast Asia	25.5	9.9	8.9	4.5	18.7	4.2	7.2
Western Asia	33.3	9.9	5.5	6.4	5.8	5.8	5.3
Northern Europe	82.5	26.4	21.3	6.0	9.0	12.2	13.3
Eastern Europe	42.6	20.1	8.7	12.8	14.5	11.8	10.2
Western Europe	84.6	29.8	12.0	6.6	10.0	12.5	11.3
Southern Europe	62.4	23.5	9.2	8.7	10.7	11.8	9.7
Australia–New Zealand	84.6	36.9	17.4	4.2	7.4	10.6	9.4
Micronesia	38.6	11.8	15.5	4.4	9.4	7.4	6.0
Polynesia	34.2	10.7	1.0	11.6	28.0	11.8	7.7

*Age adjusted to the world standard in cases per 100,000.

Data from IARC Web site. Available at: http://www-dep.iarc.fr/globocan/globocan.html.

More commonly, prevalence is derived from cross-sectional studies in which the number of individuals alive with a particular condition is identified from a survey and stated as a percentage of the total number of people who responded to the survey. Other examples of studies that yield prevalence data are those based on autopsy findings and screening tests. The frequency of previously unidentified cancers found in a series of autopsies yields data on the prevalence of occult cancer. The first application of a screening test in a previously unscreened population yields the prevalence of preclinical disease.

Cancer Survival

When the proportion of patients surviving cancer is plotted against time, the pattern often fits an exponential function. To say that survival is exponential means that the rate of death is constant over time, which can be demonstrated by plotting the logarithm of the probability of survival against time and demonstrating a straight line. Summary measures for a survival curve commonly include median survival time or the point at which 50% of the patients have died and the probability of survival at 1, 2, and 5 years.

Relative Survival   **Relative survival is defined as the ratio of the observed survival rate for the patient group to the survival rate expected for a population with similar demographic characteristics.** Relative survival rates for U.S. women diagnosed in 2000 are shown in Figure 6.3 for the major gynecologic cancers and reveal that survival is best after cancer of the corpus, worst after cancer of the ovary, and intermediate after cancer of the cervix. Five-year relative survival rates are shown in Table 6.3 by type and stage of gynecologic cancer for U.S. women.

Stage at presentation and 5-year survival are most favorable for cancer of the corpus and least favorable for cancer of the ovary. In general, African Americans tend to be diagnosed at more advanced stages and have poorer survival compared with whites, especially for cancer of the cervix and corpus.

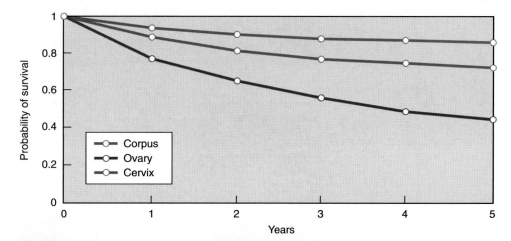

Figure 6.3 Relative survival rates for invasive cancers of the cervix, corpus, and ovaries for women diagnosed in the United States in 1995. Modified from **Ries LAG MD, Krapcho M, Stinchcomb DG, Howlader N, Horner MJ, Mariotto A, et al., eds.** *SEER Cancer Statistics Review, 1975–2005.* Bethesda, MD: National Cancer Institute. Available at http://seer.cancer.gov/csr/1975_2005/. Based on November 2007 SEER data submission posted to the SEER Web site 2008.

Table 6.3 Stage at Diagnosis for the Gynecologic Cancers[a] and 5-Year Survival Rates for U.S. Women*					
	Stage Distribution at Diagnosis (%)			*5-Year Survival Rate (%)*		
	All	**White**	**Black**	**All**	**White**	**Black**
Cervix						
All stages				71.2	72.5	61.8
Localized	51	52	44	91.7	92.6	85.9
Regional	35	34	38	55.9	56.7	47.5
Distant	10	9	8	16.6	17.5	8.9
Corpus						
All stages				82.9	84.7	61.1
Localized	69	71	54	95.5	96.2	83.7
Regional	17	17	22	67.5	69.7	45.0
Distant	9	8	17	23.6	25.3	13.9
Ovary						
All stages				45.5	45.3	38.4
Localized	19	18	17	92.7	92.7	92.5
Regional	7	7	7	71.1	71.8	58.5
Distant	67	68	67	30.6	30.9	22.7

*Data from 1996–2004. Information insufficient to stage 4% of cervical, 5% of corpus, and 7% of ovarian cases. **Ries LAG, Melbert D, Krapcho M, Stinchcomb DG, Howlader N, Horner MJ, et al., eds.** *SEER Cancer Statistics Review, 1975–2005.*

Etiologic Studies

In distinction to descriptive studies, etiologic studies examine the relationship between cancer occurrence and survival and personal factors such as diet and reproductive history. This relationship is often described by the epidemiologic parameters, relative risk, and attributable risk.

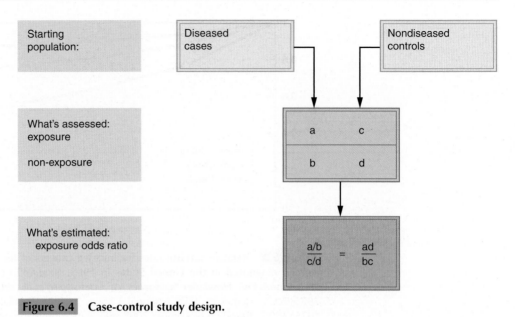

Figure 6.4   Case-control study design.

Relative risk (RR) is the risk of disease or death in a population exposed to some factor of interest divided by the risk in those not exposed. Absence of association is indicated by a RR of 1 (null value); a number greater than 1 may indicate that exposure increases the risk of disease and a number less than 1 that exposure decreases the risk of disease.

Attributable risk is the risk of disease or death in a population exposed to some factor of interest minus the risk in those not exposed. The null value is 0; a number greater than 0 may indicate that exposure increases the risk of disease and a number less than 0 that exposure decreases the risk.

Case-Control Study

In a case-control study, diseased and nondiseased populations are selected, and existing or past characteristics (exposures) are assessed to determine the possible relationship between exposure and disease. The investigator starts with diseased cases and nondiseased control subjects who are then studied to determine whether they had a particular exposure (before the illness). The odds that the cases were exposed (a/b) is compared with the odds that the control subjects were exposed (c/d) in a measure called the *exposure odds ratio* (Fig. 6.4).

Exposure Odds Ratio   **The odds of exposure among cases divided by the odds of exposure among the control subjects is the exposure odds ratio; it approximates the relative risk.** If an entire population could be characterized by its exposure and disease status, then the exposure odds ratio would be mathematically identical to the relative risk obtained in a cohort study. Because it is feasible to study only subsets of cases and control subjects, the exposure odds ratio in the sampled population approximates the relative risk, as long as the cases and control subjects actually sampled have not been preferentially selected on the basis of their exposure status.

Attributable risk cannot be directly calculated in a case-control study.

Cohort Studies

In a cohort study, the groups to be studied (the cohorts) are defined by characteristics (or exposures) that occur before the disease of interest, and the study groups are followed to observe the risk of disease in the cohorts. The investigator starts with exposed and nonexposed individuals who are monitored over time to identify the number of diseased cases that develop. The initial sizes of the cohort and the number of years cohort members are studied determine the person-time contributed by the cohorts. The investigator then calculates the rates of disease in exposed and nonexposed subjects and determines the relative or attributable risk. For rare exposures, an investigator may use the general population as the unexposed group and calculate a parameter equivalent to the relative risk that is known as the **standardized morbidity ratio** (Fig. 6.5).

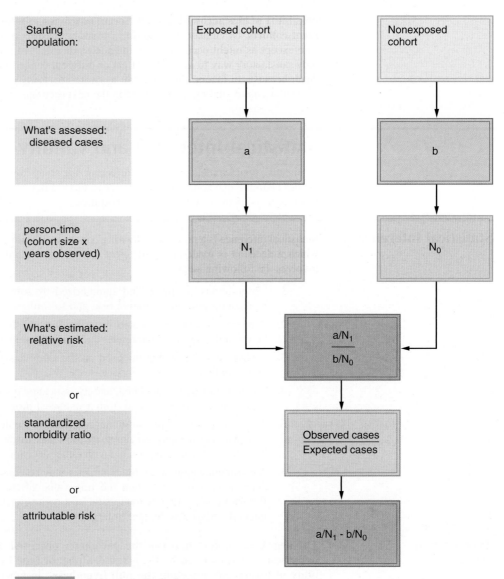

Figure 6.5   Cohort study design.

Standardized Morbidity or Mortality Ratio   **The standardized morbidity or mortality ratio (SMR) is the observed number of exposed cohort members in whom disease developed, divided by the number expected if general population disease rates had prevailed in the cohort.**

Cohort studies are further distinguished by when the exposure and outcome occurred or will occur in relation to when the investigator begins the study.

Retrospective Cohort Study   **In a retrospective cohort study, the exposures and outcomes have already occurred when the study is begun.** For example, studies of second cancers after therapeutic radiation are based on follow-up of women irradiated for cervical cancer 10 to 30 years previously. Medical records and death certificates are used to determine those who subsequently died of cancers other than cervical.

Prospective Cohort Study   **In a prospective cohort study, the relevant exposure may or may not have occurred when the study is begun, but the outcome has not yet occurred.** After the cohort is selected, the investigator must wait for the disease or outcome to appear in the cohort members. The Nurses' Health Study (4) is a good example of a prospective cohort study.

Clinical Trial   **A clinical trial is a special type of prospective cohort study in which the investigator assigns a therapy or preventive agent in randomized fashion to minimize the** possibility of bias accounting for different outcomes subsequently observed between treatment cohorts. Obviously, such studies cannot be used to assess a harmful effect of an exposure except as might occur as an unintended side effect of the therapy. Clinical trials are the only satisfactory way to assess the effect of different cancer therapies on disease recurrence or death because, in theory, they are able to overcome many of the biases that may affect case-control or cohort studies, as discussed in the next section.

Statistical Inference and Validity

Clinicians should understand issues affecting statistical significance and validity to evaluate studies claiming that some exposure causes cancer, a new therapy is superior to standard treatment, or a screening test can improve mortality.

Statistical Inference

Statistical inference is a process of drawing conclusions from data by hypothesis testing, during which a decision is made either to reject or not reject a null hypothesis. Hypothesis testing involves the following steps:

1. Observations are made and summarized by some statistical parameter such as a mean, a proportion, a relative risk, and so forth.

2. A research question is stated in terms of a null hypothesis claiming no difference between the observed parameter and some theoretical value.

3. A statistical test is chosen based on the study design and nature of the parameters being studied.

4. The test statistic is calculated, and its associated p value is read from the appropriate statistical table or generated from a statistical program.

5. A p value less than the traditional 5% leads to the decision to reject the null hypothesis, whereas a value greater than 5% leads to the decision not to reject the null hypothesis. Errors are possible with either decision.

6. A confidence interval on the parameter may be constructed from the test results and defines the range in which the true value of the parameter is expected to fall. **Precision** refers to a characteristic of a parameter falling into a narrow confidence interval, a desirable feature of large studies.

Type I Error

The degree of conflict between the parameter observed and that assumed by the null hypothesis is summarized by the p value, alpha, or type I error and indicates the probability of incorrectly rejecting the null hypothesis. In practice, an alpha level is chosen *a priori*, usually $p = 0.05$, and if the association tested has a p value less than the predetermined alpha level, then results are considered statistically significant. It is important to note, however, that when many tests are performed, some results will be observed by chance. For instance, if 100 tests are performed and the alpha level is set at 0.05, then an estimated five significant results will be observed by chance. One way to address this multiple testing issue, called **Bonferroni correction,** is to divide the alpha level by the number of tests being performed. If this method is used and 100 tests are performed, then the alpha level will be 0.05/100 or 0.0005.

Type II Error

A type II, or beta error, indicates the probability of failing to reject the null hypothesis when, in reality, it is false. To calculate a beta error, an **alternate hypothesis** must be stated.

Power

Power is 1 minus the beta error and reflects the ability of a study to detect an actual effect. More precisely, power is the ability of a test statistic to detect differences of a specified size in test parameters. In planning a clinical trial, an investigator often calculates the power that a study will have to detect an association, given a certain study size and certain assumptions about the nature of the association. Small clinical trials that find no significant difference among therapies may be cited as evidence of "no effect of therapy" when the statistical power may have been well below the accepted target of 80% for a meaningful difference in response rates.

Statistical Distributions and Tests

There are no simple rules for determining which statistical test is appropriate in every situation. The choice depends on whether the variable is qualitative (nominal) or quantitative (numerical), what assumptions are made about the distribution of the parameter being measured, what is the nature of the study question, and the number of groups or variables being studied. For example, a **chi-square test** is used to test the null hypothesis that proportions are equal or that nominal variables are independent. The unpaired *t*-test is used to compare two means from independent samples, whereas the **paired *t*-test** compares the difference or change in a numerical variable for matched or paired groups or samples.

Validity

Validity has two components: internal validity and external validity. **Internal validity means freedom from bias.** *Bias* **refers to a systematic error in the design, conduct, or analysis of a study that results in a mistaken conclusion and is commonly divided into observation bias, selection bias, and confounding. The** *external validity* **of a study refers to the ability to generalize the results observed in one study population to another.** Although there is controversy about what characteristics of a study make for generalizability, it is clear that external validity is only an issue for those studies that possess internal validity, which is the main focus of this discussion.

Observation Bias

Observation bias or misclassification occurs when subjects are classified incorrectly with respect to exposure or disease. If misclassification was equally likely to occur whether the subject was a case or control or an exposed or nonexposed cohort member, then the observation bias would be nondifferential and would cause the relative risk to be biased toward the null value, 1. Alternatively, if misclassification was more likely to occur for case than control subjects or for exposed than nonexposed cohort members, then a falsely elevated (or decreased) relative risk might occur (e.g., if cases preferentially recalled or admitted to a particular exposure compared with control subjects). Criteria for exposure or disease should be clearly defined to minimize observation bias and, whenever possible, exposure or disease confirmed from medical records. Ideally, researchers recording disease status in a cohort study or exposure status in a case-control study should be unaware of the subject's study group or blinded to key hypotheses. **In a clinical trial, observation bias may be minimized by double blindness,** when neither the subject nor investigator knows which specific treatment the subject is receiving.

Selection Bias

Selection bias is an error that results from systematic differences in the characteristics of subjects who are and are not selected for study. For example, a selection bias might occur in a case-control study if exposed cases did much better or worse than nonexposed cases. If the case group consisted of long-term survivors, then they might have a different frequency of the exposure than newly diagnosed individuals. Selection bias may also occur in the process of selecting control subjects; for example, control subjects might be selected from hospitalized patients in a disease category that may, itself, relate to the exposure. Selection bias is less likely to occur in cohort studies or in population-based case-control studies, where most cases in a particular area are studied and control subjects are selected from the general population.

Confounding

Confounding occurs when some factor not considered in the design or analysis accounts for an association because that factor is correlated with both exposure and disease. Potential confounders for any cancer study are age, ethnicity, and socioeconomic status. Confounding may be controlled during the design of a study by matching cases to control subjects on key confounding variables or during the analytic phase of the study by stratification or multivariate analysis. **Stratifying** means examining the association of interest within groups that are similar with respect to a potential confounder, whereas **multivariate analysis** is a statistical technique that controls for a number of confounders simultaneously.

In a clinical trial, confounding is avoided by randomization; that is, subjects are allocated to treatment groups by a chance mechanism such that prejudices of the investigator or preferences by the subject do not influence allocation of treatment. In practice, participant randomization assignments can be determined using computer-generated random numbers or random number tables found in most statistic textbooks (5,6). The initial table in the report of a clinical trial usually shows how the treatment groups compared with respect to age, ethnicity, or other important variables to demonstrate whether randomization indeed balanced key variables. Similar tables are helpful in case-control and cohort studies.

Other Criteria for Judging an Epidemiologic Study

In addition to validity, other criteria applied to judging an epidemiologic study include consistency, whether a dose response is present, and whether the association has biologic credibility.

Consistency	**Measurements that are in close agreement when repeated are said to be consistent.** In the context of an epidemiologic association, relative risks that are consistent among studies, especially those in which different study methods have been used, provide evidence for a causal association. However, the possibility that a systematic bias affected all the studies should also be considered. Consistency can be assessed in a formal manner by performing a study called a *metaanalysis*. **In a metaanalysis, results from independent studies examining the same exposure (or treatment) and outcome are combined so that a more powerful test of the null hypothesis may be conducted.** As part of the metaanalysis, a test for heterogeneity is performed to indicate whether there are statistical differences among the results of different studies. The metaanalysis has become an important component of evidenced-based medical reviews. For example, oral contraceptive use was less common in ovarian cancer cases compared to controls in 45 studies; when the studies results were combined in a metaanalysis, women who had ever used oral contraceptives had an estimated 17% reduction in ovarian cancer risk compared to women who had never used oral contraceptives (7).
Dose Response	*Dose response* **refers to a relationship between exposure and disease such that a change in the duration, amount, or intensity of an exposure is associated with an increase or decrease in disease risk.**
Biologic Credibility	**An association has biologic credibility if it is supported by a framework of diverse observations from the natural history or demographics of the disease and from relevant experimental models.**

Cancer Risk and Prevention

In this section, risk factors for the gynecologic cancers are discussed, along with the application of this information to cancer prevention. Table 6.4 summarizes major epidemiologic risk factors for cervical, endometrial, and ovarian cancer.

Table 6.4 Risk Factors for Gynecologic Cancers

Factor	*Cervix*	*Endometrium*	*Ovary*
Sexual	Increased risk associated with coitus at an early age, multiple partners, or "high-risk men"	Increased risk in women who have never married	Increased risk in women who have never married
Contraception	Barrier methods protective; oral contraceptives may increase risk	Oral contraceptives protective	Oral contraceptives and tubal ligation protective
Childbirth	Increasing risk with increasing parity	Decreasing risk with increasing parity	Decreasing risk with increasing parity
Age at menopause	No clear association	Late menopause increases risk	No clear association
Menopausal hormones	No clear association	Increased risk from "unopposed estrogen"	Weak increased risk with "unopposed estrogen"
Family history	Weak evidence of familial tendency	Mutations of DNA mismatch repair genes increase risk	Mutations of *BRCA1, BRCA2,* and DNA mismatch repair increase risk
Body habitus, diet	Carotene, vitamin C, and folic acid potentially protective	Obesity a strong risk factor	No clear association
Smoking	Increased risk	Decreased risk	Varies by epithelial type; increased risk of mucinous type
Other exposures	Douching may increase risk	Association with estrogen-producing tumors of the ovary, liver disease, *tamoxifen* use	Foreign bodies (talc) per vagina may increase risk; acetaminophen may decrease risk

Cervical Cancer

Invasive squamous cell carcinoma of the cervix is the end stage of a process beginning with atypical transformation of cervical epithelium at the squamocolumnar junction, leading to cervical intraepithelial neoplasia (CIN) of advancing grades and eventual invasive disease. Thus, risk factors for cervical cancer are those associated with atypical transformation and those that influence persistence and progression of disease.

Factors associated with atypical transformation largely relate to sexual practices that increase the opportunity for human papilloma virus (HPV) infection. Early age at first intercourse may also be important because adolescence is a period of heightened squamous metaplasia, and intercourse at this time may increase the likelihood of atypical transformation (8). The woman who has had intercourse with multiple partners or with a "high-risk" male who has himself had contact with multiple partners increases the likelihood of her exposure to HPV. An estimated 27% of U.S. women ages 14 to 59 have a prevalent HPV infection. Prevalence is highest among women ages 20 to 24 at 45% (9). **The link with HPV infection means that a woman can decrease her risk of cervical cancer by safe sexual practices and use of barrier methods of contraception** (10). Male circumcision would appear to decrease the risk of male HPV infection and cervical cancer in their partners (11).

The recent development of HPV vaccines offers an exciting approach to true primary prevention of this important cancer worldwide (12). It is important to note that currently available HPV vaccines only target HPV types 16 and 18, which cause an estimated 70% of cervical cancers (13,14). Consequently, screening with Papanicolaou (Pap) smears continues to be an important cervical cancer prevention strategy (14,15). Unfortunately, vaccination does not accelerate clearance of prevalent HPV infections, which means that the vaccine is not effective for women who have already been infected (16). Thus, females should receive the vaccine before sexual debut. Vaccine trials in males are ongoing because HPV vaccines may prevent not only anogenital warts and anogenital cancer but also a subset of anal, penile, oral, head, and neck cancers as well as juvenile respiratory papillomatosis in their children (17). Mathematical models suggest that male vaccination will have little impact on preventing cervical cancer in females (18). Although implementation of HPV vaccination has gone fairly smoothly in developed countries, the cost of the vaccine ($335–$360) has made distribution difficult in developing countries, where 80% of cervical cancers occur (19).

Smoking also has been associated with increased risk for cervical cancer, even after adjustment for a number of confounding factors (20). This association has biologic credibility because potentially mutagenic substances are secreted in the cervical mucus of smokers (21). In third world countries, chronic exposure to wood smoke may increase the risk for cervical cancer in HPV-infected women (22).

Besides factors that affect the risk for cervical cancer by initiating atypical transformation, others may modulate risk for cervical cancer by affecting the likelihood that a preinvasive lesion will persist or progress. A factor indisputably related to the progression of CIN is the frequency of cervical cytologic screening. **Population studies have demonstrated a correlation between cytologic screening and declining mortality from cervical cancer** (23). **Case-control studies demonstrate that women who have had Pap smears at least every 3 years have one-tenth the risk of developing invasive disease compared with women who have never had a Pap test** (24). The recent introduction of HPV testing has improved cervical cancer screening even further (described in more detail under "Screening Strategies").

Other factors that relate to disease progression may include oral contraceptive use and diet. **Long-term oral contraceptive use has been reported to increase the risk of high-grade intraepithelial lesions and invasive cervical cancer** (25)**, and a link to adenocarcinomas of the cervix has also been postulated** (26). Butterworth et al. attributed the potential harmful effects of oral contraceptives on the cervix to folate deficiency and recommended supplementation (27). More recent studies found that high homocysteine levels may correlate with risk for invasive cervical cancer, again suggesting the importance of folates and vitamins B_{12} or B_6 (28). Finally, **progression of CIN is likely to be greater in immunosuppressed women,** such as those with human immunodeficiency virus infection (29), or after kidney transplantation (30).

Endometrial Cancer

Risk for adenocarcinoma of the endometrium is largely attributed to estrogen (31). States that lead to an excess of estrogen over progesterone or increase lifetime exposure to estrogen also increase endometrial cancer risk. For instance, early age at menarche and late age at menopause increase endometrial cancer risk (32–38). Furthermore, obesity, which leads to increased estrogen production through the peripheral conversion of androstenedione, accounts for an estimated 57% of all endometrial cancers in the United States (39). Alternatively, protective factors are those associated with decreased estrogen production. Surgical castration at an early age with retention of the uterus is a strong protective factor (40). Leanness and regular exercise lower estrogen levels and protect against endometrial cancer (41). Smoking also lowers estrogen and protects against endometrial cancer but obviously cannot be encouraged as a preventive measure (42). Endometrial cancer as a consequence of decreased degradation of estrogen is illustrated by case reports of the disease in women with cirrhosis of the liver (43).

Endometrial cancer as a consequence of exogenous estrogen is demonstrated by the impressive evidence that unopposed estrogen administered for the menopause increases the risk of endometrial cancer in a dose-response fashion (44). *Tamoxifen,* with its estrogen antagonist effects in the breast and agonist effects in the uterus, has also been shown to increase the risk for endometrial cancer in clinical trial data (45). Alternatively, menopausal estrogen taken with a progestin has not been shown to increase risk (46), and past use of combination birth control pills has been reported to decrease the risk of endometrial cancer (47). Clinical trials have suggested very low rates of hyperplasia occurring with a continuous regimen of 0.625 mg of *conjugated estrogen* and 2.5 mg of *medroxyprogesterone acetate* (48).

Fitting with key roles for estrogen and progesterone in this disease, risk for endometrial cancer may be modified by genetic polymorphisms of the progesterone receptor (49), estrogen receptor alpha (50), estrogen metabolism genes (51), and aromatase, which catalyzes the conversion of androgens to estrogens (52). It is less clear how the DNA mismatch repair genes that are associated with increased risk for colorectal and endometrial cancers would operate through the "estrogen excess" model (53). Although the majority of risk factors for endometrial cancer are nicely explained by estrogen excess, the consistent observation that even inert intrauterine devices (IUDs) decrease risk suggests that immune factors related to the low-grade inflammation that occurs with IUDs may also play a role (54).

Ovarian Cancer

Ovarian cancer has been associated with a number of diverse findings with a variety of theories offered to explain them. **Consistently observed risk factors for ovarian cancer include a protective effect of pregnancy, breast-feeding, and oral contraceptive use. A popular theory to account for these findings is that these events lead to a break in monthly ovulations and, therefore, repeated disruption and healing of the surface of the ovary (incessant ovulation), which is the cause of ovarian cancer** (55). Not readily explained by this model, however, are the facts that the peak occurrence of ovarian cancer is well beyond the cessation of ovulation. In addition, very low rates of the disease are observed in Japan, where there are both low birthrates and little use of oral contraceptives.

An alternative theory to incessant ovulation is that ovarian cancer may arise from excessive gonadotropin stimulation of the ovary (56). Classic animal models for ovarian cancer involved disruption of ovarian–pituitary feedback either by prematurely destroying oocytes using radiation or chemical toxins (57,58) or by transplanting the animal's ovary to its spleen, leading to enhanced metabolism of ovarian hormones before they could exert feedback inhibition (59). A role for gonadotropins was indicated by observations that ovarian tumors did not develop in rodents who were hypophysectomized before the experimental treatment or who were given estrogen, which inhibited gonadotropin release (60,61). More recently, it has been shown that gonadal stromal tumors invariably developed in mice with a targeted deletion of the gene for the gonadotropin down regulator, α-inhibin (62), unless the mice were also incapable of secreting gonadotropins (63). Most of these experimental tumors were stromal in origin, and their relevance to the epithelial types observed in women has been debated. However, monthly ovulators, in contrast to rodents, have inclusion cysts and an abundant stromal–epithelial admixture, which might lead to epithelial proliferation as the principal manifestation of ovarian stromal stimulation in humans.

Epidemiologic data support the relevance of these models to human ovarian cancer. **Ovarian cancer incidence rises sharply between ages 45 and 54 and remains elevated for the remainder of a woman's life, paralleling gonadotropin levels over this period.** The strong protective association between oral contraceptives and ovarian cancer (64) duplicates the effects of exogenous estrogen in the animal models. Also relevant to the animal models are cohort studies that demonstrate that ovarian cancer occurs after radiation for cervical cancer after a 10- to 15-year lag period (65,66).

Parmley and Woodruff proposed that epithelial ovarian cancers might be ovarian mesotheliomas that arise from transformation of the surface lining of the ovary exposed to pelvic contaminants (67). One such contaminant might be talc used in genital hygiene, which has fairly consistently been identified as a risk factor (68). Besides talc, another pelvic "contaminant" might be the menstrual products that are believed to flow out of the fallopian tubes during menstruation to explain endometriosis (69). Indeed, prior endometriosis is a risk factor for ovarian cancer (70), especially the endometrioid and clear cell types (71). The pelvic contamination theory might also explain why tubal ligation decreases the risk of ovarian cancer (72). Other theories have suggested roles for androgens, progesterone, and inflammation and offer alternate but not necessarily competing explanations for ovarian cancer risk factors (73,74).

Uninterrupted ovulations could have immune consequences related to the surface glycoprotein and tumor marker, human mucin 1 (MUC1) (75). MUC1 is a high molecular weight protein expressed in a highly glycosylated form at low levels by many types of normal epithelial cells and in an underglycosylated form at high levels by most epithelial adenocarcinomas, including endometrial, breast, and ovarian cancer (76). In cancer patients, anti-MUC1 antibodies may correlate with a more favorable prognosis (77,78). Interestingly, anti-MUC1 antibodies are also found in healthy individuals, especially in women during pregnancy and lactation, leading to the hypothesis that a natural immunity against tumor MUC1 might develop and account for the long-term protective effect of pregnancy or breast-feeding on the risk of breast cancer (79). This led us to propose the broader theory that a variety of seemingly disparate events associated with ovarian cancer risk—including tubal ligation, mastitis, bone fracture, and possibly IUD use—may be operating by their ability to raise anti-MUC1 antibodies and enhance immunity or lower anti-MUC1 antibodies to increase immune tolerance to cancers expressing MUC1 (80).

Finally, there are a number of genetic risk factors emerging for ovarian cancer. Having a mother or sister with the disease increases a woman's risk for ovarian cancer approximately two- to threefold (81). **Specific genetic factors include mutations of the *BRCA1* and *BRCA2* as well as the DNA mismatch genes** (82). Although these genetic factors are more likely to be found in families in which a number of relatives have been affected with breast or ovarian cancer, they may be found in a surprising number of women with "sporadic" ovarian cancer: 10% in one series (83) and as much as 40% among women with a Jewish ethnic background (84).

Other Gynecologic Neoplasms

Other than clear cell adenocarcinomas of the vagina associated with maternal use of diethylstilbestrol (85), vaginal carcinoma is primarily a disease of women older than 50 years of age. Vulvar cancer has an age-incidence distribution similar to vaginal cancer. HPV infection appears to play a role in both vaginal and vulvar cancers (86–88). In a population based case-control study, HPV was detected in more than 80% of the tumor blocks from patients with *in situ* vaginal cancer and in 60% of those from invasive vaginal cancers (87). For vulvar cancer, two types of vulvar cancer have been defined (86,88). The first, which affects younger women, is associated with HPV and has a preinvasive stage. The second type occurs in older women and arises in areas with non-neoplastic epithelial disorders such as lichen sclerosis. It is not surprising that **risk factors known to exist for cervical neoplasms also pertain to vulvar and vaginal neoplasms, including sexual history and smoking** (87,89–91). Further study of dietary factors, especially folates and the carotenoids, would be worthwhile.

Trophoblastic neoplasms include complete and partial hydatidiform moles, invasive moles, and choriocarcinoma. The epidemiology of hydatidiform mole is probably better understood than that of other trophoblastic diseases, and it is likely to be relevant because of the association between molar pregnancy and subsequent invasive mole or choriocarcinoma. The prevalence of molar pregnancy varies from 1 per 100 deliveries in Asia, Indonesia, and other third world countries to 1 per 1,000 to 1,500 in the United States (92). Clearly, **the risk of having a molar pregnancy increases with maternal age** (93,94), but it is less certain whether adolescents are also at increased risk (95). A previous hydatidiform mole is also a strong risk factor; subsequent pregnancies have a 1% risk of also being a hydatidiform mole (96). The peculiar cytogenetic patterns of complete and partial hydatidiform moles are discussed in Chapter 15 and may indicate the importance of aberrant germ cells in the origin of these disorders.

Berkowitz et al. (97) suggested that deficiency of the vitamin A precursor, carotene, or of animal fats necessary for its absorption might be a factor in the cause of this disease. Vitamin A deficiency causes fetal wastage and aberrancy of epithelial development in female animals and degeneration of seminiferous epithelium with poor gamete development in male animals

(98–100). In addition, regions where molar pregnancy is common have a high incidence of night blindness (101). Interestingly, paternal blood group combinations may influence risk of a molar pregnancy. Mothers with group A blood and fathers with group A or 0 had an increased risk compared with all other blood group combinations (102–104). Oral contraceptives are associated with an increased risk of hydatidiform mole that increases with duration of use. Ten or more years of use is associated with a more than twofold increase in risk (105). Smoking also doubles the risk of hydatidiform mole and quadruples risk with ten or more years of smoking (102,106,107). The role of alcohol and infections (HPV, adenoassociated virus, and tuberculosis) have also been considered (108).

Cancer Prevention

Cancer prevention may occur at the level of **primary prevention** (the identification and modification of risk factors for disease), **secondary prevention** (the detection of the disease at earlier, more treatable stages), or **tertiary prevention** (effective treatment of clinical disease). This section addresses primary and secondary measures of prevention.

Methods of primary prevention are by no means certain, but suggestions include the following.

1. **For cervical cancer,** use of barrier methods of contraception, avoidance of tobacco, and maintaining a diet high in folates, B vitamins, and β-carotene may be beneficial. HPV vaccines have proven benefits and should be used by women before sexual debut.

2. **For endometrial cancer,** maintenance of ideal body weight, avoidance of a high-fat diet, and avoidance of unopposed estrogen therapy during menopause may be beneficial.

3. **For ovarian cancer,** use of oral contraceptives, if not medically contraindicated, and avoidance of talc in genital hygiene may be beneficial. Women known to carry a predisposing mutation should undergo prophylactic salpingo-oophorectomy after they have completed childbearing.

Secondary Prevention

Cancer deaths may also be prevented by detecting disease at a stage when it is more curable. The secondary prevention of cervical cancer has been successful, and screening programs for the other gynecologic cancers may eventually be devised. To be successful, a screening program must be directed at a "suitable" disease with a "suitable" screening test (109). A suitable disease must be one that has serious consequences, as most cancers do. Treatment must be available so that when such therapy is applied to screen-detected (preclinical) disease, it will be more effective than when applied after symptoms of the disease have appeared. Also, the preclinical phase of the disease must be long enough that the chances are good that a person will be screened. There must also be a suitable screening test as defined by simplicity, acceptability to patients, low cost, and high validity (defined by the measures in Table 6.5).

Sensitivity

The sensitivity of a test is defined as the proportion of people with a true positive screening result of all those who have the disease.

Specificity

The specificity of a test is defined as the proportion of people with a true negative screening result of all those who do not have the disease.

Predictive Value

The predictive value of a positive test is defined as the proportion of true positives out of all those who screened positive. The alternate formula shown in Table 6.5 reveals that predictive value is a function of sensitivity, specificity, and disease prevalence. This function implies that a positive screening test is more likely to indicate disease in a high-risk population than in a low-risk population (Table 6.5).

Screening Strategies

Cervical cytology represents one of the most effective screening tests for cancer ever developed; controversies relate to how to make it more efficient. Recent guidelines suggested by the American Cancer Society (110) are that the interval between screenings may be safely lengthened to 3 years in women who have had at least three consecutive negative screens and are at otherwise low risk (e.g., no history of immunosuppression). Similar guidelines were proposed by the American College of Obstetricians and Gynecologists in 2000, although the less frequent intervals were to be at the discretion of the physician (111). A recent analysis of the potential effects

Table 6.5 Measures of Validity for a Screening Procedure

Status Determined by Screening	True Disease Status		
	Positive	**Negative**	**Total**
Positive	a (true positives)	b (false positives)	a + b (all screened positives)
Negative	c (false negatives)	d (true negatives)	c + d (all screened negatives)
Total	a + c (all diseased)	b + d (all nondiseased)	N (all subjects)
Measure	*Definition*	*Formula*[a]	
Sensitivity	True positives; all diseased	$\dfrac{a}{a + c}$	
Specificity	True negatives; all nondiseased	$\dfrac{d}{b + d}$	
Predictive value of a positive screen	True positives; all screened positives	$\dfrac{a}{a + b}$ or	$\dfrac{SN(P)}{[SN(P) + (1 - SP)(1 - P)]}$

[a]SN, sensitivity; SP, specificity; P, prevalence of disease

of extending screening intervals concluded that an average excess risk of three cases of cervical cancer per 100,000 women screened would result (112). However, to avert one additional case of cancer by screening women annually for 3 years would necessitate approximately 280,000 additional Pap tests and 15,000 colposcopic examinations. HPV testing, which involves detection of HPV DNA in a cervical swab, can greatly improve the sensitivity of the traditional Pap smear. In a study of 10,154 women ages 30 to 69, the HPV test had a much higher sensitivity (95%) than the Pap smear (55%) and similar specificity (95% for HPV testing and 97% for the Pap smear). Using HPV testing together with the Pap smear increases the sensitivity to 100% (113). A cost–benefit analysis revealed that the maximum number of lives were saved when combined HPV and Pap smear screening was performed every 2 years until death (114).

Screening for endometrial cancer in asymptomatic women in the general population is not justified, but endometrial biopsies or assessment of the endometrial stripe by transvaginal ultrasound may be appropriate for perimenopausal or postmenopausal women at risk for endometrial cancer, including those who are obese, are exposed to unopposed estrogen, use *tamoxifen,* or who come from families with both colon and endometrial cancer. **Based on expert opinion only, women at high risk for ovarian cancer by virtue of a *BRCA1* or *BRCA2* mutation are recommended to have annual or semiannual screening with transvaginal ultrasound and CA125 measurements** (115). A large trial is under way in the United Kingdom to determine whether use of annual CA125 measurements with secondary ultrasonic screening would be effective at reducing ovarian cancer mortality in postmenopausal women at normal risk (116).

References

1. **Rosner BA, Colditz GA, Webb PM, Hankinson SE.** Mathematical models of ovarian cancer incidence. *Epidemiology* 2005; 16:508–515.
2. **Rothman I, Greenland S.** *Modern epidemiology.* Philadelphia: Lippincott Williams & Wilkins, 1998.
3. **Ries LAG MD, Krapcho M, Stinchcomb DG, Howlader N, Horner MJ, Mariotto A, et al., eds.** *SEER Cancer Statistics Review, 1975–2005.* Bethesda, MD: National Cancer Institute. Available at: http://seer.cancer.gov/csr/1975_2005/. Based on November 2007 SEER data submission posted to the SEER Web site 2008.
4. **Colditz GA, Hankinson SE.** The Nurses' Health Study: lifestyle and health among women. *Nat Rev Cancer* 2005;5:388–396.
5. **Rosner B.** *Fundamentals of biostatistics.* Pacific Grove, CA: Duxbury Thompson Learning, 2000.
6. **Altman DG.** *Practical statistics for medical research.* London: Chapman & Hall/CRC, 1991.
7. **Collaborative Group on Epidemiological Studies of Ovarian Cancer, Beral V, Doll R, Hermon C, Peto R, Reeves G.** Ovarian cancer and oral contraceptives: collaborative reanalysis of data from 45 epidemiological studies including 23,257 women with ovarian cancer and 87,303 controls. *Lancet* 2008;371:303–314.
8. **Singer A.** The cervical epithelium during puberty and adolescence. In: **Jordan JA SA, ed.** *The cervix.* London: WB Saunders, 1976.
9. **Dunne EF, Unger ER, Sternberg M, McQuillan G, Swan DC, Patel SS, et al.** Prevalence of HPV infection among females in the United States. *JAMA* 2007;297:813–819.
10. **Hildesheim A, Brinton LA, Mallin K, Lehman HF, Stolley P, Savitz DA, et al.** Barrier and spermicidal contraceptive methods and risk of invasive cervical cancer. *Epidemiology* 1990;1:266–272.

11. Castellsague X, Bosch FX, Munoz N, Meijer CJ, Shah KV, de Sanjose S, et al. Male circumcision, penile human papillomavirus infection, and cervical cancer in female partners. *N Engl J Med* 2002;346:1105–1112.

12. Koutsky LA, Ault KA, Wheeler CM, Brown DR, Barr E, Alvarez FB, et al. A controlled trial of a human papillomavirus type 16 vaccine. *N Engl J Med* 2002;347:1645–1651.

13. Kahn JA, Burk RD. Papillomavirus vaccines in perspective. *Lancet* 2007;369:2135–2137.

14. Savage L. Proposed HPV vaccine mandates rile health experts across the country. *J Natl Cancer Inst* 2007;99:665–666.

15. Kiviat NB, Hawes SE, Feng Q. Screening for cervical cancer in the era of the HPV vaccine—the urgent need for both new screening guidelines and new biomarkers. *J Natl Cancer Inst* 2008;100:290–291.

16. Hildesheim A, Herrero R, Wacholder S, Rodriguez AC, Solomon D, Bratti MC, et al. Effect of human papillomavirus 16/18 *L1* virus-like particle vaccine among young women with preexisting infection: a randomized trial. *JAMA* 2007;298:743–753.

17. Saslow D, Castle PE, Cox JT, Davey DD, Einstein MH, Ferris DG, et al. American Cancer Society Guideline for human papillomavirus (HPV) vaccine use to prevent cervical cancer and its precursors. *CA Cancer J Clin* 2007;57:7–28.

18. Barnabas RV, Laukkanen P, Koskela P, Kontula O, Lehtinen M, Garnett GP. Epidemiology of HPV 16 and cervical cancer in Finland and the potential impact of vaccination: mathematical modelling analyses. *PLoS Med* 2006;3:e138.

19. Cheaper HPV vaccines needed. *Lancet* 2008;371:1638.

20. Brinton LA, Barrett RJ, Berman ML, Mortel R, Twiggs LB, Wilbanks GD. Cigarette smoking and the risk of endometrial cancer. *Am J Epidemiol* 1993;137:281–291.

21. Schiffman MH, Haley NJ, Felton JS, Andrews AW, Kaslow RA, Lancaster WD, et al. Biochemical epidemiology of cervical neoplasia: measuring cigarette smoke constituents in the cervix. *Cancer Res* 1987;47:3886–3888.

22. Ferrera A, Velema JP, Figueroa M, Bulnes R, Toro LA, Claros JM, et al. Co-factors related to the causal relationship between human papillomavirus and invasive cervical cancer in Honduras. *Int J Epidemiol* 2000;29:817–825.

23. Miller AB, Lindsay J, Hill GB. Mortality from cancer of the uterus in Canada and its relationship to screening for cancer of the cervix. *Int J Cancer* 1976;17:602–612.

24. La Vecchia C, Franceschi S, Decarli A, Fasoli M, Gentile A, Tognoni G. "Pap" smear and the risk of cervical neoplasia: quantitative estimates from a case-control study. *Lancet* 1984;2:779–782.

25. Negrini BP, Schiffman MH, Kurman RJ, Barnes W, Lannom L, Malley K, et al. Oral contraceptive use, human papillomavirus infection, and risk of early cytological abnormalities of the cervix. *Cancer Res* 1990;50:4670–4675.

26. Brinton LA, Tashima KT, Lehman HF, Levine RS, Mallin K, Savitz DA, et al. Epidemiology of cervical cancer by cell type. *Cancer Res* 1987;47:1706–1711.

27. Butterworth CE, Jr., Hatch KD, Gore H, Mueller H, Krumdieck CL. Improvement in cervical dysplasia associated with folic acid therapy in users of oral contraceptives. *Am J Clin Nutr* 1982;35:73–82.

28. Weinstein SJ, Ziegler RG, Selhub J, Fears TR, Strickler HD, Brinton LA, et al. Elevated serum homocysteine levels and increased risk of invasive cervical cancer in U.S. women. *Cancer Causes Control* 2001;12:317–324.

29. Maiman M, Fruchter R, Seldlis A, Feldman J, Chen P, Burk R, et al. Prevalence, risk factors, and accuracy of cytologic screening for cervical intraepithelial neoplasia in women with the human immunodeficiency virus. *Gynecol Oncol* 1998;68:233–239.

30. Alloub MI, Barr BB, McLaren KM, Smith IW, Bunney MH, Smart GE. Human papillomavirus infection and cervical intraepithelial neoplasia in women with renal allografts. *BMJ* 1989;298:153–156.

31. Key TJ, Pike MC. The dose-effect relationship between "unopposed" oestrogens and endometrial mitotic rate: its central role in explaining and predicting endometrial cancer risk. *Br J Cancer* 1988;57:205–12.

32. Elwood JM, Cole P, Rothman KJ, Kaplan SD. Epidemiology of endometrial cancer. *J Natl Cancer Inst* 1977;59:1055–1060.

33. Kelsey JL, LiVolsi VA, Holford TR, Fischer DB, Mostow ED, Schwartz PE, et al. A case-control study of cancer of the endometrium. *Am J Epidemiol* 1982;116:333–342.

34. Ewertz M, Schou G, Boice JD, Jr. The joint effect of risk factors on endometrial cancer. *Eur J Cancer Clin Oncol* 1988;24:189–194.

35. Kalandidi A, Tzonou A, Lipworth L, Gamatsi I, Filippa D, Trichopoulos D. A case-control study of endometrial cancer in relation to reproductive, somatometric, and life-style variables. *Oncology* 1996;53:354–359.

36. Koumantaki Y, Tzonou A, Koumantakis E, Kaklamani E, Aravantinos D, Trichopoulos D. A case-control study of cancer of endometrium in Athens. *Int J Cancer* 1989;43:795–799.

37. Kvale G, Heuch I, Ursin G. Reproductive factors and risk of cancer of the uterine corpus: a prospective study. *Cancer Res* 1988;48:6217–6221.

38. McPherson CP, Sellers TA, Potter JD, Bostick RM, Folsom AR. Reproductive factors and risk of endometrial cancer. The Iowa Women's Health Study. *Am J Epidemiol* 1996;143:1195–1202.

39. Calle EE, Kaaks R. Overweight, obesity and cancer: epidemiological evidence and proposed mechanisms. *Nat Rev Cancer* 2004;4:579–591.

40. Jansen D, Ostergaard E. Clinical studies concerning the relationship of estrogens to the development of cancer of the corpus uteri. *Am J Obstet Gynecol* 1954;67:1094–1102.

41. Frisch RE, Wyshak G, Albright NL, Albright TE, Schiff I, Jones KP, et al. Lower prevalence of breast cancer and cancers of the reproductive system among former college athletes compared to non-athletes. *Br J Cancer* 1985;52:885–891.

42. Lesko SM, Rosenberg L, Kaufman DW, Helmrich SP, Miller DR, Strom B, et al. Cigarette smoking and the risk of endometrial cancer. *N Engl J Med* 1985;313:593–596.

43. Speert H. Endometrial cancer and hepatic cirrhosis. *Cancer* 1949;2:597–603.

44. Grady D, Gebretsadik T, Kerlikowske K, Ernster V, Petitti D. Hormone replacement therapy and endometrial cancer risk: a meta-analysis. *Obstet Gynecol* 1995;85:304–313.

45. Fisher B, Costantino JP, Wickerham DL, Redmond CK, Kavanah M, Cronin WM, et al. Tamoxifen for prevention of breast cancer: report of the National Surgical Adjuvant Breast and Bowel Project P-1 Study. *J Natl Cancer Inst* 1998;90:1371–1388.

46. Beresford SA, Weiss NS, Voigt LF, McKnight B. Risk of endometrial cancer in relation to use of oestrogen combined with cyclic progestagen therapy in postmenopausal women. *Lancet* 1997;349:458–461.

47. Weiss NS, Sayvetz TA. Incidence of endometrial cancer in relation to the use of oral contraceptives. *N Engl J Med* 1980;302:551–554.

48. The Writing Group for the PEPI Trial. Effects of hormone replacement therapy on endometrial histology in postmenopausal women. The Postmenopausal Estrogen/Progestin Interventions (PEPI) Trial. *JAMA* 1996;275:370–375.

49. De Vivo I, Huggins GS, Hankinson SE, Lescault PJ, Boezen M, Colditz GA, et al. A functional polymorphism in the promoter of the progesterone receptor gene associated with endometrial cancer risk. *Proc Natl Acad Sci U S A* 2002;99:12263–12268.

50. Sasaki M, Tanaka Y, Kaneuchi M, Sakuragi N, Dahiya R. Polymorphisms of estrogen receptor alpha gene in endometrial cancer. *Biochem Biophys Res Commun* 2002;297:558–564.

51. Doherty JA, Weiss NS, Freeman RJ, Dightman DA, Thornton PJ, Houck JR, et al. Genetic factors in catechol estrogen metabolism in relation to the risk of endometrial cancer. *Cancer Epidemiol Biomarkers Prev* 2005;14:357–366.

52. Paynter RA, Hankinson SE, Colditz GA, Kraft P, Hunter DJ, De Vivo I. CYP19 (aromatase) haplotypes and endometrial cancer risk. *Int J Cancer* 2005;116:267–274.

53. Watson P, Vasen HF, Mecklin JP, Jarvinen H, Lynch HT. The risk of endometrial cancer in hereditary nonpolyposis colorectal cancer. *Am J Med* 1994;96:516–520.

54. Benshushan A, Paltiel O, Rojansky N, Brzesinski A, Laufer N. IUD use and the risk for endometrial cancer. *Eur J Obstet Gynecol Reprod Biol* 2002;105:166–169.

55. Fathalla MF. Incessant ovulation—a factor in ovarian neoplasia? *Lancet* 1971;2:163.

56. **Cramer DW, Welch WR.** Determinants of ovarian cancer risk. II Inference regarding pathogenesis. *J Natl Cancer Inst* 1983; 71:717–721.

57. **Furth J, Butterworth J.** Neoplastic diseases occurring among mice subjected to general irradiation with x-rays. *Am J Cancer* 1936;71:717–721.

58. **Howell JS, Marchant J, Orr JW.** The induction of ovarian tumours in mice with 9:10-dimethyl–1:2-benzanthracene. *Br J Cancer* 1954; 8:635–646.

59. **Biskind M, Biskind G.** Development of tumors in the rat ovary after transplantation into the spleen. *Proc Soc Exp Biol Med* 1944;55: 176–179.

60. **Jull JW, Streeter DJ, Sutherland L.** The mechanism of induction of ovarian tumors in the mouse by 7,12-dimethylbenz-[alpha]anthracene. I. Effect of steroid hormones and carcinogen concentration in vivo. *J Natl Cancer Inst* 1966;37:409–420.

61. **Marchant J.** The effect of hypophysectomy on the development of ovarian tumours in mice treated with dimethylbenzanthracene. *Br J Cancer* 1961;15:821–827.

62. **Matzuk MM, Finegold MJ, Su JG, Hsueh AJ, Bradley A.** Alpha-inhibin is a tumour-suppressor gene with gonadal specificity in mice. *Nature* 1992;360:313–319.

63. **Kumar TR, Wang Y, Matzuk MM.** Gonadotropins are essential modifier factors for gonadal tumor development in inhibin-deficient mice. *Endocrinology* 1996;137:4210–4216.

64. **Schlesselman JJ.** Net effect of oral contraceptive use on the risk of cancer in women in the United States. *Obstet Gynecol* 1995;85:793–801.

65. **Boice JD Jr, Day NE, Andersen A, Brinton LA, Brown R, Choi NW, et al.** Second cancers following radiation treatment for cervical cancer. An international collaboration among cancer registries. *J Natl Cancer Inst* 1985;74:955–975.

66. **Pettersson F, Fotiou S, Einhorn N, Silfversward C.** Cohort study of the long-term effect of irradiation for carcinoma of the uterine cervix. Second primary malignancies in the pelvic organs in women irradiated for cervical carcinoma at Radiumhemmet 1914–1965. *Acta Radiol Oncol* 1985;24:145–151.

67. **Parmley TH, Woodruff JD.** The ovarian mesothelioma. *Am J Obstet Gynecol* 1974;120:234–241.

68. **Cramer DW, Liberman RF, Titus-Ernstoff L, Welch WR, Greenberg ER, Baron JA, et al.** Genital talc exposure and risk of ovarian cancer. *Int J Cancer* 1999;81:351–356.

69. **Sampson J.** the development of the implantatino theory for the origin of endometriosis. *Am J Obstet Gynecol* 1940;40:549–557.

70. **Brinton LA, Gridley G, Persson I, Baron J, Bergqvist A.** Cancer risk after a hospital discharge diagnosis of endometriosis. *Am J Obstet Gynecol* 1997;176:572–579.

71. **Mostoufizadeh M, Scully RE.** Malignant tumors arising in endometriosis. *Clin Obstet Gynecol* 1980;23:951–963.

72. **Hankinson SE, Hunter DJ, Colditz GA, Willett WC, Stampfer MJ, Rosner B, et al.** Tubal ligation, hysterectomy, and risk of ovarian cancer. A prospective study. *JAMA* 1993;270:2813–2818.

73. **Ness RB, Cottreau C.** Possible role of ovarian epithelial inflammation in ovarian cancer. *J Natl Cancer Inst* 1999;91:1459–1467.

74. **Risch HA.** Hormonal etiology of epithelial ovarian cancer, with a hypothesis concerning the role of androgens and progesterone. *J Natl Cancer Inst* 1998;90:1774–1786.

75. **Terry KL, Titus-Ernstoff L, McKolanis JR, Welch WR, Finn OJ, Cramer DW.** Incessant ovulation, mucin 1 immunity, and risk for ovarian cancer. *Cancer Epidemiol Biomarkers Prev* 2007;16:30–35.

76. **Ho SB, Niehans GA, Lyftogt C, Yan PS, Cherwitz DL, Gum ET, et al.** Heterogeneity of mucin gene expression in normal and neoplastic tissues. *Cancer Res* 1993;53:641–651.

77. **Kotera Y, Fontenot JD, Pecher G, Metzgar RS, Finn OJ.** Humoral immunity against a tandem repeat epitope of human mucin MUC-1 in sera from breast, pancreatic, and colon cancer patients. *Cancer Res* 1994;54:2856–2860.

78. **Richards ER, Devine PL, Quin RJ, Fontenot JD, Ward BG, McGuckin MA.** Antibodies reactive with the protein core of MUC1 mucin are present in ovarian cancer patients and healthy women. *Cancer Immunol Immunother* 1998;46:245–252.

79. **Agrawal B, Reddish M, Krantz M, Longenecker B.** Does pregnancy immunize against breast cancer? *Cancer Res* 1995;55: 2257–2261.

80. **Cramer DW, Titus-Ernstoff L, McKolanis JR, Welch WR, Vitonis AF, Berkowitz RS, et al.** Conditions associated with antibodies against the tumor-associated antigen MUC1 and their relationship to risk for ovarian cancer. *Cancer Epidemiol Biomarkers Prev* 2005;14:1125–1131.

81. **Kerlikowske K, Brown JS, Grady DG.** Should women with familial ovarian cancer undergo prophylactic oophorectomy? *Obstet Gynecol* 1992;80:700–707.

82. **Claus EB, Schwartz PE.** Familial ovarian cancer. Update and clinical applications. *Cancer* 1995;76:1998–2003.

83. **Rubin SC, Blackwood MA, Bandera C, Behbakht K, Benjamin I, Rebbeck TR, et al.** *BRCA1, BRCA2,* and hereditary nonpolyposis colorectal cancer gene mutations in an unselected ovarian cancer population: relationship to family history and implications for genetic testing. *Am J Obstet Gynecol* 1998;178:670–677.

84. **Lu KH, Cramer DW, Muto MG, Li EY, Niloff J, Mok SC.** A population-based study of *BRCA1* and *BRCA2* mutations in Jewish women with epithelial ovarian cancer. *Obstet Gynecol* 1999;93:34–7.

85. **Herbst AL, Kurman RJ, Scully RE, Poskanzer DC.** Clear-cell adenocarcinoma of the genital tract in young females. Registry report. *N Engl J Med* 1972;287:1259–1264.

86. **Canavan TP, Cohen D.** Vulvar cancer. *Am Fam Physician* 2002;66:1269–1274.

87. **Daling JR, Madeleine MM, Schwartz SM, Shera KA, Carter JJ, McKnight B, et al.** A population-based study of squamous cell vaginal cancer: HPV and cofactors. *Gynecol Oncol* 2002;84: 263–270.

88. **Stehman FB, Look KY.** Carcinoma of the vulva. *Obstet Gynecol* 2006;107:719–733.

89. **Crum CP, Fu YS, Levine RU, Richart RM, Townsend DE, Fenoglio CM.** Intraepithelial squamous lesions of the vulva: biologic and histologic criteria for the distinction of condylomas from vulvar intraepithelial neoplasia. *Am J Obstet Gynecol* 1982;144:77–83.

90. **Newcomb PA, Weiss NS, Daling JR.** Incidence of vulvar carcinoma in relation to menstrual, reproductive, and medical factors. *J Natl Cancer Inst* 1984;73:391–396.

91. **Brinton LA, Nasca PC, Mallin K, Baptiste MS, Wilbanks GD, Richart RM.** Case-control study of cancer of the vulva. *Obstet Gynecol* 1990;75:859–866.

92. **Bagshawe K, Lawler S. Choriocarcinoma.** In: **Schottenfeld DF FJ, ed.** *Cancer epidemiology and prevention.* Philadelphia: WB Saunders, 1982.

93. **Hayashi K, Bracken MB, Freeman DH Jr, Hellenbrand K.** Hydatidiform mole in the United States (1970–1977): a statistical and theoretical analysis. *Am J Epidemiol* 1982;115:67–77.

94. **Stone M, Bagshawe KD.** An analysis of the influences of maternal age, gestational age, contraceptive method, and the mode of primary treatment of patients with hydatidiform moles on the incidence of subsequent chemotherapy. *Br J Obstet Gynaecol* 1979;86:782–792.

95. **Jacobs PA, Hunt PA, Matsuura JS, Wilson CC, Szulman AE.** Complete and partial hydatidiform mole in Hawaii: cytogenetics, morphology and epidemiology. *Br J Obstet Gynaecol* 1982;89: 258–266.

96. **Buckley J.** Choriocarcinoma. In: **Schottenfeld D, Fraumeni JF Jr, eds.** *Cancer epidemiology and prevention,* 2nd ed. Philadelphia: Oxford University Press, 1996.

97. **Berkowitz RS, Cramer DW, Bernstein MR, Cassells S, Driscoll SG, Goldstein DP.** Risk factors for complete molar pregnancy from a case-control study. *Am J Obstet Gynecol* 1985;152:1016–1020.

98. **O'Toole BA, Fradkin R, Warkany J, Wilson JG, Mann GV.** Vitamin A deficiency and reproduction in rhesus monkeys. *J Nutr* 1974;104:1513–1524.

99. **Evans HM, Lepkovsky S, Murphy EA.** Vital need of the body for certain unsaturated fatty acids. VI. Male sterility on fat-free diets. *J Biol Chem* 1934;106:445–450.

100. **Kim HL, Picciano MF, O'Brien W.** Influence of maternal dietary protein and fat levels on fetal growth in mice. *Growth* 1981;45:8–18.

101. **McLaren DS.** Present knowledge of the role of vitamin A in health and disease. *Trans R Soc Trop Med Hyg* 1966;60:436–462.

102. **La Vecchia C, Franceschi S, Parazzini F, Fasoli M, Decarli A, Gallus G, et al.** Risk factors for gestational trophoblastic disease in Italy. *Am J Epidemiol* 1985;121:457–464.

103. **Parazzini F, La Vecchia C, Franceschi S, Pampallona S, Decarli A, Mangili G, et al.** ABO blood-groups and the risk of gestational trophoblastic disease. *Tumori* 1985;71:123–126.

104. **Parazzini F, Mangili G, La Vecchia C, Negri E, Bocciolone L, Fasoli M.** Risk factors for gestational trophoblastic disease: a separate analysis of complete and partial hydatidiform moles. *Obstet Gynecol* 1991;78:1039–1045.

105. **Palmer JR, Driscoll SG, Rosenberg L, Berkowitz RS, Lurain JR, Soper J, et al.** Oral contraceptive use and risk of gestational trophoblastic tumors. *J Natl Cancer Inst* 1999;91:635–640.

106. **Baltazar JC.** Epidemiological features of choriocarcinoma. *Bull World Health Organ* 1976;54:523–532.

107. **Ha MC, Cordier S, Bard D, Le TB, Hoang AH, Hoang TQ, et al.** Agent orange and the risk of gestational trophoblastic disease in Vietnam. *Arch Environ Health* 1996;51:368–374.

108. **Altieri A, Franceschi S, Ferlay J, Smith J, La Vecchia C.** Epidemiology and aetiology of gestational trophoblastic diseases. *Lancet* Oncol 2003;4:670–678.

109. **Cole P, Morrison AS.** Basic issues in population screening for cancer. *J Natl Cancer Inst* 1980;64:1263–1272.

110. **Saslow D, Runowicz CD, Solomon D, Moscicki AB, Smith RA, Eyre HJ, et al.** American Cancer Society guideline for the early detection of cervical neoplasia and cancer. *CA Cancer J Clin* 2002;52:342–362.

111. **ACOG Committee on Gynecologic Practice.** Committee Opinion on Routine Cancer Screening No. 247. Washington DC: American College of Obstetricians and Gynecologists, 2000.

112. **Sawaya GF, McConnell KJ, Kulasingam SL, Lawson HW, Kerlikowske K, Melnikow J, et al.** Risk of cervical cancer associated with extending the interval between cervical-cancer screenings. *N Engl J Med* 2003;349:1501–1509.

113. **Mayrand MH, Duarte-Franco E, Rodrigues I, Walter SD, Hanley J, Ferenczy A, et al.** Human papillomavirus DNA versus Papanicolaou screening tests for cervical cancer. *N Engl J Med* 2007;357:1579–1588.

114. **Mandelblatt JS, Lawrence WF, Womack SM, Jacobson D, Yi B, Hwang YT, et al.** Benefits and costs of using HPV testing to screen for cervical cancer. *JAMA* 2002;287:2372–2381.

115. **Burke W, Daly M, Garber J, Botkin J, Kahn MJ, Lynch P, et al.** Recommendations for follow-up care of individuals with an inherited predisposition to cancer. II. *BRCA1* and *BRCA2*. Cancer Genetics Studies Consortium. *JAMA* 1997;277:997–1003.

116. **Menon U, Jacobs IJ.** Ovarian cancer screening in the general population. *Curr Opin Obstet Gynecol* 2001;13:61–64.

7 Tumor Markers and Screening

Ranjit Manchanda
Ian Jacobs
Usha Menon

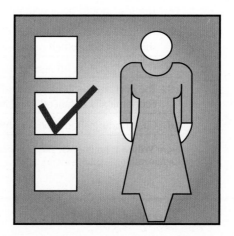

Approximately one in three women develop cancer in their lifetime (1,2), and one in four die from the disease (3,4). Gynecological malignancies account for 12% of these cancers (2). In the last 30 years, the age-standardized incidence rates of cancers in women has increased by 32% (1975–2004). However, from 1993 to 2004, the increase was limited to 3% (2). Nevertheless, even this latter figure is two- to threefold greater than the increase in cancers in men. Most of this increase has occurred in the postmenopausal population.

Among the established strategies for combating cancer in the twenty-first century is screening the asymptomatic population for premalignant conditions and early stage disease. **Such screening strategies are based on criteria laid down by the World Health Organization (WHO) (5) (Table 7.1). Mass screening for cervical cancer fulfills most of these tenets,** and organized screening programs in numerous countries have led to a significant reduction in cervical cancer mortality (6–9).

Ovarian cancer is the other gynecological malignancy that may meet the criteria of a disease for which population screening is justified (10). The disease is usually diagnosed in advanced stages when chances for long-term survival are poor. Effective treatment is available for early stage disease, and there is preliminary evidence that early detection may increase long-term survival. In a randomized controlled trial of ovarian cancer screening, a strategy incorporating sequential CA125 and transvaginal ultrasound was found to significantly increase median survival in women with ovarian cancer in the screened group (72.9 months) when compared with the control group (41.8 months) (11). Annual transvaginal ultrasonic (TVS) screening has been found to decrease disease stage at detection and increase case-specific ovarian cancer survival in a recent trial involving 25,327 women. Eighty-two percent of women who had screen-detected ovarian cancer had early stage (I or II) disease versus 34% of women in the unscreened control group ($p < 0.0001$) (12).

Mass screening for endometrial cancer is unlikely to be of benefit in the low-risk population because women present in early stages with symptomatic disease. However, screening of "high-risk" populations is recommended (13–15). Vaginal and vulvar cancers are too rare to justify screening, although it is important to raise the awareness of these conditions among the elderly population.

Table 7.1 World Health Organization Criteria for a Screening Program
1. The condition sought should be an important health problem.
2. There should be accepted treatment for patients with recognized disease.
3. Facilities for diagnosis and treatment should be available.
4. There should be a recognizable latent or early symptomatic stage.
5. There should be a suitable test or examination.
6. The test should be acceptable to the population.
7. The natural history of the condition, including development from latent to declared disease, should be adequately understood.
8. There should be an agreed policy on whom to screen.
9. The cost of case finding (including diagnosis and treatment of patients diagnosed) should be economically balanced in relation to possible expenditure on medical care as a whole.
10. Case finding should be a continuing process and not a "once and for all" project.

From **Wilson J, Jungner G.** *WHO principles and practice of screening for disease.* Geneva: World Health Organization, 1968:66–67 (5).

Tumor Markers

Tumor markers are molecules or substances produced by or in response to neoplastic proliferation that enter the circulation in detectable amounts. They indicate the likely presence of cancer or provide information about its behavior. **For screening protocols, the value of the marker depends heavily on its sensitivity (proportion of cancers detected by a positive test) and specificity (proportion of those without cancer identified by a negative test), which must be well established before it is adopted into routine practice.** An ideal tumor marker would have a 100% sensitivity, specificity, and positive predictive value. However, in practice this is never achieved. **The most limiting factor is *lack of specificity*** because the majority of markers are tumor associated rather than tumor specific and are elevated in multiple cancers as well as in benign and physiological conditions. In most diseases, tumor markers are therefore not diagnostic but contribute to differential diagnosis. They may also have an important role to play in screening, determining therapeutic efficacy, detecting recurrence, and predicting prognosis.

A wide variety of macromolecular tumor antigens—including enzymes, hormones, receptors, growth factors, biological response modifiers, and glycoconjugates—have been investigated as potential tumor markers. Innovative screening strategies using new microarray and mass-spectrometry–based technologies exploring DNA, RNA, and protein overexpression are constantly identifying novel biomarkers that could complement those previously identified by candidate gene or antibody-based techniques. This chapter will focus on the different tumor markers relevant to gynecological malignancies and their role in screening.

Despite significant research into a large variety of markers, the number of clinically useful markers is limited. Poor study design that leads to inconsistent conclusions has been cited as an important reason. General guidelines on the application and use of tumor markers have been developed by a number of multidisciplinary groups following critical appraisal of available evidence (16–20). **The National Cancer Institute's Early Detection Research Network has suggested five phases for biomarker development: preclinical exploration, clinical assays and validation, retrospective longitudinal repository studies, prospective screening studies, and conducting clinical randomized trials** for assessing end points of cancer screening. Guidelines covering methodological issues related to measurement and internal and external quality control have also been published. However, systematic reviews such as those conducted by Cochrane Collaboration are lacking in relation to tumor markers.

The evaluation of exfoliated cells has been used for many decades. In gynecology, the cervical screening program was based on nucleocytoplasmic changes detected on microscopy of Papanicolaou stained cells obtained from cervical sampling. These changes do not entirely fulfill the criteria for true tumor markers because their presence usually denotes an underlying premalignant condition—cervical intraepithelial neoplasia—rather than frank malignancy. **There are now an increasing number of sophisticated molecular techniques available for examining key events associated with the carcinogenesis, including the presence of high-risk human papilloma virus (HPV) DNA, telomerase activity, and *K-ras* mutation in cervical secretions.**

A variety of imaging modalities are in use to identify morphological characteristics of cancer. These features, although not highly specific, may serve as very sensitive markers for screening. In gynecology, real-time ultrasound is most commonly used because it has minimal side effects and provides detailed tumor morphology, which can be quantified using a variety of scoring systems. **Detailed characterization of morphology on transvaginal scanning is an important component of both ovarian and endometrial cancer screening.**

Neovascularization associated with malignancy is another marker that has been exploited in screening for genital cancers. Color-flow Doppler is used to detect altered patterns of blood flow and decreased resistance in the thin-walled new vessels in ovarian and endometrial cancers. Colposcopy exploits the same phenomenon in an entirely different manner: The abnormal new vessels are directly visualized as patterns of mosaicism and punctation.

An important aspect of screening is defining the risk groups. Even for cervical cancer, where mass screening is the norm, age is used to define the population undergoing screening. In the United Kingdom, current screening guidelines limit screening to women between ages 25 and 64 years (21). Risk groups for sporadic ovarian cancer are defined by age ($\geq$50) in clinical trials and for hereditary ovarian malignancy by family history criteria and the presence of *BRCA1* or *BRCA2* mutations. Increased risk based on family history is also the basis of defining a target population for endometrial cancer screening.

Ovarian and Fallopian Tube Cancer

Ovarian cancer accounts for 4% of cancers occurring in women, with more than 190,000 new cases diagnosed worldwide each year. Incidence rates are highest in the United States and Northern Europe and the lowest in Africa and Asia. **It is the most common gynecological cancer in England and Wales, with women having a 2.1% lifetime risk of developing the disease** (22). It is also the most lethal because of the advanced stage at which most women present. Approximately 85% of cases occur after age 50, and 80% to 85% of cancers are epithelial in origin. Traditionally, serous tumors are the most common, present at an advanced stage, and have the poorest outcome (23). However, in the reproductive age group, germ-cell tumors, granulosa cell and sex-cord tumors, and mucinous and endometrioid tumors are more common.

Deficiencies in our knowledge of the molecular and biologic events in ovarian carcinogenesis have hampered our ability to screen for this disease. **A screen-detectable precursor lesion for ovarian cancer has not been identified,** limiting the goal of screening to detection of asymptomatic, early stage disease (10). Biochemical, morphological, vascular, and cytological tumor markers have all been explored with varying success. Even though screening can detect cancers early (24), and a survival benefit has been reported, **there is as yet only preliminary evidence that ovarian cancer screening may reduce mortality** (11). In addition, it is not known whether the screen-detected early stage disease will include a significant number of high-grade serous carcinomas or just the better prognosis histological cancers. **Until a mortality impact has been reported, women in the general population should not be screened outside the context of research trials.** The ongoing trials are expected to report around 2012 to 2014 and should help address the above issues.

Biochemical Markers

CA125

CA125 is a 200-kilodalton (kd) glycoprotein recognized by the OC125 murine monoclonal antibody and first described by Bast et al. in 1981 (25). Recently on cloning, it was found to have characteristics of mucin designated as MUC16 (26). It carries two major antigenic domains, classified as A, the domain-binding monoclonal antibody OC125; and B, the domain-binding monoclonal antibody M11 (27). The first CA125 immunoassay used the OC125 antibody for both capture and detection (28,29). **The second-generation heterologous CA125 II** assay incorporates M11 and OC125 antibodies and is now widely used for measuring CA125. There are a number of CA125 assays available, most of which correlate well with each other and are clinically reliable (30). However, differences in reagent specificities and assay design can lead to variation in values obtained, and the results may not be interchangeable. **Change in methodology may require baseline samples to be retested or parallel tested using both assays (30,31). This may be of importance for patients who are undergoing serial monitoring such as in screening trials.**

CA125 is not specific to ovarian cancer and is widely distributed in adult tissues. **It is found in structures derived from the coelomic epithelium (such as endocervix, endometrium, and fallopian tube) and in tissues developed from mesothelial cells (such as pleura, pericardium, and peritoneum)** (32). It is expressed in the normal adult ovary (33) and has also been characterized in epithelial tissues of the colon, pancreas, lung, kidney, prostate, breast, stomach, and gall bladder (28,34).

CA125 levels in body fluids or ovarian cysts do not correlate well with serum levels. Serum concentration is a function not only of production of antigen by the tumor but also of other factors that affect its release into the circulation (35). **The widely adopted cutoff value of 35 U/mL is based upon the distribution of values in healthy subjects, where 99% of 888 men and women were found to have levels below 35 U/mL** (36). **However, CA125 values can show wide variation and are influenced by age, race, menstrual cycle, pregnancy, hysterectomy, and a number of benign conditions.** In postmenopausal women, CA125 levels tend to be lower than in the general population, and levels below 20 U/mL have been found (37–40). Levels fluctuate during the menstrual cycle and increase during menstruation (28,41). Levels in white women have been found to be higher than in African or Asian women (42). Caffeine intake, hysterectomy, and smoking in some (42) but not all reports (43,44) have been found to be associated with lower levels of CA125 (42).

A number of benign gynecological conditions such as endometriosis, fibroids, infections, and pelvic inflammatory disease may increase CA125. In pregnancy, peak CA125 values occur in the first trimester and postpartum (28,45–49), with wide fluctuations in levels as high as 300 U/mL, being reported at these times (28,46–48), and return to normal by 10 weeks postpartum (47). Levels of 112 U/mL and 65 U/mL have been found to correspond to the ninety-ninth percentile and the ninety-sixth percentile in the first trimester, respectively (50,51), but ideally different levels need to be defined for different stages of pregnancy and puerperium (52). **CA125 may also be elevated by nongynecological diseases causing any inflammation of the peritoneum, pleura or pericardium, pancreatitis, hepatitis, cirrhosis, ascites, tuberculosis, and other malignancies such as pancreatic, breast, colon, and lung cancer** (28,34). The benign and physiological conditions associated with an elevated CA125 can cause false positive results when CA125 is used in diagnosis or screening.

Approximately 85% of patients with epithelial ovarian cancer have CA125 levels of >35 U/mL (36,53), with elevated levels found in 50% of patients with stage I disease and more than 90% of patients with stage II to IV disease (28). CA125 levels are less frequently elevated in mucinous and borderline tumors compared to serous tumors (28,54,55).

CA125 can be elevated in the preclinical asymptomatic phase of the disease because raised levels were found in 25% of 59 stored serum samples collected 5 years before the diagnosis of ovarian cancer (38).

In a prospective ovarian cancer screening study of Swedish women, a specificity of 97% and positive predictive value (PPV) of 4.6% was achieved using CA125 (30 U/mL) in 4,290 volunteers aged 50 years and older (56). Recently published data from the Shizuoka Cohort Study on Ovarian Cancer Screening (SCSOCS) found that **the interval between the first detection of a slightly elevated CA125 level and the diagnosis of disease at surgery was significantly shorter in patients with serous-type ovarian cancer,** compared with those with nonserous-type disease (1.4 vs. 3.8 years, $p = 0.011$) (57). Although 47% nonserous-type ovarian cancers developed from slightly elevated CA125 levels between 35 and 65 U/mL, 75% serous ovarian cancers developed suddenly from a normal CA125 level (<35 U/mL) (57).

In postmenopausal women, an elevated CA125 in the absence of ovarian cancer has been found to be a risk factor for death from other malignant disease (58,59). These findings have implications when screening asymptomatic postmenopausal women.

Improving Sensitivity, Specificity, and Discriminatory Ability

Pelvic Ultrasound as a Second-Line Test

Specificity of screening with CA125 was initially improved by the addition of pelvic ultrasound as a second-line test to assess ovarian volume and morphology. Using multimodal screening incorporating sequential CA125 measurements and pelvic ultrasound, a specificity of 99.9% and PPV of 26.8% for detection of ovarian and fallopian tube cancer were achieved in 22,000 postmenopausal women (60,61). With the accumulation of data, ovarian morphology has been used to refine algorithms for the interpretation of ultrasound in postmenopausal women with elevated CA125 levels (62,63).

Risk of Ovarian Cancer Algorithm

Developing a more sophisticated approach to replace absolute cutoff levels for interpretation of CA125 titers has made further improvements to the strategy. Detailed analysis of more than 50,000 serum CA125 levels involving 22,000 volunteers followed up for a median of 8.6 years in the study by Jacobs et al. (11,61) revealed that **elevated CA125 levels in women without ovarian cancer were static or decreased with time, whereas levels associated with malignancy tended to rise. This finding has been incorporated into a computerized algorithm that uses an individual's age-specific incidence of ovarian cancer and CA125 profile to estimate her risk of ovarian cancer (ROC)** (64–66). The closer the CA125 profile to the CA125 behavior of known cases of ovarian cancer, the greater the ROC. The final result is presented as the individual's estimated risk of having ovarian cancer, so an ROC of 2% implies a risk of 1 in 50. **The ROC algorithm increases the sensitivity of CA125 compared with a single cutoff value because women with normal but rising levels are identified as being at increased risk. At the same time, specificity is improved because women with static but elevated levels are now classified as low risk.** For a target specificity of 98%, the ROC calculation achieved a sensitivity of 86% for preclinical detection of ovarian cancer (64).

When evaluated prospectively in a pilot randomized controlled trial of ovarian cancer screening, the specificity and PPV for primary invasive EOC were 99.8% (CI 99.7 to 99.9) and 19% (CI 4.1 to 45.6), respectively (67). It is part of the ongoing U.K. Collaborative Trial of Ovarian Cancer Screening (UKCTOCS) (available at: http://www.ukctocs.org.uk) (Figure 7.1).

The ROC algorithm is also being evaluated prospectively in pilot ovarian cancer screening trials in high-risk women under the auspices of the Cancer Genetics Network (CGN) and Gynecology Oncology Group (GOG) in the United States and in the Familial Ovarian Cancer Screening Study in the United Kingdom (UKFOCSS). The ROC algorithm is used to triage women into low-, intermediate-, and elevated-risk categories based on their CA125 result. Intermediate risk women have a repeat CA125 in 6 to 8 weeks, whereas those with elevated risk are referred for a TVS. An abnormal TVS leads to gynecological assessment with view to surgery.

Panel of Markers

Accurate discrimination between benign and malignant masses is essential to avoid unnecessary operations in women with benign lesions and to plan suitable surgery by appropriately trained gynecologic oncologists in tertiary care centers for those with cancer (68–72). Both prospective and retrospective data show that CA125 can be used as an adjunct in distinguishing benign and malignant masses, particularly in postmenopausal women (73–76). Using an upper limit of 35 U/mL, a sensitivity of 78%, specificity of 95%, and PPV of 82% can be achieved for ovarian cancer.

One option of improving diagnostic accuracy is using a combination or panel of markers rather than a single biomarker. However, increased sensitivity obtained is often associated with decreased specificity. TATI, CA19-9, CA72-4, and carcinoembryonic antigen (CEA) in addition to CA125 may be useful in mucinous ovarian cancer (77). Increased preoperative sensitivity for early stage disease has been reported by combining CA125 with CA72-4, CA15-3, and macrophage-colony stimulating factor (M-CSF) (78). The majority of earlier studies however reported limited ability to improve diagnostic sensitivity by the addition of other serum markers for patients with nonmucinous tumors (79–82). A panel of eight different markers—CA125, M-CSF, OVX1, lipid-associated sialic acid (LASA), CA15-3, CA72-4, CA19-9, and CA54/61—improved the sensitivity for discriminating malignant from benign pelvic masses (83). Using the same data set, a subset of four markers analyzed using an

237

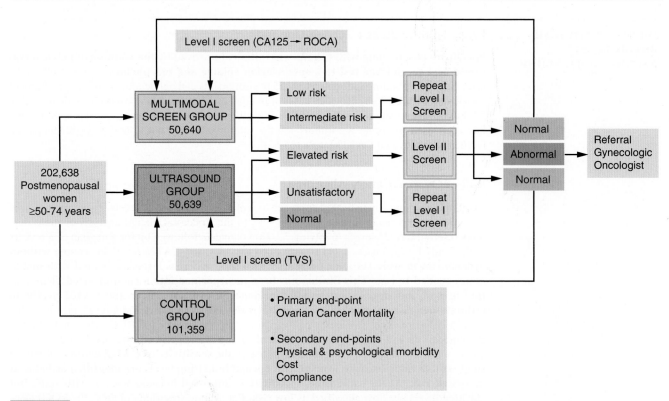

Figure 7.1   **The United Kingdom Collaborative Trial of Ovarian Cancer Screening (http://www.ukctocs.org.uk).** After a normal risk of ovarian cancer (ROC) (<1 in 2,000), a repeat CA125 level is done in 1 year: after an intermediate ROC (>1 in 2,000 to <1 in 500), a repeat CA125 level is done in 6 weeks; and after an elevated ROC (>1 in 500), a transvaginal ultrasound and CA125 level are done in 6 to 8 weeks. The primary outcome is mortality from ovarian or fallopian tube cancer. Follow-up is by postal questionnaire and the U.K. Office of National Statistics. Women in the screened arm undergo six screens, and each woman is in the trial for 7 years.

artificial neural network demonstrated improved specificity over CA125 alone (87.5% vs. 68.4%) while maintaining comparable sensitivity (79.0% vs. 82.4%) (84). In addition, greater specificity using multiple markers might be attained if serial values were employed as in the case of CA125. Preliminary data on a panel of five serum tumor markers obtained during 6 years of follow-up of 1,257 healthy women at high risk of ovarian cancer showed substantial heterogeneity of tumor marker patterns and indicated that a fixed screening cutoff level may be suboptimal to a degree that depends strongly on intraclass correlation coefficient (ICC). **Longitudinal marker levels (trends) and the ICC can lead to the development of individual-specific screening rules to improve early detection of ovarian cancer** (85).

Recently, **a preliminary report using a panel of six markers (leptin, prolactin, osteopontin, macrophage inhibitory factor, IGF-2, and CA125) found much improved sensitivity and specificity over CA125 alone** (86). Immunohistochemical data suggested that HE4 and mesothelin may be discriminatory in CA125-negative cancers (87). A recent analysis with a panel of nine markers—CA125, SMRP, HE4, CA72-4, activin, inhibin, osteopontin, epidermal growth factor, and ERBB2 (HER2)—found that the **addition of HE4 to CA125 without the use of ultrasound increased sensitivity to 76.4% at a specificity of 90% and 81% at a specificity of 90%. HE4 was found to be the single most sensitive marker and also improved detection of early stage disease** (88). The addition of HE4 may hold more promise in premenopausal women because it is elevated in ovarian cancer and not as frequently elevated in benign conditions commonly found in younger women. Further investigation of these markers in serum is underway.

Other Tumor Markers

Although a vast number of serum markers have been investigated, only a few have been validated for clinical use. Limited sensitivities and specificities constrain their use for screening purposes. In the past 5 years, significant progress has been made in developing novel tumor markers for early detection of ovarian cancer (Table 7.2). Most of these studies have used samples from women with clinically diagnosed ovarian cancer (i.e., in the differential diagnosis of ovarian cancer) as opposed to asymptomatic women with preclinical disease (i.e., early detection of ovarian cancer). Ovarian cancer tumor markers not associated with recent publications are not detailed in this chapter. They include CA15-3, CASA, CEA, tetranectin, tumor associated trypsin inhibitor (TATI), lysophosphatidic acid, LASA, lactate dehydrogenase, galactosyltransferase associated with tumor, OVX1, shed glycans, growth factors, CA130, HER-2/neu, p105, AKT2 gene, and sialyl SSEA-1 antigen.

Table 7.2 Tumor Markers That May Be Useful in Screening for Ovarian Carcinoma	
Tumor Marker	**Description**
HE4	Human epididymis protein 4 (HE4) is a glycoprotein in the epithelial cells of the epididymis. Increased HE4 serum levels and expression of the HE4 *WAP four-disulfide core domain 2 (WFCD2)* gene has been found to occur in ovarian cancer (89–93). It may also be increased in lung, pancreatic, breast, and transitional cell cancers (94). Initial reports suggest that it is a **promising new marker.** It was found to have higher specificity compared to CA125 (95) and to be of particular value in detecting early stage disease (88). **A combination of HE4 and CA125 was recently found to increase sensitivity while maintaining specificity** (88).
CA72-4 or TAG 72	**Cancer antigen 72-4 or tumor-associated glycoprotein 72** (TAG 72) is a glycoprotein surface antigen found in colon, gastric, and ovarian cancer (96). Levels are elevated in 50%–67% of ovarian cancers (96,97) with **a better sensitivity than CA125 for mucinous tumors** (98,99). CA72-4 has high specificity for ovarian malignancy and, **in combination with CA125, may increase discriminatory ability**, though reports are slightly conflicting on the impact on sensitivity (96,97,99,100). The combination of CA125II, CA72-4, and M-CSF significantly increased preoperative sensitivity for early stage disease (from 45% with CA125II alone to 70%) while maintaining 98% specificity (78).
Cytokines	A number of cytokines have been evaluated as potential tumor markers in ovarian cancers. **Macrophage-colony stimulating factor** appears to be a marker of high specificity, with levels correlating to stage. When combined with other markers, it may have a role in early detection (78,101,102). M-CSF may also be sensitive and specific for malignant germ-cell tumors of the ovary, especially dysgerminoma (103). In 187 ovarian cancer patients, **IL-7** in combination with CA125 was found to accurately predict 69% of the ovarian cancer patients without falsely classifying patients with a benign pelvic mass (104). **Immunosuppressive acidic protein** may be useful in differentiating early stage disease (105). **Soluble interleukin-2 receptor** is elevated in patients with advanced ovarian cancer (106), though reports on its utility as a discriminatory marker are conflicting (107,108). Assay of **soluble receptors of tumor necrosis factor (TNF)**—serum 55 kd and 75 kd TNFr—might have potential clinical value in detection, monitoring, and prognostic prediction (109–111).
OVX1	**Monoclonal antibody OVX1 recognizes an antigenic determinant present in ovarian and breast cancer cells** (112). A combination of OVX1, M-CSF, and CA125 can detect a greater fraction of patients with stage I ovarian cancer than CA125 alone, but this is accompanied by an additive effect on false positives (113,114).
Prostasin	**Prostasin is a serine protease that is normally present in prostatic secretions** (115). Overexpression of the prostasin gene was found to occur in ovarian cancer using gene expression profiling by cDNA microarrays and real-time quantitative polymerase chain reaction (116). Preliminary data suggest it may be of benefit in detecting early stage disease. Combining prostasin with CA125 gave a sensitivity of 92% and specificity of 94% for detecting nonmucinous ovarian cancer (116). Further studies are needed to explore and validate the potential of prostasin, either alone or in combination with CA125.

(Continued)

Table 7.2 Tumor Markers That May Be Useful in Screening for Ovarian Carcinoma *(Continued)*	
Tumor Marker	*Description*
Osteopontin	**Osteopontin is another biomarker that has been identified by exploiting gene-expression profiling techniques.** Contrary to an initial report (117), plasma osteopontin levels have been found to be higher in ovarian cancer cases compared to healthy controls, other cancers, and benign and borderline ovarian disease (118). Levels also correlate with ascites, bulky disease, and recurrence (119). In combination with CA125, it may therefore be a useful biomarker because it was found to increase its sensitivity for detecting ovarian cancer from 81% to 94% (87,120).
Cytokeratins	**Tissue polypeptide-specific (TPS) antigen** assay uses a specific monoclonal antibody against cytokeratin 18. It is better able to distinguish between different cytokeratins, leading to increased specificity. TPS is elevated in 50–77% of ovarian cancers studied with a specificity of 84–85% (121–125). Preoperatively, TPS levels have been found to correlate well with the diagnosis of cancer and the stage of disease. It has been suggested that a combination of CA125 and TPS may have an additive benefit because the former performs better in mucinous tumors (125).
Kallikrein	Kallikreins are serine proteases encoded by 15 genes (126) and are part of an enzymatic cascade pathway that is activated in ovarian cancer and other malignant diseases. Several kallikreins—4, 5, 6, 7, 8, 9, 10, 11, 13, 14, and 15—have been shown to have a role in detection, diagnosis, monitoring, and prognostication of ovarian cancer (126–145). As part of a panel of biomarkers, they may complement and improve performance of CA125. The exact role of kallikreins is evolving and is still a matter of research.
AFP	Alpha fetoprotein (AFP) is a 70-kd glycoprotein that is synthesized initially in the yolk sac, fetal liver, and intestine (146). Levels are raised in pregnancy, liver disease, and gastric, pancreatic, colon, and bronchogenic malignancies. **Elevated levels are found mainly with germ cell ovarian tumors (100% with endodermal sinus or yolk sac tumors, 33–62% with immature teratomas, and 12% with dysgerminoma and embryonal tumors)** (147,148) and rarely with ectopic production in EOC (149,150). AFP also accurately predicts the presence of yolk sac elements in mixed germ cell tumors (151).
Inhibin	**Serum inhibin is elevated in ovarian sex-cord–stromal tumors (granulosa cell tumors, or GCTs)** and has a role in differential diagnosis and surveillance of these malignancies (152–155). Both inhibin A and, more commonly, inhibin B may be secreted by GCTs (156,157). Inhibin assays that detect all inhibin forms—i.e., assays that detect the alpha subunit both as the free form and as an alphabeta subunit dimer—provide the highest sensitivity and specificity as ovarian cancer diagnostic tests (158). Total inhibin and pro-alpha C (pro-αC) immunoreactive forms are most commonly elevated, though, so pro-αC is unlikely to be a useful marker by itself (159–162). Combining pro-αC with CA125 may improve the sensitivity for detection of EOC (160). Recently, **total inhibin was found to have high sensitivity and specificity for serous and mucinous cancer; these improved in combination with CA125** (162).
Activin	Serum activin A is reported to be significantly **elevated in epithelial ovarian cancer,** with particularly high levels detected in undifferentiated tumors (156,163,164).
CA19-9	CA19-9 is a Lewis antigen derivative, and levels in pregnancy do not exceed the normal cutoff of 37 U/mL (165,166). Mucinous ovarian cancers express the antigen more frequently (76%) than serous tumors (27%) (45,167). **It is useful in detecting borderline and CA125-negative mucinous ovarian tumors** (54,168,169).
VEGF	Vascular endothelial growth factor (VEGF) is a promoter of angiogenesis and may play a pivotal role in tumor growth and metastasis. Preliminary data showed that serum VEGF on its own had a poor sensitivity (54%) and was not effective in differentiating adnexal masses (170). Subsequently, it has been **used as part of a panel of markers along with Doppler sonography to distinguish between benign and malignant ovarian masses** (171).

Newer High-Throughput Approaches

Proteomics

Proteomics is the study of the expression, structure, and function of all proteins as a function of state, time, age, and environment (172–174). **In the era of proteomics, there has been a great deal of interest in identifying global patterns of serum proteins and peptides that relate to cancer risk.** A wide range of techniques is now available for protein identification and characterization in which high sensitivity and specificity is combined with high throughput.

Mass spectrometry (MS) techniques commonly used to volatize and ionize proteins and peptides include electrospray ionization, surface-enhanced laser desorption ionization time-of-flight (SELDI-TOF) analysis, and matrix-associated laser desorption ionization time-of-flight analysis. These technologies have the potential to identify patterns or changes in thousand of proteins less than 20 kd. When combined with matrixes that selectively absorb certain serum proteins, these approaches can globally analyze almost all small proteins in complex solutions such as serum or plasma (175,176). **A combination of mass spectra generated by these new technologies and artificial-intelligence–based informatic algorithms has been used to discover small sets of key protein values that discriminate normal from ovarian cancer patients** (177). Two different proteomic approaches used include identification of a discriminatory pattern of peaks on mass spectroscopy and proteomic analysis to identify a limited number of critical markers that may then be assayed by more conventional methods. The latter seems more promising but requires further development.

A number of studies have reported better diagnostic sensitivities and specificities of MS-generated profiles compared to established biomarkers (178–181). In a preliminary study, SELDI-TOF, in combination with powerful computer algorithms, identified an ovarian cancer specific serum protein signature with a sensitivity of 100%, specificity of 95%, and PPV of 94% (178). Three potential serum biomarkers for early stage ovarian cancer were identified: apolipoprotein A1 (down regulated), a truncated form of transthyretin (down regulated), and a cleavage fragment of inter-alpha-trypsin inhibitor heavy chain H4 (ITIH4, up regulated) (179). These were subsequently validated (182). SELDI-MS and artificial intelligence technology was used to identify four distinct protein peaks in plasma samples with a sensitivity of 90% to 96.3% and specificity of 100% (183). A potential biomarker to distinguish borderline from invasive cancer was reported using MALDI-MS (184), and a recent report presented a list of 80 putative biomarkers as a base for further research (185).

The initial euphoria has been significantly moderated by a number of reports pointing out potential problems and limitations related to such things as cross-platform reliability, reproducibility, and standardization of sample handling, processing, and analytical sensitivity of minute samples (186–200). Changes in preanalytical handling variables (e.g., transportation, room temperature, incubation time) affect profiles of serum proteins, including proposed disease biomarkers (186). A different approach from healthy donors and from ovarian cancer patients has shown that CA125 remains the best single marker for nonmucinous ovarian cancer, complemented by CA15-3 or soluble mesothelin-related protein (187).

Advances in bioinformatics are leading to the development of sophisticated algorithms to analyze the large volume of preprocessed mass-spectrometric data and identify the most informative "common" peaks, but these approaches still need further refinement (188–190). The implications of such proteomic spectrum analysis for the identification of novel tumor markers are huge. Well-designed, large prospective, multicenter clinical trials are required to validate and standardize this technology (191,192). **It is likely that future early detection of ovarian cancer (and other cancers) will include markers discovered through proteomic profiling.**

Metobolomics, Epigenetics, and Epigenomics

Metabolomics refers to the rapid, high-throughput characterization and quantification of small-molecule metabolites. Metabolites are the end products of cellular regulatory processes. **Preliminary data suggest that metabolomics is a promising automated approach, in addition to functional genomics and proteomics, for analyses of molecular changes in malignant tumors.** Analysis of quantitative signatures of primary metabolites in 66 invasive ovarian carcinomas and nine borderline ovarian tumors by gas chromatography and time-of-flight mass spectrometry showed a separation of 88% of the borderline tumors from the carcinomas (193).

Epigenetic mechanisms have been shown to be extremely important in the initiation and progression of human cancer (194). DNA released from dead cancer cells varies in size, whereas DNA released from nondiseased cells undergoing apoptosis is uniformly truncated (195). Freely circulating hypermethylated tumor-derived DNA has been shown to be present in serum or plasma of patients with cancer (196,197). Circulating tumor DNA may serve as a surrogate marker for active, fast-growing invasive tumors (198). However, **before the clinical utility of circulating epigenetic markers can be determined, a number of issues related to standardization of methodology, type of assay, reproducibility, efficacy, and comparison with other markers need to be addressed** (198).

Morphological Markers

Real-time ultrasonic screening is aimed at detecting the earliest possible architectural changes in the ovary that accompany carcinogenesis. Both ovarian volume and morphology are assessed with cutoffs for volume ranging from 10 mL to 20 mL, depending on menopausal status (199). The transvaginal route is preferred because its better resolution leads to a more accurate assessment of ovarian and endometrial morphology and does not require a full bladder.

The persistence of abnormalities on repeat scanning 4 to 6 weeks after initial detection helps to reduce false positive rates (200). The lack of physiological changes in ovarian volume in postmenopausal women further decreases the number of false positives in this group compared with premenopausal women. However, even in older women, there is a high prevalence of benign ovarian lesions. In an ultrasonic and histopathological autopsy study of 52 consecutive postmenopausal women who died from causes other than gynecological or intraperitoneal cancer, 56% were found to have a benign adnexal lesion as much as 50 mm in diameter (201). Ultrasonography used in this manner can therefore lead to the detection of many benign ovarian tumors, which results in unnecessary surgery in healthy, asymptomatic women. As data accumulate with long-term follow-up of the participants of the early screening trials, it has been possible to further define the risk of ovarian cancer associated with various ultrasonic findings. **Unilocular ovarian cysts <10 cm in diameter are found in 18% of asymptomatic postmenopausal women older than 50 years and are associated with an extremely low risk of malignancy.**

Restricting the definition of abnormality to complex ovarian morphology to interpret pelvic ultrasound increases the specificity and PPV in multimodal screening (63). In contrast, complex ovarian cysts with wall abnormalities or solid areas are associated with a significant risk of malignancy (200,202).

To further decrease the number of false positives, some screening protocols use a weighted scoring system or morphological index based on ovarian volume, outline, presence of papillary projections, and cyst complexity (i.e., number of locules, wall structure, thickness of septae, and echogenicity of fluid). There is no standardized index as yet, with systems varying on the number and type of variables evaluated (203–208). Others use subjective assessment of the gray-scale images. Based on gross anatomic changes at the time of surgery, papillary projections have the highest and simple cysts and septal thickness the lowest correlation with a diagnosis of ovarian malignancy (209). **Newer modalities, such as three-dimensional (3-D) ultrasound and 3-D power Doppler (210,211), pattern-recognition computer models, and artificial neural networks (212–215) may increase the reproducibility of results and improve ultrasonic performance.**

Subjective evaluation using gray scale and Doppler (pattern recognition) by an experienced examiner has been found to be better than either CA125 alone (216) or mathematical logistic regression models (215) in discriminating between benign and malignant disease. Recently, the International Ovarian Tumor Analysis (IOTA) study reported a logistic regression model incorporating 12 variables that included ultrasound-based pattern recognition and found that it was superior to CA125 alone for discriminating benign from malignant ovarian masses. Addition of CA125 values to the model did not improve its performance (217,218). **Ovarian histoscanning** is another ultrasound-based technique that may hold promise for the future (219). These technologies need external validation and further comparison with other established models.

Other second-line tests have been explored to reduce the false positive rate and facilitate discrimination between benign and malignant ovarian lesions. **The risk of malignancy index (RMI) combines serum CA125 values with ultrasonic-detected ovarian morphology and** menopausal status and has been widely used as a discriminatory tool for the primary evaluation of patients with an adnexal mass (220). It was initially reported to have a sensitivity of 85% and a specificity of 97% (220) and has been validated both retrospectively and prospectively in gynecological oncology and general gynecological units (221–229), with prospective studies reporting slightly lower sensitivity, specificity, and PPV (228,229). A recent comparison found it performed as well as most logistic regression models or artificial neural networks (230). Patients with an elevated RMI score had an average 42-fold increase in the background risk of ovarian cancer (220). A higher RMI sensitivity can be achieved by increasing the RMI cutoff (223–225), using artificial neural networks (213), or modifying the RMI calculation (226,227). In women with an RMI cutoff between 25 and 1,000, the addition of specialist ultrasound and magnetic resonance imaging improved sensitivity (94%) and specificity (90%) (231). Ultrasonic assessment for an "ovarian crescent sign" in women with an RMI above 200 has also been shown to improve accuracy (232).

There is a move toward conservative management of adnexal cysts judged to be benign at transvaginal ultrasonic examination when they are incidentally detected in post-menopausal women (233). Follow-up data on such women in ongoing randomized screening trials will be important in determining optimal strategies for operative intervention in screening.

Vascular Markers

Neovascularization is an obligate early event in tumor growth and neoplasia (234). Fast-growing tumors contain many new vessels that have less smooth muscle in their walls and therefore provide less resistance to blood flow when compared with vessels within benign ovarian tumors. **Color-flow Doppler imaging uses these altered blood-flow patterns as markers to differentiate malignant from physiologic and benign lesions.** It has been used both as a first-line screening test in combination with transvaginal ultrasound (235,236) and as a second-line test following an abnormal ultrasound (237,238) in both general and high-risk population screening.

The early promise of Doppler to differentiate between malignant and benign ovarian masses and therefore improve the specificity of ultrasound (235,236) **was initially not confirmed in subsequent studies** (208,239,240). Although it was demonstrated that the mean pulsatility index of vessels supplying ovarian cancers is lower than that of vessels supplying benign ovarian tumors, the overlap in vascular resistance between these two groups may prevent reliable separation of malignant from benign disease. However, more **recently, the International Ovarian Tumor Analysis (IOTA) group proposed a logistic regression model to distinguish between malignant and benign masses that incorporates both color Doppler flow indexes and tumor morphology assessed by gray-scale imaging.** A sensitivity of 93% and a specificity of 76% were achieved at a probability of 0.10 (217). This model was subsequently prospectively validated in a multicenter study (218).

It has been reported that lack of blood flow in an ovarian tumor, as detected by color Doppler, may preclude cancer (240). This was not substantiated in data from the Kentucky screening trial in which 6% of ovarian tumors without blood flow were malignant (208). Even when Doppler examinations were simplified and limited to the expression of internal color flow, gray-scale sonography was a more sensitive indicator of malignancy than Doppler sonography (241).

Key issues with regard to Doppler examination as a possible second-line study for ultrasound-based ovarian cancer screening protocols are (i) whether the examination should focus on quantitative or qualitative differences in blood flow within complex masses and (ii) the difficulties with interobserver variation and standardization. **Pattern-recognition models using a combination of gray-scale and color Doppler ultrasound have been found to be better than CA125 alone at discriminating between benign and malignant adnexal masses** (216). However, the effectiveness of a screening strategy that incorporates Doppler evaluation of ovarian masses in addition to gray-scale sonography has yet to be established. The UKCTOCS trial is collecting Doppler data on abnormal adnexal masses detected on ultrasonic screening, although these are not being used in the screening algorithm (http://www.ukctocs.org.uk). Recently, some studies have shown that three-dimensional power Doppler examinations may be more accurate than two-dimensional Doppler examinations (210,242), although this is also controversial (243).

Target Populations

Two distinct populations are at increased risk for ovarian cancer: the general population and a high-risk population.

General Population

The majority of ovarian cancers are sporadic and occur in the general population. **More than 90% of sporadic cancers occur in women older than 50 years,** so screening studies in the general population usually target this group. Some of the **other known risk factors** in the general population such **as oral contraceptive use, parity, and hysterectomy** can be used for determining risk. Groups are also currently investigating the role of **single nucleotide polymorphisms** in low-penetrance genes (244). In the future, it may be possible to identify women with increased susceptibility for sporadic ovarian cancer by virtue of their genetic profiles.

High-Risk Population

Hereditary syndromes account for approximately 5% to 10% of ovarian cancers. Female relatives of affected members from ovarian, breast, breast and ovarian, or Lynch syndrome (LS) families who have a greater than 10% lifetime risk of developing ovarian cancer are considered to be high risk. Much of this risk results from mutations arising in the *BRCA1, BRCA2,* and mismatch repair (*MMR*) genes. A recent metaanalysis indicated that **the average cumulative risk by age 70 years for ovarian cancer is 40% (35% to 46%) in *BRCA1* mutation carriers and 18% (13% to 23%) in *BRCA2* mutation carriers** (162). *MMR* gene-mutation carriers have a lifetime risk of ovarian cancer of approximately 10% to 12% (246).

In women with strong evidence of a hereditary predisposition, screening from the age of 35 is frequently advocated, although the efficacy of such surveillance has not yet been established (247). Screening premenopausal women can be problematic because this population has a variety of both physiological (e.g., menstrual cycle variations) and benign (e.g., endometriosis, ovarian cysts) conditions that can give rise to false positive abnormalities on ultrasound and CA125. Hence, criteria for interpretation of the screening tests need to be different from those developed for postmenopausal women in the general population.

To date, 24 studies have reported on screening for familial ovarian cancer (Table 7.3). More than 17,000 women have been screened, and 76 primary invasive epithelial ovarian and peritoneal cancers have been detected using mainly ultrasonography and CA125 levels as first-line tests. Criteria for interpreting the test results vary, and screening protocols are not always clearly reported. **Most studies have used a combination of absolute CA125 levels and ultrasound.** Ten of the studies have reported interval cancers, which presented between 2 and 46 months following the last screen (199,248–256). In addition, multifocal primary peritoneal cancer is probably a phenotypic variant of familial ovarian cancer, and neither CA125 nor ultrasound are reliable in detecting early stage disease (250,257).

Annual screening using this modality has not been found effective in detecting early stage disease (251,252,258). A modified premenopausal version of the ROC algorithm is being piloted in phase 2 of the UKFOCSS and in the CGN and GOG trials in the United States. These trials are evaluating more frequent 3- to 4-month screening and are likely to report in 2012. **Women in the high-risk population who request screening should be counseled about the current lack of evidence for the efficacy of both CA125 and ultrasonic screening and the associated false positive rates.** Many still opt for screening despite understanding the risks and limitations. **The recommended first-line option for these women is risk-reducing salpingo-oophorectomy after completion of their families** (259–261).

Current Ovarian Cancer Screening Trials

Two distinct screening strategies have emerged, one based on ultrasonography and the other on measurement of the serum tumor marker CA125 with ultrasonography as the secondary test (multimodal screening) (199,262–270). Overall, the data from large prospective studies of screening for ovarian cancer in the general population (Table 7.4) suggest that sequential multimodal screening has superior specificity and PPV compared with strategies based on transvaginal ultrasound alone. However, ultrasonography as a first-line test may offer greater sensitivity for early stage disease.

Trials in the General Population

Ongoing randomized controlled trials (RCT) in the general population aim to assess the impact of screening on ovarian cancer mortality. **In the UKCTOCS trial, more than 202,638 postmenopausal women are randomized to either control or annual screening**

Table 7.3 Prospective Ovarian Cancer Screening Studies in Women with a Family History of Ovarian or Breast Cancer or a Personal History of Breast Cancer

Study	Population	Screening Protocol	No. Screened (Premenopausal %)	No. Referred for Diagnostic Tests[a] (%)	No. of Invasive EOC Detected (Borderline Tumors)	Cancers in Screen-Negative Women
Bourne et al. 1994 (247)	Aged >17 (mean 47) FH Ov cancer	TVS then CDI	1,502 (60)	62 (3.8)	4 (3) 2 stage I	2: PP (2–8 mths) 4: EOC (24–44 mths)
Weiner et al. 1993 (271)	PH Br cancer	TVS and CDI	600	12 (3)	3 1 stage I	Not stated
Muto et al. 1993 (272)	Aged >25 FH Ov cancer	TVS and CA125	384 (85.4)	15 (3.9)	0	Not stated
Schwartz et al. 1995 (273)	Aged >30 FH Ov cancer	TVS and CDI and CA125	247	1 (0.4)	0	Not stated
Belinson et al. 1995 (274)	Aged >23 (mean 43) FH Ov cancer	TVS and CDI and CA125	137	2 (1.5)	1	Not stated
Menkiszak et al. 1998 (275)	Aged >20 FH Br, Ov cancer	TVS and CA125 (6 monthly)	124	Not available	1 (3)	Not available
Karlan et al. 1993 (276) Karlan et al. 1999 (250)	Aged >35 FH Ov, Br, Endo, Colon cancer PH Br cancer	TVS and CDI and CA125 (6 monthly until 1995, then annually)	597[b] (75) 1,261	10 (1.7) Not stated	0 (1) 1 EOC, 3 PP (2) 1 stage 1	Not stated 4 PP (5, 6, 15, 16 mths)
Dorum et al. 1996 (277)	Aged >25 (mean 43)	TVS and CA125	180[b]	16 (8.9)	4 (3)[b]	2[c]
Dorum et al. 1999 (249)	Strict criteria for FH Br, Ov cancer		803	Not stated	16 (4)	Not stated
Van Nagell et al. 2000 (199)	FH Ov cancer	TVS and CDI and CA125	3,299	Not stated	3 EOC (1) 2 stage 1	2 (12, 14 mths)
Scheuer et al. 2002 (278)	Aged >35 *BRCA1, BRCA2* mutation carriers	TVS and CA125 (6 monthly)	62	22 (35.5) 10 had surgery	5 4 EOC, 1 PP 3 stage I	0[d]
Laframboise et al. 2002 (279)	Age >22 (mean 47) Strict criteria for FH Br, Ov cancer	TVS and CA125 (6 monthly)	311	9 (3)	1	Not stated
Liede et al. 2002 (280)	Mean age 47 Jewish FH Br, Ov cancer	TVS and CA125 (6 monthly)	290	Not stated	1EOC 2PP 1 stage 1	Not stated
Tailor 2003 (255)	Age>17 (mean 47) FH Ov cancer	TVS and CDI	2,500 (65)	104 (3)	6 EOC (4) 4 stage 1	2 PP(20–40 mths) 7EOC (9–46 mths)

(Continued)

					No. of Invasive	
				No. Referred	EOC Detected	Cancers in
		Screening	No. Screened	for Diagnostic	(Borderline	Screen-Negative
Study	Population	Protocol	(Premenopausal %)	Tests[a] (%)	Tumors)	Women
Fries et al. 2004 (281)	Age>28 (mean 53) FH Br, Ov cancer	TVS and CA125 (6 monthly)	53	3 (6)	0	Not stated
Stirling et al. 2005 (254) cancer	Strict criteria for FH Br, Ov	TVS and CA125 (annually)	1,110	39 (4)	9 EOC (1) 2 stage 1	3 (2,4,12 mths)
Vasen et al. 2005 (256)	BRCA1, BRCA2 carriers, relatives	TVS and CA125 (annually)	138	Not stated	5	1 (11 months)
Meeuwissen et al. 2005 (282)	Age >18 (mean 42) Strict criteria for FH Br, Ov cancer	TVS and CA125 (annually)	383	20 (5)	0	0
Oei et al. 2006 (283)	Age >20 (mean 40) Strict criteria for FH Br, Ov cancer	TVS and CA125 (annually)	512	24 (4.7)	1 EOC	0
Garenstroom et al. 2006 (251)	Age >27 (mean 45) Strict criteria for FH Br, Ov cancer	TVS and CA125 (annually)	269	26 (9.6)	3 EOC (1) 2 PP 1 stage 1	2 (8, 10 months)
Bosse et al. 2006 (284)	Median 40–45 Strict criteria for FH Br, Ov cancer 85 BRCA carriers	TVS and CA125 (6 monthly)	676 (77)	10 (1.5)	1 EOC Stage 1	0
Hermsen et al. 2007 (252)	>35 BRCA1, BRCA2 mutation carriers	TVS and CA125 (annually)	888	25 (4)	10 EOC 1 stage 2	5 (3–10 mths)
Skates et al. (253) 2007	Strict criteria for FH Br, Ov cancer	TVS and CA125 (3 monthly) ROC algorithm	2343	38	2 EOC (2) 1 PP 1 stage 1	1

PH, personal history; FH, family history; Ov, ovarian; Br, breast; Endo, endometrial; EOC, epithelial ovarian cancer; PP, primary peritoneal cancer; TVS, transvaginal ultrasound; CDI, color Doppler imaging; ROC, risk of ovarian cancer.

[a]Following positive secondary screens.

[b]Not included in total because there are more recent updates on the trial.

[c]Further 13 women underwent oophorectomy for breast cancer; two had ovarian cancer not detected by TVS.

[d]Two women who opted for oophorectomy with normal scans and CA125 had stage I ovarian cancer.

with ultrasonography or a multimodal strategy in a 2:1:1 fashion. In the multimodal group, the ROC algorithm is used to triage women into low-, intermediate-, and elevated-risk categories based on their CA125 result. Intermediate risk women have a repeat CA125 in 12 weeks, whereas those with elevated risk are referred for a TVS and repeat CA125 in 6 weeks. Apart from ovarian cancer mortality, the study also addresses the issues of target population, compliance,

Table 7.4 Prospective Ovarian Cancer Screening Studies in the General Population

Study	Main Features	Screening Strategy	No. Screened	No. of Invasive Epithelial Ovarian Cancers Detected[a]	No. of Positive Screens	No. of Operations, Cancer Detected
CA125 Alone						
Einhorn et al. 1992 (56)	Age ≥40 years	Serum CA125	5,550	6 2 stage I	175[b]	29[b]
Multimodal Approach: CA125 (Level 1 Screen), then USS (Level 2 Screen)						
Menon et al. 2005 (67)	Age ≥50 years Postmenopausal	Serum CA125 ROCA, TVS if ROC↑	6532	3 (1) 2 stage I	16	3
Jacobs et al. 1993 (60) 1996 (61)	Age ≥45 years (median 56) Postmenopausal	Serum CA125 TAS, if CA125↑	22,000	11 4 stage I	41	3.7
Jacobs et al. 1999 (11)	Age ≥45 years (median 56) Postmenopausal	RCT Serum CA125 TAS/TVS, if CA125↑	10,958 3 annual screens	6 3 stage I	29	4.8
Grover et al. 1995 (266)	Age ≥40 years (median 51) or with family history (3%)	Serum CA125 TAS/TVS, if CA125↑	2,550	1 0 stage I	16	16
Adonakis et al. 1996 (262)	Age ≥45 years (mean 58)	Serum CA125 TVS, if CA125↑	2,000	1 (1) 1 stage I	15	15
USS-Only Approach: USS (Level 1 Screen), then Repeat USS (Level 2 Screen)						
De Priest et al. 1997 (264)	Age ≥50 years and post-menopausal or ≥30 with FH	TVS Annual screens Mean 4 screens per woman	6,470	6 5 stage I	90	18
van Nagell et al. 2000 (199) van Nagell et al. 2007 (12)	Postmenopausal >50 and >25 with FH of ovarian cancer	TVS (annual) CA125 and CDI if TVS persistent positive	14,469 25,312	11 (3) 1 PP 29 (10) 14 stage 1	180 364	16.3 12.5
Sato et al. 2000 (285)	Part of general screening program	TVS TVS + markers at level 2	51,550	22 17 stage I	324	14.7
Hayashi et al. 1999 (267)	Age ≥50 years	TVS	23,451	3 (3)	258	[c]
Tabor et al. 1994 (270)	Aged 46–65 years	TVS	435	0	9	—
Campbell et al. 1989 (263)	Age ≥45 years (mean 53) or with family history (4%)	TAS 3 screens at 18 monthly intervals	5,479	2 (3) 2 stage I	326	163

(Continued)

Table 7.4 Prospective Ovarian Cancer Screening Studies in the General Population (*Continued*)

Study	Main Features	Screening Strategy	No. Screened	No. of Invasive Epithelial Ovarian Cancers Detected[a]	No. of Positive Screens	No. of Operations, Cancer Detected
Millo et al. 1989 (269)	Age ≥45 years or post-menopausal (mean 54)	USS (mode not specified)	500	0	11	—
Goswamy et al. 1983 (265)	Age 39–78 Postmenopausal	TAS	1,084	1 1 stage I		
USS and CDI(Level 1 Screen)						
Kurjak et al. 1995 (268)	Aged 40–71 years (mean 45)	TVS and CDI	5,013	4 4 stage I	38	9.5
Vuento et al. 1995 (236)	Aged 56–61 years (mean 59)	TVS and CDI	1,364	(1)	5	—
USS (Level 1) and Other Tests (Level 2 Screen)						
Parkes et al. 1994 (238)	Aged 50–64 years	TVS then CDI if TVS positive	2,953	1 1 stage I	15[d]	15
Holbert et al. 1994 (286)	Postmenopausal Aged 30–89 years	TVS then CA125 if TVS positive	478	1 1 stage I	33[e]	33
USS and CA125						
Buys et al. 2005 (272)	Postmenopausal Aged 55–74 years	TVS and CA125 (annual)	28,816	18 (9) 2 stage 1 1 PP	1,706[b] (570: surgery)	28.5
Kobayashi et al. 2007 (24)	Postmenopausal >50 years	TVS and CA125 (annual)	41,688	27	4,744[b] (305: surgery)	11.3

RCT, randomized controlled trial; ROC, risk of ovarian cancer; TAS, transabdominal ultrasound; TVS, transvaginal ultrasound; USS, ultrasound; CDI, color Doppler imaging.

[a]Primary invasive epithelial ovarian cancers. The borderline and granulosa tumors detected are shown in parentheses.

[b]Not all of these women underwent surgical investigation because the study design involved intensive surveillance rather than surgical intervention.

[c]Only 95 women consented to surgery, and there are no follow-up details on the remaining.

[d]86 women had abnormal USS before CDI.

[e]Only 11 of these women underwent surgery.

health economics, and physical and psychological morbidity of screening. Results are expected around 2013 (http://www.ukctocs.org.uk).

The Prostate, Lung, Colorectal, and Ovarian (PLCO) Cancer Screening Trial has enrolled 78,000 women aged 55 to 74 at 10 screening centers in the United States with balanced randomization to intervention and control arms (Figure 7.2). **For ovarian cancer, women are screened using both serum CA125 and transvaginal ultrasonography for 3 years and CA125 alone for a further 2 years.** Follow-up will continue for at least 13 years from randomization to assess health status and cause of death (287). Recently published prevalence screen results in 28,816 screened women reported 29 neoplasms, of which 20 were invasive and

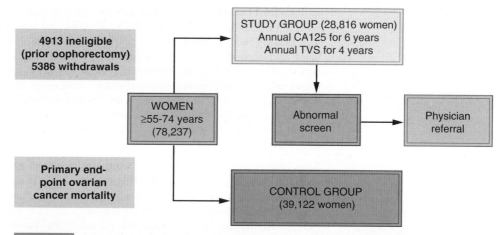

Figure 7.2 The National Institutes of Health Prostrate, Lung, Colorectal, and Ovarian (NIH-PLCO) Cancer Screening Study (287). Ovarian screening is part of the study, and the primary outcome measure is mortality from ovarian cancer. All women will be followed up until 2013 by postal questionnaire.

9 borderline. Of all screened women, 4.7% had an abnormal scan and 1.4% an abnormal CA125. The PPV for invasive cancer was 3.7%, 1%, and 23.5% for abnormal CA125, TVS, and both CA125 and TVS, respectively (288).

The Japanese Shizuoka Cohort Study of Ovarian Cancer Screening RCT, using an annual ultrasound and absolute CA125-based strategy in 82,487 low-risk postmenopausal women, did not find a statistically significant difference in the number of screen-detected ovarian cancers ($n = 27$) and those in the control arm ($n = 32$). Eight additional interval cancers occurred in the screened arm. The proportion of stage I ovarian cancers was greater in the screened (63%) than in the control group (38%), although this did not reach statistical significance ($p = 0.2285$). Ovarian cancer detection rates of 0.31 per 1,000 at prevalent screen and 0.38 to 0.74 per 1,000 at subsequent screens were found (24).

Trials in a High-Risk Population

The sensitivity and effectiveness of screening in the younger high-risk population is still not established (289). **Annual screening does not seem effective, hence, ongoing trials in the United Kingdom and United States are piloting a more frequent 3- to 4-month approach to screening using the ROC algorithm. The UK Familial Ovarian Cancer Screening Study** is a prospective study based on annual transvaginal ultrasonography and CA125 titers every 4 months (290). This ongoing trial has recruited more than 3,700 women from 31 centers in the United Kingdom. **Similar trials are under way in the United States under the auspices of the National Cancer Institute's CGN and the GOG** (291), with the scope for metaanalysis in the future. In the U.S. trials, screening is based on 3-month serum CA125 levels, which are interpreted using the ROC algorithm. Preliminary results from 2,343 high-risk women in the U.S.-based CGN trial reported that 38 women underwent surgery following 6,284 screens. Five ovarian cancers were detected: two prevalent (one early, one late stage) and three incident (three early) cases, resulting in a PPV of 13%. Three further occult cancers were detected at risk-reducing salpingo-oophorectomy, and one woman developed an interval (late-stage) cancer (253).

Endometrial Cancer

Endometrial cancer is a disease mainly seen in postmenopausal women. Just 7% occur in the reproductive age group and are mainly linked to familial predisposition, obesity, or polycystic ovarian syndrome (PCOS). The prevalence of endometrial cancer in asymptomatic women is low, and the overall prognosis is good as women present in early stages with abnormal bleeding. **Most endometrial cancers (77%) are diagnosed at an early, favorable stage.** The consensus is that screening for endometrial cancer is not warranted for women who have no identifiable risk factors (292–297). **The only trial to support mass screening for**

endometrial cancer is from Tohoku University, Japan. The study reported that early stage (88.1% vs. 65.3%), low-grade (74.7% vs. 61.0%), and 5-year survival (94% vs. 84.3%) were significantly more frequent in 126 cases of endometrial cancer detected by mass screening using endometrial smears compared with the 1,069 cases diagnosed clinically during the period 1987 to 1997 (298). However, even in women at increased risk as a result of unopposed use of estrogen, *tamoxifen* therapy, nulliparity, infertility or anovulation, obesity, diabetes, or hypertension, **the American Cancer Society Working Group does not recommend screening for endometrial cancer.** As is the case with average-risk women, individuals at increased risk who develop endometrial cancer tend to present with symptoms at an early, favorable stage.

Screening is only recommended in women with or at high risk for hereditary nonpolyposis colon cancer (HNPCC) or Lynch syndrome. LS is an autosomal dominant syndrome characterized by the development of a number of different cancers, the most common of which are colorectal and endometrial cancers. Historically, HNPCC has been diagnosed on the basis of strict family-history–based clinical criteria called the **Amsterdam criteria.** It is caused by a mutation in one of the DNA mismatch repair genes: *MLH1, MSH2, MSH6, PMS1,* and *PMS2.* **Individuals from LS or HNPCC families have a 30% to 60% lifetime risk of endometrial cancer** (246,299–302).

Various strategies have been used to screen for endometrial cancer in women with Lynch syndrome, but the efficacy of endometrial screening in these women remains unproven. The main modalities used include TVS and endometrial sampling. The latter has been used both alone and in combination with hysteroscopy. However, available data are limited, and the **evidence to recommend any particular method of screening is lacking.** Interval cancers occur despite screening, and the impact of screening on morbidity and mortality is unknown.

Although TVS has been used as a first-line screening tool, there is lack of consensus on an appropriate cutoff value for endometrial thickness (ET) in asymptomatic premenopausal women, and interval cancers are known to occur (303–304). **Pipelle** endometrial biopsy is a well-established method for endometrial sampling and is well tolerated by women as an outpatient procedure. However, it has a tissue yield and procedure failure rate of approximately 10% (305,306), and inadequate samples are more common in the postmenopausal age group. **The diagnostic accuracy of pipelle is higher in postmenopausal women.** A large metaanalysis of the use of pipelle reported a 99% sensitivity for the diagnosis of endometrial cancer and 81% for the diagnosis of hyperplasia in postmenopausal women. In premenopausal women, the sensitivity for endometrial cancer was 91% with a specificity of >98% (305).

Hysteroscopy-directed endometrial sampling is now routinely performed as an outpatient procedure. Hysteroscopy may permit directed biopsy from a focal lesion and can detect polyps and submucous fibroids that may be missed by both ultrasound and pipelle (307,308). The efficacy and patient acceptability of outpatient hysteroscopy is similar to the in-patient procedure. Overall, five endometrial cancers have been recently reported in two prospective series using annual hysteroscopy for endometrial surveillance in 119 high-risk women (306,309). Outpatient hysteroscopy failure rates of 8% and 11% were found in these two series, respectively.

The largest reported series of ET screening in high-risk women is from Finland. Eleven screen-detected and two interval cancers were found in 175 Finnish women undergoing annual surveillance with ultrasound and endometrial biopsies (304). The interval cancers occurred in symptomatic women at 3 and 31 months after a surveillance visit. Transvaginal scans alone would have missed six of the cancers in this cohort. In addition, complex atypical hyperplasia was found in four, complex hyperplasia without atypia in eight, and simple hyperplasia in two women undergoing surveillance. Prospectively collected data in women undergoing screening suggest that cancers may present with abnormal bleeding for as long as 3 months before diagnosis (306,309). This emphasizes the importance of counseling women undergoing screening about reporting any abnormal menstrual symptoms or bleeding patterns and subsequently investigating them.

Data show that screening can lead to the detection of endometrial cancers in high-risk women. Notwithstanding the reported shortcomings, screening may have a role in women who wish to delay or avoid preventative surgery. Women in this high-risk group should be counseled about the risks and symptoms of endometrial cancer and the potential benefits, risks, and limitations of endometrial cancer screening. **For women with Lynch syndrome opting for**

endometrial screening, most current guidelines recommend a strategy of TVS and endometrial sampling from the age of 30 to 35 years (13–15). Hysteroscopically directed sampling may have the added benefit of diagnosing focal premalignant lesions in asymptomatic women. Prophylactic hysterectomy and bilateral salpingo-oophorectomy is the recommended alternative for prevention of endometrial and ovarian cancer in LS women who have completed their families (310).

Morphological Markers

The most commonly used tumor marker is endometrial thickness, which is measured using transvaginal ultrasound. It is defined as the distance from the proximal to the distal interface of the hypoechoic halo that surrounds the more echogenic myometrium. It is conventional to measure double thickness (thickness of both endometrial layers) at the thickest point in the midsagittal view. Cutoffs of 12 mm in premenopausal women and 5 mm in postmenopausal women have been used in earlier trials, but there is no consensus on this, and interval cancers have been known to occur. Any abnormality such as a polyp should be investigated irrespective of endometrial thickness.

In symptomatic patients with postmenopausal bleeding who are not on hormone-replacement therapy (HRT), a cutoff for endometrial thickness of >4.0 mm has a sensitivity for detection of endometrial cancer of 98% and a negative predictive value of 99% (311). The Postmenopausal Estrogen and Progestin Interventions trial found that a ET threshold of 5 mm yielded a PPV of 9%, NPV of 99%, sensitivity of 90%, and specificity of 48% for detecting endometrial hyperplasia or cancer (312). A subsequent metaanalysis suggested an endometrial thickness of 5 mm as a cutoff for investigating postmenopausal bleeding. A negative test would reduce the likelihood of endometrial cancer to 2.5% (313). Even though these cutoffs effectively exclude endometrial atrophy, they fail to differentiate between hyperplasia and carcinoma (314). The endometrial thickness for women using sequential HRT is greater than that for those using a continuous combined preparation. The Scottish Intercollegiate Guidelines Network recommends using 3 mm as a cutoff for women in the following circumstances: (i) those on continuous combined HRT, (ii) those who have not used HRT for a year, and (iii) those who have never taken HRT. They recommend a cut off of 5 mm in women on a sequential preparation (315).

As a tumor marker in asymptomatic postmenopausal women, endometrial thickness has the same poor positive predictive value but high negative predictive value for the detection of serious endometrial disease (312). Screening studies using conventional and color Doppler ultrasonography in apparently healthy postmenopausal women have established that endometrial carcinomas can be detected at a preclinical stage (235,316,317) and that transvaginal ultrasonography is more sensitive than blind endometrial biopsy (318). However, in the absence of symptoms, repeat sampling is not warranted in patients with a thickened endometrium and negative findings at initial biopsy (319). Endometrial fluid accumulation is detected in 12% of asymptomatic elderly postmenopausal women and is rarely a sign of malignancy (317). Other techniques that are under investigation and not part of routine protocols include 3-D ultrasonography for the measurement of endometrial volume and power Doppler analysis (320–322) and saline infusion sonohysterography (323,324). The ability of 3-D sonography to distinguish between hyperplasia and cancer is still limited. Saline-infusion sonohysterography may be better than standard TVS at evaluating intrauterine pathology such as polyps or fibroids, but it has limited value in diagnosing hyperplasia or carcinoma (325).

Women on *tamoxifen* are more prone to develop endometrial polyps or hyperplasia and have a four- to fivefold higher risk of endometrial cancer. In asymptomatic women on long-term *tamoxifen*, abnormal ultrasonographic findings are common in the absence of underlying endometrial pathology. The apparent increase in thickness observed on ultrasound probably results from *tamoxifen*-induced changes in endometrial stroma and myometrium (326,327). The sensitivity and specificity of TVS as a screening tool is therefore considerably reduced, and the ideal endometrial thickness cutoff for women on *tamoxifen* is not known (315). Prompt investigation of abnormal vaginal bleeding rather than screening is probably the best option in this group (328,329). There may be a role for pretreatment assessment of the endometrium before *tamoxifen* therapy, though this needs further investigation. Limited data suggest that women at risk for severe atypical hyperplasia can be identified on the basis of hyperplastic lesions detected on endometrial biopsy before starting *tamoxifen* (330). No development of atypical lesions has been reported on subsequent follow-up of lesions treated before *tamoxifen* therapy (331).

Cytological Markers

Although the Papanicolaou stained cervical smear was designed to detect cervical cancers, it can detect the presence of malignancy in women with endometrial malignancy. The presence of normal as well as abnormal-looking endometrial cells in cervical smears in the second half of the menstrual cycle or in postmenopausal women should alert the clinician to the possibility of underlying endometrial disease. In a **retrospective analysis, 13.5% of postmenopausal women with normal endometrial cells on routine smear, 23% of those with atypical cells, and 77% of those with suspicious cells had either endometrial hyperplasia or carcinoma** (332). Among premenopausal women, three of 57 with normal endometrial cells in the secretory phase of the menstrual cycle had endometrial hyperplasia, whereas one of two with atypical cells had endometrial polyps, and both with cells suspicious of carcinoma had endometrial carcinoma (332). **A PPV of 64% for the later diagnosis of endometrial malignancy was obtained on follow-up of 359 women who received a cytologic report of endometrial malignancy from the Victorian Cytology Service from 1982 to 1987** (333). In another series, 13.5% of women with endometrial cells of some type on Pap smears had endometrial carcinoma (334). The presence of glandular abnormalities and high-grade squamous intraepithelial lesions on smear is also associated with an increased risk of endometrial carcinoma (334–337). **The sensitivity of cervical cytology performed within 2 years of the diagnosis of endometrial malignancy is 28%** (333).

The low sensitivity of cytology using conventional Pap smears that indirectly sample the endometrium can be improved by directly sampling the endometrial cavity using a variety of commercially available sampling devices. Although these techniques are simple and have low risk and good yield, they are associated with technical difficulties because of cervical stenosis and varying degrees of patient discomfort. **Their use in screening asymptomatic women is probably best limited to those with a positive result on first-line ultrasonic screening** (338). However, they have a low positive predictive value and a lower diagnostic accuracy than pipelle biopsy (305,339).

Molecular Markers

Polymerase-chain-reaction–based technology has made possible the detection of mutations and other key events in small numbers of cancer cells scattered among large numbers of normal cells. **Mutations in oncogenes and tumor suppressor genes have been used as molecular markers to detect endometrial carcinoma from cervical smears.** *K-ras* mutations were found to be present as many as 5 months before the diagnosis of endometrial cancer. **In addition to *K-ras* mutations, which may be present in 10% to 30% of tumors, mutations have also been found in *p53* (20% cancers) and *PTEN/MMACI* genes (34% cancers)** (340,341). However, some of these may be late events in endometrial carcinogenesis and may not be suitable for screening. Telomerase is expressed by normal cycling endometrium (342) and preferentially expressed in most malignant tissues, including endometrial carcinoma (343,344). It has been cited as a possible marker for endometrial hyperplasia and carcinoma in postmenopausal women because activity is normally absent or weak in postmenopausal atrophic endometrium (343,345–348).

Microsatellite instability (MSI) and immunohistochemistry are other molecular markers that may have potential in predicting the development of endometrial cancer in HNPCC-positive women (349–351). **MSI may occur in as many as 75% of HNPCC- and LS-related (352–355) and 33% of sporadic endometrial tumors (353,355–358). DNA methylation has also been implicated in sporadic endometrial cancer and is the cause of MSI in these tumors** (359). Endometrial hyperplasia has been shown to demonstrate MSI and to precede endometrial cancer (349,350). MSI was demonstrated in cases of endometrial cancer but not in women with normal endometrium in a pilot study (360).

DNA for molecular analysis is possible on a sample of endometrial cells obtained from pipelle (blind biopsy) (360), cervical smears (361), and even noninvasively from tampons and sanitary towels (362,363). The yield of DNA using pipelle endometrial biopsy has been found to compare well with the recovery rates of DNA from stool samples (364). The ability to obtain sufficient DNA for analysis was not found to be affected by the time of the menstrual cycle, but extraction was less effective if the sample was heavily blood stained (360). **DNA screening may well serve as a useful adjunct to screening protocols in the future, but further research is needed before this can be achieved.**

Other Serum Biomarkers

A host of serological markers has been investigated for a role in endometrial cancer such as CA125, CEA, SCC, CA15-3, CA125, CA19-9, CA72-4, CASA AST, ALT, SAP, gamma-GT, OVX1 antigen, CYFRA 21-1, placental protein 4, UGF, and M-CSF. However, none of them has a well-established role in screening or clinical management. Preliminary data recently suggested YKL-40 as a promising new marker for detection and prognosis (365). **Proteomic studies** using mass-spectrometric technologies have identified a panel of promising biomarkers including **pyruvate kinase, chaperonin, and alpha-1-antitrypsin,** which give a high sensitivity (0.85–0.95), specificity (0.93–0.95), and PPV (0.88–0.95) for endometrial cancer (366,367). However, these observations require further validation, and their clinical value remains to be determined.

Until the ideal tumor marker for endometrial cancer is described, screening tests will continue to be characterized by low false negative but high false positive rates. Although screening is inappropriate for the general population, a strategy of early evaluation of post-menopausal bleeding with judicious use of hysteroscopy and endometrial biopsy is important for the early detection of endometrial cancer.

Cervical Cancer

Cervical cancer is the major cause of death from gynecological cancer worldwide, with most deaths occurring in the developing world. More than 90% of the cases of carcinoma *in situ* occur in women under 45, with the peak incidence being in the 25 to 29 age group. In contrast, the occurrence of invasive cervical cancer is fairly evenly spread across age groups older than 25, with approximately 42% to 46% occurring in the reproductive age (22,368).

Screening for cervical cancer is one of the most prevalent and successful public health measures for the prevention of cancer. **Protection against cervical cancer offered by cervical screening ranges from approximately 60% to 85%** (8). **It is slightly lower in the age group younger than 40 than older than 40.** Primary screening has traditionally involved a repetitive exfoliative cytology-based program with colposcopy as a second-line test. This has led to a significant decrease in cervical cancer incidence in the United Kingdom and the rest of the Western world. It has been suggested that an overall coverage of 80% can potentially decrease associated mortality rates by 95%. **Although cytological screening may be less effective against cervical adenocarcinoma (15% of cervical cancers), it does have a substantial impact even in this subgroup.** An audit of smear histories in women younger than 70 years with cervical cancer revealed that 49% occurred despite adequate cytological screening and follow-up in the 5 years before diagnosis (369). Although cervical cancer is a preventable disease and completely curable if detected at an early stage, **cytological screening alone may not eradicate the disease.**

Cervical Cytology

Sensitivity and specificity of cervical cytology has been reported to range between 30% to 87% and 86% to 100%, respectively (370). The traditional method of obtaining cytological specimens—**the Papanicolou smear—is being replaced by liquid-based cytology (LBC) in a number of centers** (371). Several LBC systems such as SurePath, ThinPrep, Cytoscreen, and Labonard Easy Prep are commercially available. **LBC leads to the preparation of more homogenous easier-to-read slides and a more efficient automated laboratory-sample–handling process, resulting in increased productivity. However, LBC lacks formal criteria used for defining smear adequacy.** Data suggest that compared to Pap smears, **LBC is associated with increased sensitivity for abnormal smears and fewer inadequate or unsatisfactory smears** (371). An English pilot study reported increased sensitivity of 2.8% to 12% and an 87% reduction in inadequate smears from 9% to 1.6% with LBC while maintaining specificity. It also found a reduction in the glandular neoplasms detected from 0.08% to 0.04%, though follow-up data showed no change in the number of adenocarcinomas (371). The sensitivity for low-grade smears may be higher than high-grade ones. A number of systematic reviews have advocated a preference for LBC (372–374), whereas others have found no difference between LBC and conventional Pap smears (375,376). **A recent metaanalysis of all studies using colposcopic-directed biopsy as the gold standard found that sensitivity and specificity of LBC was not significantly different from Pap smears** (377).

Human Papilloma Virus DNA

A well-established causal link has been found between HPV and all grades of cervical intraep-ithelial neoplasia (CIN) and invasive cervical cancer (166,378). HPV DNA has been found in 99.7% of cervical cancers, and cancer can develop 5 to 30 years after the primary infection. There is considerable worldwide variation in the distribution of high-risk viral types, but approximately 70% of cancers have been linked to HPV types 16 and 18 (379–381). Low-risk HPV types 6 and 11 are responsible for genital warts, low-grade cervical lesions, and respira-tory papillomatosis. Multiple infections may be more common below age 30 but less common between ages 30 and 64 (381).

Recent systematic reviews and metaanalyses have shown that HPV DNA testing can accurately pick up treatment failures earlier, and its performance can exceed that of cytological follow-up (382–384). **High-risk HPV DNA testing has been shown to have a higher sensitivity but slightly lower specificity (of the order of 8% to 12%) than cytology alone for detecting high-grade disease** (382). A combination of HPV testing and cytology is associated with an even higher sensitivity (382) and may save additional years of life at reasonable costs compared with cytology testing alone (385). Modeling studies show that a screening strategy of HPV DNA testing and cytology every 2 to 3 years provides a greater reduction in cancer and is less costly than annual conventional cytology (386). Women who test negative for high-risk HPV DNA and have a normal cytology are extremely unlikely to develop CIN or cancer in the next 5 to 10 years (387,388). High-risk HPV-DNA–negative women with a smear that is borderline or shows atypical squamous cells of undetermined significance (ASC-US) have a <2% risk of high-grade CIN or cancer in the next 2 years, which is similar to women with a negative smear (389). A positive high-risk HPV DNA test in the presence of a severely dyskaryotic smear and high-grade disease at colposcopy suggests a 60% to 80% risk of CIN 3 or worse in the next 2 years (390,391).

HPV DNA testing has been recommended in triaging ASC-US (Atypical squamous cells of undetermined significance) cytology or borderline smears, predicting posttreatment recur-rence risk, and the identification of women with abnormal cytology and low-grade histol-ogy needing postcolposcopic follow-up (371,392,394). It helps identify a group of women who are more likely to develop high-grade CIN or cancer. The value of HPV typing may be further increased by subtyping because **some variants of HPV 16 confer a 6.5-fold increase in risk of CIN 2 or CIN 3 compared with other HPV 16 variants** (395). Thus, compared to cytology alone, high-risk HPV testing can improve risk stratification and increase the efficiency of cervical cancer screening. However, it may not be as effective in adolescent women because of a low PPV resulting from a high prevalence of HPV infection and a low incidence of progres-sive precancerous lesions in this age group (396,397). **High-risk HPV DNA testing has been incorporated into the recently published 2006 consensus guidelines adopted by the American Society for Colposcopy and Cervical Pathology and has been recommended as a co-test with cytology for routine screening in women older than 30 (392,393).**

Other Screening Strategies

Various other strategies such as naked eye visual inspection of the cervix after application of acetic acid (VIA), visual inspection after Lugol's iodine (VILI), visual inspection with a magnifying glass (VIAM), and HPV DNA testing are emerging as effective screening options, especially for developing countries that have limited resources and lack estab-lished efficient screening programs. A recent metaanalysis (398) of five screening strategies from 11 studies involving 58,000 women showed that VIA, VILI, and VIAM had a high sensi-tivity (79%) and specificity (85%) for high-grade disease. Pap smears had a lower sensitivity (57%) but higher specificity (93%). A large RCT showed that the VIA-based screening strat-egy is effective and can lead to decreased mortality in the screened arm (high risk of 0.65) (399). However, sensitivity reported with strategies such as VIA may be slightly inflated because of a gold standard (colposcopic-directed biopsy) misclassification error (400).

DNA Imaging Cytometry

DNA imaging cytometry is a novel, automated slide-reading method that measures the amount of DNA in the cell nuclei using an automated image cytometer, thus minimizing the need for skilled cytotechnologists. Preliminary data suggest that it can successfully detect high-grade lesions (401,402). When combined with conventional cytology and HPV DNA testing as part of a multimodal strategy, it was found to increase PPV and the identification of low-grade lesions likely to progress (403). **Hyperspectral imaging,** which uses novel algorithms for spectral and spatial differences to distinguish among normal, precancerous, and cancerous cells, is also being investigated (404).

Molecular Markers

Although telomerase expression is reported to be a discriminatory marker of premalignant and malignant squamous cell lesions, its clinical utility is still under evaluation. It was detected in as much as 100% of cervical cancer and 62% to 96% of high-grade CIN specimens (347,405,406): 88% to 100% of invasive smears and 40% to 59% of abnormal cytologyic specimens in women with CIN (407–410) as well as in five cases of CIN with no cytological abnormality (411). However, conflicting data showing poor (4.5% to 25%) sensitivity for high-grade CIN (405,409) and increased expression in 46% to 56% benign lesions have also been reported (347,412,413). **A recent systematic review of ten studies reported the diagnostic odds ration of a positive telomerase test to be 3.2** (1.9, 5.6) **for low-grade squamous intraepithelial lesion (LSIL), 5.8** (3.1, 10) **for high-grade squamous intraepithelial lesion (HSIL), 8.1** (3.1, 20.3) **for cervical cancer versus HSIL, and 40.9** (18.2, 91) **for cervical cancer versus LSIL.** The catalytic subunit of telomerase protein–human telomerase reverse transcriptase is the rate-limiting determinant of telomerase activity. It has also shown promise in determining high-grade CIN in cervical screening and predicting progressive disease (414,415).

Another approach that has been investigated for reducing the false negative rate of cytology includes immunostaining of smears using antibodies against proteins that regulate DNA replication such as CDC6 and MCM5 (416). Recently, a combination of LR67 and VEGF-C have also been found to be of value in detecting high-grade CIN, but this needs further evaluation and validation in cytological samples before they can be considered for screening purposes (417).

Serological Markers

No serological markers have been found to be sufficiently sensitive (especially for early-stage cervical cancer) or specific for screening purposes. However, a variety of serum markers have been investigated in assessing prognosis, monitoring response to treatment, and detecting recurrence.

Summary

One of the established strategies for combating cancer in the twenty-first century is screening the asymptomatic population for premalignant conditions and early-stage disease. The effectiveness of ovarian cancer screening is being addressed by ongoing research trials both in the high and low-risk populations. These trials are expected to report by 2012–14. Screening outside the context of research trials is not recommended. Despite the vast number of serum markers studied, only a few have been validated for clinical use and limited sensitivities/specificities constrain their use for screening purposes. Serum CA125 remains clinically the most widely used marker for epithelial ovarian cancer. New imaging technologies and related algorithms may serve as useful adjuncts in distinguishing benign from malignant adnexal masses. Given the heterogeneity of cancer, a combination of modalities such as risk of ovarian cancer algorithm, transvaginal ultrasonic pattern recognition and multiple marker models may provide maximum advantage. Genomic, epigenetic, metabolomic and proteomic technologies hold tremendous promise for the future. However, they require further research and validation before this promise is realized.

Screening for endometrial cancer in the low-risk population is not recommended. The ideal method for screening asymptomatic high-risk women has not been established. While a number of molecular markers and biomarkers are under investigation for screening purposes, none has made it to clinical practice.

Well established, effective cytologic/colposcopic based screening programs for cervical cancer exist in the developed world. Significant changes have occurred over the last few years such as the introduction of liquid based cytology (LBC) and HPV DNA testing. Newer methods such as VIA/VILI/VIAM/HPV DNA testing hold potential for the developing world. No serological markers have been found to be effective in screening for cervical cancer. **Despite the availability of HPV vaccination and its promise for the future, there are still a number of unresolved issues, and an effective screening program will remain the cornerstone of any preventive strategy for cervical cancer for many years to come.**

References

1. **Jemal A, Siegel R, Murray T, Hao Y, Xu J, Murray T, Thun MJ.** Cancer statistics, 2009. *CA Cancer J Clin* 2009;published online. doi:10.3322/caac.20006.

2. **Cancer Research UK.** CancerStats Key Facts All Cancers. Available at: http://info.cancerresearchuk.org/cancerstats/incidence/. Accessed August 2007.

3. **Cancer Research UK.** Cancer in the EU: incidence and mortality in the European Union. Available at: http://info.cancerresearchuk.org/cancerstats/geographic/cancerineu/incidenceandmortality. Accessed January 2008.

4. **Cancer Research UK.** UK cancer mortality statistics for common cancers. Available at: http://info.cancerresearchuk.org/cancerstats/mortality/cancerdeaths/. Accessed January 2008.

5. **Wilson J, Jungner G.** *Principles and practice of screening for disease.* Public Health Papers no. 34. Geneva: World Health Organization, 1968:66–67.

6. **Mahlck CG, Jonsson H, Lenner P.** Pap smear screening and changes in cervical cancer mortality in Sweden. *Int J Gynaecol Obstet* 1994;44:267–272.

7. **Sasieni P, Adams J.** Effect of screening on cervical cancer mortality in England and Wales: analysis of trends with an age period cohort model. *BMJ* 1999;318:1244–1245.

8. **Sasieni P, Adams J, Cuzick J.** Benefit of cervical screening at different ages: evidence from the UK audit of screening histories. *Br J Cancer* 2003;89:88–93.

9. **Taylor RJ, Morrell SL, Mamoon HA, Wain GV.** Effects of screening on cervical cancer incidence and mortality in New South Wales implied by influences of period of diagnosis and birth cohort. *J Epidemiol Community Health* 2001;55:782–788.

10. **Menon U, Jacobs I.** The current status of screening for ovarian cancer. In: **Jacobs I, Shepherd JH, Oram D, Blackett AL, DM, Berchuck A, Hudson C, eds.** *Ovarian cancer.* London: Oxford University Press, 2002:171–178.

11. **Jacobs IJ, Skates SJ, MacDonald N, Menon U, Rosenthal AN, Davies AP, et al.** Screening for ovarian cancer: a pilot randomised controlled trial. *Lancet* 1999;353:1207–1210.

12. **van Nagell JR, Jr., Depriest PD, Ueland FR, DeSimone CP, Cooper AL, McDonald JM, et al.** Ovarian cancer screening with annual transvaginal sonography: findings of 25,000 women screened. *Cancer* 2007;109:1887–1896.

13. **Hendriks YM, de Jong AE, Morreau H, Tops CM, Vasen HF, Wijnen JT, et al.** Diagnostic approach and management of Lynch syndrome (hereditary nonpolyposis colorectal carcinoma): a guide for clinicians. *CA Cancer J Clin* 2006;56:213–225.

14. **Lindor NM, Petersen GM, Hadley DW, Kinney AY, Miesfeldt S, Lu KH, et al.** Recommendations for the care of individuals with an inherited predisposition to Lynch syndrome: a systematic review. *JAMA* 2006;296:1507–1517.

15. **Vasen HF, Möslein G, Alonso A, Bernstein I, Bertario L, Blanco I, et al.** Guidelines for the clinical management of Lynch syndrome (hereditary non-polyposis cancer). *J Med Genet* 2007;44:353–362.

16. **Duffy MJ, Bonfrer JM, Kulpa J, Rustin JG, Soletormos G, Torre GC, et al.** CA125 in ovarian cancer: European Group on Tumor Markers guidelines for clinical use. *Int J Gynecol Cancer* 2005;15:679–691.

17. **Sturgeon C.** Practice guidelines for tumor marker use in the clinic. *Clin Chem* 2002;48:1151–1159.

18. **Aebi S, Castiglione M.** Epithelial ovarian carcinoma: ESMO clinical recommendations for diagnosis, treatment and follow-up. *Ann Oncol* 2008;19 Suppl 2:ii14–6.

19. Practice Guidelines and Recommendations for Use of Tumor Markers in the Clinic. In: **Diamandis EP, Sturgeon C, Hoffman B, eds.** *NACB: Laboratory Medicine Practice Guidelines (LMPG).* Washington, DC: The National Academy of Clinical Biochemistry, 2005. Available at: http://www.aacc.org/members/nacb/LMPG/OnlineGuide/DraftGuidelines/TumorMarkers/Pages/TumorMarkersPDF.aspx.

20. **Duffy MJ, McGing P.** *Guidelines for the use of tumor markers.* 3rd ed. Dublin: Association of Clinical Biochemists in Ireland (ACBI), 2005. Available at: http://www.acbi.ie/acbi-tmk.html.

21. **Colposcopy and Programme Management.** *Guidelines for the NHS Cervical Screening Programme.* Sheffield, UK: NHS Cancer Screening Programmes, 2004.

22. **Cancer Research UK.** *Latest UK summary—Cancer incidence 2004 and mortality 2005.* Available at: http://info.cancerresearchuk.org/images/pdfs/2004inc2005mortpdf. Accessed January 2008.

23. **Seidman JD, Horkayne-Szakaly I, Haiba M, Boice CR, Kurman RJ, Ronnett BM.** The histologic type and stage distribution of ovarian carcinomas of surface epithelial origin. *Int J Gynecol Pathol* 2004;23:41–44.

24. **Kobayashi H, Yamada Y, Sado T, Sakata M, Yoshida S, Kawaguchi R, et al.** A randomized study of screening for ovarian cancer: a multicenter study in Japan. *Int J Gynecol Cancer* 2008; 18:414–420. Epub 2007 July 21.

25. **Bast RC, Jr., Feeney M, Lazarus H, Nadler LM, Colvin RB, Knapp RC.** Reactivity of a monoclonal antibody with human ovarian carcinoma. *J Clin Invest* 1981;68:1331–1337.

26. **Yin BW, Lloyd KO.** Molecular cloning of the CA125 ovarian cancer antigen: identification as a new mucin, MUC16. *J Biol Chem* 2001;276:27371–27375.

27. **Nustad K, Bast RC, Jr., Brien TJ, Nilsson O, Seguin P, Suresh MR, et al.** Specificity and affinity of 26 monoclonal antibodies against the CA125 antigen: first report from the ISOBM TD-1 workshop. International Society for Oncodevelopmental Biology and Medicine. *Tumour Biol* 1996;17:196–219.

28. **Jacobs I, Bast RC Jr.** The CA125 tumour-associated antigen: a review of the literature. *Hum Reprod* 1989;4:1–12.

29. **Bast RC Jr, Xu FJ, Yu YH, Barnhill S, Zhang Z, Mills GB.** CA125: the past and the future. *Int J Biol Markers* 1998;13:179–187.

30. **Davelaar EM, van Kamp GJ, Verstraeten RA, Kenemans P.** Comparison of seven immunoassays for the quantification of CA125 antigen in serum. *Clin Chem* 1998;44:1417–1422.

31. **Mongia SK, Rawlins ML, Owen WE, Roberts WL.** Performance characteristics of seven automated CA125 assays. *Am J Clin Pathol* 2006;125:921–927.

32. **Kabawat SE, Bast RC Jr, Bhan AK, Welch WR, Knapp RC, Colvin RB.** Tissue distribution of a coelomic-epithelium-related antigen recognized by the monoclonal antibody OC125. *Int J Gynecol Pathol* 1983;2:275–285.

33. **Nouwen EJ, Hendrix PG, Dauwe S, Eerdekens MW, De Broe ME.** Tumor markers in the human ovary and its neoplasms. A comparative immunohistochemical study. *Am J Pathol* 1987;126: 230–242.

34. **Tuxen MK, Soletormos G, Dombernowsky P.** Tumor markers in the management of patients with ovarian cancer. *Cancer Treat Rev* 1995;21:215–245.

35. **Fleuren GJ, Nap M, Aalders JG, Trimbos JB, de Bruijn HW.** Explanation of the limited correlation between tumor CA125 content and serum CA125 antigen levels in patients with ovarian tumors. *Cancer* 1987;60:2437–2442.

36. **Bast RC, Jr., Klug TL, St John E, Jenison E, Niloff JM, Lazarus H, et al.** A radioimmunoassay using a monoclonal antibody to monitor the course of epithelial ovarian cancer. *N Engl J Med* 1983;309:883–887.

37. **Bon GG, Kenemans P, Verstraeten R, van Kamp GJ, Hilgers J.** Serum tumor marker immunoassays in gynecologic oncology: establishment of reference values. *Am J Obstet Gynecol* 1996;174: 107–114.

38. **Zurawski VR Jr, Orjaseter H, Andersen A, Jellum E.** Elevated serum CA125 levels prior to diagnosis of ovarian neoplasia: relevance for early detection of ovarian cancer. *Int J Cancer* 1988;42:677–680.

39. **Alagoz T, Buller RE, Berman M, Anderson B, Manetta A, DiSaia P.** What is a normal CA125 level? *Gynecol Oncol* 1994;53:93–97.

40. **Bonfrer JM, Korse CM, Verstraeten RA, van Kamp GJ, Hart GA, Kenemans P.** Clinical evaluation of the Byk LIA-mat CA125 II assay: discussion of a reference value. *Clin Chem* 1997;43: 491–497.

41. **Grover S, Koh H, Weideman P, Quinn MA.** The effect of the menstrual cycle on serum CA125 levels: a population study. *Am J Obstet Gynecol* 1992;167:1379–1381.

42. **Pauler DK, Menon U, McIntosh M, Symecko HL, Skates SJ, Jacobs IJ.** Factors influencing serum CA125II levels in healthy postmenopausal women. *Cancer Epidemiol Biomarkers Prev* 2001;10:489–493.

43. **Green PJ, Ballas SK, Westkaemper P, Schwartz HG, Klug TL, Zurawski VR, Jr.** CA 19-9 and CA125 levels in the sera of normal blood donors in relation to smoking history. *J Natl Cancer Inst* 1986;77:337–341.

44. **Tuxen MK, Soletormos G, Petersen PH, Schioler V, Dombernowsky P.** Assessment of biological variation and analytical imprecision of CA125, CEA, and TPA in relation to monitoring of ovarian cancer. *Gynecol Oncol* 1999;74:12–22.

45. **Gocze PM, Szabo DG, Than GN, Csaba IF, Krommer KF.** Occurrence of CA125 and CA 19-9 tumor-associated antigens in sera of patients with gynecologic, trophoblastic, and colorectal tumors. *Gynecol Obstet Invest* 1988;25:268–272.

46. **Fiegler P, Kazmierczak W, Fiegler-Mecik H, Wegrzyn P.** Why do we observe a high concentration of CA125 in mother's serum during pregnancy? *Ginekol Pol* 2005;76:209–213.

47. **Spitzer M, Kaushal N, Benjamin F.** Maternal CA-125 levels in pregnancy and the puerperium. *J Reprod Med* 1998;43:387–392.

48. **Takahashi K, Yamane Y, Yoshino K, Shibukawa T, Matsunaga I, Kitao M.** Studies on serum CA125 levels in pregnant women. *Nippon Sanka Fujinka Gakkai Zasshi* 1985;37:1931–1934.

49. **Urbancsek J, Hauzman EE, Lagarde AR, Osztovits J, Papp Z, Strowitzki T.** Serum CA-125 levels in the second week after embryo transfer predict clinical pregnancy. *Fertil Steril* 2005;83:1414–1421.

50. **El-Shawarby SA, Henderson AF, Mossa MA.** Ovarian cysts during pregnancy: dilemmas in diagnosis and management. *J Obstet Gynaecol* 2005;25:669–675.

51. **Sarandakou A, Protonotariou E, Rizos D.** Tumor markers in biological fluids associated with pregnancy. *Crit Rev Clin Lab Sci* 2007;44:151–178.

52. **Aslam N, Ong C, Woelfer B, Nicolaides K, Jurkovic D.** Serum CA125 at 11–14 weeks of gestation in women with morphologically normal ovaries. *Br J Obstet Gynaecol* 2000;107:689–690.

53. **Canney PA, Moore M, Wilkinson PM, James RD.** Ovarian cancer antigen CA125: a prospective clinical assessment of its role as a tumour marker. *Br J Cancer* 1984;50:765–769.

54. **Tamakoshi K, Kikkawa F, Shibata K, Tomoda K, Obata NH, Wakahara F, et al.** Clinical value of CA125, CA19-9, CEA, CA72-4, and TPA in borderline ovarian tumor. *Gynecol Oncol* 1996;62:67–72.

55. **Vergote IB, Bormer OP, Abeler VM.** Evaluation of serum CA125 levels in the monitoring of ovarian cancer. *Am J Obstet Gynecol* 1987;157:88–92.

56. **Einhorn N, Sjövall K, Knapp RC, Hall P, Scully RE, Bast RC Jr, et al.** Prospective evaluation of serum CA125 levels for early detection of ovarian cancer. *Obstet Gynecol* 1992;80:14–18.

57. **Kobayashi H, Ooi H, Yamada Y, Sakata M, Kawaguchi R, Kanayama S, et al.** Serum CA125 level before the development of ovarian cancer. *Int J Gynaecol Obstet* 2007;99:95–99. Epub 2007 July 23.

58. **Jeyarajah AR, Ind TE, MacDonald N, Skates S, Oram DH, Jacobs IJ.** Increased mortality in postmenopausal women with serum CA125 elevation. *Gynecol Oncol* 1999;73:242–246.

59. **Sjovall K, Nilsson B, Einhorn N.** The significance of serum CA125 elevation in malignant and nonmalignant diseases. *Gynecol Oncol* 2002;85:175–178.

60. **Jacobs I, Davies AP, Bridges J, Stabile I, Fay T, Lower A, et al.** Prevalence screening for ovarian cancer in postmenopausal women by CA125 measurement and ultrasonography. *BMJ* 1993;306:1030–1034.

61. **Jacobs IJ, Skates S, Davies AP, Woolas RP, Jeyarajah A, Weidemann P, et al.** Risk of diagnosis of ovarian cancer after raised serum CA125 concentration: a prospective cohort study. *BMJ* 1996;313:1355–1358.

62. **Menon U, Talaat A, Jeyarajah AR, Rosenthal AN, MacDonald ND, Skates SJ, et al.** Ultrasound assessment of ovarian cancer risk in postmenopausal women with CA125 elevation. *Br J Cancer* 1999;80:1644–1647.

63. **Menon U, Talaat A, Rosenthal AN, MacDonald N, Jeyarajah A, Skates SJ, et al.** Performance of ultrasound as a second line test to serum CA125 in ovarian cancer screening. *Br J Obstet Gynaecol* 2000;107:165–169.

64. **Skates SJ, Menon U, MacDonald N, Rosenthal AN, Oram DH, Knapp RC, et al.** Calculation of the Risk of Ovarian Cancer From Serial CA-125 Values for Preclinical Detection in Postmenopausal Women. *J Clin Oncol* 2003;21:206s–210s.

65. **Skates SJ PD, Jacobs IJ.** Screening based on the risk of cancer calculation from Bayesian hierarchical change point and mixture models of longitudinal markers. *J Am Stat Assoc2001* 2001;96:429–435.

66. **Skates SJ, Xu FJ, Yu YH, Sjövall K, Einhorn N, Chang Y, et al.** Toward an optimal algorithm for ovarian cancer screening with longitudinal tumor markers. *Cancer* 1995;76:2004–2010.

67. **Menon U, Skates SJ, Lewis S, Rosenthal AN, Rufford B, Sibley K, et al.** Prospective study using the risk of ovarian cancer algorithm to screen for ovarian cancer. *J Clin Oncol* 2005;23:7919–7926.

68. **Earle CC, Schrag D, Neville BA, Yabroff KR, Topor M, Fahey A, et al.** Effect of surgeon specialty on processes of care and outcomes for ovarian cancer patients. *J Natl Cancer Inst* 2006;98:172–180.

69. **Engelen MJ, Kos HE, Willemse PH, Aalders JG, de Vries EG, Schaapveld M, et al.** Surgery by consultant gynecologic oncologists improves survival in patients with ovarian carcinoma. *Cancer* 2006;106:589–598.

70. **Giede KC, Kieser K, Dodge J, Rosen B.** Who should operate on patients with ovarian cancer? An evidence-based review. *Gynecol Oncol* 2005;99:447–461.

71. **Olaitan A, Weeks J, Mocroft A, Smith J, Howe K, Murdoch J.** The surgical management of women with ovarian cancer in the south west of England. *Br J Cancer* 2001;85:1824–1830.

72. **Paulsen T, Kjaerheim K, Kaern J, Tretli S, Trope C.** Improved short-term survival for advanced ovarian, tubal, and peritoneal cancer patients operated at teaching hospitals. *Int J Gynecol Cancer* 2006;16 Suppl 1:11–17.

73. **Finkler NJ.** Clinical utility of CA125 in preoperative diagnosis of patients with pelvic masses. *Eur J Obstet Gynecol Reprod Biol* 1993;49:105–107.

74. **Jacobs IJ, Rivera H, Oram DH, Bast RC Jr.** Differential diagnosis of ovarian cancer with tumour markers CA125, CA 15-3 and TAG 72.3. *Br J Obstet Gynaecol* 1993;100:1120–1124.

75. **Mogensen O, Mogensen B, Jakobsen A.** Tumour-associated trypsin inhibitor (TATI) and cancer antigen 125 (CA125) in mucinous ovarian tumours. *Br J Cancer* 1990;61:327–329.

76. **Schutter EM, Kenemans P, Sohn C, Kristen P, Crombach G, Westermann R, et al.** Diagnostic value of pelvic examination, ultrasound, and serum CA125 in postmenopausal women with a pelvic mass. An international multicenter study. *Cancer* 1994;74:1398–1406.

77. **Stenman UH, Alfthan H, Vartiainen J, Lehtovirta P.** Markers supplementing CA125 in ovarian cancer. *Ann Med* 1995;27:115–120.

78. **Skates SJ, Horick N, Yu Y, Xu FJ, Berchuck A, Havrilesky LJ, et al.** Preoperative sensitivity and specificity for early stage ovarian cancer when combining cancer antigen CA-125II, CA 15-3, CA 72-4, and macrophage colony-stimulating factor using mixtures of multivariate normal distributions. *J Clin Oncol* 2004;22:4059–4066.

79. **de Bruijn HW, van der Zee AG, Aalders JG.** The value of cancer antigen 125 (CA125) during treatment and follow-up of patients with ovarian cancer. *Curr Opin Obstet Gynecol* 1997;9:8–13.

80. **Padungsutt P, Thirapagawong C, Senapad S, Suphanit I.** Accuracy of tissue polypeptide specific antigen (TPS) in the diagnosis of ovarian malignancy. *Anticancer Res* 2000;20:1291–1295.

81. **Sehouli J, Akdogan Z, Heinze T, Könsgen D, Stengel D, Mustea A, et al.** Preoperative determination of CASA (Cancer Associated Serum Antigen) and CA-125 for the discrimination between benign and malignant pelvic tumor mass: a prospective study. *Anticancer Res* 2003;23:1115–1118.

82. **Senapad S, Neungton S, Thirapakawong C, Suphanit I, Hangsubcharoen M, Thamintorn K.** Predictive value of the combined serum CA125 and TPS during chemotherapy and before second-look laparotomy in epithelial ovarian cancer. *Anticancer Res* 2000;20:1297–1300.

83. **Woolas RP, Conaway MR, Xu F, Jacobs IJ, Yu Y, Daly L, et al.** Combinations of multiple serum markers are superior to individual assays for discriminating malignant from benign pelvic masses. *Gynecol Oncol* 1995;59:111–116.

84. **Zhang Z, Barnhill SD, Zhang H, Xu F, Yu Y, Jacobs I, et al.** Combination of multiple serum markers using an artificial neural

network to improve specificity in discriminating malignant from benign pelvic masses. *Gynecol Oncol* 1999;73:56–61.

85. **Crump C, McIntosh MW, Urban N, Anderson G, Karlan BY.** Ovarian cancer tumor marker behavior in asymptomatic healthy women: implications for screening. *Cancer Epidemiol Biomarkers Prev* 2000;9:1107–1111.

86. **Visintin I, Feng Z, Longton G, Ward DC, Alvero AB, Lai Y, et al.** Diagnostic Markers for Early Detection of Ovarian Cancer. *Clin Cancer Res* 2008;14:1065–1072.

87. **Rosen DG, Wang L, Atkinson JN, Yu Y, Lu KH, Diamandis EP, et al.** Potential markers that complement expression of CA125 in epithelial ovarian cancer. *Gynecol Oncol* 2005;99:267–277. Epub 2005 Aug 2.

88. **Moore RG, Brown AK, Miller MC, Skates S, Allard WJ, Verch T, et al.** The use of multiple novel tumor biomarkers for the detection of ovarian carcinoma in patients with a pelvic mass. *Gynecol Oncol* 2008;108:402–408. Epub 200 7 Dec 3.

89. **Schummer M, Ng WV, Bumgarner RE, Nelson PS, Schummer B, Bednarski DW, et al.** Comparative hybridization of an array of 21,500 ovarian cDNAs for the discovery of genes overexpressed in ovarian carcinomas. *Gene* 1999;238:375–385.

90. **Ono K, Tanaka T, Tsunoda T, Kitahara O, Kihara C, Okamoto A, et al.** Identification by cDNA microarray of genes involved in ovarian carcinogenesis. *Cancer Res* 2000;60:5007–5011.

91. **Wang K, Gan L, Jeffery E, Gayle M, Gown AM, Skelly M, et al.** Monitoring gene expression profile changes in ovarian carcinomas using cDNA microarray. *Gene* 1999;229:101–108.

92. **Drapkin R, von Horsten HH, Lin Y, Mok SC, Crum CP, Welch WR, et al.** Human epididymis protein 4 (HE4) is a secreted glycoprotein that is overexpressed by serous and endometrioid ovarian carcinomas. *Cancer Res* 2005;65:2162–2169.

93. **Grisaru D, Hauspy J, Prasad M, Albert M, Murphy KJ, Covens A, et al.** Microarray expression identification of differentially expressed genes in serous epithelial ovarian cancer compared with bulk normal ovarian tissue and ovarian surface scrapings. *Oncol Rep* 2007;18:1347–1356.

94. **Galgano MT, Hampton GM, Frierson HF, Jr.** Comprehensive analysis of HE4 expression in normal and malignant human tissues. *Mod Pathol* 2006;19:847–853.

95. **Hellström I, Raycraft J, Hayden-Ledbetter M, Ledbetter JA, Schummer M, McIntosh M, et al.** The HE4 (WFDC2) protein is a biomarker for ovarian carcinoma. *Cancer Res* 2003;63:3695–3700.

96. **Guadagni F, Roselli M, Cosimelli M, Ferroni P, Spila A, Cavaliere F, et al.** CA 72-4 serum marker—a new tool in the management of carcinoma patients. *Cancer Invest* 1995;13:227–238.

97. **Scambia G, Benedetti Panici P, Perrone L, Sonsini C, Giannelli S, Gallo A, et al.** Serum levels of tumour associated glycoprotein (TAG 72) in patients with gynaecological malignancies. *Br J Cancer* 1990;62:147–151.

98. **Negishi Y, Iwabuchi H, Sakunaga H, Sakamoto M, Okabe K, Sato H, et al.** Serum and tissue measurements of CA72-4 in ovarian cancer patients. *Gynecol Oncol* 1993;48:148–154.

99. **Hasholzner U, Baumgartner L, Stieber P, Meier W, Reiter W, Pahl H, et al.** Clinical significance of the tumour markers CA125 II and CA 72-4 in ovarian carcinoma. *Int J Cancer* 1996;69:329–334.

100. **Schutter EM, Sohn C, Kristen P, Möbus V, Crombach G, Kaufmann M, et al.** Estimation of probability of malignancy using a logistic model combining physical examination, ultrasound, serum CA 125, and serum CA 72-4 in postmenopausal women with a pelvic mass: an international multicenter study. *Gynecol Oncol* 1998;69:56–63.

101. **Suzuki M, Ohwada M, Aida I, Tamada T, Hanamura T, Nagatomo M.** Macrophage colony-stimulating factor as a tumor marker for epithelial ovarian cancer. *Obstet Gynecol* 1993;82:946–950.

102. **Suzuki M, Ohwada M, Sato I, Nagatomo M.** Serum level of macrophage colony-stimulating factor as a marker for gynecologic malignancies. *Oncology* 1995;52:128–133.

103. **Suzuki M, Kobayashi H, Ohwada M, Terao T, Sato I.** Macrophage colony-stimulating factor as a marker for malignant germ cell tumors of the ovary. *Gynecol Oncol* 1998;68:35–37.

104. **Lambeck AJ, Crijns AP, Leffers N, Sluiter WJ, ten Hoor KA, Braid M, et al.** Serum cytokine profiling as a diagnostic and prognostic tool in ovarian cancer: a potential role for interleukin 7. *Clin Cancer Res* 2007;13:2385–2391.

105. **Castelli M, Battaglia F, Scambia G, Panici PB, Ferrandina G, Mileo AM, et al.** Immunosuppressive acidic protein and CA125 levels in patients with ovarian cancer. *Oncology* 1991;48:13–17.

106. **Barton DP, Blanchard DK, Michelini-Norris B, Roberts WS, Hoffman MS, Fiorica JV, et al.** Serum soluble interleukin-2 receptor alpha levels in patients with gynecologic cancers: early effect of surgery. *Am J Reprod Immunol* 1993;30:202–206.

107. **Ferdeghini M, Gadducci A, Prontera C, Marrai R, Malgnino G, Annicchiarico C, et al.** Serum soluble interleukin-2 receptor (sIL-2R) assay in cervical and endometrial cancer. Preliminary data. *Anticancer Res* 1993;13:709–713.

108. **Hurteau JA, Woolas RP, Jacobs IJ, Oram DC, Kurman CC, Rubin LA, et al.** Soluble interleukin-2 receptor alpha is elevated in sera of patients with benign ovarian neoplasms and epithelial ovarian cancer. *Cancer* 1995;76:1615–1620.

109. **Gadducci A, Ferdeghini M, Castellani C, Annicchiarico C, Gagetti O, Prontera C, et al.** Serum levels of tumor necrosis factor (TNF), soluble receptors for TNF (55- and 75-kDa sTNFr), and soluble CD14 (sCD14) in epithelial ovarian cancer. *Gynecol Oncol* 1995;58:184–188.

110. **Grosen EA, Granger GA, Gatanaga M, Ininns EK, Hwang C, DiSaia P, et al.** Measurement of the soluble membrane receptors for tumor necrosis factor and lymphotoxin in the sera of patients with gynecologic malignancy. *Gynecol Oncol* 1993;50:68–77.

111. **Rzymski P, Opala T, Wilczak M, Wozniak J, Sajdak S.** Serum tumor necrosis factor alpha receptors p55/p75 ratio and ovarian cancer detection. *Int J Gynaecol Obstet* 2005;88:292–298.

112. **Xu FJ, Yu YH, Li BY, Moradi M, Elg S, Lane C, et al.** Development of two new monoclonal antibodies reactive to a surface antigen present on human ovarian epithelial cancer cells. *Cancer Res* 1991;51:4012–4019.

113. **van Haaften-Day C, Shen Y, Xu F, Yu Y, Berchuck A, Havrilesky LJ, et al.** OVX1, macrophage-colony stimulating factor, and CA-125-II as tumor markers for epithelial ovarian carcinoma: a critical appraisal. *Cancer* 2001;92:2837–2844.

114. **Woolas RP, Xu FJ, Jacobs IJ, Yu YH, Daly L, Berchuck A, et al.** Elevation of multiple serum markers in patients with stage I ovarian cancer. *J Natl Cancer Inst* 1993;85:1748–1751.

115. **Yu JX, Chao L, Chao J.** Prostasin is a novel human serine proteinase from seminal fluid. Purification, tissue distribution, and localization in prostate gland. *J Biol Chem* 1994;269:18843–18848.

116. **Mok SC, Chao J, Skates S, Wong K, Yiu GK, Muto MG, et al.** Prostasin, a potential serum marker for ovarian cancer: identification through microarray technology. *J Natl Cancer Inst* 2001;93:1458–1464.

117. **Tiniakos DG, Yu H, Liapis H.** Osteopontin expression in ovarian carcinomas and tumors of low malignant potential (LMP). *Hum Pathol* 1998;29:1250–1254.

118. **Kim JH, Skates SJ, Uede T, Wong KK, Schorge JO, Feltmate CM, et al.** Osteopontin as a potential diagnostic biomarker for ovarian cancer. *JAMA* 2002;287:1671–1679.

119. **Brakora KA, Lee H, Yusuf R, Sullivan L, Harris A, Colella T, Seiden MV.** Utility of osteopontin as a biomarker in recurrent epithelial ovarian cancer. *Gynecol Oncol* 2004;93:361–365.

120. **Nakae M, Iwamoto I, Fujino T, Maehata Y, Togami S, Yoshinaga M, et al.** Preoperative plasma osteopontin level as a biomarker complementary to carbohydrate antigen 125 in predicting ovarian cancer. *J Obstet Gynaecol Res* 2006;32:309–314.

121. **Salman T, el-Ahmady O, Sawsan MR, Nahed MH.** The clinical value of serum TPS in gynecological malignancies. *Int J Biol Markers* 1995;10:81–86.

122. **Shabana A, Onsrud M.** Tissue polypeptide-specific antigen and CA125 as serum tumor markers in ovarian carcinoma. *Tumour Biol* 1994;15:361–367.

123. **Sliutz G, Tempfer C, Kainz C, Mustafa G, Gitsch G, Koelbl H, et al.** Tissue polypeptide specific antigen and cancer associated serum antigen in the follow-up of ovarian cancer. *Anticancer Res* 1995;15:1127–1129.

124. **Tempfer C, Hefler L, Haeusler G, Reinthaller A, Koelbl H, Zeisler H, et al.** Tissue polypeptide specific antigen in the follow-up of ovarian and cervical cancer patients. *Int J Cancer* 1998;79: 241–244.

125. **Harlozinska A, Sedlaczek P, Van Dalen A, Rozdolski K, Einarsson R.** TPS and CA125 levels in serum, cyst fluid and ascites of patients with epithelial ovarian neoplasms. *Anticancer Res* 1997;17:4473–4478.

126. **Diamandis EP, Yousef GM.** Human tissue kallikreins: a family of new cancer biomarkers. *Clin Chem* 2002;48:1198–1205.

127. **Davidson B, Xi Z, Klokk TI, Tropé CG, Dørum A, Scheistrøen M, et al.** Kallikrein 4 expression is up-regulated in epithelial ovarian carcinoma cells in effusions. *Am J Clin Pathol* 2005;123:360–368.

128. **Diamandis EP, Yousef GM, Soosaipillai AR, Bunting P.** Human kallikrein 6 (zyme/protease M/neurosin): a new serum biomarker of ovarian carcinoma. *Clin Biochem* 2000;33:579–583.

129. **Paliouras M, Borgoño C, Diamandis EP.** Human tissue kallikreins: the cancer biomarker family. *Cancer Lett* 2007;249:61–79.

130. **Diamandis EP.** Proteomic patterns in serum and identification of ovarian cancer. *Lancet* 2002;360:170; author reply 170–171.

131. **Borgoño CA, Kishi T, Scorilas A, Harbeck N, Dorn J, Schmalfeldt B, et al.** Human kallikrein 8 protein is a favorable prognostic marker in ovarian cancer. *Clin Cancer Res* 2006;12:1487–1493.

132. **Chang A, Yousef GM, Jung K, Rajpert-De Meyts E, Diamandis EP.** Identification and molecular characterization of five novel kallikrein gene 13 (*KLK13; KLK-L4*) splice variants: differential expression in the human testis and testicular cancer. *Anticancer Res* 2001;21:3147–3152.

133. **Diamandis EP, Borgoño CA, Scorilas A, Harbeck N, Dorn J, Schmitt M.** Human kallikrein 11: an indicator of favorable prognosis in ovarian cancer patients. *Clin Biochem* 2004;37:823–829.

134. **Diamandis EP, Okui A, Mitsui S, Luo LY, Soosaipillai A, Grass L, et al.** Human kallikrein 11: a new biomarker of prostate and ovarian carcinoma. *Cancer Res* 2002;62:295–300.

135. **Diamandis EP, Scorilas A, Fracchioli S, Van Gramberen M, De Bruijn H, Henrik A, et al.** Human kallikrein 6 (hK6): a new potential serum biomarker for diagnosis and prognosis of ovarian carcinoma. *J Clin Oncol* 2003;21:1035–1043.

136. **Dong Y, Kaushal A, Bui L, Chu S, Fuller PJ, Nicklin J, et al.** Human kallikrein 4 (KLK4) is highly expressed in serous ovarian carcinomas. *Clin Cancer Res* 2001;7:2363–2371.

137. **Hoffman BR, Katsaros D, Scorilas A, Diamandis P, Fracchioli S, Rigault de la Longrais IA, et al.** Immunofluorometric quantitation and histochemical localisation of kallikrein 6 protein in ovarian cancer tissue: a new independent unfavourable prognostic biomarker. *Br J Cancer* 2002;87:763–771.

138. **Kim H, Scorilas A, Katsaros D, Yousef GM, Massobrio M, Fracchioli S, et al.** Human kallikrein gene 5 (KLK5) expression is an indicator of poor prognosis in ovarian cancer. *Br J Cancer* 2001;84:643–650.

139. **Kishi T, Grass L, Soosaipillai A, Scorilas A, Harbeck N, Schmalfeldt B, et al.** Human kallikrein 8, a novel biomarker for ovarian carcinoma. *Cancer Res* 2003;63:2771–2774.

140. **Kurlender L, Yousef GM, Memari N, Robb JD, Michael IP, Borgoño C, et al.** Differential expression of a human kallikrein 5 (KLK5) splice variant in ovarian and prostate cancer. *Tumour Biol* 2004;25:149–156.

141. **Luo LY, Bunting P, Scorilas A, Diamandis EP.** Human kallikrein 10: a novel tumor marker for ovarian carcinoma? *Clin Chim Acta* 2001;306:111–118.

142. **Obiezu CV, Scorilas A, Katsaros D, Massobrio M, Yousef GM, Fracchioli S, et al.** Higher human kallikrein gene 4 (KLK4) expression indicates poor prognosis of ovarian cancer patients. *Clin Cancer Res* 2001;7:2380–2386.

143. **Yousef GM, Polymeris ME, Grass L, Soosaipillai A, Chan PC, Scorilas A, et al.** Human kallikrein 5: a potential novel serum biomarker for breast and ovarian cancer. *Cancer Res* 2003;63: 3958–3965.

144. **Yousef GM, Polymeris ME, Yacoub GM, Scorilas A, Soosaipillai A, Popalis C, et al.** Parallel overexpression of seven kallikrein genes in ovarian cancer. *Cancer Res* 2003;63:2223–2227.

145. **Yousef GM, Scorilas A, Katsaros D, Fracchioli S, Iskander L, Borgoño C, et al.** Prognostic value of the human kallikrein gene 15 expression in ovarian cancer. *J Clin Oncol* 2003;21:3119–3126.

146. **Gitlin D, Perricelli A, Gitlin GM.** Synthesis of fetoprotein by liver, yolk sac, and gastrointestinal tract of the human conceptus. *Cancer Res* 1972;32:979–982.

147. **Lu KH, Gershenson DM.** Update on the management of ovarian germ cell tumors. *J Reprod Med* 2005;50:417–425.

148. **Kawai M, Kano T, Kikkawa F, Morikawa Y, Oguchi H, Nakashima N, et al.** Seven tumor markers in benign and malignant germ cell tumors of the ovary. *Gynecol Oncol* 1992; 45:248–253.

149. **Maida Y, Kyo S, Takakura M, Kanaya T, Inoue M.** Ovarian endometrioid adenocarcinoma with ectopic production of alpha-fetoprotein. *Gynecol Oncol* 1998;71:133–136.

150. **Onsrud M.** Tumour markers in gynaecologic oncology. *Scand J Clin Lab Invest Suppl* 1991;206:60–70.

151. **Olt G, Berchuck A, Bast RC Jr.** The role of tumor markers in gynecologic oncology. *Obstet Gynecol Surv* 1990;45:570–577.

152. **Boggess JF, Soules MR, Goff BA, Greer BE, Cain JM, Tamimi HK.** Serum inhibin and disease status in women with ovarian granulosa cell tumors. *Gynecol Oncol* 1997;64:64–69.

153. **Cooke I, O'Brien M, Charnock FM, Groome N, Ganesan TS.** Inhibin as a marker for ovarian cancer. *Br J Cancer* 1995;71: 1046–1050.

154. **Jobling T, Mamers P, Healy DL, MacLachlan V, Burger HG, Quinn M, et al.** A prospective study of inhibin in granulosa cell tumors of the ovary. *Gynecol Oncol* 1994;55:285–289.

155. **Lappohn RE, Burger HG, Bouma J, Bangah M, Krans M, de Bruijn HW.** Inhibin as a marker for granulosa-cell tumors. *N Engl J Med* 1989;321:790–793.

156. **Petraglia F, Luisi S, Pautier P, Sabourin JC, Rey R, Lhomme C, Bidart JM.** Inhibin B is the major form of inhibin/activin family secreted by granulosa cell tumors. *J Clin Endocrinol Metab* 1998;83:1029–1032.

157. **Yamashita K, Yamoto M, Shikone T, Minami S, Imai M, Nishimori K, Nakano R.** Production of inhibin A and inhibin B in human ovarian sex cord stromal tumors. *Am J Obstet Gynecol* 1997;177:1450–1457.

158. **Robertson DM, Stephenson T, Pruysers E, Burger HG, McCloud P, Tsigos A, et al.** Inhibins/activins as diagnostic markers for ovarian cancer. *Mol Cell Endocrinol* 2002;191:97–103.

159. **Burger HG, Robertson DM, Cahir N, Mamers P, Healy DL, Jobling T, Groome N.** Characterization of inhibin immunoreactivity in post-menopausal women with ovarian tumours. *Clin Endocrinol (Oxf)* 1996;44:413–418.

160. **Lambert-Messerlian GM, Steinhoff M, Zheng W, Canick JA, Gajewski WH, Seifer DB, et al.** Multiple immunoreactive inhibin proteins in serum from postmenopausal women with epithelial ovarian cancer. *Gynecol Oncol* 1997;65:512–516.

161. **Menon U, Riley SC, Thomas J, Bose C, Dawnay A, Evans LW, et al.** Serum inhibin, activin and follistatin in postmenopausal women with epithelial ovarian carcinoma. *Bjog* 2000;107: 1069–1074.

162. **Tsigkou A, Marrelli D, Reis FM, Luisi S, Silva-Filho AL, Roviello F, et al.** Total inhibin is a potential serum marker for epithelial ovarian cancer. *J Clin Endocrinol Metab* 2007;92:2526–2531. Epub 2007 May 1.

163. **Michiel DF, Oppenheim JJ.** Cytokines as positive and negative regulators of tumor promotion and progression. *Semin Cancer Biol* 1992;3:3–15.

164. **Welt CK, Lambert-Messerlian G, Zheng W, Crowley WF Jr, Schneyer AL.** Presence of activin, inhibin, and follistatin in epithelial ovarian carcinoma. *J Clin Endocrinol Metab* 1997;82: 3720–3727.

165. **Hohlfeld P, Dang TT, Nahoul K, Daffos F, Forestier F.** Tumour-associated antigens in maternal and fetal blood. *Prenat Diagn* 1994;14:907–912.

166. **Kobayashi F, Sagawa N, Nanbu Y, Nakamura K, Nonogaki M, Ban C, et al.** Immunohistochemical localization and tissue levels of tumor-associated glycoproteins CA125 and CA 19-9 in the decidua and fetal membranes at various gestational ages. *Am J Obstet Gynecol* 1989;160:1232–1238.

167. **Terracciano D, Mariano A, Macchia V, Di Carlo A.** Analysis of glycoproteins in human colon cancers, normal tissues and in human colon carcinoma cells reactive with monoclonal antibody NCL-19-9. *Oncol Rep* 2005;14:719–722.

168. **Ayhan A, Guven S, Guven ES, Kucukali T.** Is there a correlation between tumor marker panel and tumor size and histopathology in well staged patients with borderline ovarian tumors? *Acta Obstet Gynecol Scand* 2007;86:484–490.

169. **Gadducci A, Cosio S, Carpi A, Nicolini A, Genazzani AR.** Serum tumor markers in the management of ovarian, endometrial and cervical cancer. *Biomed Pharmacother* 2004;58:24–38.

170. **Obermair A, Tempfer C, Hefler L, Preyer O, Kaider A, Zeillinger R, et al.** Concentration of vascular endothelial growth factor (VEGF) in the serum of patients with suspected ovarian cancer. *Br J Cancer* 1998;77:1870–1874.

171. **Czekierdowski A.** Studies on angiogenesis in the benign and malignant ovarian neoplasms with the use of color and pulsed Doppler sonography and serum CA-125, CA-19.9, CA-72.4 and vascular endothelial growth factor measurements. *Ann Univ Mariae Curie Sklodowska [Med]* 2002;57:113–131.

172. **Reynolds T.** For proteomics research, a new race has begun. *J Natl Cancer Inst* 2002;94:552–554.

173. **Wilkins MR, Sanchez JC, Gooley AA, Appel RD, Humphery-Smith I, Hochstrasser DF, et al.** Progress with proteome projects: why all proteins expressed by a genome should be identified and how to do it. *Biotechnol Genet Eng Rev* 1996;13:19–50.

174. **Wilkins MR, Sanchez JC, Williams KL, Hochstrasser DF.** Current challenges and future applications for protein maps and post-translational vector maps in proteome projects. *Electrophoresis* 1996;17:830–838.

175. **Baak JP, Path FR, Hermsen MA, Meijer G, Schmidt J, Janssen EA.** Genomics and proteomics in cancer. *Eur J Cancer* 2003;39:1199–1215.

176. **Mills GB, Bast RC Jr, Srivastava S.** Future for ovarian cancer screening: novel markers from emerging technologies of transcriptional profiling and proteomics. *J Natl Cancer Inst* 2001;93:1437–1439.

177. **Plebani M.** Proteomics: the next revolution in laboratory medicine? *Clin Chim Acta* 2005;357:113–122.

178. **Petricoin EF, Ardekani AM, Hitt BA, Levine PJ, Fusaro VA, Steinberg SM, et al.** Use of proteomic patterns in serum to identify ovarian cancer. *Lancet* 2002;359:572–577.

179. **Zhang Z, Bast RC Jr, Yu Y, Li J, Sokoll LJ, Rai AJ, et al.** Three biomarkers identified from serum proteomic analysis for the detection of early stage ovarian cancer. *Cancer Res* 2004;64:5882–5890.

180. **Rai AJ, Zhang Z, Rosenzweig J, Shih IeM, Pham T, Fung ET, et al.** Proteomic approaches to tumor marker discovery. *Arch Pathol Lab Med* 2002;126:1518–1526.

181. **Lopez MF, Mikulskis A, Kuzdzal S, Golenko E, Petricoin EF 3rd, Liotta LA, et al.** A novel, high-throughput workflow for discovery and identification of serum carrier protein-bound peptide biomarker candidates in ovarian cancer samples. *Clin Chem* 2007;53:1067–1074.

182. **Moore LE, Fung ET, McGuire M, Rabkin CC, Molinaro A, Wang Z, et al.** Evaluation of apolipoprotein A1 and posttranslationally modified forms of transthyretin as biomarkers for ovarian cancer detection in an independent study population. *Cancer Epidemiol Biomarkers Prev* 2006;15:1641–1646.

183. **Lin YW, Lin CY, Lai HC, Chiou JY, Chang CC, Yu MH, et al.** Plasma proteomic pattern as biomarkers for ovarian cancer. *Int J Gynecol Cancer* 2006;16 Suppl 1:139–146.

184. **Lemaire R, Menguellet SA, Stauber J, Marchaudon V, Lucot JP, Collinet P, et al.** Specific MALDI imaging and profiling for biomarker hunting and validation: fragment of the 11S proteasome activator complex, Reg alpha fragment, is a new potential ovary cancer biomarker. *J Proteome Res* 2007;6:4127–4134.

185. **Gortzak-Uzan L, Ignatchenko A, Evangelou AI, Agochiya M, Brown KA, St Onge P, et al.** A proteome resource of ovarian cancer ascites: integrated proteomic and bioinformatic analyses to identify putative biomarkers. *J Proteome Res* 2008;7:339–351.

186. **Timms JF, Arslan-Low E, Gentry-Maharaj A, Luo Z, T'Jampens D, Podust VN, et al.** Preanalytic influence of sample handling on SELDI-TOF serum protein profiles. *Clin Chem* 2007;53:645–656. Epub 2007 Feb 15.

187. **Skates SJ, Horick NK, Moy JM, Minihan AM, Seiden MV, Marks JR, et al.** Pooling of case specimens to create standard serum sets for screening cancer biomarkers. *Cancer Epidemiol Biomarkers Prev* 2007;16:334–341.

188. **Bast RC Jr, Badgwell D, Lu Z, Marquez R, Rosen D, Liu J, et al.** New tumor markers: CA125 and beyond. *Int J Gynecol Cancer* 2005;15 Suppl 3:274–281.

189. **Fushiki T, Fujisawa H, Eguchi S.** Identification of biomarkers from mass spectrometry data using a "common" peak approach. *BMC Bioinformatics* 2006;7:358.

190. **Oh JH, Gao J, Nandi A, Gurnani P, Knowles L, Schorge J.** Diagnosis of early relapse in ovarian cancer using serum proteomic profiling. *Genome Inform* 2005;16:195–204.

191. **van der Merwe DE, Oikonomopoulou K, Marshall J, Diamandis EP.** Mass spectrometry: uncovering the cancer proteome for diagnostics. *Adv Cancer Res* 2007;96:23–50.

192. **Chan DW, Semmes OJ, Petricoin EF, Liotta LA, van der Merwe DE, Diamandis EP.** *National Academy of Clinical Biochemistry Guidelines: The use of MALDI-TOF mass spectrometry profiling to diagnose cancer, 2006.* Available at: http://www.aacc.org/NR/rdonlyres/45357D4E-FA88-4997-B8A6-74BFE31A3D49/0/chp4b_mass_spec.pdf. Accessed January 2008.

193. **Denkert C, Budczies J, Kind T, Weichert W, Tablack P, Sehouli J, et al.** Mass spectrometry-based metabolic profiling reveals different metabolite patterns in invasive ovarian carcinomas and ovarian borderline tumors. *Cancer Res* 2006;66:10795–10804.

194. **Jones PA, Baylin SB.** The fundamental role of epigenetic events in cancer. *Nat Rev Genet* 2002;3:415–428.

195. **Giacona MB, Ruben GC, Iczkowski KA, Roos TB, Porter DM, Sorenson GD.** Cell-free DNA in human blood plasma: length measurements in patients with pancreatic cancer and healthy controls. *Pancreas* 1998;17:89–97.

196. **Jen J, Wu L, Sidransky D.** An overview on the isolation and analysis of circulating tumor DNA in plasma and serum. *Ann N Y Acad Sci* 2000;906:8–12.

197. **Laird PW.** The power and the promise of DNA methylation markers. *Nat Rev Cancer* 2003;3:253–266.

198. **Widschwendter M, Menon U.** Circulating methylated DNA: a new generation of tumor markers. *Clin Cancer Res* 2006;12:7205–7208.

199. **van Nagell JR Jr, DePriest PD, Reedy MB, Gallion HH, Ueland FR, Pavlik EJ, et al.** The efficacy of transvaginal sonographic screening in asymptomatic women at risk for ovarian cancer. *Gynecol Oncol* 2000;77:350–356.

200. **Bailey CL, Ueland FR, Land GL, DePriest PD, Gallion HH, Kryscio RJ, et al.** The malignant potential of small cystic ovarian tumors in women over 50 years of age. *Gynecol Oncol* 1998;69:3–7.

201. **Valentin L, Skoog L, Epstein E.** Frequency and type of adnexal lesions in autopsy material from postmenopausal women: ultrasound study with histological correlation. *Ultrasound Obstet Gynecol* 2003;22:284–289.

202. **Modesitt SC, Pavlik EJ, Ueland FR, DePriest PD, Kryscio RJ, van Nagell JR Jr.** Risk of malignancy in unilocular ovarian cystic tumors less than 10 centimeters in diameter. *Obstet Gynecol* 2003;102:594–599.

203. **Ferrazzi E, Zanetta G, Dordoni D, Berlanda N, Mezzopane R, Lissoni AA.** Transvaginal ultrasonographic characterization of ovarian masses: comparison of five scoring systems in a multicenter study. *Ultrasound Obstet Gynecol* 1997;10:192–197.

204. **Lerner JP, Timor-Tritsch IE, Federman A, Abramovich G.** Transvaginal ultrasonographic characterization of ovarian masses with an improved, weighted scoring system. *Am J Obstet Gynecol* 1994;170:81–5.

205. **Mol BW, Boll D, De Kanter M, Heintz AP, Sijmons EA, Oei SG, et al.** Distinguishing the benign and malignant adnexal mass: an external validation of prognostic models. *Gynecol Oncol* 2001;80:162–167.

206. **Sassone AM, Timor-Tritsch IE, Artner A, Westhoff C, Warren WB.** Transvaginal sonographic characterization of ovarian disease: evaluation of a new scoring system to predict ovarian malignancy. *Obstet Gynecol* 1991;78:70–76.

207. **Timmerman D, Bourne TH, Tailor A, Collins WP, Verrelst H, Vandenberghe K, et al.** A comparison of methods for preoperative discrimination between malignant and benign adnexal masses: the development of a new logistic regression model. *Am J Obstet Gynecol* 1999;181:57–65.

208. **Ueland FR, DePriest PD, Pavlik EJ, Kryscio RJ, van Nagell JR Jr.** Preoperative differentiation of malignant from benign ovarian tumors: the efficacy of morphology indexing and Doppler flow sonography. *Gynecol Oncol* 2003;91:46–50.

209. **Granberg S, Wikland M, Jansson I.** Macroscopic characterization of ovarian tumors and the relation to the histological diagnosis: criteria to be used for ultrasound evaluation. *Gynecol Oncol* 1989; 35:139–144.

210. **Cohen LS, Escobar PF, Scharm C, Glimco B, Fishman DA.** Three-dimensional power Doppler ultrasound improves the diagnostic accuracy for ovarian cancer prediction. *Gynecol Oncol* 2001; 82:40–48.

211. **Kurjak A, Kupesic S, Sparac V, Kosuta D.** Three–dimensional ultrasonographic and power Doppler characterization of ovarian lesions. *Ultrasound Obstet Gynecol* 2000;16:365–371.

212. **Clayton RD, Snowden S, Weston MJ, Mogensen O, Eastaugh J, Lane G.** Neural networks in the diagnosis of malignant ovarian tumours. *Br J Obstet Gynaecol* 1999;106:1078–1082.

213. **Tailor A, Jurkovic D, Bourne TH, Collins WP, Campbell S.** Sonographic prediction of malignancy in adnexal masses using an artificial neural network. *Br J Obstet Gynaecol* 1999;106:21–30.

214. **Timmerman D, Verrelst H, Bourne TH, DeMoor B, Collins WP, Vergote I, et al.** Artificial neural network models for the preoperative discrimination between malignant and benign adnexal masses. *Ultrasound Obstet Gynecol* 1999;13:17–25.

215. **Valentin L, Hagen B, Tingulstad S, Eik-Nes S.** Comparison of "pattern recognition" and logistic regression models for discrimination between benign and malignant pelvic masses: a prospective cross validation. *Ultrasound Obstet Gynecol* 2001;18:357–365.

216. **Van Calster B, Timmerman D, Bourne T, Testa AC, Van Holsbeke C, Domali E, et al.** Discrimination between benign and malignant adnexal masses by specialist ultrasound examination versus serum CA-125. *J Natl Cancer Inst* 2007;99:1706–1714.

217. **Timmerman D, Testa AC, Bourne T, Ferrazzi E, Ameye L, Konstantinovic ML, et al.** Logistic regression model to distinguish between the benign and malignant adnexal mass before surgery: a multicenter study by the International Ovarian Tumor Analysis Group. *J Clin Oncol* 2005;23:8794–8801.

218. **Timmerman D, Van Calster B, Jurkovic D, Valentin L, Testa AC, Bernard JP, et al.** Inclusion of CA-125 does not improve mathematical models developed to distinguish between benign and malignant adnexal tumors. *J Clin Oncol* 2007;25:4194–4200. Epub 2007 Aug 13.

219. **Bleiberg H, Akakpo J, Granberg S, et al.** *HistoScanning, a new device to enhance ultrasound's contribution to clinical assessment of pelvic masses.* American Society of Clinical Oncology (ASCO) 2006. Available at: http://www.histoscanning.com/ASCO.pdf.

220. **Jacobs I, Oram D, Fairbanks J, Turner J, Frost C, Grudzinskas JG.** A risk of malignancy index incorporating CA125, ultrasound and menopausal status for the accurate preoperative diagnosis of ovarian cancer. *Br J Obstet Gynaecol* 1990;97:922–929.

221. **Andersen ES, Knudsen A, Rix P, Johansen B.** Risk of malignancy index in the preoperative evaluation of patients with adnexal masses. *Gynecol Oncol* 2003;90:109–112.

222. **Aslam N, Tailor A, Lawton F, Carr J, Savvas M, Jurkovic D.** Prospective evaluation of three different models for the pre-operative diagnosis of ovarian cancer. *Bjog* 2000;107:1347–1353.

223. **Bailey J, Tailor A, Naik R, Lopes A, Godfrey K, Hatem HM, et al.** Risk of malignancy index for referral of ovarian cancer cases to a tertiary center: does it identify the correct cases? *Int J Gynecol Cancer* 2006;16 Suppl 1:30–34.

224. **Davies AP, Jacobs I, Woolas R, Fish A, Oram D.** The adnexal mass: benign or malignant? Evaluation of a risk of malignancy index. *Br J Obstet Gynaecol* 1993;100:927–931.

225. **Ma S, Shen K, Lang J.** A risk of malignancy index in preoperative diagnosis of ovarian cancer. *Chin Med J (Engl)* 2003;116: 396–399.

226. **Manjunath AP, Pratapkumar, Sujatha K, Vani R.** Comparison of three risk of malignancy indices in evaluation of pelvic masses. *Gynecol Oncol* 2001;81:225–229.

227. **Morgante G, la Marca A, Ditto A, De Leo V.** Comparison of two malignancy risk indices based on serum CA125, ultrasound score and menopausal status in the diagnosis of ovarian masses. *Br J Obstet Gynaecol* 1999;106:524–527.

228. **Tingulstad S, Hagen B, Skjeldestad FE, Onsrud M, Kiserud T, Halvorsen T, et al.** Evaluation of a risk of malignancy index based on serum CA125, ultrasound findings and menopausal status in the pre-operative diagnosis of pelvic masses. *Br J Obstet Gynaecol* 1996;103:826–831.

229. **Ulusoy S, Akbayir O, Numanoglu C, Ulusoy N, Odabas E, Gulkilik A.** The risk of malignancy index in discrimination of adnexal masses. *Int J Gynaecol Obstet* 2007;96:186–191.

230. **Van Holsbeke C, Van Calster B, Valentin L, Testa AC, Ferrazzi E, Dimou I, et al.** External validation of mathematical models to distinguish between benign and malignant adnexal tumors: a multicenter study by the International Ovarian Tumor Analysis Group. *Clin Cancer Res* 2007;13:4440–4447.

231. **van Trappen PO, Rufford BD, Mills TD, Sohaib SA, Webb JA, Sahdev A, et al.** Differential diagnosis of adnexal masses: risk of malignancy index, ultrasonography, magnetic resonance imaging, and radioimmunoscintigraphy. *Int J Gynecol Cancer* 2007;17: 61–67.

232. **Yazbek J, Aslam N, Tailor A, Hillaby K, Raju KS, Jurkovic D.** A comparative study of the risk of malignancy index and the ovarian crescent sign for the diagnosis of invasive ovarian cancer. *Ultrasound Obstet Gynecol* 2006;28:320–324.

233. **Valentin L, Akrawi D.** The natural history of adnexal cysts incidentally detected at transvaginal ultrasound examination in postmenopausal women. *Ultrasound Obstet Gynecol* 2002;20: 174–180.

234. **Folkman J, Watson K, Ingber D, Hanahan D.** Induction of angiogenesis during the transition from hyperplasia to neoplasia. *Nature* 1989;339:58–61.

235. **Kurjak A, Shalan H, Kupesic S, Kosuta D, Sosic A, Benic S, et al.** An attempt to screen asymptomatic women for ovarian and endometrial cancer with transvaginal color and pulsed Doppler sonography. *J Ultrasound Med* 1994;13:295–301.

236. **Vuento MH, Pirhonen JP, Makinen JI, Laippala PJ, Gronroos M, Salmi TA.** Evaluation of ovarian findings in asymptomatic postmenopausal women with color Doppler ultrasound. *Cancer* 1995;76:1214–1218.

237. **Bourne TH, Campbell S, Reynolds KM, Whitehead MI, Hampson J, Royston P, et al.** Screening for early familial ovarian cancer with transvaginal ultrasonography and colour blood flow imaging. *BMJ* 1993;306:1025–1029.

238. **Parkes CA, Smith D, Wald NJ, Bourne TH.** Feasibility study of a randomised trial of ovarian cancer screening among the general population. *J Med Screen* 1994;1:209–214.

239. **Brown DL, Frates MC, Laing FC, DiSalvo DN, Doubilet PM, Benson CB, et al.** Ovarian masses: can benign and malignant lesions be differentiated with color and pulsed Doppler US? *Radiology* 1994;190:333–336.

240. **Timor-Tritsch LE, Lerner JP, Monteagudo A, Santos R.** Transvaginal ultrasonographic characterization of ovarian masses by means of color flow-directed Doppler measurements and a morphologic scoring system. *Am J Obstet Gynecol* 1993;168:909–913.

241. **Valentin L.** Pattern recognition of pelvic masses by gray-scale ultrasound imaging: the contribution of Doppler ultrasound. *Ultrasound Obstet Gynecol* 1999;14:338–347.

242. **Kurjak A, Kupesic S, Sparac V, Prka M, Bekavac I.** The detection of stage I ovarian cancer by three-dimensional sonography and power Doppler. *Gynecol Oncol* 2003;90:258–264.

243. **Guerriero S, Alcazar JL, Ajossa S, Lai MP, Errasti T, Mallarini G, et al.** Comparison of conventional color Doppler imaging and power doppler imaging for the diagnosis of ovarian cancer: results of a European study. *Gynecol Oncol* 2001;83:299–304.

244. **Ramus SJ, Vierkant RA, Johnatty SE, Pike MC, Van Den Berg DJ, Wu AH, et al.** Consortium analysis of 7 candidate SNPs for ovarian cancer. *Int J Cancer* 2008;123:380–388.

245. **Chen S, Parmigiani G.** Meta-analysis of *BRCA1* and *BRCA2* penetrance. *J Clin Oncol* 2007;25:1329–1333.

246. **Aarnio M, Sankila R, Pukkala E, Salovaara R, Aaltonen LA, de la Chapelle A, et al.** Cancer risk in mutation carriers of DNA-mismatch-repair genes. *Int J Cancer* 1999;81:214–218.

247. **Nelson HD, Huffman LH, Fu R, Harris EL.** Genetic risk assessment and *BRCA* mutation testing for breast and ovarian cancer susceptibility: systematic evidence review for the U.S. Preventive Services Task Force. *Ann Intern Med* 2005;143:362–379.

248. **Bourne TH, Campbell S, Reynolds K, Hampson J, Bhatt L, Crayford TJ, et al.** The potential role of serum CA125 in an ultrasound-based screening program for familial ovarian cancer. *Gynecol Oncol* 1994;52:379–385.

249. **Dorum A, Heimdal K, Løvslett K, Kristensen G, Hansen LJ, Sandvei R, et al.** Prospectively detected cancer in familial breast/ovarian cancer screening. *Acta Obstet Gynecol Scand* 1999; 78:906–911.

250. **Karlan BY, Baldwin RL, Lopez-Luevanos E, Raffel LJ, Barbudo D, Narod S, et al.** Peritoneal serous papillary carcinoma, a phenotypic variant of familial ovarian cancer: implications for ovarian cancer screening. *Am J Obstet Gynecol* 1999;180:917–928.

251. **Gaarenstroom KN, van der Hiel B, Tollenaar RA, Vink GR, Jansen FW, van Asperen CJ, et al.** Efficacy of screening women at high risk of hereditary ovarian cancer: results of an 11-year cohort study. *Int J Gynecol Cancer* 2006;16 Suppl 1:54–59.

252. **Hermsen BB, Olivier RI, Verheijen RH, van Beurden M, de Hullu J, Massuger LF, et al.** No efficacy of annual gynaecological screening in *BRCA1/2* mutation carriers; an observational follow-up study. *Br J Cancer* 2007;96:1335–1342.

253. **Skates SJ, Drescher CW, Isaacs C, Schildkraut JM, Armstrong DK, Buys SS, et al.** *A prospective multi-center ovarian cancer screening study in women at increased risk.* American Society of Clinical Oncology 2007, Chicago, IL: 276s.

254. **Stirling D, Evans DG, Pichert G, Shenton A, Kirk EN, Rimmer S, et al.** Screening for familial ovarian cancer: failure of current protocols to detect ovarian cancer at an early stage according to the international Federation of gynecology and obstetrics system. *J Clin Oncol* 2005;23:5588–5596.

255. **Tailor A, Bourne TH, Campbell S, Okokon E, Dew T, Collins WP.** Results from an ultrasound-based familial ovarian cancer screening clinic: a 10-year observational study. *Ultrasound Obstet Gynecol* 2003;21:378–385.

256. **Vasen HF, Tesfay E, Boonstra H, Mourits MJ, Rutgers E, Verheyen R, et al.** Early detection of breast and ovarian cancer in families with *BRCA* mutations. *Eur J Cancer* 2005;41:549–554.

257. **Schorge JO, Muto MG, Welch WR, Bandera CA, Rubin SC, Bell DA, et al.** Molecular evidence for multifocal papillary serous carcinoma of the peritoneum in patients with germline *BRCA1* mutations. *J Natl Cancer Inst* 1998;90:841–845.

258. **Hogg R, Friedlander M.** Biology of epithelial ovarian cancer: implications for screening women at high genetic risk. *J Clin Oncol* 2004;22:1315–1327.

259. **Finch A, Beiner M, Lubinski J, Lynch HT, Moller P, Rosen B, et al.** Salpingo-oophorectomy and the risk of ovarian, fallopian tube, and peritoneal cancers in women with a *BRCA1* or *BRCA2* Mutation. *JAMA* 2006;296:185–192.

260. **Kauff ND, Barakat RR.** Risk-reducing salpingo-oophorectomy in patients with germline mutations in *BRCA1* or *BRCA2*. *J Clin Oncol* 2007;25:2921–2927.

261. **Kauff ND, Satagopan JM, Robson ME, Scheuer L, Hensley M, Hudis CA, et al.** Risk-reducing salpingo-oophorectomy in women with a *BRCA1* or *BRCA2* mutation. *N Engl J Med* 2002;346:1609–1615.

262. **Adonakis GL, Paraskevaidis E, Tsiga S, Seferiadis K, Lolis DE.** A combined approach for the early detection of ovarian cancer in asymptomatic women. *Eur J Obstet Gynecol Reprod Biol* 1996;65:221–225.

263. **Campbell S, Bhan V, Royston P, Whitehead MI, Collins WP.** Transabdominal ultrasound screening for early ovarian cancer. *BMJ* 1989;299:1363–1367.

264. **DePriest PD, Gallion HH, Pavlik EJ, Kryscio RJ, van Nagell JR Jr.** Transvaginal sonography as a screening method for the detection of early ovarian cancer. *Gynecol Oncol* 1997;65:408–414.

265. **Goswamy RK, Campbell S, Whitehead MI.** Screening for ovarian cancer. *Clin Obstet Gynaecol* 1983;10:621–643.

266. **Grover S, Quinn MA, Weideman P, Koh H, Robinson HP, Rome R, et al.** Screening for ovarian cancer using serum CA125 and vaginal examination: report on 2550 females. *Int J Gynecol Cancer* 1995;5:291–295.

267. **Hayashi H, Yaginuma Y, Kitamura S, Saitou Y, Miyamoto T, Komori H, et al.** Bilateral oophorectomy in asymptomatic women over 50 years old selected by ovarian cancer screening. *Gynecol Obstet Invest* 1999;47:58–64.

268. **Kurjak A, Kupesic S.** Transvaginal color Doppler and pelvic tumor vascularity: lessons learned and future challenges. *Ultrasound Obstet Gynecol* 1995;6:145–159.

269. **Millo R, Facca MC, Alberico S.** Sonographic evaluation of ovarian volume in postmenopausal women: a screening test for ovarian cancer? *Clin Exp Obstet Gynecol* 1989;16:72–78.

270. **Tabor A, Jensen FR, Bock JE, Hogdall CK.** Feasibility study of a randomised trial of ovarian cancer screening. *J Med Screen* 1994;1:215–219.

271. **Weiner Z, Beck D, Shteiner M, Borovik R, Ben-Shachar M, Robinzon E, et al.** Screening for ovarian cancer in women with breast cancer with transvaginal sonography and color flow imaging. *J Ultrasound Med* 1993;12:387–393.

272. **Muto MG, Cramer DW, Brown DL, Welch WR, Harlow BL, Xu H, et al.** Screening for ovarian cancer: the preliminary experience of a familial ovarian cancer center. *Gynecol Oncol* 1993;51:12–20.

273. **Schwartz PE, Chambers JT, Taylor KJ.** Early detection and screening for ovarian cancer. *J Cell Biochem Suppl* 1995;23:233–237.

274. **Belinson JL, Okin C, Casey G, Ayoub A, Klein R, Hart WR, et al.** The familial ovarian cancer registry: progress report. *Cleve Clin J Med* 1995;62:129–134.

275. **Menkiszak J, Jakubowska A, Gronwald J, Rzepka-Gorska I, Lubinski J.** [Hereditary ovarian cancer: summary of 5 years of experience]. *Ginekol Pol* 1998;69:283–287.

276. **Karlan BY, Raffel LJ, Crvenkovic G, Smrt C, Chen MD, Lopez E, et al.** A multidisciplinary approach to the early detection of ovarian carcinoma: rationale, protocol design, and early results. *Am J Obstet Gynecol* 1993;169:494–501.

277. **Dorum A, Kristensen GB, Abeler VM, Trope CG, Moller P.** Early detection of familial ovarian cancer. *Eur J Cancer* 1996;32A:1645–1651.

278. **Scheuer L, Kauff N, Robson M, Kelly B, Barakat R, Satagopan J, et al.** Outcome of preventive surgery and screening for breast and ovarian cancer in *BRCA* mutation carriers. *J Clin Oncol* 2002;20:1260–1268.

279. **Laframboise S, Nedelcu R, Murphy J, Cole DE, Rosen B.** Use of CA-125 and ultrasound in high-risk women. *Int J Gynecol Cancer* 2002;12:86–91.

280. **Liede A, Karlan BY, Baldwin RL, Platt LD, Kuperstein G, Narod SA.** Cancer incidence in a population of Jewish women at risk of ovarian cancer. *J Clin Oncol* 2002;20:1570–1577.

281. **Fries MH, Hailey BJ, Flanagan J, Licklider D.** Outcome of five years of accelerated surveillance in patients at high risk for inherited breast/ovarian cancer: report of a phase II trial. *Mil Med* 2004;169:411–416.

282. **Meeuwissen PA, Seynaeve C, Brekelmans CT, Meijers-Heijboer HJ, Klijn JG, Burger CW.** Outcome of surveillance and prophylactic salpingo-oophorectomy in asymptomatic women at high risk for ovarian cancer. *Gynecol Oncol* 2005;97:476–482.

283. **Oei AL, Massuger LF, Bulten J, Ligtenberg MJ, Hoogerbrugge N, de Hullu JA.** Surveillance of women at high risk for hereditary ovarian cancer is inefficient. *Br J Cancer* 2006;94:814–819.

284. **Bosse K, Rhiem K, Wappenschmidt B, Hellmich M, Madeja M, Ortmann M, et al.** Screening for ovarian cancer by transvaginal ultrasound and serum CA125 measurement in women with a familial predisposition: a prospective cohort study. *Gynecol Oncol* 2006;103:1077–1082.

285. **Sato S, Yokoyama Y, Sakamoto T, Futagami M, Saito Y.** Usefulness of mass screening for ovarian carcinoma using transvaginal ultrasonography. *Cancer* 2000;89:582–588.

286. **Holbert TR.** Screening transvaginal ultrasonography of postmenopausal women in a private office setting. *Am J Obstet Gynecol* 1994;170:1699–1703; discussion 1703–1704.

287. **Hasson MA, Fagerstrom RM, Kahane DC, Walsh JH, Myers MH, Caughman C, et al.** Design and evolution of the data management systems in the Prostate, Lung, Colorectal and Ovarian (PLCO) Cancer Screening Trial. *Control Clin Trials* 2000;21:329S–348S.

288. **Buys SS, Partridge E, Greene MH, Prorok PC, Reding D, Riley TL, et al.** Ovarian cancer screening in the Prostate, Lung, Colorectal and Ovarian (PLCO) cancer screening trial: findings from the initial screen of a randomized trial. *Am J Obstet Gynecol* 2005;193:1630–1639.

289. **Jacobs I.** Screening for familial ovarian cancer: the need for well-designed prospective studies. *J Clin Oncol* 2005;23:5443–5445.

290. United Kingdom Familial Ovarian Cancer Screening Study (protocol). London: Gynaecological Cancer Research Centre, EGA Institute for Women's Health, University College London, United Kingdom.

291. **Greene MH, Piedmonte M, Alberts D, Gail M, Hensley M, Miner Z, et al.** A prospective study of risk-reducing salpingo-oophorectomy and longitudinal CA-125 screening among women at increased genetic risk of ovarian cancer: design and baseline characteristics: a gynecologic oncology group study. *Cancer Epidemiol Biomarkers Prev* 2008;17:594–604.

292. **Fleischer AC, Wheeler JE, Lindsay I, Hendrix SL, Grabill S, Kravitz B, et al.** An assessment of the value of ultrasonographic screening for endometrial disease in postmenopausal women without symptoms. *Am J Obstet Gynecol* 2001;184:70–75.

293. **Gerber B, Krause A, Müller H, Reimer T, Külz T, Kundt G, et al.** Ultrasonographic detection of asymptomatic endometrial cancer in postmenopausal patients offers no prognostic advantage over symptomatic disease discovered by uterine bleeding. *Eur J Cancer* 2001;37:64–71.

294. **Gottlieb S.** No advantage in screening for endometrial cancer. *BMJ* 2000;321:1039A.

295. **Korhonen MO, Symons JP, Hyde BM, Rowan JP, Wilborn WH.** Histologic classification and pathologic findings for endometrial biopsy specimens obtained from 2964 perimenopausal and postmenopausal women undergoing screening for continuous hormones as replacement therapy (CHART 2 Study). *Am J Obstet Gynecol* 1997;176:377–380.

296. **Smith RA, von Eschenbach AC, Wender R, Levin B, Byers T, Rothenberger D, et al.** American Cancer Society guidelines for the early detection of cancer: update of early detection guidelines for prostate, colorectal, and endometrial cancers. Also: update 2001—testing for early lung cancer detection. *CA Cancer J Clin* 2001;51:38–75; quiz 77–80.

297. **Sonoda Y, Barakat RR.** Screening and the prevention of gynecologic cancer: endometrial cancer. *Best Pract Res Clin Obstet Gynaecol* 2006;20:363–377.

298. **Nakagawa-Okamura C, Sato S, Tsuji I, Kuramoto H, Tsubono Y, Aoki D, et al.** Effectiveness of mass screening for endometrial cancer. *Acta Cytol* 2002;46:277–283.

299. **Dunlop MG, Farrington SM, Carothers AD, Wyllie AH, Sharp L, Burn J, et al.** Cancer risk associated with germline DNA mismatch repair gene mutations. *Hum Mol Genet* 1997;6:105–110.

300. **Quehenberger F, Vasen HF, van Houwelingen HC.** Risk of colorectal and endometrial cancer for carriers of mutations of the *hMLH1* and *hMSH2* gene: correction for ascertainment. *J Med Genet* 2005;42:491–496.

301. **Vasen HF, Watson P, Mecklin JP, Jass JR, Green JS, Nomizu T, et al.** The epidemiology of endometrial cancer in hereditary nonpolyposis colorectal cancer. *Anticancer Res* 1994;14:1675–1678.

302. **Watson P, Lynch HT.** Cancer risk in mismatch repair gene mutation carriers. *Fam Cancer* 2001;1:57–60.

303. **Dove-Edwin I, Boks D, Goff S, Kenter GG, Carpenter R, Vasen HF, et al.** The outcome of endometrial carcinoma surveillance by ultrasound scan in women at risk of hereditary nonpolyposis colorectal carcinoma and familial colorectal carcinoma. *Cancer* 2002;94:1708–1712.

304. **Rijcken FE, Mourits MJ, Kleibeuker JH, Hollema H, van der Zee AG.** Gynecologic screening in hereditary nonpolyposis colorectal cancer. *Gynecol Oncol* 2003;91:74–80.

305. **Dijkhuizen FP, Mol BW, Brolmann HA, Heintz AP.** The accuracy of endometrial sampling in the diagnosis of patients with endometrial carcinoma and hyperplasia: a meta-analysis. *Cancer* 2000;89:1765–1772.

306. **Lécuru F, Le Frère Belda MA, Bats AS, Tulpin L, Metzger U, Olschwang S, et al.** Performance of office hysteroscopy and endometrial biopsy for detecting endometrial disease in women at risk of human non-polyposis colon cancer: a prospective study. *Int J Gynecol Cancer* 2008 Jan 23 [Epub ahead of print].

307. **Pasqualotto EB, Margossian H, Price LL, Bradley LD.** Accuracy of preoperative diagnostic tools and outcome of hysteroscopic management of menstrual dysfunction. *J Am Assoc Gynecol Laparosc* 2000;7:201–209.

308. **Tahir MM, Bigrigg MA, Browning JJ, Brookes ST, Smith PA.** A randomised controlled trial comparing transvaginal ultrasound, outpatient hysteroscopy and endometrial biopsy with inpatient hysteroscopy and curettage. *Br J Obstet Gynaecol* 1999;106:1259–1264.

309. **Lécuru F, Metzger U, Scarabin C, Le Frère Belda MA, Olschwang S, Laurent Puig P.** Hysteroscopic findings in women at risk of HNPCC. Results of a prospective observational study. *Fam Cancer* 2007;6:295–299.

310. **Schmeler KM, Lynch HT, Chen LM, Munsell MF, Soliman PT, Clark MB, et al.** Prophylactic surgery to reduce the risk of gynecologic cancers in the Lynch syndrome. *N Engl J Med* 2006;354:261–269.

311. **Ferrazzi E, Torri V, Trio D, Zannoni E, Filiberto S, Dordoni D.** Sonographic endometrial thickness: a useful test to predict atrophy in patients with postmenopausal bleeding. An Italian multicenter study. *Ultrasound Obstet Gynecol* 1996;7:315–321.

312. **Langer RD, Pierce JJ, O'Hanlan KA, Johnson SR, Espeland MA, Trabal JF, et al.** Transvaginal ultrasonography compared with endometrial biopsy for the detection of endometrial disease. Postmenopausal estrogen/progestin interventions trial. *N Engl J Med* 1997;337:1792–1798.

313. **Gupta JK, Chien PF, Voit D, Clark TJ, Khan KS.** Ultrasonographic endometrial thickness for diagnosing endometrial pathology in women with postmenopausal bleeding: a meta-analysis. *Acta Obstet Gynecol Scand* 2002;81:799–816.

314. **Fistonic I, Hodek B, Klaric P, Jokanovic L, Grubisic G, Ivicevic-Bakulic T.** Transvaginal sonographic assessment of premalignant and malignant changes in the endometrium in postmenopausal bleeding. *J Clin Ultrasound* 1997;25:431–435.

315. **SIGN.** *Investigation of postmenopausal bleeding—A national clinical guideline.* Scottish Intercollegiate Guidelines Network, 2002.

316. **Vuento MH, Pirhonen JP, Mäkinen JI, Tyrkkö JE, Laippala PJ, Grönroos M, et al.** Screening for endometrial cancer in asymptomatic postmenopausal women with conventional and colour Doppler sonography. *Br J Obstet Gynaecol* 1999;106:14–20.

317. **Vuento MH, Stenman UH, Pirhonen JP, Mäkinen JI, Laippala PJ, Salmi TA.** Significance of a single CA125 assay combined with ultrasound in the early detection of ovarian and endometrial cancer. *Gynecol Oncol* 1997;64:141–146.

318. **Shipley CF 3rd, Simmons CL, Nelson GH.** Comparison of transvaginal sonography with endometrial biopsy in asymptomatic postmenopausal women. *J Ultrasound Med* 1994;13:99–104.

319. **Brooks SE, Yeatts-Peterson M, Baker SP, Reuter KL.** Thickened endometrial stripe and/or endometrial fluid as a marker of pathology: fact or fancy? *Gynecol Oncol* 1996;63:19–24.

320. **Gruboeck K, Jurkovic D, Lawton F, Savvas M, Tailor A, Campbell S.** The diagnostic value of endometrial thickness and volume measurements by three-dimensional ultrasound in patients with postmenopausal bleeding. *Ultrasound Obstet Gynecol* 1996;8:272–276.

321. **Mercé LT, Alcazar JL, Lopez C, Iglesias E, Bau S, Alvarez de los Heros J, et al.** Clinical usefulness of 3-dimensional sonography and power Doppler angiography for diagnosis of endometrial carcinoma. *J Ultrasound Med* 2007;26:1279–1287.

322. **Odeh M, Vainerovsky I, Grinin V, Kais M, Ophir E, Bornstein J.** Three-dimensional endometrial volume and 3-dimensional power Doppler analysis in predicting endometrial carcinoma and hyperplasia. *Gynecol Oncol* 2007;106:348–353.

323. **Schwartz LB, Snyder J, Horan C, Porges RF, Nachtigall LE, Goldstein SR.** The use of transvaginal ultrasound and saline infusion sonohysterography for the evaluation of asymptomatic postmenopausal breast cancer patients on *tamoxifen. Ultrasound Obstet Gynecol* 1998;11:48–53.

324. **Markovitch O, Tepper R, Aviram R, Fishman A, Shapira J, Cohen I.** The value of sonohysterography in the prediction of endometrial pathologies in asymptomatic postmenopausal breast cancer *tamoxifen*-treated patients. *Gynecol Oncol* 2004;94:754–759.

325. **Montgomery BE, Daum GS, Dunton CJ.** Endometrial hyperplasia: a review. *Obstet Gynecol Surv* 2004;59:368–378.

326. **Bornstein J, Auslender R, Pascal B, Gutterman E, Isakov D, Abramovici H.** Diagnostic pitfalls of ultrasonographic uterine screening in women treated with *tamoxifen. J Reprod Med* 1994;39:674–678.

327. **Cecchini S, Ciatto S, Bonardi R, Mazzotta A, Grazzini G, Pacini P, et al.** Screening by ultrasonography for endometrial carcinoma in postmenopausal breast cancer patients under adjuvant *tamoxifen*. *Gynecol Oncol* 1996;60:409–411.

328. **Fung MF, Reid A, Faught W, Le T, Chenier C, Verma S, et al.** Prospective longitudinal study of ultrasound screening for endometrial abnormalities in women with breast cancer receiving *tamoxifen*. *Gynecol Oncol* 2003;91:154–159.

329. **Love CD, Muir BB, Scrimgeour JB, Leonard RC, Dillon P, Dixon JM.** Investigation of endometrial abnormalities in asymptomatic women treated with *tamoxifen* and an evaluation of the role of endometrial screening. *J Clin Oncol* 1999;17:2050–2054.

330. **Berliere M, Charles A, Galant C, Donnez J.** Uterine side effects of *tamoxifen*: a need for systematic pretreatment screening. *Obstet Gynecol* 1998;91:40–44.

331. **Garuti G, Grossi F, Centinaio G, Sita G, Nalli G, Luerti M.** Pretreatment and prospective assessment of endometrium in menopausal women taking *tamoxifen* for breast cancer. *Eur J Obstet Gynecol Reprod Biol* 2007;132:101–106.

332. **Yancey M, Magelssen D, Demaurez A, Lee RB.** Classification of endometrial cells on cervical cytology. *Obstet Gynecol* 1990;76:1000–1005.

333. **Mitchell H, Giles G, Medley G.** Accuracy and survival benefit of cytological prediction of endometrial carcinoma on routine cervical smears. *Int J Gynecol Pathol* 1993;12:34–40.

334. **Kerpsack JT, Finan MA, Kline RC.** Correlation between endometrial cells on Papanicolaou smear and endometrial carcinoma. *South Med J* 1998;91:749–752.

335. **Leeson SC, Inglis TC, Salman WD.** A study to determine the underlying reason for abnormal glandular cytology and the formulation of a management protocol. *Cytopathology* 1997;8:20–26.

336. **Viikki M, Pukkala E, Hakama M.** Risk of endometrial, ovarian, vulvar, and vaginal cancers after a positive cervical cytology followed by negative histology. *Obstet Gynecol* 1998;92:269–273.

337. **Zweizig S, Noller K, Reale F, Collis S, Resseguie L.** Neoplasia associated with atypical glandular cells of undetermined significance on cervical cytology. *Gynecol Oncol* 1997;65:314–318.

338. **Tsuda H, Kawabata M, Yamamoto K, Inoue T, Umesaki N.** Prospective study to compare endometrial cytology and transvaginal ultrasonography for identification of endometrial malignancies. *Gynecol Oncol* 1997;65:383–386.

339. **Koss LG, Schreiber K, Oberlander SG, Moussouris HF, Lesser M.** Detection of endometrial carcinoma and hyperplasia in asymptomatic women. *Obstet Gynecol* 1984;64:1–11.

340. **Berchuck A.** Biomarkers in the endometrium. *J Cell Biochem Suppl* 1995;23:174–178.

341. **Risinger JI, Hayes AK, Berchuck A, Barrett JC.** *PTEN/MMAC1* mutations in endometrial cancers. *Cancer Res* 1997;57:4736–4738.

342. **Kyo S, Takakura M, Kohama T, Inoue M.** Telomerase activity in human endometrium. *Cancer Res* 1997;57:610–614.

343. **Maida Y, Kyo S, Kanaya T, Wang Z, Tanaka M, Yatabe N, et al.** Is the telomerase assay useful for screening of endometrial lesions? *Int J Cancer* 2002;100:714–718.

344. **Zheng PS, Iwasaka T, Yamasaki F, Ouchida M, Yokoyama M, Nakao Y, et al.** Telomerase activity in gynecologic tumors. *Gynecol Oncol* 1997;64:171–175.

345. **Brien TP, Kallakury BV, Lowry CV, Ambros RA, Muraca PJ, Malfetano JH, et al.** Telomerase activity in benign endometrium and endometrial carcinoma. *Cancer Res* 1997;57:2760–2764.

346. **Saito T, Schneider A, Martel N, Mizumoto H, Bulgay-Moerschel M, Kudo R, et al.** Proliferation-associated regulation of telomerase activity in human endometrium and its potential implication in early cancer diagnosis. *Biochem Biophys Res Commun* 1997;231:610–614.

347. **Shroyer KR, Thompson LC, Enomoto T, Eskens JL, Shroyer AL, McGregor JA.** Telomerase expression in normal epithelium, reactive atypia, squamous dysplasia, and squamous cell carcinoma of the uterine cervix. *Am J Clin Pathol* 1998;109:153–162.

348. **Yokoyama Y, Takahashi Y, Morishita S, Hashimoto M, Niwa K, Tamaya T.** Telomerase activity in the human endometrium throughout the menstrual cycle. *Mol Hum Reprod* 1998;4:173–177.

349. **de Leeuw WJ, Dierssen J, Vasen HF, Wijnen JT, Kenter GG, Meijers-Heijboer H.** Prediction of a mismatch repair gene defect by microsatellite instability and immunohistochemical analysis in endometrial tumours from HNPCC patients. *J Pathol* 2000;192:328–335.

350. **Ichikawa Y, Tsunoda H, Takano K, Oki A, Yoshikawa H.** Microsatellite instability and immunohistochemical analysis of *MLH1* and *MSH2* in normal endometrium, endometrial hyperplasia and endometrial cancer from a hereditary nonpolyposis colorectal cancer patient. *Jpn J Clin Oncol* 2002;32:110–112.

351. **Sutter C, Dallenbach-Hellweg G, Schmidt D, Baehring J, Bielau S, von Knebel Doeberitz M, et al.** Molecular analysis of endometrial hyperplasia in HNPCC-suspicious patients may predict progression to endometrial carcinoma. *Int J Gynecol Pathol* 2004;23:18–25.

352. **Berends MJ, Wu Y, Sijmons RH, van der Sluis T, Ek WB, Ligtenberg MJ, et al.** Toward new strategies to select young endometrial cancer patients for mismatch repair gene mutation analysis. *J Clin Oncol* 2003;21:4364–4370.

353. **Broaddus RR, Lynch HT, Chen LM, Daniels MS, Conrad P, Munsell MF, et al.** Pathologic features of endometrial carcinoma associated with HNPCC: a comparison with sporadic endometrial carcinoma. *Cancer* 2006;106:87–94.

354. **Modica I, Soslow RA, Black D, Tornos C, Kauff N, Shia J.** Utility of immunohistochemistry in predicting microsatellite instability in endometrial carcinoma. *Am J Surg Pathol* 2007;31:744–751.

355. **Risinger JI, Berchuck A, Kohler MF, Watson P, Lynch HT, Boyd J.** Genetic instability of microsatellites in endometrial carcinoma. *Cancer Res* 1993;53:5100–5103.

356. **Catasus L, Machin P, Matias-Guiu X, Prat J.** Microsatellite instability in endometrial carcinomas: clinicopathologic correlations in a series of 42 cases. *Hum Pathol* 1998;29:1160–1164.

357. **Kobayashi K, Sagae S, Kudo R, Saito H, Koi S, Nakamura Y.** Microsatellite instability in endometrial carcinomas: frequent replication errors in tumors of early onset and/or of poorly differentiated type. *Genes Chromosomes Cancer* 1995;14:128–132.

358. **Lax SF.** Molecular genetic pathways in various types of endometrial carcinoma: from a phenotypical to a molecular-based classification. *Virchows Arch* 2004;444:213–223.

359. **Esteller M, Levine R, Baylin SB, Ellenson LH, Herman JG.** *MLH1* promoter hypermethylation is associated with the microsatellite instability phenotype in sporadic endometrial carcinomas. *Oncogene* 1998;17:2413–2417.

360. **Hewitt MJ, Wood N, Quinton ND, Charlton R, Taylor G, Sheridan E, et al.** The detection of microsatellite instability in blind endometrial samples—a potential novel screening tool for endometrial cancer in women from hereditary nonpolyposis colorectal cancer families? *Int J Gynecol Cancer* 2006;16:1393–1400.

361. **Al-Jehani RM, Jeyarajah AR, Hagen B, Hogdall EV, Oram DH, Jacobs IJ.** Model for the molecular genetic diagnosis of endometrial cancer using *K-ras* mutation analysis. *J Natl Cancer Inst* 1998;90:540–542.

362. **Fiegl H, Gattringer C, Widschwendter A, Schneitter A, Ramoni A, Sarlay D, et al.** Methylated DNA collected by tampons—a new tool to detect endometrial cancer. *Cancer Epidemiol Biomarkers Prev* 2004;13:882–888.

363. **Tong TR, Chan OW, Chow TC, Yu V, Leung KM, To SH.** Detection of human papillomavirus in sanitary napkins: a new paradigm in cervical cancer screening. *Diagn Cytopathol* 2003;28:140–141.

364. **Ahlquist DA.** Stool-based DNA tests for colorectal cancer: clinical potential and early results. *Rev Gastroenterol Disord* 2002;2 Suppl 1:S20–26.

365. **Diefenbach CS, Shah Z, Iasonos A, Barakat RR, Levine DA, Aghajanian C, et al.** Preoperative serum YKL-40 is a marker for detection and prognosis of endometrial cancer. *Gynecol Oncol* 2007;104:435–442.

366. **DeSouza LV, Grigull J, Ghanny S, Dubé V, Romaschin AD, Colgan TJ, et al.** Endometrial carcinoma biomarker discovery and verification using differentially tagged clinical samples with multidimensional liquid chromatography and tandem mass spectrometry. *Mol Cell Proteomics* 2007;6:1170–1182.

367. **Dubé V, Grigull J, DeSouza LV, Ghanny S, Colgan TJ, Romaschin AD, et al.** Verification of endometrial tissue biomarkers previously discovered using mass spectrometry-based proteomics by means of immunohistochemistry in a tissue microarray format. *J Proteome Res* 2007;6:2648–2655.

368. Ries LAG, Melbert D, Krapcho M, Mariotto A, Miller BA, Feuer EJ, et al. *SEER Cancer Statistics Review, 1975–2004.* Bethesda, MD: National Cancer Institute. Available at: http://seer.cancer.gov/csr/1975_2004/. Based on November 2006 SEER data submission posted to the SEER Web site 2007.

369. Sasieni PD, Cuzick J, Lynch-Farmery E. Estimating the efficacy of screening by auditing smear histories of women with and without cervical cancer. The National Coordinating Network for Cervical Screening Working Group. *Br J Cancer* 1996;73:1001–1005.

370. Nanda K, McCrory DC, Myers ER, Bastian LA, Hasselblad V, Hickey JD, et al. Accuracy of the Papanicolaou test in screening for and follow-up of cervical cytologic abnormalities: a systematic review. *Ann Intern Med* 2000;132:810–819.

371. National Institute for Clinical Excellence. *Guidance on the use of liquid-based cytology for cervical screening.* London: National Institue for Clinical Excellence, 2003.

372. Abulafia O, Pezzullo JC, Sherer DM. Performance of ThinPrep liquid-based cervical cytology in comparison with conventionally prepared Papanicolaou smears: a quantitative survey. *Gynecol Oncol* 2003;90:137–144.

373. Bernstein SJ, Sanchez-Ramos L, Ndubisi B. Liquid-based cervical cytologic smear study and conventional Papanicolaou smears: a metaanalysis of prospective studies comparing cytologic diagnosis and sample adequacy. *Am J Obstet Gynecol* 2001;185:308–317.

374. Bishop JW, Marshall CJ, Bentz JS. New technologies in gynecologic cytology. *J Reprod Med* 2000;45:701–719.

375. Davey E, Barratt A, Irwig L, Chan SF, Macaskill P, Mannes P, et al. Effect of study design and quality on unsatisfactory rates, cytology classifications, and accuracy in liquid-based versus conventional cervical cytology: a systematic review. *Lancet* 2006;367:122–132.

376. Sulik SM, Kroeger K, Schultz JK, Brown JL, Becker LA, Grant WD. Are fluid-based cytologies superior to the conventional Papanicolaou test? A systematic review. *J Fam Pract* 2001;50:1040–1046.

377. Arbyn M, Bergeron C, Klinkhamer P, Martin-Hirsch P, Siebers AG, Bulten J. Liquid compared with conventional cervical cytology: a systematic review and meta-analysis. *Obstet Gynecol* 2008;111:167–177.

378. Richart RM, Masood S, Syrjänen KJ, Vassilakos P, Kaufman RH, Meisels A, et al. Human papillomavirus. International Academy of Cytology Task Force summary. Diagnostic Cytology Towards the 21st Century: An International Expert Conference and Tutorial. *Acta Cytol* 1998;42:50–58.

379. Bhatla N, Lal N, Bao YP, Ng T, Qiao YL. A meta-analysis of human papillomavirus type-distribution in women from South Asia: Implications for vaccination. *Vaccine* 2008.

380. Clifford GM, Gallus S, Herrero R, Muñoz N, Snijders PJ, Vaccarella S, et al. Worldwide distribution of human papillomavirus types in cytologically normal women in the International Agency for Research on Cancer HPV prevalence surveys: a pooled analysis. *Lancet* 2005;366:991–998.

381. Sargent A, Bailey A, Almonte M, Turner A, Thomson C, Peto J, et al. for ARTISTIC Study Group. Prevalence of type-specific HPV infection by age and grade of cervical cytology: data from the ARTISTIC trial. *Br J Cancer* 2008;98:1704–1709. Epub 2008 Apr 8.

382. Koliopoulos G, Arbyn M, Martin-Hirsch P, Kyrgiou M, Prendiville W, Paraskevaidis E. Diagnostic accuracy of human papillomavirus testing in primary cervical screening: a systematic review and meta-analysis of non-randomized studies. *Gynecol Oncol* 2007;104:232–246.

383. Paraskevaidis E, Arbyn M, Sotiriadis A, Diakomanolis E, Martin-Hirsch P, Koliopoulos G, et al. The role of HPV DNA testing in the follow-up period after treatment for CIN: a systematic review of the literature. *Cancer Treat Rev* 2004;30:205–211.

384. Zielinski GD, Bais AG, Helmerhorst TJ, Verheijen RH, de Schipper FA, Snijders PJ, et al. HPV testing and monitoring of women after treatment of CIN 3: review of the literature and meta-analysis. *Obstet Gynecol Surv* 2004;59:543–553.

385. Mandelblatt JS, Lawrence WF, Womack SM, Jacobson D, Yi B, Hwang YT, et al. Benefits and costs of using HPV testing to screen for cervical cancer. *JAMA* 2002;287:2372–2381.

386. Goldie SJ, Kim JJ, Wright TC. Cost-effectiveness of human papillomavirus DNA testing for cervical cancer screening in women aged 30 years or more. *Obstet Gynecol* 2004;103:619–631.

387. Kjaer S, Høgdall E, Frederiksen K, Munk C, van den Brule A, Svare E, et al. The absolute risk of cervical abnormalities in high-risk human papillomavirus-positive, cytologically normal women over a 10-year period. *Cancer Res* 2006;66:10630–10636.

388. Sherman ME, Lorincz AT, Scott DR, Wacholder S, Castle PE, Glass AG, et al. Baseline cytology, human papillomavirus testing, and risk for cervical neoplasia: a 10-year cohort analysis. *J Natl Cancer Inst* 2003;95:46–52.

389. Safaeian M, Solomon D, Wacholder S, Schiffman M, Castle P. Risk of precancer and follow-up management strategies for women with human papillomavirus-negative atypical squamous cells of undetermined significance. *Obstet Gynecol* 2007;109:1325–1331.

390. Walker JL, Wang SS, Schiffman M, Solomon D. Predicting absolute risk of CIN 3 during post-colposcopic follow-up: results from the ASCUS-LSIL Triage Study (ALTS). *Am J Obstet Gynecol* 2006;195:341–348.

391. Wang SS, Walker JL, Schiffman M, Solomon D. Evaluating the risk of cervical precancer with a combination of cytologic, virologic, and visual methods. *Cancer Epidemiol Biomarkers Prev* 2005;14:2665–2668.

392. Wright TC, Jr., Massad LS, Dunton CJ, Spitzer M, Wilkinson EJ, Solomon D. 2006 consensus guidelines for the management of women with abnormal cervical cancer screening tests. *Am J Obstet Gynecol* 2007;197:346–355.

393. Wright TC, Jr., Massad LS, Dunton CJ, Spitzer M, Wilkinson EJ, Solomon D. 2006 consensus guidelines for the management of women with cervical intraepithelial neoplasia or adenocarcinoma *in situ.* *Am J Obstet Gynecol* 2007;197:340–345.

394. van den Akker-van Marie ME, van Ballegooijen M, Rozendaal L, Meijer CJ, Habbema JD. Extended duration of the detectable stage by adding HPV test in cervical cancer screening. *Br J Cancer* 2003;89:1830–1833.

395. Xi LF, Koutsky LA, Galloway DA, Kuypers J, Hughes JP, Wheeler CM, et al. Genomic variation of human papillomavirus type 16 and risk for high grade cervical intraepithelial neoplasia. *J Natl Cancer Inst* 1997;89:796–802.

396. Castle PE, Sideri M, Jeronimo J, Solomon D, Schiffman M. Risk assessment to guide the prevention of cervical cancer. *Am J Obstet Gynecol* 2007;197:356 e1–e6.

397. Moscicki AB, Shiboski S, Hills NK, Powell KJ, Jay N, Hanson EN, et al. Regression of low-grade squamous intra-epithelial lesions in young women. *Lancet* 2004;364:1678–1683.

398. Arbyn M, Sankaranarayanan R, Muwonge R, Keita N, Dolo A, Mbalawa CG, et al. Pooled analysis of the accuracy of five cervical cancer screening tests assessed in eleven studies in Africa and India. *Int J Cancer* 2008;123:153–160.

399. Sankaranarayanan R, Esmy PO, Rajkumar R, Muwonge R, Swaminathan R, Shanthakumari S, et al. Effect of visual screening on cervical cancer incidence and mortality in Tamil Nadu, India: a cluster-randomised trial. *Lancet* 2007;370:398–406.

400. Pretorius RG, Bao YP, Belinson JL, Burchette RJ, Smith JS, Qiao YL. Inappropriate gold standard bias in cervical cancer screening studies. *Int J Cancer* 2007;121:2218–2224.

401. Sun XR, Che DY, Tu HZ, Li D, Wang J. Assessment of cervical intraepithelial neoplasia (CIN) lesions by DNA image cytometry. *Zhonghua Zhong Liu Za Zhi* 2006;28:831–835.

402. Sun XR, Wang J, Garner D, Palcic B. Detection of cervical cancer and high grade neoplastic lesions by a combination of liquid-based sampling preparation and DNA measurements using automated image cytometry. *Cell Oncol* 2005;27:33–41.

403. Bollmann R, Bankfalvi A, Griefingholt H, Trosic A, Speich N, Schmitt C, et al. Validity of combined cytology and human papillomavirus (HPV) genotyping with adjuvant DNA-cytometry in routine cervical screening: results from 31031 women from the Bonn-region in West Germany. *Oncol Rep* 2005;13:915–922.

404. Siddiqi AM, Li H, Faruque F, Williams W, Lai K, Hughson M, et al. Use of hyperspectral imaging to distinguish normal, precancerous, and cancerous cells. *Cancer* 2008;114:13–21.

405. Gorham H, Yoshida K, Sugino T, Marsh G, Manek S, Charnock M, et al. Telomerase activity in human gynaecological malignancies. *J Clin Pathol* 1997;50:501–504.

406. Yashima K, Ashfaq R, Nowak J, Von Gruenigen V, Milchgrub S, Rathi A, et al. Telomerase activity and expression of its RNA component in cervical lesions. *Cancer* 1998;82:1319–1327.

407. **Iwasaka T, Zheng PS, Yokoyama M, Fukuda K, Nakao Y, Sugimori H.** Telomerase activation in cervical neoplasia. *Obstet Gynecol* 1998;91:260–262.

408. **Kyo S, Takakura M, Ishikawa H, Sasagawa T, Satake S, Tateno M, et al.** Application of telomerase assay for the screening of cervical lesions. *Cancer Res* 1997;57:1863–1867.

409. **Wisman GB, Hollema H, de Jong S, ter Schegget J, Tjong-A-Hung SP, Ruiters MH, et al.** Telomerase activity as a biomarker for (pre)neoplastic cervical disease in scrapings and frozen sections from patients with abnormal cervical smear. *J Clin Oncol* 1998;16:2238–2245.

410. **Zheng PS, Iwasaka T, Yokoyama M, Nakao Y, Pater A, Sugimori H.** Telomerase activation in in vitro and in vivo cervical carcinogenesis. *Gynecol Oncol* 1997;66:222–226.

411. **Ngan HY, Cheung AN, Liu SS, Liu KL, Tsao SW.** Telomerase assay and HPV 16/18 typing as adjunct to conventional cytological cervical cancer screening. *Tumour Biol* 2002;23:87–92.

412. **Mutirangura A, Sriuranpong V, Termrunggraunglert W, Tresukosol D, Lertsaguansinchai P, Voravud N, et al.** Telomerase activity and human papillomavirus in malignant, premalignant and benign cervical lesions. *Br J Cancer* 1998;78:933–939.

413. **Rosa MI, Medeiros LR, Bozzetti MC, Fachel J, Wendland E, Zanini RR, et al.** Accuracy of telomerase in cervical lesions: a systematic review. *Int J Gynecol Cancer* 2007;17:1205–1214.

414. **Takakura M, Kyo S, Kanaya T, Tanaka M, Inoue M.** Expression of human telomerase subunits and correlation with telomerase activity in cervical cancer. *Cancer Res* 1998;58:1558–1561.

415. **Saha B, Chaiwun B, Tsao-Wei DD, Groshen SL, Naritoku WY, Atkinson RD, et al.** Telomerase and markers of cellular proliferation are associated with the progression of cervical intraepithelial neoplasia lesions. *Int J Gynecol Pathol* 2007;26:214–222.

416. **Williams GH, Romanowski P, Morris L, Madine M, Mills AD, Stoeber K, et al.** Improved cervical smear assessment using antibodies against proteins that regulate DNA replication. *Proc Natl Acad Sci U S A* 1998;95:14932–14937.

417. **Branca M, Ciotti M, Giorgi C, Santini D, Di Bonito L, Costa S, et al.** Predicting high-risk human papillomavirus infection, progression of cervical intraepithelial neoplasia, and prognosis of cervical cancer with a panel of 13 biomarkers tested in multivariate modeling. *Int J Gynecol Pathol* 2008;27:265–273.

DISEASE SITES

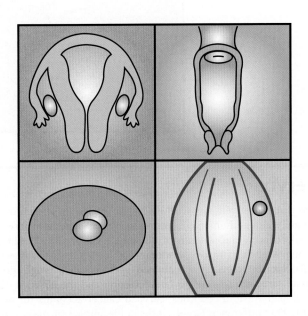

8

Preinvasive Disease

Michael J. Campion

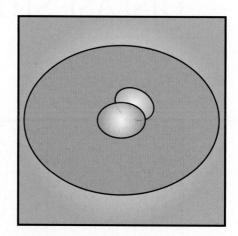

Cervix

Cervical cancer remains worldwide the second most common cancer among women and is, uniquely among human cancers, entirely attributable to infection. It accounts for 15% of all female cancers and a tenth of all female cancer deaths (1). It is the most common cancer among women in many developing countries, constituting 20% to 30% of female cancers (2,3). Societal impact is accentuated by the young average age at death (4). This is due to inadequate screening leading to late detection and the absence of standard treatment options. In developed Western countries, cervical cancer accounts for only 4% to 6% of female cancers (5,6). This difference largely reflects the impact of mass screening using cervical cytologic methods (7–9).

The primary goal of cervical screening is to prevent cervical cancer. This is achieved by the detection, eradication, and follow-up of preinvasive cervical lesions (10–12). The ability to detect preinvasive cervical disease, coupled with comparatively easy access to the cervix for screening and assessment, have contributed greatly to the understanding of cervical carcinogenesis and to the definition of the precursor lesions to cervical cancer. Modern understanding that almost all cervical cancers are caused by persistent infection with approximately 15 types of human papillomavirus (HPV) has led to promising new approaches to cervical cancer prevention (13–15).

Classification of Preinvasive Cervical Disease (Precancer)

The proposal that invasive squamous carcinoma of the cervix arises through progression of a preinvasive lesion as opposed to a *de novo* event was initially postulated by Schauenstein in 1908 (16). The term "carcinoma *in situ*" was later introduced to describe cancerous changes confined to the epithelium (17).

The Dysplasia Terminology

Although referred to earlier by Papanicolaou and Traut (18), Reagan and Hamonic in 1956 (19) described cytologic differences between "carcinoma *in situ*" and a group of "less anaplastic" lesions, for which they introduced the term **dysplasia** (20). In 1975, the World Health Organization defined dysplasia as a "lesion in which part of the epithelium is replaced by cells showing varying degrees of atypia." Dysplastic changes were graded as mild, moderate, and severe, but precise guidelines for these subdivisions were not defined, and grading always remained highly subjective (21–24).

A dual terminology for epithelial abnormalities of the cervix developed, leading to irrational treatment policies. If a diagnosis of "dysplasia" was made, this was considered a nonspecific change, and the patient was subjected to a cone biopsy. If the diagnosis of "carcinoma *in situ*" was made, this was considered a "preinvasive cancer," and the patient underwent an obligatory hysterectomy (23–25).

Cervical Intraepithelial Neoplasia

Invasive squamous cell carcinoma of the cervix was demonstrated to be the end result of progressive intraepithelial dysplastic atypia occurring within the metaplastic epithelium of the cervical transformation zone (26). The classification of lesions from mild dysplasia to carcinoma *in situ* did not truly reflect either the morphologic or biologic continuum of preinvasive cervical disease. The diagnosis was highly subjective and was not reproducible. After pioneering research into the natural history of cervical cancer precursors, **Richart** (27) **proposed the term "cervical intraepithelial neoplasia" (CIN)** to describe the biologic spectrum of cervical preinvasive squamous disease. **Three grades of CIN were described, specifically, CIN 1 (mild dysplasia), CIN 2 (moderate dysplasia), and CIN 3 (severe dysplasia/carcinoma *in situ*).** This system was consistent with biologic evidence that strongly implied a single process of cervical squamous carcinogenesis (27–33).

Forty years' experience with the CIN terminology, coupled with recent advances in the understanding of the role of human papillomavirus (HPV) in the causation of cervical neoplasia (32–38), has led to critical reappraisal of this model. It has also led to further reclassification of the terminology for reporting cytologic abnormalities consistent with preinvasive disease (39–46). **The CIN grading is very subjective. No reproducible cytologic or histologic distinction at the lower end of the CIN continuum exists between CIN 1 and HPV infection alone.** Both interobserver and intraobserver consistency in diagnosis are poor (45–48). Separating CIN 2 from CIN 3 is again often not reproducible (49–52). In reality, **the two critical questions in the assessment of the cervical epithelium are: (i) do the changes represent a cancer precursor; and (ii) is the lesion invasive cancer?**

In histologic terms, CIN 3 is clearly established as a *bona fide* cancer precursor. CIN 3 is a reliable and reproducible morphological diagnosis, with undifferentiated cells with fixed genetic abnormalities replacing almost the full thickness of the cervical epithelium (48,49). CIN 3 is reliably distinguished from recently acquired HPV infection and is a genuine surrogate marker of subsequent cancer risk. **There still exists uncertainty in relation to the progressive potential of less severe dysplastic lesions** (53,54).

CIN 1 is increasingly viewed as an insensitive histologic marker of HPV infection. The diagnosis includes errors of processing and interpretation of colposcopically directed biopsies (48). **Standardized for positivity for a given high-risk HPV type, a diagnosis of CIN 1 does not predict a meaningfully higher risk of CIN 3 than does a negative biopsy** (53). Histologically confirmed CIN 1 lesions confer a lower risk of developing cervical cancer than does a Pap smear report of low-grade squamous intraepithelial lesion (53).

Recent data indicate considerable heterogeneity in the microscopic diagnosis, biology, and clinical behavior of CIN 2 lesions (54). CIN 2 can be produced by noncarcinogenic HPV types and is equivocal in cancer potential (55). Some represent acute HPV infection with a more severe microscopic appearance and are destined to regress. Others are incipient precancer and will persist and progress with an attendant high risk of future invasion if left untreated. The clinical dilemma remains the inability to reliably predict those lesions less severe than CIN 3 that are at greatest risk of progression to cancer and those that are likely to regress. New molecular markers hold promise in this regard (56–58), but prospective validation to determine risk of invasion is unethical.

Cervical Precancer – Modern Concepts

The stepwise progression of increasingly severe cervical intraepithelial neoplasia to invasive cancer, implicit in the CIN continuum, remains an important histopathological concept to assist clinical management. Two decades of epidemiologic and preventive research focused on the HPV cervical cancer model have revolutionized our understanding of cervical precancer (15).

HPV infection is a broad transition state between normal and precancer. A defined precancerous lesion remains the target of screening and preventive treatment programs and represents a genuine surrogate for cancer risk (59). With increasing detection of smaller and less serious lesions in cervical screening programs and the inclusion of such lesions in the precancer continuum, the likelihood of diagnosing a precancerous lesion as a surrogate predictor of invasive cancer risk has declined. This has altered the effect and assessment of cervical cancer prevention programs.

CIN 3, particularly full thickness carcinoma *in situ,* shares the same HPV-type spectrum and cofactor profile as invasive cancer. CIN 3 lesions demonstrate the same aneuploid DNA content and genetic instability as seen in invasive cancer. CIN 3 is the most certain surrogate marker of cancer risk. Some CIN 3 lesions are small; some will regress, particularly after biopsy and the eventual risk of invasion for such lesions is less certain. At this time there is no reliable predictor of CIN 3 lesions likely to progress to cancer and as such all are managed as definite precancer.

CIN 2 demonstrates greater heterogeneity in biology and definition (54). It can be caused by low-risk HPV types rarely found in cancer and has a greater regression potential. A diagnosis of CIN 2 is not a reliable surrogate for cancer risk. Although of equivocal malignant potential, in the absence of reliable predictors of risk of progression, CIN 2 lesions tend to be managed as precancer to provide a further safety margin against development of cancer.

A histological diagnosis of low-grade cervical intraepithelial lesions (HPV infection/CIN 1) is increasingly viewed as not representing precancer. Persistence of oncogenic HPV types is strongly linked to precancer (60–62). Incident HPV infection might not be associated with any microscopic abnormality while most low-grade abnormalities will regress (63,64), particularly among young women (65). Only a fraction of precancers arise from HPV infection in the absence of mild or equivocal microscopic abnormalities.

High-grade lesions are commonly found within a broader field of low-grade disease, suggesting that CIN 3 may develop in high-risk HPV-infected epithelium independent of and within a CIN 1 lesion, rather than as a classical stepwise progression. The reported progressive potential of low-grade lesions is small but definite, varying from 12% to 33% (25,26,66–68).

Understanding the Cervical Transformation Zone

Embryogenesis

The cervix and vagina are derived from the müllerian ducts and are initially lined by a single layer of müllerian-derived columnar epithelium. At 18 to 20 weeks of gestation, this columnar epithelium lining the vaginal tube is colonized by the upward growth of stratified squamous epithelium derived from cloacal endoderm.

Original Squamocolumnar Junction

The junction in fetal life between the stratified squamous epithelium of the vagina and ectocervix, and the columnar epithelium of the endocervical canal is called the original squamocolumnar junction (69). Original squamous epithelium extends from Hart's line or the mucocutaneous, vulvovaginal junction to the original squamocolumnar junction. The position of the original squamocolumnar junction is variable, lying on the ectocervix in 66%, within the endocervical canal in 30%, and on the vaginal fornices in 4% of female infants (70). The position of the original squamocolumnar junction determines the extent of cervical squamous metaplasia (70,71). Squamous metaplasia is a pivotal process in cervical carcinogenesis. Embryogenesis, in determining the distribution of native squamous and columnar epithelia, is an important early influence in determining future risk of neoplastic transformation (Fig. 8.1).

New Squamocolumnar Junction

The volume of the cervix alters throughout a woman's life in response to hormonal stimulation (69,70). Increased estrogen secretion, particularly with puberty and with the first pregnancy, causes an increase in cervical volume and an eversion of endocervical columnar epithelium to an ectocervical location (70). This eversion of columnar epithelium onto the ectocervix is called an ectropion. An ectropion is often mistakenly referred to as an erosion.

The estrogen surge of puberty results in the establishment of lactobacilli as part of the normal flora of the vagina. These microorganisms produce lactic acid, reducing the vaginal pH to 4 or less (70). Everted endocervical columnar epithelium is exposed in the postpubertal years to the acidity of the vaginal environment. Damage to the everted columnar epithelium caused by vaginal acidity results in proliferation of a stromal reserve cell underlying the columnar epithelium. This results in replacement of the columnar epithelium with an immature, undifferentiated, stratified, squamous, metaplastic epithelium (70,71). Immature squamous metaplasia then undergoes a maturation process, producing a mature, stratified squamous metaplastic epithelium distinguishable only with difficulty from the original squamous epithelium.

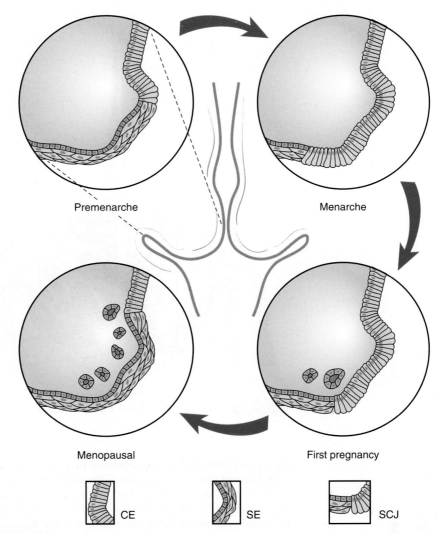

Figure 8.1 **Location of squamocolumnar junction at various times in a woman's life.** *CE,* columnar epithelium; *SE,* squamous epithelium; *SCJ,* squamocolumnar junction.

The original linear junction between squamous and columnar epithelium is replaced by a zone of squamous metaplasia at varying degrees of maturation. At the upper or cephalad margin of this zone is a sharp demarcation between epithelium, which appears morphologically squamous, and villous epithelium, which appears colposcopically columnar. This colposcopic junction is called the **new squamocolumnar junction.**

The Transformation Zone	**The transformation zone is defined as that area lying between the original squamocolumnar junction and the colposcopic new squamocolumnar junction** (28,29). The initial clinical assessment for most women is in the postpubertal years. Mature squamous metaplastic epithelium has often replaced the distal or caudad limit of the columnar epithelium. As the transformation zone matures, the original squamocolumnar junction becomes impossible to delineate. Only the presence of Nabothian follicles and gland openings hint at the original columnar origin of mature squamous metaplasia.

Cervical neoplasia almost invariably originates within the transformation zone. Understanding squamous metaplasia is the key to understanding the concepts of the cervical transformation zone and its role in cervical carcinogenesis (Fig. 8.2). For reasons that are poorly understood, persistent HPV infection causes cancers mainly at the transformation zone between different kinds of epithelia (e.g., cervix, anus, and oropharynx) (2). Carcinogenic HPV infection is equally common in the cervical and vaginal epithelia (72). Cervical cancer is the second most common cancer among women while vaginal cancer is rare. This reflects the pivotal importance of the metaplastic epithelium of the transformation zone in cervical carcinogenesis (73).

271

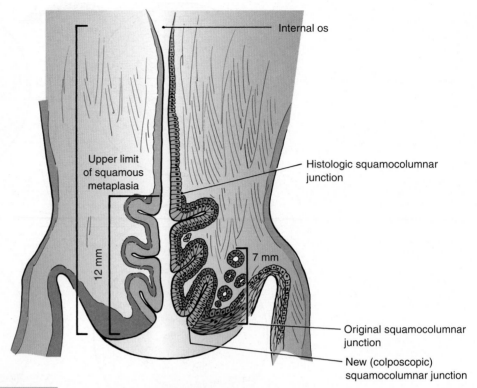

Figure 8.2   The anatomy of the transformation zone.

Squamous metaplasia is a permanent process but is not continuous. It occurs in "spurts," with greatest activity during puberty and the first pregnancy. During the maturation phase, the columnar villi fuse, losing the distinctive appearance of columnar epithelium and producing a myriad of cytologic, colposcopic, and histologic appearances. The process fluctuates in response to hormonal influences but ultimately produces a mature, glycogenated squamous epithelium. **The presence of a subepithelial inflammatory infiltrate in biopsy specimens of immature squamous metaplasia may lead to a histologic misdiagnosis of chronic cervicitis.** The presence of such inflammatory white cells is a normal part of the metaplastic process and is not a response to an infectious organism. A histologic diagnosis of "chronic cervicitis" is often misleading and should not be accepted as a satisfactory explanation for an abnormal Papanicolaou (Pap) smear (Fig. 8.3).

If the new squamocolumnar junction is seen in its entirety in the absence of premalignant disease, the incidence of squamous disease above or cephalad to the new squamocolumnar junction is virtually nil, and **the colposcopic examination of the cervix is described as satisfactory.** If the new squamocolumnar junction is not seen in its entirety, the colposcopic examination is described as unsatisfactory. The transformation zone further defines the distal limit of high-grade glandular intraepithelial neoplasia, the precursor lesion to invasive adenocarcinoma of the cervix.

Upper Limit of Squamous Metaplasia

The new squamocolumnar junction is an unstable boundary. Serial colposcopic assessments of the cervix frequently show the new squamocolumnar junction to have moved cephalad. Careful colposcopic assessment of columnar villi immediately above the new squamocolumnar junction reveals opaque, opalescent tips and early villous fusion (Fig. 8.4). Histologic study of colposcopically directed biopsy specimens reveals reserve cell hyperplasia and early immature squamous metaplasia occurring in epithelium, which appears colposcopically columnar. This early immature squamous metaplasia can extend as far as 10 mm above the new squamocolumnar junction.

The immature metaplastic epithelium cephalad to the new squamocolumnar junction is not included in the modern definition of the transformation zone but represents the

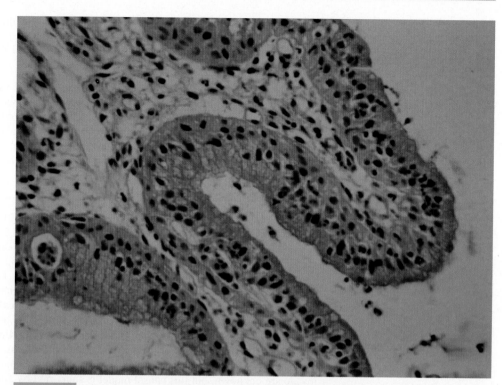

Figure 8.3   Histology of immature squamous metaplasia (chronic cervicitis).

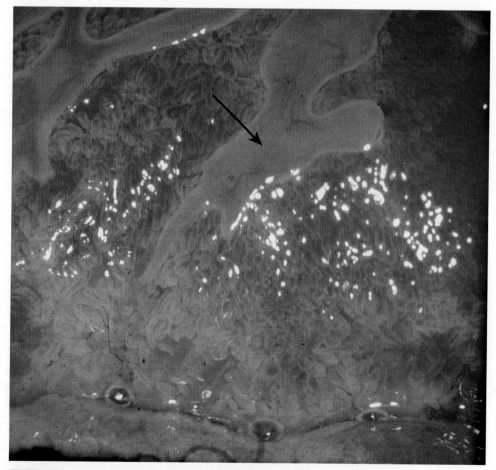

Figure 8.4   Colposcopic appearance of immature squamous metaplasia.

epithelium at greatest risk for future neoplastic transformation. During dynamic phases of metaplasia, occurring particularly with puberty and the first pregnancy, the immature metaplastic cells are actively phagocytic (70). **The most critical phase is the initiation of squamous metaplasia at puberty and in early adolescence.**

Age of coitarche is an important epidemiologic variable in determining risk of cervical neoplasia (74–78). The lifetime risk for development of cervical cancer is increased 26-fold if age at first intercourse is within 1 year of menarche, as opposed to 23 years of age or older (76). Potential carcinogens in the vaginal environment at times of active metaplasia can deviate early metaplastic transformation along a neoplastic pathway. Mature metaplastic epithelium exposed to the same mutagen is at less risk of neoplastic transformation.

Human Papillomaviruses and Cervical Neoplasia

Extensive molecular biologic and epidemiologic research confirms certain HPV types to be carcinogenic in humans (13–15,79–85). Infections with HPV cause approximately 5% of the global burden of human cancers and at least 500,000 deaths annually (1). Infection with specific HPV types is necessary for the development of the vast majority of cervical cancers (>99.7%) and the immediate precursor lesion (CIN 3) (85). The magnitude of the association between HPV and cervical cancer is higher than the association between smoking and lung cancer. **The four major steps in the development of cervical cancer are (i) infection of the metaplastic epithelium of the transformation zone with one or more carcinogenic HPV types; (ii) viral persistence rather than clearance reflecting the host immune response; (iii) clonal progression of persistently infected epithelium to cervical precancer (CIN 3); and (iv) invasion.** The precise molecular events which lead HPV-infected cervical cells to invade are unknown, but this causal model is supported by a large volume of epidemiological and laboratory data.

Taxonomy and Biology

Papillomaviruses are small, nonenveloped, double-stranded DNA viruses encased in a 72-sided icosahedral protein capsid. The HPV genome consists of circular, double-stranded DNA of approximately 7,900 nucleotide base pairs. Papillomaviruses are a divergent group of evolutionarily related viruses with similar biologic characteristics but enormous differences in species specificity, site of predilection, and oncogenic potential (86,87). **More than 100 types of HPV have been fully sequenced.**

HPV types are divided into phylogenetic trees based on DNA sequence and protein homologies which assist in understanding HPV classification and behaviour (88,89). Four major groups are recognized: two infecting genital skin, generally acquired through sexual intercourse, and two infecting nongenital skin acquired from shed virus (87). At each site, one group causes warts which rarely become malignant and the other includes oncogenic types associated with induction of cancer. Within the four broad groups of HPVs, genetic sequencing defines clades of viruses which produce similar pathology (87). Viruses of clades A7 and A9 are most commonly associated with anogenital cancers (14). In addition to those that infect only humans, there is a large number of other species-specific papillomaviruses affecting other mammalian species, including cattle, horses, sheep, dogs, rabbits, monkeys, pigs, and deer.

The HPV genome is usually maintained as a stable viral episome, independent of the host cell genome, in the nucleus of infected cells. It codes for only eight genes (90). In some high-grade CIN lesions, and more frequently in cervical cancer, HPV genomes are covalently bonded or integrated into the host chromosomes (91–94). This integration event occurs at random within the host cell genome but is highly specific in relation to the viral genome, involving the *E1* and *E2* genes, with important consequences for regulation of viral gene expression (Fig. 8.5) (95,96). **This integration of the HPV genome into the host genome is associated with invasive cancer and might serve as an important biomarker to distinguish HPV infection from precancer** (97). Viral integration may not be necessary for invasion as not all women with invasive cancer have measurable integration (94,98). Continued transcriptional activity of HPV oncogenes is required to maintain the cancer (99).

The late genes, *L1* and *L2,* the sequences of which are highly conserved among all papillomaviruses, encode the common capsid proteins. These viral proteins reflect late viral gene

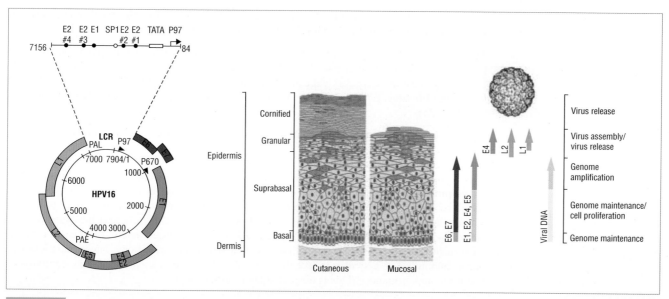

Figure 8.5   **The HPV genome and its expression within the epithelium.** The HPV genome consists of approximately 8,000 base pairs of single-stranded, circular DNA. HPV genes are designated as E or L according to their expression in early or late differentiation stage of the epithelium: *E1, E2, E5, E6,* and *E7* are expressed early in the differentiation, *E4* is expressed throughout, and *L1* and *L2* are expressed during the final stages of differentiation. The viral genome is maintained at the basal layer of the epithelium, where HPV infection is established. Early proteins are expressed at low levels for genome maintenance (raising the possibility of a latent state) and cell proliferation. As the basal epithelial cells differentiate, the viral life cycle enters successive stages of genome amplification, virus assembly and virus release, with a concomitant shift in expression patterns from early genes to late genes, including *L1* and *L2,* which assemble into viral capsid. (Reproduced with permission from **Schiffman M, Castle PE, Jeronimo J, Rodriguez AC, Wacholder S.** Human papillomavirus and cervical cancer. *The Lancet* 2007; 370;890–907).

expression and are exclusively present in well-differentiated keratinocytes (100). Both proteins play an important role in mediating efficient virus infectivity.

The proteins encoded by the *E6* and *E7* genes of high-risk HPV types, particularly HPV 16 (clade A9) and 18 (clade A7), are directly involved in cellular transformation in the presence of an active oncogene (84,101). **E6 and E7 are the primary HPV oncoproteins with numerous cellular targets** (90,101–103). Both E6 and E7 proteins can immortalize primary keratinocytes from cervical epithelium and can influence transcription from viral and cellular promoters (104). The activity of these viral oncoproteins results in genomic instability, leading to the malignant phenotype. **E6 proteins of high-risk HPV types bind the tumor suppressor protein p53** (105,106). This induces ubiquitination and degradation of p53, removing the p53-dependent control of the host cell cycle (107–111). The role of E6 as an antiapoptotic protein is of key significance in the development of cervical cancer as it compromises the effectiveness of the cellular DNA damage response and allows the accumulation of secondary mutations to go unchecked.

E6 also increases telomerase activity in keratinocytes through increased transcription of the *telomerase catalytic subunit* **gene (hTERT) through induction of** *c-myc* (112,113). Telomerase activity is usually absent in somatic cells, leading to shortening of *telomeres* with successive cell divisions and to eventual cell senescence. **E6 mediation of telomerase activity may predispose to long-term infection and the development of cancer.** Recently E6 and E7 viral oncogenes have been shown to antagonize *BRCA*-mediated inhibition of the hTERT promoter (114).

The *E7* **gene product is a nuclear phosphoprotein that associates with the product of the** *retinoblastoma* **gene (pRb), which is a tumor suppressor gene important in the negative control of cell growth** (115–117). **E7 is the primary transforming protein.** Degradation of p53 by E6 and the functional inactivation of pRb by E7 represent the main mechanisms whereby expression of HPV E6 and E7 oncoproteins subverts the function of the negative regulators of the cell cycle (118–120). **Deregulated expression of the viral oncogenes is a predisposing factor to the development of HPV-associated cancers**.

The products of the *E2* gene are involved in transcriptional regulation of the HPV genome. The process of HPV integration into the cellular genome, which occurs in some high-grade CIN lesions and most invasive cervical cancers, disrupts the *E2* gene (84). This results in increased levels of E6 and E7 expression, correlating with increased immortalization activity (84,122–125).

Both E6 and E7 proteins are expressed at low levels in the process of HPV infection. At some undefined point in neoplastic transformation and the development of precancer, E6 and E7 expression is deregulated by genetic or epigenetic influence. This leads to overexpression in CIN 3 lesions. **Aberrant expression of high-risk viral oncogenes can predispose to the development of cervical cancer but their expression alone is not sufficient** (90). HPV-mediated oncogenesis requires accumulation of additional genetic mutations over time. The average age of women with invasive cervical cancer is 50 years, whereas the mean age for women with CIN 3 is 28 years. This suggests a long precancerous state in most cases of invasive cancer that allows the accumulation of secondary genetic mutations. These mutations can occur randomly but may also reflect the influence of cofactors such as smoking carcinogens and hormonal influences. This is discussed later in this chapter.

Human Papillomavirus Type–Specific Disease Pattern

Differing genomic nucleotide sequences of specific HPV types are responsible for the specific anatomic tropism of each HPV type. There are more than 30 genital HPV types. These transfect the mucous membranes of the genital tract most efficiently, but may also be present in the keratinized epithelium of the vulva, perineum, penis, and anorectal areas. Genital HPV types are also occasionally associated with oropharyngeal, conjunctival, and subungual lesions. The genital HPV types are divided into groups based on the frequency of association with malignant tumors and presumed oncogenic potential. **The International Agency for Research on Cancer (IARC) reassessed the carcinogenicity of HPV in 2005 and revised these groupings so that the list of high-risk HPV's includes thirteen types, specifically HPV types 16, 18, 31, 33, 35, 39, 45, 51, 52, 56, 58, 59, and 66** (86).

Low-risk HPV types, particularly HPVs 6 and 11 (clade A10), are associated with condylomata acuminata of the genital tract in both sexes. HPV 6 and 11 are also detected alone in low-grade cervical lesions (exophytic condylomata acuminata, subclinical HPV infection, CIN 1 and some CIN 2 lesions). Using more reliable HPV detection techniques, not a single cervical cancer has been shown to be associated with low-risk HPV types, and HPVs 6 and 11 in particular. These viruses do not appear to induce malignant transformation; they are unable to integrate into the human genome. The E6 and E7 proteins of "low-risk" HPV types only weakly bind p53 and pRb and thus do not immortalize keratinocytes *in vitro*.

Human papillomavirus 16 is the HPV type universally detected with greatest frequency in high-grade intraepithelial neoplasia and invasive cancers. HPV 16 is associated with 50% of cervical squamous cancers and more than 30% of adenocarcinomas (14,126–127). It is present in more than 80% of high-grade cervical, vaginal, vulvar, perianal, and penile preinvasive lesions. It is detected in more than 25% of low-grade cervical lesions, 40% of subclinical vulvar HPV infections, and 10% of genital condylomata acuminata, particularly the recalcitrant lesions (14,127–129).

HPV 18 is the second most common (25%) **HPV type in invasive cervical cancer,** but is uncommon (5%) in preinvasive cervical lesions (130,131). The association of HPV 18 with aggressive adenocarcinomas, particularly in younger women, and the underrepresentation of this viral type in preinvasive lesions have raised concerns that HPV 18 may be associated with "rapid-transit" cancers that escape reliable cytologic detection (132,133). Although this remains a controversial issue (134), epidemiologic and molecular data support the hypothesis (135,136). **HPV 18 DNA is detected 2.6 times more frequently in invasive cervical cancers occurring within 1 year of a negative smear** (133). The average age of patients with HPV 18–containing cancers is 8 to 12 years younger, and recurrence rates are higher (45% vs. 16%) than for patients with HPV 16–containing cancers (137). The lack of HPV 18-induced squamous precancerous lesions contributes to the failed detection of glandular and endocervical lesions in well-screened populations with the attendant increased proportion of adenocarcinoma.

Human Papillomavirus and Cervical Cancer: A Causal or Casual Association

Although the true prevalence of cervical HPV infection is unknown, it is the most common sexually transmitted infection, with most sexually active women younger than 35 years of age exposed (138). The 2-year cumulative incidence for first time genital HPV infection for young women is 32% (139). Incidences are similar for virgins and nonvirgins from the time of acquisition of a new partner. For monogamous women, the risk of acquiring HPV after sexual debut is 46% at 3 years (140). Smoking, oral contraceptive use, and report of a new male sexual partner are predictive of incident infection. **Male condom usage is not protective** (141). Infection in virgins is rare, but any nonpenetrative sexual contact is associated with an increased risk (139). Basal cells of the cervical epithelium are inoculated with the virus at sites of microtrauma. HPV prevalence and incidence peak in women under 20 years of age and decline in women over 30, secondary to HPV clearance, with most women in the world exposed to one or more genital HPV types during their sexual life (138,142).

Most HPV infections, whether associated with a cytological abnormality or not, are transient, usually being cleared or suppressed by cell-mediated immunity, within several months to 2 years (143). The median time to clearance of HPV infection in an immunocompetent woman is 6 to 18 months (average of 12 months) with **90% of women clearing a specific HPV-type after 2 years of observation** (144). Humoral and cellular immune responses to genital HPV types are difficult to detect, possibly because the virus is nonlytic to infected cells and does not spread systemically. **Viral clearance is not often associated with reappearance of the same HPV type.** Occasionally the same HPV type will reappear (145). It is unclear whether this represents reinfection or resurgence from a latent state in the basal cells of the epithelium with very low viral copy numbers and without late viral expression.

The high rate of HPV infection among immunosuppressed HIV-infected women supports the concept of latency (146–148). However, HIV-infected women with normal CD4 counts demonstrate increased high-risk HPV persistence compared with HIV-uninfected women, suggesting HPV clearance is generally impaired in this group (149). **Secondary peaks of HPV infection in older and postmenopausal women suggest the possibility of reactivation of a latent reservoir due to senescence of cell-mediated immunity,** although this could also be explained by sexual behavior (of women or partners).

The longer a specific HPV type persists in the epithelium, the lower the probability of clearance within a defined period, and the greater the risk of precancer (144). Clinical strategies which require repeated specific HPV type detection over 12 months or longer before referral for diagnostic workup take advantage of this natural history to separate transient infections from persistent lesions which carry a greater risk to the patient (61,150,151).

Only persistent high-risk HPV infection of the cervical epithelium appears to trigger neoplastic progression (150–154) (Table 8.5) (Fig. 8.6). There is no accepted definition of clinically significant persistence. Follow-up strategies suggest persistence beyond 1 year and certainly beyond 2 years defines a greater risk to patients (151). The small proportion of high-risk HPV infections (about 10%) which persist for several years is strongly linked to a high risk of developing CIN 3 (89). **The risk factors for HPV persistence and progression to CIN 3 are not fully understood. HPV type is the strongest factor affecting risk of viral persistence** (89). HPV 16 is highly carcinogenic with an absolute risk of CIN 3 approaching 40% at 3 to 5 years (38). The risks of progression to CIN 3 with other HPV types are several-fold lower. More than 20% to 30% of women with cervical HPV associated disease, regardless of degree of CIN, have more than one HPV type (155). Women infected with multiple HPV types have a further increased risk but it is not clear if the risk is equal to or greater than the cumulative risk associated with each of the individual HPV types. It is also unknown whether infection with multiple HPV types interferes with persistence of a given HPV type or with risk of progression to CIN 3 (145,155,156).

Viral burden or the amount of HPV DNA in the cervical epithelium appears to have an independent effect on CIN incidence as a surrogate for HPV persistence, but does not independently predict future risk of CIN 3 or cancer (157). Low viral load is associated with normal microscopic findings and a low risk of neoplastic progression. **High viral loads do not generally imply an increased prospective risk of cancer, except for HPV 16** (158,159). Recently acquired low-grade cervical lesions contain some of the highest viral loads, analogous to condylomata acuminata, and frequently regress (160). Cervical cancers have low amounts of intact virus, probably associated with genomic integration. Infection with multiple HPV types is a

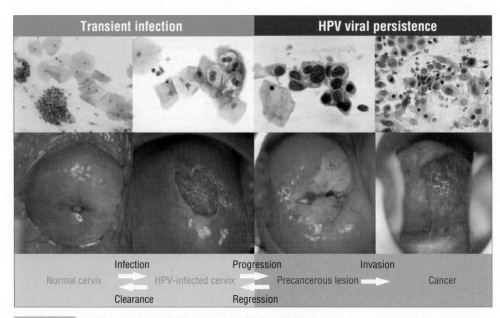

Figure 8.6 **Major steps in the development of cervical cancer.** Incident HPV infection is best measured by molecular tests. Most HPV infections show no concurrent cytological abnormality. Approximately 30% of infections produce concurrent cytopathology, usually non-classical (equivocal) changes. Most HPV infections clear within 2 years. Ten percent persist for 2 years and are highly linked to development of precancer. (Reproduced with permission from **Schiffman M, Castle PE, Jeronimo J, Rodriguez AC, Wacholder S.** Human papillomavirus and cervical cancer. *The Lancet* 2007;370;890–907).

further complicating factor as this will affect viral load but cervical cancer typically is a monoclonal event related to a specific single HPV type. **The role of viral load in the natural history of HPV infection is unclear and viral load measurement is not clinically useful** (15).

The modal time from HPV infection to CIN 3 is 7 to 15 years, with infection occurring in the late teens or early twenties and CIN 3 diagnosis peaking at 25 to 30 years (127,161). The average age of diagnosis of CIN 3 depends on average societal age of first intercourse, a proxy for initial HPV exposure, and age of onset and intensity of screening. **The time from HPV infection to the development of CIN 3 can be short, often within 5 years** (162). CIN 3 has been diagnosed within 2 years of coitarche and CIN 2-3 has been documented to rapidly develop within several months of an incident HPV infection (78,163). The biological significance and risk of invasion associated with these early CIN 3 lesions is uncertain. It is plausible that many might regress but prospective follow-up of these lesions is unethical.

CIN 3 lesions are a homologous population of aneuploid lesions, mostly associated with oncogenic HPVs, and are genuine cancer precursors. The transit time to invasive cancer is variable, taking as little as 12 to 18 months or as long as several decades. Most cervical abnormalities do not transform to invasive cancer. The median age of women with invasive cancer is two to three decades later than for CIN 3 and is older still in poorly screened communities. Invasive cervical cancers detected through screening are often earlier stage and are detected among women at least 10 years older than those with CIN 3. This suggests generally a long average transit time for CIN 3 to invasive cancer. Rapid onset invasive cancers, often occurring in young women are rare, but are sometimes fatal and have a disproportionate impact on screening and preventive strategies (15).

Cervical neoplasia can be viewed as the result of a complex interplay between a "seed," that is, high-risk HPV types, and a "soil," that is, the immature, metaplastic epithelium of the cervical transformation zone. Exposure to specific high-risk HPV types, in the presence of cofactor activity, may deviate the metaplastic process along a neoplastic pathway. Disease expression begins at the new squamocolumnar junction. The initial abnormality produced is usually a low-grade cervical lesion. Such lesions represent a heterologous mixture of genuine cancer precursors and benign HPV infections (164). The most critical step in cervical carcinogenesis is not acquisition of an HPV infection but progression to CIN 3. **HPV infection alone is**

necessary but not sufficient to induce carcinoma in an immunocompetent host. HPV infection with oncogenic viral types is much more common than cervical neoplasia, indicating the necessity of cofactors in the process of cervical carcinogenesis (165).

Cofactor Interaction with Human Papillomavirus

Plausible cofactors in cervical and lower genital tract carcinogenesis include **the use of tobacco products, infection by other microbial agents, specific vitamin deficiencies, hormonal influences, and immunosuppression.**

Cigarette Smoking

Cigarette smoking has been demonstrated to be a risk factor for cervical and vulvar carcinoma (167–172). An increased risk of developing a high-grade squamous intraepithelial lesion (HSIL) has been demonstrated among high-risk HPV positive women who smoke or who are passive smokers. The detection of high levels of genotoxic breakdown products of cigarette smoke—including nicotine, cotinine, hydrocarbons, and tars—in cervical secretions of smokers and the demonstration of mutagenic activity of these products in cervical cells, similar to that observed in lung cells, point to an important role for these compounds in cervical carcinogenesis. The association between smoking and HPV persistence is less consistent.

Cigarette smoking influences epithelial immunity by decreasing the numbers of antigen-presenting Langerhans cells in the genital epithelium (173,174). Cervical HPV infection and CIN are associated with diminished numbers of intraepithelial Langerhans cells. Such local immunologic depletion could favor viral persistence, contributing to malignant transformation. Cigarette smoke concentrates have been demonstrated *in vitro* to transform HPV-16–immortalized endocervical cells (169), although no increased risk of adenocarcinoma has been identified in association with use of tobacco products. The increased risk associated with passive smoking is as strong as that observed in association with personal cigarette smoking (167,168). The high levels of nitrosamines inhaled in passive smoking may be relevant.

Smoking cessation promotes resolution of HPV-associated abnormalities in Pap smears with probable enhancement of cellular immunity.

Infection by Other Microbial Agents

Genital HPV infection and cervical neoplasia are more common among individuals who have had multiple sexual partners or whose partner has had multiple sexual partners (175,176). An increased incidence of other sexually transmitted diseases has been reported in association with genital HPV infection and cervical neoplasia (176). **Disruption of epithelial integrity and reparative metaplasia associated with acute cervicitis that is due to** *Chlamydia trachomatis,* *Neisseria gonorrhoeae,* **herpes simplex virus (HSV), or** *Trichomonas vaginalis* **may increase susceptibility to genital HPV infection.** No clear picture has emerged from epidemiologic studies addressing these associations (177–181). The role of chronic inflammation due to coinfection with *Chlamydia trachomatis* is also unclear but chlamydial infection appears to be associated with increased persistence of high-risk HPV infection (182). Chlamydial infection in HPV-positive women is also associated with development of high-grade CIN and invasive cancer suggesting a possible cofactor role (183,184).

Sex Hormonal Influences

Condylomata acuminata increase rapidly in size and number in pregnancy. This could suggest that maternal estrogen status is permissive for HPV replication, although it may reflect the immunosuppressive effect of pregnancy. Increased detection of HPV DNA in cervical cytologic samples in pregnancy, including detection of oncogenic HPV types in up to 27% of pregnant women, suggests hormonally induced active viral replication (185,186).

CIN and cervical cancer are more frequently found in women with increased parity (187–189) and in women on oral contraceptives independent of sexual activity (189–195). **Epidemiologic studies have shown an increased risk of CIN in long-term oral contraceptive pill (OCP) users,** rising to twofold for 5 or more years of OCP use. OCP-induced folate deficiency with reduced metabolism of mutagens is a proposed mechanism for increased risk (196). Prospective follow-up of high-risk HPV-positive women does not demonstrate an increased risk of CIN 3 among OCP users (189). **There has been no demonstrable clinical value to ceasing oral contraceptives in the management of HPV-associated disease.**

Protective benefits of barrier contraception remain unclear (197). An earlier association between condom use and decreased persistence of high-risk and low-risk HPV types and reduced risk of progression to CIN 3 among high-risk HPV-positive women has been confirmed in recent studies (198,199). Increased HPV clearance and low-grade CIN regression with condom use has also been reported (200).

Exogenous and Endogenous Immunosuppression

Iatrogenic induction of immunosuppression in renal transplant recipients increases the rate of CIN to 16 times that of the general community (201). The risk of CIN and cervical cancer is increased in human immunodeficiency virus (HIV)–infected women, and failure rates of treatment for preinvasive lesions are increased (202–206). HPV prevalence and persistence are increased in HIV-positive women. HIV infection has a lesser influence on the probability of developing invasive cancer but the risk is increased (206). Systemic immune suppression from diseases such as Hodgkin's disease, leukemia, and collagen vascular diseases are associated with an increased incidence and recalcitrancy of HPV-associated disease.

Dietary Factors

Dietary deficiencies of vitamin A or beta-carotene may increase the risk of CIN and cervical cancer (208). Higher dietary consumption of vitamins A, C, and E as well as β-carotene and increased circulating levels of certain micronutrients may be protective against cervical neoplasia (209–211). Higher levels of dietary vitamin A and carotenoids, reflected in higher dietary vegetable intake and increased circulating levels of cis-lycopene, are associated with a greater than 50% reduction in persistence of high-risk HPV DNA (211). There is a possible protective association between higher folate levels and risk of high-grade CIN. Low socioeconomic status appears to remain a risk factor among HPV infected women even when standardized for available medical care.

Human Papillomavirus Vaccines

The HPV vaccine is a major scientific and public health advance in the prevention of cervical cancer (212,213). Most invasive cervical cancers and CIN lesions are attributable to high-risk HPV infection (15). It is estimated that the annual financial burden of HPV-associated disease in the United States is over $5 billion and 90% of this is spent in the follow-up of abnormal Pap smears and treatment of precancerous lesions (215,216). **A prophylactic or therapeutic vaccine against HPV has the potential to have a substantial impact on HPV infection and rates of CIN and cervical cancer** (217). HPVs cannot be grown in the laboratory so standard approaches to vaccine development, such as inactivation of live virus or development of attenuated virus, are not possible. Prophylactic vaccines have been produced using recombinant DNA technology. HPV prophylactic vaccines, designed to prevent HPV infection, are based on viruslike particle (VLP) technology developed through the pioneering research of Zhou and Fraser in Brisbane, Australia (218,219).

Fraser describes this process as the major capsid protein of the virus being expressed in eukaryotic cells and self assembling to produce empty viral capsids (212). VLPs are three-dimensional structures similar to papillomavirus particles and produced by expression of L1 and L2 HPV viral capsid proteins. These DNA-free VLPs are empty capsids and contain no oncogenic or infectious materials. Viruslike particles resemble the virus immunologically and induce HPV type-specific antibody on administration (220,221).

The immunogenicity of HPV involves presentation of the major capsid protein L1 to the immune system. L1 VLP vaccines induce strong cell-mediated as well as humoral immune responses (222–224). Such vaccines have demonstrated prophylactic efficacy in animal models (225) and then in human clinical trials (220,221, reviewed 213). Two vaccine products have been developed, a quadrivalent vaccine incorporating HPVs 16, 18, 6, and 11 (*Gardasil;* approved by the U.S. Food and Drug Administration [FDA] in June 2006) and a bivalent vaccine incorporating HPVs 16 and 18 (*Cervarix;* currently under review by FDA).

Vaccine Efficacy

Clinical trials demonstrate that HPV vaccines are effective and safe (220,221,226–229). For ethical and scientific reasons, surrogate end points were prevention of HPV acquisition, long-term viral persistence, development of genital neoplasia and genital warts as opposed to development of cervical cancer. Studies were largely undertaken among sexually active women 16 to 25 years of age although recent studies have been extended to include women up to 45 years (e.g., FUTURE III). Age groups where new HPV infection is uncommon include male and female children ages 9 to 15 years where antibody levels produced are on average substantially higher than in 16- to 24-year-old women (230). Women ages 25 to 45 years also have a lower level of new HPV infection and the antibody response is lower (231,232), but the quadrivalent vaccine does prevent 90% of new high-risk HPV infections in this 24- to 45-year-old female age group (233).

The quadrivalent vaccine demonstrates, following exact clinical protocols, 100% efficacy in preventing condylomata and vulvovaginal precancerous lesions and 98% efficacy in preventing high-grade cervical lesions among young sexually active women (212,213). In trial populations which include less strenuously defined criteria, such as including women with known infection or disease associated with vaccine types prior to vaccination, the quadrivalent vaccine is 44% effective in preventing CIN 2-3 and 73% effective in preventing condylomata and other HPV associated vulvovaginal lesions (213). In strict protocol studies, the bivalent vaccine demonstrates 100% efficacy in preventing persistent high risk HPV cervical infection and development of vaccine type CIN lesions (220,234,235).

For women recruited under less strict protocol conditions, who received at least one vaccine dose and who tested negative for high-risk HPV types or had no cytologic abnormality at a screening visit within 90 days of enrollment, the quadrivalent vaccine efficacy was 94% in preventing persistent high-risk HPV infections at 12 months and 96% in preventing abnormal Pap smears (236). **No therapeutic effects have been demonstrated in women with vaccine-type existing HPV infection or HPV-related disease,** with lesions regressing or progressing at similar rates in vaccine and placebo recipients (237).

Follow-up studies of women vaccinated with both vaccines have demonstrated sustained efficacy for at least 5 years. Three administrations of vaccine induce peak antibody levels 20 times higher than those seen with natural HPV infection (212). Antibody levels fall significantly in the first 2 years after immunisation but remain above those stimulated by natural infection for at least 5 years (238). These levels are associated with continued protection against infection. A modeling study suggests antibody levels will remain above those associated with natural infection for 12 years or more (239). Immunological memory is retained and a single booster dose given 60 months post-completion of the HPV vaccination protocol has been shown to produce a strong anamnestic increase in antibody titres, not seen in nonimmune subjects, with continued sustained efficacy typical of many vaccines (238).

Immunization with HPV 16 and 18 VLPs provides some protection against other high-risk HPV types and development of associated disease. The bivalent HPV 16/18 vaccine has been demonstrated to provide significant protection against HPV 45 infection and partial protection against HPV 33 infection (220). The quadrivalent (HPV 6/11/16/18) vaccine showed 27% protection against new high-grade cervical lesions associated with 10 nonvaccine HPV types (212). The real level of cross protection with current vaccines is not sufficient at this time to justify change to current clinical practice and **vaccinated women should continue conventional screening for cervical neoplasia** (240,241).

The immunogenicity and clinical efficacy of HPV vaccines in immunosuppressed women and in women with chronic disease is uncertain but is under study. The quadrivalent vaccine appears safe in pregnant women with no increased rates of spontaneous pregnancy loss or fetal abnormalities compared to placebo risks. The vaccine is classified Category B in terms of pregnancy risk and vaccination during pregnancy is not recommended (240,242). **Women who become pregnant during the vaccination schedule should be reassured that adverse consequence for the pregnancy related to vaccination is most unlikely.**

Vaccine Safety

No serious adverse affects attributable to vaccination were seen in placebo controlled trials (227,228,234,243–245). Local reactogenicity at the immunization site, systemic malaise and fever were slightly more common than with placebo but did not lead to discontinuation of the vaccination schedule. Redness and swelling at the vaccination site was increased with the bivalent vaccine adjuvanted with monophosphoryl Lipid A compared to placebo (234). Since vaccine licensure, over 12 million doses of the quadrivalent vaccine have now been given to young women. The vaccine adverse events reporting service indicates no rare, serious adverse events occurring with greater frequency among vaccine recipients than might be expected in the age-matched unvaccinated population (212,213). **Fainting after vaccination is the most common adverse event.**

Vaccine Deployment

The quadrivalent HPV vaccine is currently licensed in over 80 countries and the bivalent vaccine in 2 countries. Vaccination is approved for young women up to the age of 26 years. **The greatest public health benefit is achieved by vaccination of girls and young women prior to sexual initiation as the vaccines are prophylactic** (246). The U.S. Advisory Committee on Immunization Practices (ACIP) recommends routine vaccination with the quadrivalent HPV vaccine of all 11- to 12-year-old girls, "catch-up" vaccination of all 13- to 26-year-old girls and women (240). Modeling suggests this will have the most immediate impact on prevention of CIN detected through existing screening programs (212,247,248). Vaccination of 9 to 10-year-old girls should be at the providers' discretion.

Vaccination of young sexually active women may still provide some protection. Routine performance of Pap smears or HPV DNA testing prior to vaccination is not recommended, although such screening may be appropriate for sexually active women. **Cervical cancer screening should continue for the immunized population to screen for disease caused by nonvaccine HPV types,** to monitor the continued efficacy of the vaccination program (which may not be 100%), and to screen HPV infected women as the vaccine is not therapeutic.

The optimal vaccine dosing schedule is three doses at 0, 2, and 6 months. Accelerated delivery schedules over 4 months are being used in some countries. The U.S. Advisory Committee on Immunization Practices (ACIP) recommends (240):

1. First and second doses must be separated by at least 4 weeks.
2. Second and third doses must be separated by at least 12 weeks.
3. If the dosing schedule is interrupted, the vaccine series is not restarted but the required dose is given as soon as possible.

All studies examining cost effectiveness suggest that vaccinating 12-year-old girls against HPV is cost effective (247–252), followed by either annual screening starting at age 18 or even 3 yearly screening starting at age 25. The costs of lost productivity due to cervical cancer related illness and death, which will further improve cost effectiveness of prevention, are not factored into these studies. Cost savings are achieved in reducing abnormal Pap smear results, colposcopy referrals, cervical biopsies and treatment procedures, as well as reducing the costs of diagnosis and treatment of genital warts. **The costs, both financial and personal, associated with the complications of treatment procedures among young women, including the obstetric morbidity related to impaired cervical function in pregnancy such as premature delivery, low birth weight babies, and premature rupture of membranes will also be reduced.** Divergent findings have been reported in assessment of the cost effectiveness of vaccinating females and males (247,251), though no efficacy data exists yet for vaccination of young men.

The HPV vaccine can be administered with other age-appropriate vaccines such as those for meningococcus, tetanus, diphtheria, and pertussis. Lactating and immunocompromised women can receive the vaccine but it is not recommended in pregnancy due to insufficient data supporting safety (240). Most cervical disease in older women results from persistence of preexisting HPV infection. The vaccines do not treat existing HPV infection or associated disease. New high-risk HPV infections occur throughout life but with reduced frequency. Cross-protection against infection with other nonvaccine HPV types is partial (253) or nonexistent (221). **The benefit of vaccination in preventing cervical cancer falls with increasing age** (241,246). The relevant benefit of cervical cancer screening increases. At a still undetermined age, the benefits and cost effectiveness of screening may outweigh those of vaccination.

The reduction in cervical cancer risk with vaccination will be determined by the number of oncogenic HPV types included in the vaccine, the proportion of the population vaccinated, the durability of protection and the continued compliance by women and providers with screening guidelines. The possible 70% reduction in risk of cervical cancer associated with the current vaccines cannot be assessed for several decades, as young girls currently vaccinated begin to reach the median age of cervical cancer diagnosis of 48 years. **Premature relaxation of existing cancer control measures could see cervical cancer rates rise** offsetting some of the benefits of vaccination.

Widespread HPV vaccination will decrease the prevalence of CIN 2-3 in the population, causing the positive predictive value of Pap smear screening tests for detection of precancer to decrease and negative predictive value to increase. With a lowered incidence of disease in the community, there will be a need for more sensitive screening tests. In this context, HPV 16 and HPV 18 type-specific screening tests are likely to alter screening recommendations for vaccinated and unvaccinated women in the future. At this time, vaccinated women should continue to be screened according to recommendations, with close monitoring of changes in test performance characteristics.

The development of an effective HPV vaccine could provide a powerful strategy for the control of cervical cancer in resource-poor regions and underserved populations in developed countries. Cytologic screening programs have been relatively ineffective in poor countries throughout the world and have underperformed among minority groups in developed regions. The reasons for this failure are complex. They reflect racial, ethnic, and socioeconomic disparities in participation in the screening program, in addition to the relative insensitivity of a single Pap smear, and the multivisit model for diagnosis and treatment.

The success of HPV vaccination programs in poor regions will depend on cost of vaccine, HPV epidemiology, sociocultural environment, and the commitment of national and international health organizations to the logistical challenges of implementing widespread HPV vaccination programs weighed against other health priorities. An international effort is currently underway to make HPV vaccination globally available in an affordable manner.

The politics surrounding a vaccine directed against a sexually transmitted disease and aimed at prevention of a related disease in women alone, possibly years later, are extremely challenging (254,255). Concerns have been raised that protecting girls and young women from later development of HPV-associated disease by vaccination may increase unsafe sexual behavior and premature sexual activity ("behavioral disinhibition") (256–259). This has been seen as a potential barrier to vaccine acceptance and implementation, as well as to parental and provider acceptance. The basis for these concerns is the perception that fear of HPV infection is a motivation for abstinence or for safe sex practices among adolescents. In reality, the understanding of HPV as a sexually transmitted disease is extremely limited among male and female adolescents (260) and even among adults (261). Overall, HPV vaccine acceptance among young women, parents and providers is very high (259) influenced by the vaccines' high efficacy and safety, the risks and severity of the targeted diseases and the support by professional organizations. Controversial issues remain surrounding mandatory vaccination, affordability, access, impact on screening behavior and influence on sexual behavior (262–266).

According to the American Cancer Society's Guideline for HPV Vaccine Use (240), the limitations of current vaccines are: (i) the vaccines do not protect against all carcinogenic HPV types; (ii) the vaccines do not treat existing HPV infections; (iii) the duration of protection and the length of protection required to prevent cancer are unknown; (iv) the cost of vaccination and the possible need for booster doses may limit vaccine use among poor and uninsured women; and (v) the three-dose regimen may not be feasible in poor and medically underserved populations.

The Guideline suggests further research is required for: (i) long-term data on duration of vaccine-induced immunity; (ii) vaccine safety data including reproductive toxicity and side effects of HPV vaccination with other adolescent vaccines; (iii) registry data to assess vaccine coverage; (iv) surveillance data to assess population-based vaccine efficacy; (v) data for population-based and lesion-based changes in type-specific HPV prevalence across the full spectrum of HPV-associated disease, and (vi) qualitative and quantitative data on vaccine acceptability and the impact on sexual behavior and screening practices.

Vaccination against a subset of high-risk HPV types may not have the same long-term protective effect as destruction or excision of the transformation zone among women with established CIN lesions. Prevention will avoid the trauma, costs, and morbidity associated with the detection, diagnosis, and management of CIN lesions. There is a critical need to understand the likely impact of vaccination on screening, including the performance characteristics of cytology and high-risk HPV-DNA testing as well as on women's screening behavior and providers recommendations regarding screening. **The combination of vaccination of adolescents and young women with primary HPV DNA screening in older women could**

283

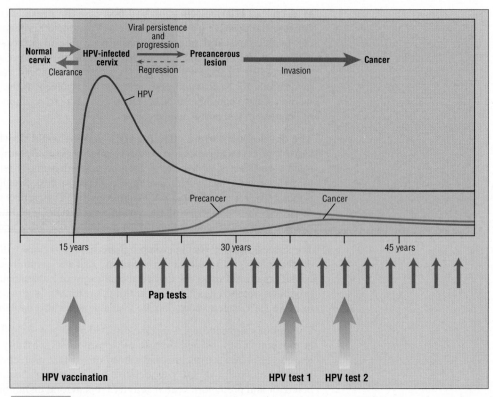

Figure 8.7   **HPV Vaccination and the Natural History of HPV Infection in Cervical Cancer Prevention.** Peak prevalence of transient infections with carcinogenic types of HPV (blue line) occurs among women during their teens and 20s after initiation of sexual activity. Peak prevalence of cervical precancer occurs approximately 10 years later (green line). Peak prevalence of invasive cancer occurs at 40 to 50 years of age (red line). The conventional model of cervical-cancer prevention is based on repeated rounds of cytologic examination, including Papanicolaou smears, and colposcopy (small blue arrows). Alternative strategies include HPV vaccination of adolescents (large beige arrow), one or two rounds of HPV screening at the peak ages of treatable precancerous conditions and early cancer (large reddish-brown arrows), or both. (Reproduced with permission from **Schiffman M, Castle PE**. The promise of global cervical-cancer prevention. *N Engl J Med* 2005;353;2101–2104).

substantially decrease the incidence of cervical cancer whilst requiring a limited lifetime number of patient visits. Such an approach needs validation before widespread adoption (Fig. 8.7).

Screening for Cervical Neoplasia

Incidence and mortality rates for cervical cancer in the United States have steadily decreased since the 1950s (267). Although the incidence of cervical cancer in Western countries was beginning to decline before the introduction of screening efforts, the significant decreases in cervical cancer incidence and mortality can be largely attributed to the success of widespread screening (267–270). **The Pap smear is widely recognized as the most cost-effective cancer screening test yet devised, and serves as a model for screening for other malignancies.**

A cohort effect for cervical cancer incidence and mortality has been clearly demonstrated (271). **Women who entered their early reproductive years at times of great social upheaval, such as during World Wars I and II, remained at high risk for cervical neoplasia all their lives.** Women in their early reproductive years in the two decades after the end of World War II, a period of reversion to very traditional sexual and social mores in many Western countries, appear to have been at low risk for development of cervical cancer. There has been an increasing incidence of cervical cancer in young women in many Western countries since the 1970s in spite of dramatic increases in diagnosis and treatment of preinvasive cervical disease (5,271–273).

Test Performance Characteristics of Conventional Cervical Cytologic Screening

The accuracy of the Pap smear has never been tested in a prospective, double-blinded study. Only relatively recently has the accuracy of the Pap smear been questioned (273), although **it has long been apparent that it has a definite false-negative rate** for invasive cancer and its precursors (274–278).

Sensitivity of Cervical Cytologic Screening

Sensitivity levels reported by experts under research conditions are not reproducible in routine clinical practice. Reasonable test performance using a competent laboratory results in false-negative rates of 15% to 30% for high-grade lesions (HGLs) (CIN 2 to 3) (279–282). False-negative rates for invasive cervical cancer can be even higher, approaching 50% in some series, because of obscuring effects of blood, inflammatory exudate, and necrotic debris. In Western countries, many women in whom invasive cancer develops have never been screened but up to 50% have been screened yet still develop cancer (283,284). This occurs more frequently among younger women with invasive cancer and reflects the inherent suboptimal sensitivity of conventional cytologic screening (Fig. 8.8).

A false-negative cytologic result occurs when the smear report does not predict the presence of any grade of cervical neoplasia. This consists of "true" false-negative results (70%) and laboratory errors (30%) (285,286). **True false-negative smears are free of abnormal cells, even on review of the slide, in the presence of histologically proven cervical disease.** The main factors contributing to the false-negative rate are (i) specimen collection; (ii) laboratory error; and (iii) deficiencies in laboratory quality assurance mechanisms.

Specimen Collection   The accuracy of cytologic diagnosis is highly sensitive to sample-to-sample variation in number of cells per smear. The quality of sample taking is the major factor contributing to this variability. **The cervix may desquamate unpredictably.** A large, four-quadrant HGL may fail to provide representative cells despite conscientious sampling.

The patient should be informed to refrain from douching or using tampons or intravaginal medications for at least 48 hours before the scheduled examination. She should also avoid intercourse for 48 hours before the visit and should reschedule if menstrual bleeding occurs. **Best results are obtained by paired use of the Ayre's spatula and cytobrush or sampling devices that adequately sample both endocervix and ectocervix.**

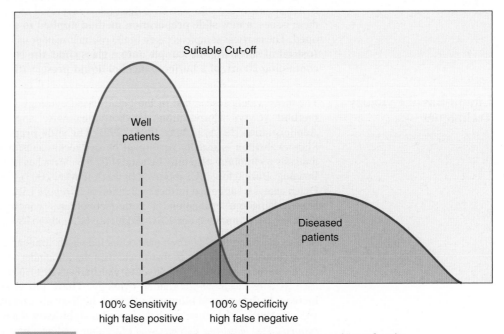

Figure 8.8   **Sensitivity and specificity of screening test as reciprocal ratios.**

Laboratory Error   **One-third of false-negative smear reporting is attributable to laboratory error** (280, 285). In response to medical and media pressure to address this problem, there has been a significant increase in the number of smears reported as showing minor abnormalities. The effect of this has been to decrease the specificity of cytologic methodology without significantly increasing the sensitivity of the test for high-grade lesions and cancer (282,286–289).

Quality Assurance   **Laboratories in the United States are required to rescreen 10% of randomly selected negative cases.** This strategy has been of uncertain value because it provides limited assurance of quality given the relatively low prevalence of high-grade lesions and cancer. The Health Care Financing Agency has restricted the number of cervical smears that a cytopathologist can evaluate to 80 slides per day.

Specificity of Cervical Cytologic Screening

Historically, the primary aim of cervical screening was the detection of clinically occult cervical cancer. High specificity was required at the cost of reduced sensitivity. The recognition that cytologic screening prevents cervical cancer by detection of preinvasive disease has shifted this balance, favoring increased sensitivity. Cytologic criteria for HGLs and invasive cancer were formulated when specificity was demanded, and **competent laboratories operate with a very low false-positive rate, usually between 2% and 5%, for the diagnosis of high-grade disease** (290). The specificity of cytologic screening has been eroded by cytologic overcall of low-grade disease (270). **Colposcopic assessment of women with low-grade cytologic abnormalities reveals no disease in as many as 30% of cases** (287).

Liquid-Based, Thin-Layer Cervical Cytology

A meta-analysis of 28 studies in which conventional cytology was evaluated for accuracy as a screening test reported a mean sensitivity and specificity of 58% and 69%, respectively (281). A large U.S. study concluded that estimates of the sensitivity of the conventional smear were biased in most studies (287). **Based on the least biased studies, they concluded the sensitivity of conventional cytology was 51%, much lower than generally believed.**

Sampling and preparation errors are responsible for more than 70% of false-negative Pap smears (289). Up to 80% of cervical cells are discarded with collection devices used in taking conventional smears (288,290). **When abnormal cells are present on the slide, they may be difficult to identify and interpret in conventional smears because of the obscuring effects of air-drying artifact, excess blood, mucus, and inflammatory debris, or areas of thick cellularity** where there may be insufficient permeation of the fixative.

When previous negative Pap smears of women diagnosed with cancer of the cervix are reviewed, many are shown to have been falsely reported as negative (283,284,291). To address these issues, **a new slide preparation method applied to gynecologic specimens was developed.** The cervical sample is taken in the routine manner using conventional sampling devices. **Instead of smearing the sample onto a glass slide, the collection device is rinsed in a vial containing 20 mL of a buffered alcohol liquid preservative.**

Liquid-Based Cytology Techniques

The most widely researched of the liquid-based cytology (LBC) techniques is the *ThinPrep* **method** (Cytyc Corporation, Boxborough, MA; approved by the Food and Drug Administration [FDA] in May 1996) (292). **The slide preparation technique is automated.** Slide evaluation is usually performed by cytotechnicians/cytologists, but **automated image analysis technology also may be used** (Fig. 8.9). Another LBC technique, *SurePath* (TripPath Imaging, Burlington, NC; approved by FDA in May 2003), is available for gynecologic use. A Dutch analysis suggested further evaluation of *Surepath* LBC was necessary (293), whereas the United Kingdom evaluation of both technologies concluded that there was insufficient evidence to recommend one LBC product over another (294–296).

Studies assessing the *ThinPrep* method include both split-sample studies (295–298), in which a conventional smear is first prepared and then the remainder of the specimen is rinsed into a vial for thin-layer preparation, and direct-to-vial studies (299–302), in which the thin-layer sample is used as a replacement for routine cytology. **These initial studies suggested a substantial increase in detection of biopsy-confirmed, high-grade cervical abnormalities, ranging from 16% to 100%. The same studies showed a significant decrease in "unsatisfactory" smear reports.** The *ThinPrep* Pap test was FDA approved as a replacement for the conventional Pap smear on the basis that the test was significantly more effective than the conventional smear for the detection of low-grade and more severe cervical abnormalities in a variety of populations.

A

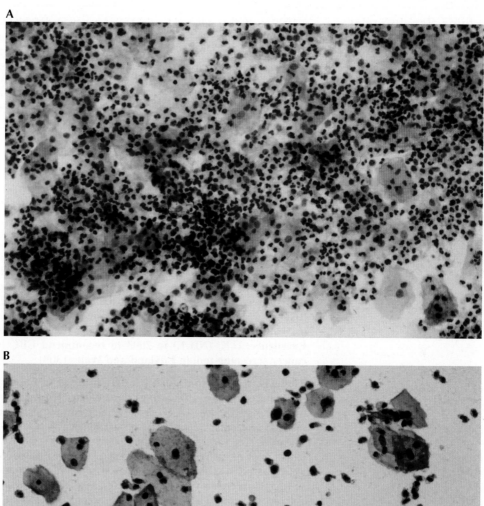

B

Figure 8.9   Comparison of (A) standard Papanicolaou smear with (B) mono-layer preparation.

In the United States, there has been rapid adoption of LBC for cervical screening over the past decade. Most cervical smears in the United States are taken into solution despite the lack of large randomized studies (303). Recent technological improvements in automation of processing and assessment of LBC specimens, particularly the use of an automated imager, are likely to increase this utilization (304). **The ability to test LBC specimens for HPV DNA and other sexually transmitted organisms further enhances the clinical appeal of this technology.**

The challenging questions asked by screening programs around the world are (i) Is LBC more sensitive and specific than conventional cytology; and (ii) Is implementation of LBC cost effective? Screening programs rely on analyses that adopt a population-based model as opposed to limited laboratory and clinical studies of specific clinical populations. The results of these analyses have been as varied as the screening programs (305–312).

Liquid-Based Cytology: Clinical Efficacy and Cost Effectiveness

A 1999 analysis conducted for the U.S. Agency for Health Care Policy and Research (AHCPR) assessed the efficiency and cost effectiveness of new cervical cytologic screening technologies based on a metaanalysis of published research (287). **This study reported that the *ThinPrep* test was the most cost effective new cervical cytologic screening technology.** The report indicated an improved sensitivity for LBC as opposed to conventional cytology but found no precise estimates for the effect on specificity, particularly with reported increased detection of atypical squamous cells of undetermined significance (ASC-US) and low-grade squamous intraepithelial lesions (LSIL). It reported there was insufficient evidence to make recommendations for adopting LBC and suggested further study.

Following an extensive literature review and assessment, **the American Cancer Society reported in 2002 that LBC (ThinPrep) was more sensitive but possibly less specific than conventional cytology for the detection of HSIL** (313). The revised guidelines of the ACS recommended liquid-based cytology as an alternative to conventional smears with screening to be performed every two years.

The United Kingdom experience lent strong support to the claim that LBC offers improved clinical performance in cervical screening. The 2001 Scottish Cervical Screening Programme pilot study reported that use of LBC increased detection of HSIL and significantly reduced unsatisfactory smear rates when compared with the conventional smear (311). **LBC was subsequently introduced into the Scottish Cervical Screening Programme.** Similar findings were reported in England after interim clinical assessment of the pilot conducted by the U.K. National Screening Program (308). **This led the National Institute for Clinical Excellence, U.K. (NICE) in 2003 to recommend LBC be used as the primary cervical cancer screening tool in England and Wales** (309).

The U.K. experience argued strongly in favor of improved clinical effectiveness of LBC (314). Introduction of LBC will be complete in the United Kingdom in 2008 following an implementation pilot (315). The desired end points are to reduce the rate of inadequate samples and increase screening capacity. This has been achieved and specificity has been maintained (316). There has been some increase in detection rates (317) but increased sensitivity was not a specific aim of implementation. **Cost effectiveness will be influenced by a number of additional variables,** such as availability and implementation of automated screening devices, increased screening intervals with increased screening sensitivity, reduction in unsatisfactory smear rates, colposcopic referral guidelines, introduction of HPV DNA testing in older age groups to further increase safe screening intervals, use of reflex HPV DNA testing for triage of equivocal LBC results, and use of LBC specimens for broader testing for other sexually transmitted diseases.

More recent systematic reviews have concluded that the evidence about liquid-based cytology was not good enough to judge LBC performance relative to conventional cytology. The U.S. Preventive Services Task Force, reporting in 2003, concluded there was insufficient evidence to make a recommendation to adopt LBC (312). Recent metaanalyses of the performance of LBC, based on nonrandomized trials, have reached conflicting conclusions (303,318–320).

In 2007, Ronco and colleagues reported the first large randomized, controlled comparison of conventional cytology with liquid based cytology in over 45,000 women presenting for primary screening in 9 centers in Europe (321). The same cytologists read both types of slides and abnormal results were checked by a panel of cytologists. Histologic confirmation of CIN or worse in a colposcopically directed biopsy was the principle end point with pathologists blinded to cytologic results. Sensitivity and specificity could not be calculated as patients with normal cytology did not have colposcopy. The frequency of abnormal findings was greater with liquid-based cytology than conventional cytology (6.3% vs. 3.8%). **Liquid-based cytology showed significantly increased sensitivity for CIN1 but not for CIN3 or invasive cancer.** LBC was slightly more sensitive in detection of CIN2 lesions but this was not significant. **Detection of high-grade disease and invasive cancer was similar in both groups suggesting sensitivity and frequency of false-negative results were also similar.** The probability of histologically confirmed CIN after a positive result was lower in the LBC group suggesting lower specificity, lower positive-predictive value and higher false-positive rates. LBC also reported proportionately more slides as atypical squamous cells of undetermined significance.

The finding of lower sensitivity of LBC for high-grade CIN and worse in this large, well designed randomized study was surprising and at odds with manufacturer claims that LBC is "significantly more sensitive" than conventional cytology for detecting cervical neoplasia.

A further recent large, Dutch, prospective randomized comparison of LBC against conventional cytology showed no statistically significant difference in cytologic test positivity rates but significantly fewer unsatisfactory tests (322). **Lower unsatisfactory test reporting, the ability to perform additional testing on the liquid-based sample and laboratory benefits such as automation and time savings will need to be weighed against the potential physical and psychological trauma to women associated with false positive results** (318,320,323).

The 2001 Bethesda System

The Bethesda System for reporting cervical/vaginal cytological diagnoses was originally developed in 1988 at a United States National Cancer Institute (Bethesda, MD) workshop (41). The recommendations of the 1988 workshop rapidly gained widespread acceptance in laboratory practice in the United States and beyond. In 1991, a second NCI-sponsored workshop reviewed and modified the Bethesda System on the basis of laboratory and clinical experience (43) (Fig. 8.10).

A cervical-vaginal smear report using the revised 1991 Bethesda system had three components: (i) **a description of smear adequacy;** (ii) **a general categorization** (i.e., "within normal limits" or "not within normal limits"); and (iii) **description of the cytologic abnormality**, specifying whether squamous or glandular. Abnormal morphology that may represent preinvasive squamous disease falls into three descriptive categories: **ASC-US, LSIL, and HSIL.**

With the increased utilization of new cervical cancer screening technologies and in response to recent research findings, in 2001, the NCI sponsored a further multidisciplinary workshop to reevaluate and update the Bethesda System (45). The most clinically relevant changes are described in Chapter 6.

ASCUS-LSIL Triage Study (The ALTS Trial)

In the United States, more than 55 million Papanicolaou tests are performed annually. Five percent are reported as ASC-US and 2% as LSIL. The clinical dilemma is the need to identify the small number of women with CIN 3 and invasive cancer weighed against the high prevalence of ASC-US and LSIL reporting (324,325). Effective colposcopic triage strategies are

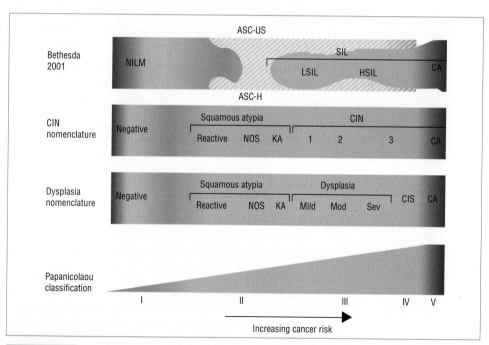

Figure 8.10 **Comparison of terminolgy for classification of HPV-associated squamous disease. Top: The Bethesa System.** Equivocal interpretations of ASC-US (atypical squamous cells of undetermined significance) and ASC-H (atypical squamous cells, cannot rule out high-grade squamous intraepithelial lesions) are noted with stippling, the amount and colour of which suggests the expected frequencies within the differential diagnosis. **2.** The CIN Classification **3.** The Dysplasia Classsification and **Bottom** the old Papanicolaou system. (Reproduced with permission from **Schiffman M, Castle PE, Jeronimo J, Rodriguez AC, Wacholder S.** Human papillomavirus and cervical cancer. *The Lancet* 2007;370;890–907.)

needed to identify the minority of women with clinically significant disease while avoiding excessive intervention for others.

The ASC-US/LSIL Triage Study (ALTS) (48,54,55,326–331) was a multicenter, randomized trial comparing the sensitivity and specificity of the following management strategies to detect CIN 3 among women referred with ASC-US and LSIL smear reports: (i) **immediate colposcopy** (considered to be the reference standard); (ii) **triage to colposcopy based on enrollment HPV DNA testing results** from Hybrid Capture 2 (HC 2) and thin-layer LBC results with a colposcopy referral threshold of HSIL; or (iii) **conservative management with triage based on repeat cytology results alone** at a referral threshold of HSIL. The trial had a majority of young women with a mean age of 29 years and included 2-year follow-up with exit colposcopy. Loop electrosurgical excision procedure (LEEP) was offered to women with histologic diagnoses of CIN 2 or CIN 3 at any visit or persistent CIN 1 at exit.

ALTS Trial: ASCUS Results

There were 3,488 women recruited with a community-based referral smear report of ASC-US. ASC-US interpretation was not highly reproducible, with only 32.4% of women having repeat ASC-US reported on enrollment LBC (54,326). **The overall percentage of CIN 2-3 in the ASC-US study population was 15.4%.** The 2-year cumulative diagnosis of CIN 3 was 8% to 9% in all study arms (329,330). **A single enrollment HPV DNA test identified 92% of women ultimately diagnosed with CIN 3 with 53% of women with an ASC-US smear report being referred for colposcopy.** Only 1.4% of women who were HPV negative at enrollment were ultimately found to have CIN 3 over 2 years. Serial cytology with a repeat ASC-US result as threshold for referral required two visits to achieve similar sensitivity (95%) and would have referred 67% of women to colposcopy. **HPV triage is at least as sensitive as immediate colposcopy for detecting CIN 3 but refers approximately half as many women to colposcopy.** Repeat cytology is sensitive at an ASC-US referral threshold, but requires two follow-up visits and more colposcopic examinations than HPV triage.

The ALTS trial demonstrates that testing for cancer-associated HPV-DNA is a viable option in the management of women with ASC-US. The American Society for Colposcopy and Cervical Pathology (ASCCP) 2001 Consensus Management Guidelines state that reflex HPV testing is the preferred triage for an ASC-US smear result when LBC methods are used (332).

The 2001 Bethesda System did not specifically endorse HPV DNA testing. Simultaneous reporting of the cytology and HPV DNA results is recommended but not always feasible.

ALTS Trial: LSIL Results

There were 1,572 women recruited with a community-based referral smear report of LSIL (331). **A cytologic interpretation of LSIL was more reproducible and was associated with a 25% risk of CIN 2-3 within 2 years.** There were five invasive cancers and one case of adenocarcinoma *in situ* detected. No intermediate triage strategy significantly decreased the need for colposcopic referral. **Most (more than 85%) LSIL cases are oncogenic HPV DNA positive, and the use of HPV DNA testing for the initial triage of LSIL is discouraged.**

Repeat cytology with an HSIL threshold for referral for colposcopy required only 19% of women to be referred for colposcopy but detected only 48% of cumulative CIN 3 cases. This strategy is not sufficiently sensitive for the timely detection of CIN 3. If the referral threshold was decreased to a single ASCUS result or above on repeat cytology, more than 80% of women were referred, achieving 90% sensitivity in detection of CIN 3. **Three sequential cytologic examinations with a referral threshold of LSIL demonstrated acceptable sensitivity (93%) and referral rate (69%). High patient retention is critical to this strategy, requiring a commitment from patient and provider to obtain quality cervical samples every 6 months.** Two-thirds of women would still be eventually referred for colposcopy.

If compliance can be achieved, cytologic follow-up of LSIL might be considered in selected populations such as adolescents who are at high risk of HPV infection and abnormal smear results but at low risk of cancer. Loss to follow-up of patients remains a major concern. **The ALTS data suggest that there is currently no efficient triage for LSIL. In general, the level of risk of CIN 2-3 warrants colposcopic evaluation.**

In both the ASC-US and LSIL study groups, the cumulative 2-year detection rates of CIN 3 did not vary significantly by study arm. However, in both study groups, the cumulative detection of CIN 2 was significantly reduced among women who were followed by 6-monthly conventional cytology compared with those referred for immediate colposcopy. This implies significant regression of missed prevalent cases of CIN 2 over the 2 years. **CIN 2 may represent a heterogeneous group of lesions, only some of which are incipient CIN 3.** CIN 2 lesions are currently treated. To avoid possible overtreatment, **it would be useful to determine those lesions likely to regress, possibly through identification of biomarkers of cancer risk among CIN 2 cases.**

ALTS Trial: Performance of Colposcopy

The strategy of immediate colposcopy was included as an arm in the ALTS study as the reference standard of optimal sensitivity and safety. **Of significant concern was the finding that immediate colposcopy in response to either an ASC-US or LSIL smear report was only 56% sensitive for the cumulative CIN 3 detected during the trial** (330). Some of the CIN 3 lesions may have developed after enrollment to be appropriately detected at follow-up visits. Review of CIN 3 cases suggested that many represented prevalent cases missed at initial colposcopic examination. Some of the CIN 3 lesions were detected in LEEP specimens at exit from the study.

Prospective follow-up of CIN 3 lesions is not ethically justifiable. If the goal of cervical screening is the timely detection of CIN 3, **the ALTS trial suggests that colposcopically directed biopsy is not a gold standard of absolute sensitivity.**

ALTS Trial: Risk of CIN 2-3

The 2-year cumulative risk of CIN 2-3 was virtually the same for women with LSIL and HPV-positive ASC-US (27.6% and 26.7%, respectively) (332). Women with HPV-positive ASC-US were more likely to have negative colposcopy or negative histology on reporting of colposcopically directed biopsies. Both LSIL and HPV-positive ASC-US had an 18% risk of detection of CIN 2-3 at initial colposcopically directed biopsy, which underlies the need for identical initial colposcopic management as indicated in the 2001 ASCCP Management Consensus Guidelines.

Women with documented CIN 1 are most commonly managed expectantly by intermittent colposcopy and repeat cytology. Women with negative findings at colposcopy and biopsy tend to be followed by cytology alone. Women with CIN 1 detected at initial colposcopic workup are presumed to be at higher risk of subsequent CIN 2-3 than women who have no pathology confirmed, but **the 2-year follow-up of women in the ALTS study revealed no difference in the subsequent risk of CIN 2-3 between women with no disease documented at initial colposcopy and women with documented CIN 1.** This reinforces the need for follow-up of the majority of women (82%) with LSIL or HPV-positive ASC-US smear reports and who have CIN 1 or less diagnosed from the initial colposcopic assessment.

The ALTS longitudinal data were reviewed to determine the most efficient follow-up strategy for detection of prevalent high-grade disease in women referred with LSIL or HPV-positive ASC-US and who had CIN 1 or less at initial colposcopy. **An HPV DNA test at 12 months was the single test with the highest sensitivity and lowest referral to repeat colposcopy.** HPV DNA testing at the 6-month follow-up examination was equally sensitive, but referred 13% more patients for repeat colposcopy (62.4% vs. 55.0%). Addition of cytology to the HPV test only marginally increased sensitivity but significantly increased referral. Three repeat cytologic tests at a threshold of ASC-US and without HPV testing achieved marginally higher sensitivity but referred a much higher percentage of women for colposcopy and required multiple office visits.

ALTS Trial: Cost-Effectiveness Model

A comprehensive cost-effectiveness analysis of alternative strategies based on the ALTS trial was conducted (333). A policy of ignoring equivocal smear results significantly reduced the effectiveness of cervical cancer screening and was not considered a viable alternative. The three management strategies of repeat cytology, immediate colposcopy, and oncogenic HPV DNA testing produce extremely small differences in cancer incidence reduction, although repeat cytology was less effective than both alternative strategies under all model conditions. Costs associated with each management strategy differed substantially. **Reflex HPV DNA testing was always less costly than repeat cytology, as it eliminates the need for repeat clinical examination to obtain a further cervical specimen and reduces the number of colposcopic examinations by 40% to 60%.** Referral of all women with ASC-US smears for colposcopy was always more costly than repeat cytology or HPV DNA testing.

ALTS Trial: Implications for Screening

The model then assessed the most efficient screening options by considering alternative strategies to manage equivocal smear results while simultaneously varying screening frequencies and types of cytological tests (334). **Triennial screening using liquid-based cytology with reflex HPV DNA testing for ASC-US smear results appeared the most cost-effective model.**

In part because of these findings and citing lack of direct evidence that annual screening leads to better outcomes than wider interval screening, the U.S. Preventive Services Task Force recommended that screening for cervical cancer be performed "at least every three years" rather than every year (335). **The American Cancer Society Guidelines suggest 3-yearly screening interval for women 30 years of age and older who have had negative results on three or more consecutive cervical smears (313). A combined cytologic and HPV DNA test was also recommended by the American Cancer Society** as a reasonable alternative to cytologic testing alone **for women 30 years of age or older,** with an explicit recommendation that the testing not be performed more often than every three years.

An analysis of data from the National Breast and Cervical Cancer Early Detection Program administered by the Centers for Disease Control and Prevention (CDC) concluded that "women 30 to 64 years of age with three or more previous negative smears who are screened three-yearly (once every three years) after the last negative test rather than annually have an excess risk of cancer of no more than 3 in 100,000" (335). Swedish investigators reported an annual incidence of squamous cervical cancer of 0.8 per 100,000 women with at least one previous negative test (336).

In part because of these findings, **the CDC program changed its screening policy, in line with the other national organizations, increasing the interval between screenings to 3 years after three consecutive negative tests.** More than 80% of women in the United States have undergone cervical screening in the past three years.

Human Papillomavirus Testing in Primary Screening

Large HPV DNA screening studies, employing both cross-sectional and longitudinal study designs, provide compelling evidence supporting the adjunctive use of HPV DNA testing in routine screening in women older than 30 years and for younger women in certain settings (337–350). These studies demonstrate that **HPV DNA testing using clinically available detection tools can identify almost all patients with CIN 3, high-grade glandular neoplasia, and invasive cancer.** Addition of LBC to HPV DNA testing increases sensitivity by 5%. **Combination HPV DNA testing and LBC has 90% to 100% sensitivity for CIN 3 and invasive cancer. The negative predictive value of such combined testing is above 99% in all studies and approaches 100% in most.**

A negative HPV DNA test virtually excludes any risk of underlying disease even in the presence of a reported cytologic abnormality. In response to this collective experience, **HPV DNA testing was approved as a primary screening tool in conjunction with cytology in women aged more than 30 years by the FDA in 2003.**

Although the high sensitivity and the high negative predictive value are obvious advantages of the HPV test, **its use as a primary screening tool is potentially hampered by low specificity and risk of overtreatment of HPV DNA–positive women** (351). Specificity and positive predictive value is further decreased when HPV DNA testing is combined with LBC, reflecting the inverse relationship between sensitivity and specificity in screening methodology.

HPV DNA testing identifies many transient HPV infections not associated with high-grade CIN, particularly in younger women. This is the main contributing factor to reduced specificity. **Women who are HPV DNA positive but who have a normal cervical smear or have no clinical evidence of HPV-related disease are at greatest risk of developing cervical neoplasia prospectively** (352,353). Such women should not be viewed as having "false-positive" tests but require close follow-up and repeat testing. For HPV testing to be cost effective in primary screening, an efficient policy is required for the management of women who test positive for high-risk HPV-DNA but who have negative or equivocal cytologic reporting (354). This strategy would use HPV DNA testing alone as primary screening and cytology would be used to triage HPV DNA–positive women.

The HART Study

The HART (HPV in Addition to Routine Testing) study from the United Kingdom recruited 11,085 women attending 161 U.K. family practices for routine cervical screening (343). **This** study confirmed HPV DNA testing to be a more sensitive primary screening technique than conventional (not liquid-based) cytology for detecting high-grade CIN (97.1% vs. 76.6%). High-risk HPV DNA detection combined with conventional cytology had 100% sensitivity for high-grade CIN lesions and above. HPV DNA testing was significantly less specific than conventional cytology (93.3% vs. 95.8%) and had a positive predictive value of 12.8%, less than that of an equivocal or worse conventional smear (15.8%). **The high rate of positive HPV DNA testing in women with no significant histologic abnormality in this study appears to be an impediment to the use of HPV DNA testing in primary screening.**

The authors estimated that referral rates for colposcopy would be reduced if (i) women with equivocal (and possibly with LSIL) smear reports but who were HPV DNA negative were returned to routine screening; (ii) HPV DNA–positive women with negative or equivocal smears were retested at 12 months; and (iii) the screening interval was extended to 5 years.

Three recent large European population-based, randomized, controlled trials of HPV DNA testing for primary cervical cancer screening have been reported from the Netherlands (355), Sweden (356), and Italy (357,358). In each study, the combination of HPV DNA testing and cytology was compared with conventional cytology alone for the detection of cervical neoplasia.

In the Dutch study (355), implementation of HPV DNA testing in addition to conventional cytology led to a 70% increase in the number of histologically confirmed lesions reported as CIN 3 or worse in the baseline screening round. At the second round of screening, 55% fewer women in the combined screening group had CIN 3 or worse detected compared to the cytology alone group. Similar results were reported for CIN 2 lesions which are usually treated when identified. **The decreased detection of high-grade precursor lesions in the second round of screening suggest earlier detection of high-grade lesions** which would have persisted rather than a subset of regressive lesions. This is supported by the finding that the decrease in the number of lesions detected at the second round was almost the same as the increase seen at baseline.

This early detection of a substantial proportion of persistent CIN 3 lesions leads to greater protection against invasive cervical cancer from a single round of screening. This would permit safe extension of the screening interval with probable decreased costs and improved participation. **Nonparticipation in screening is still the greatest risk factor for future development of cervical cancer.** Women who are high-risk HPV DNA negative but have an abnormal smear had a negligible risk of CIN 3 or worse, supporting the model of primary screening with HPV DNA testing and cytology as triage of HPV DNA positive women. **Conservative follow-up of HPV DNA positive women with normal cytology led to few referrals for colposcopy and may have avoided detection of rapidly regressive low-grade lesions.** Women in this trial were recruited from age 30 years onwards as is the norm in the Netherlands.

The large Italian randomized, controlled trial of HPV DNA testing versus conventional cytology also demonstrated a substantial gain in sensitivity of HPV DNA testing over cytology in detection of CIN 2-3 with only a small reduction in positive predictive value for women aged 35 to 60 years (357,358). Among younger women, 25 to 34 years of age, HPV DNA testing had an even higher sensitivity for detection of CIN 2-3 compared to cytology than with the older age group. Intensive screening and referral for colposcopy of HPV DNA positive young women and teenagers led to the detection of a high incidence of CIN 2-3 lesions soon after initial HPV infection. The difference in detection rates of high-grade CIN among young women when all HPV DNA positive women were referred for colposcopy versus only those who also had an associated cytological abnormality of ASC-US or worse was interpreted by the authors to suggest that most abnormalities, including CIN 2-3 lesions, in young women are destined to regress. Confirmation will require further screening cycles. This raises concerns in relation to increased referral of young women for colposcopy and treatment of high-grade CIN with associated increased risk of pregnancy related morbidity. **The recommendation from the study is that young women under 35 years who are HPV DNA positive should only be referred to colposcopy if cytology is abnormal or if HPV positivity persists after 1 year.**

The Swedish population based randomized controlled trial of HPV DNA testing versus conventional cytology among women aged 32 to 38 years demonstrated a 51% greater detection of CIN 2-3 or cancer among those screened using HPV DNA testing (356). At subsequent screening rounds, the HPV DNA screened group had a 42% lower detection of CIN 2 or worse and a 47% decrease in CIN 3 or worse. Women with persistent HPV DNA detection in later screening rounds remained at high risk of CIN 2-3 or worse after referral for colposcopy. The authors concluded that the improved sensitivity of HPV-based cervical cancer screening was not overdiagnosis, but attributable to earlier detection of high-grade lesions which do not regress.

Based on currently available data, the combination of HPV DNA testing with cytology significantly increases screening sensitivity. Women with "double-negative" results can be screened safely at longer intervals, offsetting the increased cost of the initial screen (350). **The duration of low-risk after a negative HPV DNA test is unknown.** Patients identified as being at increased risk on the basis of a positive HPV DNA test but who do not have identifiable disease should be monitored more closely.

There is no consensus regarding the appropriate age for cessation of screening. Lifetime screening continues to save lives but the benefits for regularly screened women beyond age 65 years are minimal. The probability of a false-positive cervical smear result is much greater than a true-positive result after age 65 years for regularly screened women. **The high negative predictive value of HPV DNA testing could be used as an additional means of safely exiting women from routine screening beyond a certain age.**

The wider use of HPV DNA testing in the primary screening setting will inevitably hinge on the acceptability of testing for a sexually transmitted virus to the target population and the provision of HPV DNA testing at low cost (359). **The anticipated lower incidence of disease developing among a younger generation who have received the cervical cancer vaccine as they enter the screening age groups will require the most sensitive screening tests. High-risk HPV DNA testing may become the preferred primary screening test** in this population due to the greater sensitivity and high negative predictive value.

HPV testing may have an important role in primary cervical screening in developing countries (360,361). The crude incidence rate of cervical cancer in some developing countries is as high as 100 cases per 100,000 women, compared with approximately 4 to 10 per 100,000 in developed countries. The simplicity of taking the sample, the stability of the transport medium, and the ability to automate the processing of the specimens are all advantages in developing countries.

Systematic Approach to Colposcopy

Colposcopy is the examination of the epithelia of the cervix, lower genital tract, and anogenital area using magnified illumination after the application of specific solutions to detect abnormal appearances consistent with neoplasia or to affirm normality. Integral to the procedure is targeting biopsies to areas of greatest abnormality.

Indications for Colposcopy

Colposcopy is most frequently performed in response to an abnormal cervical smear. Abnormal findings on adjunctive screening tests, such as HPV testing, can also be the indication for colposcopy. If the cervix is clinically abnormal or suspicious on naked-eye examination, colposcopy is also indicated. Abnormal and unexplained intermenstrual or postcoital bleeding and unexplained, persistent vaginal discharge may also be assessed by colposcopy to exclude a neoplastic cause. Other indications include a personal history of *in utero diethylstilbestrol (DES)* exposure, vulvar or vaginal neoplasia, or condylomata acuminata, and possibly sexual partners of patients with genital tract neoplasia or condylomata acuminata.

There are no absolute contraindications to colposcopy. The examination may be deferred until after bleeding ceases for women who are menstruating. **Acute cervicitis or vulvovaginitis should be evaluated and treated before colposcopy is performed** unless poor patient compliance is anticipated. The colposcopic procedure is modified in pregnancy, with a less liberal use of biopsy in the absence of warning signs of high-grade disease or cancer and avoidance of endocervical curettage. **Postmenopausal women who are not taking hormone replacement may benefit from a 3-week course of topical or oral estrogen before colposcopy.** Patients should avoid use of all intravaginal products for 24 hours before the examination.

Initial Clinical Workup

The patient should be prepared for the examination by a comprehensive explanation of the indication for colposcopy and a thorough verbal description of the procedure.

A complete medical history and general examination should be obtained. A history of previous premalignant cervical disease or cervical treatment should be determined. A history of endogenous or exogenous immune suppression is relevant. A social history of smoking or other "recreational" drug use should be obtained.

A clinical and speculum examination of the cervix, vagina, vulva, and perianal areas should be performed before the colposcopic examination. Squamous neoplasia may be multicentric (involving more than one genital tract site, i.e., cervix, vagina, or vulva) or multifocal (involving several areas at one site).

A bimanual pelvic and rectal examination should be performed, usually on completion of the colposcopy, to exclude clinically apparent coexistent gynecologic or pelvic disease. Uncommonly, abnormal cervical smears are caused by palpable malignancies of the endocervix, uterine body, adnexae, or bowel.

Locating the Source of Abnormal Cells

Colposcopy is performed in the dorsal lithotomy position with a drape covering the patient's legs. The cervix is visualized using a standard speculum. The colposcopic examination involves the application of three standard solutions to the cervix to determine the source of the abnormal cells in the cervical smear.

1. **Normal saline is initially applied to remove obscuring mucus and debris, to moisten the cervix, and to examine the cervix unaltered by subsequent solutions.** The two abnormal colposcopic findings detected after application of normal saline are **hyperkeratosis** (leukoplakia) and **atypical vessels.** Hyperkeratosis is a white, thickened epithelial area of the cervix (or lower genital tract) that is clinically apparent before application of acetic acid. Biopsy is indicated to exclude an underlying neoplastic process. Atypical vessels are the colposcopically apparent bizarre vascular abnormalities that occur in association with invasive cancer. **Green-filter examination of the cervix enhances the angioarchitecture.**

2. **A 3% to 5% acetic acid solution is then liberally applied to the cervix using soaked swabs or a spray technique. The abnormal colposcopic findings after application of acetic acid are acetowhite epithelium and abnormal vascular patterns.** Abnormal vascular patterns, reflecting the underlying capillary distribution, are **mosaicism and punctation.** Tissue swelling associated with the initial application of acetic acid compresses subepithelial capillaries, rendering vascular patterns less distinct. As the acetic acid reaction fades, mosaicism and punctation become vivid against the whiter background.

3. **Lugol's iodine (one-quarter strength) application to the cervix (if the patient is not allergic to iodine) is called a Schiller's test.** Normal ectocervical and vaginal squamous epithelium contains glycogen and stains mahogany brown after application of iodine solution. Normal columnar epithelium and immature squamous metaplastic or neoplastic epithelium do not contain glycogen, are not stained by iodine solution, and appear mustard yellow. Iodine solution application is considered an optional colposcopic procedure and is not uniformly performed, but is invaluable in the assessment of the vaginal mucosa.

Delineating the Margins of the Lesion

Once the source of abnormal cells in a cervical smear is located, the peripheral and distal margins of the lesion should be determined.

Distal Margin

The distal or peripheral margin of the lesion is usually readily identified. Occasionally, the lesion may extend onto the vaginal fornices, especially in the *DES*-exposed patient.

Proximal Margin

Delineation of the proximal or upper margin of the lesion requires the colposcopic visualization of the new squamocolumnar junction, which establishes the colposcopy as satisfactory or unsatisfactory. Failure accurately to delineate the position of the new squamocolumnar junction represents one of the most common colposcopic triage errors. An endocervical speculum may be helpful if the proximal margin is within the canal.

Endocervical Curettage

Endocervical curettage is performed to exclude an occult cancer in the canal (362). With the increasing incidence of cervical adenocarcinoma *in situ* (AIS) and invasive adenocarcinoma, many of which are associated with squamous CIN lesions, endocervical curettage may provide a safeguard against missing such lesions.

Routine performance of endocervical curettage is controversial. **When the entire new squamocolumnar junction can be visualized, it is reasonable to omit the routine endocervical curettage.** A negative endocervical curettage from a patient with an abnormal high-grade cytology and an unsatisfactory colposcopy does not exclude occult endocervical cancer, arid excisional cone biopsy remains mandatory. **When specifically indicated, collection of an endocervical sample using a cytobrush has been shown to be a more sensitive sampling device than endocervical curettage for endocervical squamous and glandular disease.** Specificity, however, is decreased (364).

Colposcopically Directed Cervical Biopsy

Cervical biopsies should be directed to the most significant lesions. **Multiquadrant lesions may require multiple biopsies.** Any area suspicious for occult invasion must be carefully sampled. The most reliable method of ensuring the accuracy of targeted biopsies is to grade lesions by deriving a colposcopic score. Cervical biopsies should be taken through the colposcope. The colposcopic grading score of the lesions and the biopsy sites should be carefully recorded.

Documentation of Colposcopic Findings

The findings of the colposcopic examination should be carefully documented. **Photodocumentation can be extremely valuable.** A system for recording patient information, laboratory results, management plan, and tracking log should be established and maintained to ensure appropriate patient care and follow-up. **Modern computerized systems provide for many of these needs in a most effective manner.**

The Abnormal Transformation Zone

If the transformation zone is deviated along a neoplastic pathway, epithelial and vascular alterations produce the characteristic morphologic appearances of the abnormal transformation zone (365). The colposcopic signs of the abnormal transformation zone are described in Table 8.1.

Squamous metaplasia, repair and regeneration, inflammation, and infection may all produce abnormal colposcopic transformation zone findings, such as acetowhite epithelium and abnormal vessels. Significant changes in the hormonal milieu such as accompany pregnancy, oral contraceptive pill use, estrogen withdrawal, and estrogen replacement can produce abnormal colposcopic signs in the absence of cervical disease. Atypical vessels, considered one of the colposcopic hallmarks of invasive cancer, can also occur in association with benign conditions, including immature metaplasia, nabothian follicles, inflammation, radiation treatment, and granulation tissue.

Table 8.1 Colposcopic Signs of the Abnormal Transformation Zone

Appearance	Cause
Epithelial abnormalities	
Leukoplakia	Abnormal keratin production from an inflammatory, viral, or neoplastic process
	Thickening of superficial epithelium in response to trauma
Acetowhite epithelium	Increased cellular and nuclear density
	Intracellular protein agglutination
	Abnormal intracellular keratins
	Intracellular dehydration
Vascular abnormalities	
Abnormal vessel patterns: mosaic and punctation	Alterations in the epithelial capillaries due to: 1. Normal metaplastic transformation 2. Capillary proliferative effect of human papillomavirus 3. Intraepithelial pressure created by expanding neoplastic tissue 4. Tumor angiogenesis factor
Atypical blood vessels	Tumor angiogenesis factor

Colposcopic Grading Systems

The basis of colposcopic management decision making is the process of cytologic–colposcopic–histologic correlation, with each component affording certain safeguards. **There are four basic colposcopic diagnoses: (i) normal; (ii) low-grade disease (HPV infection/CIN 1)i (iii) high-grade disease (CIN 2 or 3)i and (iv) invasive cancer.** Colposcopic grading systems have been developed to provide an objective, accurate, reproducible, and clinically meaningful prediction of the severity of CIN lesions based on discriminatory analysis of specific colposcopic signs (366–369).

Routine determination of a colposcopic diagnosis permits quality-control measures to be implemented in colposcopy (370,371). In colposcopic quality control programs, the colposcopist is required to achieve at least an 80% accuracy rate in colposcopic–histologic correlation or receive remedial training in colposcopic assessment of cervical lesions (372).

In current colposcopic experience, the Reid Colposcopic Index represents the most reproducible and clinically valid means of standardizing the evaluation of cervical lesions (368,369) (Table 8.2).

Reid Colposcopic Index   The Reid Colposcopic Index uses four colposcopic features of premalignant cervical lesions to achieve predictive accuracy. The colposcopic index permits accurate differentiation of low-grade from high-grade disease. It is not designed to differentiate premalignant from malignant cervical neoplasia. **The four colposcopic criteria used are (i) the margin of the lesion; (ii) the color of the acetowhitening; (iii) the type of vascular pattern; and (iv) the iodine staining reaction.**

The four colposcopic signs are scored individually and sequentially. The value of these colposcopic signs is maximized by combining them into a weighted scoring system. Scores of 0, 1, or 2 are assigned for each criterion, as described in Table 8.2. The total score is then reported as a ratio, the denominator of which is constant at 8. The numerator is the score derived from adding the four scores derived from evaluation of the four colposcopic signs and fluctuates as the

Table 8.2 Scoring System for Deriving the Colposcopic Index

Colposcopic Sign	Score		
	Zero Points	**One Point**	**Two Points**
Margin	Exophytic condylomas; areas showing a micropapillary contour Lesions with distinct edges Feathered, scalloped edges Lesions with an angular, jagged shape "Satellite" areas and acetowhitening distal to the original squamocolumnar junction	Lesions with a regular (circular or semicircular) shape, showing smooth, straight edges	Rolled, peeling edges Any internal demarcation between areas of differing colposcopic appearance
Color	Shiny, snow-white color Areas of faint (semitransparent) whitening	Intermediate shade (shiny, but gray-white)	Dull reflectance with oyster-white color
Vessels	Fine-caliber vessels, poorly formed patterns	No surface vessels	Definite, coarse punctation or mosaic
Iodine	Any lesion staining mahogany brown; mustard-yellow staining by a minor lesion (by first three criteria)	Partial iodine staining (mottled pattern)	Mustard-yellow staining of a significant lesion (an acetowhite area scoring 3 or more points by the first three criteria)

Adapted from **Reid R, Scalzi P.** Genital warts and cervical cancer: VII. An improved colposcopic index for differentiating benign papillomaviral infections from high-grade cervical intraepithelial neoplasia. *Am J Obstet Gynecol* 1985;153:611–618.

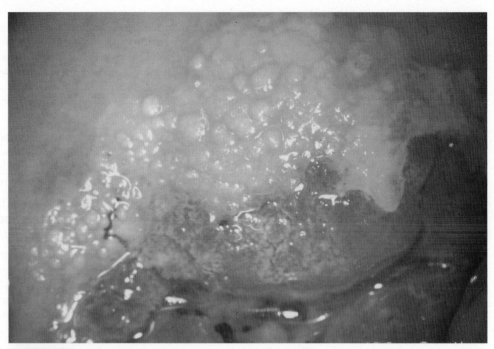

Figure 8.11   Colposcopy of low-grade cervical lesions showing acetowhite epithelium with fine abnormal vascular pattern.

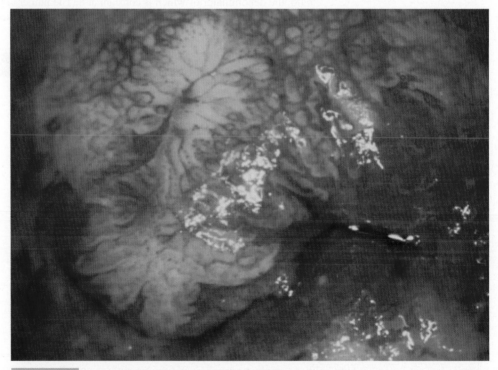

Figure 8.12   Colposcopy of high-grade cervical lesion showing dense acetowhite epithelium and coarse abnormal vascular pattern.

predictor of disease severity. **Scores of 0 to 2 are predictive of low-grade lesions (HPV infection/CIN 1;** Fig. 8.11). **Scores of 6 to 8 usually denote high-grade lesions** (CIN 2 to 3; Fig. 8.12). Scores of 3 to 5 represent an area of overlap between low-grade and high-grade lesions.

The overall predictive accuracy of the index exceeds 90% after a short training period. The colposcopic index permits a significantly more accurate colposcopic–histologic agreement than can be achieved by less systematic approaches to colposcopic diagnosis.

Table 8.3 Colposcopic Warning Signs of Invasive Cancer

1. Yellow, degenerate, friable epithelium particularly with contact bleeding

2. Irregular surface contour, particularly when occurring in a high-grade colposcopic abnormality (RCI score >6 points)

3. Surface ulceration or true "erosion," particularly when occurring in a high-grade colposcopic abnormality (RCI score >6 points)

4. Atypical blood vessels (coarse, varicose, bizarre subepithelial vessels with irregular caliber and nondichotomous branching or long, unbranched course)

5. Extremely coarse abnormal vascular patterns (i.e., mosaicism and punctation), especially with wide and irregular intercapillary distances and umbilication

6. Large, complex, high-grade lesions (RCI score >6 points) occupying three or four cervical quadrants

7. High-grade colposcopic lesions extending into cervical canal either >5 mm or beyond colposcopic view

CI, Reid Colposcopic Index.

Colposcopic Warning Signs of Invasive Cancer

Although a rare event in many colposcopic settings, invasive cancer must not be missed and still remains the major challenge to the colposcopist. Clinicians working in oncologic settings may over time acquire significant experience in the colposcopy of occult and overt cervical cancer. Although most invasive cancers are clinically apparent and do not require colposcopy for identification, early invasive lesions may be clinically occult. Exclusion of invasive cancer demands both a high index of suspicion and knowledge of warning signs. Colposcopic warning signs are shown in Table 8.3.

Other warning signs for invasive cancer include:

1. **Any cytologic evidence of possible squamous carcinoma, adenocarcinoma, or AIS or recurrent high-grade cytologic findings in a patient previously treated for CIN 3**

2. **Any histologic evidence of invasive cancer or CIN 2 or 3 in a tangentially sectioned punch biopsy in which the basement membrane cannot be adequately defined**

3. **High-grade cytologic abnormality in a postmenopausal or previously irradiated woman**

ASCCP 2006 Consensus Guidelines

In 2001, the American Society for Colposcopy and Cervical Pathology (ASCCP) Consensus Guidelines were developed to assist in the management of women with cytological abnormalities (332) and in the management of cervical cancer precursors (373), in part in response to the 2001 Bethesda System.

Since 2001, improved understanding of the pathogenesis and natural history of cervical HPV infection and cervical cancer precursors, of the future pregnancy implications of treatment for CIN among young women, and of the management of adenocarcinoma *in situ* has led to a critical review of the earlier Guidelines (374,375). The ASCCP 2006 Consensus Guidelines are presented in Figs. 8.13 and 8.14. Although the Guidelines have been developed for the U.S. setting, most of the recommendations are relevant internationally.

Summary of Key Aspects of the ASCCP 2006 Consensus Guidelines

Management of Women with CIN 1 Preceded by ASC-US, ASC-H, or LSIL Cytology

Women with a histological diagnosis of CIN I (usually implying previous referral for colposcopy and colposcopically directed biopsy), **preceded by ASC-US, ASC-H, or LSIL cytology should be followed by yearly HPV-DNA testing or 6- to 12-month Pap smears** (Fig. 8.14A). If HPV DNA testing remains positive or if repeat cytology is reported as ASC-US or greater, repeat colposcopy is recommended. **If the HPV DNA test is negative or two consecutive Pap smears are reported as negative, return to routine screening is recommended.** If CIN 1 persists for 2 years or more, continued follow-up or treatment is appropriate. Treatment can be ablative or excisional. If colposcopy is unsatisfactory, the endocervical sample is positive for CIN or the patient has been previously treated, a diagnostic excisional procedure is recommended.

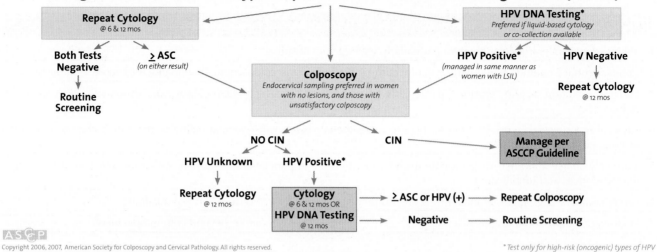

A Management of Women with Atypical Squamous Cells of Undetermined Significance (ASC-US)

*Test only for high-risk (oncogenic) types of HPV

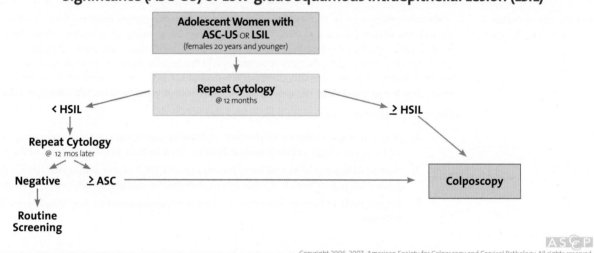

B Management of Adolescent Women with Either Atypical Squamous Cells of Undetermined Significance (ASC-US) or Low-grade Squamous Intraepithelial Lesion (LSIL)

C Management of Women with Atypical Squamous Cells: Cannot Exclude High-grade SIL (ASC - H)

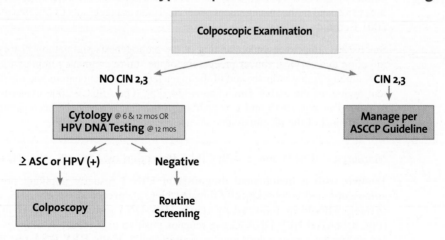

Figure 8.13 A–J   Algorithms from the 2006 Consensus Guidelines for the Management of Women with Cervical Cytological **Abnormalities.** (Reprinted from *The Journal of Lower Genital Tract Disease* Vol. 11, Issue 4, with the permission of ASCCP © American Society for Colposcopy and Cervical Pathology 2007. No copies of the algorithms may be made without the prior consent of ASCCP.)

D

Management of Women with Low-grade Squamous Intraepithelial Lesion (LSIL) *

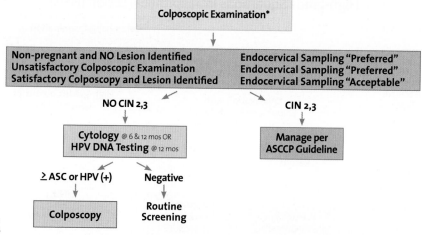

Colposcopic Examination*

Non-pregnant and NO Lesion Identified	Endocervical Sampling "Preferred"
Unsatisfactory Colposcopic Examination	Endocervical Sampling "Preferred"
Satisfactory Colposcopy and Lesion Identified	Endocervical Sampling "Acceptable"

NO CIN 2,3   CIN 2,3

Cytology @ 6 & 12 mos OR
HPV DNA Testing @ 12 mos   Manage per ASCCP Guideline

≥ ASC or HPV (+)   Negative

Colposcopy   Routine Screening

Management options may vary if the woman is pregnant, postmenopausal, or an adolescent - (see text)

E

Management of Pregnant Women with Low-grade Squamous Intraepithelial Lesion (LSIL)

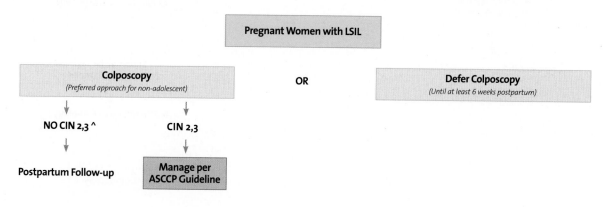

Pregnant Women with LSIL

Colposcopy
(Preferred approach for non-adolescent)   OR   Defer Colposcopy
(Until at least 6 weeks postpartum)

NO CIN 2,3 ^   CIN 2,3

Postpartum Follow-up   Manage per ASCCP Guideline

^ In women with no cytological, histological, or suspected CIN 2,3 or cancer

F

Management of Women with High-grade Squamous Intraepithelial Lesion (HSIL) *

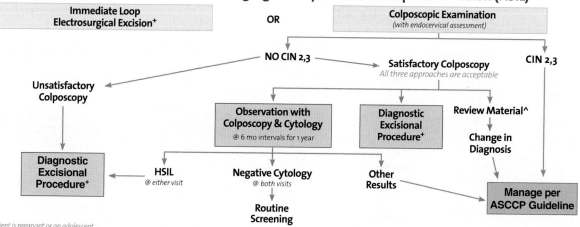

Immediate Loop Electrosurgical Excision+   OR   Colposcopic Examination
(with endocervical assessment)

NO CIN 2,3   Satisfactory Colposcopy   CIN 2,3
All three approaches are acceptable

Unsatisfactory Colposcopy

Observation with Colposcopy & Cytology @ 6 mo intervals for 1 year   Diagnostic Excisional Procedure+   Review Material^

Change in Diagnosis

Diagnostic Excisional Procedure+   HSIL @ either visit   Negative Cytology @ both visits   Other Results   Manage per ASCCP Guideline

Routine Screening

+ Not if patient is pregnant or an adolescent
^ Includes referral cytology, colposcopic findings, and all biopsies
* Management options may vary if the woman is pregnant, postmenopausal, or an adolescent

Figure 8.13 A–J   Continued

G

Management of Adolescent Women (20 Years and Younger) with High-grade Squamous Intraepithelial Lesion (HSIL)

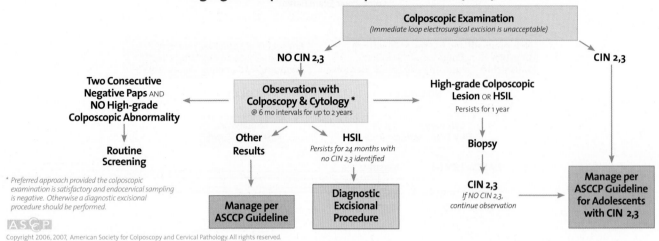

H

Initial Workup of Women with Atypical Glandular Cells (AGC)

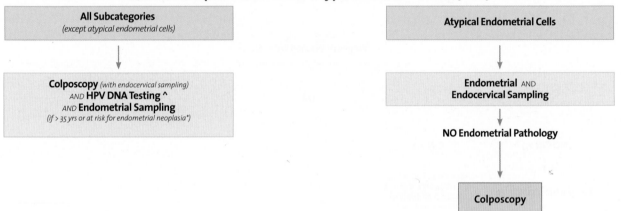

I

Subsequent Management of Women with Atypical Glandular Cells (AGC)

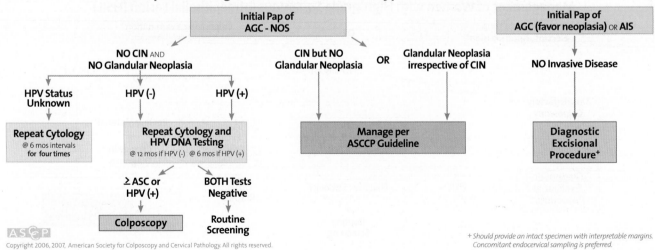

Figure 8.13 A–J   *Continued*

J

Use of HPV DNA Testing * as an Adjunct to Cytology for Cervical Cancer Screening in Women 30 Years and Older

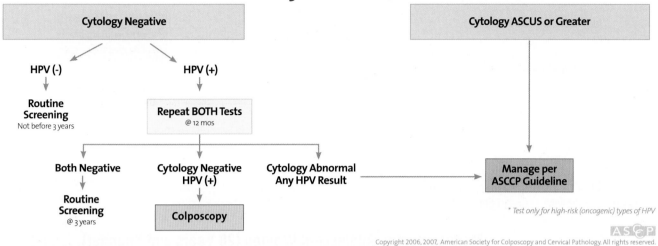

Figure 8.13 A–J   Continued

Two consecutive negative Pap smear reports in prospective follow-up of low-grade lesions, whilst statistically reassuring, does not necessarily represent disease regression and is no guarantee against disease progression.

Management of Women with CIN 1 Preceded by HSIL or AGC-NOS Cytology

Women with a histological diagnosis of CIN 1 which has been diagnosed in the assessment of abnormal Pap smears reported as HSIL (CIN 2-3) or atypical glandular cells not otherwise specified (AGC-NOS) can be managed by either **an excisional diagnostic procedure or 6-monthly colposcopy and cytology for 1 year** (Fig. 8.14B). This is provided women with a cytological finding of AGC-NOS have a satisfactory colposcopic examination and negative endocervical sampling. A full review of the cytological, colposcopic, and histological results can also be undertaken with management according to the guidelines for any revised diagnosis.

A

Management of Women with a Histological Diagnosis of Cervical Intraepithelial Neoplasia Grade 1 (CIN 1) Preceded by ASC-US, ASC-H, or LSIL Cytology

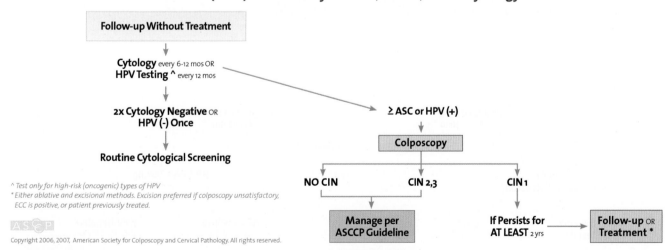

Figure 8.14 A–F   Algorithms from the 2006 Consensus Guidelines for the Management of Women with Cervical Histological Abnormalities. (Reprinted from *The Journal of Lower Genital Tract Disease* Vol. 11, Issue 4, with the permission of ASCCP © American Society for Colposcopy and Cervical Pathology 2007. No copies of the algorithms may be made without the prior consent of ASCCP.)

B Management of Women with a Histological Diagnosis of Cervical Intraepithelial Neoplasia - Grade 1 (CIN 1) Preceded by HSIL or AGC-NOS Cytology

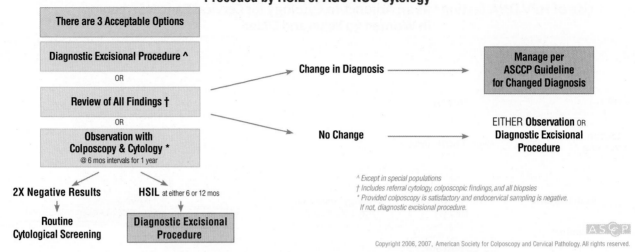

There are 3 Acceptable Options

Diagnostic Excisional Procedure ^

OR

Review of All Findings †

OR

Observation with Colposcopy & Cytology *
@ 6 mos intervals for 1 year

Change in Diagnosis → **Manage per ASCCP Guideline for Changed Diagnosis**

No Change → EITHER **Observation** OR **Diagnostic Excisional Procedure**

2X Negative Results → Routine Cytological Screening

HSIL at either 6 or 12 mos → **Diagnostic Excisional Procedure**

^ Except in special populations
† Includes referral cytology, colposcopic findings, and all biopsies
* Provided colposcopy is satisfactory and endocervical sampling is negative. If not, diagnostic excisional procedure.

C

Management of Adolescent Women (20 Years and Younger) with a Histological Diagnosis of Cervical Intraepithelial Neoplasia - Grade 1 (CIN 1)

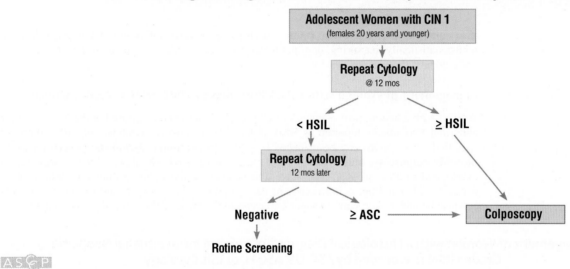

Adolescent Women with CIN 1
(females 20 years and younger)

Repeat Cytology
@ 12 mos

< HSIL / ≥ HSIL

Repeat Cytology
12 mos later

Negative / ≥ ASC → **Colposcopy**

Rotine Screening

D

Management of Women with a Histological Diagnosis of Cervical Intraepithelial Neoplasia - (CIN 2,3) *

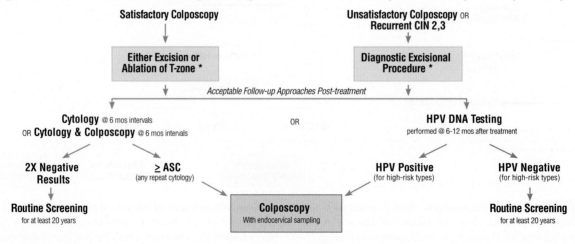

Satisfactory Colposcopy

Unsatisfactory Colposcopy OR Recurrent CIN 2,3

Either Excision or Ablation of T-zone *

Diagnostic Excisional Procedure *

Acceptable Follow-up Approaches Post-treatment

Cytology @ 6 mos intervals
OR **Cytology & Colposcopy** @ 6 mos intervals

OR

HPV DNA Testing
performed @ 6-12 mos after treatment

2X Negative Results

≥ ASC
(any repeat cytology)

HPV Positive
(for high-risk types)

HPV Negative
(for high-risk types)

Routine Screening
for at least 20 years

Colposcopy
With endocervical sampling

Routine Screening
for at least 20 years

* Management options will vary in special circumstances

Figure 8.14 A–F *Continued*

E

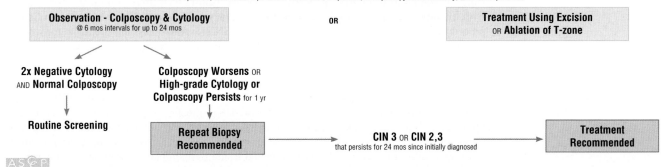

Management of Adolescent and Young Women
with a Histological Diagnosis of Cervical Intraepithelial Neoplasia - Grade 2,3 (CIN 2,3)

Adolescents and Young Women with CIN 2,3

Either treatment or observation is acceptable, provided colposcopy is satisfactory.
When CIN 2 is specified, observation is preferred. When CIN 3 is specified, or colposcopy is unsatisfactory, treatment is preferred.

Observation - Colposcopy & Cytology
@ 6 mos intervals for up to 24 mos

OR

Treatment Using Excision
OR **Ablation of T-zone**

2x Negative Cytology
AND **Normal Colposcopy**

Colposcopy Worsens OR
High-grade Cytology or
Colposcopy Persists for 1 yr

Routine Screening

Repeat Biopsy
Recommended

CIN 3 OR **CIN 2,3**
that persists for 24 mos since initially diagnosed

Treatment
Recommended

F

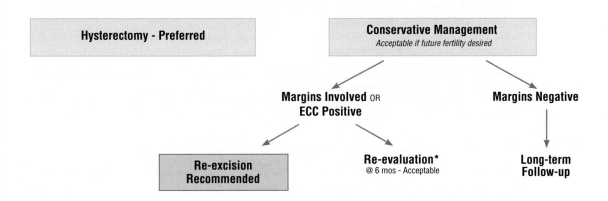

Management of Women with Adenocarcinoma *in-situ* (AIS)
Diagnosed from a Diagnostic Excisional Procedure

Hysterectomy - Preferred

Conservative Management
Acceptable if future fertility desired

Margins Involved OR
ECC Positive

Margins Negative

Re-excision
Recommended

Re-evaluation*
@ 6 mos - Acceptable

Long-term
Follow-up

* Using a combination of cytology, HPV testing, and colposcopy with endocervical sampling

Figure 8.14 A–F   *Continued*

If prospective observation is selected, a diagnostic excisional procedure is recommended if the repeat cytology at either 6 or 12 months is reported as HSIL or AGC-NOS. If histology of a colposcopically directed biopsy taken in prospective follow-up confirms high-grade CIN, management is according to guidelines irrespective of the cytology result. **After two consecutive "negative for intraepithelial neoplasia or malignancy" results in prospective follow-up, woman can return to routine cytological screening.** The same warning applies in relation to the implications of negative Pap smears in the follow-up of histologically proven CIN although, in this situation, colposcopy has been included in the follow-up regimen, affording a higher level of reassurance. If CIN 1 is preceded by HSIL or AGC-NOS cytology and colposcopy is unsatisfactory, a diagnostic excisional procedure is recommended except in special populations such as pregnant women.

CIN 1 in Adolescence and Pregnancy

For adolescents with CNI 1, **follow-up with annual cytology is recommended** (Fig. 8.14C). Only those with HSIL or greater at 12 months should be referred for colposcopy. At 24 months, those with ASC-US or greater should be referred. Prospective follow-up by **HPV DNA testing in this age group is of no value** due to the frequency of positive results.

305

Management of Women with CIN 2, 3

The heterogeneity of CIN 2 lesions is significant and regression rates are higher than for CIN 3. The histological distinction between CIN 2 and CIN 3 remains subjective and these diagnoses remain combined in the 2006 Consensus Guidelines to define the threshold for treatment for squamous intraepithelial lesions.

Both excisional and ablative procedures are acceptable treatment modalities for women with histologically proven CIN 2-3 with satisfactory colposcopy (Fig. 8.14D). An excisional procedure is recommended for residual/recurrent CIN 2-3. Ablation is unacceptable for women with a histological diagnosis of CIN 2-3 and unsatisfactory colposcopy. Cytologic and colposcopic follow-up of CIN 2-3 is unacceptable except in specific circumstances.

Acceptable posttreatment follow-up options include 6-monthly cytology alone, 6 monthly combined cytology and coloposcopy, and HPV DNA testing at 6 to 12 months. If HPV DNA testing is positive or if the repeat cytology is ASC-US or greater, very common situations particularly at a 6-month posttreatment examination, referral for colposcopy and endocervical sampling is recommended. If HPV DNA testing is negative or if two consecutive posttreatment cytology results are "negative for intraepithelial lesion or malignancy," routine screening for at least 20 years is recommended and should be annual for at least 5 years. The power of a negative HPV DNA test as a predictor of normality posttreatment for CIN 2-3 should be emphasized.

If CIN 2-3 is reported histologically at the margins of an excised specimen or in an endocervical sample obtained immediately after the procedure, 4 to 6 monthly cytologic follow-up with endocervical sampling is preferred. The role of colposcopy in this follow-up option is not clearly defined in the Guidelines. In practice, cytology and colposcopy will be performed in most clinical settings. **A repeat diagnostic excisional procedure is acceptable.** The Guidelines allow for hysterectomy if a repeat diagnostic, excisional procedure is not feasible although great care should be taken to exclude an undisclosed invasive cancer within the endocervical canal prior to hysterectomy.

For women with histologically proven residual/recurrent CIN 2-3, the Guidelines permit a repeat excisional procedure or hysterectomy. If a repeat excisional procedure is not feasible, our practice is to perform a modified radical hysterectomy.The specimen is evaluated intraoperatively, if necessary by frozen section, to determine any need for lymphadenectomy.

CIN 2, 3 in Adolescence and Pregnancy

For adolescents with a histological diagnosis of CIN 2-3 not otherwise specified, the Guidelines state that either treatment or 6-monthly observation by cytology and colposcopy for up to 24 months is acceptable provided colposcopy is satisfactory (Fig. 8.14E). Allowing for the subjectivity in this histological distinction, observation is preferred for a diagnosis of CIN 2 alone but treatment is acceptable. Treatment is recommended for a specified histological diagnosis of CIN 3 or if colposcopy is unsatisfactory. Although invasive cervical cancer is very rare in this age group, prospective follow-up of a histological diagnosis of CIN 2-3, not otherwise specified, in young women should be limited to those women likely to be compliant with the recommendations. After two consecutive "negative for intraepithelial lesion or malignancy" results, implying negative cytology and colposcopy with satisfactory colposcopic examinations, these adolescents and young women can return to routine cytologic screening. An annual screening interval should be recommended. **Treatment is recommended if CIN 3 is diagnosed histologically or if CIN 2-3 persists for 24 months.**

Management of Women with Cervical Adenocarcinoma *In Situ* (AIS)

Hysterectomy remains the preferred management recommendation for women with a histological diagnosis of AIS on a specimen from a diagnostic excisional procedure (Fig. 8.14F). A histological diagnosis of AIS from a punch biopsy or a cytologicaldiagnosis of AIS is not sufficient to justify hysterectomy without a diagnostic excisional procedure. The difficulty in defining colposcopic limits of AIS lesions, the frequent extension of disease to within the endocervical canal and the presence of multifocal, "skip lesions" (i.e., lesions which are not contiguous) compromise conservative excisional procedures.

Negative margins in an excisional specimen do not mean the lesion is completely excised. If future fertility is desired, conservative excisional management is acceptable. The overall failure

Table 8.4 Triage Rules for Ablative Therapy for Cervical Intraepithelial Neoplasia

1. Visualization of the entire new squamocolumnar junction, that is, 360 degrees of normal columnar epithelium seen with no significant disease extension within the endocervical canal

2. No colposcopic warning signs of invasive cancer

3. No cytologic or histologic evidence of invasive cancer

4. Concordance to within 1 degree of severity between the cytology and the histology of colposcopically directed biopsies

5. No evidence of high-grade disease on endocervical curettage

6. No cytologic or histologic suspicion of high-grade glandular neoplasia

rate of excision is less than 10%. Margin status is a useful clinical predictor of residual disease as is endocervical sampling at the time of excision. If a conservative excisional procedure is performed and margins are involved or the endocervical sample at the time of excision shows AIS or CIN, reexcision is recommended. A reassessment at six months using a combination of cytology, colposcopy, HPV DNA testing, and endocervical sampling is acceptable. Long-term follow-up is recommended for women who do not undergo hysterectomy for AIS.

Treatment of Cervical Intraepithelial Neoplasia

Historically, Anderson (376) from the United Kingdom in 1965 and Kolstad and Klem (377) from the Norwegian Radium Institute in 1969, demonstrated that **cone biopsy was as effective as hysterectomy in preventing the progression of carcinoma in situ to invasive cervical cancer.** In 1973, Stafl and Mattingly (378) from Wisconsin demonstrated that **colposcopically directed punch biopsies, taken by an experienced colposcopist, were as accurate as cone biopsy in obtaining a histologic diagnosis in women with an abnormal cervical smear.** This facilitated the use of physical modalities to destroy the abnormal transformation zone in selected patients.

Subsequently, high primary cure rates with minimal morbidity were reported for ablative techniques such as cryosurgery (379), electrocoagulation diathermy (380), and the carbon dioxide laser (381). Patient selection is based on a set of triage rules (Table 8.4). **Diagnostic conization is now performed only for specific indications** in which there remains a genuine risk of undisclosed invasive cancer.

In the 1990s, loop electrosurgical excision procedures (LEEP) gained in popularity because of concerns regarding the occurrence of invasive cervical cancer in patients who had undergone ablative treatment (382). Invasive cancer has been reported after each of the ablative modalities (383). **When cancer occurred after ablative therapy, it occurred within 12 months in 66% of cases and within 2 years in 90%.** This suggested that a triage error was made in the initial assessment and invasive cancer was missed. Reports of a low incidence of misclassification of invasive cervical cancer or high-grade glandular neoplasia as squamous intraepithelial disease have raised concerns about the safety of ablation of high-grade squamous lesions (384–386).

LEEP allows for excision of the transformation zone with removal of a volume of tissue similar to that removed by ablative procedures, and with no greater morbidity. **When the procedure is performed by an inexperienced operator, adequate histologic evaluation can be difficult** because of diathermy artifact and orientation difficulties.

Pregnancy-Related Morbidity Associated with Treatment for CIN

All **excisional procedures** used in the treatment of cervical intraepithelial neoplasia **are associated with adverse obstetric morbidity. Recent research and metaanalyses have confirmed that excisional procedures for CIN are associated with an increased risk of preterm delivery and low birth weight babies in future pregnancies** (387–394).

The greatest increased risk is associated with cold-knife conization where there are significantly increased risks of perinatal mortality, extreme preterm delivery and very low birth weight infants (388,392). A recent Norwegian population based cohort study reported a 17.2%

incidence of preterm delivery among women who gave birth after cervical conisation versus 6.7% among women who gave birth before cervical conisation and 6.2% in women who had never undergone cervical conisation (392). The excess risk was highest for late abortion and for preterm delivery prior to 33 weeks.

Large loop excision is also associated with an increased risk of preterm delivery and low birth weight babies, but is not associated with increased perinatal mortality, or with extreme preterm delivery (reviewed 388,393). It is probable that loop excision procedures that remove large amounts of cervical tissue would have the same negative impact as cold-knife conization. Clinicians should inform women of the risks of adverse pregnancy related outcomes associated with excisional treatment procedures.

Ablative procedures are associated with fewer adverse pregnancy outcomes than excisional procedures (388), although radical diathermy treatment is associated with significant pregnancy related morbidity. **Treatment should be avoided where possible for young women and adolescents, particularly with low-grade lesions, which have a high rate of spontaneous regression. The "see-and-treat" approach, combining diagnosis and treatment in one visit, is now not generally recommended due to the potential for unnecessary treatment** (394).

Treatment Modalities

The treatment modalities for preinvasive cervical disease are ablative procedures and include cryosurgery, electrocoagulation diathermy, and CO_2 laser; and excisional procedures, including LEEP, cervical (excisional) conization, CO_2 laser excision, and hysterectomy. A Cochrane Database of Systematic Review (2003) examined surgical treatment modalities for cervical intraepithelial neoplasia (395). The evidence from 28 randomized controlled trials suggested that **there is no overwhelmingly superior technique for eradicating CIN. Cryotherapy is an effective treatment of LSIL but not HSIL.**

Cryosurgery

Cryosurgery is a simple, effective, inexpensive, and relatively easy therapeutic option for treatment of selected patients with CIN. Cervical cryosurgery, which was **first introduced in 1968,** involves the destruction by cryonecrosis of the lesion, including the entire transformation zone. Hypothermia is produced by the evaporation of liquid refrigerants. Compressed nitrous oxide (N_2O) is allowed to expand through a small jet, producing an iceball at the surface of a metal probe placed in contact with the surface of the tissues to be frozen. **Crystallization of intracellular water results in cell death.**

The most appropriate cryoprobe tips are the 19-mm and 25-mm minicone. A water-soluble gel is used to coat the probe tip before the procedure. Temperatures achieved at the cryotip using N_2O are recorded at $-65°C$ to $-85°C$. Cell death occurs in the range of $-20°C$ to $-30°C$. **The lethal zone during cryosurgery begins 2 mm proximal to the iceball margin,** with the temperature at the margin of the iceball equal to $0°C$. **To ensure a 5-mm depth of freezing, a total lateral spread of freeze of 7 mm is required.** For cervical cryosurgery, **the probe must cover the lesion and the entire transformation zone.**

If the transformation zone is large, successive overlapping treatments are required, increasing the duration and discomfort of the procedure. **Cryosurgery is therefore used mainly for smaller, ectocervical lesions.** It is usually used for low-grade lesions (LGLs) without extension to within the endocervical canal.

Technique   The procedure is performed under colposcopic supervision without anesthesia. Prophylactic premedication with nonsteroidal antiinflammatory drugs 30 to 60 minutes before the procedure may reduce pain and cramping associated with prostaglandin release from dying cells. The procedure should not be performed in pregnancy or during the menstrual period. The procedure is performed as follows:

1. **The cervix is exposed using a speculum, and a careful colposcopy is performed to check the topography of the lesion and to ensure that the triage rules are fulfilled.**

2. **A warm cryotip is chosen that best conforms to the topography of the cervix, and a water-soluble gel is applied thinly to the tip.**

3. **The cryotip is positioned at room temperature on the cervix, with care taken to cover the entire lesion and the transformation zone.** The probe must be clear of the vaginal walls. The procedure is initiated by activating a trigger on the cryogun. If the probe comes into contact with the vagina, the treatment is ceased and then reinitiated.

Table 8.5 Comparison of Therapeutic Modalities for Cervical Intraepithelial Neoplasia				
Procedure Rates	*Technical Ease*	*Equipment Cost*	*Complication Rates*	*Primary Cure*
Cryosurgery	+++	+++	++	80%
Loop electrosurgical excision procedures	+++	++	+++	95%
Laser ablation	++	+	+++	95%
Laser excision	+	+	++	95%
Cold-knife conization	++	+++	++	98%

+, low benefit; ++, medium benefit; +++, high benefit.

4. **Crystallization begins on the back of the probe and proceeds until the ice ball is seen to extend 7 mm laterally beyond the edge of the probe.** This visual landmark is the indicator of the depth of the freeze (approximately 5 mm) and is the method for determining the duration of the procedure.

5. **The probe is defrosted completely and then disengaged from the cervix.**

A freeze–thaw–freeze technique is commonly used. This technique was reported by Creasman et al. (396) to reduce the failure rate from 29% to 7%, although others claimed similar results from a single freeze (397,398). The second freeze is not commenced until the tissues have visibly thawed from the initial treatment.

Patients experience a watery, malodorous, blood-tinged discharge for 2 to 3 weeks after the procedure. This can be decreased by debridement of the bullous, necrotic tissue using a ring forceps and gauze 48 hours after the procedure. The patient should abstain from vaginal intercourse and tampon use for 4 weeks after the procedure.

Primary cure rates in excess of 90% have been reported for cryosurgical management of CIN lesions. The larger the lesion, the lower the primary cure rate. Cryosurgery for large ectocervical lesions covering the ectocervix is associated with failure rates as high as 42%. Endocervical glandular involvement increases the failure rate from 9% to 27%. Decreasing cure rates with increasing severity of disease, specifically 94% for CIN 1, 93% for CIN 2, and 84% for CIN 3, have also been reported (399). This may in part reflect the increased size of HGLs, which more frequently occupy two or more quadrants of the cervix (400) (Table 8.5).

Loop Electrosurgical Excision Procedure

To minimize the risk of failed detection of early invasive cancer and high-grade glandular neoplasia at the time of colposcopic triage, LEEP of the transformation zone has become a widely used and valuable therapeutic option. The equipment is relatively inexpensive, and the surgical skills are readily acquired. **The procedure combines the advantages of conservative ablative procedures in preserving cervical tissue with the safety of histologic assessment of the entire lesion.**

Cartier originally developed an electrosurgical method for management of CIN using 5-mm rectangular, thin wire loops to sample and treat the cervix by removing the epithelium and underlying stroma in multiple 5-mm strips (401). The process was time consuming, and thermal injury at the edge of the strips frequently compromised the specimen.

Prendiville et al. (402,403) introduced larger loop electrodes, 1 to 2 cm in width and 0.7 to 1.5 cm in depth, for excision of the entire transformation zone, usually in a single pass. The combination of very thin wire loops and modern electrosurgical generators capable of delivering high powers (35 to 55 W) has allowed electrosurgical cutting with little associated thermal injury.

The technique for electrosurgical loop excision is as follows:

1. **The cervix is visualized using a nonconductive nylon or plastic-coated speculum with suction attached.** For parous patients, a nonconductive vaginal lateral wall retractor is advisable to improve access to the cervix and to minimize the risk of inadvertent injury to the vaginal sidewall.

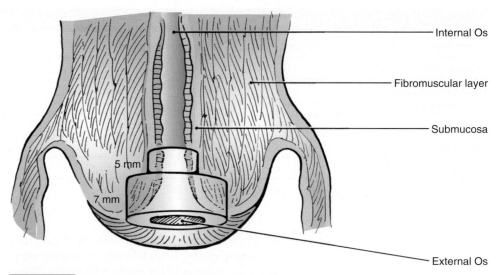

Internal Os

Fibromuscular layer

Submucosa

External Os

5 mm

7 mm

Figure 8.15   **"Cowboy-hat" configuration for LEEP.**

2. **The cervix is evaluated colposcopically to determine the distribution of the lesion and the transformation zone.** The appropriate loop size is chosen. Lugol's iodine solution helps demarcate the outer margin of excision. The procedure is performed under colposcopic control.

3. **The cervix is infiltrated with 4 to 6 mL of local anesthetic (1% to 2% *lidocaine* with *epinephrine*) using a dental syringe with a 27-gauge needle.** The local anesthetic is injected as a slow subepithelial infiltrate at the 3, 6, 9, and 12 o'clock positions after a test dose of 1 mL is observed for side effects.

4. **A grounding pad is attached to the patient's thigh, with care taken to ensure proper adherence.**

5. **The electrosurgical generator is set at an appropriate power setting for the size of loop chosen for the procedure, usually 35 to 55 W of either pure cutting or blended current.**

6. **Suction is attached to the speculum.**

7. **The specimen is excised by activating the generator with a foot pedal or hand switch with the loop 2 mm from the tissue.** The loop is advanced perpendicularly into the cervix 2 to 3 mm lateral to the lesion and transformation zone to a depth of 5 to 7 mm and drawn across the cervix until 2 mm lateral to the opposite side of the transformation zone. The excised specimen is usually dome shaped, 5 to 6 mm deep at the lateral margins, and 7 to 10 mm deep in the center. **Larger lesions may require more than a single pass with the electrode.** The central portion of the lesion should be excised first and remaining lesional tissue excised with additional passes (Fig. 8.15). More peripheral CIN tissue can be destroyed with the ball electrode provided a directed biopsy is taken and the triage rules for ablation are fulfilled.

8. **The base of the crater is lightly fulgurated using the 5-mm ball electrode with the electrosurgical generator at 40 to 60 W of coagulation current.** This is intended to stop bleeding but not to char the tissue in the crater, which devitalizes a significant volume of tissue and increases the risk of postoperative bleeding and infection.

9. **An endocervical curettage, sampling, or "cowboy hat" biopsy should be performed if one has not been previously performed.**

10. **Monsel's solution is applied to the cervix to maintain hemostasis.**

Complications are minimal, comparing favorably with those associated with CO_2 laser procedures (395). **Postoperative bleeding occurs in 2% to 5% of patients.** Postoperative infection is uncommon. **Clinically significant cervical stenosis and cervical incompetence are rare complications,** but the patient must be made aware of the possibility of such adverse reproductive sequelae. **Cure rates** are comparable with those achieved with CO_2 laser procedures and with "cold-knife" conization, **often in excess of 95%** (395).

Electrosurgical loop excision offers several advantages over CO_2 laser ablation. The procedure is quicker and easier. However, ease of use carries an attendant risk of overuse. Patient acceptance is improved and intraoperative pain is decreased. The submission of the entire specimen for histologic study increases the probability that unsuspected cancer will be detected and not ablated. In many large studies of LEEP, the unsuspected invasive cancer and high-grade glandular disease rate has been as high as 1% to 2% (404–407).

Another potential advantage of LEEP is the ability to "see-and-treat" at one visit. However, histologic study of loop-excised specimens removed at a "see-and-treat" approach revealed no disease in 5% to 40% of specimens, particularly in young women referred with minor cytologic abnormalities (408).

Carbon Dioxide Laser Ablation of the Transformation Zone

The CO_2 laser is the ideal choice for vaporizing sharply defined tissue volumes to a precisely determined depth (409–411). To achieve optimal vaporization with minimal lateral thermal injury, the CO_2 laser should be used at the highest power output with which the surgeon is comfortable. This should be a minimum of 25 W but preferably above 60 W. The cautious use of low-power outputs is one of the most common CO_2 laser surgery errors causing thermal injury.

Most gynecologists treating cervical preinvasive lesions with the CO_2 laser have access to a laser providing 50 W maximum power or less. As such, the laser is best used in *continuous mode* for the ablation of cervical lesions. However, in addition to using the highest controllable power output, thermal conduction can be further minimized by the choice of *rapid superpulse* as the temporal mode. The main advantage of higher-powered lasers is the higher average power achieved in rapid superpulse settings. This offers a distinct advantage in situations where control of thermal injury is critical, such as the *DES*-exposed, breastfeeding, postmenopausal, or postirradiated patient. For transformation zone ablative procedures, the average power density must be kept within the range of 750 to 2,000 W/cm^2 (412).

Surgical Control of the CO_2 Laser

The CO_2 laser can be readily controlled by the surgeon at any power setting provided the appropriate Y-beam geometry is selected (see later in this chapter). For cervical transformation zone ablation, a high-power laser setting is selected. The spot diameter is progressively enlarged by defocusing the beam using the micromanipulator until a point is found where the impact crater (tested on a moistened wooden tongue blade) is hemispherical. This permits controlled tissue vaporization with minimal lateral heat conduction. The higher the average power setting on the laser, the larger the spot size or impact crater in a Y-beam geometry. For transformation zone ablation, this affords the advantage of minimizing thermal conduction and associated tissue damage. The laser energy is delivered in short bursts either by use of the mechanical timer in the laser console or, preferably, by gating the laser pulses using the foot pedal. This permits precise, controlled tissue vaporization.

CO_2 laser ablation of the transformation zone should always be performed using a micromanipulator attached to a colposcope or operating microscope. Careful colposcopy is required at the time of transformation zone ablation to determine the lateral extent of disease. **The entire transformation zone must be treated, as selective ablation of areas of disease results in much lower primary cure rates.**

A major advantage of CO_2 laser ablation is the ability to destroy tissue to a precisely controlled depth. The maximum depth of gland involvement with CIN is 5.2 mm, whereas the maximum depth of uninvolved glands is 7.9 mm. Frequency and depth of gland crypt involvement increase with the grade of CIN. **The transformation zone is usually destroyed to a depth of 7 to 10 mm.**

Control of Intraoperative Pain and Bleeding

CO_2 laser ablation of the transformation zone is usually performed under local anesthesia. The cervix is infiltrated with 4 to 6 mL of local anesthetic such as 1% *lidocaine,* with or without a vasospastic agent. The infiltration is best performed as a slow, subepithelial infiltrate using a dental syringe with a 27-gauge dental needle. A deeper, paracervical block does not always provide adequate anesthesia and its administration is associated with more discomfort and bleeding.

Laser ablation is usually associated with minimal bleeding. Should a small vessel such as an arteriole be encountered, hemostasis is readily achieved by using direct pressure from a moistened cotton-tipped applicator and lasing immediately onto the applicator tip at the site of the vessel. Monsel's solution is applied to the cervix on completion of the procedure to minimize the risk of postoperative bleeding. CO_2 laser ablation of the transformation zone is an excellent treatment for selected patients with CIN, achieving **primary cure rates of up to 95%, with minimal morbidity** (395).

Sequelae of Conservative Treatment Procedures

Patients can expect **a vaginal discharge for up to 3 weeks** after the procedure. **Infection is rare,** but persistence of an offensive discharge or development of postoperative pelvic pain warrants assessment. **Minor spotting** may occur in the first two postoperative weeks but usually settles promptly. If bleeding is heavier and does not settle quickly, the patient should be examined and hemostasis secured using Monsel's solution. Rarely, sutures may be required to secure hemostasis with **secondary bleeding.** The patient should refrain from tampon use, douching, and vaginal intercourse for 3 to 4 weeks after surgery.

Repeat Pap smears and colposcopy should be performed at 6 and 12 months posttreatment. If these assessments are normal, the patient may return to annual screening, particularly if a high-risk HPV DNA test is negative. **A significant proportion of patients continue to show minor abnormalities on cervical smears in the first 12 months after treatment,** reflecting reparative changes or continued expression of minimally developed HPV-induced changes. These patients rarely require further treatment.

Excisional Cervical Conization

Excisional conization performed with a scalpel, sometimes referred to as a "cold-knife conization," was traditionally the standard response to cytologic abnormalities (413) and remains an important therapeutic option in the management of CIN. It is both diagnostic and therapeutic. The geometry of the conization should adapt to the size and shape of the lesion as well as the geometry of the cervix (Fig. 8.16). The procedure is performed in the following manner:

1. **Careful colposcopic examination is performed** to delineate the lateral margins of the lesion and transformation zone. Lugol's iodine solution aids in this determination.
2. **Lateral sutures are placed** on the side of the cervix at the 3 and 9 o'clock positions to provide traction and hemostasis.
3. **The cervix may be infiltrated with a vasospastic agent** to decrease intraoperative bleeding.
4. **The endocervical canal is sounded** to guide the direction and depth of the excision.
5. **The specimen is excised using a no. 11 scalpel blade,** preferably with a cylinder-shaped geometry.
6. **The excised specimen is tagged at the 12 o'clock position** using suture to allow for proper orientation by the pathologist.
7. **A fractional curettage (or biopsy) of the endocervical canal and endometrium is performed** to exclude residual squamous or glandular disease of the upper endocervical canal or disease of the endometrium.
8. **On completion of the procedure, the base of the surgical site can be cauterized** to secure or maintain hemostasis, or hemostatic sutures can be placed. The traditional Sturmdorf sutures are not advisable because of the risk of burying residual disease. Simple U-sutures placed anteriorly and posteriorly may be used if bleeding persists.

Cervical conization achieves cure rates for high-grade CIN in excess of 95%. **The risk of cervical stenosis and cervical incompetence is higher** for cervical conization performed with a scalpel than for CO_2 laser and electrosurgical excisional conization. This in part reflects the fact that cervical conization performed with a scalpel has been traditionally used for the most severe lesions, when invasive cancer has not been excluded or when colposcopy has been unsatisfactory, often with significant disease extension to within the endocervical canal (414).

Hysterectomy

Hysterectomy is rarely indicated in the primary management of CIN. The most common indication is **coexistence of a gynecologic condition that warrants hysterectomy.** Such conditions include dysfunctional uterine bleeding, fibroids, uterovaginal prolapse, or patient request for sterilization.

Before any hysterectomy, colposcopic assessment is important. If the entire lesion and transformation zone is not seen, if there is any cytologic, colposcopic, or histologic suspicion of

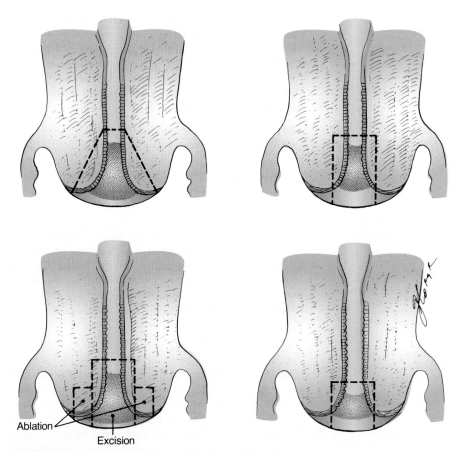

Ablation

Excision

Figure 8.16 Tissue excised for cervical conization procedures depending on the extent of disease and the anatomy and shape of the cervix.

invasive cancer, if an endocervical specimen is positive for high-grade neoplasia, or if there is any evidence of high-grade glandular neoplasia, **an excisional conization must be performed to exclude invasive cancer before hysterectomy is performed.**

In 2% to 3% of patients with high-grade CIN, the disease extends to the vaginal vault (415). If the vaginal cuff is not carefully fashioned in these patients, preferably using a vaginal approach, neoplastic epithelium may be sutured into the vaginal vault. High-grade vaginal intraepithelial neoplasia (VAIN) occurs in the vaginal vault in 1% to 7% of patients who have undergone hysterectomy to treat CIN. Coppleson and Reid (416) reported 38 cases of invasive cancer occurring in the vaginal vault after hysterectomy among 8,998 women (0.4%).

If hysterectomy is performed for the management of CIN, the patient should have vault cytologic testing and colposcopy performed on two occasions in the 18 months after surgery. **She should be screened by vaginal vault smears on an annual basis thereafter.**

Cervical Adenocarcinoma *In Situ*

The reported incidence of cervical glandular neoplasia has increased, predominantly among nulliparous and primiparous women in the reproductive age groups with up to 30% of cases occurring in women younger than 35 years of age (417–421).

These changes in the clinical profile of cervical cancer have focused much attention toward AIS. **There is convincing evidence that AIS is a precursor lesion** (422–426). The mean age of diagnosis of AIS is 15 years younger than that for invasive adenocarcinoma (427,428). AIS frequently coexists with invasive adenocarcinoma in histologic specimens. **Patients who have a cone biopsy performed in response to cytologic evidence of AIS already have invasive cancer in up to one-third of cases.** Women diagnosed with cervical adenocarcinoma frequently have had previous cytologic evidence of endocervical atypia on smears for intervals of 2 to 10 years.

Specific HPV types, in particular HPV 18, are strongly implicated in the etiology of high-grade glandular neoplasia (131). Persistent high-risk HPV infection, particularly with HPV 18, is the greatest risk factor for developing AIS. Prolonged oral contraceptive usage, beyond 5 years, may be a cofactor in the development of glandular neoplasia, particularly in young women (131,429). **Widespread vaccination against HPV 16 and 18 which are associated with 90% of glandular neoplasms, should significantly decrease the incidence of both AIS and adenocarcinoma** (15,212,213).

The relationship between AIS and lesser degrees of cervical glandular neoplasia is more controversial. No prospective study of glandular dysplasia has been undertaken, and the neoplastic potential of these lesions remains uncertain. Glandular dysplasia, less than adenocarcinoma *in situ,* represents a heterogeneous group of lesions with variable progressive potential. Glandular dysplasia is much less predictably associated with high-risk HPV types when compared to AIS, further confusing understanding of the significance of such lesions.

Clinical Presentation

Adenocarcinoma *in situ* is usually diagnosed after an abnormal Pap test result. The abnormal smear may predict the presence of high-grade glandular disease. Only 38% to 69% of AIS cases are detected by cytology prior to conization. The diagnosis increases to 85% following colposcopy, biopsy, and endocervical sampling. **Because AIS coexists with high-grade squamous CIN in 50% of cases, the abnormal smear will frequently predict only the squamous lesion** (430). The diagnosis of AIS is often a coincidental finding in the histologic assessment of an excised specimen taken in the management of high-grade CIN, which is a compelling argument for the routine excision of high-grade CIN.

The 2001 Bethesda system includes a category for atypical glandular cells (AGC). **Patients with AGC smear reports have a 30% to 50% risk of having high-grade cervical disease** and are at much higher risk of significant disease than those with ASC smear reports (431–435). An AGC smear report is an indication for referral for colposcopy and careful endocervical assessment. The underlying lesion is most frequently high-grade squamous CIN, which occurs in up to 25% of patients. AIS, cervical adenocarcinoma, and endometrial disease, including hyperplasia and carcinoma, occur in up to 20% of patients (431–435).

The colposcopic features of AIS and early adenocarcinoma are widely seen as nonspecific. A minority view is that most high-grade glandular lesions do have specific colposcopic features. Discrete or extensive stark acetowhitening of individual or fused columnar villi may be seen surrounded by normal villiform structures (Fig. 8.17). Prominent atypical vessels may also be seen, particularly in association with early invasion. Although colposcopy should be performed in response to cytologic or clinical suspicion of glandular neoplasia, **excisional conization is mandatory for definitive diagnosis.**

Management

The potential for AIS to involve the entire endocervical canal and the frequent association with invasive carcinoma demands formal excisional conization in the management of AIS (436). AIS is often unifocal and is located at the transformation zone (437). The cone biopsy should be fashioned as a cylinder of at least 2.5 cm in depth and be performed with a cold knife to avoid thermal injury to the specimen. Care must be taken in particular with excision of the apex of the cone to avoid traumatic or thermal distortion. If the conization margins are clear of disease, more than 80% of patients have negative cytologic and colposcopic follow-up beyond 12 months from treatment (438–441). However, **even when excision margins are clear, 6% to 25% of women who proceed to hysterectomy are reported to have persistent disease** in the specimen (442). For this reason, **hysterectomy is still considered the gold standard for women with AIS who do not desire fertility preservation** (443,444).

Younger women may be managed by excisional conization alone if margins of excision are clear. Careful cytologic and colposcopic **follow-up is important**, with recurrent AIS being detected in 7% to 10% and squamous and glandular preinvasive disease in as many as 33% of such patients (445,446). Invasive cancer has been reported as late as 7 years postconization (436,446–449).

If the margins of excision are positive, more than 50% of patients have residual disease at hysterectomy (443,446). **Patient with positive conization margins and/or a positive endocervical curettage require repeat excisional conization with further endocervical sampling to exclude invasive cancer.** If the repeat cone biopsy is negative for invasive cancer, hysterectomy is indicated in the older patient and should be seriously considered in the younger patient.

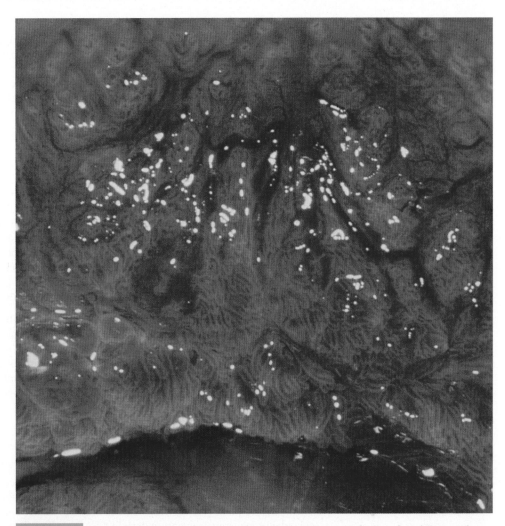

Figure 8.17   Colposcopic appearance of adenocarcinoma *in situ* lesion showing prominent atypical vessels.

In modern clinical practice, up to 50% of patients with AIS are diagnosed following the histologic assessment of a loop excision specimen. The appropriate management of such cases is controversial. The standard approach has been to proceed to cold-knife conization regardless of margin status. **Recent studies have reported follow-up of these women if the margins are clear** (440,450,451). A recent metaanalysis comparing cold-knife conization and loop excision showed no difference in the probability of obtaining negative margins, and no difference in the probability of residual disease or subsequent development of cervical adeno-carcinoma (452). Further prospective studies are required to determine the safety of conservative management of young women desiring to preserve fertility, who have had AIS diagnosed following a loop excision procedure. HPV DNA testing is a valuable test of cure following conservative treatment of cervical AIS (453).

Vagina

Classification of Vaginal Intraepithelial Neoplasia

Vaginal intraepithelial neoplasia is classified similarly to cervical lesions: VAIN 1 (mild dysplasia), VAIN 2 (moderate dysplasia), and VAIN 3 (severe dysplasia/carcinoma *in situ*). **VAIN 3 is a premalignant lesion,** but the natural history of the lesser degrees of VAIN has not been submitted to prospective study. VAIN 1 is an HPV-induced change without an established progressive potential but is associated with high-risk HPV types in 64% to 84% of cases (454). Management should be conservative, usually by observation. **Most of high-grade VAIN and vaginal cancer is caused by high-risk HPV types.**

Clinical Profile

Since the 1970s, the diagnosis of high-grade VAIN has been made with increasing frequency. The mean age at diagnosis has decreased to 35 years, but patients with high-grade VAIN are older on average than those diagnosed with high-grade CIN. **The increased rate of diagnosis of high-grade VAIN is due to increased clinical awareness, improved screening, and an absolute increase in incidence.** The rarity of primary vaginal squamous cancer, accounting for 1% to 2% of female genital tract cancers, suggests that the malignant potential of VAIN is low, but progression to invasive cancer does occur (455).

High-grade VAIN usually occurs in association with high-grade CIN, which extends onto the vaginal fornices in approximately 3% of cases, but primary foci of high-grade VAIN also occur (456,457). **VAIN 2-3 involves the upper third of the vagina in more than 70% of cases** and less commonly the lower third, with the middle third infrequently involved. Occasionally, multifocal disease can extend throughout the vagina, particularly in the presence of extensive multicentric intraepithelial neoplasia. This reflects the **"field effect"** of squamous carcinogenesis in the lower genital tract related to HPV 16 in particular (458). This is further supported by the more rapid development of VAIN among women with a prior history of **anogenital neoplasia.** A prior history of treatment for **cervical cancer and cigarette smoking** are major risk factors for development of high grade VAIN (455,459), as is **immunosuppression,** e.g., following organ transplantation or due to concurrent HIV infection (455).

High-grade VAIN lesions are asymptomatic and are usually diagnosed by colposcopy and biopsy following abnormal cytologic screening (460). Among women who have not had a hysterectomy, concomitant or antecedent high-grade CIN is detected in over two-thirds of patients with high-grade VAIN. Cervical cytologic testing is therefore usually positive in the presence of VAIN. **The vaginal vault, in particular, and the vaginal walls should be inspected at the time of colposcopy.** In addition, certain specific indications require careful vaginal colposcopy (Table 8.6).

Patients with VAIN have a 10% incidence of coexisting high-grade VIN. Careful vulvar colposcopy should be performed for all women with VAIN.

Diagnosis

High-grade VAIN is generally diagnosed by histology of colposcopically directed biopsies. Lesions are usually flat and inconspicuous before application of acetic acid, although occasionally raised pink, red, or white lesions may be seen. Clinically apparent hyperkeratosis or leukoplakia may represent an underlying VAIN lesion. Peeling or ulceration of the vaginal epithelium, particularly in the perimenopausal and postmenopausal patient, may be an indicator of underlying high-grade VAIN. **Occasionally, recalcitrant condylomatous lesions of the vagina reveal a high-grade dysplastic morphology.**

VAIN 2 to 3 has a colposcopic appearance similar to that of high-grade CIN (Figs. 8.18, 8.19) **after application of 5% acetic acid** (461). The reaction takes longer to develop than for CIN, and the rugosity of the vagina further impairs detection. **Vascular patterns are usually**

Table 8.6 Indications for Vaginal Colposcopy
1. Abnormal cytology after apparently successful treatment of CIN
2. Abnormal vaginal vault cytology posthysterectomy
3. Abnormal cytology al the presence of colposcopically normal cervix, particularly if colposcopy is satisfactory
4. Confirmed high-grade CIN in an immunosuppressed patient
5. Confirmed diagnosis of high-grade vulvar intraepithelial neoplasia
6. Abnormal gross vaginal examination
7. Confirmed or suspected intrauterine diethylstilbestrol exposure
8. Diagnosis and treatment of multicentric human papillomavirus infection, particularly if recalcitrant to conservative treatment

CIN, cervical intraepithelial neoplasia.

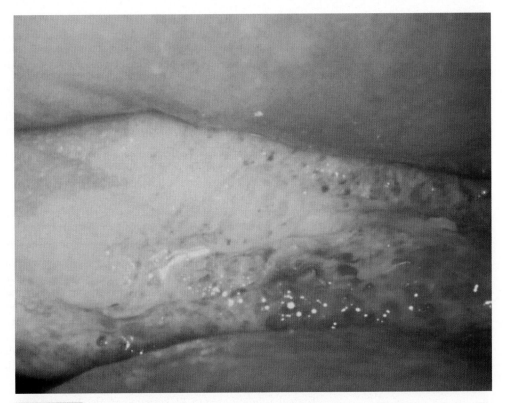

Figure 8.18   Colposcopic appearance of high-grade vaginal intraepithelial neoplasia with acetic acid.

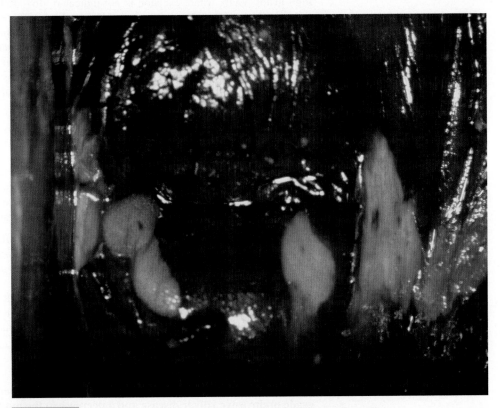

Figure 8.19   Colposcopic appearance after staining with Lugol's Iodine.

indistinct or absent. A fine capillary punctation is often seen with high-grade VAIN as the acetic acid reaction fades. Prominent abnormal vascular patterns develop late in the neoplastic process. **Widely spaced, varicose punctation and, less frequently, mosaicism occurring in an area of high-grade VAIN are highly suspicious for invasive cancer.**

The ability reliably to predict the probable histologic status of vaginal colposcopic lesions is a challenge for the most experienced colposcopist. A lesion may appear inconspicuous and trivial but reveal high-grade dysplasia on biopsy. **Examination under general or regional anesthesia may be required, particularly in the presence of extensive disease,** to permit accurate diagnosis.

The difficulty in colposcopic assessment of the vagina renders examination after application of aqueous iodine solution invaluable. Poorly differentiated vaginal epithelium is unglycogenated and rejects iodine staining. High-grade VAIN lesions appear mustard yellow against the mahogany-brown staining of normal surrounding mucosa. This assists in the mapping of significant lesions and in obtaining accurate biopsies. The application of aqueous iodine is mandatory for delineation of treatment margins.

Treatment of High-Grade Vaginal Intraepithelial Neoplasia

Vaginal intraepithelial neoplasia can be very difficult to treat, particularly in the presence of extensive, multifocal disease or when the vaginal vault is involved posthysterectomy. **Surgical excision, often requiring partial vaginectomy, or vaginal irradiation were historically used as the main treatment modalities.** Significant morbidity is associated with both approaches. **The CO_2 laser is regarded as the treatment of choice for most VAIN cases** (462,463). The vaginal wall is relatively thin compared with other genital tract sites, with vital organs in close proximity. Surgical access is, at times, difficult. The CO_2 laser provides the surgeon with the ability to treat to a precisely controlled depth and achieve very high cure rates for selected patients (464).

Topical *5-fluorouracil (5-FU)* **cream can also be used with good effect for carefully selected patients** (465,466). *5-FU* cream produces chemoinflammation and chemoulceration that often adequately treats VAIN lesions. Care is required to protect the vulvar skin and to avoid persistent denudation of the vaginal mucosa, particularly in the posterior fornix.

Application of 5% *imiquimod* **cream may be considered as an alternative treatment for high-grade VAIN** where excision is not indicated (467–469). Although the data are limited, *imiquimod* cream has been demonstrated to achieve high clearance and response rates for VAIN. Recurrence rates are no greater than for other topical treatments and it appears to be safe and well tolerated by most patients. *Imiquimod* **has been used for management of extensive, multifocal VAIN lesions, both as primary treatment, as well as with the aim of decreasing the extent of disease before ablation** (469). Conservative ablative therapy requires expert colposcopy, liberal use of directed biopsies, and no cytologic, colposcopic, or histologic evidence of invasive cancer.

Carbon dioxide laser treatment for high-grade VAIN is best performed using a high-powered superpulse or ultrapulse laser. The beam is defocused to an appropriate beam geometry (see vulvar section) and controlled by a micromanipulator attached to a colposcope or operating microscope. **The vaginal mucosa is destroyed to the depth of the lamina propria, which is at most 2 to 3 mm.** Because the vaginal mucosa contains no gland crypts or skin appendages, superficial treatment only is required. Conservatism is important because delayed healing and scarring occur after overenthusiastic destruction of vaginal mucosa.

Treatment of high-grade VAIN in the vaginal vault represents a particular surgical challenge. Woodman et al. (470) reported results of vaginal vault laser surgery for VAIN following hysterectomy in 23 patients who were followed for a mean period of 30 months. Only six patients remained disease free, and invasive cancer developed in two patients. Hoffman et al. (471) reported 32 patients who underwent upper vaginectomy for VAIN 3. Occult invasive cancer was found in nine patients (28%). This very difficult problem is increasingly viewed as an indication for surgical excision, although CO_2 laser ablation may have a role if the patient is young and reliable.

Vulva and Perianal Area

Since approximately 1970, there has been a marked increase in the incidence of high-grade preinvasive vulvar disease and a decrease in the modal age of diagnosis (473). There has been a much smaller increase in the incidence of invasive vulvar cancer, presumably because the preinvasive disease is actively treated (474–476). Although more than 95% of cervical malignancies (15) and up to 90% of high grade VIN lesions are HPV-associated (454), **HPV DNA is detected only in approximately 50% of vulvar cancers** (477). Many of the HPV-negative cancers, particularly in older women, are associated with lichen sclerosus (478–484).

Classification

Preinvasive neoplasia of the vulva has been recognized for more than 75 years, but the descriptive terminology has been confusing. **Vulvar carcinoma *in situ* has been described as Bowen's disease, erythroplasia of Queyrat, carcinoma *in situ* simplex, bowenoid papulosis, kraurosis vulvae,** and **leukoplakia.** This confusion was compounded by the use of similar terms to describe a group of nonneoplastic vulvar diseases to which Jeffcoate (485) in 1966 assigned the term **chronic vulvar dystrophy.** In 1986, the International Society for the Study of Vulvar Disease (ISSVD) agreed on a new classification of vulvar epithelial disorders (Table 8.7) (486).

Although this classification represented a significant advance in rationalizing previously confusing terminology, significant shortcomings existed. The vulvar intraepithelial neoplasia (VIN) terminology was introduced for uniformity and consistency with the grade classification for CIN. Although this seemed logical, there existed an established biologic continuum from CIN 1 to CIN 3. **The neoplastic biologic continuum from VIN 1 through VIN 3 to invasive cancer has not been established** (454).

Although the progression rate of VIN 3 to invasive cancer remains controversial, the malignant potential is undisputed (487–492). By contrast, **there is no direct evidence that VIN 1 has any malignant potential.** The detection of high risk HPV-DNA types in 30% to 40% of VIN 1 lesions, a considerably higher rate than in condylomata acuminata, has been advanced as an argument for retaining low-grade lesions within the VIN diagnosis (454), but the inclusion of such lesions in the neoplastic continuum creates pressure for a more aggressive therapeutic approach and **there is a compelling argument for excluding low-grade VIN from the "intraepithelial neoplasia" category** (493). When mild squamous atypia is seen in vulvar skin, usually limited to the lower epidermis, the lesion is more likely to be nonneoplastic

Table 8.7 Classification of Epithelial Vulvar Disorders
Nonneoplastic epithelial disorders of skin and mucosa
Lichen sclerosus (formerly lichen sclerosus et atrophicus)
Squamous hyperplasia (formerly hyperplastic dystrophy)
Other dermatoses (e.g., psoriasis)
Intraepithelial neoplasia
Squamous intraepithelial neoplasia
VIN, usual type
a. VIN, warty type
b. VIN, basaloid type
c. VIN, mixed (warty/basaloid) type
VIN, differentiated type
Nonsquamous intraepithelial neoplasia
Paget's disease
Tumors of the melanocytes, noninvasive (melanoma *in situ*)
Mixed nonneoplastic and neoplastic epithelial disorders
Invasive tumors

VIN, vulvar intraepithelial neoplasia.

From Committee on Terminology, International Society for the Study of Vulvar Disease, 2004.

reactive atypia. Considerable inter- and intraobserver variation occurs with the VIN 1 diagnosis and this diagnostic category is not reproducible (494).

Most histologic VIN lesions are categorized as VIN 2-3 and good histologic agreement is obtained when VIN 2-3 are combined as a single high-grade VIN diagnosis (494). **Careful histologic and molecular review in the 1990s,** particularly by Kurman and associates, **led to a reclassification of VIN 3 into three histologic subtypes, namely basaloid, warty (or bowenoid) and differentiated (or carcinoma simplex)** (495–496). Further clinical correlation refined the high-grade VIN diagnosis to include two distinct lesions which have different morphology, biology and clinical features (494).

VIN, usual type, is seen adjacent to 30% of both warty (condylomatous) and basaloid types of invasive squamous vulvar cancers. It is mostly high-risk HPV related, as are the associated cancers. It has a definite invasive potential, particularly in women over 30 years of age. A variant of VIN, usual type, is the multifocal, pigmented, papular lesion seen in younger women, often of non-European background, associated with genital warts and sometimes seen in pregnancy. These lesions can regress spontaneously and although there is a definite potential to progress, close prospective follow-up is justified (495,496).

The less-common VIN, differentiated type, is seen in older women, often adjacent to invasive keratinizing squamous cell carcinoma of the vulva (494,497,498). It may occur with chronic vulvar dermatoses, particularly lichen sclerosus, but also with squamous cell hyperplasia, lichen simplex chronicus and erosive lichen planus. **VIN, differentiated type, is not HPV associated nor is the associated keratinizing squamous cell cancer.** Clinically, these lesions are difficult to distinguish against a dystrophic background. A keratotic nodule or shallow ulcer may be the only clinical indicator.

In 2004, the ISSVD recommended the following modifications to the terminology for squamous vulvar intraepithelial neoplasia (494):

1. **The term VIN 1 is no longer used** and is replaced with flat condyloma acuminatum or HPV effect. The term "atypia" is this context is discouraged.

2. **The term VIN applies to histologic high-grade squamous intraepithelial lesions (VIN 2-3).**

3. **Two categories of VIN exist:**
   a) The more common **VIN, usual type** encompassing VIN 2, VIN 3 and the older clinical and histologic terms: Bowen's disease, bowenoid papulosis, dysplasia, and carcinoma *in situ*. These lesions are associated with high-risk HPV types, particularly HPV 16. VIN, usual type, is **subcategorized histologically as warty** (condylomatous), **basaloid, or mixed.**
   b) The less-common **VIN, differentiated type.** These lesions are not associated with HPV but frequently occur against a background of a vulvar dermatosis, particularly lichen sclerosus.

4. The occasional VIN lesion that cannot be classified as VIN, usual or differentiated types is termed **VIN, unclassified type** (or VIN, NOS). (This includes the rare pagetoid VIN.)

5. Classification is on the basis of histologic morphology only and not clinical appearance or HPV type.

The 2004 ISSVD classification of VIN is shown in Table 8.7.

Paget's Disease

Paget's disease of the vulva is an uncommon intraepithelial lesion. It is sometimes associated with underlying invasive carcinoma. These conditions are discussed in Chapter 13.

Clinical Profile of High-Grade Vulvar Intraepithelial Neoplasia

The increased incidence of VIN 3 in recent decades reflects increased clinical awareness, improved diagnostic accuracy, and an absolute increase in disease incidence. **Specific genital HPV types, in particular HPV 16, are strongly implicated in the causation of high-grade VIN** (454,499–502). Other vulvar HPV-induced lesions, including condylomata acuminata and subclinical HPV infection, frequently either coexist with or predate the diagnosis of VIN 3. **Cigarette smoking, nutritional deficiency, poor personal hygiene, granulomatous vulvar diseases, endogenous and exogenous systemic immune suppression including HIV infection,** previous radiation therapy, and pregnancy have been implicated as cofactors in the pathogenesis of VIN 3 (474,489). There is a strong association between VIN 3 and sexually transmitted disease, with rates varying from 20% to 60%.

Distribution

High-grade VIN lesions tend to be localized and unifocal in the older patient. A higher malignant potential is presumed for such lesions because invasive vulvar cancer occurs predominantly in the older age groups. However, many of the invasive cancers in elderly women occur against a background of lichen sclerosis and without a prior history of VIN 3 or coexisting histologic evidence of VIN 3.

In younger patients, high-grade VIN lesions are frequently multifocal and extensive. Lesions may remain discrete or coalesce to develop a large field of disease. Lesions may extend laterally from the inner aspect of the mucous membranes of the labia minora to the hair-bearing skin of the labia majora and from the clitoris, periclitoral area, and mons pubis anteriorly to the perineum and perianal area posteriorly. Difficult-to-access sanctuary sites, such as the urethra, clitoris, vagina, and anal canal, need to be carefully inspected.

Symptoms

More than 30% of women with VIN 3 experience vulvar symptomatology. The most common symptoms are pruritus, burning, pain, and dysuria (503). Vulvar symptoms are often exacerbated by voiding. Patients may present reporting a localized lump or thickening in the vulvar skin, or they may notice an area of increased or decreased pigmentation. The patient may present with a history of recalcitrant vulvar condylomata acuminata.

Delay in diagnosis of high-grade VIN, even in symptomatic patients, is common (473,489,503). Opportunistic inspection of the vulva, particularly at the time of colposcopy for abnormal cervical cytology, is recommended.

Clinical Appearance

The clinical appearance of VIN 3 lesions varies according to patient age and skin color, as well as the location of the lesions in the vulva and perianal region (Figs. 8.20, 8.21). In both the hair-bearing and non–hair-bearing keratinized vulvar skin, **lesions tend to be raised or papular. They may be white, red, or brown in color.** White lesions are due to hyperkeratosis or dehydration of the outer keratinized layer. Red lesions result from increased vascularity, reflecting either an inflammatory response or increased blood vessel formation secondary to angiogenic factors of neoplasia. Brown or pigmented lesions, which occur in more than 10% of patients, result from melanin incontinence, usually in the keratinized squamous epithelium. **On the mucosal surfaces and less frequently on the keratinized surfaces, VIN 3 lesions may be flat or macular.** Occasionally, such macular lesions are evident through associated erythema or pigmentation. **Usually, macular lesions are subclinical and are detected on colposcopic examination** after application of 5% acetic acid solution.

The clinical appearance of VIN 3 in dark-skinned women is similar when detected on mucosal surfaces but may differ in keratinized and hair-bearing areas. Relative hypopigmentation may occur, producing pink or erythematous plaques. Such lesions may blanch densely acetowhite after application of acetic acid solution. Unifocal, localized lesions in older women less frequently involve the mucous membranes. **Care must be taken in the assessment of suspicious vulvar lesions in older women because of the increased risk of undisclosed invasive cancer.** Warning signs of an occult invasive lesion include yellow discoloration, nodularity, ulceration, thick scale, and abnormal vascularity.

Vulvar intraepithelial neoplasia grade 3 is often found on biopsy of recalcitrant and abnormal appearing condylomata acuminata. **VIN 3 is reported in biopsies from 30% of patients with large, persistent condylomatous lesions, particularly if the lesions are pigmented or coalescent and sessile with a micropapilliferous surface.** Condylomatous lesions exhibiting a severely dysplastic morphology on biopsy frequently harbor high-risk HPV types, with HPV 16 and 18 detected in more than 70% of such lesions (500).

Diagnosis

Colposcopy is now an accepted standard in the diagnostic assessment of preinvasive vulvar disease. After application of 5% acetic acid solution and colposcopic assessment using a magnification of at least 7, lesions appear as clearly demarcated, dense acetowhite areas. The multifocal distribution is usually evident. The acetic acid reaction is best seen in lesions that are nonpigmented or red. Pigmented lesions often develop an acetowhite hue or a rim of acetowhitening. Initial clinical examination may identify clinically apparent lesions.

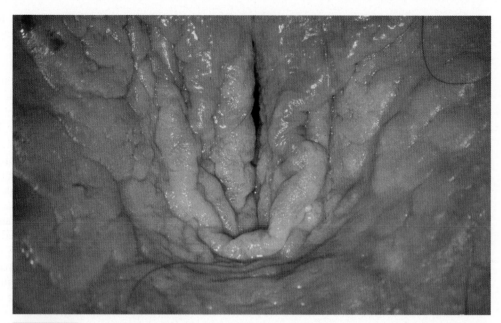

Figure 8.20   Clinical appearance of vulvar intraepithelial neoplasia showing hyperkeratotic papular lesions.

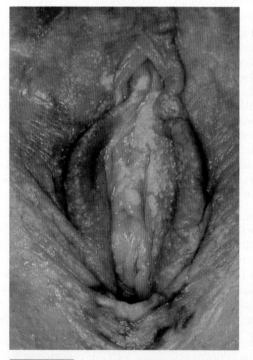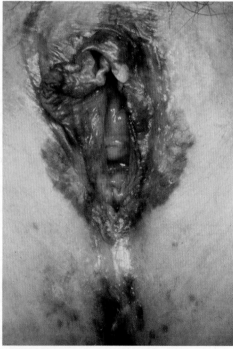

Figure 8.21   *Left:* Multifocal VIN 3 lesion with multiple hyperpigmented and hyperkeratotic lesions. *Right:* Multifocal VIN 3 with confluent hyperpigmented areas on the vulva extending to the perineum and perianal areas.

Colposcopy may permit identification of previously unidentified, subclinical lesions and better define the distribution of clinically evident disease.

In high-grade vulvar preinvasive lesions, vascular patterns are often inconspicuous or absent, particularly in the presence of hyperkeratosis. Macular lesions on the mucous membranes may reveal a capillary punctation pattern, and a fine punctation is sometimes observed in papular lesions. **Marked vascular abnormalities** characterized by a varicose, widely spaced punctation and, rarely, mosaicism **represent a definite warning sign of invasive cancer,** and the lesion must be excised. Colposcopic warning signs of vulvar cancer occur late in the neoplastic process, limiting the sensitivity of colposcopy for the identification of early invasive cancer. **Histologic evidence of VIN 3 may be seen outside colposcopically identified margins of disease, particularly laterally in the hair-bearing areas.**

Diagnosis ultimately depends on liberal use of directed biopsy. This is particularly the case if ablative treatment is being considered, either alone or in combination with excisional procedures. **Biopsies are best taken with a Keyes biopsy instrument** under local anesthesia in the office setting.

Natural History of High-Grade Vulvar Intraepithelial Neoplasia

Vulvar intraepithelial neoplasia grade 3 coexists with invasive cancer in 30% to 50% of cases. Vulvar dystrophy occurs in up to 50% of specimens, with lichen sclerosus and squamous hyperplasia equally represented. There is no coexistent disease in 10% to 15% of specimens (473,489,503).

Few studies have examined the natural history of untreated VIN. Jones and Rowan from New Zealand (488) reported in 1994 on the follow-up of 113 women with VIN 3 diagnosed between 1961 and 1993. **Of 105 women whose disease was treated, 4 (3.8%) developed invasive cancer** 7 to 18 years after treatment. **Of eight untreated cases of VIN 3, progression to invasive cancer was reported in seven patients (87.5%)** within 8 years, and the disease regressed spontaneously in the remaining patient. This very high incidence of progression within a reasonably short time is troubling. More recent studies, with much shorter follow-up of untreated women, suggest a lower progression rate (487,491).

A more recent study from New Zealand reported women who experienced spontaneous regression of VIN 2-3 (495). These women had a median age of 19 years, an initial presentation through a sexual health clinic, and a previous history of condylomata acuminata. Most had multifocal, pigmented lesions. Median time to regression was 9.5 months.

The occurrence, usually in younger women, of multifocal, pigmented, papular vulvar lesions reported histologically as VIN 3 is well recognized and has been described as **"bowenoid papulosis"** (504). Reports of spontaneous regression, especially associated with pregnancy, suggested distinctive epidemiologic features for bowenoid papulosis, but the term has been abandoned by the International Society for the Study of Vulvar Disease and the International Society for Gynecologic Pathologists. **High-grade VIN is a disease with a varied and individual clinical profile and histologic appearance.** This range encompasses the entity previously described as "bowenoid papulosis."

Treatment of High-Grade Vulvar Intraepithelial Neoplasia

Treatment is aimed at control of symptoms and prevention of progression to invasive cancer. Many treatment modalities have been used and, historically, vulvar carcinoma *in situ* was managed by simple vulvectomy (505). Such a radical approach is unjustified and is associated with significant morbidity, particularly for young women, including scarring, dyspareunia, urinary stream difficulties, loss of elasticity for vaginal delivery, and a "castration-like" self-image.

Since the 1970s, there has been a trend toward more conservative therapy, initially using excisional approaches and more recently, ablative modalities (506,507).

The risk of occult malignancy occurring in association with VIN 3 is too low to mandate complete excision of disease in all patients but too high to allow routine ablation. Women undergoing excisional treatment for VIN 3 are reported to have a 15% to 23% incidence of unsuspected invasive squamous cell carcinoma on histologic examination of the excised specimen(s) (503,508,509).

The clinical profile of VIN, including a broad age range and marked variability in extent, distribution, and symptomatology, demands individualization of the therapeutic approach for each patient. A period of close prospective follow-up without treatment may be appropriate for young, immunocompetent women with multifocal disease, particularly if they are pregnant. The patient must comply with close follow-up and understand and accept the risks of treatment delay.

Wide Local Excision, Skin Flap Procedures, and Superficial (Skinning) Vulvectomy

Localized high-grade VIN lesions are best managed by local, superficial excision. The lesion should be excised with a disease-free margin of at least 5 mm. Wide, local excision is ideal for unifocal and lateral lesions or for hemorrhoids involved with high-grade intraepithelial neoplasia. It is mandatory if a lesion has warning signs of possible invasive cancer. **Primary closure of the defect usually achieves uncomplicated healing and a very satisfactory cosmetic and functional outcome.** The elasticity of the vulvar skin permits preservation of sexual and reproductive functions, of particular importance in the young patient.

The surgical specimen should be submitted to careful histologic evaluation to exclude invasive disease and to ensure clear margins of excision. **Surgical excision with disease-free surgical margins achieves a 90% cure rate for localized disease. If the margins of excision are involved with disease, the cure rate falls to 50%,** demanding very close follow-up. **As long as all macroscopic disease has been removed, reexcision is not justified for positive margins.** Most recurrences occur within three years of treatment, although late recurrence and progression to cancer can occur. Development of symptoms should prompt urgent review.

Large, confluent lesions or extensive multifocal disease, particularly in the presence of colposcopic warning signs of early invasion, require more extensive excisional procedures with rotational flaps to fill the defect, or superficial (skinning) vulvectomy with a split-thickness skin graft (510,511). Primary closure of a large vulvar wound may not be possible without undue tension leading to wound breakdown or excessive scarring. Cutaneous flaps with no muscle component have been used for cases of extensive excision of VIN (512–514). Perineal flaps of skin and fascial tissue rotated around a perforating branch of the internal iliac artery have been used to close larger vulvo-vaginal defects (512). Thin skin flaps with less than 1cm of underlying fat can be raised from the buttock and rotated medially to close vulvar defects (513). Good postoperative healing is usually achieved without significant morbidity or long-term negative impact on sexual functioning.

"Skinning" vulvectomy was introduced by Rutledge and Sinclair (510) **for extensive VIN lesions,** particularly in the hair-bearing skin where the skin appendages may be involved. Lesions are carefully mapped and a shallow layer of vulvar skin is excised, preserving the subcutaneous tissues. The vulvar skin at risk is replaced with epidermis from a donor site on the inner aspect of the thigh or buttock. The clitoris is preserved, with lesions on the prepuce or glans being superficially excised or laser ablated. The epithelium regenerates without loss of sensation.

DiSaia (511) reported a 39% recurrence rate in patients with VIN 3 treated by skinning vulvectomy with split-thickness skin grafting. There were no recurrences in grafted areas, although such recurrence has been reported. Although this procedure has been largely outmoded by CO_2 laser treatment for many patients with extensive disease, it remains an important therapeutic option when there is an increased risk of occult invasive cancer.

CO_2 Laser Surgery

Vulvar intraepithelial neoplasia is occurring more frequently in young women, and the disease may be very extensive, involving the hair-bearing area of the labia majora in more than 30% of cases. **Excision of such wide areas, even with skin grafting, can cause significant scarring and anatomic distortion.** With careful, expert colposcopy and liberal use of directed biopsy, the undisclosed cancer risk in selected patients is low.

Some consider an ablative procedure in these young patients using the CO_2 laser to be the treatment of choice (515–519). The morbidity associated with ablation of large areas of VIN 3 has been found to be unacceptable in some studies. The initial 2 weeks following more extensive laser ablative procedures will be associated with significant pain, particularly with micturition. The use of appropriate laser technology and settings, advanced surgical expertise with careful control of depth of ablation, and appropriate postoperative care will mitigate much of the potential morbidity. **CO_2 laser ablation is particularly useful in patients with periclitoral and perianal disease, where the preservation of anatomy and function is a substantial benefit.**

Physical Principles Governing Vulvar Laser Surgery

1. **Choice of appropriate laser wavelength:** The CO_2 laser is the only laser proven to be safe and effective for the management of high-grade VIN.

2. **Rapid delivery of the required energy dose:** Vulvar laser surgery demands minimization of lateral thermal injury to prevent scarring and morbidity. The surgeon must be able to control higher powers to permit precise, rapid ablation. For ablative

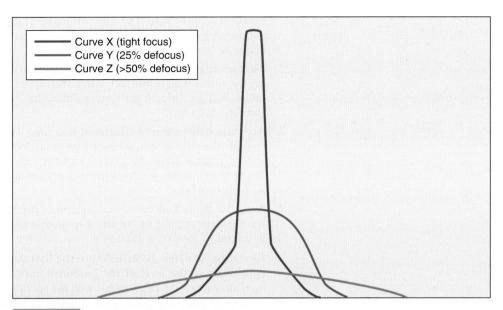

Figure 8.22   Diagrammatic representation of CO_2 laser beam geometry.

procedures, **powers of less than 50 W in continuous mode are associated with an increased risk of thermal injury** and should be avoided.

3. **Choice of appropriate temporal mode:** The option of choosing **rapid super-pulse or the newer ultrapulse technology** affords a definite therapeutic advantage in CO_2 laser ablation of vulvar lesions. The ability precisely to vaporize diseased tissue under visual control with minimal heat propagation to adjacent tissue is the key to nonmorbid laser surgery.

4. **Choice of appropriate power density:** CO_2 laser ablation requires power densities in the range of 800 to 1,400 W/cm^2.

5. **Choice of appropriate beam geometry:** The incident laser beam produces a conical impact crater with marked variation in intensity of the beam from point to point in the focal spot. The clinical importance of the concept of beam geometry is that the crater shape mirrors the intensity profile of the incident energy (Fig. 8.22). When the incident laser beam is highly focused, the vaporization crater is a narrow, deep "drill hole." This reflects the high power density and is arbitrarily designated as the *X-beam geometry.* The X-beam geometry is for cutting or for excisional procedures. If the incident laser beam is flattened completely, it will simply coagulate a broad zone of tissue at the impact site but will not have sufficient power to vaporize tissue. The wide, flattened spot size produces the *Z-beam geometry.* In contrast, **defocusing the laser beam to an intermediate, round beam geometry produces a round, shallow vaporization crater at the impact site. This is designated the** *Y-beam geometry* and permits controlled tissue vaporization to a relatively uniform and predictable depth.

   For ablative treatment of VIN, a high-power laser setting is selected. The spot diameter is progressively enlarged by defocusing the beam using the micromanipulator until a point is found where the impact crater is hemispherical. This permits controlled tissue vaporization with minimal lateral heat conduction. The laser should be first tested on a moistened tongue blade to defocus the beam to the hemispherical Y-beam geometry before use on the skin.

6. **Intermittent gated pulsing:** CO_2 laser surgery to the vulvar skin requires training and skill in the use of the foot pedal to deliver the laser energy in short bursts to control the depth of ablation.

Surgical Strategies Governing Vulvar CO_2 Laser Surgery

1. **Choice of appropriate beam delivery system:** For ablative procedures, the laser must be controlled using a micromanipulator through a colposcope or operating microscope with a 300-mm objective to produce a relatively large spot size with

excellent depth of field. The angle of impact of the laser is controlled by traction on the skin. A handheld mirror may occasionally be required to reflect the beam to difficult-to-access sites.

2. **Minimization of thermal injury:** Thermal injury can be further minimized by chilling the vulvar skin, before and during surgery, with laparotomy packs soaked in iced saline solution. This simple strategy diminishes postoperative pain and swelling and promotes healing.

3. **Accurate delineation of treatment margins:** The laser is used under colposcopic control. The possible extension of high-grade VIN beyond areas that are colposcopically evident indicates the need for treatment margins of several spot sizes. The laser can be used initially to circumscribe the distribution of the lesions before the acetic acid reaction fades.

4. **Accurate depth control:** Determination of depth of ablation is best achieved by a precise understanding of the visual landmarks of the surgical planes of the vulva as described by Reid et al. (516,517).

   First surgical plane **Destruction to the first surgical plane removes the surface epithelium to the level of the basement membrane.** The laser beam is rapidly oscillated across the target tissue with the spot describing a series of roughly parallel lines. When the impact debris is wiped away with a moistened swab, the moist "sand-grain" appearance of the papillary dermis will be evident.

   Second surgical plane **Ablation to the second plane removes the epidermis and the superficial papillary dermis.** This plane is achieved by a slightly slower oscillation of the laser beam across the first surgical plane, scorching but not penetrating the papillary dermis. The visual effect is a shrinking of the target tissue because of dehydration, and a finely roughened, yellowish surface similar in appearance to chamois cloth is produced. Ablation extends to the deep papillary dermis with minimal thermal injury to the underlying reticular dermis. **The second surgical plane is the preferred depth of ablation for condylomata acuminata treated with the CO_2 laser.**

   Third surgical plane **Destruction to the third surgical plane removes the epidermis, papillary dermis, and superficial reticular dermis containing the upper portions of the skin appendages,** specifically the pilosebaceous ducts and hair follicles. This is achieved by a slower, purposeful movement of the laser beam across the second surgical plane. The tissue is seen to relax and separate as the midreticular dermis is exposed as moistened gray-white fibers representing coarse collagen bundles. **Healing occurs from the base of the skin appendages, and scarring is absent or minimal. Ablative procedures for VIN 3 should be carried to the depth of the third surgical plane** (Fig. 8.23).

   The skin appendages are involved with the VIN process in more than 50% of cases (517). Depth of hair follicle involvement is usually less than 1 mm but may extend to 2 mm. Measured sweat gland involvement has been more than 3 mm in depth. Beyond 3 mm, the equivalent of a third-degree thermal defect is created, resulting in delayed healing, scarring, and alopecia. The implications of residual disease after treatment of VIN are different from those of residual CIN, which may be buried and escape detection. Although the surgeon should be aware of vulvar skin appendage involvement, this is not an indication to destroy beyond the midreticular dermis.

   Fourth surgical plane **Destruction of the reticular dermis creates a thermal injury extending to the subcutaneous tissues and must be avoided.**

5. **Control of intraoperative and postoperative pain and bleeding:** CO_2 laser procedures for high-grade VIN are performed under general or regional anesthesia unless the disease is localized. Subcutaneous injection of a long-acting local anesthetic on completion of the procedure diminishes pain in the immediate postoperative period.

   Narcotic analgesia is usually required in the immediate postoperative period or, alternatively, prolonged epidural analgesia can be used. Regular sitz baths followed by topical application of a mixture of equal parts 1% *lidocaine* and 2% *silver sulfadiazine* creams to the surgical site aid in pain relief. The postoperative discomfort is often most severe on the third to the sixth postoperative days. Patients should have available appropriate oral narcotic analgesics to provide relief after discharge from hospital.

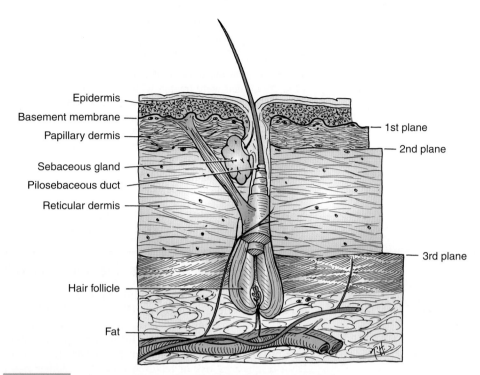

Figure 8.23 Diagrammatic representation of three surgical planes.

Long-Term Follow-up

Regardless of treatment modality, **recurrence of VIN is common.** Even with modern treatment and management of VIN, invasive cancer will still develop in 3% to 5% of women, considerably higher than the risk of cervical cancer post treatment of CIN. Recurrent VIN is a significant problem and represents both incomplete primary treatment and disease recurrence. **Lifelong vigilance is an important component of the management of high-grade VIN.**

Immune Response Modifiers: *Imiquimod*

Surgery is the treatment of choice for high-grade VIN, to remove visible lesions, relieve symptoms, and prevent invasive cancer. However, the margins of excised specimens are positive for disease in 24% to 68% of cases and disease recurrence is common. Surgery does not eradicate HPV, the primary cause of most cases of VIN. The discovery that VIN 2-3 lesions, particularly multifocal lesions in younger women, are strongly HPV associated, argues for the possible efficacy of immune response modifiers in treatment of high-grade VIN (375,376).

Imiquimod (Aldara) is an imidazoquinoline, a novel synthetic compound that **is a topical immune response stimulator.** It enhances both the innate and acquired immune pathways, particularly the T helper cell type 1–mediated immune response, resulting in antiviral, antitumor, and immunoregulatory activities (520,521). *Imiquimod* causes cytokine induction in the skin, which up-regulates the host immune system to recognize the presence of a viral infection or tumor, theoretically leading to eradication of the lesion. It also stimulates activation, maturation, and migration of Langerhans cells, the major antigen-presenting cells of the skin, which are depleted by HPV infection (521,522).

A patient-applied topical 5% *imiquimod cream* **is clinically efficacious and safe in the management of condylomata acuminata** (523–526). It was licensed in 1997 for the treatment of anogenital condylomata acuminata and is recommended for this application in sexually transmitted disease guidelines from the U.S. Centers for Disease Control and Prevention, as well as guidelines from Europe, Latin America, and Australia.

The beneficial effects, patient acceptability, and low morbidity of *imiquimod* **in the treatment of genital condylomata acuminata have led to its recent evaluation in the treatment of VIN 2-3.** Case reports demonstrated efficacy against VIN 2-3, including in an immune-suppressed lung transplant patient (527). Pilot studies, applying *imiquimod* one to three times a week at night, have reported a 30% complete response rate and 60% partial response after

327

6 to 30 weeks of treatment (469,528). **In contrast to surgical treatment,** *imiquimod* **focuses on the cause of many VIN cases, and preserves the anatomy and function of the vulva.** Exclusion of invasive cancer is an important aspect of pretreatment assessment.

In a recent placebo controlled, randomized trial of *imiquimod* in the treatment of high-grade VIN, 26 women were treated with the active cream (529). Over an observation period of one year, 9 women (35%) showed complete response and 12 (46%) showed a partial response. Regression from VIN 2-3 to low grade disease was seen in 18 of 26 patients treated (69%) and 15 of these tested negative for HPV DNA after treatment. Three patients developed early invasive cancer to a depth less than 1 mm, two after placebo treatment and one after *imiquimod,* reinforcing the need for close follow-up. Patients reported good symptom relief and there was no reported adverse influence on health-related quality of life, body images, or sexuality. *Imiquimod* is well tolerated and less invasive than surgery.

No treatment modality is ideal for every woman. Treatment should be individualized according to age, distribution, severity, associated disease, and previous treatment.

Multicentric Lower Genital Tract Neoplasia

The concept of multicentricity of lower genital tract neoplasia is well established (530) reflecting the "field effect" of high-risk HPV types (531,532). Multiple primary preinvasive or invasive lesions involving the cervix, vagina, vulva, and/or anus can occur synchronously or metachronously in this region. **Multicentric preinvasive disease has a higher recurrence rate after treatment than unicentric disease** (533). Continued detection of high-risk HPV DNA results in a risk of recurrence of 45%. Other risk factors for recurrence include age, immunosuppression, smoking, choice of treatment modality, and positive surgical margins.

High-grade *perianal intraepithelial neoplasia (PAIN)* **occurs in more than 30% of patients with VIN 3 or multicentric squamous neoplasia.** High-grade PAIN may occur in recalcitrant perianal condylomata acuminata or as thickened, hyperkeratotic, often pigmented papular lesions usually visible to the naked eye. Proctoscopic examination using the colposcope after application of acetic acid may reveal high-grade squamous preinvasive disease extending to above the dentate line. Squamous cancer of the anus remains an uncommon disease (534), although its incidence has increased significantly in homosexual men (535,536). Viral analysis confirms a strong association with HPV 16 (537).

High-grade PAIN is managed similarly to VIN 3. Conservation of normal tissues by careful colposcopic delineation of diseased areas is important. The CO_2 laser may afford some therapeutic advantage in this area because disruption of nerve fibers with full-thickness excision can lead to diminished ability to differentiate feces and flatus, leading to a degree of anal incontinence. Disease may also extend posteriorly to the anus and onto the natal cleft. Although considerable postoperative care is required for pain control and wound care, **modern CO_2 laser surgery is usually the treatment of choice in this difficult situation** after exclusion of invasive cancer. **Topical** *imiquimod* **cream may be a useful primary treatment** or adjuvant in difficult to access sites.

References

1. **Parkin DM, Bray F, Ferlay J, Pisani P.** Global cancer statistics, 2002. *CA Cancer J Clin* 2005;55:74–108.
2. **Parkin DM, Bray F.** Chapter 2: the burden of HPV-related cancers. *Vaccine* 2006;24:S11–S25.
3. **Ferlay J, Bray f, Pisani P, Parkin DM.** GLOBOCAN 2002: cancer incidence, mortality and prevalence worldwide. IARC Cancer Base No. 5 Version 2.0 IARC Press. Available at: http://www-depdb.iarc.fr/globocan/GLOBOCAN2002.HTM
4. **Yang BH, Bray FI, Parkin DM, Sellors JW, Zhang ZF.** Cervical cancer as a priority for prevention in different world regions: an evaluation using years of life lost. *Int J Cancer* 2004;109:418–424.
5. **U.S. Cancer Statistics Working Group.** United States Cancer Statistics: 2004 Incidence and Mortality. Atlanta: U.S. Department of Health and Human Services, Centers for Disease Control and Prevention and National Cancer Institute; 2007. Accessed at:

http://www.cdc.gov/cancer/npcr/npcrpdfs/US_Cancer_Statistics_2004_Incidence_and_Mortality.pdf.
6. **Swan J, Breen N, Coates RJ, Rimer BK, Lee NC.** Progress in cancer screening practices in the United States: results from the 2000 National Health Interview Survey. *Cancer* 2003;97:1528–1540.
7. **Nieminen P, Kallio M, Hakama M.** The effect of mass screening on incidence and mortality of squamous and adenocarcinoma of cervix uteri. *Obstet Gynecol* 1995;85:1017–1021.
8. **Sawaya GF, Brown AD, Washington AE, Garber AM.** Current approaches to cervical cancer screening. *N Engl J Med* 2001;344:1603–1607.
9. **Solomon D, Breen N, McNeel T.** Cervical cancer screening rates in the United States and the potential impact of implementation of screening guidelines. *CA Cancer J Clin* 2007;57:105–111.

10. **Pund ER, Nieburgs H, Nettles JB, Caldwell JD.** Preinvasive carcinoma of the cervix in seven cases in which it was detected by examination of routine endocervical smears. *Pathol Lab Med* 1947;44: 571–577.

11. **Barron BA, Richart RM.** Screening protocols for cervical neoplastic disease. *Gynecol Oncol* 1981;12:S156–S167.

12. **Sasieni PD, Cuzick J, Lynch-Farmery E.** Estimating the efficacy of screening by auditing smear histories of women with and without cervical cancer. The National Co-ordinating Networth for Cervical Screening Working Group. *Br J Cancer* 1996;73:1001–1005.

13. **Cogliano V, Baan R, Straif K, Grosse Y, Secretan B, El Ghissassi F.** Carcinogenicity of human papillomaviruses, *Lancet Oncol* 2005;6:204.

14. **Munoz N, Castellsague X, Berrington de Gonzalez A, Gissmann L.** HPV in the aetiology of human cancer. *Vaccine* 2006;24(suppl 3):1–10.

15. **Schiffman M, Castle PE, Jeronimo J, Rodriguez AC, Wacholder S.** Human papillomavirus and cervical cancer. *Lancet* 2007;370: 890–907.

16. **Schauenstein W.** Histologische untersuchunges uber atypisches plattiepethel an der portio an der innerflache der cervix uteri. *Arch Gynakol* 1908;85:576.

17. **Weid GL.** Exfoliative cytology. In: Weid GL, ed. *Proceedings of the 1st International Congress on Exfoliative Cytology.* Philadelphia: JB Lippincott, 1961:283–295.

18. **Papanicolaou G, Traut RF.** *The diagnosis of uterine cancer by the vaginal smear.* New York: Commonwealth Fund, 1943.

19. **Reagan JW, Hamonic MJ.** The cellular pathology in carcinoma-in-situ: cytohistopathologic correlation. *Cancer* 1956;9:385–402.

20. **Reagan JW, Patten SE.** Dysplasia: a basic reaction to injury of the uterine cervix. *Ann N Y Acad Sci* 1962;97:622–629.

21. **Reagan JW, Patten SE.** Analytic study of cellular changes in carcinoma-*in-situ*, squamous cell cancer and adenocarcinoma of the uterine cervix. *Clin Obstet Gynecol* 1961;4:1097–1106.

22. **Koss LG, Stewart FW, Foote FW, Jordan MJ, Bader GM, Day E.** Some histological aspects of behavior of epidermoid carcinoma *in situ* and related lesions of the uterine cervix. *Cancer* 1963;16: 1160–1211.

23. **Koss LG.** Dyplasia: a real concept or a misnomer? *Obstet Gynecol* 1978;51:374–379.

24. **Langley FA, Crompton AC.** Epithelial abnormalities of the cervix uteri. *Recent Results Cancer Res* 1973;2–5,141–143.

25. **Richart RM.** Natural history of cervical intraepithelial neoplasia. *Clin Obstet Gynecol* 1968;10:748–784.

26. **Richart RM, Barron BA.** A follow-up of patients with cervical dysplasia. *Am J Obstet Gynecol* 1969;105:386–393.

27. **Richart RM.** Cervical intraepithelial neoplasia. *Pathology Ann* 1973;8:301–328.

28. **Coppleson M, Reid BL.** Aetiology of squamous carcinoma of the cervix. *Obstet Gynecol* 1968;32:432–436.

29. **Coppleson M, Reid BL.** Interpretation of changes of the uterine cervix. *Lancet* 1969;2:216–217.

30. **Richart RM.** Causes and management of cervical intraepithelial neoplasia. *Cancer* 1987;60:1951–1959.

31. **Oster AG.** Natural history of CIN: a critical review. *Int J Gynecol Pathol* 1993;12:186–192.

32. **Duggan MA, McGregor SE, Stuart GC, Morris S, Chang-Poon V, Schepansky A, et al.** The natural history of CIN 1 lesions. *Eur J Gynaecol Oncol* 1998;19:338–344.

33. **Holowaty P, Miller AB, Rohan T, To T.** Natural history of dysplasia of the uterine cervix. *J Natl Cancer Inst* 1999;91:252–258.

34. **Melnikow J, Nuovo J, Willan AR, Chan BK, Howell LP.** Natural history of cervical squamous intraepithelial lesions: a meta-analysis. *Obstet Gynecol* 1998;92:727–735.

35. **Hildesheim A, Schiffman MH, Gravitt PE, Glass AG, Greer CE, Zhang T, et al.** Persistence of type-specific human papillomavirus infection among cytologically normal women. *J Infect Dis* 1994;169:235–240.

36. **Herrero R, Schiffman MH, Bratti C, Hildesheim A, Balmaceda I, Sherman ME, et al.** Design and methods of a population-based natural history study of cervical neoplasia in a rural province of Costa Rica: the Guanacaste Project. *Rev Panam Salud Publica* 1997;1:362–375.

37. **Manos MM, Kinney WK, Hurley LB, Sherman MF, Shiel-Ngai J, Kurman RJ, et al.** Identifying women with cervical neoplasia:

38. **Moscicki A-B, Schiffman M, Kjaer S, Villa LL.** Chapter 5: updating the natural history of HPV and anogenital cancer. *Vaccine* 2006;24(supp 3):S42–S51.

39. **Koutsky LA, Holmes KK, Critchlow CW, Stevens CE, Paavonen J, Becicman AM.** A cohort study of the risk of cervical intraepithelial neoplasia grade 2 or 3 in relation to papillomavirus infection. *N Engl J Med* 1992;327:1272–1278.

40. **Ho GY, Bierman R, Beardsley L, Chang CJ, Burk RD.** Natural history of cervicovaginal papillomavirus infection in young women. *N Engl J Med* 1998;338:423–428.

41. **National Cancer Institute Workshop.** The 1988 Bethesda system for reporting cervical/vaginal cytological diagnoses. *JAMA* 1989; 262:931–934.

42. **Schiffman MH.** Recent progress in defining the epidemiology of human papillomavirus infection and cervical neoplasia. *J Natl Cancer Inst* 1992;84:394–398.

43. **National Cancer Institute Workshop.** The Bethesda System for reporting cervical/vaginal cytologic diagnoses: revised after second National Cancer Institute Workshop (April 29–30, 1991). *Acta Cytol* 1993;37:115–124.

44. **Kurman RJ, Henson DE, Herbst AL, Noller KL, Schiffman MH.** Interim guidelines for management of abnormal cervical cytology. *JAMA* 1994;271:1866–1869.

45. **Solomon D, Davey D, Kurman R, Moriarty A, O'Connor D, Prey M, et al.** The 2001 Bethesda System: terminology for reporting results of cervical cytology. *JAMA* 2002;287:2114–2119.

46. **Stoler MH.** New Bethesda terminology and evidence-based management guidelines for cervical cytology findings. *JAMA* 2002;287:2140–2141.

47. **Wright Jr TC, Massad LS, Dunton CJ, Spitzer M, Wilkinson EJ, Solomon D, (for the 2006 ASCCP–sponsored Consensus Conference).** 2006 consensus guidelines for the management of women with abnormal cervical cancer screening tests. *Am J Obstet Gynecol* 2007;197:346–355.

48. **Stoler MH, Schiffman M.** Interobserver reproducibility of cervical cytologic and histologic interpretations: realistic estimates from the ASCUS-LSIL Triage Study. *JAMA* 2001;285:1500–1505.

49. **Melnikow J, Nuovo J, Willan AR, Chan BK, Howell LP.** Natural history of cervical squamous intraepithelial lesions: a meta-analysis, *Obstet Gynecol* 1998;92:727–735.

50. **Robertson AJ, Anderson JM, Beck JS et al.** Observer variability in histopathological reporting of cervical biopsy specimens, *J Clin Pathol* 1989;42:231–238.

51. **Mitchell MF, Tortolero-Luna G, Wright T, et al.** Cervical human papillomavirus infection and intraepithelial neoplasia: a review, *J Natl Cancer Inst Monogr* 1996;21:17–25.

52. **Wright Jr TC.** Pathology of HPV infection at the cytologic and histologic levels: basis for a 2-tiered morphologic classification system. *Int J Gynaecol Obstet* 2006;94:S22–S31.

53. **Cox JT, Schiff man M, Solomon D.** Prospective follow-up suggests similar risk of subsequent cervical intraepithelial neoplasia grade 2 or 3 among women with cervical intraepithelial neoplasia grade 1 or negative colposcopy and directed biopsy. *Am J Obstet Gynecol* 2003;188:1406–1412.

54. **ASCUS-LSIL Triage Study (ALTS) Group.** Results of a randomized trial on the management of cytology interpretations of atypical squamous cells of undetermined significance. *Am J Obstet Gynecol* 2003;188:1383–1392.

55. **Castle PE, Stoler MH, Solomon D, Schiffman M.** The relationship of community biopsy-diagnosed cervical intraepithelial neoplasia grade 2 to the quality control pathology-reviewed diagnoses: an ALTS report. *Am J Clin Pathol* 2007;127:805–815.

56. **von Knebel DM.** New markers for cervical dysplasia to visualise the genomic chaos created by aberrant oncogenic papillomavirus infections. *Eur J Cancer* 2002;38:2229–2242.

57. **Sindos M, Ndisang D, Pisal N, Chow C, Singer A, Latchman DS.** Measurement of Brn-3a levels in Pap smears provides a novel diagnostic marker for the detection of cervical neoplasia. *Gynecol Oncol* 2003;90:366–371.

58. **Middleton K, Peh W, Southern S, Griffin H, Sotlar K, Nakahara T, et al.** Organization of human papillomavirus productive cycle during neoplastic progression provides a basis for selection of diagnostic markers. *J Virol* 2003;77:10186–10201.

using human papillomavirus DNA testing for equivocal Papanicolaou results. *JAMA* 1999;281:1605–1610.

59. **Castle PE, Sideri M, Jeronimo J, Solomon D, Schiffman M.** Risk assessment to guide the prevention of cervical cancer. *Am J Obstet Gynecol* 2007;356.e1–356.e6.

60. **Schiffman M, Herrero R, Desalle R, et al.** The carcinogenicity of human papillomavirus types reflects viral evolution. *Virology* 2005;337:76–84.

61. **Kjaer S, Hogdall E, Frederiksen K, et al.** The absolute risk of cervical abnormalities in high-risk human papillomavirus-positive, cytologically normal women over a 10-year period. *Cancer Res* 2006;66:10630–10636.

62. **Khan MJ, Castle PE, Lorincz AT, et al.** The elevated 10-year risk of cervical precancer and cancer in women with human papillomavirus (HPV) type 16 or 18 and the possible utility of type-specific HPV testing in clinical practice. *J Natl Cancer Inst* 2005;97:1072–1079.

63. **Nobbenhuis MA, Helmerhorst TJ, van den BruleAJ, et al.** Cytological regression and clearance of high-risk human papillomavirus in women with an abnormal cervical smear, *Lancet* 2001;358:1782–1783.

64. **Schlecht NF, Platt RW, Duarte-Franco E, et al.** Human papillomavirus infection and time to progression and regression of cervical intraepithelial neoplasia, *J Natl Cancer Inst* 2003;95:1336–1343.

65. **Moscicki AB, Shiboski S, Hills NK, et al.** Regression of low-grade squamous intra-epithelial lesions in young women, *Lancet* 2004;364:1678–1683.

66. **Campion MJ, McCance DJ, Cuzick J, Singer A.** Progressive potential of mild cervical atypia: prospective cytological, colposcopic, and virological study. *Lancet* 1986;2:237–240.

67. **Reid R.** Biology and colposcopic features of human papillomavirus-associated cervical disease. *Obstet Gynecol Clin North Am* 1993;20:123–151.

68. **Greenberg MD, Reid R, Schiffman M, Campion MJ, Precop SL, Berman NR, et al.** A prospective study of biopsy-confirmed cervical intraepithelial neoplasia grade I: colposcopic, cytological and virological risk factors for progression. *Journal of Lower Genital Tract Disease* 1999;3:104–109.

69. **Pixley E.** Morphology of the fetal and prepubertal cervicovaginal epithelium. In: Jordan JA, Singer A, eds. *The cervix*. Philadelphia: WB Saunders, 1976:75–87.

70. **Coppleson M, Pixley E, Reid BL.** *Colposcopy: a scientific approach to the cervix uteri in health and disease*. Springfield, IL: Charles C Thomas, 1986.

71. **Kolstad P, Stafl A.** *Atlas of colposcopy*. Baltimore: University Park Press, 1982.

72. **Castle PE, Schiffman M, Bratti MC, et al.** A population-based study of vaginal human papillomavirus infection in hysterectomized women. *J Infect Dis* 2004;190:458–467.

73. **Castle PE, Jeronimo J, Schiffman M, et al.** Age-related changes of the cervix influence human papillomavirus type distribution. *Cancer Res* 2006;66:1218–1224.

74. **Brinton LA.** Current epidemiologic studies: emerging hypothesis. *Banbury Report* 1986;21:17–28.

75. **Brock KE, Berry G, Brinton LA, Kerr C, MacLennan R, Mock PA, et al.** Sexual, reproductive and contraceptive risk factors for carcinoma-in-situ of the uterine cervix in Sydney. *Med J Aust* 1989;150:125–130.

76. **Edebiri AA.** Cervical intraepithelial neoplasia: the role of age at first intercourse in its etiology. *J Reprod Med* 1990;35:225–259.

77. **Murthy NS, Mathew M.** Risk factors for pre-cancerous lesions of the cervix. *Eur J Cancer* 2000;9:5–18.

78. **Rodriguez AC, Burk RD, Herrero R, et al.** The natural history of HPV infection and cervical intraepithelial neoplasia among young women in the Guanacaste cohort shortly after initiation of sexual life. *Sex Transm Dis* 2007;34:494–502.

79. **Munoz MM, Bosch FX, Shah V, Meheus A, eds.** *The epidemiology of cervical cancer and human papillomavirus.* IARC Scientific Publications no. 119. Lyon, France: International Agency for Research on Cancer, 1992.

80. **Schiffman MH, Bauer HM, Hoover RN, Glass AG, Cadell DM, Rush BB, et al.** Epidemiologic evidence showing that human papillomavirus infection causes most cervical intraepithelial neoplasia. *J Natl Cancer Inst* 1993;85:958–964.

81. **International Agency for Research on Cancer.** *IARC monograph on the evaluation of carcinogenic risks to humans, vol. 64: human papillomaviruses.* Lyon, France: IARC Scientific Publications, 1995.

82. **zur Hausen H.** Immortalisation of human cells and their malignant conversion by high risk human papillomavirus genotypes. *Semin Cancer Biol* 1999;9:405–411.

83. **zur Hausen H.** Papillomaviruses causing cancer: evasion from host-cell control in early events in carcinogenesis. *J Natl Cancer Inst* 2000;92:690–698.

84. **Fehrmann F, Laimins LA.** Human papillomaviruses: targeting differentiating epithelial cells for malignant transformation. *Oncogene* 2003;22:5201–5207.

85. **Smith JS, Lindsay L, Hoots B, et al.** Human papillomavirus type distribution in invasive cervical cancer and high-grade cervical lesions: a meta-analysis update. *Int J Cancer* 2007;121:621–632.

86. **Bernard HU.** The clinical importance of the nomenclature, evolution and taxonomy of human papillomaviruses. *J Clin Virol* 2005;32:S1–S6.

87. **de Villiers EM, Fauquet C, Broker TR, Bernard HU, zur Hausen H.** Classification of papillomaviruses. *Virology* 2004;324:17–27.

88. **Doorbar J.** Papillomavirus life cycle organization and biomarker selection. *Dis Markers* 2007;23:297–313.

89. **Schiffman M, Herrero R, Desalle R, Hildesheim A, Wacholder S, Rodriguez AC, et al.** The carcinogenicity of human papillomavirus types reflects viral evolution. *Virology* 2005;337:76–84.

90. **Doorbar J.** Molecular biology of human papillomavirus infection and cervical cancer. *Clin Sci* (London) 2006;110:525–541.

91. **Durst M, Kleinheinz A, Hotz M, Gissman L.** The physical state of human papillomavirus type 16 DNA in benign and malignant genital tumours. *J Gen Virol* 1985;66:1515–1522.

92. **Cullen AP, Reid R, Campion MJ, Lorincz AT.** Analysis of the physical state of different human papillomavirus DNAs in intraepithelial and invasive cervical neoplasms. *J Virol* 1991;65:606–612.

93. **Fujii T., Masumoto N., Saito M, et al.** Comparison between *in situ* hybridization and real-time PCR technique as a means of detecting the integrated form of human papillomavirus 16 in cervical neoplasia. *Diagn Mol Pathol* 2005;14:103–108.

94. **Pirami L, Giache V, Becciolini A.** Analysis of HPV16, 18, 31, and 35 DNA in pre-invasive and invasive lesions of the uterine cervix. *J Clin Pathol* 1997;50:600–604.

95. **Bernard HU, Chan SY, Delius H.** Evolution of papillomaviruses. *Curr Top Microbiol Immunol* 1994;186:33–54.

96. **Einstein MH, Goldberg GL.** Human papillomavirus and cervical neoplasia. *Cancer Invest* 2002;20:1080–1085.

97. **Peitsaro P, Johansson B, Syrjanen S.** Integrated human papillomavirus type 16 is frequently found in cervical cancer precursors as demonstrated by a novel quantitative real-time PCR technique. *J Clin Microbiol* 2002;40:886–891.

98. **Arias-Pulido H, Peyton CL, Joste NE, Vargas H, Wheeler CM.** Human papillomavirus type 16 integration in cervical carcinoma *in situ* and in invasive cervical cancer. *J Clin Microbiol* 2006;44:1755–1762.

99. **Wentzensen N, Vinokurova S, von Knebel DM.** Systematic review of genomic integration sites of human papillomavirus genomes in epithelial dysplasia and invasive cancer of the female lower genital tract. *Cancer Res* 2004;64:3878–3884.

100. **Doorbar J, Ely S, Sterling J, McLean C, Crawford L.** Specific interaction between HPV-16 E1-E4 and cytokeratins results in collapse of the epithelial cell intermediate filament network. *Nature* 1991;352:824–827.

101. **Munger K, Phelps WC, Bubb V, Howley PM, Schlegal R.** The E6 and E7 genes of the human papillomavirus type 16 together are necessary and sufficient for transformation of human primary keratinocytes. *J Virol* 1989;63:4417–4421.

102. **Munger K, Basile JR, Duensing S, et al.** Biological activities and molecular targets of the human papillomavirus E7 oncoprotein. *Oncogene* 2001;20:7888–7898.

103. **Mantovani F, Banks L.** The human papillomavirus E6 protein and its contribution to malignant progression. *Oncogene* 2001;20:7874–7887.

104. **McCance DJ, Kopan R, Fuchs E, Laimins LA.** Human papillomavirus type 16 alters epithelial cell differentiation in vitro. *Proc Natl Acad Sci USA* 1988;85:7169–7173.

105. **Scheffner M, Werness BA, Huibregtse JM, Levine AJ, Howley PM.** The E6 oncoprotein encoded by human papillomavirus types 16 and 18 promotes the degradation of p53. *Cell* 1990;63:1129–1136.

106. **Paquette RL, Lee YY, Wilczynski SP, Karmakar A, Kizaki M, Miller CW, et al.** Mutations of p53 and human papillomavirus infection in cervical carcinoma. *Cancer* 1993;72:1272–1280.

107. Scheffner M, Takahashi T, Huibregtse JM, Minna JD, Howley PM. Interaction of the human papillomavirus type 16 E6 oncoprotein with wild-type and mutant p53 oncoprotein. *J Virol* 1992;66: 5100–5105.

108. Busby-Earle RMC, Steele CM, Williams AR, Cohen B, Bird CC. Papillomaviruses, p53 and cervical cancer. *Lancet* 1992;339: 1350–1366.

109. Milde-Langosch K, Albrecht K, Joram S, Schlechte H, Giessing M, Loning T. Presence and persistence of HPV infection and p53 mutation in cancer of the cervix uteri and the vulva. *Int J Cancer* 1995;63:639–645.

110. Bosch FX, Lorincz A, Munoz N, Meijer CJ, Shah KV. The causal relation between human papillomavirus and cervical cancer. *J Clin Pathol* 2002;55:244–265.

111. Duensing S, Munger K. Human papillomaviruses and centrosome duplication errors: modeling the origins of genomic instability. *Oncogene* 2002;21:6241–6248.

112. Klingelhutz A J, Foster SA and McDougall J K. Telomerase activation by the *E6* gene product of human papillomavirus type 16. *Nature* (London) 1996;380:79–82.

113. McMurray HR, McCance DJ. Human papillomavirus type 16 E6 activates TERT gene transcription through induction of *c-myc* and release of USF-mediated repression. *J Virol* 2003;77:9852–9861.

114. Zhang Y, Fan S, Meng Q, et al. *BRCA1* interaction with human papillomavirus oncoproteins. *J Biol Chem* 2005;280:33165–33177.

115. Dyson N, Howley PM, Munger K, Harlow E. The human papillomavirus-16E-oncoprotein is able to bind the retinoblastoma gene product. *Science* 1989;243:934–937.

116. Gage JR, Meyers C, Wettstein F O. The E7 proteins of the nononcogenic human papillomavirus type 6b (HPV-6b) and of the oncogenic HPV-16 differ in retinoblastoma protein binding and other properties. *J Virol* 1990;64:723–730.

117. Berezutskaya E, Yu B, Morozov A, Raychaudhuri P, Bagchi S. Differential regulation of the pocketdomains of the retinoblastoma family proteins by the HPV16 E7 oncoprotein. *Cell Growth Differ* 1997;8:1277–1286.

118. Boyer SN, Wazer DE, Band V. E7 protein of human papilloma virus-16 induces degradation of retinoblastoma protein through the ubiquitin-proteasome pathway. *Cancer Res* 1996;56:4620–4624.

119. Helt AM, Galloway DA. Mechanisms by which DNA tumor virus oncoproteins target the *Rb* family of pocket proteins. *Carcinogenesis* 2003;24:159–169.

120. Balsitis SJ, Sage J, Duensing S, Munger K, Jacks T, Lambert PF. Recapitulation of the effects of the human papillomavirus type 16 E7 oncogene on mouse epithelium by somatic *Rb* deletion and detection of pRb-independent effects of E7 in vivo. *Mol Cell Biol* 2003; 23:9094–9103.

121. De Villiers EM. Human pathogenic papillomavirus types: an update. *Curr Top Microbiol Immunol* 1994;186:13–31.

122. Woodworth CD, Doniger J, diPaola JA. Immortalization of human keratinocytes by various human papillomavirus DNAs corresponds to their association with cervical carcinoma. *J Virol* 1989;63: 159–164.

123. Barbosa MS, Shiegel R. The *E6* and *E7* genes of HPV 18 are sufficient for inducing two stage in vitro transformation of human keratinocytes. *Oncogene* 1990;43:1529–1532.

124. Fournier, N., Raj, K., Saudan, P. et al. Expression of human papillomavirus 16 E2 protein in *Schizosaccharomyces pombe* delays the initiation of mitosis. *Oncogene* 1999;18:4015–4021.

125. Nishimura A, Ono T, Ishimoto A, et al. Mechanisms of human papillomavirus E2-mediated repression of viral oncogene expression and cervical cancer cell growth inhibition. *J Virol* 2000;74: 3752–3760.

126. Bosch FX, Manos MM, Munoz N, Sherman M, Jansen AM, Peto J, et al. Prevalence of human papillomavirus in cervical cancer: a worldwide perspective. *J Natl Cancer Inst* 1995;87:796–802.

127. Bosch FX, de Sanjose S. The epidemiology of human papillomavirus infection and cervical cancer. *Dis Markers* 2007;23:213–227.

128. Reid R, Greenberg MD, Jenson AB, Husain M, Willet J, Daoud Y, et al. Sexually transmitted papillomaviral infections: 1. The anatomic distribution and pathologic grade of neoplastic lesions associated with different viral types. *Am J Obstet Gynecol* 1987;156:212–222.

129. Lorincz AT, Reid R, Jenson AB, Kurman RT. Human papillomavirus infection of the cervix: relative risk associations of 15 common anogenital types. *Obstet Gynecol* 1992;79:328–337.

130. Duggan MA, Benoit JL, McGregor SE, Nation JG, Inoue M, Stuart GC. The human papillomavirus status of 114 endocervical adenocarcinoma cases by dot-blot hybridization. *Hum Pathol* 1993;24:121–125.

131. Castellsague X, Diaz M, de Sanjose S, et al. Worldwide human papillomavirus etiology of cervical adenocarcinoma and its cofactors: implications for screening and prevention. *J Natl Cancer Inst* 2006;98:303–315.

132. Kurman RJ, Schiffman MH, Lancaster WD, Reid R, Jenson AB, Temple GF, et al. Analysis of individual human papillomavirus types in cervical neoplasia: a possible role for type 18 in rapid progression. *Am J Obstet Gynecol* 1988;159:293–296.

133. Barnes W, Woodworth G, Waggoner S, Stoler M, Jenson AB, Delgado G, et al. Rapid dysplastic transformation of human genital cells by human papillomavirus type 18. *Gynecol Oncol* 1990;38: 343–346.

134. Hildesheim A, Hadjimichael O, Schwartz PE, Wheeler CM, Barnes W, Lowell DM, et al. Risk factors for rapid-onset cervical cancer. *Am J Obstet Gynecol* 1999;180:571–577.

135. Berrington de Gonzalez A, Green J. Comparison of risk factors for invasive squamous cell carcinoma and adenocarcinoma of the cervix: collaborative reanalysis of individual data on 8097 women with squamous cell carcinoma and 1374 women with adenocarcinoma from 12 epidemiological studies. *Int J Cancer* 2007;120:885–91.

136. Stoler MH, Rhodes CR, Whitbeck A, Chow LT, Broker TR. Gene expression of HPV types 16 and 18 in cervical neoplasia. *UCLA Symp Mol Cell Biol New Ser* 1990;124A:1–11.

137. Winkelstein W, Selvin S. Cervical cancer in young Americans [Letter]. *Lancet* 1989;1:1385.

138. Burchell AN, Winer RL, de Sanjose S, Franco EL. Chapter 6: epidemiology and transmission dynamics of genital HPV infection. *Vaccine* 2006;24(suppl 3):S52–61.

139. Winer RL, Lee S-K, Hughes JP, Adam DE, Kiviat NB, Koutsky LA. Genital human papillomavirus infection: incidence and risk factors in a cohort of female university students. *Am J Epidemiol* 2003;157:218–226.

140. Collins S, Mazloomzadeh S, Winter H, Blomfield P, Bailey A, Young LS, et al. High incidence of cervical human papillomavirus infection in women during their first sexual relationship. *Br J Obstet Gynaecol* 2002;109:96–98.

141. Manhart LE, Koutsky LA. Do condoms prevent genital HPV infection, external genital warts, or cervical neoplasia? A meta-analysis. *Sex Transm Dis* 2002;29:725–735.

142. Baseman JG, Koutsky LA. The epidemiology of human papillomavirus infections. *J Clin Virol* 2005;32:S16–24.

143. Stanley M. Immune responses to human papillomavirus. *Vaccine* 2006;24:S16–22.

144. Plummer M, Schiffman M, Castle PE, Maucort-Boulch M, Wheeler CM. A 2-year prospective study of HPV persistence among women with ASCUS or LSIL cytology. *J Infect Dis* 2007;195: 1582–1589.

145. Schiffman M, Kjaer SK. Chapter 2: natural history of anogenital human papillomavirus infection and neoplasia. *J Natl Cancer Inst Monogr* 2003;31:14–19.

146. Strickler HD, Burk RD, Fazzari M, Anastos H, Minkoff H, Massad LS, et al. Natural history and possible reactivation of human papillomavirus in human immunodeficiency virus-positive women. *J Natl Cancer Inst* 2005;97:577–586.

147. Palefsky JM, Gillison ML, Strickler HD. Chapter 16: HPV vaccines in immunocompromised women and men. *Vaccine* 2006; 24:S140–146.

148. Harris TG, Burk RD, Palefsky JM, et al. Incidence of cervical squamous intraepithelial lesions associated with HIV serostatus, CD4 cell counts, and human papillomavirus test results. *JAMA* 2005;293:1471–1476.

149. Clifford GM, Goncalves MA, Franceschi S. Human papillomavirus types among women infected with HIV: a meta-analysis. *AIDS* 2006;20:2337–2344.

150. Castle PE, Solomon D, Schiffman M, Wheeler CM. Human papillomavirus type 16 infections and 2-year absolute risk of cervical precancer in women with equivocal or mild cytologic abnormalities. *J Natl Cancer Inst* 2005;97:1066–1071.

151. Bulkmans NW, Berkhof J, Bulk S, et al. High-risk HPV type-specific clearance rates in cervical screening. *Br J Cancer* 2007; 96:1419–1424.

152. **Remmick AJ, Walboomers JM, Helmerhorst TJ, Voorhofst FJ, Rosenthal L, Risse EKJ, et al.** The presence of persistent high-risk genotypes in dysplastic cervical lesions is associated with progressive disease: natural history up to 36 months. *Int J Cancer* 1995;61:306–311.

153. **Koshiol J, Lindsay L, Pimenta JM, Poole C, Jenkins D, Smith JS.** Persistent human papillomavirus infection and cervical neoplasia: a systematic review and meta-analysis. *Am J Epidem* 2008;168:123–137.

154. **Castle PE, Schiffman M, Herrero R, et al.** A prospective study of age trends in cervical human papillomavirus acquisition and persistence in Guanacaste, Costa Rica. *J Infect Dis* 2005;191:1808–1816.

155. **Moscicki AB, Ellenberg S, Farhat S, Xu J.** Persistenec of human papillomavirus infection in HIV-infected and -uninfected adolescent girls: risk factors and differences by phylogenetic type. *J Infect Dis* 2004;190:37–45.

156. **Castle PE, Wacholder S, Sherman ME, et al.** Absolute risk of a subsequent abnormal pap among oncogenic human papillomavirus DNA-positive, cytologically negative women. *Cancer* 2002;95:2145–2151.

157. **Lorincz AT, Castle PE, Sherman ME, et al.** Viral load of human papillomavirus and risk of CIN3 or cervical cancer. *Lancet* 2002;360:228–229.

158. **Ylitalo N, Sorensen P, Josefsson AM, et al.** Consistent high viral load of human papillomavirus 16 and risk of cervical carcinoma *in situ*: a nested case-control study. *Lancet* 2000;355:2194–2198.

159. **Josefsson AM, Magnusson PK, Ylitalo N, et al.** Viral load of human papilloma virus 16 as a determinant for development of cervical carcinoma *in situ*: a nested case-control study. *Lancet* 2000;355:2189–2193.

160. **Sherman ME, Wang SS, Wheeler CM, et al.** Determinants of human papillomavirus load among women with histological cervical intraepithelial neoplasia 3: dominant impact of surrounding low-grade lesions. *Cancer Epidemiol Biomarkers Prev* 2003;12:1038–1044.

161. **Bosch FX, de Sanjose S.** Chapter 1: human papillomavirus and cervical cancer – burden and assessment of causality. *J Natl Inst Monogr* 2003;31:3–13.

162. **Woodman CB, Collins S, Winter H, et al.** Natural history of cervical human papillomavirus infection in young women: a longitudinal cohort study. *Lancet* 2001;357:1831–1836.

163. **Richardson H, Kelsall G, Tellier P, et al.** The natural history of type-specific human papillomavirus infections in female university students. *Cancer Epidemiol Biomarkers Prev* 2003;12:485–490.

164. **Greenberg MD, Reid R, Schiffman M, Campion MJ, Precop SL, Berman NR, et al.** A prospective study of biopsy-confirmed cervical intraepithelial neoplasia grade I: colposcopic, cytological and virological risk factors for progression. *Journal of Lower Genital Tract Disease* 1999;3:104–109.

165. **Wang SS, Hildesheim A.** Viral and host factors in human papillomavirus persistence and progression. *J Natl Cancer Inst* 2003;35–40.

166. **Marshall JR, Graham S, Byers T, Swanson M, Brasure J.** Diet and smoking in the epidemiology of cancer cervix. *J Natl Cancer Inst* 1983;70:847–851.

167. **Slattery ML, Robison LM, Schuman KI, French TK, Abbott TM, Overall JC Jr, et al.** Cigarette smoking and exposure to passive smoke are risk factors for cervical cancer. *JAMA* 1989;261:1593–1598.

168. **Coker AL, Bond SM, Williams A, Gerasimova T, Pirisi L.** Active and passive smoking, high-risk papillomavirus and cervical neoplasia. *Cancer Detect Prev* 2002;26:121–128.

169. **Yang X, Jin G, Nakao Y, Rahimtula M, Pater MM, Pater A.** Malignant transformation of HPV 16-immortalized human endocervical cells by cigarette smoke condensate and characterization of multistage carcinogenesis. *Int J Cancer* 1996;65:338–344.

170. **Ho GY, Kadish AS, Burk RD, Basu J, Palan PR, Mikhail M, et al.** HPV 16 and cigarette smoking as risk factors for high-grade cervical intraepithelial neoplasia. *Int J Cancer* 1998;78:281–285.

171. **International Collaboration of Epidemiological Studies of Cervical Cancer.** Carcinoma of the cervix and tobacco smoking: collaborative reanalysis of individual data on 13 541 women with carcinoma of the cervix and 23 017 women without carcinoma of the cervix from 23 epidemiological studies. *Int J Cancer* 2006;118:1481–1495.

172. **Vaccarella S, Herrero R, Snijders PJ, Min D, Thomas JO, Nguyen TH, et al.** Smoking and human papillomavirus infection: pooled analysis of the International Agency for research on Cancer HPV Prevalence Surveys. *Int J Epidem* 2008;37:536–546.

173. **Hawthorn RJ, Murdoch JB, McLean AB, McKie RM.** Langerhan's cells and subtypes of human papillomavirus in cervical intraepithelial neoplasia. *BMJ* 1988:297:643–646.

174. **Viac J, Guerin-Reverchon I, Chardonnet Y, Bremond A.** Langerhan's cells and epithelial modifications in cervical intraepithelial neoplasia: correlation with human papillomavirus infection. *Immunobiology* 1990;180:328–338.

175. **Syrajanen K, Varyrynen M, Casren O, Yliskoski M, Mantijarvi R, Pyrhonen S, et al.** Sexual behavior of women with human papillomavirus (HPV) lesions of the uterine cervix. *Br J Vener Dis* 1984;60:243–248.

176. **Herrero R, Brinton LA, Reeves WC.** Sexual behaviour, venereal diseases, hygiene practices and invasive cervical cancer in a high risk population. *Cancer* 1990;65:380–386.

177. **Castle PE, Giuliano AR.** Chapter 4: genital tract infections, cervical inflammation and antioxidant nutrients-assessing their roles as human papillomavirus cofactors. *J Natl Inst Monogr* 2003;31:29–34.

178. **Zur Hausen H.** Human genital cancer: synergism between two virus infections or synergism between virus infection and initiating events? *Lancet* 1982;2:1370–1372.

179. **Tran-Thanh D, Provencher D, Koushik A, Duarte-Franco E, Kessous A, Drouin P, et al.** Herpes simplex virus type II is not a cofactor to human papillomavirus in cancer of the uterine cervix. *Am J Obstet Gynecol* 2003;188:129–134.

180. **Matsumoto K, Yasugi T, Oki A, Hoshiai H, Taketani Y, Kawana T.** Are smoking and chlamydial infection risk factors for CIN? Different results after adjustment HPV DNA and antibodies. *Br J Cancer* 2003;89:831–833.

181. **Dhanwada KR, Garrett L, Smith P, Thompson KD, Doster A, Jones C.** Characterization of human keratinocytes transformed by high risk human papillomavirus types 16 or 18 and herpes simplex virus type 2. *J Gen Virol* 1993;74:955–963.

182. **Samoff E, Koumans EH, Markowitz LE, Sternberg M, Sawyer MK, Swan D, et al.** Association of *Chlamydia trachomatis* with persistence of high-risk human papillomavirus in a cohort of female adolescents. *Am J Epidemiol* 2005;162:668–675.

183. **Castle PE, Escoffery C, Schachter J, Rattray C, Schiffman M, Moncada J, et al.** Chlamydia trachomatis, herpes simplex virus 2, and human T-cell lymphotrophic virus type 1 are not associated with grade of cervical neoplasia in Jamaican colposcopy patients. *Sex Transm Dis* 2003;30:575–580.

184. **Smith JS, Bosetti C, Munoz N, et al.** Chlamydia trachomatis and invasive cervical cancer: a pooled analysis of the IARC multicentric case-control study. *Int J Cancer* 2004;111:431–439.

185. **Schneider A, Holtz M, Gissmann L.** Increased prevalence of human papillomavirus in the lower genital tract of pregnant women. *Int J Cancer* 1987;40:198–201.

186. **Rando RF, Lindheim S, Hasty L, Sedlacek TV, Woodland M, Eder C.** Increased frequency of detection of human papillomavirus deoxyribonucleic acid in exfoliated cervical cells during pregnancy. *Am J Obstet Gynecol* 1989;161:50–55.

187. **Brinton LA, Reeves WC, Brenes MM, Herrero R, de Britton RC, Gaitan E, et al.** Parity as a risk for cervical cancer. *Am J Epidemiol* 1989;130:486–496.

188. **Munoz N, Franceschi S, Bosetti C, Moreno V, Herrero R, Smith JS, et al.** Role of parity and human papillomavirus in cervical cancer: the IARC multicentric case-control study. *Lancet* 2002;359:1093–1101.

189. **Castle PE, Walker JL, Schiffman M, Wheeler CM.** Hormonal contraceptive use, pregnancy and parity, and the risk of cervical intraepithelial neoplasia 3 among oncogenic HPV DNA-positive women with equivocal or mildly abnormal cytology. *Int J of Cancer* 2005;117:1007–1012.

190. **Hildesheim A, Reeves WC, Brinton LA, Lavery C, Brenes M, De La Guardia ME, et al.** Association of oral contraceptive use and human papilloma viruses in invasive cervical cancer. *Int J Cancer* 1990;45:860–864.

191. **Ye Z, Thomas DB, Ray RM.** Combined oral contraceptive and risk of cervical carcinoma *in situ*: WHO collaborative study of neoplasia and steroid contraceptives. *Int J Epidemiol* 1995;24:19–26.

192. **Moreno V, Bosch FX, Munoz N, Meijer CJ, Shah KV, Walboomers JM, Herrero R, Franceschi S.** Effect of oral contraceptives on risk of cervical cancer in women with human papillomavirus infection: the IARC multicentric case-control study. *Lancet* 2002;359:1085–1092.

193. **Smith JS, Green J, Berrington DG, Appleby P, Peto J, Plummer M, Franceschi S, Beral V.** Cervical cancer and use of hormonal contraceptives: a systematic review. *Lancet* 2003;361:1159–1167.

194. **Castellsague X, Munoz N.** Chapter 3: cofactors in human papillomavirus carcinogenesis – role of parity, oral contraceptives, and tobacco smoking. *J Natl Cancer Inst Monogr* 2003;20–28.

195. **Anon.** Cervical cancer and hormonal contraceptives: collaborative reanalysis of individual data for 16,573 women with cervical cancer and 35,509 without cervical cancer from 24 epidemilogical studies. *Lancet* 2007;370:1609–1621.

196. **de Villiers EM.** Relationship between steroid hormone contraceptives and HPV, cervical intraepithelial neoplasia and cervical carcinoma. *Int J Cancer* 2003;103:705–708.

197. **Coker AL, Hulka BS, McCann MF, Walton LA.** Barrier methods of contraception and cervical intraepithelial neoplasia. *Contraception* 1992;45:1–10.

198. **Richardson H, Abrahamowicz M, Tellier PP, Kelsall G, Hansson, du BR, Ferenczy A, et al.** Modifiable risk factors associated with clearance of type-specific cervical human papillomavirus infections in a cohort of university students. *Cancer Epidemiol Biomarkers Prev* 2005;14:1149–1156.

199. **Shew ML, Fortenberry JD, Tu W, Juliar BE, Batteiger BE, Qadadri B, et al.** Association of condom use, sexual behaviors, and sexually transmitted infections with the duration of genital HPV infection among adolescent women. *Arch Pediatr Adolesc Med* 2006;160:151–156.

200. **Hogewoning CJ, Bleeker MC, van den Brule AJ, Voorhurst FJ, Snijders PJ, Berkhof J, et al.** Condom use promotes regression of cervical intraepithelial neoplasia and clearance of human papillomavirus: a randomised clinical trial. *Int J Cancer* 2003;107:811–816.

201. **Sillman F, Stanek A, Sedlis A, Rosenthal J, Lanks KW, Buchhagen D, et al.** The relationship between human papillomavirus and lower genital intraepithelial neoplasia in immunosuppressed women. *Am J Obstet Gynecol* 1984;150:300–308.

202. **Schafer A, Friedmann W, Mielke M, Schwartlander B, Bell JA.** The increased frequency of cervical dysplasia-neoplasia in women infected with the human immunodeficiency virus is related to the degree of immunosuppression. *Am J Obstet Gynecol* 1991;164:593–599.

203. **Conley LJ, Ellerbrook TV, Bush TJ, Chiasson MA, Sawo D, Wright TC.** HIV-1 infection and risk of vulvovaginal and perianal condylomata acuminata and intraepithelial neoplasia: a prospective cohort study. *Lancet* 2002;359:108–113.

204. **Harris TG, Burk RD, Palefsky JM, et al.** Incidence of cervical squamous intraepithelial lesions associated with HIV serostatus, CD4 cell counts, and human papillomavirus test results. *JAMA* 2005;293:1471–1476.

205. **Palefsky JM, Gillison ML, Strickler HD.** Chapter 16: HPV vaccines in immunocompromised women and men. *Vaccine* 2006;24:S140–146.

206. **Clifford GM, Goncalves MA, Franceschi S.** Human papillomavirus types among women infected with HIV: a meta-analysis. *AIDS* 2006;20:2337–2344.

207. **Wylie-Rosett JA, Romney SL, Slagle NS, Wassertheil-Smoller S, Miller GL, Palan PR, et al.** Influence of vitamin A on cervical dysplasia and carcinoma *in situ*. *Nutr Cancer* 1984;6:49–57.

208. **Garcia-Closas R, Castellsague X, Bosch X, Gonzalez CA.** The role of diet and nutrition in cervical carcinogenesis: a review of recent evidence. *Int J Cancer* 2005;117:629–637.

209. **Ziegler RG, Brinton LA, Hamman RF, Lehman HF, Levine RS, Mallin K, et al.** Diet and the risk of invasive cancer among white women in the United States. *Am J Epidemiol* 1990;132:432–445.

210. **Butterworth CE, Hatch KD, Macaluso M, Cole P, Sauberlich HE, Soong SJ, et al.** Folate deficiency and cervical dysplasia. *JAMA* 1992;267:528–533.

211. **Sedjo RL, Papenfuss MR, Craft NE, Giuliano AR.** Effect of plasma micronutrients on clearance of oncogenic human papillomavirus (HPV) infection (United States). *Cancer Causes Control* 2003;14:319–326.

212. **Frazer IH.** HPV vaccines and the prevention of cervical cancer. *Update on Cancer Therapeutics* 2008;3:43–48.

213. **Barr E, Sings HL.** Prophylactic HPV vaccines: new interventions for cancer control. *Vaccine* 2008;26:6844–6857.

214. **Hughes JP, Garnett GP, Koutsky L.** The theoretical population-level impact of a prophylactic human papilloma virus vaccine. *Epidemiology* 2002;13:631–639.

215. **Chesson HW, Blandford JM, Gift TL, Tao G, Irwin KL.** The estimated direct medical cost of sexually transmitted diseases among American youth, 2000. *Perspect Sex Reprod Health* 2004;36:11–19.

216. **Lacey C, Lowndes CM, Shah KV.** Chapter 4: burden and management of non-cancerous HPV-related conditions: HPV-6/11 disease. *Vaccine* 2006;24:S35–41.

217. **Hughes JP, Garnett GP, Koutsky L.** The theoretical population-level impact of a prophylactic human papilloma virus vaccine. *Epidemiology* 2002;13:631–639.

218. **Zhou J, Sun XY, Stenzel DJ, Frazer IH.** Expression of vaccinia recombinant HPV 16 L1 and L2 ORF proteins in epithelial cells is sufficient for assembly of HPV virion-like particles. *Virology* 1991;185:251–257.

219. **Kirnbauer R, Taub J, Greenstone H, Roden R, Durst M, Gissmann L, et al.** Efficient self-assembly of human papillomavirus type 16 L1 and L1–L2 into virus-like particles. *J Virol* 1993;67(12, Dec.):6929–6936.

220. **Harper DM, Franco EL, Wheeler CM, Moscicki AB, Romanowski B, Roteli-Martins CM, et al.** Sustained efficacy up to 4.5 years of a bivalent L1 virus-like particle vaccine against human papillomavirus types 16 and 18: follow-up from a randomised control trial. *Lancet* 2006;367:1247–1255.

221. **Mao C, Koutsky LA, Ault KA, Wheeler CM, Brown DR, Wiley DJ, et al.** Efficacy of human papillomavirus-16 vaccine to prevent cervical intraepithelial neoplasia: a randomized controlled trial. *Obstet Gynecol* 2006;107:18–27.

222. **Wilderoff L, Schiffman M, Haderer P, Armstrong A, Greer CE, Manos MM, et al.** Seroactivity to human papillomavirus types 16, 18, 31 and 45 virus-like particles in a case-control study of cervical squamous intraepithelial lesions. *J Infect Dis* 1999;180:1424–1428.

223. **Harro CD, Pang YY, Roden RB, Hildesheim A, Wang Z, Reynolds MJ, et al.** Safety and immunogenicity trial in adult volunteers of human papillomavirus 16 L1 virus-like particle vaccine. *J Natl Cancer Inst* 2001;93:284–292.

224. **Pinto LA, Edwards J, Castle PE, Harro CD, Lowy DR, Schiller JT, et al.** Cellular immune responses to human papillomavirus (HPV)-16 L1 in healthy volunteers immunized with recombinant HPV-16 L1 virus-like particles. *J Infect Dis* 2003;188:327–338.

225. **Jansen KU, Rosolowsky M, Schultz LD, Markus HZ, Cook JC, Donnelly JJ, et al.** Vaccination with yeast-expressed cottontail rabbit papillomavirus (CRPV) virus-like particles protects rabbits from CRPVinduced papilloma formation. *Vaccine* 1995;13:1509–1514.

226. **Villa LL, Costa RLR, Petta CA, Andrade RP, Ault KA, Giuliano AR, et al.** Prophylactic quadrivalent human papillomavirus (types 6, 11, 16 and 18) L1 virus-like particle vaccine in young women: a randomised double-blind placebocontrolled multicentre phase II efficacy trial. *Lancet Oncol* 2005;6:271–278.

227. **Garland SM, Hernandez-Avila M, Wheeler CM, Perez G, Harper DM, Leodolter S, et al.** Quadrivalent vaccine against human papillomavirus to prevent anogenital diseases. *N Engl J Med* 2007;356:1928–1943.

228. **The FUTURE II Study Group.** Quadrivalent vaccine against human papillomavirus to prevent high-grade cervical lesions. *N Engl J Med* 2007;356:1915–1927.

229. **Barr E, Gause CK, Bautista OM.** Impact of a prophylactic quadrivalent human papillomavirus (types 6, 11, 16, 18) L1 virus-like particle vaccine in a sexually active population of North American women. *Am J Obstet Gynecol* 2008;198:261.e1–261.e11.

230. **Gardasil package insert.** Released June 2006. Accessed at: http://wwwfdagov/cber/label/hpvmer060806LBhtm 2006.

231. **Markowitz LE.** Quadrivalent HPV vaccine update. ACIP 2007 February 22, 2007. Available at: http://www.cdc.gov/vaccines/recs/acip/slidesfeb07.htm. Accessed August 2008.

232. **T.F. Schwarz, G. Dubin, the HPV Vaccine Study Investigators for Adult Women.** Human papillomavirus (HPV) 16/18 L1 AS04 virus-like particle (VLP) cervical cancer vaccine is immunogenic and well-tolerated 18 months after vaccination in women up to age 55 years [abstract]. *J Clin Oncol* 2007 ASCO Annual Meeting Proceedings Part I 2007;25. Abstract 3007.

233. **Luna J, Saah A, Hood S, Bautista O, Barr E.** Safety, efficacy, and immunogenicity of quadrivalent HPV vaccine (Gardasil) in women aged 24–45. 24th International Papillomavirus Congress 2007 November 3–9. China: Beijing, 2007.

234. **Harper DM, Franco EL, Wheeler C, Ferris DG, Jenkins D, Schuind A, et al.** Efficacy of a bivalent L1 virus-like particle vaccine in prevention of infection with human papillomavirus types 16 and 18 in young women: a randomised controlled trial. *Lancet* 2004;364:1757–1765.

235. **Wright TC, Bosch FX, Franco EL, Cuzick J, Schiller JT, Garnett GP, Meheus A.** Chapter 30: HPV vaccines and screening in the prevention of cervical cancer; conclusions from a 2006 workshop of international experts. *Vaccine* 2006;24:251–261.

236. **Ault KA.** Effect of prophylactic human papillomavirus L1 virus-like-particle vaccine on risk of cervical intraepithelial neoplasia grade 2, grade 3, and adenocarcinoma *in situ:* a combined analysis of four randomised clinical trials. *Lancet* 2007;369:1861–1868.

237. **Hildesheim A, Herrero R, Wacholder S, Rodriguez AC, Solomon D, Bratti MC, et al.** Effect of human papillomavirus 16/18 L1 virus-like particle vaccine among young women with preexisting infection: a randomized trial. *JAMA* 2007;298:743–753.

238. **Olsson S-E, Villa LL, Costa R, Petta C, Andrade R, Malm C, et al.** Induction of immune memory following administration of a prophylactic quadrivalent human papillomavirus (HPV) types 6/11/16/18 L1 virus-like-particle vaccine. *Vaccine* 2007;25: 4931–4939.

239. **Fraser C, Tomassini JE, Xi L, Golm G, Watson M, Giuliano AR, Barr E, Ault K.** Modeling the long-term antibody response of a human papillomavirus (HPV) virus-like particle (VLP) type 16 prophylactic vaccine. *Vaccine* 2007;25:4324–4333.

240. **Saslow D, Castle PE, Cox JT, Davey DD, Einstein MH, Ferris DG, et al.** American Cancer Society Guideline for human papillomavirus (HPV) vaccine use to prevent cervical cancer and its precursors. *CA Cancer J Clin* 2007;57:7–28.

241. **Zimet GD, Shew ML, Kahn JA.** Appropriate use of cervical cancer vaccine. *Annual Review of Medicine* 2008;59:223–236.

242. **Centers for Disease Control and Prevention.** 2007. Quadrivalent human papillomavirus vaccine: recommendations of the Advisory Committee on Immunization Practices (ACIP). *MMWR* 56(No. RR-2): 1–26.

243. **Villa LL, Ault K, Giuliano AR, Costa RLR, Petta CA, Andrade RP, et al.** Immunologic responses following administration of a vaccine targeting human papillomavirus types 6, 11, 16 and 18. *Vaccine* 2006;24:5571–5583.

244. **Block SL, Nolan T, Sattler C, Barr E, Giacoletti KE, Marchant CD, et al.** Comparison of the immunogenicity and reactogenicity of a prophylactic quadrivalent human papillomavirus (types 6, 11, 16, and 18) L1 virus-like particle vaccine in male and female adolescents and young adult women. *Pediatrics* 2006;118:2135–2145.

245. **Reisinger KS, Block SL, Lazcano-Ponce E, Samakoses R, Esser MT, Erick J, et al.** Safety and persistent immunogenicity of a quadrivalent human papillomavirus types 6, 11, 16, 18 L1 virus-like particle vaccine in preadolescents and adolescents: a randomized controlled trial. *Ped Infect Dis J* 2007;26:201–209.

246. **Wright TC, Huh WK, Monk BJ, Smith JS, Ault K, Herzog TJ.** Age considerations when vaccinating against HPV. *Gynecol Oncol* 2008;109:S40–S47.

247. **Elbasha EH, Dasbach EJ, Insinga RP.** Model for assessing human papillomavirus vaccination strategies. *Emerg Infect Dis* 2007;13: 28–41.

248. **Garnett GP, Kim JJ, French K, et al.** Chapter 21: modelling the impact of HPV vaccines on cervical cancer and screening programmes. *Vaccine* 2006;24:178–186.

249. **Kulasingam SL, Myers ER.** Potential health and economic impact of adding a human papillomavirus vaccine to screening programs. *JAMA* 2003;290:781–789.

250. **Sanders GD, Taira AV.** Cost effectiveness of a potential vaccine for human papillomavirus. *Emerg Infect Dis* 2003;9:37–48.

251. **Taira AV, Neukermans CP, Sanders GD.** Evaluating human papillomavirus vaccination programs. *Emerg Infect Dis* 2004;10: 1915–1923.

252. **Kim JJ, Goldie SJ.** Health and economic implications of HPV vaccination in the United States. *N Eng J Med* 2008;359:821–832.

253. **Joura EA, Leodolter S, Hernandez-Avila M, et al.** Efficacy of a quadrivalent prophylactic human papillomavirus (types 6, 11, 16, and 18) L1 virus-like-particle vaccine against high-grade vulval and vaginal lesions: a combined analysis of three randomised clinical trials. *Lancet* 2007;369:1693–1702.

254. **Garnett P, Waddell H.** Public health paradoxes and the epidemiological impact of an HPV vaccine. *J Clin Virol* 2000;19:101–111.

255. **Stanley MA.** Progress in prophylactic and therapeutic vaccines for human papillomavirus infection. *Expert Rev Vaccines* 2003;2: 381–389.

256. **Zimet GD, Liddon N, Rosenthal SL, et al.** Chapter 24: psychosocial aspects of vaccine acceptability. *Vaccine* 2006;24(suppl 3): 201–209.

257. **Liddon N.** *Record of the meeting of the Advisory Committee on Immunization Practices: behavioral issues related to HPV vaccination.* 2006. Available at http://www.cdc.gov/nip/ACIP/minutes/ acip_min_feb06.pdf.

258. **Lo B.** HPV vaccine and adolescents' sexual activity. *BMJ* 2006; 332:1106–1107.

259. **Constantine NA, Jerman P.** Acceptance of human papillomavirus vaccination among Californian parents of daughters: a representative statewide analysis. *J Adolesc Health* 2007;40:108–115.

260. **Dell DL, Chen H, Ahmad F, Stewart DE.** Knowledge about HPV among adolescents. *Obstet Gynecol* 2000;96:653–656.

261. **Waller J, McCaffery K, Forrest S, et al.** Awareness of HPV among women attending a well woman clinic. *Sex Trans Infect* 2003;79: 320–322.

262. **Colgrove J.** The ethics and politics of compulsory HPV vaccination. *N Eng J Med* 2006;355:2389–2391.

263. **Zimmerman RK.** Ethical analysis of HPV vaccine policy options. *Vaccine* 2006;24:4812–4820.

264. **Charo RA.** Politics, parents, and prophylaxis—mandating HPV vaccination in the United States. *N Engl J Med* 2007;356:1905–1908.

265. **Gostin LO, DeAngelis CD.** Mandatory HPV vaccination: public health vs private wealth. *JAMA* 2007;297:1921–1923.

266. **Javitt G, Berkowitz D, Gostin LO.** Assessing Mandatory HPV vaccination: who should call the shots. *J Law Med Ethics* 2008; 36:384–395.

267. **Ponten J, Adami HO, Bergstrom R, Dillner J, Friberg LG, Gustafsson L, et al.** Strategies for global control of cervical cancer. *Int J Cancer* 1995;60:1–26.

268. **Gustafsson L, Ponten J, Bergstrom R, Adami HO.** International incidence rates of invasive cervical cancer before cytological screening. *Int J Cancer* 1997;71:159–165.

269. **Anon.** *Cervix cancer screening.* Lyon: IARC Press, IARC Handbooks of Cancer Prevention, 2005.

270. **Kitchener HC, Castle PE, Cox JT.** Chapter 7: achievements and limitations of cervical cytology screening. *Vaccine* 2006;24: S63–70.

271. **Cook GA, Draper GJ.** Trends in cervical cancer and carcinoma-in-situ in Great Britain. *Br J Cancer* 1984;503:67–75.

272. **Carmichael JA, Clarke DH, Moher D.** Cervical cancer in women aged 34 years and younger. *Am J Obstet Gynecol* 1989;154:264–269.

273. **Koss L.** The Papanicolaou test for cervical cancer detection: a triumph and a tragedy. *JAMA* 1989;261:737–743.

274. **Figge DC, Bennington JL, Schweid AI.** Cervical cancer after initial negative and atypical vaginal cytology. *Am J Obstet Gynecol* 1970; 108:422–428.

275. **Gay JD, Donaldson LD, Goellner JR.** False negative results in cervical cytologic studies. *Acta Cytol* 1985;29:1043–1046.

276. **Janerich DT, Hadjimichael O, Schwartz PE, Lowell DM, Meigs JW, Merino MJ, et al.** The screening histories of women with invasive cancer, Connecticut. *Am J Public Health* 1995;85:791–794.

277. **Schwartz PE, Hadjimichael O, Lowell DM, Merino MJ, Janerich D.** Rapidly progressive cervical cancer: the Connecticut experience. *Am J Obstet Gynecol* 1996;175:1105–1109.

278. **Hildesheim A, Hadjimichael O, Schwartz PE, Wheeler CM, Barnes W, Lowell DM, et al.** Risk factors for rapid-onset cervical cancer. *Am J Obstet Gynecol* 1999;180:571–577.

279. **U.S. Preventive Services Task Force.** Screening for cervical cancer. *Ann Intern Med* 1990;113:214–226.

280. **Wilkinson EJ.** Pap smears and screening for cervical neoplasia. *Clin Obstet Gynecol* 1990;33:817–825.

281. **Fahey MT, Irwig L, Macaskill P.** Meta-analysis of Pap-test accuracy. *Am J Epidemiol* 1995;141:680–689.

282. **Nanda K, McCrory DC, Myers ER, et al.** Accuracy of the Papanicolaou test in screening for and follow-up of cervical cytologic abnormalities: a systematic review. *Ann Intern Med* 2000;132:810–819.

283. **Bjerre B.** Invasive cervical cancer in a thoroughly screened population. *J Exp Clin Res* 1990;9(suppl):276.

284. **Kristensen GB, Skyggebjerg KD, Holund B, Holm K, Hansen MK.** Analysis of smears obtained within three years of diagnosis of invasive cervical cancer. *Acta Cytol* 1991;35:47–50.

285. **Boscha MC, Rietweld-Scheffers PEM, Boon ME.** Characteristics of false-negative smears in the normal screening population. *Acta Cytol* 1992;36:711–716.

286. **Sherman ME, Kelly D.** High-grade squamous intraepithelial lesions and invasive cancer following the report of three negative Papanicolaou smears: screening failure or rapid progression. *Mod Pathol* 1992;5:327–342.

287. **Agency for Health Care Policy and Research.** Evaluation of cervical cytology: evidence report/technology assessment (no. 5) Rockville, MD: AHCPR, January 1999. Online monograph: http://www.ahcpr.gov/clinic/epcsums/cervsumm.htm.

288. **Martin-Hirsch P, Lilford R, Jarvis G, Kitchener HC.** Efficacy of cervical-smear collection devices: a systematic review and meta-analysis. *Lancet* 1999;354:1763–1770.

289. **Sawaya GF, Kerlikowske K, Lee NC, Gildengorin G, Washington AE.** Frequency of cervical smear abnormalities within 3 years of normal cytology. *Obstet Gynecol* 2000;96:219–223.

290. **Corkill M, Knapp D, Hutchinson ML.** Improved accuracy for cervical cytology with the ThinPrep method and the endocervical brush-spatula collection procedure. *Journal of Lower Genital Tract Disease* 1998;2:12–16.

291. **Vikki M, Pakkala E, Hakama M.** Risk of cervical cancer after a negative Pap smear. *J Med Screen* 1999;6:103–107.

292. **Klinkhamer PJ, Meerding WJ, Rosier PF, Hanselaar AG.** Liquid-based cervical cytology: a review of the literature with methods of evidence-based medicine. *Cancer (Cancer Cytopathol)* 2003;99: 263–271.

293. **Coste J, Cochand-Priollet B, de Cremoux P, Le Gales C, Cartier I, Molinie V, et al.** Cross sectional study of conventional cervical smear, monolayer cytology, and human papillomavirus DNA testing for cervical cancer screening. *BMJ* 2003;326:733–737. Available online at http://bmj.com/cgi/reprint/326/7392/733.pdf.

294. **Payne N, Chilcott J, McCoogan E.** *Liquid-based cytology in cervical screening: a report by the School of Health and Related Research (ScHARR), the University of Sheffield, for the NCCHTA on behalf of NICE.* Sheffield, UK: Trent Institute for Health Services Research, 2000.

295. **Sheets EE, Constantine NM, Dinisco S, Dean B, Cibas ES.** Colposcopically-directed biopsies provide a basis for comparing the accuracy of Thinprep and Papanicolaou smears. *J Gynecol Tech* 1995;1:27–34.

296. **Lee KR, Ashfaq R, Birdsong GG, Corkill ME, McIntosh KM, Inhorn SL.** Comparison of conventional Papanicolaou smears and a fluid-based, thin layer system for cervical cancer screening. *Obstet Gynecol* 1997;90:278–284.

297. **Roberts JM, Gurley AM, Thurloe JK, Bowditch R, Laverty CR.** Evaluation of the ThinPrep test as an adjunct to the conventional Pap smear. *Med J Aust* 1997;167:466–469.

298. **Papillo JL, Zarka MA, St. John TL.** Evaluation of the ThinPrep Pap test in clinical practice: a seven-month 16,314 case experience in northern Vermont. *Acta Cytol* 1998;42:203–208.

299. **Hutchinson ML, Zahniser DJ, Sherman ME, Herrero R, Alfaro M, Bratti MC, et al.** Utility of liquid-based cytology for cervical carcinoma screening: results of a population-based study conducted in a region of Costa Rica with a high incidence of cervical carcinoma. *Cancer* 1999;87:48–55.

300. **Diaz-Rosario LA, Kabawat SE.** Performance of a fluid-based, thin-layer Papanicolaou smear method in the clinical setting of an independent laboratory and an outpatient screening population in New England. *Arch Pathol Lab Med* 1999;123:817–821.

301. **Park IA, Lee SN, Chae SW, Park KH, Kim JW, Lee HP.** Comparing the accuracy of ThinPrep Pap tests and conventional Papanicolaou smears on the basis of the histologic diagnosis: a clinical study of women with cervical abnormalities. *Acta Cytol* 2001;45:519–524.

302. **Limaye A, Connor AJ, Huang X, Luff R.** Comparative analysis of conventional Papanicolaou tests and a fluid-based thin-layer method. *Arch Pathol Lab Med* 2003;127:200–204.

303. **Davey E, Barratt A, Irwig L, Chan SF, Macaskill P, Mannes P, et al.** Effect of study design and quality on unsatisfactory rates, cytology classifications, and accuracy in liquid-based versus conventional cervical cytology: a systematic review. *Lancet* 2006;367: 122–132.

304. **Davey E, Irwig L, Macaskill P, D'Assuncoa J, Richards A, Farnsworth A.** Accuracy of reading liquid based cytology slides using the ThinPrep Imager compared with conventional cytology: prospective study. *BMJ* 2007;335:31–5.

305. **Australian Health Technology Advisory Committee.** Review of automated and semi-automated cervical screening devices (monograph online). Canberra: Commonwealth Department of Health and Family Services, 1988. Available online at http://www.csp.nsw.gov.au/downloads/review_automated_sem.pdf.

306. **Broadstock M.** Effectiveness and cost effectiveness of automated and semi-automated cervical screening devices: a systematic review. New Zealand health technology assessment report, vol. 3 (monograph outline). Christchurch, NZ: Clearing House for Health Outcomes and Health Technology Assessment, 2000. Available online at http://nzhta.chmeds.ac.nz.nzhtainfo/csv3n1.pdf.

307. **National Institute for Clinical Excellence.** Final appraisal consultation document: guidance on the use of liquid-based cytology for cervical screening (review of existing guidance Number 5) (monograph online). London: NICE, 2003. Available online at http://www.nice.org.uldDocref.asp?d=82877.

308. **National Institute for Clinical Excellence.** Guidance on the use of liquid based cytology for cervical screening. London: NICE, 2002. (Technology appraisal guidance No 5.) http://www.nice.org.uk/page.aspx?o=82877

309. **National Institute Clinical Excellence.** Liquid based cytology in cervical screening: an updated rapid and systematic review. London: NICE, 2003. (Technology appraisal guidance No 69.) http://guidance.nice.org.uk/page.aspx?o=65586

310. **Noorani HZ.** Assessment of techniques for cervical cancer screening (monograph online). Ottawa, ON: Canadian Coordinating Office for Health Technology Assessment, 1997. Available online at http://www.ccohta.ca/entry_e.html.

311. **Scottish Cervical Screening Programme.** Steering group report on the feasibility of introducing liquid-based cytology (monograph online). Edinburgh: Scottish Cervical Screening Programme, 2002. Available online at http://www.omni.ac.uk/browse/mesh/detail/C0010818L0010818.html.

312. **U.S. Preventive Services Task Force.** Screening cervical cancer: update, 2003 release (monograph online). Rockville, MD: Agency for Healthcare Research and Quality, 2003. Available online at http://www.ahrq.gov/clinic/uspstf/uspcerv.htm.

313. **Saslow D, Runowicz C, Solomon D, Moscicki AB, Smith RA, Eyre HJ, et al.** American Cancer Society cervical cancer screening guidelines 2002. *CA Cancer J Clin* 2002;52:375–376.

314. **Colgan TJ.** Programmatic assessments of the clinical effectiveness of gynecologic liquid-based cytology: the ayes have it. *Cancer (Cancer Cytopathol)* 2003;99:259–262.

315. **Moss SM, Gray A, Marteau T, Legood R, Henstock E, Maissi E.** Evaluation of HPV/LBC cervical screening pilot studies. Report to the Department of Health, October 2004. Available at http://www.cancerscreening.nhs.uk/cervical/evaluation-hpv-2006feb.pdf.

316. **NHS Information Centre.** Cervical screening programme. December 2006. Available at http://www.ic.nhs.uk/pubs/csp0506

317. **Williams AR.** Liquid-based cytology and conventional smears compared over two 12-month periods. *Cytopathology* 2006; 17:82–85.

318. **Sawaya GF, Sox HC.** Trials that matter: liquid-based cervical cytology: disadvantages seem to outweigh advantages. *Ann Intern Med* 2007;147:668–669.

319. **Arbyn M, Bergeron C, Klinkhamer P, Martin-Hirsch P, Siebers AG, Bulten J.** Liquid compared with conventional cervical cytology:

a systematic review and meta-analysis. *Obstet Gynecol* 2008;111; 167–177.

320. **Editorial.** Evidence-based medicine versus liquid-based cytology. *Obstet Gynecol* 2008;111;2–3.

321. **Ronco G, Cuzick J, Pierotti P, Cariaggi MP, Palma PD, Naldoni C, et al.** Accuracy of liquid based cytology versus conventional cytology: overall results of the new technologies for cervical screening (NTCC) randomised controlled trial. *BMJ* 2007;335:28–31.

322. **Siebers AG, Klinkhamer PJ, Arbyn M, Raifu AO, Massuger L F, Bulten J.** Cytologic detection of cervical abnormalities using liquid-based compared with conventional cytology: a randomized controlled trial. *Obstet Gynecol* 2008;112:1327–1334.

323. **Denton KJ.** Liquid based cytology in cervical cancer screening. *BMJ* 2007;335;1–2.

324. **Wright TC, Sun XW, Koulos J.** Comparison of management algorithms for the evaluation of women with low-grade cytologic abnormalities. *Obstet Gynecol* 1995;85:202–210.

325. **Kinney WK, Manos MM, Hurley LB, Ransley JE.** Where's the high grade cervical neoplasia? The importance of minimally abnormal Papanicolaou diagnoses. *Obstet Gynecol* 1998;91:973–976.

326. **Stoler MH, Schiffman M.** Interobserver reproducibility of cervical cytologic and histologic interpretations: realistic estimates from the ASCUS-LSIL Triage Study. *JAMA* 2001;285:1500–1505.

327. **Sherman ME, Solomon D, Schiffman M.** Qualification of an ASCUS: a comparison of equivocal LSIL and equivocal HSIL cervical cytology in the ASCUS LSIL Triage Study. *Am J Clin Pathol* 2001;116:386–394.

328. **Sherman ME, Schiffman M, Cox JT.** Effects of age and human papilloma viral load on colposcopy triage: date from the randomized Atypical Squamous Cells of Undetermined Significance/Low-Grade Squamous Intraepithelial Lesion Triage Study (ALTS). *J Natl Cancer Inst* 2002;94:102–107.

329. **Schiffman M, Solomon D.** Findings to date from the ASCUS-LSIL Triage Study (ALTS). *Arch Pathol Lab Med* 2003;127:946–949.

330. **Cox JT, Schiffman M, Solomon D.** Prospective follow-up suggests similar risk of subsequent cervical intraepithelial neoplasia grade 2 or 3 among women with cervical intraepithelial neoplasia grade 1 or negative colposcopy and directed biopsy. *Am J Obstet Gynecol* 2003;188:1406–1412.

331. **Guido R, Schiffman M, Solomon D, Burke L.** Postcolposcopy management strategies for women referred with low-grade squamous intraepithelial lesions or human papillomavirus DNA-positive atypical squamous cells of undetermined significance: a two-year prospective study. *Am J Obstet Gynecol* 2003;188:1401–1405.

332. **Wright TC Jr, Cox JT, Massad LS, Twiggs LB, Wilkinson EJ.** 2001 consensus guidelines for the management of women with cervical cytological abnormalities. *JAMA* 2002;287:2120–2129.

333. **Kim JJ, Wright TC, Goldie SJ.** Cost-effectiveness of alternative triage strategies for atypical squamous cells of undetermined significance. *JAMA* 2002;287:2382–2390.

334. **Cervical cancer-screening.** Rockville, MD: Preventive Services Task Force, 2003. Available online at http://www.ahrq.gov/clinic/uspstf/uspcerv.htm.

335. **Sawaya GF, McConnell KJ, Kulasingam SL, Lawson HW, Kerlikowske K, Melnikow JL, et al.** Risk of cervical cancer associated with extending the interval between cervical-cancer screenings. *N Engl J Med* 2003;349:1501–1509.

336. **Stenkvist B, Soderstrom J.** Reasons for cervical cancer despite extensive screening. *J Med Screen* 1996;3:204–207.

337. **Nobbenhuis MA, Walboomers JM, Helmerhorst TJ, Rozendaal L, Remmink AJ, Risse EK, et al.** Relation of human papillomavirus status to cervical lesions and consequences for cervical-cancer screening: a prospective study. *Lancet* 1999;354:20–25.

338. **Schiffman M, Herrero R, Hildesheim A, Sherman ME, Bratti M, Wacholder S, et al.** HPV DNA testing in cervical cancer screening: results from women in a high-risk province of Costa Rica. *JAMA* 2000;283:87–93.

339. **Schneider A, Hoyer H, Lotz B, Leistritza S, Kuhne-Heid R, Nindl I, et al.** Screening for high-grade cervical intraepithelial neoplasia and cancer by testing for high-risk HPV, routine cytology or colposcopy. *Int J Cancer* 2000;89:529–534.

340. **Bory JP, Cucherousset J, Lorenzato M, Gabriel R, Quereux C, Birembaut C, et al.** Recurrent human papillomavirus infection detected with the Hybrid Capture II assay selects women with

normal cervical smears at risk for developing high grade cervical lesions: a longitudinal study of 3,091 women. *Int J Cancer* 2002; 102:519–525.

341. **Castle PE, Wacholder S, Lorincz AT, Scott DR, Sherman ME, Glass AG, et al.** A prospective study of high-grade cervical neoplasia risk among human papillomavirus infected women. *J Natl Cancer Inst* 2002;94:1406–1414.

342. **Sherman ME, Lorincz AT, Scott DR, Wacholder S, Castle PE, Glass AG, et al.** Baseline cytology, human papillomavirus testing and risk for cervical neoplasia: a 10-year cohort analysis. *J Natl Cancer Inst* 2003;95:46–52.

343. **Cuzick J, Szarewski A, Cubie H, Hulman G, Kitchener H, Luesley D, et al.** Management of women who test positive for high-risk types of human papillomavirus: the HART study. *Lancet* 2003;362:1871–1876.

344. **Wright TC Jr, Schiffman M.** Adding a test for human papillomavirus DNA to cervical-cancer screening. *N Engl J Med* 2003;348:489–490.

345. **Sherman ME, Lorincz AT, Scott DR, et al.** Baseline cytology, human papillomavirus testing, and risk for cervical neoplasia: a 10-year cohort analysis. *J Natl Cancer Inst* 2003;95:46–52.

346. **Clavel C, Cucherousset J, Lorenzato M, et al.** Negative human papillomavirus testing in normal smears selects a population at low risk for developing high-grade cervical lesions. *Br J Cancer* 2004;90:1803–1808.

347. **Bulkmans NW, Rozendaal L, Voorhorst FJ, Snijders PJ, Meijer CJ.** Long-term protective effect of high-risk human papillomavirus testing in population-based cervical screening. *Br J Cancer* 2005;92:1800–1802.

348. **Hoyer H, Scheungraber C, Kuehne-Heid R, et al.** Cumulative 5-year diagnoses of CIN2, CIN3 or cervical cancer after concurrent high-risk HPV and cytology testing in a primary screening setting. *Int J Cancer* 2005;116:136–143.

349. **Datta SD, Koutsky LA, Ratelle S, Unger ER, Shlay J, McClain T, et al.** Human Papillomavirus Infection and Cervical Cytology in Women Screened for Cervical Cancer in the United States, 2003–2005. *Ann Intern Med* 2008;148;493–500.

350. **Dillner J, Rebolj M, Birembaut P, Petry K-U, Szarewski A, Munk C, et al.** Long term predictive values of cytology and human papillomavirus testing in cervical cancer screening: joint European cohort study. *BMJ* 2008;337;a1754–a1754.

351. **Kulasingam SL, Hughes JP, Kiviat NB, Mao C, Weiss NS, Kuypers JM, et al.** Evaluation of human papillomavirus testing in primary screening for cervical abnormalities: comparison of sensitivity, specificity, and frequency of referral. *JAMA* 2002;288:1749–1757.

352. **Schlecht NF, Platt RW, Duarte-Franco E, Costa MC, Sobrinho JP, Prado JC, et al.** Human papillomavirus infection and time to progression and regression of cervical intraepithelial neoplasia. *J Natl Cancer Inst* 2003;95:1336–1343.

353. **Tachezy R, Salakova M, Hamsikova E, Kanka J, Havrankova A, Vonka V.** Prospective study on cervical neoplasia: presence of HPV DNA in cytological smears precedes the development of cervical neoplastic lesions. *Sex Trans Infect* 2003;79:191–196.

354. **Lorincz AT, Richard RM.** Human papillomavirus DNA testing as an adjunct to cytology and cervical screening programs. *Arch Pathol Lab Med* 2003;127:959–968.

355. **Bulkmans NW, Berkhof J, Rozendaal L, van Kemenade FJ, Boeke AJ, Bulk S, et al.** Human papillomavirus DNA testing for the detection of cervical intraepithelial neoplasia grade 3 and cancer: 5-year follow-up of a randomised controlled implementation trial. *Lancet* 2007;370:1764–72.

356. **Naucler P, Ryd W, Tornberg S, Strand A, Wadell G, Elfgren K, et al.** Human papillomavirus and Papanicolaou tests to screen for cervical cancer. *N Engl J Med* 2007;357:1589–1597.

357. **Ronco G, Giorgi-Rossi P, Carozzi F, Dalla Palma P, Del Mistro A, De Marco L, et al.** Human papillomavirus testing and liquid-based cytology in primary screening of women younger than 35 years: results at recruitment for a randomised controlled trial. *Lancet Oncol* 2006;7:547–555.

358. **Ronco G, Segnan N, Giorgi-Rossi P, Zappa M, Casadei GP, Carozzi F, et al.** Human papillomavirus testing and liquid-based cytology: results at recruitment from the new technologies for cervical cancer randomized controlled trial. *J Natl Cancer Inst* 2006; 98:765–774.

359. Sasieni P, Cuzick J. Could HPV testing become the sole primary screening test? *J Med Screen* 2002;9:49–51.

360. Kuhn L, Denny L, Pollack A, Lorincz A, Richart RM, Wright TC. Human papillomavirus DNA testing for cervical cancer screening in low-resource settings. *J Natl Cancer Inst* 2000;92:818–825.

361. Mandelblatt JS, Lawrence WF, Gaffikin L, Limpahayom KK, Lumbiganon P, Warakamin S, et al. Costs and benefits of different strategies to screen for cervical cancer in less developed countries. *J Natl Cancer Inst* 2002;94:1469–1483.

362. Urcuyo R, Rome RM, Nelson JH Jr. Some observations on the value of endocervical curettage performed as an integral part of colposcopic examination of patients with abnormal cervical cytology. *Am J Obstet Gynecol* 1977;128:787–792.

363. Kobak WH, Roman LD, Felix JC, Muderspach LI, Schlaerth JB, Morrow CP. The role of endocervical curettage at cervical conization for high-grade dysplasia. *Obstet Gynecol* 1995;85:197–201.

364. Weitzman GA, Korhonen MO, Reeves KO, Irwin JF, Carter TS, Kaufman RH. Endocervical brush cytology: an alternative to endocervical curettage? *J Reprod Med* 1988;33:677–683.

365. Walker P, Dexeus S, De Palo G, Barrasso R, Campion M, Girardi F, et al. International terminology of colposcopy: an updated report from the International Federation for Cervical Pathology and Colposcopy. *Obstet Gynecol* 2003;101:175–177.

366. Coppleson M. Colposcopic features of papillomaviral infection and premalignancy on the lower genital tract. *Obstet Gynecol Clin North Am* 1987;14:471–494.

367. Reid R, Herschman BR, Crum CP, Fu YS, Braun L, Shah KV, et al. Genital warts and cervical cancer: V. The tissue basis of colposcopic change. *Am J Obstet Gynecol* 1984;149:293–303.

368. Reid R, Stanhope CR, Herschman BR, Crum CP, Agronow SJ. Genital warts and cervical cancer: IV. A colposcopic index for differentiating subclinical papillomaviral infection from cervical intraepithelial neoplasia. *Am J Obstet Gynecol* 1984;149:815–823.

369. Reid R, Scalzi P. Genital warts and cervical cancer. VII. An improved colposcopic index for differentiating benign papillomaviral infections from high-grade cervical intraepithelial neoplasia. *Am J Obstet Gynecol* 1985;153:611–618.

370. Luesley DM. *Standards and quality in colposcopy.* Sheffield, UK: NHS Cervical Screening Programme, 1996.

371. Ferris DG, Cox JT, Burke L, Campion MJ, Litaker MS, Harper DM. Colposcopy quality control: establishing colposcopy criterion standards for the National Cancer Institute ALTS trial using cervigrams. *Journal of Lower Genital Tract Disease* 1998;9:973–976.

372. Massad LS, Collins YC. Strength of correlations between colposcopic impression and biopsy histology. *Gynecol Oncol* 2003;89:424–428.

373. Wright YC Jr, Cox JT, Massad LS, Carlson J, Twiggs LB, Wilkinson EJ. 2001 consensus guidelines for the management of women with cervical intraepithelial neoplasia. *Am J Obstet Gynecol* 2003;189:295–304.

374. Wright TC, Massad LS, Dunton CJ, Spitzer M, Wilkinson EJ, Solomon D. 2006 American Society for Colposcopy and Cervical Pathology-sponsored Consensus Conference. 2006 consensus guidelines for the management of women with abnormal cervical cancer screening tests. *Am J Obstet Gynecol* 2007;197:346–355.

375. Wright TC, Massad LS, Dunton CJ, Spitzer M, Wilkinson EJ, Solomon D. 2006 American Society for Colposcopy and Cervical Pathology-sponsored Consensus Conference. 2006 consensus guidelines for the management of women with cervical intraepithelial neoplasia or adenocarcinoma-in-situ. *Am J Obstet Gynecol* 2007;197:340–345.

376. Anderson F. Treatment and follow up of noninvasive cancer of the uterine cervix: report on 205 cases (1948–57). *J Obstet Gynaecol Br Commonw* 1965;72:172–177.

377. Kolstad P, Klem V. Long-term follow-up of 1,121 cases of carcinoma-in-situ. *Obstet Gynecol* 1979;48:125–129.

378. Staff A, Mattingly RE. Colposcopic diagnosis of cervical neoplasia. *Obstet Gynecol* 1973;41:168–176.

379. Anderson ES, Thorup K, Larsen G. Results of cryosurgery for cervical intraepithelial neoplasia. *Gynecol Oncol* 1988:30:21–25.

380. Chanen W, Rome RM. Electrocoagulation diathermy for cervical dysplasia and carcinoma-in-situ: a 15-year survey. *Obstet Gynecol* 1983;61:673–679.

381. Burke L. The use of the carbon dioxide laser in the therapy of cervical intraepithelial neoplasia. *Am J Obstet Gynecol* 1982;144:337–340.

382. Luesley DM, Cullimore J, Redman CW, Lawton FG, Emens JM, Rollason TP, et al. Loop diathermy excision of the cervical transformation zone in patients with abnormal cervical smears. *BMJ* 1990;300:1690–1693.

383. Soutter WP, de Barros Lopes A, Fletcher A, Monaghan JM, Duncan ID, Paraskevaidis E, et al. Invasive cervical cancer after conservative therapy for cervical intraepithelial neoplasia. *Lancet* 1997;349:978–980.

384. Benedet JL, Anderson GH, Boyes DA. Colposcopic accuracy in the diagnosis of microinvasive and occult invasive carcinoma of the cervix. *Obstet Gynecol* 1985;65:562–577.

385. Howe DT, Vincenti AC. Is large loop excision of the transformation zone (LLETZ) more accurate than colposcopically directed biopsy in the diagnosis of cervical intraepithelial neoplasia? *BJOG* 1991;98:588–591.

386. Anderson ES, Nielsen K, Pedersen B. The reliability of preconization diagnostic evaluation in patients with cervical intraepithelial neoplasia and microinvasive carcinoma. *Gynecol Oncol* 1995;59:143–147.

387. Sadler L, Saftlas A, Wang W, Exeter M, Whittaker J, McCowan L. Treatment for cervical intraepithelial neoplasia and risk of preterm delivery. *JAMA* 2004;291:2100–2106.

388. Kyrgiou M, Koliopoulos G, Martin-Hirsch P, Arbyn M, Prendiville W, Paraskevaidis E. Obstetric outcomes after conservative treatment for intraepithelial or early invasive cervical lesions: systematic review and meta-analysis. *Lancet* 2006;367:489–498.

389. Bruinsma F, Lumley J, Tan J, Quinn M. Precancerous changes in the cervix and risk of subsequent preterm birth. *BJOG* 2007;114:70–80.

390. Jakobsson M, Gissler M, Sainio S, Paavonen J, Tapper AM. Preterm delivery after surgical treatment for cervical intraepithelial neoplasia. *Obstet Gynecol* 2007;109:309–313.

391. Jakobsson M, Gissler M, Tiitinen A, Paavonen J, Tapper AM. Treatment for cervical intraepithelial neoplasia and subsequent IVF deliveries. *Hum Reprod* 2008; online Jul 16; doi: 10.1093/humrep/den271.

392. Albrechtsen S, Rasmussen S, Thoresen S, Irgens LM, Iversen OE. Pregnancy outcome in women before and after cervical conisation. *BMJ* 2008;337:a1343.

393. Arbyn M, Kyrgiou M, Simoens C, Raifu AO, Koliopoulos G, Martin-Hirsch P, et al. Perinatal mortality and other severe adverse pregnancy outcomes associated with treatment of cervical intraepithelial neoplasia: meta-analysis. *BMJ* 2008;337:a1284.

394. Jakobsson M, Bruinsma F. Editorial. Adverse pregnancy outcomes after treatment for cervical intraepithelial neoplasia. *BMJ* 2008;337:a1350.

395. Martin-Hirsch PL, Paraskevaidis E, Kitchener H. The Cochrane Database of Systematic Reviews. Surgery for cervical intraepithelial neoplasia. *The Cochrane Library* 2003;3:1–40.

396. Creasman WT, Weed JC, Curry SL, Johnston WW, Parker RT. Efficacy of cryosurgical treatment of severe cervical intraepithelial neoplasia. *Obstet Gynecol* 1973;41:501–505.

397. Popkin DR, Scall V, Ahmed MN. Cryosurgery for the treatment of cervical intraepithelial neoplasia. *Am J Obstet Gynecol* 1978;130:551–554.

398. Kaufman RH, Irwin JF. The cryosurgical therapy of cervical intraepithelial neoplasia: III. Continuing follow-up. *Am J Obstet Gynecol* 1978;131:381–388.

399. Benedet JL, Miller DM, Nickerson KG, Anderson GH. Efficacy of cryosurgical treatment of cervical intraepithelial neoplasia at one, five and ten years. *Am J Obstet Gynecol* 1987;157:268–273.

400. Tidbury P, Singer A, Jenkins D. CIN 3: the role of lesion size in invasion. *BJOG* 1992;99:583–586.

401. Cartier R. The role of colposcopy in the diagnosis and treatment of dysplasias and interepithelial carcinomas of the uterine cervix. *Bull Cancer* 1979;66:447–454.

402. Prendiville W, Cullimore J. Excision of the transformation zone using the low voltage diathermy (LVD) loop: a superior method of treatment. *Colposc Gynecol Laser Surg* 1987;122S:1–15.

403. Prendiville W, Cullimore J, Norman S. Large loop excision of the transformation zone (LLETZ): a new method of management for women with cervical intraepithelial neoplasia. *BJOG* 1989;96:1054–1060.

404. Phipps JH, Gunasekara PC, Lewis BY. Occult cervical carcinoma revealed by large loop diathermy. *Lancet* 1989;2:453–454.

405. **Chappatte OA, Bryne DL, Raju KS, Nayagam M, Kenny A.** Histological differences between colposcopic-directed biopsy and loop excision of the transformation zone (LLETZ): a cause for concern. *Gynecol Oncol* 1991;43:46–50.

406. **Murdoch JB, Grimshaw RN, Morgan PR, Monaghan JM.** The impact of loop diathermy on management of early invasive cervical cancer. *Int J Gynecol Cancer* 1992;2:129–133.

407. **Burger MPM, Hollema H.** The reliability of the histologic diagnosis in colposcopically directed biopsies: a plea for LLETZ. *Int J Gynecol Cancer* 1993;3:385–390.

408. **Howells REJ, O'Mahony F, Tucker H, Millinship J, Jones PW, Redman CWE.** How can the incidence of negative specimens resulting from large loop excision of the cervical transformation zone (LLETZ) be reduced? An analysis of negative LLETZ specimens and development of a predictive model. *BJOG* 2000;107;1075–1082.

409. **Reid R.** Physical and surgical principles governing expertise with the carbon dioxide laser. *Obstet Gynecol Clin North Am* 1987; 14:513–535.

410. **Reid R.** Symposium on cervical neoplasia. V. Carbon dioxide laser ablation. *Colposc Gynecol Laser Surg* 1984;1:291–297.

411. **Reid R.** Physical and surgical principles of laser surgery in the lower genital tract. *Obstet Gynecol Clin North Am* 1991;18:429–474.

412. **Fuller TA.** Laser tissue interaction: the influence of power density. In: Baggish M, ed. *Basic and advanced laser surgery and gynecology.* New York: Appleton-Century-Crofts, 1985:51–60.

413. **Bjerre B, Eliasson G, Linell F, Soderberg H, Sjoberg NO.** Conization as only treatment of carcinomain-situ of the uterine cervix. *Am J Obstet Gynecol* 1976;15:143–151.

414. **Luesly DM, McCann A, Terry PB, Wade-Evans T, Nicholson HD, Mylotte MJ, et al.** Complications of cone biopsy related to the dimensions of the cone and the influence of prior colposcopic assessment. *BJOG* 1985;92:158–162.

415. **Benedet JL, Saunders BH.** Carcinoma *in situ* of the vagina. *Am J Obstet Gynecol* 1984;148:695–699.

416. **Coppleson M, Reid B.** Treatment of preclinical carcinoma of the cervix. In: Coppleson M, Reid B, eds. *Preclinical carcinoma of the cervix.* Oxford: Pergamon Press, 1967:1–321.

417. **Boon ME, Baak JP, Kurver PJ, Overdiep SH, Verdonk GW.** Adenocarcinoma *in situ* of the cervix: an underdiagnosed lesion. *Cancer* 1981;48:768–773.

418. **Anton-Culver H, Bloss JD, Bringman D, Lee-Feldstein A, DiSaia P, Manetta A.** Comparison of adenocarcinoma and squamous cell carcinoma of the uterine cervix: a population-based epidemiologic study. *Am J Obstet Gynecol* 1992;166:1507–1514.

419. **Vizcaino AP, Moreno V, Bosch FX, Munoz N, Barros-Dios XM, Parkin DM.** International trends in the incidence of cervical cancer: I. Adenocarcinoma and adenosquamous cell carcinomas. *Int J Cancer* 1998;75;536–545.

420. **Sasieni P, Adams J.** Changing rates of adenocarcinoma and adenosquamous carcinoma of the cervix in England. *Lancet* 2001; 357;1490–1493.

421. **Wang SS, Sherman ME, Hildesheim A, Lacey JV Jr, Devesa S.** Cervical adenocarcinoma and squamous cell carcinoma incidence trends among white women and black women in the United States for 1976–2000. *Cancer* 2004;100;1035–1044.

422. **Schoolland M, Segal A, Allpress S, Miranda A, Frost FA, Sterrett GF.** Adenocarcinoma *in situ* of the cervix. *Cancer* 2002;96;330–337.

423. **Smith HO, Padilla LA.** Adenocarcinoma *in situ* of the cervix: sensitivity of detection by cervical smear: will cytologic screening for adenocarcinoma *in situ* reduce incidence rates for adenocarcinoma? *Cancer* 2002;96;319–322.

424. **Kinney W, Sawaya GF, Sung HY, Kearney KA, Miller M, Hiatt RA.** Stage at diagnosis and mortality in patients with adenocarcinoma and adenosquamous carcinoma of the uterine cervix diagnosed as a consequence of cytologic screening. *Acta Cytol* 2003;47; 167–171.

425. **Syrjanen K.** Is improved detection of adenocarcinoma *in situ* by screening a key to reducing the incidence of cervical adenocarcinoma? *Acta Cytol* 2004;48;591–594.

426. **Herzog TJ, Monk BJ.** Reducing the burden of glandular cancers of the uterine cervix. *Am J Obstet Gynecol* 2007;197:566–571.

427. **Kjaer SK, Brinton LA.** Adenocarcinomas of the uterine cervix: the epidemiology of an increasing problem. *Epidemiol Rev* 1993;15: 486–498.

428. **Schoolland M, Segal A, Allpress S, Miranda A, Frost FA, Sterrett GE.** Adenocarcinoma *in situ* of the cervix. *Cancer* 2002;96: 330–337.

429. **Ursin G, Peters RK, Henderson BE, d'Ablaing G III, Monroe KR, Pike MC.** Oral contraceptive use and adenocarcinoma of cervix. *Lancet* 1994;344:1390–1394.

430. **van Aspert-van Erp AJ,Smedts FM,Vooijs GP.** Severe cervical glandular cell lesions with coexisting squamous cell lesions. *Cancer* 2004;102;218–227.

431. **Kennedy AW, Salmieri SS, Wirth SL, Biscotti CV, Tuason LJ, Travarca MJ.** Results of the clinical evaluation of atypical glandular cells of undetermined significance (AGCUS) detected on cervical cytology screening. *Gynecol Oncol* 1996;63:14–18.

432. **Nasuti JF, Fleisher SR, Gupta PK.** Atypical glandular cells of undetermined significance (AGUS): clinical considerations and cytohistologic correlation. *Diagn Cytopathol.* 2002;26:186–190.

433. **Raab SS.** Can glandular lesions be diagnosed in pap smear cytology? *Diagn Cytopathol* 2000;23;127–133.

434. **Jeng CJ, Liang HS, Wang TY, Shen J, Yang YC, Tzeng CR.** Cytologic and histologic review of atypical glandular cells (AGC) detected during cervical cytology screening. *Int J Gynecol Cancer* 2003;13;518–521.

435. **MattoSinho de Castro Ferraz Mda G, Focchi J, Stavale JN, Nicolau SM, Rodrigues de Lima G, Baracat EC.** Atypical glandular cells of undetermined significance: cytologic predictive value for glandular involvement in high-grade squamous intraepithelial lesions. *Acta Cytol* 2003;47:154–158.

436. **Christopherson W, Nealon N, Gray LA.** Noninvasive precursor lesions of adenocarcinoma and mixed adenosquamous carcinoma of the cervix uteri. *Cancer* 1979, 44;975–983.

437. **Bertrand M, Lickrish GB, Colgan TJ.** The anatomic distribution of cervical adenocarcinoma *in situ:* implications for treatment. *Am J Obstet Gynecol* 1987;137:21–25.

438. **Brand E, Berek JS, Hacker NF.** Controversies in the management of cervical adenocarcinoma. *Obstet Gynecol* 1988;71:261–269.

439. **Poynor EA, Barakat RR, Hoskins WJ.** Management and follow-up of patients with adenocarcinoma *in situ* of the uterine cervix. *Gynecol Oncol* 1995;57:158–164.

440. **Soutter WP, Haidopoulos D, Gornall RJ, McIndoe GA, Fox J, Mason WP, et al.** Is conservative treatment for adenocarcinoma *in situ* of the cervix safe? *BJOG* 2001;108:1184–1189.

441. **Bull-Phelps SL, Garner EI, Walsh CS, Gehrig PA, Miller DS, Schorge JO.** Fertility-sparing surgery in 101 women with adenocarcinoma *in situ* of the cervix. *Gynecol Oncol* 2007;107;316–319.

442. **Krivak TC, Rose GS, McBroom JW, Carlson JW, Winter WE, Kost ER.** Cervical adenocarcinoma *in situ:* a systematic review of therapeutic options and predictors of persistent or recurrent disease. *Obstet Gynecol Surv* 2001;56;567–575.

443. **Young JL, Jazaeri AA, Lachance JA, et al.** Cervical adenocarcinoma *in situ:* the predictive value of conization margin status. *Am J Obstet Gynecol* 2007;197:195.e1–195.e8.

444. **Dedecker F, Graesslin O, Bonneau S, Quéreux C.** Persistence and recurrence of *in situ* cervical adenocarcinoma after primary treatment. About 121 cases. *Gynécologie Obstétrique & Fertilité* 2008; 36;616–622.

445. **Cullimore JE, Luesley DM, Rollason TP, Byrne P, Buckley CH, Anderson M, et al.** A prospective study of conization of the cervix in the management of cervical intraepithelial glandular neoplasia (CIGN)-a preliminary report. *BJOG* 1992;99:314–317.

446. **Wolf JK, Levenback C, Malpica A, Morris M, Burke T, Mitchell MF.** Adenocarcinoma *in situ* of the cervix: significance of cone biopsy margins. *Obstet Gynecol* 1996;88:82–86.

447. **Hocking GR, Hayman JA, Ostor AG.** Adenocarcinoma *in situ* of the uterine cervix progressing to invasive adenocarcinoma, *Aust N Z J Obstet Gynecol* 1996;36;218–220.

448. **Azodi M, Chambers SK, Rutherford TJ, Kohorn EI, Schwartz PE, Chambers JT.** Adenocarcinoma *in situ* of the cervix: management and outcome. *Gynecol Oncol* 1999;73:348–353.

449. **Cohn DE, Morrison CD, Zanagnolo VL, Goist MM, Copeland LJ.** Invasive cervical adenocarcinoma immediately following a cone biopsy for adenocarcinoma *in situ* with negative margins, *Gynecol Oncol* 2005;98:158–160.

450. **Purcell K, Cass I, Natarajan S, Dadmanesh F, Aoyama C, Holschneider C.** Cold knife cone superior to loop electrosurgical

excision procedure for conservative management of cervical adeno-carcinoma *in situ. Obstet Gynecol* 2003;101(suppl 1):S104–S105.

451. **Bryson P, Stulberg R, Shepherd L, McLelland K, Jeffrey J.** Is electrosurgical loop excision with negative margins sufficient treatment for cervical AIS? *Gynecol Oncol* 2004;93;465–468.

452. **Salani R, Puri I, Bristow RE.** Adenocarcinoma *in situ* of the uterine cervix: a metaanalysis of 1278 patients evaluating the predictive value of conization margin status. *Am J Obstet Gynecol* 2009;200:182.e1–182.e5.

453. **Costa S, Negri G, Sideri M, Santini D, Martinelli G, Venturoli S, et al.** Human papillomavirus (HPV) test and PAP smear as predictors of outcome in conservatively treated adenocarcinoma *in situ* (AIS) of the uterine cervix. *Gynecol Oncol* 2007;106;170–176.

454. **Srodon M, Stoler MH, Baber GB, et al.** The distribution of low and high-risk HPV types in vulvar and vaginal intraepithelial neoplasia (VIN and VaIN). *Am J Surg Pathol* 2006;30:1513–1518.

455. **Sillman FH, Fruchter RG, Chen YS, Camilien L, Sedlis A, McTigue E, et al.** Vaginal intraepithelial neoplasia: risk factors for persistence, recurrence, and invasion and its management. *Am J Obstet Gynecol* 1997;176:93–99.

456. **Dorsey JH, Baggish MS.** Multifocal vaginal intraepithelial neoplasia with uterus *in situ*. In: Sharp F, Jordan JA, eds. *Gynaecological laser surgery: proceedings of the 15th study group of the Royal College of Obstetricians and Gynaecologists.* Ithaca, NY: Perinatology Press, 1985:173.

457. **Dodge JA, Eltabbakh GH, Mount SL, Walker RP, Morgan A.** Clinical features and risk of recurrence among patients with vaginal intraepithelial neoplasia. *Gynecol Oncol* 2001;83:363–369.

458. **Campion MJ.** Clinical manifestations and natural history of genital human papillomavirus infections. *Dermatol Clin* 1991;9:235–249.

459. **Sherman JF, Mount SL, Evans MF, Skelly J, Simmons-Arnold L, Eltabbakh GH.** Smoking increases the risk of high-grade vaginal intraepithelial neoplasia in women with oncogenic human papillomavirus. *Gynecol Oncol* 2008;110:396–401.

460. **Bosquet EG, Torres A, Busquets M ,Esteva C,Munoz-Almagro C, Lailla JM.** Prognostic factors for the development of vaginal intraepithelial neoplasia. *Eur J Gynecol Oncol* 2008;29:43–45.

461. **Gagné HM.** Colposcopy of the Vagina and Vulva. *Obstet Gynecol Clin North Am* 2008;35;659–669.

462. **Staff A, Wilkinson EJ, Mattingly RF.** Laser treatment of cervical and vaginal neoplasia. *Am J Obstet Gynecol* 1977;128:128–136.

463. **Yalcin OT, Rutherford TJ, Chambers SK, Chambers JT, Schwartz PE.** Vaginal intraepithelial neoplasia: treatment by carbon dioxide laser and risk factors for failure. *Eur J Obstet Gynecol Reprod Biol* 2003;106:64–68.

464. **Diakomanolis E, Stefanidis K, Rodolakis A, Haidopoulos D, Sindos M, Chatzipappas I, et al.** Vaginal intraepithelial neoplasia: report of 102 cases. *Eur J Gynaecol Oncol* 2002;23:457–459.

465. **Sillman FH, Sedlis A, Boyce JIG.** A review of lower genital intraepithelial neoplasia and the use of topical *5-fluorouracil. Obstet Gynecol Surv* 1985;40:190–220.

466. **Krebs HB.** Prophylactic topical *5-fluorouracil* following treatment of human papillomavirus-associated lesions of the vulva and vagina. *Obstet Gynecol* 1986;68:837–841.

467. **Diakomanolis E, Haidopoulos D, Stefanidis K.** Treatment of high-grade vaginal intraepithelial neoplasia with *imiquimod* cream. *New Engl J Med* 2002;347;374.

468. **Haidopoulos D, Diakomanolis E, Rodolakis A, Voulgaris Z, Vlachos G, Antsaklis A.** Can local application of *imiquimod* cream be an alternative mode of therapy for patients with high-grade intraepithelial lesions of the vagina? *Int J Gynecol Cancer* 2005;15:898–902.

469. **Iavazzo C, Pitsouni E, Athanasiou S, Falagas ME.** Imiquimod for treatment of vulvar and vaginal intraepithelial neoplasia. *Int J Gynecol Obstet* 2008;101;3–10.

470. **Woodman CB, Jordan JA, Wade-Evans T.** The management of vaginal intraepithelial neoplasia after hysterectomy. *BJOG* 1984;91:707–711.

471. **Hoffman NIS, DeCesare SL, Roberts WS, Fiorica JU, Finan MA, Cavanaugh D.** Upper vaginectomy for *in situ* and occult superficially invasive carcinoma of the vagina. *Am J Obstet Gynecol* 1992;166:30–33.

472. **Gardner HL, Friedrich EC Jr, Kaufman RH, Woodruff JD.** The vulvar dystrophies, atypias, and carcinoma *in situ*: an invitational symposium. *J Reprod Med* 1976;17:111–117.

473. **Hart W.** Vulvar intraepithelial neoplasia: historical aspects and current status. *Int J Gyn Path* 2001;20;16–30.

474. **Sturgeon S, Britnon L, Devesa S, Kurman R.** *In situ* and invasive vulvar cancer incidence trends (1973 to 1987). *Am J Obstet Gynecol* 1992;166:1482–1485.

475. **Iversen T, Tretli S.** Intraepithelial and invasive squamous cell neoplasia of the vulva: trends in incidence, recurrence, and survival rate in Norway, *Obstet Gynecol* 1998;91;969–972.

476. **Joura EA, Losch A, Haider-Angeler MG, Breitenecker G, Leodolter, S.** Trends in vulvar neoplasia. Increasing incidence of vulvar intraepithelial neoplasia and squamous cell carcinoma of the vulva in young women. *J Reprod Med* 2000;45;613–615.

477. **Rusk D, Sutton GP, Look KY, Roman A.** Analysis of invasive squamous cell carcinoma, the vulva and vulvar intraepithelial neoplasia for the presence of human papillomaviral DNA. *Obstet Gynecol* 1991;77:918–922.

478. **Rodke G, Friedrich EG, Wilkinson E.** Malignant potential of mixed vulvar dystrophy (lichen sclerosis associated with squamous cell hyperplasia). *J Reprod Med* 1988;33:545–550.

479. **Bloss JD, Liao SY, Wilczynski SP, Macri C, Walker J, Peake M, et al.** Clinical and histologic features of vulvar carcinomas analyzed for human papillomavirus status: evidence that squamous cell carcinoma of the vulva has more than one etiology. *Hum Pathol* 1991;22:711–718.

480. **Toki T, Kurman RJ, Park JS, Kessts T, Daniel RW, Shah KV.** Probable nonpapillomaviral etiology of squamous cell carcinoma of the vulva in older women: a clinicopathologic study using *in situ* hybridization and polymerase chain reaction. *Int J Gynecol Pathol* 1991;10:107–125.

481. **Park JS, Kurman R, Schiffman M.** Basaloid and warty carcinoma of the vulva: distinctive types of squamous carcinoma with human papillomavirus. *Lab Invest* 1991;1:62–68.

482. **Hording U, Junge J, Daugaard S, Lundvall F, Poulsen H, Bock JE.** Vulvar squamous cell carcinoma and papillomaviruses: indications for two different etiologies. *Gynecol Oncol* 1994;52:241–246.

483. **Trimble CL, Hildesheim A, Brinton LA, Shah KV, Kurman RJ.** Heterogeneous etiology of squamous carcinoma of the vulva. *Obstet Gynecol* 1996;87:59–64.

484. **Kim YT, Thomas NF, Kessis TD, Wilkinson EJ, Hedrick L, Cho KR.** p53 mutations and clonality in vulvar carcinomas and squamous hyperplasias: evidence suggesting that squamous hyperplasias do not serve as direct precursors of human papillomavirus-negative vulvar carcinomas. *Hum Pathol* 1996;27:389–395.

485. **Jeffcoate TNA.** Chronic vulval dystrophies. *Am J Obstet Gynecol* 1966;95:61–74.

486. **Committee on Terminology, International Society for the Study of Vulvar Disease.** New nomenclature for vulvar disease. *Int J Gynecol Pathol* 1989;8:83–84.

487. **Herod JJ, Shafi MI, Rollason TP, Jordan, JA, Luesley DM.** Vulvar intraepithelial neoplasia: long term follow up of treated and untreated women, *Br J Obstet Gynaecol* 1996;103:446–452.

488. **Jones RW, Rowan DM.** Vulvar intraepithelial neoplasia: III. A clinical study of outcome in 113 cases with relation to later development of invasive vulvar carcinoma. *Obstet Gynecol* 1994;83:741–745.

489. **McNally OM, Mulvany NJ, Pagano R, Quinn MA, Rome RM.** VIN 3: a clinicopathologic review, *Int J Gynecol Cancer* 2002;12;490–495.

490. **Jones RW, Rowan DM, Stewart AW.** Vulvar intraepithelial neoplasia: aspects of the natural history and outcome in 405 women, *Obstet Gynecol* 2005;106;1319–1326.

491. **Van Seter M, Van Beurden M, de Craen AJ.** Is the assumed natural history of vulvar intraepithelial neoplasia III based on enough evidence? A systematic review of 3322 published patients, *Gynecol Oncol* 2005;97:645–651.

492. **Preti M, Van Seters M, Sideri M, Van Beurden M.** Squamous vulvar intraepithelial neoplasia, *Clin Obstet Gynecol* 2005;48:845–861.

493. **Shylasree TS, Karanjgaokar V, Tristram A, Wilkes AR, MacLean AB, Fiander AN.** Contribution of demographic, psychological and disease-related factors to quality of life in women with high-grade vulval intraepithelial neoplasia. *Gynecol Oncol* 2008;110;185–189.

494. **Sideri M, Jones RW, Wilkinson EJ, Preti M, Heller D, Scurry J, et al.** Squamous vulvar intraepithelial neoplasia: 2004 Modified Terminology, ISSVD Vulvar Oncology Subcommittee. *J Reprod Medicine* 2005;50:807–810.

495. **Jones RW, Rowan DM.** Spontaneous regression of vulvar intraepithelial neoplasia 2–3. *Obstet Gynecol* 2000;96;470–472.

496. **Jones RW, MacLean AB.** Re: "Is the assumed natural history of vulvar intraepithelial neoplasia III based on enough evidence? A systematic review of 3322 published patients." *Gynecol Oncol* 2006;101;371–372.

497. **Kurman RJ, Toki T, Schiffman MH.** Basaloid and warty carcinoma of the vulva. *Am J Surg Pathol* 1993;17:133–145.

498. **Kaufman RH.** Vulvar intraepithelial neoplasia. *Gynecol Oncol* 1995;56:8–21.

499. **Haefner HK, Tate JE, McLachlin CM, Crum CP.** Vulvar intraepithelial neoplasia: age, morphologic phenotype, papillomavirus DNA and coexisting invasive carcinoma. *Hum Pathol* 1995;26: 147–154.

500. **van Beurdren M, ten Kate FJW, Smits HL, Berkhout RJ, de Craen AJ, van der Vange N, et al.** Multifocal vulvar intraepithelial neoplasia grade III and multicentric lower genital tract neoplasia is associated with transcriptionally active human papilloma virus. *Cancer* 1995;75:2879–2884.

501. **Van Beurden M, Kate FW, Tjong A, de Craen AJ, van der Vange N, Lammes FB, et al.** Human papillomavirus DNA in multicentric vulvar intraepithelial neoplasia. *Int J Gynecol Pathol* 1998;17: 12–16.

502. **Davidson EJ, Sehr P, Faulkner RL, Parish JL, Gaston K, Moore RA, et al.** Human papillomavirus type 16 E2- and L1-specific serological and T-cell responses in women with vulval intraepithelial neoplasia, *J Gen Virol* 2003;84;2089–2097.

503. **Thuis YN, Campion M, Fox H, Hacker NF.** Contemporary experience with the management of vulvar intraepithelial neoplasia. *Int J Gynecol Cancer* 2000;10:223–227.

504. **Berger BW, Hori V.** Multicentric Bowen's disease of the genitalia: spontaneous regression of lesions. *Arch Dermatol* 1978;114: 1698–1699.

505. **Forney JP.** Management of carcinoma-*in-situ* of the vulva. *Am J Obstet Gynecol* 1977;127:801–806.

506. **Rodolakis A, Diakomanolis E, Vlachos G, Iconomou T, Protopappas A, Stefanidis C, et al.** Vulvar intraepithelial neoplasia (VIN)-diagnostic and therapeutic challenges. *Eur J Gynaecol Oncol* 2003;24:317–322.

507. **McFadden K, Cruickshank M.** New developments in the management of VIN. *Rev in Gyn Pract* 2005;5;102–108.

508. **Modesitt SC, Waters AB, Walton L, Van Le L.** Vulvar intraepithelial neoplasia 111: occult cancer and the impact of margin status on recurrence. *Obstet Gynecol* 1998;92:962–966.

509. **Sykes P, Smith N, McCormick P, Frizelle FA.** High-grade vulval intraepithelial neoplasia (VIN 3): a retrospective analysis of patient characteristics, management, outcome and relationship to squamous cell carcinoma of the vulva 1989–1999. *Aust N Z J Obstet Gynaecol* 2002;42:69–74.

510. **Rutledge F, Sinclair M.** Treatment of intraepithelial neoplasia of the vulva by skin excision and graft. *Am J Obstet Gynecol* 1968;102: 806–812.

511. **DiSaia P.** Management of superficially invasive vulvar carcinoma. *Clin Obstet Gynecol* 1985;28:196–203.

512. **Yii NW, Niranjan NS.** Lotus petal flaps in vulvo-vaginal reconstruction. *Br J Plast Surg* 1996;49:547–554.

513. **Davison PM, Sarhanis P, Shroff JF, Kilby M, Redman CW.** A new approach to reconstruction following vulval excision. *Br J Obstet Gynaecol* 1996;103;475–477.

514. **Narayansingh GV, Cumming GP, Parkin DP, McConnell DT, Honey E., Kolhe PS.** Flap repair: an effective strategy for minimising sexual morbidity associated with the surgical management of vulval intra epithelial neoplasia, *J R Coll Surg Edinb* 2000;45;81–84.

515. **Reid R.** Superficial laser vulvectomy: I. The efficacy of extended superficial ablation for refractory and very extensive condylomas. *Am J Obstet Gynecol* 1985;151:1047–1052.

516. **Reid R, Elfont EA, Zirkin RM, Fuller TA.** Superficial laser vulvectomy: II. The anatomic and biophysical principles permitting accurate control of the depth of thermal destruction with the carbon-dioxide laser. *Am J Obstet Gynecol* 1985;152:261–271.

517. **Reid R.** Superficial laser vulvectomy: III. A new surgical technique for appendage-conserving ablation of refractory condylomas and vulvar intraepithelial neoplasia. *Am J Obstet Gynecol* 1985:152: 504–509.

518. **Reid R, Greenberg MD, Lorincz A, Daoud Y, Pizzuti D, Stoler M.** Superficial laser vulvectomy: IV. Extended laser vaporization and adjunctive *5-fluorouracil* therapy of human papillomavirus-associated vulvar disease. *Obstet Gynecol* 1990;76:439–448.

519. **Reid R, Greenberg MD, Pizzuti DJ, Omoto KH, Rutledge LH, Soo W.** Superficial laser vulvectomy: V. Surgical debulking is enhanced by adjuvant systemic interferon. *Am J Obstet Gynecol* 1992;166:815–820.

520. **Friedman-Kien AE, Eron LJ, Conant M, Growdon W, Badiak H, Bradstreet PW, et al.** Natural interferon alpha for treatment of condylomata acuminata. *JAMA* 1988;259:533–538.

521. **Hengge UR, Benninghoff B, Ruzicka T, Goos M.** Topical immunomodulators: progress towards treating inflammation, infection and cancer. *Lancet Infect Dis* 2001;1:189–198.

522. **Tyring SK.** Immune-response modifiers: a new paradigm in the treatment of human papillomavirus. *Curr Ther Res Clin Exp* 2000; 61:584–596.

523. **Garland SM.** *Imiquimod. Curr Opin Infect Dis* 2003;16:85–89.

524. **Beutner KR, Tyring SK, Trofatter KF, Douglas JM Jr, Spruance S, Owens ML, et al.** *Imiquimod,* a patient-applied immune-response modifier for treatment of external genital warts. *Antimicrob Agents Chemother* 1998;42:789–794.

525. **Edwards L, Ferenczy A, Eron L, Baker D, Owens ML, Fox TL, et al.** Self-administered topical 5% *imiquimod* cream for external anogenital warts. HPV Study Group. Human Papilloma Virus. *Arch Dermatol* 1998;134:25–30.

526. **Garland SM, Sellors JW, Wilkstrom A, Petersen CS, Aranda C, Aractingi S, et al.** *Imiquimod* 5% cream is a safe and effective self-applied treatment for anogenital warts: results of an open-label, multicentre Phase IIIB trial. *Int J STD AIDS* 2001;12:722–729.

527. **Travis LB, Weinberg JM, Krumholz BA.** Successful treatment of vulvar intraepithelial neoplasia with topical *imiquimod* 5% cream in a lung transplanted patient. *Acta Derm Venereol* 2002;82: 475–476.

528. **van Seters M, Fons G, van Beurden M.** *Imiquimod* in the treatment of multifocal vulvar intraepithelial neoplasia 2/3. Results of a pilot study. *J Reprod Med* 2002;47:701–705.

529. **Van Seters M, van Beurden M, ten Kate FJW, Beckman I, Ewing PC, Eijkemans MJ, et al.** Treatment of vulvar intraepithelial neoplasia with topical *imiquimod. New Engl J Med* 2008;358; 1465–1473.

530. **Campion MJ, Clarkson P, McCance DJ.** Squamous neoplasia of the cervix in relation to other genital tract neoplasia. *Clin Obstet Gynecol* 1985;12:265–280.

531. **Spitzer M, Krumholz BA, Seltzer VL.** The multicentric nature of disease related to human papillomavirus infection of the female lower genital tract, *Obstet Gynecol* 1989;73;303–307.

532. **Vinokurova S, Wentzensen N, Einenkel J, et al.** Clonal history of papillomavirus-induced dysplasia in the female lower genital tract, *J Natl Cancer Inst* 2005;97;1816–1821.

533. **Menguellet SA, Collinet P, Debarge VH, Nayama M, Vinatier D, Leroy J-L.** Management of multicentric lesions of the lower genital tract. *Eur J Obstet Gynecol Reprod Bio* 2007;132:116–120.

534. **McConnell EM.** Squamous carcinoma of the anus: a review of 96 cases. *Br J Surg* 1970;57:89–92.

535. **Daling JR, Weiss NS, Klopfenstein LL, Cochran LE, Chow WH, Daifuku R.** Correlates of homosexual behavior and the incidence of anal cancer. *JAMA* 1982;247:1988–1990.

536. **Frazer IH, Medley G, Crapper RM, Brown TC, Mackay IR.** Association between anorectal dysplasia, human papillomavirus, and human immunodeficiency virus infection in homosexual men. *Lancet* 1986;2:657–660.

537. **Ogunbiyi OA, Scholefield JH, Robertson G, Smith JH, Sharp F, Rogers K.** Anal human papillomavirus infection and squamous neoplasia in patients with invasive vulvar cancer. *Obstet Gynecol* 1994;83:212–216.

9 Cervical Cancer

Neville F. Hacker
Michael L Friedlander

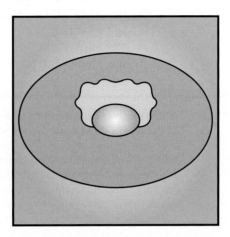

Cervical cancer is the second most common cancer in women worldwide and the most common female cancer in many developing countries. Annual global estimates for the year 2000 were 470,600 new cases and 233,400 deaths (1). Both the incidence and mortality rates are likely to be underestimated in underresourced countries because of poor registry reporting. In the United States, 11,270 new cases with 4,070 deaths were anticipated in 2009 (2).

The mean age for cervical cancer is 51.4 years, with the number of patients fairly evenly divided between the age groups 30 to 39 and 60 to 69 years (1). There is a trend toward increasing stage with increasing age, suggesting that older patients are not being screened as often as younger patients (1).

In recent years, molecular biology has firmly established a **causal relationship between persistent infection with high-risk human papilloma virus (HPV) genotypes and cervical cancer.** In a study of almost 1,000 cases of cervical cancer worldwide, the prevalence of HPV infection was 99.7% (3). This causal relationship has led to the promise of global cervical cancer prevention using both primary prevention through vaccination against HPV in young women and secondary prevention by screening directly for carcinogenic HPV in older women (4). Two HPV vaccines are currently approved by the FDA: the quadrivalent *Gardasil* and the bivalent *Cervarix*.

Cervical cancer progresses slowly from preinvasive cervical intraepithelial neoplasia (CIN) to invasive cancer, and screening asymptomatic women with regular Papanicolaou (Pap) smears allows diagnosis of the readily treatable preinvasive phase. Hence, appropriate screening programs are an important public health issue. **In developed countries, most cases of cervical cancer occur in women who have not had regular Pap smear screening.**

In low-resource countries, facilities for screening asymptomatic women are not readily available, and cultural attitudes and lack of public education also discourage early diagnosis. Hence, **most patients in developing countries present with advanced disease that may have already eroded into the bladder, rectum, pelvic nerves, or bone.** Because radiation therapy and palliative care facilities are also usually inadequate in these countries, many of these women die as social outcasts, with severe pain and a foul-smelling vaginal discharge. Most of these women have dependent children, so the social devastation caused by this disease can be readily appreciated.

Even in the United States, nearly 9% of women receive no therapy for their disease (5). Trimble et al. reported that this was particularly common in older, unmarried women, who presented with late-stage disease. Obstacles to treatment were postulated to include lack of access to treatment facilities, inability to pay, and inadequate social support.

Diagnosis

Early diagnosis of cervical cancer can be extremely challenging because of three factors:

1. **the frequently asymptomatic nature of early-stage disease;**
2. **the origin of some tumors from within the endocervical canal or beneath the epithelium of the ectocervix,** making visualization on speculum examination impossible; and
3. **the significant false negative rate for Pap smears,** even in women having regular screening

Symptoms

Abnormal vaginal bleeding is the most common presenting symptom of invasive cancer of the cervix. In sexually active women, this usually includes postcoital bleeding, but there may also be intermenstrual or postmenopausal bleeding. Unlike endometrial cancer, which usually bleeds early, **cervical cancer often is asymptomatic until quite advanced in women who are not sexually active.** Large tumors commonly become infected, and a vaginal discharge, sometimes malodorous, may occur before the onset of bleeding. In very advanced cases, pelvic pain, pressure symptoms pertaining to the bowel or bladder, and occasionally vaginal passage of urine or feces may be presenting symptoms.

In a review of 81 patients diagnosed with cervical cancer in southern California, Pretorius et al. (6) reported that 56% presented with abnormal vaginal bleeding, 28% with an abnormal Pap smear, 9% with pain, 4% with vaginal discharge, and 4% with other symptoms. Patients presenting with an abnormal Pap smear had smaller tumors and earlier-stage disease.

Cytology

The presence of malignant cells in a background of necrotic debris, blood, and inflammatory cells is typical of invasive carcinoma (Fig. 9.1). Differentiation between squamous and glandular cells is usually possible except for poorly differentiated lesions. **The false negative rate for Pap smears in the presence of invasive cancer is up to 50%, so a negative Pap smear should never be relied on in a symptomatic patient** (7).

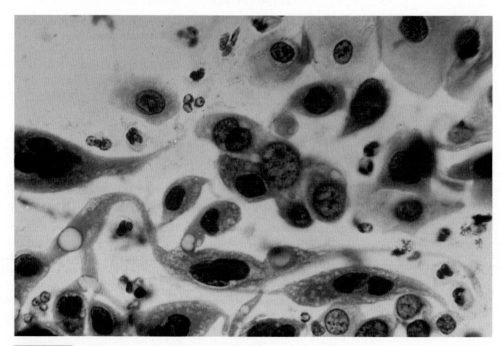

Figure 9.1   Pap smear of cervical squamous cell carcinoma. Malignant squamous cells, singly and in groups, show nuclear pleomorphism. A "tadpole" cell is present on the left. (Original magnification 165×.)

Signs

Physical examination should include palpation of the liver, supraclavicular, and groin nodes to exclude metastatic disease. On speculum examination, the primary lesion may be exophytic, endophytic, ulcerative, or polypoid. If the tumor arises beneath the epithelium or in the endocervical canal, the ectocervix may appear macroscopically normal. Direct extension to the vagina is usually grossly apparent, but the infiltration may be subepithelial and suspected only on the basis of obliteration of the vaginal fornices or the presence of apical stenosis. In the latter situation, it may be difficult to visualize the cervix. On palpation, the cervix is firm (except during pregnancy) and usually expanded. **The size of the cervix is best determined by rectal examination, which is also necessary for the detection of any extension of disease into the parametrium.**

Biopsy

Any obvious tumor growth or ulceration should undergo office punch biopsy or diathermy loop excision for histologic confirmation. Any cervix that is unusually firm or expanded should also undergo biopsy and endocervical curettage (ECC).

If the patient has a normal-appearing cervix but is symptomatic or has an abnormal Pap smear, then colposcopy should be performed. If a definitive diagnosis of invasive cancer cannot be made on the basis of an office biopsy, then diagnostic conization may be necessary.

Colposcopy for Invasive Cancer

Colposcopic detection of a microinvasive carcinoma depends on its size and location. Very small lesions may be missed, although the likelihood of having early stromal invasion increases with the surface extent of the preinvasive lesion (8). If the microinvasive carcinoma is entirely within the endocervical canal, then the ectocervix may be colposcopically normal.

Ectocervical microcarcinomas are classically associated with atypical vessels, which are prone to bleed. **Atypical vessels show a completely irregular and haphazard disposition, great variation in caliber, and abrupt changes in direction, often forming acute angles** (Fig. 9.2). The intercapillary distance is increased and tends to be variable (8).

Frankly invasive cancers can usually be seen with the naked eye, but the colposcope highlights their surface irregularity and highly atypical blood vessels (Fig. 9.3). Endophytic tumors may present as an "erosion," the true nature of which can be recognized only by their papillary

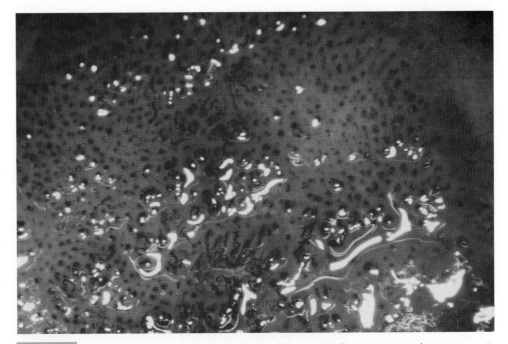

Figure 9.2   Colposcopic appearance of microinvasive cervical cancer. Note the severe varicose vascular abnormality with course punctation and transitional forms to atypical vessels.

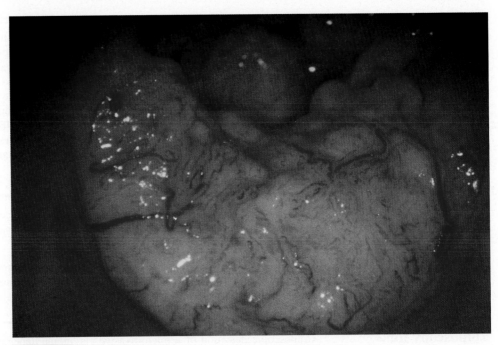

Figure 9.3   Colposcopic appearance of invasive cervical cancer. Note the surface irregularity and dilated atypical vessels.

surface and atypical vessels. A keratotic surface may mask the colposcopic features of an endophytic lesion, so biopsy of areas of keratosis is mandatory.

Adenocarcinomas present no specific features. They often occur in association with squamous CIN, and all of the vascular changes described previously may be seen with these lesions.

Staging

Cervical cancer is staged clinically because most patients worldwide are treated only with radiation therapy.

The 1994 staging system of the International Federation of Gynecology and Obstetrics (FIGO) is shown in Table 9.1 (9). **For updated FIGO surgical staging tables (2008), see table 9.1A on page 665.** A comparison of the FIGO staging and the TNM (tumor, nodes, metastasis) classification is shown in Table 9.2.

Clinical Staging

Clinical staging is often inaccurate in defining the extent of disease. The Gynecologic Oncology Group (GOG) (10), in a study of 290 patients with surgically staged cervical cancer, reported errors in FIGO clinical staging ranging from 24% in stage IB to 67% for stage IVA disease. **Most patients were upstaged on the basis of surgical exploration, with the most likely sites of occult metastases being the pelvic and paraaortic lymph nodes.** Other sites of occult disease were the parametrium, peritoneum, and omentum. As many as 14% of patients may also be downstaged (11), usually because a benign pathologic process is discovered, such as pelvic inflammatory disease, endometriosis, or fibroids.

Noninvasive Diagnostic Studies

Because information about the extent of disease is critical for treatment planning, various imaging studies have been used to define more accurately the extent of disease.

Computed Tomography   Computed tomography (CT) has been used to help stage pelvic cancers since the mid 1970s. In addition to the lymph nodes, a pelvic and abdominal CT scan allows an evaluation of the liver, urinary tract, and bony structures. **A CT can detect only changes in the size of the nodes, those greater than 1 cm in diameter usually being considered positive.** Normal-sized nodes containing microscopic deposits give false negative results, whereas nodal enlargement from inflammatory or hyperplastic changes gives false positive results. If nodes greater than 1.5 cm in diameter are considered positive, then the sensitivity of the test is improved at the expense of the specificity.

Table 9.1 Carcinoma of the Cervix Uteri: FIGO Nomenclature (Montreal, 1994)	
Stage 0	Carcinoma *in situ*, cervical intraepithelial neoplasia 3 (CIN 3).
Stage I	The carcinoma is strictly confined to the cervix (extension to the corpus would be disregarded).
IA	Invasive carcinoma that can be diagnosed only by microscopy. All macroscopically visible lesions—even with superficial invasion—are allotted to stage IB carcinomas.
	Invasion is limited to a measured stromal invasion with a maximal depth of 5.0 mm and a horizontal extension of ≤7.0 mm.
	Depth of invasion should not exceed 5.0 mm from the base of the epithelium of the original tissue superficial or glandular. The involvement of vascular spaces—venous or lymphatic—should not change the stage allotment.
IA1	Measured stromal invasion of ≤3.0 mm in depth and extension of 7.0 mm.
IA2	Measured stromal invasion of >3.0 mm and ≤5.0 mm with an extension of ≤7.0 mm.
IB	Clinically visible lesions limited to the cervix uteri or preclinical cancers greater than stage IA.
IB1	Clinically visible lesions ≤4 cm.
IB2	Clinically visible lesions >4 cm.
Stage II	Cervical carcinoma invades beyond the uterus but not to the pelvic wall or to the lower third of the vagina.
IIA	No obvious parametrial involvement.
IIB	Obvious parametrial involvement.
Stage III	The carcinoma has extended to the pelvic wall. On rectal examination, there is no cancer-free space between the tumor and the pelvic wall. The tumor involves the lower one-third of the vagina. All cases with hydronephrosis or a nonfunctioning kidney are included, unless they are known to result from another cause.
IIIA	Tumor involves lower one-third of the vagina, with no extension to the pelvic wall.
IIIB	Extension to the pelvic wall or hydronephrosis or nonfunctioning kidney.
Stage IV	The carcinoma extends beyond the true pelvis or involves (biopsy proven) the mucosa of the bladder or rectum. A bullous edema, as such, does not permit a case to be allotted to stage IV.
IVA	Spread of the growth to adjacent organs.
IVB	Spread to distant organs.

For the updated Carcinoma of the Cervix Uteri 2008 FIGO staging, see Table 9.1A, on page 665.

FIGO, International Federation of Gynecology and Obstetrics.

The following "Rules for Classification" are reproduced from the 24th volume of the *Annual Report on the Results of Treatment in Gynaecological Cancer* (8).

Clinical-Diagnostic Staging

Staging of cervical cancer is based on clinical evaluation; therefore, careful clinical examination should be performed in all cases, preferably by an experienced examiner and under anesthesia. The clinical staging must not be changed because of subsequent findings. When there is doubt as to which stage a particular cancer should be allocated, the earlier stage is mandatory. The following examinations are permitted: palpation, inspection, colposcopy, endocervical curettage, hysteroscopy, cystoscopy, proctoscopy, intravenous urography, and x-ray examination of the lungs and skeleton. Suspected bladder or rectal involvement should be confirmed by biopsy and histologic evidence. Conization or amputation of the cervix is regarded as a clinical examination. Invasive cancers so identified are to be included in the reports. Findings of optional examinations (e.g., lymphangiography, arteriography, venography, laparoscopy, ultrasound, computed tomographic scan, and magnetic resonance imaging) are of value for planning therapy but, because these are not generally available and the interpretation of results is variable, the findings of such studies should not be the basis for changing the clinical staging. Fine-needle aspiration of scan-detected suspicious lymph nodes may be helpful in treatment planning.

Postsurgical Treatment-Pathologic Staging

In cases treated by surgical procedures, the pathologist's findings in the removed tissues can be the basis for extremely accurate statements on the extent of disease. The findings should not be allowed to change the clinical staging but should be recorded in the manner described for the pathologic staging of disease. The TNM nomenclature is appropriate for this purpose. Infrequently, hysterectomy is carried out in the presence of unsuspected extensive invasive cervical carcinoma. Such cases cannot be clinically staged or included in therapeutic statistics, but it is desirable that they be reported separately.

As in all gynecological cancers, staging is determined at the time of the primary diagnosis and cannot be altered, even at recurrence.

Only if the rules for clinical staging are strictly observed will it be possible to compare results among clinics and by differing modes of therapy.

FIGO Stage	T	N	M
Table 9.2 Carcinoma of the Cervix Uteri: Stage Grouping			
		UICC	
	T	**N**	**M**
0	Tis	N_0	M_0
IA1	T_1a_1	N_0	M_0
IA2	T_1a_2	N_0	M_0
IB1	T_11b_1	N_0	M_0
IB2	T_1b_2	N_0	M_0
IIA	T_{2a}	N_0	M_0
IIB	T_{2b}	N_0	M_0
IIIA	T_{3b}	N_0	M_0
IIIB	T_1	N_1	M_0
	T_2	N_1	M_0
	T_{3a}	N_1	M_0
	T_{3b}	any N	M_0
IVA	T_4	any N	M_0
IVB	any T	any N	M_1

FIGO, International Federation of Gynecology and Obstetrics; UICC, International Union Against Cancer; T, tumor; N, nodes; M, metastasis.

In a review of the literature, Hacker and Berek (12) reported that the overall accuracy for the detection of paraaortic lymph node metastases was 84.4%, with a false positive rate of approximately 21% (9 of 41 positive readings) and a false negative rate of approximately 13% (13 of 99 negative readings).

Magnetic Resonance Imaging   Because CT cannot discriminate between cancer and normal soft tissue of the cervix and uterus, it is limited in the evaluation of early cervical cancer. Magnetic resonance imaging (MRI), which has been used since the early 1980s, has high-contrast resolution and multiplanar imaging capability and is **a valuable modality for determining tumor size, degree of stromal penetration, vaginal extension, corpus extension, parametrial extension, and lymph node status** (13) (Figure 9.4).

Subak et al. (14) evaluated CT or MRI before surgical exploration in 79 patients with FIGO stage IB, IIA, or IIB cervical carcinoma. They reported that **MRI estimated tumor size to within 0.5 cm of the surgical specimen in 64 of 69 patients (93%) and had an accuracy of 78% for measuring depth of stromal invasion.** By contrast, CT was unable to evaluate tumor size or depth of invasion. For the evaluation of stage of disease, MRI had an accuracy of 90% compared with 65% for CT ($p < 0.005$), and it was also more accurate in assessing parametrial invasion (94% vs. 76%, $p < 0.005$). Both modalities were comparable for the evaluation of lymph node metastases (each 86% accurate).

Narayan and colleagues from Melbourne reported that the cervical diameter determined by EUA correlated poorly with the MRI diameter, but the MRI diameter correlated strongly with the pathologic diameter after surgical removal of the specimen ($p < 0.0001$) (15). **The ability of MRI to more accurately determine tumor diameter and parametrial infiltration, particularly in patients with bulky cervical tumors, makes it a useful adjunct to clinical evaluation in treatment planning (16). MRI is also appropriate for the evaluation of pregnant patients because it poses no risk to the fetus** (17).

A metaanalysis comparing the utility of lymphangiogram, CT, and MRI for the detection of pelvic and paraaortic lymph node metastases in patients with cervical cancer concluded that the three imaging modalities performed comparably (18).

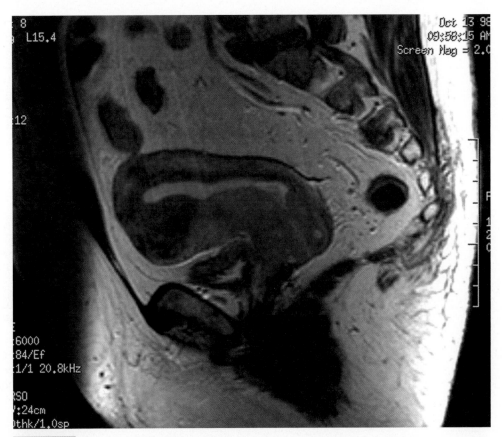

Figure 9.4 **MRI Scan showing a moderate sized cervical tumor with extension to the uterine corpus.** (Scan courtesy of Dr Kailash Narayan, Melbourne, Australia.)

Positron Emission Tomography   The positron emission tomgraphy (PET) imaging technique has been available in some centers since the mid-1990s. It depends on metabolic, rather than anatomic, alteration for the detection of disease. PET uses radionuclides, which decay with the emission of positrons (positively charged particles). Because cancer cells are avid users of glucose, a radionuclide-labeled analogue of glucose, 2-[18F] fluoro-2-deoxy-D-glucose (FDG), can be used to detect sites of malignancy by identifying sites of increased glycolysis. **The PET scan has the potential to delineate more accurately the extent of disease, particularly in lymph nodes that are not enlarged** and in distant sites that are undetectable by conventional imaging studies.

Rose et al. (19) performed PET scanning on 32 patients with stages IIB to IVA cervical cancer before surgical staging lymphadenectomy. For the paraaortic lymph nodes, PET scanning had a sensitivity of 75%, a specificity of 92%, a positive predictive value of 75%, and negative predictive value of 92%. In a study aimed at determining whether PET scanning could obviate the need for surgical staging, Narayan et al. reported a sensitivity of 83%, specificity of 92%, positive predictive value of 91%, and negative predictive value of 85% for 24 patients evaluable for pelvic nodal status (20). However, PET detected only four of seven (57%) cases of positive paraaortic nodes. All histologically confirmed nodes not visualized on PET were <1 cm in diameter.

Grigsby et al. retrospectively compared the results of CT lymph node staging with whole-body FDG–PET in 101 consecutive patients with cervical cancer who were referred for primary radiation therapy (21). CT demonstrated abnormally enlarged pelvic lymph nodes in 20 patients (20%) and paraaortic lymph nodes in seven (7%). PET demonstrated abnormal FDG uptake in pelvic nodes in 67 patients (67%), in paraaortic nodes in 21 patients (21%), and in supraclavicular nodes in eight patients (8%). For the 94 patients with negative paraaortic nodes on CT scan, the 2-year progression-free survival (PFS) was 64% in PET-negative patients and 18% in PET-positive patients ($p < 0.0001$) (Fig. 9.5). **A multivariate analysis demonstrated that the most significant factor for PFS was the presence of positive paraaortic lymph nodes as detected by PET imaging** ($p = 0.025$).

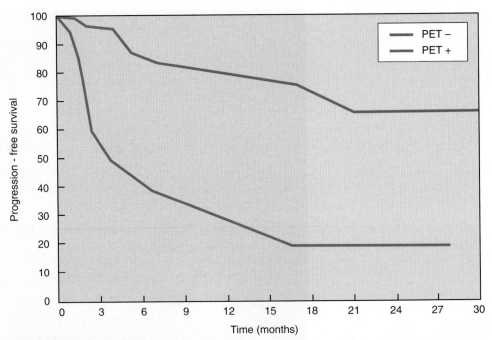

Figure 9.5 Survival curves for patients with a negative CT scan in relation to PET scan status of the paraaortic lymph nodes. (Reproduced with permission from **Grigsby PW, Siegel BA, Dehdashti F.** Lymph node staging by positron emission tomography in patients with carcinoma of the cervix. *J Clin Oncol* 2001;19:3745–3749.)

The combined use of MRI and PET for pretreatment staging of nonoperable cervical cancer has led to a better understanding of the relationship between FIGO stage tumor volume and nodal metastases (22).

Extension of cervical cancer into the uterus can be readily detected by MRI. In univariate analysis, Narayan et al. reported a significant association between nodal involvement and both FIGO stage ($p = 0.018$) and uterine body involvement; in multivariate analysis, however, **only uterine body extension was independently related to the risk of lymph node involvement** (21). PET-documented pelvic node positivity was 75% (39 of 52) in patients with uterine extension as compared with 11% (2 of 18) in those without ($p < 0.001$).

A recent analysis of 15 published PET studies in cervical cancer reported that the pooled sensitivity of FDG–PET for paraaortic lymph node metastases in cervical cancer was 84% [95% confidence interval (CI), 68%–94%], **and the specificity 95%** (95% CI, 89%–98%) (23).

Fine-Needle Aspiration Cytology   If pelvic or abdominal masses or enlarged lymph nodes are detected during physical examination or imaging studies, fine-needle aspiration may be performed under CT or ultrasonic guidance. The procedure is performed under local anesthesia and is free of major complications, even in the presence of clotting problems or perforation of a hollow viscus. The reported accuracy for abdominopelvic nodes ranges from 74% to 95% (24,25). **Only a positive cytologic diagnosis should be used as a basis for therapeutic decision making.**

Surgical Staging

The inability of available noninvasive diagnostic tests to detect small lymph node metastases led many investigators in the 1970s to undertake pretreatment staging laparotomies to identify patients with positive paraaortic nodes. These patients were then treated with extended-field radiation to encompass the involved nodes.

The initial approach used was transperitoneal, but this was associated with a significant risk of postoperative adherent, fixed loops of bowel, and increased postradiation morbidity (26). Of the first 33 patients staged with this approach at the University of California, Los Angeles (UCLA), ten (30.3%) subsequently had small bowel complications requiring surgical correction (27). The complications included enterovaginal fistulas in five patients, small bowel obstruction in nine, and radiation enteritis in six.

After this experience, the UCLA group introduced the extraperitoneal approach (27). Although originally described through a left lateral J-shaped incision, it is most readily performed through a midline incision, which facilitates easy access to both sides of the pelvis. **When closed with running PDS or Maxon Smead-Jones sutures, the midline incision does not delay the onset of radiation therapy.** Before the node dissection, the peritoneum is opened, and a thorough exploration of the peritoneal cavity is carried out. The peritoneum is then stripped off the anterior and lateral abdominal wall to expose the pelvic sidewall on each side. Each round ligament must be transected extraperitoneally to facilitate exposure. The dissection may be extended cephalad as far as necessary by extending the lower midline incision around the umbilicus to the epigastrium.

Surgical complications of staging laparotomies include damage to the great vessels, particularly the inferior vena cava, and ureteric injury, but are infrequent in the hands of an experienced surgeon. In the GOG report of almost 300 patients (10), the operative mortality was 0.3% (one case), intraoperative injuries to the vein or ureter occurred in four cases (1.6%), and a postoperative urinary fistula or bowel obstruction occurred in seven patients (2.9%).

In the 1990s, some investigators proposed laparoscopic staging (28). This is discussed in Chapter 21.

In spite of the theoretical advantages of surgical staging, the benefits in terms of patient outcomes remain unproven. Lai et al., from Taipei, conducted a randomized trial to compare clinical with surgical staging for patients with locally advanced cervical cancer (29). Patients in the surgical arm were randomly allocated to either a laparoscopic or an extraperitoneal approach. Although paraaortic nodal metastases were documented in 25% of patients in the surgical arm, patient accrual was terminated after 61 patients were entered because interim analysis showed a significantly worse outcome in terms of progression-free survival ($p = 0.003$) and overall survival ($p = 0.024$) for patients in the surgical arm.

A retrospective review of three phase III Gynecologic Oncology Group studies (GOG 85, 120, and 165) was undertaken to compare the outcome for patients who had negative paraaortic lymph nodes by pretreatment surgical staging with that of patients who had only radiographic (CT or MRI) exclusion of paraaortic nodal disease before pelvic chemoradiation (30). There were 555 in the surgical staging group, and 130 in the radiographic group. **In multivariate analysis, radiographic staging was associated with a poorer prognosis both for disease progression [hazard ratio (HR) 1.35; 95% CI, 1.01–1.81] and for death (HR 1.46; 95% CI, 1.08–1.99).**

The results from the ongoing collaborative study of PET, MRI, and surgical staging being conducted by the American College of Radiology Imaging network and the GOG will help clarify whether or not there is any ongoing role for surgical staging in the PET scan era (available at http://www.clinicaltrials.gov). By constructing a mathematical model from the available literature, Petereit et al. predicted that surgical staging would save 2.6, 6, and 7 lives per 100 patients treated, for stages IB, IIB, and IIIB, respectively (31).

Patterns of Spread

Cervical cancer spreads by the following means:

1. **direct invasion** into the cervical stroma, corpus, vagina, and parametrium
2. **lymphatic permeation and metastasis**
3. **hematogenous dissemination**

Direct Infiltration

Invasive cervical cancer, whether squamous or glandular, arises from intraepithelial neoplasia. Malignant cells penetrate the basement membrane, then progressively infiltrate the underlying stroma. They may progressively infiltrate laterally to involve the cardinal and uterosacral ligaments, superiorly to involve the uterine corpus, inferiorly to involve the vagina, anteriorly to involve the bladder, and posteriorly to involve the peritoneum of the pouch of Douglas and the rectum.

Lymphatic Spread

Cervical cancer can spread to all pelvic node groups, although the obturator nodes are most frequently involved. The parametrial nodes are not necessarily involved before the nodes on the pelvic sidewall. Although tumor cells can reach the common iliac and paraaortic nodes directly by the posterior cervical trunk (32), this is very uncommon, and **lymph node spread in cervical**

Table 9.3 Incidence of Pelvic Lymph Node Metastases in Stage IB Cervical Cancer			
Author	**Patients**	**Positive Nodes**	**%**
Zander *et al.*, 1981 (34)	860	163	18.9
Fuller *et al.*, 1982 (35)	280	42	15.0
Timmer *et al.*, 1984 (36)	119	18	15.1
Inoue and Okamura, 1984 (37)	362	47	13.0
Creasman *et al.*, 1986 (38)	258	36	14.0
Finan *et al.*, 1986 (39)	229	49	21.4
Artman *et al.*, 1987 (40)	153	13	8.5
Monaghan *et al.*, 1990 (41)	494	102	20.6
Samlal *et al.*, 1997 (42)	271	53	19.6
Total	3,026	523	17.3

cancer almost invariably occurs in an orderly fashion from the nodes on the pelvic sidewall to the common iliac and then the paraaortic group. From the paraaortic nodes, spread can occasionally occur through the thoracic duct to the left scalene nodes (29). The incidence of pelvic lymph node metastases in stage IB cervical cancer is shown in Table 9.3. The incidence of paraaortic nodal metastases in stages II and III cervical cancer is shown in Table 9.4.

The concept of sentinel node identification for cervical cancer was first introduced by Dargent in 2000 (52). Using a combination of patent blue dye and radiolabeled colloid injected into the cervix preoperatively, several authors have subsequently confirmed the ability to identify sentinel nodes in 70% to 100% of patients (53–56) (see Chapter 21). Sentinel nodes have usually been located in the hypogastric, external iliac, or obturator nodal groups but have also been reported in the common iliac and paraaortic region. In one patient, a sentinel node was found in the left groin (57).

Lymphatic invasion by tumor cells is commonly seen in the primary tumor, and tumor cells are also seen occasionally in lymphatic channels in the parametrium. Burghardt and Girardi (58) believe that tumor emboli are sometimes held up in a lymphatic vessel and grow to become foci of discontinuous parametrial involvement.

Table 9.4 Incidence of Paraaortic Lymph Node Metastases in Stages II and III Cervical Cancer						
	Stage II			**Stage III**		
Author	**Explored**	**Positive**	**%**	**Explored**	**Positive**	**%**
Nelson *et al.*, 1977 (26)	63	9	14.3	39	15	38.5
Delgado *et al.*, 1977 (43)	18	8	44.4	13	5	38.5
Piver and Barlow, 1977 (44)	46	6	13.0	49	18	36.7
Sudarsanam *et al.*, 1978 (45)	43	7	16.3	19	3	15.8
Buchsbaum, 1979 (46)	19	1	5.3	104	34	32.7
Hughes *et al.*, 1980 (47)	80	14	17.5	96	23	24.0
Ballon *et al.*, 1981 (48)	48	9	18.8	24	4	16.7
Welander *et al.*, 1981 (49)	63	13	20.6	38	10	26.3
Berman *et al.*, 1984 (50)	265	43	16.2	180	45	25.0
Potish *et al.*, 1985 (51)	47	5	10.6	11	4	36.4
La Polla *et al.*, 1986 (11)	47	6	12.8	38	14	36.8
Total	739	121	16.4	611	175	28.6

Ovarian involvement by cervical cancer is rare but most likely occurs through the lymphatic connection between the uterus and the adnexal structures (59). In a study of patients with clinical stage IB cervical cancer, the GOG reported ovarian spread in four of 770 patients (0.5%) with squamous carcinoma and in two of 121 patients (1.7%) with adenocarcinoma. All six patients with ovarian metastases had other evidence of extracervical spread (60).

Hematogenous Spread

Although spread to virtually all parts of the body has been reported, the most common organs for hematogenous spread are the lungs, liver, and bone.

Treatment

Treatment of invasive cancer involves appropriate management for both the primary lesion and potential sites of metastatic disease. Both surgery and radiation therapy may be used for primary treatment, although definitive surgery is usually limited to patients with stages I or early IIA disease. Some European and Asian centers also treat patients with stage IIB disease with primary surgery (61–63).

Microinvasive Carcinoma

The term **microcarcinoma of the uterine cervix** was first introduced by Mestwerdt (64) in the German literature in 1947. He suggested that 5 mm was the deepest penetration acceptable. Since then, both terminology and treatment have been the subject of much debate.

In 1961, the Cancer Committee of FIGO recommended that clinical stage I cervical cancer should be subdivided into stage IA and stage IB, and stage IA was vaguely defined as a preclinical cancer with early stromal invasion. This did little to clarify even the definition.

In 1974, the Committee on Nomenclature of **the Society of Gynecologic Oncologists (SGO) in the United States proposed that microinvasive carcinoma should be defined as a lesion that invaded below the basement membrane to a depth of 3 mm or less, and in which there was no evidence of lymph-vascular space invasion.** Although this definition provided no horizontal dimension, patients whose disease fulfilled these criteria were shown to have virtually no risk of lymph node metastases and to be adequately treated by either hysterectomy or cone biopsy (65–67).

In 1985, FIGO included measurements in the definition of stage IA disease for the first time (68). The new definition stated that stage IA was a preclinical carcinoma (i.e., diagnosed only by microscopy) and should be divided into two groups: stage IA1, in which there was minimal stromal invasion, and stage IA2, in which the depth of stromal invasion should not exceed 5 mm and the horizontal spread should not exceed 7 mm. Vascular space invasion did not influence the staging. This definition still failed to define the border between stage IA1 and IA2 lesions.

A more precise definition of microinvasive carcinoma was adopted by FIGO in 1995. Stage IA1 was defined as a tumor that invaded to a depth of 3 mm or less, whereas stage IA2 referred to a tumor that invaded to a depth greater than 3 mm and up to 5 mm. In both stages, the horizontal spread should not exceed 7 mm. Lymph-vascular space invasion was not included as part of the definition.

Stage IA1: Squamous Carcinoma

Although stromal invasion can be seen in small punch biopsies, a definitive diagnosis of microinvasion can be made only in conization (or hysterectomy) specimens (69). The conization specimen must be thoroughly sampled, not only to make the correct diagnosis but also to be certain about the margins.

In an extensive review of the literature, Ostor (70) reported that of 2,274 squamous lesions with invasion of less than 1 mm only three were cases of lymph node metastases (0.1%) and invasive recurrence developed in eight cases (0.4%). Among 1,324 squamous lesions invading between 1 and 3 mm, there were seven cases with lymph node metastases (0.5%) and 26 cases in which invasive recurrence developed (2%). No horizontal limitation was placed on these lesions, so they do not strictly fit the current FIGO definition of stage IA1 disease, and most of the cases were treated without lymph node dissection.

Studies of stage IA disease in patients meeting the 1995 FIGO definition are limited. Elliott and colleagues from Sydney reported 476 such patients (71). There were 418 (88%) squamous and

58 (12%) glandular tumors. Of 180 patients undergoing lymphadenectomy, the incidence of positive nodes in patients with stage IA1 disease was 0.8% (1 of 121 cases). Lee et al. (72) from South Korea reported positive nodes in three of 116 patients (2.6%) undergoing lymphadenectomy for stage 1A1 squamous cell carcinoma of the cervix.

Roman et al. (73) reported 87 cases of microinvasive carcinoma diagnosed on cone biopsy and followed by either repeat cone biopsy or hysterectomy. Significant predictors of residual invasion included status of the internal margin (residual invasion present in 22% of women with dysplasia at the margin vs. 3% with a negative margin; $p < 0.03$) and the combined status of the internal margin and the postconization ECC (residual invasion 4% if both negative, 13% if one positive, and 33% if both positive; $p < 0.015$). Depth of invasion and the number of invasive foci were not significant. The researchers concluded that **if either the internal margin or the postconization ECC contained dysplasia or carcinoma, then the risk of residual invasion was high and warranted repeat conization before definitive treatment planning.**

A study from Chang Mai, Thailand, confirmed these findings (74). Histopathology studies were reviewed from 129 patients who underwent hysterectomy following a cone biopsy that showed microinvasive squamous cell carcinoma. All had high-grade CIN or invasive carcinoma at the cone margins. Of the 129 patients, 77 (59.7%) had residual disease in the hysterectomy specimen, of whom 20 patients (15.5%) had residual invasive cancer: 18 were microinvasive and two were frankly invasive. **Factors that significantly affected the risk of residual disease**

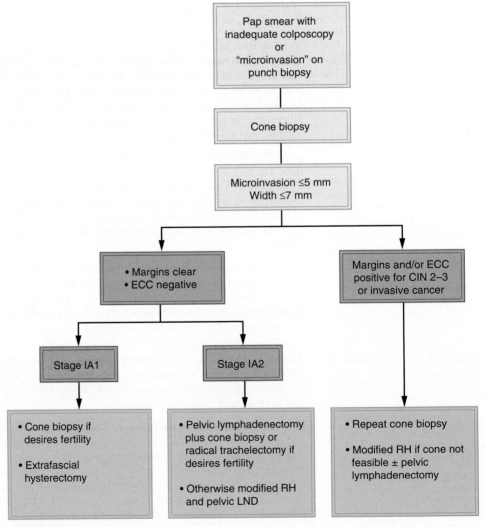

Figure 9.6 Algorithm for the management of patients with a high-grade Pap smear and inadequate colposcopy or with microinvasive cervical carcinoma on punch biopsy.

included positive postconization endocervical curettage (*p* = 0.001), positive cone margins for invasive cancer (*p* = 0.003), and depth of stromal invasion >1mm (*p* = 0.014). They also recommended repeat conization to determine the exact severity of the lesion before planning definite treatment.

In view of these considerations, a cone biopsy with clear surgical margins and a negative ECC should be considered adequate treatment for a patient with stage IA1 squamous carcinoma of the cervix. If future childbearing is not required, then extrafascial hysterectomy may be considered. **If the cone margins or postconization ECC reveal high-grade dysplasia or microinvasive carcinoma, then a repeat conization should be performed before proceeding to simple hysterectomy because more extensively invasive disease may be present.**

Lymph-vascular space invasion is uncommon in stage IA1 lesions, with Ostor (70) reporting an incidence of 15% from a literature review. Elliott et al. (71) reported lymph-vascular space invasion in 8.5% of tumors invading 1 mm or less, 19% between 1.1 and 2 mm, 29% between 2.1 and 3 mm, and 53% between 3.1 and 5 mm. Lee et al. (72) also found a **positive correlation between depth of invasion and the presence of lymph-vascular space invasion** but found **no definite correlation between lymph-vascular space invasion (LVSI) and lymph node metastases,** only two of their four patients with positive nodes having LVSI (72). Its significance in microinvasive cervical cancer remains controversial, and it is not mentioned in the FIGO definition. It probably should be disregarded when planning treatment, unless it is extensive. A proposed algorithm for the management of microinvasive cervical cancer is shown in Fig. 9.6.

Stage IA2: Squamous Carcinoma

In spite of the extensive literature on microinvasive cervical carcinoma, there is limited information available on lesions 3 to 5 mm deep with as much as 7 mm of horizontal spread (i.e., 1995 FIGO stage IA2 lesions). The 1985 FIGO definition of stage IA2 included all cases other than those with early stromal invasion, which usually meant approximately 1 mm of invasion. Hence, some large European studies of this group of patients would have underestimated the risk of lymph node metastases and invasive recurrence for patients whose tumors invaded 3 to 5 mm. For example, Kolstad (75), in a review of 411 patients with 1985 FIGO stage IA2 squamous carcinoma of the cervix, reported only four cancer-related deaths (1%) and 12 local recurrences (2.9%). Similarly, Burghardt et al. (76) reported two pelvic sidewall recurrences after abdominal hysterectomy among 89 patients (2.2%). A local recurrence developed in three other patients (3.4%). Four of the five recurrences had vascular space invasion.

Investigators in the United States have tended to separate lesions with invasion of 3 mm or less and no vascular space involvement from stage IA2 lesions because such cases met the SGO criteria for conservative management. Therefore, a few publications, mainly from the United States, have reported cases with stromal invasion of 3 to 5 mm, although most have not included the horizontal dimension currently required in the FIGO definition. The overall incidence of lymph node metastases in such cases was 7.1%, although it varied from 0% to 13.8% (Table 9.5). The incidence of invasive recurrence was 3.6%, and 2.9% of patients died of their disease. Most patients were treated by radical hysterectomy and pelvic lymph node dissection.

Table 9.5 Incidence of Lymph Node Metastases with Stromal Invasion of 3 to 5 mm—Horizontal Dimension Not Stated

Author	No.	Nodal Metastases	Invasive Recurrences	Dead of Disease
Van Nagell *et al.*, 1983 (77)	32	3 (9.4%)	3	2
Hasumi *et al.*, 1980 (78)	29	4 (13.8%)	NS	NS
Simon *et al.*, 1986 (67)	26	1 (3.8%)	0	0
Maiman *et al.*, 1988 (79)	30	4 (13.3%)	0	0
Buckley *et al.*, 1996 (80)	94	7 (7.4%)	5	4
Creasman *et al.*, 1998 (81)	51	0 (0.0%)	0	0
Takeshima *et al.*, 1999 (82)	73	5 (9.6%)	3	3
Total	335	24 (7.1%)	11 (3.6%)	9 (2.9%)

NS, not stated.

Takeshima et al. (82) **reported that, of 73 patients with depth of invasion between 3 and 5 mm, the incidence of lymph node metastasis was 3.4% for tumors with a horizontal spread of 7 mm or less and 9.1% for those with greater than 7 mm spread.** Elliott et al. also reported positive nodes in 3.4% of patients (2 of 59) with stage IA2 cervical cancer (71).

It is apparent that more data are needed for this group of patients, and it is hoped that the Cancer Committee of FIGO will not change the current definition of microinvasion so that more information can be obtained about the risk of lymph node metastases and the risk of recurrence with various treatment approaches.

Our **recommended treatment for stage IA2 squamous carcinoma of the cervix is modified radical hysterectomy and pelvic lymph node dissection. In a medically unfit patient, intracavitary radiation may be used.**

Many patients with early cervical cancer are young, and preservation of fertility is a major concern. Consequently, surgical approaches that remove the primary lesion and regional lymph nodes, while conserving the corpus for future childbearing, have been explored.

Cone biopsy and extraperitoneal lymphadenectomy have been used in the past, but in 1994 Dargent et al. pioneered the use of **radical trachelectomy and laparoscopic pelvic lymphadenectomy** (83). A nonabsorbable cervical cerclage is usually placed around the uterine isthmus at the time of the trachelectomy. Several other groups have subsequently confirmed that the operation is feasible in experienced hands, that cure rates are high, and that subsequent pregnancies can be carried to viability in many cases (See Table 21.3). Covens et al. (84) reported an actuarial conception rate at 12 months of 37% following radical trachelectomy on 30 patients with stage IA–early IB disease (85).

Radical abdominal trachelectomy was first reported by Smith et al. **in 1997** (85). One advantage of this approach is that the anatomy is more familiar to most gynecologic oncologists. Although the procedure has not yet gained wide acceptance, successful pregnancy outcomes have been reported (86).

Although radical trachelectomy is associated with less operative time and short-term morbidity than radical hysterectomy, **there are some long-term morbidities.** In a retrospective review of 29 patients undergoing radical trachelectomy, the group from St. Bartholomew's Hospital in London reported **dysmenorrhea in 24%, irregular menstruation in 17%, recurrent candidiasis in 14%, cervical suture problems in 14%, isthmic stenosis in 10%, and prolonged amenorrhea in 7% of patients** (87).

A critical issue for trachelectomy by either route is the extent of tumor extension up the endocervical canal. An adequate endocervical surgical margin is mandatory if local recurrence is to be avoided, so some type of preoperative imaging is desirable. **Magnetic resonance imaging appears to be highly sensitive and specific for the determination of tumor extension beyond the internal os** (88).

Microinvasive Adenocarcinoma

Although the concept of microinvasive squamous carcinoma is well accepted, the concept for the glandular counterpart is more controversial, partly because of the lack of available data, but also because of the difficulty in accurately determining the true extent of glandular lesions. Microinvasion has usually been reported as depth of invasion or tumor thickness of 5 mm or less, the measurement being taken from the mucosal surface (89,90) or from the base of the surface epithelium (91). Width and volume of tumor involvement have varied considerably, and only recently have reports looked specifically at microinvasion as now defined by the FIGO staging.

Most cases arise adjacent to the transformation zone, although Teshima et al. (92) reported that three of 30 cases (10%) arose outside the transformation zone. Adenocarcinoma *in situ* may extend up the entire endocervical canal, and invasion may occur at any point (92). Lee and Flynn (93), in a study of 40 cases of adenocarcinoma invasive to 5 mm or less, reported that in 78% of the cases, the midpoint of the invasive focus was in the region of the transformation zone. **The endometrioid variant was particularly likely to arise higher in the canal.**

Whereas squamous lesions are usually unifocal, glandular lesions are sometimes multifocal. Ostor et al. (90) reported that 21 of 77 cases (27.3%) were multicentric, meaning that both cervical lips were affected, without continuity around the "edges" at 3 and 9 o'clock. They reported no "skip" lesions, which they arbitrarily defined as separation between discrete microinvasive adenocarcinomas in the same lip of greater than 3 mm. More than one focus of invasive disease was present in four of 40 cases (10%) reported by Lee and Flynn (93).

Positive lymph nodes have rarely been reported in FIGO stage IA1 lesions, although Elliott reported a solitary nodal metastasis in a patient with <1 mm stromal invasion (71). Berek and co-workers (89), in a report of 102 patients with primary adenocarcinoma of the cervix from UCLA, reported no lymph node metastases in patients whose tumor was less than 2 cm in diameter, although two of 18 patients (11.1%) with 2 to 5 mm of invasion had positive nodes. Kaku et al. (91) reported recurrences at the vaginal vault in two of 30 patients (6.7%) with less than 5 mm of invasion. One patient had a tumor volume of 1,222 mm^3, but the other had a tumor with a depth of 3.9 mm and a width of 4.9 mm (i.e., FIGO stage IA2). The only adeno-carcinoma recurrence in the 77 patients reported by Ostor et al. (90) involved a patient whose tumor invaded to a depth of 3.2 mm but was 21 mm in length (i.e., stage IB1).

A study from Melbourne reported 29 patients with stage IA1 and 9 with stage IA2 microinva-sive adenocarcinoma of the cervix (94). A variety of treatment methods were used. Cone biopsy of the cervix was performed in 18 patients, including two with stage IA2 disease. No recur-rences were noted during an average follow-up of 72 months. **In a literature review**, the same authors noted **positive nodes in 12 of 814 patients (1.5%) undergoing pelvic lymph node dissection for microinvasive adenocarcinoma of the cervix.** Lymph-vascular space invasion was present in 25 patients (3%), all without lymph node involvement (94).

The Surveillance, Epidemiology, and End Results (SEER) database was used to identify 131 cases of stage IA1 and 170 cases of stage IA2 adenocarcinoma of the cervix treated between 1988 and 1997 (95). There was no histologic review, and patients were treated in a variety of ways from cone biopsy to radical hysterectomy and pelvic lymphadenectomy. Simple hysterectomy alone was used for 118 patients (39.2%). **With a mean follow-up of 46.5 months, the censored survival was 99.2% for patients with stage IA1 disease and 98.2% for stage IA2.**

In view of these observations, **it seems reasonable to treat the disease in a similar manner to its squamous counterpart. A cone biopsy with negative margins appears to be adequate treatment for the primary lesion if fertility is desired** (96), **particularly in the absence of lymph-vascular space invasion. The cone biopsy should be a cold knife proce-dure;** loop excision procedures obscure depth of invasion, and margins and are not acceptable either for diagnosis or therapy (97). Following childbearing, it seems reasonable to recom-mend hysterectomy because Pap smears and colposcopy are less reliable, and Poynor et al. (98) reported that ECC was positive before cervical conization in only 43% of patients with glandular lesions.

Stage IB1 and Early Stage IIA Cervical Cancer

In 1994, FIGO recognized the prognostic significance of tumor size by subdividing stage IB disease into stage IB1 (primary lesion ≤4 cm diameter) and stage IB2 (primary lesion >4 cm diameter).

Patients with stage IB1 are universally regarded as being ideal candidates for radical hysterectomy and pelvic lymphadenectomy, although equal cure rates may be obtained with primary radiation therapy (99). The choice of modality should depend mainly on the availability of the appropriate expertise. Since the introduction of fellowship training in gyne-cologic oncology, expertise in radical pelvic surgery has become widely available in the United States and most developed countries. The Patterns of Care study in the United States suggests that the same may not be true for radiation oncology, particularly outside of tertiary referral units (100). If both surgical and radiotherapeutic expertise are available, then radiation is usually reserved for the surgically unfit patient. **Chronologic age should not be considered a contraindication to radical surgery because elderly patients experience morbidity similar to that of younger patients** (101).

Primary surgery has the advantage of removing the primary disease and allowing accu-rate surgical staging, thereby allowing any adjuvant therapy to be more accurately targeted. In addition, it avoids the possible chronic radiation damage to the bladder, small and large bowel, and vagina, which is difficult to manage. Surgical injuries to the same organs are more readily repaired because the blood supply is not compromised. Sexual dysfunction is, in general, underreported but is a problem for many patients who have had both external-beam therapy and brachytherapy because of vaginal atrophy, fibrosis, and stenosis (102). Although the vagina is shortened by approximately 1.5 cm after radical hysterectomy, it is more elastic; in premenopausal patients, ovarian function can be preserved. In postmenopausal patients, the nonirradiated vagina responds much better to estrogen therapy.

Influence of Diagnostic Conization

The influence of previous cone biopsy on the morbidity of radical hysterectomy is controversial. Samlal et al. (103) reported no significant difference in morbidity, but the conization–radical hysterectomy interval in their study was 6 weeks. They believed that delaying the definitive surgery may allow the tissue reaction to subside, thereby decreasing morbidity. Others have found that the interval between the conization and radical hysterectomy has no influence on morbidity, and they recommend proceeding without delay (104). Our policy is to proceed immediately with radical hysterectomy if the surgical margins of the cone biopsy are involved but to postpone surgery for 6 weeks if the cone margins are clear.

Types of Radical Hysterectomy

In 1974, Piver et al. (105) described the following five types of hysterectomy: extrafascial, modified radical, radical, extended radical, and partial exenteration.

Extrafascial Hysterectomy (Type I)   This is a simple hysterectomy and is suitable for stage IA1 cervical carcinoma.

Modified Radical Hysterectomy (Type II)   This is basically the hysterectomy described by Ernst Wertheim (106). The uterine artery is ligated where it crosses the ureter, and the medial half of the cardinal ligaments and proximal uterosacral ligaments are resected. Piver et al. (105) described removal of the upper one-third of the vagina, but this is rarely necessary unless vaginal intraepithelial neoplasia (VAIN) 3 is extensive. The operation described by Wertheim involved selective removal of enlarged nodes rather than systematic pelvic lymphadenectomy. **The modified radical hysterectomy is appropriate for stage IA2 cervical cancer.**

Radical Hysterectomy (Type III)   The most commonly performed operation for stage IB cervical cancer is that originally described by Meigs in 1944 (107). The uterine artery is ligated at its origin from the superior vesicle or internal iliac artery, allowing removal of the entire width of the cardinal ligaments. Piver (105) originally described excision of the uterosacral ligaments at their sacral attachments and resection of the upper half of the vagina. Such extensive dissection of the uterosacral ligaments and vagina is seldom required for stage IB cervical cancer.

Extended Radical Hysterectomy (Type IV)   This differs from the type III operation in three aspects: (i) The ureter is completely dissected from the vesicouterine ligament, (ii) the superior vesicle artery is sacrificed, and (iii) three-fourths of the vagina is excised. The risk of ureteric fistula is increased with this procedure, which Piver (105) used for selected small central recurrences after radiation therapy.

Partial Exenteration (Type V)   The indication for this procedure was removal of a central recurrence involving a portion of the distal ureter or bladder. The relevant organ was partially excised and the ureter reimplanted into the bladder. This procedure is occasionally performed if cancer is found to be unexpectedly encasing the distal ureter at the time of radical hysterectomy. Alternatively, the operation may be aborted and the patient treated with primary radiation.

A new classification for radical hysterectomy was described following a consensus meeting in Kyoto, Japan, which was arranged by Shingo Fujii in February 2007 (108). **The classification is based only on the lateral extent of the resection.** Four basic types are described, A–D, adding when necessary a few subtypes that consider nerve preservation and paracervical lymphadenectomy. **Lymph node dissection is considered separately,** and four levels (1–4) are defined according to the corresponding arterial anatomy and the radicality of the procedure. A description of the procedures from the original paper by Querleu and Morrow is given below.

Type A: Minimum Resection of Paracervix

This is an extrafascial hysterectomy. The paracervix is transected medial to the ureter but lateral to the cervix. The uterosacral and vesicouterine ligaments are not transected at a distance from the uterus. Vaginal resection is generally at a minimum, routinely less than 10 mm, without removal of the vaginal part of the paracervix (paracolpos).

Type B: Transection of the Paracervix at the Ureter

This type has two levels:

B1—Without removal of lateral paracervical lymph nodes
B2—With removal of lateral paracervical nodes

Partial resection of the uterosacral and vesicouterine ligaments is a standard part of this category. The ureter is unroofed and rolled laterally, permitting transection of the paracervix at the level of the ureteral tunnel. The neural component of the paracervix caudal to the deep uterine vein is not resected. At least 10mm of the vagina from the cervix or tumor is resected.

The operation corresponds to the modified or proximal radical hysterectomy and is adapted to early cervical cancer. The radicality of this operation can be improved without increasing postoperative morbidity by lymph node dissection of the lateral part of the paracervix, thus defining two subtypes—B1 and B2—with additional removal of the lateral paracervical lymph nodes.

The border between paracervical and iliac or parietal lymph node dissection is defined arbitrarily as the obturator nerve: Paracervical nodes are medial and caudal. The combinatiuon of paracervical and parietal dissections is simply a comprehensive pelvic node dissection. The lateral part of the paracervix has traditionally been resected fully in so-called types III to IV or distal radical hysterectomy.

The morbidity of type B2 does not differ from that of B1, although the combination of B1 with paracervical lymph node dissection may be equivalent to that of type C1 resection.

Type C

In type C, the paracervix is transected at the junction with the internal iliac vascular system and has two types:

C1—With nerve preservation
C2—Without preservation of autonomic nerves

This type involves transection of the uterosacral ligament at the rectum and vesicouterine ligament at the bladder. The ureter is mobilized completely, and 15–20 mm of vagina from the tumor or cervix and the corresponding paracolpos is resented routinely, depending on vaginal and paracervical extent and on surgeon choice.

Type C corresponds to variants of classical radical hysterectomy. By contrast with types A and B, in which the autonomic nerve supply to the bladder is not threatened, the issue of nerve preservation is crucial. Two subcategories are defined: C1 with nerve preservation and C2 without preservation of autonomic nerves. In C1, the uterosacral ligament is transected after separation of the hypogastric nerves. The bladder branches of the pelvic plexus are preserved in the lateral ligament of the bladder (i.e., lateral part of bladder pillar). If the caudal part of the paracervix is transected, then careful identification of bladder nerves is needed.

For C2, the paracervix is transected completely, including the part caudal to the deep uterine vein.

Type D

In type D, the entire paracervix is resected:

D1—Resection of the entire paracervix along with the hypogastric vessels
D2—Resection of the entire paracervix, along with the hypogastric vessels and adjacent fascial or muscular structure

This group of rare operations feature additional ultraradical procedures, mostly indicated at the time of pelvic exenteration. Type D1 is resection of the entire paracervix at the pelvic sidewall along with the hypogastric vessels, exposing the roots of the sciatic nerve. There is total resection of the vessels of the lateral part of the paracervix. These vessels (i.e., inferior gluteal, internal pudendal, and obturator vessels) arise from the internal iliac system.

Type D2 is D1 plus resection of the entire paracervix with the hypogastric vessels and adjacent fascial or muscular structures. This resection corresponds to the LEER (laterally extended endopelvic resection) procedure (109).

Lymph Node Dissection

Lymph node dissection has four levels:

> **Level 1—External and internal iliac**
> **Level 2—Common iliac (including presacral)**
> **Level 3—Aortic inframesenteric**
> **Level 4—Aortic infrarenal**

This classification ignores the widely used pelvic versus paraaortic dissection, in which the limit of the pelvis dissection is around the midcommon iliac area.

Within every level, and independently from each other, several types of lymph node dissection must be defined to describe adequately the radicality of the procedure: diagnostic (minimum sampling of sentinel node only, removal of enlarged nodes only, or random sampling); systematic lymph node dissection; and debulking (resection of all nodes >2cm) (110).

Technique for Radical Hysterectomy

The patient is given prophylactic antibiotics for 24 hours, and pneumatic calf compressors are used during and after surgery until the patient is fully mobilized. In addition, prophylactic subcutaneous *heparin* is given for 5 days after surgery.

Incision   The abdomen may be opened either through a lower midline incision extending to the left of the umbilicus or through a low transverse **Maylard or Cherney** incision. The low transverse incision, which is described in Chapter 20, requires division of the rectus abdominis muscle but provides excellent exposure of the primary tumor and pelvic sidewalls. The midline incision, which can be readily extended, provides better exposure of the paraaortic region, but this is seldom necessary for early stage cervical cancer.

Exploration   After entering the peritoneal cavity, all organs are systematically palpated, and any evidence of metastatic spread is documented by frozen section. The vesicouterine fold and pouch of Douglas peritoneum are examined for evidence of tumor infiltration, and the tubes and ovaries are examined for any abnormalities. Any bulky pelvic or paraaortic nodes are removed and frozen sections obtained to differentiate between inflammatory and malignant changes.

Radical Hysterectomy   With the uterus under traction, the retroperitoneum is entered through the round ligaments bilaterally. The ureter is identified as it crosses the pelvic rim, and the pelvic sidewall spaces are developed by a combination of sharp and blunt dissection (Figs. 9.6, 9.7).

The **paravesicle space** (Fig. 9.7) is bordered by:

1. the obliterated umbilical artery (a continuation of the superior vesicle artery) running along the bladder medially
2. the obturator internus muscle laterally
3. the cardinal ligament or paracervix posteriorly
4. the pubic symphysis anteriorly

The **pararectal space** is bordered by:

1. the rectum medially
2. the hypogastric artery laterally
3. the cardinal ligament or paracervix anteriorly
4. the sacrum posteriorly

The floor of the spaces is formed by the levator ani muscle.

Bladder Takedown   The vesicouterine fold of peritoneum is opened and the bladder dissected off the anterior cervix and upper vagina. This should be done before any blood supply is ligated, because occasionally tumor may infiltrate into the bladder base, making hysterectomy impossible. Rather than resecting the relevant section of the bladder in this situation, the abdomen is usually closed and the patient treated with primary radiation.

Ligation of the Uterine Artery   The uterine artery usually arises from the superior vesicle artery, close to its origin from the hypogastric artery. The artery is ligated at its origin in a type III or type C radical hysterectomy, or at the point where it crosses the ureter in the modified or

Round ligament   Branch to bladder   Paravesical space

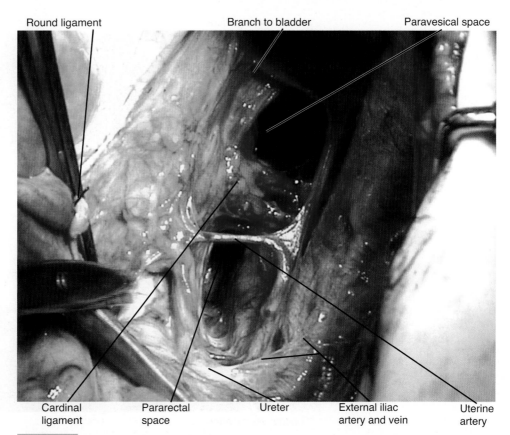

Cardinal   Pararectal   Ureter   External iliac   Uterine
ligament   space   artery and vein   artery

Figure 9.7   **Paravesicle and pararectal spaces.**

type B radical hysterectomy, then mobilized over the ureter by gentle traction and dissection. The uterine veins must be identified and clipped or troublesome bleeding will occur.

Dissection of the Ureter   The roof of the ureteric tunnel is the anterior vesicouterine ligament. This can be taken down in a piecemeal fashion bilaterally (Fig. 9.8), thereby avoiding the troublesome venous bleeding that can occur by blindly advancing a right-angled forceps into the tunnel. Each ureter is mobilized off its peritoneal attachment fairly low in the pelvis to avoid unnecessary stripping from its peritoneal blood supply. It is also mobilized off the side of the uterus. This exposes the posterior or caudal vesicouterine ligament, which is also divided in a type III hysterectomy but not in a type II procedure. The anterolateral surface of the distal ureter is left attached to the bladder in a further effort to preserve the blood supply. If the caudal vesicouterine ligament is transected, then it is desirable to identify and preserve the bladder branch from the inferior hypogastric plexus (111,112).

Posterior Dissection   The peritoneum across the pouch of Douglas is incised and the recto-vaginal space identified by posterior traction on the rectum. The rectum is taken off the posterior vagina and the uterosacral ligaments using sharp and blunt dissection, and the latter are divided at the rectum (type III or C) or closer to the cervix (type II or B) (Fig. 9.9).

Lateral Dissection   After division of the uterosacral ligaments, the cardinal ligaments (para-cervix) are clamped at the level of the pelvic sidewall (type III or C) or more medially (type II or B), after which two more clamps are usually required across the paravaginal tissues to reach the vagina. If the ovaries are to be removed, then the infundibulopelvic ligaments are divided at this stage. If they are to be retained, then they are freed from the fundus by transecting the ovarian ligament and fallopian tube.

Vaginal Resection   The length of vagina to be removed depends on the nature of the primary lesion and the colposcopic findings in the vagina. If the primary lesion is confined to the cervix and there is no evidence of VAIN, it is necessary to resect only 1.5 to 2 cm of upper vagina. This is achieved by entering the vagina anteriorly and transecting it with a knife or scissors. The vault is closed, making sure to avoid "dog ears." The vaginal angles are sutured to the paravaginal tissues and uterosacral ligaments.

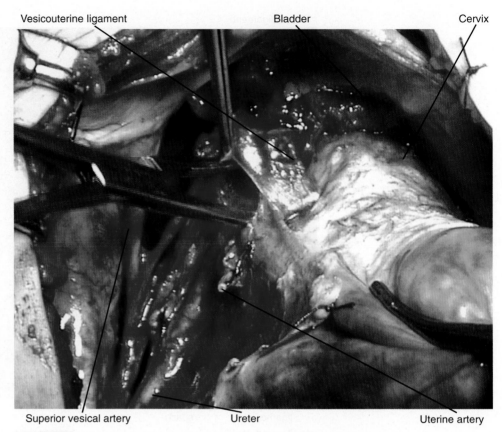

Vesicouterine ligament   Bladder   Cervix

Superior vesical artery   Ureter   Uterine artery

Figure 9.8   Piecemeal dissection of anterior vesicouterine ligament.

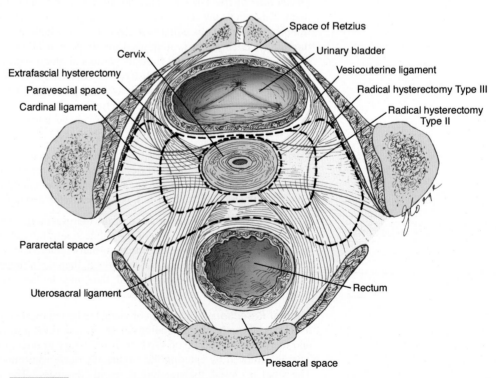

Cervix

Space of Retzius

Urinary bladder

Vesicouterine ligament

Radical hysterectomy Type III

Radical hysterectomy
Type II

Extrafascial hysterectomy
Paravescial space
Cardinal ligament

Pararectal space

Uterosacral ligament

Rectum

Presacral space

Figure 9.9   The pelvic ligaments and spaces.

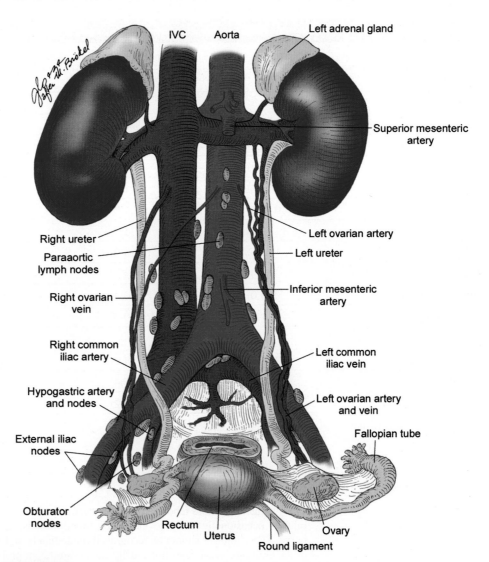

Figure 9.10   The pelvic and paraaortic lymph nodes and their relationship to the major retroperitoneal vessels.

Pelvic Lymphadenectomy   Once the uterus has been removed, the pelvic sidewall exposure is excellent. **If there are any bulky positive pelvic or paraaortic lymph nodes confirmed by frozen section, our policy is to remove only the enlarged nodes and rely on external-beam radiation to sterilize any micrometastases.** If there are no suspicious nodes, then full pelvic lymphadenectomy is performed (Fig. 9.10). Using sharp dissection with Metzenbaum scissors, all fatty tissue is stripped off the vessels from the midcommon iliac region to the circumflex iliac vein distally, preserving the genitofemoral nerve on the psoas muscle. The obturator fossa is entered by retracting the external iliac artery and vein medially, then stripping the fatty tissue off the pelvic sidewall. All fatty tissue is then sharply dissected out of the obturator fossa, taking care particularly to avoid the obturator nerve, which enters the fossa at the bifurcation of the common iliac vein. An accessory obturator vein is seen in at least 30% of patients and is easily torn if not identified. It enters the distal external iliac vein inferiorly.

Postextirpation   The peritoneal cavity is irrigated with warm water or saline. The pelvic peritoneum is not closed, and no drains are used unless there is concern about hemostasis. When the retroperitoneal space is left open and prophylactic antibiotics are used, drains may actually increase febrile morbidity, pelvic cellulitis, and length of postoperative ileus (113). A suprapubic catheter is placed in the bladder and the abdomen closed with a continuous mass closure technique.

	Pikaat et al. (114)	Samlall et al. (115)	Sivanesaratnam et al. (116)	
Table 9.6 Postoperative Complications of Radical Hysterectomy				
Complication	n = 156 (%)	n = 271 (%)	n = 397 (%)	Total (%)
Early				
Urinary tract infection	10 (6.4)	NS	36 (9.1)	46/553 (8.3)
Venous thrombosis	1 (0.6)	6 (2.2)	9 (2.3)	16/824 (1.9)
Pulmonary embolism	2 (1.2)	1 (0.4)	2 (0.5)	5/824 (0.6)
Ureterovaginal fistula	1 (0.6)	5 (1.8)	1 (0.3)	7/824 (0.8)
Vesicovaginal fistula	0 (0.0)	2 (0.7)	2 (0.5)	4/824 (0.5)
Fever	11 (7.1)	10 (3.7)	2 (0.5)	23/824 (2.8)
Lymphocyst	1 (0.6)	8 (3.0)	3 (0.8)	12/824 (1.5)
Ileus	3 (1.9)	9 (3.3)	NS	12/427 (2.8)
Burst abdomen	0 (0.0)	1 (0.4)	1 (0.2)	2/824 (0.2)
Ureteral obstruction	2 (1.2)	1 (0.4)	0 (0.0)	3/824 (0.4)
Late				
Bladder atony	13 (8.3)	14 (5.2)	3 (0.8)	30/824 (3.6)
Lymphedema	1 (0.6)	20 (7.4)	4 (1.0)	25/824 (3.0)
Sexual dysfunction	NS	6 (2.2)	NS	6/271 (2.2)

[a]Pelvic abscess, pelvic cellulitis, atelectasis, wound infection, psoas abscess.

NS, not stated.

Complications of Radical Hysterectomy

Intraoperative

The average blood loss reported is usually between 500 (114) and 1,500 dL (115). Intraoperative injuries occasionally occur to the pelvic blood vessels, ureter, bladder, rectum, or obturator nerve. These injuries should be recognized immediately and repaired. Even complete severance of the obturator nerve does not usually cause significant problems with walking.

Postoperative Complications

Detailed information about postoperative morbidity is infrequently supplied. Table 9.6 gives data from three series from which detailed information is available. It can be seen that urinary tract infection is the most common complication, related to the need for prolonged catheter drainage. Other febrile morbidity from such causes as atelectasis or wound infection is also relatively common. **Prolonged ileus occasionally occurs and, in our experience, may result from lymphatic ascites that can develop following lymphadenectomy** (117). It may require repeated paracenteses but will eventually settle completely. Venous thrombosis is undoubtedly underdiagnosed, but with proper prophylactic measures, pulmonary embolism is infrequent. Vesicovaginal or ureterovaginal fistulas occur in approximately 1% of cases.

Late Complications

Bladder Dysfunction   **The most distressing late complication is prolonged bladder dysfunction, necessitating voiding by the clock with the aid of the abdominal muscles, and, in some cases, self-catheterization.** Covens and colleagues (118) reported a significant difference in the incidence of bladder dysfunction at 3 months among different surgeons at the University of Toronto. Twenty-one percent of patients reported objective or subjective bladder dysfunction, but the range among the eight surgeons concerned varied from 0% to 44%. Samlal et al. (115) from Amsterdam, using a more radical dissection of the cardinal ligaments than is usually done in the United States (Okabayashi technique), reported a 5.2% incidence of this complication.

Voiding difficulties and bowel dysfunction are inevitable in the immediate postoperative period, and suprapubic or urethral catheter drainage and laxatives are desirable for at least

the first 5 days. If cystometry is performed to evaluate bladder dysfunction, two abnormal patterns are found (119). The hypertonic bladder with elevated urethral pressure is most common. The hypotonic bladder occurs much less frequently. Patients with a hypertonic pattern have the normal bladder-filling sensation and the usual discomfort of a full bladder. The condition is self-limiting, usually within 3 weeks of surgery. The prognosis is much worse for patients with a hypotonic bladder, and some of these patients eventually require lifelong self-catheterization.

Sexual Dysfunction   A large Swedish study of sexuality in cervical cancer survivors reported sexual dysfunction in 55% of patients treated by radical hysterectomy alone (120). Problems included insufficient lubrication, reduced genital swelling at arousal, reduced vaginal length and elasticity, and dyspareunia. The addition of preoperative brachytherapy or external beam radiation yielded no excess risk of sexual dysfunction.

This is in marked contrast to our own experience at the Royal Hospital for Women, where Grumann et al., in a more detailed study of a much smaller group of patients, reported that radical hysterectomy was not associated with major sexual sequelae (121).

The differences between the two groups may be explained by the radicality of the surgery. We do not take more than 1.5 cm of normal vagina at radical hysterectomy, so reports of vaginal shortness are very unusual.

Other studies have also reported a favorable outcome in terms of sexual function following radical hysterectomy (122,123), and the nerve sparing operation is likely to further enhance sexual function, particularly in terms of orgasmic sensation and vaginal lubrication.

To avoid bowel, bladder, and sexual dysfunction, a nerve-sparing radical hysterectomy has been developed (111, 112,124,125,126). The operation seems to be associated with prompt recovery of bladder function and minimal need for self-catheterization (127,128). From the superior hypogastric plexus located over the sacral promontory, two hypogastric nerves containing sympathetic fibers run into the small pelvis beneath the ureter and are responsible for such functions as bladder compliance, urinary continence, and small muscle contractions at orgasm. The hypogastric nerves fuse with parasympathetic fibers of the pelvic splanchnic nerves, coming from sacral roots 2.3 and 4, to form the inferior hypogastric plexus, which is situated in the dorsal part of the parametrium and the dorsal vesicouterine ligament. The parasympathetic fibers are responsible for vaginal lubrication and genital swelling during sexual arousal, detrusor contractility, and various rectal functions.

Performance of the nerve-sparing operation, as described by Trimbos and colleagues (112), involves three basic steps: (i) **The hypogastric nerve is identified and preserved** as it runs in a loose sheath beneath the ureter and lateral to the uterosacral ligament, (ii) **the inferior hypogastric plexus is lateralized and avoided during parametrial dissection,** and (iii) **the most distal part of the inferior hypogastric plexus is preserved during the dissection of the posterior or caudal part of the vesicouterine ligament.**

Nerve sparing occurs inevitably with a more conservative type of radical hysterectomy. A prospective, randomized study of type II versus type III radical hysterectomy for stages IB to IIA cervical cancer was reported by Landoni et al. (131). There was no significant difference in recurrence rate (24% type II vs. 26% type III) or the number of patients dead of disease (18% type II vs. 20% type III) for the two procedures, but urologic morbidity was significantly reduced with the less radical operation (13% vs. 28%).

Tumors less than 2 cm in diameter, with <10mm of stromal invasion, no vascular space invasion and negative lymph nodes have <10% risk of parametrial invasion (132,133). Further study is warranted to determine the feasibility of omitting parametrectomy in these low-risk patients (133).

Lymphedema   As a late complication of pelvic lymphadenectomy, lymphedema is underreported in the medical literature. In a study of 233 patients having pelvic lymphadenectomy in our center, 47 (20.2%) developed lymphedema (134). The onset of the swelling was within 3 months in 53%, within 6 months in 71%, and within 12 months in 84% of patients. The addition of pelvic radiation postoperatively increased the risk of lymphedema.

Stage IB2 Cervical Carcinoma

Optimal management of patients with primary tumors greater than 4 cm in diameter is controversial. Local, regional, and distant failure are more likely than for stage IB1 lesions

whatever primary modality of treatment is chosen. Most patients are cured, so quality of life is an important issue, and properly randomized trials are necessary to determine the best approach.

Primary Radiation Therapy

There is a strong correlation between tumor size and outcome for patients with stage IB cervical cancer (135). Perez and colleagues from St. Louis reported 10-year disease-free survival rates of 90% for stage IB tumors <2 cm, 76% for 2–4 cm, 61% for 4.1–5 cm, and 47% for >5 cm (136). For lesions <2 cm doses of 75 Gray (Gy) to point A resulted in pelvic failure rates of 10%, whereas for more extensive lesions, even doses of 85 Gy resulted in 35–50% pelvic failure rates (136). A recent study from Cambridge reported a local control rate of only 66.7% for 12 patients with stage IB2 cervical cancer, yet three patients (25%) had grade 3 or 4 late toxicity (137).

Bulky tumors require aggressive radiotherapy, and complication rates are high. Perez et al. (138), in a study of 552 patients with stages IB to IIA cervical cancer treated with radiation alone, reported grade 3 morbidity in 7% of cases with grade 2 morbidity in a further 10% of cases. Grade 3 morbidity included six rectovaginal fistulae, one rectouterine fistula, five vesicovaginal fistulae, one enterocolic fistula, one enterocutaneous fistula, one sigmoid perforation, seven rectal strictures, ten ureteral strictures, and ten small bowel obstructions. Montana et al. (139) reported grade II and III morbidity in 8% of cases of stage IB squamous carcinoma treated with radiation alone and noted a relationship between the dose to point A and the dose to the bladder and rectum, as well as the incidence of complications.

Currently, chemoradiation is usually given in line with reports for advanced cervical cancer (140).

Radiation and Extrafascial Hysterectomy

In 1969, Durrance et al. (141) initially reported that central failure could be reduced from 15% (14 of 94 patients) to 2.6% (1 of 39 patients) by the addition of extrafascial hysterectomy following primary pelvic radiation. The GOG recently reported the results of a trial of 256 eligible patients with tumors ≥4 cm diameter who were randomized between radiation alone ($n = 124$) and attenuated radiation followed by extrafascial hysterectomy ($n = 132$) (142). Twenty-five percent of patients had tumors ≥7 cm diameter. There was a lower incidence of local relapse in the hysterectomy group (27% vs. 14% at 5 years), although outcomes were not statistically different. Their conclusions were somewhat ambiguous: "Overall, there was no clinically important benefit with the use of extrafascial hysterectomy. However, there is good evidence to suggest that patients with 4, 5, and 6 cm tumors may have benefited from extrafascial hysterectomy."

Chemoradiation and Extrafascial Hysterectomy

A 1999 GOG study (143) of bulky (≥4 cm) cervical cancers randomly assigned patients to be treated with radiation therapy (external beam and intracavitary cesium) and adjuvant extrafascial hysterectomy 3 to 6 weeks later, with or without weekly *cisplatin* during the external radiation. *Cisplatin* was to be delivered at a dose of 40 mg/m^2 (maximum dose, 70 mg/week) weekly for 6 weeks. There were 374 patients entered into the study. Residual cancer in the hysterectomy specimen was significantly reduced in the group receiving *cisplatin* (47% vs. 57%). Survival at 24 months was significantly improved by the addition of *cisplatin* (89% vs. 79%), as was recurrence-free survival (81% vs. 69%). Grades 3 and 4 hematologic and gastrointestinal toxicities were more frequent in the group receiving *cisplatin,* whereas other toxicities were equivalent in both treatment arms.

Neoadjuvant Chemotherapy

In 1993, Sardi et al. (144) reported the results of a randomized trial of neoadjuvant chemotherapy for patients with bulky stage IB cervical cancer. In the control arm (75 patients), a Wertheim-Meigs operation followed by adjuvant whole-pelvic radiation was carried out, whereas in the neoadjuvant group (76 patients), the same procedures were preceded by three cycles of chemotherapy with the "quick" *vincristine, bleomycin,* and *cisplatin* (VBP) regimen. The chemotherapy protocol consisted of *cisplatin* 50 mg/m^2 on day 1, *vincristine* 1 mg/m^2 on day 1, and *bleomycin* 25 mg/m^2 on days 1, 2, and 3 (the latter given as a 6-hour infusion). Three cycles were given at 10-day intervals. Survival and progression-free interval were significantly improved for patients with an echographic volume greater than 60 dL, mainly because of a decrease in the incidence of locoregional failures. In the control group, pelvic recurrences were observed in 24.3% of patients compared with 7.6% of patients in the neoadjuvant group.

A 2002 metaanalysis was reported using updated individual patient data from five randomized controlled trials conducted worldwide between 1988 and 1999 that compared neoadjuvant chemotherapy plus surgery with radiotherapy alone (145). There were 872 patients in the metaanalysis and 368 deaths. The overall results showed a highly significant benefit for the neoadjuvant chemotherapy and surgery arm with a 36% reduction in the risk of death

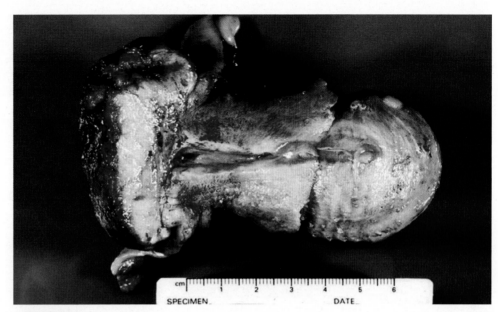

Figure 9.11   Radical hysterectomy specimen from a patient with an exophytic stage IB2 cervical cancer.

and an absolute improvement in survival of 15% at 5 years. An updated metaanalysis using data from 28 trials and more than 3,000 patients revealed that favorable outcomes were only obtained if the chemotherapy cycle length was 14 days or shorter or the *cisplatin* dose intensity was at least 25 mg/m^2 per week (146).

Primary Radical Hysterectomy and Tailored Postoperative Radiation

Our preferred option for the management of stage IB2 carcinoma of the cervix is primary radical hysterectomy and postoperative adjuvant radiation, with or without chemotherapy, depending on the operative findings (Fig. 9.11). This philosophy is also applied to patients with stage IIA disease, provided the tumor does not come down the anterior vaginal wall. Our approach to stage IB or IIA cervical cancer is shown in Fig. 9.12. **Older patients tolerate radical surgery remarkably well, although approximately 10% of patients older than 70 years of age have a medical contraindication to surgery** (101). Radiation tolerance in elderly patients is controversial. Although comparable outcomes to younger patients have been reported (147), others have indicated that comorbid conditions in the elderly necessitate more frequent treatment breaks and less ability to deliver intracavitary therapy, thereby impairing overall prognosis (148).

There are several advantages to a primary surgical approach. First, it allows for accurate staging of the disease, thereby allowing adjuvant therapy to be modified according to needs (149). **Second, it allows resection of bulky positive lymph nodes,** thereby improving the prognosis significantly (110,150). **Third, it allows removal of the primary cancer,** thereby avoiding the difficulty of determining whether there is viable residual disease after the cervix has responded to radiation. **Finally, for most premenopausal patients, it allows preservation of ovarian function.** A primary surgical approach is mandatory in patients with acute or chronic pelvic inflammatory disease, anatomic problems making optimal radiation therapy difficult, or an undiagnosed coexistent pelvic mass (151).

In a retrospective study comparing radical hysterectomy for stage IB1 versus IB2 disease, Finan et al. (39) reported no significant increase in morbidity for patients with stage IB2 disease. They noted positive nodes in 15.5% of patients (28 of 181) with stage IB1 disease versus 43.8% (21 of 48) with stage IB2. Positive paraaortic nodes were present in 1.8% of patients having paraaortic dissection for stage IB1 disease (2 of 111) versus 6.3% of patients with stage IB2 (2 of 32). These patients cannot be salvaged without extended-field radiation (47).

In addition, **approximately half of the patients with positive nodes have bulky nodal metastases. These patients are also unlikely to be salvaged without resection of the bulky nodes, but if the bulky nodes are resected and the patient is given adjuvant radiation, then the prognosis is converted to that of a patient with nodal micrometastases** (110,150).

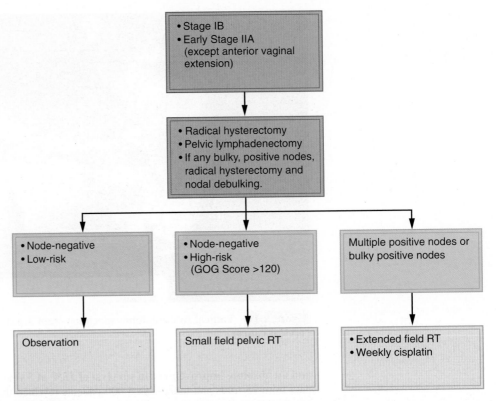

Figure 9.12   Algorithm for the management of stages IB and early IIA carcinoma of the cervix. RT, radiation therapy; GOG, Gynecologic Oncology Group.

In the report by Finan et al. (39), positive surgical margins were noted in 5.0% of patients (9 of 181) with stage IB1 disease versus 12.5% of patients (6 of 48) with stage IB2. In addition, 77% of patients (27 of 35) with stage IB2 disease had more than 15 mm of stromal invasion compared with 27.3% of patients (30 of 110) with stage IB1.

Although the optimal management of patients with stage IB2 disease awaits further randomized, prospective studies, our own experience and that of others (151–157) suggests that good survival rates with tolerably low morbidity can be achieved with a primary surgical approach, giving tailored postoperative radiation in the majority of cases.

In the only randomized, prospective study looking at radical surgery versus primary radiation for stage IB to IIA cervical cancer, Landoni et al. (99) reported that for patients with a cervical diameter larger than 4 cm, the rate of pelvic relapse in the group treated with radiation therapy was more than twice the rate of distant relapse (30% vs. 13%). In addition, there was a significantly higher rate of pelvic relapse among those who had radiation alone (16 of 54; 30%) compared with those who had surgery plus adjuvant radiation (9 of 46; 20%).

To determine the cost-effectiveness of the three common strategies for managing stage IB2 squamous carcinoma of the cervix, Rocconi et al. created a decision-analysis model (158). They chose a hypothetical cohort of 10,000 patients, which they estimated to be the number of new cases of stage IB2 cervical cancer diagnosed in the United States every 5 years. They assumed all patients were diagnosed and clinically staged by a gynecologic oncologist and that each patient underwent a CT scan of the pelvis and abdomen to exclude advanced disease. A literature review was undertaken to determine grades 3 and 4 complication and disease-free survival rates for each modality, and costs were calculated for each 10,000 patient cohort.

Radical hysterectomy with pelvic and paraaortic lymphadenectomy and tailored chemoradiation for high-risk patients was the least expensive strategy, with a cost of $284 million per 10,000 women and a 5-year disease-free survival of 69% (158). Neoadjuvant chemotherapy followed by radical hysterectomy and tailored chemoradiation for high-risk patients had an estimated cost of $299 million (DFS 69.3%), whereas primary chemoradiation had an estimated cost of $508 million and a disease-free survival of 70%. **They concluded that**

Table 9.7 Survival after Radical Hysterectomy for Stages IB and IIA Cervical Cancer

Author	No.	5-Year Survival Rate (%)		
		Negative Nodes	Positive Nodes	Overall
Langley *et al.*, 1980 (159)	204	94	65	87
Benedet *et al.*, 1980 (160)	202	81	66	73
Kenter *et al.*, 1989 (161)	213	94	65	87
Lee *et al.*, 1989 (162)	954	88	73	86
Monaghan *et al.*, 1990 (163)	498	91	51	83
Ayhan *et al.*, 1991 (164)	278	91	63	84
Averette *et al.*, 1993 (165)	978	96	64	90
Samlal *et al.*, 1997 (42)	271	95	76	90
Kim *et al.*, 2000 (166)	366	95	78	88

primary surgery was the most cost-effective strategy and that neoadjuvant chemotherapy would cost approximately $500,000 per additional survivor, and primary chemoradiation an additional $2.2 million per additional survivor.

Prognostic Factors for Stages IB to IIA

The major prognostic factors for patients having radical hysterectomy and pelvic lymphadenectomy for stages IB to IIA cervical cancer are as follows:

1. status of the lymph nodes
2. size of the primary tumor
3. depth of stromal invasion
4. presence or absence of lymph-vascular space invasion
5. presence or absence of parametrial extension
6. histologic cell type
7. status of the vaginal margins

Lymph Node Status

The most important prognostic factor is the status of the lymph nodes. Survival data for patients with positive nodes are shown in Table 9.7. The influence of the number of positive nodes is shown in Table 9.8. Patients with a single positive node below the common iliac bifurcation have a prognosis similar to that of patients with negative nodes (166,169,170). Patients with positive paraaortic nodes treated with extended-field radiation have a 5-year survival rate of approximately 50% (110,171).

Tumor Size, Depth of Stromal Invasion, Lymph-Vascular Space Invasion

In 1989, the GOG (170) published the results of a prospective clinicopathologic study of 732 patients with stage IB cervical carcinoma treated by radical hysterectomy and bilateral pelvic lymphadenectomy. Of these, 645 patients had no gross disease beyond the cervix or uterus and negative paraaortic nodes. One hundred patients had micrometastases in pelvic nodes, but their survival was not significantly different from patients with negative nodes.

Table 9.8 Five-Year Survival Rate (%) versus Number of Positive Pelvic Nodes in Stage IB Cervical Carcinoma

Author	Patients	No. of Positive Nodes		
		1	1–3	>4
Noguchi *et al.*, 1987 (167)	177	—	54	43
Lee *et al.*, 1989 (162)	954	62	—	44
Inoue and Morita, 1990 (168)	484	91	—	50

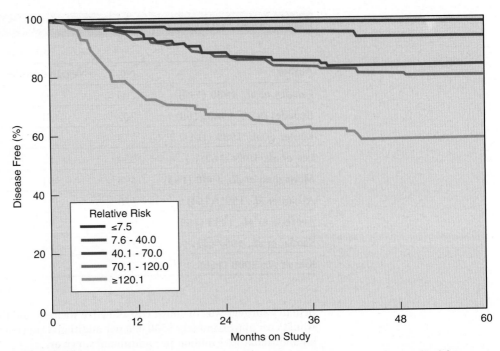

Figure 9.13 Disease-free survival for patients with cervical cancer after radical hysterectomy and bilateral pelvic lymphadenectomy. (From **Delgado G, Bundy B, Zaino R, Sevin B-U, Creasman WT, Major F.** Prospective surgical-pathological study of disease-free interval in patients with stage IB squamous cell carcinoma of the cervix: a Gynecologic Oncology Group study. *Gynecol Oncol* 1990;38:352–357, with permission.)

There were three independent prognostic factors:

1. **the clinical size of the tumor**
2. **the presence or absence of lymph-vascular space invasion**
3. **the depth of tumor invasion**

A relative risk (RR) was calculated for each prognostic variable and an overall estimate of risk determined by multiplying the appropriate RR for the three independent variables. For example, a tumor 4 cm in diameter was estimated to have a RR of 2.9. If it invaded 12 mm into the outer third of the cervix, then the RR was estimated to be 37. Lymph-vascular space invasion conferred a RR of 1.7. The overall estimate of risk was therefore $2.9 \times 37 \times 1.7 = 182.4$. The latter figure may be termed the *GOG score.* Disease-free survival curves were constructed for several RR groups (Fig. 9.13). It can be seen that the likelihood of recurrence for a patient with a GOG score greater than 120 is 40% at 3 years.

The extent of lymph-vascular space invasion varies markedly between tumors, and Roman et al. (172) have shown that **the quantity of lymph-vascular space invasion correlates significantly with the risk of nodal metastases in women with early stage cervical cancer. The quantity of LVSI,** as defined by the percentage of all histologic sections with LVSI and the total number of foci with LVSI, **has also been shown to be an independent prognostic factor for time to recurrence** in women with early stage squamous carcinoma of the cervix (173).

Parametrial Invasion

Burghardt et al. (174) analyzed 1,004 cases of stage IB, IIA, or IIB cervical carcinoma treated by radical hysterectomy at Graz, Munich, and Erlangen, with all surgical specimens processed as giant sections. This processing technique allows accurate assessment of tumor volume and parametrial extension. The 5-year survival rate for 734 patients with no parametrial extension was 85.8% compared with 62.4% for 270 patients with parametrial extension.

The group at Yale (175) reported that patients with parametrial extension, regardless of lymph node status, had a significantly shorter disease-free interval than patients with positive nodes alone, with 12 of 19 such patients (63%) recurring in the pelvis. By contrast, a Japanese study of 117 patients with stages IB to IIB disease and parametrial invasion after radical hysterectomy were divided into two groups based on the status of the pelvic lymph nodes. Five-year overall survival for node-positive and node-negative patients was 52% and 89%, respectively ($p = 0.0005$) (176). Extrapelvic recurrence was more common in patients with positive nodes ($p = 0.005$).

Histologic Cell Type

Small-cell carcinoma of the cervix is uncommon but has an unequivocally poor prognosis (177).

The prognostic significance of adenocarcinoma histologic type is more controversial. These tumors usually arise in the endocervical canal and diagnosis is often delayed, so it is difficult to be certain that lesions of comparable size are being compared. **Many centers report adenocarcinoma histologic type as a poor prognostic factor in multivariate analysis** (166,178,179), but Shingleton et al. (180) were unable to confirm this. In a patient care evaluation study of the American College of Surgeons, they evaluated 11,157 patients from 703 hospitals with cervical cancer treated in 1984 and 1990. There were 9,351 cases of squamous carcinoma (83.8%), 1,405 cases of adenocarcinoma (12.6%), and 401 cases of adenosquamous carcinoma (3.6%). In a multivariate analysis of patients with clinical stage IB disease, histologic type had no significant effect on survival.

The prognostic significance of adenosquamous carcinoma of the cervix is also controversial, with some authors reporting a significantly worse prognosis for patients with these tumors (181,182), whereas others report no difference from squamous lesions with respect to metastatic potential or outcome (183,184). Farley et al. investigated 185 women with pure adenocarcinomas (AC) and 88 women with adenosquamous carcinomas (ASC) (185). They reported no difference in survival for patients with FIGO stage I disease (AC, 89%; ASC 86%; $p = 0.64$) but a significantly decreased median and overall survival for adenosquamous carcinoma in patients with advanced disease (FIGO stages II to IV).

Close Vaginal Margins

Investigators at the Jackson Memorial Hospital in Miami, Florida, reviewed the charts of 1,223 patients with stages IA2, IB, or IIA cervical cancer who had undergone radical hysterectomy (165). Fifty-one patients (4.2%) had positive or close vaginal margins, the latter being defined as tumor no more than 0.5 cm from the vaginal margin of resection. Twenty-three of these cases had negative nodes and no parametrial involvement, and 16 of the 23 (69.6%) received postoperative radiation. The 5-year survival rate was significantly improved by the addition of adjuvant radiation (81.3% vs. 28.6%; $p < 0.05$). They recommended that close vaginal margins without other high-risk factors should be considered a poor prognostic variable.

Newer Markers

Several newer markers have been reported to have prognostic value in early stage cervical cancer.

Serum Squamous Cell Carcinoma Antigen Level   The group at Groningen, the Netherlands, have demonstrated that increased pretreatment serum squamous cell carcinoma antigen (SCC-Ag) levels correlate strongly with FIGO stage, tumor size, deep stromal invasion, and lymph node metastases (186). Even in node-negative patients, the risk of recurrence was three times higher if the SCC-Ag level was elevated before surgery. A Japanese study recommended routine SCC-Ag monitoring following treatment because **the overall survival was higher when recurrence was predicted on the basis of tumor marker elevation than when diagnosed by other modalities** ($p = 0.03$) (187). The prediction of isolated paraaortic lymph node recurrence significantly correlated with SCC-Ag elevation as an initial sign ($p = 0.001$).

Human Papilloma Virus Genotype   Cervical tumors associated with HPV type 18 have been associated with an increased risk of recurrence and death in patients with surgically treated cervical cancer (188,189). It has also been suggested that HPV-18–containing tumors may progress to invasion without a prolonged preinvasive phase (190).

Microvessel Density   Because angiogenesis is considered essential for tumor growth and the development of metastases, it is not surprising that high microvessel density has been reported adversely to influence survival in clinical stage IB cervical cancer and to identify patients with negative nodes at risk for relapse (191).

Postoperative Radiation

Adjuvant pelvic radiation following radical hysterectomy should be given in two circumstances: (i) patients with positive nodes, positive parametria, or positive surgical margins; and (ii) patients with negative nodes but high-risk features in the primary tumor.

Patients with Positive Nodes, Positive Parametria, or Positive Surgical Margins

In 2000, the Southwest Oncology Group (SWOG) and Gynecologic Oncology Group reported results of a randomized study of women with FIGO stages IA2, IB, and IIA carcinoma of the cervix found to have positive pelvic lymph nodes, positive parametrial involvement, or positive surgical margins at the time of primary radical hysterectomy and pelvic lymphadenectomy (192). Patients had to have confirmed negative paraaortic nodes. The regimens were as follows:

Regimen I—external pelvic radiation with *cisplatin* and *5-fluorouracil* (5-FU) infusion
Regimen II—external pelvic radiation

Patients on regimen I received intravenous *cisplatin* 70 mg/m^2 followed by a 96-hour continuous intravenous infusion of 5-FU (4,000 mg/m^2) every 3 weeks for four courses. Radiation therapy in both arms delivered 4,930 centiGray (cGy) to the pelvis using a four-field box technique. Patients with metastatic disease in high common iliac nodes also received 4,500 cGy to a paraaortic field.

The 3-year survival rate for women on the adjuvant chemotherapy plus radiation arm was 87%, compared with 77% for women receiving adjuvant radiation alone. This difference was statistically significant.

A follow-up report was published in 2005 (193). **The absolute improvement in 5-year survival for adjuvant chemotherapy in patients with tumors ≤2 cm was only 5%** (77% versus 82%), whereas for tumors >2 cm it was 19% (58% versus 77%). Similarly, **the absolute 5-year survival benefit was less evident among patients with one nodal metastasis (79% vs. 83%)** than when at least two nodes were positive (55% vs. 75%).

Patients with Negative Nodes but High-Risk Features in the Primary Tumor

Although patients with negative nodes have an 85% to 90% survival rate after radical hysterectomy and pelvic lymphadenectomy, they contribute approximately 50% of the treatment failures, with most of the failures (about 70%) occurring in the pelvis (194).

In 1999, the GOG reported the results of a randomized study of adjuvant whole-pelvic radiation at a dose of 50.4 Gy versus no further treatment after radical hysterectomy for patients with high-risk, node-negative stage IB cervical cancer (195). To be eligible for the study, patients had to have at least two of the following risk factors: greater than one-third stromal invasion, lymph-vascular space invasion, and large tumor size (usually ≥4 cm). There were 277 patients entered into the study. **The addition of radiation significantly reduced the risk of recurrence with a recurrence-free rate of 88% for radiation versus 79% for observation at 2 years.** Severe (GOG grades 3 to 4) gastrointestinal or urologic toxicity occurred in 6.2% of patients receiving radiation versus 1.4% of controls.

An update of this GOG study was reported in 2006, which included seven additional recurrences and 19 additional deaths (196). **The radiation therapy arm continued to show a statistically significant reduction in risk of recurrence, but the improvement in overall survival with radiation did not reach statistical significance (HR = 0.70, 90% CI 0.45–1.05; p = 0.074).** Postoperative radiation appeared to be particularly beneficial for patients with adeno or adenosquamous histologies.

The group from Leiden University in the Netherlands identified 51 patients (13%) who had two of the three high-risk factors identified by the GOG, among 402 patients who underwent radical hysterectomy for early stage cervical cancer (197). They compared 34 patients (66%) who received postoperative pelvic radiation with 17 patients (33%) who did not. **A statistically significant difference was found in 5-year cancer-specific survival in favor of the high-risk group treated with pelvic radiation (86% versus 57%).**

Radiation morbidity is highly correlated with the target volume, and a clinical review of our experience in patients with stage IB, node-negative, cervical cancer at the Royal Hospital for Women in Sydney revealed that 87% of recurrences occurred in the central pelvis (vaginal vault or paravaginal soft tissues). We therefore decided to pilot a study involving a radiation field focused on the central pelvis to see if the central failure rate could be decreased without causing significant morbidity. The results were reported in 1999 (198). The portals for the standard and small-pelvic radiation fields used on patients treated at the Royal Hospital for Women are shown in Table 9.9 (Fig. 9.14). **The small field decreases the amount of small and large bowel that is irradiated.**

Table 9.9 Anteroposterior and Lateral Portals for Standard and Small-Field Pelvic Radiation Used for Patients from the Royal Hospital for Women, Sydney

	Standard Field	*Small Field*
Anteroposterior		
Superior	L4–5 junction	S1–2 junction
Inferior	Inferior obturator foramen	Midobturator foramen
Lateral	1.5 cm lateral to pelvic brim	Bony pelvic brim
Lateral		
Anterior	Outer edge of pubic symphysis	1 cm posterior to pubic tubercle
Posterior	Ischial tuberosities	Anterior sacral plane

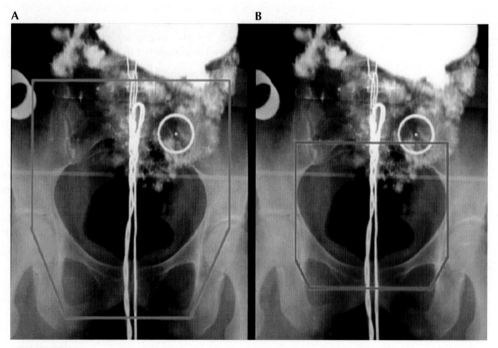

A   B

Figure 9.14   **Comparison between (A) standard field and (B) small field for pelvic radiation.**

High-risk, node-negative patients were selected on the basis of a GOG score of at least 120 (Fig. 9.13). Twenty-five consecutive patients were selected with a mean GOG score of 166 (range 120 to 263). With a mean follow-up of 32 months (range 12 to 64 months), there was only one recurrence (4%) at 16 months. A log-rank analysis demonstrated a significant improvement in the 5-year disease-free survival rate when this group was compared with the high-risk patients in the GOG study (GOG score >120) who were observed without postoperative radiation ($p = 0.005$) (198). No major morbidity occurred, but minor morbidity was recorded in four patients: lymphedema in three and mild rectal incontinence in one.

A **2003 Japanese study compared adjuvant small-field pelvic radiation** for 42 patients with high-risk, node-negative stage I or II cervical cancer **with whole-pelvic radiation** for 42 patients with node-positive disease (199). **The 5-year pelvic control rate was 93% in the small-pelvic field cohort and 90% in the whole-pelvic field group.** They concluded that small-pelvic field radiation appeared to be adequate for high-risk node-negative patients. The same group subsequently reported decreased haematologic and gastrointestinal toxicity with the small field technique (200).

Adjuvant Chemotherapy after Radical Hysterectomy

Japanese workers have reported a favorable outcome for intermediate and high-risk patients treated with adjuvant chemotherapy following radical hysterectomy (201). *Intermediate risk* was defined as stromal invasion >50% (*n* = 30), whereas *high risk* was defined as positive surgical margins, parametrial invasion, or lymph node metastases, (*n* = 35). Three courses of *bleomycin, vincristine, mitomycin C,* and *cisplatin* were given for intermediate risk cases, and 5 courses for high-risk cases. Estimated 5-year disease-free survival was 93.3% for the 30 patients with intermediate-risk tumors, and 85.7% for the 35 with high-risk tumors. The incidence of locoregional recurrence was 3.3% in the intermediate-risk group and 8.6% in the high-risk group.

Stages IIB to IVA Disease

Primary Radiation Therapy

Radiation therapy can be used to treat all stages of cervical cancer, but for early stage disease it is usually reserved for medically unfit patients. Radical external-beam radiation therapy plus brachytherapy is the gold standard for advanced disease, but as the volume of the primary lesion increases, the likelihood of sterilizing it with radiation decreases. Increasing the dose of radiation increases the late morbidity to the bowel, bladder, and vaginal vault, so **various strategies have been investigated to try to improve local control.**

Strategies that have been investigated include:

1. **hyperfractionation** of the radiation
2. **neoadjuvant chemotherapy before radiation**
3. **use of hypoxic cell radiation sensitizers**
4. **concurrent use of radiation and chemotherapy** (chemoradiation)

Hyperfractionated radiation has not been adequately studied for cervical cancer (202), **and trials of neoadjuvant chemotherapy followed by radiation have generally been disappointing.** A metaanalysis from the United Kingdom looked at updated individual patient data from 18 randomized controlled trials conducted worldwide between 1982 and 1995 (203). There was a high level of statistical heterogeneity, although trials using a higher dose intensity of *cisplatin* and shorter cycle length appeared to increase survival, whereas a lower dose intensity and longer cycle length appeared to reduce survival.

***Hydroxyurea* and *misonidazole* are the best-studied radiation sensitizers** (204), **but they have been shown to be inferior to *cisplatin*-based chemoradiation** (140).

Concurrent Chemotherapy and Radiation

Three large randomized prospective trials, all reported in 1999, have established chemoradiation as the treatment of choice for patients with advanced cervical cancer.

The GOG reported the results of a phase III randomized study of external-beam pelvic radiation and intracavitary radiation combined with concomitant *hydroxyurea* versus weekly *cisplatin* versus 5 FU-*cisplatin* and *hydroxyurea* (HFC) in 526 patients with stages IIB, III, and IVA cervical cancer who had undergone extraperitoneal surgical sampling of the paraaortic lymph nodes. Women with intraperitoneal disease or disease metastatic to the paraaortic lymph nodes were ineligible (140). Chemotherapy regimens were as follows:

Regimen I—weekly *cisplatin* 40 mg/m^2/week for 6 weeks
Regimen II—*hydroxyurea* orally 2 mg/m^2 twice weekly for 6 weeks, **5-FU** 1,000 mg/m^2/day as a 96-hour infusion on days 1 and 29, *cisplatin* 50 mg/m^2 days 1 and 29
Regimen III—*hydroxyurea* orally 3 g twice weekly

Both platinum-containing regimens improved the PFS compared with *hydroxyurea* alone (*p* <0.005). The percentage of patients recurrence free at 24 months was 70% for weekly *cisplatin*, 67% for HFC, and 50% for *hydroxyurea*. Grade 3 or 4 leukopenia and grade 4 gastrointestinal toxicity were increased with HFC compared with weekly *cisplatin* or *hydroxyurea* (*p* = 0.0001 and *p* = 0.02, respectively). The investigators concluded that weekly *cisplatin* was more effective than *hydroxyurea* and more tolerable than HFC as a concomitant chemoradiation regimen for locally advanced cervical cancer.

Long-term follow-up of these patients confirmed improved progression-free and overall survival for both *cisplatin* containing arms compared with *hydroxyurea* (p <0.001) (205). The relative risk of progression of disease or death was 0.57 (95% CI, 0.43 to 0.75) with *cisplatin* and 0.51 (95% CI, 0.38 to 0.67 with *cisplatin*-based combination chemotherapy compared with *hydroxyurea*. The improved survival occurred collectively and individually for patients with stages IIB and III disease.

The Radiation Therapy Oncology Group (RTOG) randomized 403 patients with advanced cervical cancer confined to the pelvis between pelvic and paraaortic radiation, and pelvic radiation with concurrent *cisplatin* and *5-fluorouracil* (206). With a median follow-up of 43 months, the actuarial survival at 5 years was 73% among patients having chemoradiation and 58% among those having radiation alone (p = 0.004). Disease-free 5-year survivals were 67% in the chemoradiation arm and 40% in the radiation alone arm, respectively (p <0.001). The rates of distal metastases and locoregional recurrences were significantly higher among patients treated with radiation alone.

The GOG–SWOG groups randomized 388 patients with FIGO stages IIB, III, or IVA disease and negative paraaortic nodes at retroperitoneal paraaortic lymph node sampling between standard pelvic radiation with *hydroxyurea* and standard pelvic radiation with *5-fluorouracil* and *cisplatin* (207). Both progression-free (p = 0.03) and overall survival (p = 0.02) were significantly better for patients randomized to receive 5 FU-*cisplatin*.

Since publication of these clinical trials and the NCI clinical announcement in 1999, there has been a significant change in the management of cervical cancer in the United States, with the number of patients receiving concurrent chemoradiation increasing from 20% in 1997 to 72% in 2001 (208).

The optimal regimen for the chemotherapy is yet to be defined, but single-agent *cisplatin* at a dose of 40 mg/m^2 given weekly during external beam therapy is widely used. The high rates of chemotherapy completion achieved in multiinstitutional trials can be difficult to reproduce in standard practice, and toxicity may be higher than reported, possibly because patients on trials are younger and have less comorbidity (209).

Stage IIIB Cervical Cancer with Hydronephrosis	There are two criteria for the diagnosis of stage IIIB cervical cancer: (i) tumor fixation to the pelvic sidewall or (ii) the presence of hydronephrosis. When the tumor is not fixed to the pelvic sidewall and the level of ureteric obstruction is above the main tumor mass, it is most likely the result of external ureteric compression from enlarged pelvic or paraaortic lymph nodes. **Resection of these nodes via an extraperitoneal approach before radiation therapy can markedly improve survival** (110,150).

If bulky nodal metastases are not resected, survival is significantly compromised. Data from the Mallindkrodt Institute of Radiology in St. Louis reveal that PFS at 5 years was 35% in patients with hydronephrosis and tumor fixed to the pelvic sidewall but decreased to 23% for 16 patients who presented with hydronephrosis without sidewall fixation (p <0.001) (210). **When the level of ureteric obstruction was below the pelvic brim, 5-year PFS was 39%, but this fell to 22% when the obstruction was above the brim** (p = 0.02).

Patients with bilateral hydronephrosis and a creatinine clearance <50 mL/min should be considered for elective ureteral stenting before the commencement of radiation therapy (211).

Extended-Field Radiation	Clinical staging fails to detect extension of disease to the paraaortic lymph nodes in approximately 7% of patients with stage IB disease, 17% with stage IIB, and 29% with stage III (Table 9.4). Such patients will have a "geographic" treatment failure if standard radiation therapy ports are used.

As a routine procedure, operative staging has failed to realize its intended goal of substantially increasing survival. There are three principal reasons for this. First, **patients with positive paraaortic nodes often have occult distant metastases** and therefore require an effective systemic chemotherapy. Second, **failure to control the pelvic disease has contributed significantly to the poor overall survival for this group of patients** (Table 9.10). Finally, if it is assumed that approximately 25% of patients will have positive paraaortic nodes

Table 9.10 Sites of Recurrence in Patients with Cervical Cancer Having Extended-Field Radiation for Positive Paraaortic Nodes			
Author	Patients	Distinct Metastases	Pelvic Recurrence
Nelson et al., 1977 (26)	23	12 (52%)	NS
Piver et al., 1981 (212)	31	14 (45%)	NS
Welander et al., 1981 (49)	31	17 (55%)	12 (38%)
Tewfik et al., 1982 (213)	23	10 (44%)	5 (22%)
Berman et al., 1984 (50)	90	32 (36%)	25 (28%)
Rubin et al., 1984 (171)	14	5 (36%)	2 (14%)
La Polla et al., 1986 (11)	13	8 (62%)	7 (54%)
Vigliotti et al., 1992 (214)	43	23 (53%)	20 (46%)
Total	268	121 (45.1%)	71/214 (33.1%)

NS, not stated.

Modified from **Hacker NF.** Clinical and operative staging of cervical cancer. *Baillieres Clin Obstet Gynaecol* 1988;2:747–759, with permission.

and approximately 25% of these will benefit from extended-field radiation (Table 9.11), it is evident that **only 6% or so of patients undergoing a staging laparotomy will have a survival benefit as a consequence of the altered therapy.** Greater survival benefits will accrue to patients with earlier stage disease because of the better pelvic disease control.

Because of the demonstrated high incidence of positive paraaortic lymph nodes in patients with advanced cervical cancer, prophylactic extended-field radiation may be justified in view of the acceptable incidence of complications in the absence of previous laparotomy (215).

The RTOG in the United States conducted a randomized trial of prophylactic paraaortic radiation (4,500 cGy) in 330 patients with stages IB and IIA (>4 cm) or IIB cervical cancer (216). Patients with lymphangiographic or surgical evidence of paraaortic nodal involvement were excluded. **Significantly better 5-year survival rates (66% vs. 55%) were demonstrated for the patients receiving extended-field radiation therapy.** In addition,

Table 9.11 Survival after Extended-Field Radiation		
Author	Patients	5-Year Survival Rate (%)
Buchsbaum, 1979 (46)	21	23.0
Hughes et al., 1980 (47)	22	29.0
Ballon et al., 1981(48)	18	23.0
Piver et al., 1981 (212)	31	9.6
Welander et al., 1981 (49)	31	25.8
Rubin et al., 1984 (171)	14[a]	57.1
Potish et al., 1985 (51)	17	40.0
La Polla et al., 1986 (11)	16	30.0
Vigliotti et al., 1992 (214)	43	28.0
Total	213	27.2

[a]All patients had stage IB or IIA disease.

Modified from **Hacker NF.** Clinical and operative staging of cervical cancer. *Baillieres Clin Obstet Gynaecol* 1988;2:747–759, with permission.

patients treated with pelvic radiation alone had a higher risk of distant failure (32% vs. 25%). Severe gastrointestinal morbidity was more common in the group receiving extended-field therapy but was mainly seen in patients having previous abdominal surgery.

The GOG conducted a trial of extended-field chemoradiation for patients with biopsy-proven paraaortic lymph node metastases (217). The radiation dose to the paraaortic area was 4,500 cGy, and the chemotherapeutic regime was *5-fluorouracil* 1,000 mg/m^2/day for 96 hours and *cisplatin* 50 mg/m^2 in weeks 1 and 5. There were 86 evaluable patients with stages IB to IVA disease, and the 3-year overall and progression-free survivals were 39% and 34%, respectively. Severe acute toxicity was mainly gastrointestinal (18.6%) and hematologic (15%), and the major late morbidity was gastrointestinal (14% actuarial risk at 4 years). **This trial demonstrated the feasibility of extended-field chemoradiation and confirmed that not all patients with paraaortic nodal metastases have systemic disease.**

For patients without proven paraaortic nodal disease, the RTOG study reported in 1999 demonstrated that pelvic radiation plus concurrent chemotherapy was superior to prophylactic extended-field radiation without chemotherapy (206).

Our practice is to still give extended-field chemoadiation to the level of the superior border of *L1* for patients with proven common iliac or paraaortic lymph node metastases, although the dose of *cisplatin* frequently has to be reduced. Extended-field intensity and modulated radiation with concurrent *cisplatin* has been reported to give good locoregional control, with distant metastases being the predominant mode of failure (218).

Plan of Management for Advanced Cervical Cancer

In view of the aforementioned results, our current approach to patients with advanced cervical cancer at the Royal Hospital for Women in Sydney is summarized in Fig. 9.15. All patients are subjected to a chest, pelvic, and abdominal CT scan and a PET scan. If there are systemic metastases, palliative pelvic radiation is given. **Pretreatment laparotomy is undertaken if there is (i) adnexal pathology, (ii) pelvic or paraaortic lymph nodes at least 2 cm diameter, and (iii) no systemic metastases. Enlarged nodes are resected by an extraperitoneal approach because of the evidence strongly suggesting that such an approach converts the prognosis to that of patients with micrometastases** (110,150). Patients with bulky positive nodes that have been resected from the pelvic or paraaortic area are given

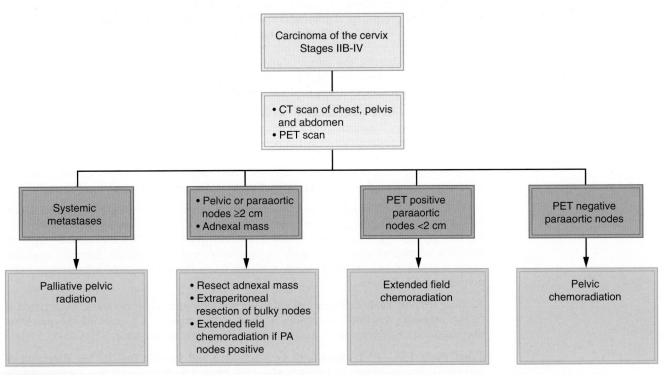

Figure 9.15 Algorithm for the management of patients with advanced cervical cancer. RT, radiation therapy.

Table 9.12 Carcinoma of the Cervix Uteri: Patients treated in 1999 to 2001: Survival by FIGO Stage (*n* = 11,639)

Overall Survival Rates (%)

Stage	Patients	1-Year	2-Year	3-Year	4-Year	5-Year
Stage IA1	829	99.8	99.5	98.3	97.5	97.5
Stage IA2	275	98.5	96.9	95.2	94.8	94.8
Stage IB1	3,020	98.2	95.0	92.6	90.7	89.1
Stage IB2	1,090	95.8	88.3	81.7	78.8	75.7
Stage IIA	1,007	96.1	88.3	81.5	77.0	73.4
Stage IIB	2,510	91.7	79.8	73.0	69.3	65.8
Stage IIIA	211	76.7	59.8	54.0	45.1	39.7
Stage IIIB	2,028	77.9	59.5	51.0	46.0	41.5
Stage IVA	326	51.9	35.1	28.3	22.7	22.0
Stage IVB	343	42.2	22.7	16.4	12.6	9.3

From **Quinn MA, Benedet J, Odicino F, et al.** Carcinoma of the cervix uteri: annual report on the results of treatment in gynecological cancer. *Int J Gynecol Obstet* 2006;95:543–S103 with permission.

extended-field radiation with weekly *cisplatin* 30–40 mg/m^2, and all other patients are given pelvic chemoradiation.

Stage IVA Disease with Vesicovaginal or Rectovaginal Fistula   An occasional patient in Western countries has a vesicovaginal or rectovaginal fistula at presentation. If a CT scan of the chest, pelvis, and abdomen or a PET scan demonstrates no evidence of systemic disease, then these patients are suitable for primary pelvic exenteration.

Prognosis

The survival of patients with cervical cancer according to the *Annual Report on the Results of Treatment in Gynaecological Cancer* is shown in Table 9.12. Older patients have a lower survival for any given stage. Differences resulting from case mix, age group, type of tumor, and other factors may be responsible for variations or differences between centers.

Posttreatment Surveillance

After radiation therapy, the patient should be monitored monthly for the first 3 months. Regression may continue throughout the period, but if any progression of disease occurs, histologic confirmation should be obtained and consideration given to surgery.

After the immediate postradiation surveillance or postoperative checkup, patients are usually seen every 3 months until 2 years, every 6 months until 5 years, and annually thereafter. The role of routine follow-up has been questioned because most recurrences are detected at self-referral because of symptoms (219). Nevertheless, follow-up also allows psychosocial support for the patient as well as data collection; in a Dutch study, 32% of all cases of recurrence were diagnosed at routine follow-up (219). The mean disease-free interval was 18 months.

At each visit, patients should be questioned about symptoms, and physical examination should include assessment of the supraclavicular and inguinal nodes, as well as abdominal and rectovaginal examination. A Pap smear should be obtained at each visit. Chen et al. (220) reported that 72% of vaginal recurrences were asymptomatic, and most had an abnormal cytologic smear. The others were detected by noting ulceration on visual inspection or by palpation of a nodule or cuff induration.

Because the only realistic chance of cure is in patients with a central pelvic recurrence, it is not necessary routinely to obtain a chest radiograph or CT scan of the pelvis or abdomen. Any symptoms (e.g., cough) should be promptly investigated.

Whole-body FDG–PET appears to be a sensitive and specific tool for the detection of recurrent cervical cancer in patients who have clinical findings suspicious for recurrence (221). It has also been reported to be **a sensitive modality for the detection of recurrent cervical cancer in asymptomatic patients.** A study of 121 consecutive patients from the

Republic of Korea reported a sensitivity of 96.1%, a specificity of 84.4%, and an accuracy of 91.7% for detection of recurrent disease (222). These authors suggested that the earlier diagnosis may have a favorable impact on survival. **The PET scan has limitations in the detection of lesions less than 1 cm^3** (223).

Nonsquamous Histologic Types

Adenocarcinoma

Adenocarcinomas currently represent 20% to 25% of cervical cancers in the industrialized countries. In the United States, the age-adjusted incidence rates for adenocarcinoma have increased by 29.1% since the mid-1970s, and the proportion of adenocarcinomas relative to squamous carcinomas has increased by 95.2% (224). Age-adjusted cervical adenocarcinoma incidence rates have also increased throughout Europe, particularly in younger women (225).

Most of this relative increase is related to a decreasing incidence of squamous carcinomas secondary to screening programs, but **oral contraceptive use has been implicated in the absolute increase in adenocarcinomas in women younger than 35 years of age** (226).

In England, the substantial increase in adenocarcinomas in recent years has been largely attributed to a birth-cohort effect, presumably associated with greater exposure to human papilloma virus after the sexual revolution of the 1960s (227). **A Canadian study reported HPV in 70% of cases (53 of 77) with HPV 16 the predominant type** (228). There was no correlation between HPV status and outcome. It is likely that HPV vaccination (229) and better cytologic and HPV screening (230) will reverse this trend in the future.

Adenocarcinomas are generally regarded as being more radioresistant than squamous carcinomas. **In the Italian randomized study of radical surgery versus radiation therapy for stages IB to IIA cervical cancer,** 46 of 343 patients (13.4%) had adenocarcinomas (99). Surgery and radiation therapy were found to be identical in terms of 5-year survival and disease-free survival rates for the entire group, but **for patients with adenocarcinomas, surgery was significantly better in terms of both overall survival (79% vs. 59%, $p = 0.05$) and disease-free survival rates (66% vs. 47%, $p = 0.02$).**

Workers in the Netherlands have shown that pretreatment serum CA125 levels are of prognostic significance for adenocarcinomas (231). The 5-year survival rate for stage IB adenocarcinomas was 52.4% when CA125 levels were elevated versus 95.6% when normal levels were present ($p < 0.01$). Similarly, 42% of patients with elevated serum CA125 levels had lymph node metastases versus 4% when normal levels were found ($p = 0.012$). Although the prognostic significance of adenocarcinoma is somewhat controversial, the presence of lymph node metastases seems to portend a much worse prognosis for patients with adenocarcinomas than squamous carcinomas (115,224,232).

Adenosquamous Carcinoma

Adenosquamous carcinomas represent approximately 20% to 30% of all adenocarcinomas of the cervix. **Most studies report a poorer outcome, although interpretation of the literature is confounded by a failure of investigators to adopt uniform criteria for diagnosis.** The main issue is whether to include poorly differentiated squamous cell carcinomas in which the glandular elements are identified only by the use of mucin stains.

In the largest series of surgically staged IB cases, Helm et al. (233) matched 38 patients with adenosquamous carcinomas with patients with other histologic subtypes of adenocarcinoma with respect to stage, lesion size, nodal status, grade of adenocarcinoma, and age at diagnosis. Diagnosis was based on hematoxylin and eosin staining without use of mucin staining. Glassy cell carcinomas were included. **Overall 5-year survival and disease-free survival rates for the matched adenosquamous and adenocarcinomas were not significantly different (83% vs. 90% and 78% vs. 81%, respectively), but the mean time to recurrence was significantly shorter in the adenosquamous group: 11 versus 32 months ($p = 0.003$).** In addition, six patients with adenosquamous carcinomas could not be matched. Five of these had positive nodes in association with lesions measuring between 2 and 4 cm in diameter, and one had an 8-cm lesion with negative nodes.

Similar findings were reported from the M.D. Anderson Cancer Center comparing 29 patients with stage IB1 adenosquamous carcinoma with 97 patients with stage IB1 adenocarcinoma of the cervix undergoing radical hysterectomy. The authors reported no difference in recurrence rates between the two histologic groups, but the **time to recurrence was shorter for patients with adenosquamous carcinoma (7.9 months vs. 15 months;** $p = 0.01$ **) (184).**

Glassy Cell Carcinoma

In 1956, Glucksman and Cherry (234) defined "glassy cell" carcinoma of the cervix as **a poorly differentiated adenosquamous carcinoma, the cells of which had a moderate amount of cytoplasm and a typical "ground glass" appearance.** Survival was poor, regardless of the mode of therapy. In 1982, Maier and Norris (235) suggested that **poorly differentiated large-cell, nonkeratinizing squamous carcinomas have a similar histologic appearance.** Subsequently, Tamimi et al. (236) reviewed their experience with undifferentiated large-cell nonkeratinizing carcinomas of the cervix at the University Hospital in Seattle, Washington, and reported 29 cases over an 8-year period. The mean age of the patients was 31 years, and all cases were stage IB. All but one case was treated by radical hysterectomy, and the survival rate was 55%. In all but one case, the interval to recurrence was less than 8 months. The researchers concluded that **the poor prognosis ascribed to the classically defined glassy cell carcinoma also holds true for this extended group of large-cell undifferentiated cervical cancers that display similar histologic features.**

A contemporary series of 22 patients from the University of Washington suggests a better prognosis than previously reported (237). The overall survival for the series was 73%, with the overall survival for patients having stage I disease being 86% (12 of 14). Pelvic relapse was associated with lymph-vascular space invasion, deep stromal invasion, and large tumor size.

Adenoma Malignum

The term **adenoma malignum of the cervix** was first used in 1870 by Gusserow to describe a very highly differentiated adenocarcinoma. McKelvey and Goodlin (238) reported five cases in 1963, four of which were fatal within 4 years of presentation. They pointed out the deceptively benign histologic appearance of the tumor and stated that **"if a lesion can be recognized as malignant by the usual criteria for adenocarcinoma of the cervix, it should be excluded from the adenoma malignum group."** McKelvey and Goodlin suggested that these tumors were radioresistant.

In 1975, Silverberg and Hurt (239) reported five additional cases. All patients were treated by modern radiotherapeutic techniques, and four of the five were long-term survivors. The authors believed that, with proper therapy, the tumor was no more malignant than might be expected for a highly differentiated adenocarcinoma, and they suggested the name **minimal deviation adenocarcinoma.**

An association has been noted with Peutz-Jeghers syndrome, as well as with sex-cord tumors with annular tubules, a distinctive ovarian neoplasm with features intermediate between those of the granulosa and Sertoli cell type (240).

These tumors represent approximately 1% of adenocarcinomas of the cervix and occur mainly in the fifth and sixth decades (241). **Diagnosis is often delayed because Pap smears may be normal or show very minor abnormalities.**

Clinically, patients usually present with a watery or mucous discharge or with abnormal uterine bleeding. On physical examination, the cervix is usually firm and indurated (242). **Punch biopsy is not helpful, and deep wedge or cone biopsy is necessary to demonstrate the depth of glandular penetration.**

Radical hysterectomy, bilateral salpingo-oophorectomy, and pelvic lymphadenectomy is the treatment of choice for operable cases, and the prognosis for such cases appears to be very good (242). For more advanced cases, lymph node metastases are common, and the overall prognosis is poor, with only three of 22 patients (14%) alive and disease free at 2 years in one large series (243).

Adenoid Cystic Carcinoma

Adenoid cystic carcinoma is a rare tumor that occurs most frequently in the salivary glands but also in the respiratory tract, skin, mucous membranes of the head and neck, and the breast. **In the female genital tract, it occurs in Bartholin's gland, the endometrium, and the cervix** (244). Ultrastructural features of both squamous and glandular epithelium are seen, leaving the issue of the etiology of these tumors unresolved. Approximately half the tumors have associated squamous carcinoma or dysplasia (245), whereas adenocarcinoma has a less-frequent association.

These tumors usually occur in postmenopausal black women of high parity (244,246). Most present with postmenopausal bleeding, but some may be suspected by the presence of small "undifferentiated" cells on a routine Pap smear (244). Approximately half the cases are stage I at presentation, but **overall survival is poor.** Prempree et al. (246), in a review of the literature, reported a 3- to 5-year survival rate of only 56.3% (9 of 16) for patients with stage I disease, regardless of the type of treatment. The survival rate for stage II disease was 27.3% (3 of 11), and no patient with stage III or IV disease survived. **Lung metastases are common, whereas the tumors spread locally by direct tissue invasion and perineural infiltration.**

Adenoid Basal Carcinoma

This is a rare tumor with an excellent prognosis. Most adenoid basal carcinomas have coexistent *in situ* or invasive squamous carcinoma, and 50% have coexistent *in situ* or invasive adenocarcinoma (247). The disease is almost invariably confined to the cervix, and in a review of 26 cases reported in the literature, only one died of disease (with lung metastases) (248). Invasion is usually superficial, and extrafascial or radical hysterectomy without lymphadenectomy is a reasonable treatment option.

Clear Cell Adenocarcinoma

Clear cell adenocarcinoma of the cervix was rare until 1970, when the incidence rose because of its association with *in utero* exposure before the eighteenth week of pregnancy to *diethylstilbestrol* and related nonsteroidal estrogens (249). The tumor occurs in two distinct age groups: those younger than 24 years and those older than 45 years (250). The latter are unrelated to *in utero diethylstilbestrol* exposure, but **even in young women, there is no history of hormone exposure in 25% of cases.** Treatment should be similar to that for other adenocarcinomas. **Unlike clear cell carcinoma of the endometrium, which carries a much worse prognosis, clear cell adenocarcinoma of the cervix has a prognosis comparable to that of other adenocarcinomas** (250,251).

Villoglandular Papillary Adenocarcinoma

This uncommon lesion tends to occur in younger women and to have a more favorable prognosis. Young and Scully (252) reviewed their consultation files to report 13 cases. The patients' ages ranged from 23 to 54 years (average 33 years). Two of the patients were pregnant. Both were asymptomatic, both had a grossly abnormal-appearing cervix, and one had an abnormal Pap smear. Treatment ranged from cone biopsy for very superficial cases to radical hysterectomy and pelvic lymphadenectomy. With follow-up of 2 to 14 years, no recurrences were seen.

In the largest reported series by Jones et al. (253), none of 24 cases had lymph-vascular invasion or lymph node metastases, and all patients remained free of disease with 7 to 77 months of follow-up. A review of seven cases by Kaku et al. (254) revealed lymph-vascular invasion in two patients, both of whom had pelvic lymph node metastasis. One of the two had recurrence at 30 months and died at 46 months.

Because of their generally excellent prognosis and young age at presentation, conservative management may be justified in selected patients who want to retain fertility (253).

Small-Cell Carcinoma

Small-cell cancers are a rare, heterogeneous group of tumors, representing 0.5% to 5% of all invasive cervical cancers (255). In a thorough evaluation of 2,201 invasive cervical cancers at the University of Kentucky Medical Center, Van Nagell et al. (177) noted 25 cases (1.1%) of small-cell carcinoma. They were characterized by a nuclear area of 160 μm^2 or less and a maximum nuclear diameter of 16.2 μm. **Thirty-three percent of the small-cell carcinomas stained positively for the neuroendocrine markers (neuron-specific enolase and chromogranin), whereas the remainder stained only for epithelial markers such as cytokeratin and epithelial membrane antigen. Both types of small-cell cancers had a higher frequency of lymph-vascular space invasion, a significantly higher rate of recurrence, particularly to extrapelvic sites, and a lower survival rate.**

The neuroendocrine tumors arise from the argyrophil cells or APUD cells (**a**mine **p**recursor **u**ptake and **d**ecarboxylation) in the cervix (255). None of the neuroendocrine tumors in the Kentucky series had clinical signs of a paraendocrine syndrome, **although these tumors may sometimes present with carcinoid syndrome, and the patients then have elevated levels of 5-hydroxy-indoleacetic acid in the urine.**

An epidemiological study using population-based data reported to the Surveillance, Epidemiology, and End Results program in the United States compared 239 cases of endocrine tumors of the cervix with 18,458 squamous cell carcinomas (256). Mean age at diagnosis was 49 years for the endocrine tumors versus 52 years for the squamous carcinomas ($p < 0.01$). Endocrine tumors were more likely to present at a later FIGO stage ($p < 0.01$) and to have lymph node involvement at diagnosis (57% vs. 18%, $p < 0.01$). At all stages of disease, survival was worse for the women with endocrine tumors.

A later study reviewing SEER data from 1977 to 2003 identified 290 women (0.9%) with small-cell carcinoma of the cervix, 27,527 (83.3%) with squamous cell carcinoma, and 5231 patients (15.8%) with adenocarcinoma (257). **Five-year survival for small-cell carcinoma (35.7%) was worse compared with squamous cell carcinoma (60.5%) and adenocarcinoma (69.7%).** They noted that small-cell carcinomas had a predilection for nodal and distant metastases, but there was decreased survival even in early stage, node-negative patients.

Because of the small-cell carcinomas' propensity for early systemic spread, chemotherapy is usually advocated in addition to surgery or radiation therapy. The group at the Chang Gung Memorial Hospital in Taiwan administered adjuvant chemotherapy to 23 consecutive patients with stage IB to II small-cell cervical cancer who had been treated primarily with radical hysterectomy (258). Ten of 14 patients (71.4%) who received a combination of *vincristine, doxorubicin,* and *cyclophosphamide* alternating with *cisplatin* and *etoposide* had no evidence of disease during a median follow-up of 41 months, whereas only 3 of 9 (33.3%) who received *cisplatin, vinblastine,* and *bleomycin* (PVB) survived. The survival rate was 70% for patients with negative lymph nodes and 35% for those with positive nodes ($p = 0.05$). All patients who died of disease had extrapelvic metastases.

The group in Buenos Aires (259) reported 20 patients with neuroendocrine cervical carcinoma. Patients with stages IA2 (one) or IB1 (four) were treated by radical hysterectomy and pelvic lymphadenectomy with or without adjuvant chemotherapy, and all patients survived. Thirteen patients with stages IB2 to IVA disease received neoadjuvant chemotherapy with the quick VBP scheme (*vincristine* 1 mg/m^2/day on day 1, *bleomycin* 25 mg/m^2/day on days 1 to 3, and *cisplatin* 50 mg/m^2/day on day 1, for 3 courses with 10-day intervals). Treatment was completed by 5,000 cGy whole-pelvic adjuvant radiation. Response to neoadjuvant chemotherapy was greater than 50% in 9 of 13 patients (69.4%), and complete response occurred in two of 13 patients (15.3%). When residual tumor was less than 2 cm after neoadjuvant chemotherapy, the overall survival was 58%, compared with 21% when it was greater than 2 cm ($p < 0.05$). For patients with negative nodes, the overall survival was 72%, compared with 11% for those with positive nodes ($p < 0.01$).

Papillary Serous Carcinoma

This tumor resembles microscopically its counterparts elsewhere in the female genital tract and peritoneum. Zhou and colleagues reported a series of 17 cases (260). There was a bimodal age distribution, with one peak occurring before the age of 40 years and the second peak after 65 years. Eight patients (47%) had a polypoid or exophytic mass, two patients (12%) had an ulcerated lesion, and no abnormality was detected in 7 patients (41%). Two tumors were stage IA, 12 were stage IB, two were stage II, and one was stage III. Seven tumors (41%) were mixed with another histologic subtype of cervical adenocarcinoma, most commonly low-grade villoglandular adenocarcinoma. Eight patients (47%) were alive without evidence of disease with a mean follow-up of 56 months. The researchers concluded that **the tumors can behave aggressively with supradiaphragmatic metastases and a rapidly fatal course when diagnosed at an advanced stage, but the outcome for patients with stage I tumors was similar to that of patients with cervical adenocarcinomas of the usual type.**

Sarcoma

A literature review by Rotmensch et al. (261) in 1983 identified 105 reported cases of cervical sarcomas. They classified them as shown in Table 9.13. A variety of therapies had been used in the management of cervical sarcomas, and the overall prognosis was poor, except for the adenosarcomas. The authors concluded that more rigid criteria for diagnosis were needed to allow evaluation of the various therapies.

Sarcoma Botryoides

In 1988, Daya and Scully (262) reviewed 13 cases of this rare tumor. The patient ages ranged from 12 to 26 years, with a mean of 18 years. All had polypoid lesions and presented with vaginal bleeding, "something" protruding from the introitus, or both. The patients were treated with a variety of operative procedures, with or without adjuvant chemotherapy, the operative procedures ranging from cervical polypectomy to hysterectomy with pelvic and paraaortic node dissection. Twelve of the 13 patients (92%) were alive and well 1 to 8 years after surgery.

Results from the Intergroup Rhabdomyosarcoma Study Group's four treatment protocols were summarized by Arndt et al. in 2001 (263). There were 151 patients entered into the four protocols,

Table 9.13 Classification of Cervical Sarcomas		
Tumor Type	*No. Reported*	*Average Age (Year)*
I Leiomyosarcoma	18	47
II Stromal sarcoma		
A Homologous	12	54
B Heterologous (liposarcoma)	1	59
C Sarcoma botryoides	61	27
D Adenosarcoma	4	31
E Malignant mixed müllerian tumor	9	54

Modified from **Rotmensch J, Rosenshein NB, Woodruff JD.** Cervical sarcoma: a review. *Obstet Gynecol Surv* 1983;38:456–460, with permission.

and 23 tumors (15%) arose from the cervix. **The modern approach to management is conservative surgery and chemotherapy—primarily *vincristine, actinomycin D,* and *cyclophosphamide*—with or without radiation therapy.** The overall 5-year survival for the 151 patients was 82%. For patients with localized embryonal botryoid tumors, there was no significant difference in 5-year survival among patients with tumors at different sites. **Patients with more advanced disease should be treated initially with chemotherapy, and surgical excision should attempt to conserve the function of the bladder, rectum, vagina, and ovaries if possible (264).**

Malignant Mixed Müllerian Tumor

There have only been 40 or so cases of this rare tumor reported in the English literature. Sharma and colleagues from the University of Iowa (265) reported five cases with a mean age of 49.6 years. Most patients presented with abnormal vaginal bleeding. Two patients had stage IB1 disease, two had stage IB2, and one had stage IVB. The four patients with disease confined to the cervix were treated with radical hysterectomy, with or without postoperative radiation, and all were alive and free of disease at 28, 35, 42, and 65 months, respectively.

Lymphoma

Cervical lymphomas are rare. Of 9,500 women with lymphomas reported by the Armed Forces Institute of Pathology, only 6 (0.06%) had primary cervical lesions (266).

Patients usually present with abnormal vaginal bleeding, and clinically the cervix is expanded by a subepithelial mass without ulceration or fungation.

Histologic diagnosis is difficult. Harris and Scully (267) reported that only 15 of 25 cases (55%) referred for consultation were correctly diagnosed by the referring pathologist. Komaki et al. (268) emphasized the importance of distinguishing malignant lymphoma from undifferentiated carcinoma or sarcoma because **cervical lymphoma can be successfully treated in spite of locally advanced disease.**

Perrin et al. (269) reviewed the literature in 1992 and found 72 cases of lymphoma of the cervix or upper vagina reported since 1963. Interpretation of the data was hindered by outdated methods of histologic classification in approximately half the cases. Staging information, if given, tended to be reported according to the FIGO classification rather than according to the Ann Arbor classification used routinely in lymphoma practice.

The researchers concluded that the outcome for cervical and vaginal lymphomas was unpredictable but that excellent results could be achieved even if the tumor was high grade, bulky, or extensive. **They stressed the need for thorough staging, including CT scan of the chest, pelvis, and abdomen; bone marrow aspiration; hematologic analysis; and biochemistry.**

Regarding treatment, they **found no evidence that radical gynecologic surgery was advantageous** (269). For localized (Ann Arbor stage IE) and nonbulky disease (FIGO stage I and II) of low and intermediate grade, they recommended pelvic radiation therapy or modern combination chemotherapy. For more extensive disease (stage IIE), bulky locally advanced disease (FIGO stages III and IV), or disease of high grade, they recommended modern chemotherapy, possibly in conjunction with radiation therapy.

Verrucous Carcinoma

This slow-growing, locally aggressive, papillomatous lesion was first reported in the cervix in 1972 (270).

In a literature review in 1988, Crowther et al. (271) reported 34 cases of cervical verrucous carcinoma, although they believed that some of these should be considered papillomas that had undergone malignant change to squamous cell carcinomas. The age of the women ranged from 30 to 84 years (average 51 years), and only two had a past history of genital warts. Symptoms included vaginal discharge (42%) and abnormal bleeding (50%), whereas 35% had an abnormal Pap smear. **Colposcopy was not helpful because the lesion looked like a large condyloma acuminatum.** The lesions were confined to the cervix in 41% of cases, involved the vagina in 36%, and the parametrium in 23%. One case invaded the bladder.

Radical surgery is the mainstay of treatment. Radicality of surgery varied in the cases reviewed by Crowther et al. (271), but of 14 patients having radical hysterectomy (with vaginectomy in 3 cases), recurrence occurred in six (43%). Three of the recurrences were salvaged with radiation therapy or exenterative surgery. **Radiation therapy was used as a primary or secondary treatment in 17 cases, and failures occurred in ten of these (59%).** Anaplastic change was not noted. Lymph node metastases were found in two patients and pulmonary metastases in a third, but careful histologic evaluation at autopsy showed nests of classic squamous carcinoma cells invading the stroma in two of these cases. Overall, recurrent or persistent disease was noted in 21 of the 34 cases (62%), with 82% of relapses occurring within 8 months.

Schwade et al. (272) reported anaplastic transformation and rapid clinical deterioration following radiation therapy in 10.7% of verrucous carcinomas, but suggested that many of these lesions were large and may have already contained occult areas of squamous cell carcinoma.

Melanoma

Malignant melanoma of the cervix is a rare entity, and it is important to exclude a metastatic lesion. Literature reviews and case studies have been reported by Mordel et al. (273) in 1989 and Santosa et al. (274) in 1990. These tumors have in general been reported to occur in the seventh and eighth decades of life, and most lesions present with abnormal vaginal bleeding. **Macroscopically, the tumors are strongly colored, polypoid masses, and most patients have FIGO stage I or II disease at diagnosis.** Recommended treatment is usually radical hysterectomy with or without pelvic lymphadenectomy. **Adjuvant radiation may improve local control if the surgical margins are close.** The 5-year survival rate is poor, not exceeding 40% for stage I disease and reaching only 14% in stage II (273).

Metastatic Carcinoma

Metastasis of malignant epithelial tumors to the uterine cervix is a rare occurrence. Lemoine and Hall (275) reviewed the surgical pathology files of the London Hospital for the 65 years from 1919 to 1984 and found only 33 acceptable cases. Cases that involved direct extension from a primary site, such as the endometrium or rectum, were excluded. They also reviewed the literature for individual case reports and small series. Documented primary sites of diseases included stomach (25 cases), ovary (23), colon (21), breast (14), kidney (1), renal pelvis (1), carcinoid (1), and pancreas (1).

The patients almost invariably present with vaginal bleeding, and the histologic features of the cervical biopsy lead to a search for an asymptomatic primary tumor.

Cancer of the Cervical Stump

Subtotal hysterectomy is less commonly performed today than in the past, but when invasive cancer arises in a cervical stump, the principles of treatment are the same as those for an intact uterus. The technique for abdominal radical trachelectomy is essentially the same as for radical hysterectomy, the only difficulty being the maintenance of adequate traction on the stump. Sometimes the bladder may be adherent over the stump, necessitating careful dissection. **The ability to deliver an adequate dose of radiation to patients with advanced disease depends on the length of the cervical canal and is compromised if the canal is less than 2 cm long.** Although 5-year survival rates compare favorably to those in patients with an intact uterus, complication rates are higher because of the previous surgery and the sometimes compromised methods of radiation therapy (276).

Invasive Cancer Found after Simple Hysterectomy

When invasive cervical cancer is discovered after simple hysterectomy, **the treatment options include full pelvic radiation or radical surgery consisting of radical parametrectomy, upper vaginectomy, and pelvic lymphadenectomy.**

Our preference is to perform radical surgery, as long as a CT scan of the chest, pelvis, and abdomen or a PET scan shows no evidence of metastatic disease and there are no high-risk features in the hysterectomy specimen (i.e., positive surgical margins, tumor deeply infiltrating, or prominent vascular space invasion). In the presence of high-risk features, we prefer primary pelvic radiation.

The operation is considerably more difficult than a radical hysterectomy, the main difficulty being the identification of the bladder, which is usually adherent over the vaginal vault. Operating in the low lithotomy position to allow use of a metal instrument (e.g., narrow malleable retractor) to push up on the vault from below facilitates identification of the bladder boundaries. Kinney et al. (277) from the Mayo Clinic reported 27 patients undergoing reoperation. Ureterovaginal fistulas developed in two of the 27 cases (7%), but the 5-year absolute survival rate was 82%. The group at Irvine, California, reported 18 patients with a median follow-up of 72 months (278). The overall actuarial survival was 89%. Morbidity was comparable to that of patients undergoing primary radical hysterectomy.

Hopkins et al. (279) reported 92 patients who were treated by primary radiation therapy. Prognosis was similar to that for patients treated initially by radical surgery or radiation therapy for squamous lesions. Fifty-seven patients with stage I squamous cell carcinoma had a 5-year survival rate of 85%, whereas 27 patients with stage I adenocarcinoma had a 5-year survival rate of 42%. The researchers suggested that alternative approaches should be investigated for adenocarcinomas.

A study from South Korea reported 64 patients who were treated by primary external beam radiation therapy or intracavitary radiation (280). Overall 5-year survival was 75.8%. For patients in retrospect stages IA, IB, and IIB (gross residual after surgery), overall 5-year survival rates were 90.9%, 88.8%, and 27.9% respectively.

A study from Chandigarh, India, reported 105 patients who were found to have invasive cervical cancer following total ($n = 82$) or subtotal ($n = 23$) hysterectomy (281). All patients were treated with external beam radiation, with or without intracavitary radiation. The 5-year overall survival, disease-free survival, and pelvic control rates for all patients were 55.2%, 53.3%, and 72%, respectively. **Adverse prognostic factors included absence of brachytherapy, hemoglobin <10 g%, and interval between surgery and radiation >80 days.**

Coexistent Pelvic Mass

A pelvic mass may be identified clinically or on a staging CT scan of the pelvis and abdomen. Solid masses of uterine origin are usually leiomyomas and do not need further investigation.

If the preferred treatment is radiation, any coexistent pyometra or hematometra must be drained, using ultrasonic guidance if necessary. Repeated dilatation of the cervix and aspiration of pus may be necessary every 2 to 3 days if there is ultrasonic evidence of a further collection. Broad-spectrum antibiotics should be used to cover *Bateroides,* anaerobic *Streptococcus,* and aerobic coliforms. **Active infection decreases the response to radiation and may be exacerbated into a systemic infection if brachytherapy rods are packed into the uterus.**

Coexistent adnexal masses must be explored and a histologic diagnosis obtained. A laparoscopic approach may be appropriate if the risk of malignancy is low. Benign adnexal masses can be surgically excised. Inflammatory masses can be excised and an omental carpet used to prevent bowel adhesions. Malignant masses require surgical staging or cytoreductive surgery, depending on the individual case.

Cervical Bleeding

Torrential bleeding may occasionally follow biopsy or pelvic examination, particularly with friable, advanced cancer. **A wide gauze bandage, soaked in Monsel's solution (ferric subsulfate) and tightly packed against the cervix, usually controls the bleeding.** It should be changed after 48 hours. If control of the bleeding is not achieved, then consideration should be given to embolization of the hypogastric or uterine arteries (282), although this approach may increase tumor hypoxia, thereby decreasing radiosensitivity.

Commencement of external-beam therapy controls the bleeding within a few days. Daily fractions may be increased to 300 to 500 cGy for 2 or 3 days, or transvaginal orthovoltage treatment may be given if a suitable machine is available.

Recurrent Cervical Cancer

Treatment of recurrent disease depends on the mode of primary therapy and the site of recurrence. **If the disease recurs in the pelvis after primary radiation therapy, most patients require some type of pelvic exenteration** (see Chapter 22), although an occasional patient may be salvaged by radical hysterectomy.

Eifel et al. investigated the time course of central pelvic recurrence in 2,997 patients treated with radiation therapy for stages I and II squamous cell carcinoma of the cervix at the M.D. Anderson Cancer Center in Houston, Texas (283). Recurrence rates were 6.8%, 7.8%, and 9.6% at 5, 10, and 20 years, respectively. **The risk of central pelvic recurrence was independently correlated with tumor size ($p < 0.0001$) but not with FIGO stage.** Although after 3 years the risk of central recurrence was low, it continued to be slightly greater for patients with tumors ≥ 5 cm than for those with smaller tumors ($p = 0.001$). **Patients with recurrence after 36 months had a significantly better survival following salvage therapy.**

With pelvic recurrence after primary surgery, radiation therapy is the treatment of first choice. Grigsby reported 36 patients who received external beam and brachytherapy for recurrent cervical cancer following radical hysterectomy (284). Tumor was recurrent in the central pelvis in 33 patients (92%) and on the pelvic sidewall in three cases. The overall 5- and 10-year survivals were 74% and 50%, respectively. Ten patients (28%) developed a further recurrence after irradiation, and seven (70%) of these had a pelvic component to the failure. Severe complications developed in four patients (11.1%), including one hip fracture, one bowel obstruction requiring a colostomy, and two fistulae. Using radiation with concurrent chemotherapy (*5-fluorouracil* with or without *mitomycin C*), Thomas et al. reported eight of 17 patients (47%) alive and disease free 21 to 58 months after therapy. The recurrent disease was present in the pelvis alone or pelvis and paraaortic nodes, and seven of the eight survivors had a component of pelvic sidewall disease (285).

Pulmonary metastases following primary radical hysterectomy have been reported in 6.4% of patients (24 of 377) with negative pelvic nodes and 11.3% of patients (16 of 142) with positive pelvic nodes (286). When the lung was the only site of recurrence, a 5-year survival of 46% was achieved by surgical resection followed by chemotherapy in 12 patients who initially had negative pelvic nodes and who now had one to three pulmonary metastases. Surgery was performed in the presence of unilateral or bilateral metastases.

Radical Hysterectomy for Recurrence

Selected patients with limited persistent or recurrent disease in the cervix after primary radiation therapy may be suitable for radical hysterectomy, with or without partial resection of bowel, bladder, or ureter. The morbidity rate is high, but some patients can be cured without the need for a stoma.

Rutledge et al. (287) from London, Ontario, reported data on 41 patients who underwent conservative surgery for postradiation recurrent or persistent cervical cancer. Thirteen patients who initially had FIGO stage IB or IIA disease underwent radical abdominal or radical vaginal hysterectomy. The 5-year survival rate for this group was 84%, and major morbidity occurred in 31% of cases. A second group of 20 patients had more advanced initial disease, and all underwent radical abdominal hysterectomy. This group had a 49% 5-year survival rate and a major morbidity rate of 50%. A third group of eight patients required an extended Wertheim's operation to encompass locally advanced disease involving the bladder base or parametrium. This group had a 5-year survival rate of 25% but experienced a 75% rate of major morbidity, including two treatment-related deaths. Fistula formation occurred in 26% of patients overall.

An Italian study of 34 patients reported an actuarial 5-year survival of 49% for the whole group, with major complications in 44% of cases and a fistula rate of 15% (252). Patients with FIGO stage IB–IIA disease at primary diagnosis, no clinical parametrial involvement, and small (≤ 4 cm) tumor diameter at the time of recurrence had a survival of 65% (11 of 17).

It would appear that conservative surgery is realistic only for patients with small disease confined to the cervix, preferably detected on biopsy 4 to 6 months after primary radiation for bulky stage IB or IIA cervical cancer.

Chemotherapy

Patients with recurrent or metastatic cervical cancer are commonly symptomatic and may experience pain, anorexia, weight loss, vaginal bleeding, cachexia, and dyspnoea, among other symptoms. The role of chemotherapy in such patients is palliation, with the primary objective to relieve symptoms and improve quality of life. A secondary objective is to prolong survival.

Many factors influence the likelihood of response to chemotherapy, and these include performance status, patient age, histological subtype, site of recurrence (lung vs. pelvis), number of metastatic sites, previous radiotherapy or chemotherapy, and the interval from initial radiotherapy or chemoirradiation (289,290). These factors should be taken into consideration when making treatment decisions because they can all influence the choice of treatment as well as the response rate.

A number of chemotherapic agents have activity in patients with metastatic cervical cancer, and the response rates for single agents are summarized in Table 9.14 (291). These studies span the last 20 years and are a composite of many trials that included very different patient subsets, making interpretation difficult. In general, the most active single agents include cisplatin, paclitaxel, topotecan, vinorelbine, gemcitabine, and ifosfamide (289,290,292,293).

Table 9.14 Single Conventional Agent Chemotherapy in Cervical Carcinoma

Drugs	Patients (Response/Treated)	Response (%)
Alkylating agents		
Cyclophosphamide	36/271	13
Chlorambucil	11/44	25
Melphalan	4/20	20
Antimetabolites		
5-fluorouracil	36/270	13
Methotrexate	12/73	16
Antibiotics		
Doxorubicin	32/172	19
Bleomycin	19/176	11
Mitomycin C	5/23	22
Plant alkaloids		
Vincristine	10/58	17
Vinblastine	2/20	10
Vinorelbine	13/76	17
Miscellaneous		
Cisplatin*	238/968	25
Carboplatin*	50/250	20
Ifosfamide	34/93	37
Paclitaxel*	27/113	24
Topotecan*	13/84	15

Modified and updated from **Vermorken JB.** The role of chemotherapy in squamous cell carcinoma of the uterine cervix: a review. *Int J Gynecol Cancer* 1993;3:129, with permission.

*Agents commonly used in combination chemotherapeutic regimens

Cisplatin **is the single most active agent for squamous cell carcinoma, and its preferred dose and schedule of administration is 50 mg/m^2 every 3 weeks, intravenously** (291). Although the response rate is higher with 100 mg/m^2 (31.4%) than 50 mg/m^2 (20.7%), this is achieved at the cost of significant toxicity, and there is no difference in response duration, progression-free interval, or overall survival (294). The duration of response remains disappointing (4 to 6 months).

The response rates with combination chemotherapy are generally double that seen with single agents, although the majority of responses are partial and of short duration (4 to 6 months) (289,290,292,293). **Long-term remissions occasionally occur,** and anecdotally we have seen three long-term durable complete responses ($>$10 years): one in a patient with multiple pulmonary metastases, one in a patient with a supraclavicular lymph node metastasis diagnosed on fine-needle aspiration cytology, and, most unusually, one in a patient with a pelvic recurrence after neoadjuvant chemotherapy and radiation who presented with a large fixed pelvic recurence with almost complete obstruction of the rectum and was not suitable for exenteration. The first two patients were treated with single agent *cisplatin* and *carboplatin* and the third with *carboplatin* and *paclitaxel*. Interestingly, the group from Memorial Sloan Kettering recently reported three cases of recurrent metastatic cervical cancer in which the patients remain disease free many years after completing salvage chemotherapy and surgery (295).

A large number of phase II studies and a smaller number of phase III studies have investigated a variety of *cisplatin*-based combinations in the treatment of patients with metastatic cervical cancer, and these have been reviewed by several authors (289,290,292). There has also been a recent systematic review of all the randomized trials (293). Response rates or time to progression are traditionally the end points of phase II studies whereas progression-free survival and overall survival are the primary end points of phase III trials. **Relatively few studies in the past incorporated quality of life as an endpoint, but this is now recognized as an important measure and should be included in all phase III trials.**

Response rates as high as 75% have been reported with some combinations in phase II trials. On average, the median progression-free survival has been 6 to 8 months (289,290,292). The combination regimens have generally included *cisplatin* in addition to one or two other agents. Long has recently reviewed the published literature on the activity of these *cisplatin* doublets, triplets, and four-drug regimens and concluded that, although response rates were doubled and progression-free survival was also increased, this was not associated with any prolongation of overall survival in most studies (289).

There have been very high response rates reported with three drug regimens, but these high response rates have not been confirmed in randomized trials. For example, the combination of **bleomycin, ifosfamide,** and *cisplatin* was reported to have a response rate of 69% and a median survival of 10 months in a phase II study of 49 patients (296). However, when the GOG compared this regimen with *cisplatin* and *ifosfamide,* the response rates were the same in both arms (approximately 32%), which is in the same range as that achieved with *cisplatin* alone (297).

The most active doublet regimens include *cisplatin* in combination with *paclitaxel, gemcitabine, vinorelbine,* or *topotecan*. The GOG reported data on *cisplatin* and *paclitaxel* as first-line therapy for advanced and recurrent squamous cell carcinoma (298). Of 41 evaluable patients, five (12.2%) had a complete response and 14 (34.1%) had a partial response, for an **overall response rate of 46.3%.** The median progression-free interval was $>$5.4 months (range of 0.3 to $>$22 months), with a median survival of $>$10.0 months (range 0.9 to 22.2 months). **Response rates were higher in patients with disease in nonirradiated sites** (70% vs. 23%; $p = 0.008$), a common finding in many studies.

The combination of *cisplatin* and *gemcitabine* has also been reported to have a particularly high response rate. *Cisplatin* was administered as an i.v. infusion on day 1 (70 mg/m^2), and *gemcitabine* was administered as an i.v. infusion over 30 minutes on days 1 and 8 (1,250 mg/m^2) in a 21-day cycle (299). Forty patients who either had previous pelvic radiation or were stage 4 at presentation were evaluable, and the authors reported that three of 40 (7.5%) had a complete response, 27 of 40 (67.5%) a partial response, and five of 40 (12.5%) had stable disease. Five of 40 (12.5%) progressed on treatment. The median time to progression was 8.3 months, and the median survival was 9.6 months. Thirty percent of the patients were alive at 12 months.

The GOG reported a phase II study of *cisplatin* and *vinorelbine* in 73 patients with advanced or recurrent squamous cell carcinoma of the cervix (300). The initial doses administered were *cisplatin* 75 mg/m^2 every 4 weeks and *vinorelbine* 30 mg/m^2 weekly. The overall response rate was 30% (5 complete and 15 partial responses). The overall median response duration was >5.5 months. The major toxicity was neutropenia: 16% grade 3 and 67% grade 4. Gastrointestinal and neurotoxicity were infrequent and mild.

Fiorica et al. reported a phase II trial of *cisplatin* and *topotecan* as first-line therapy for patients with persistent or recurrent squamous and nonsquamous cervical cancer (301). There were 32 evaluable patients, and the overall response rate was 28% (9 of 32), with three complete responses (9%). Response rates were the same in irradiated and nonirradiated tissues. Median duration of response was 5 months (range 2 to >15 months), and the median survival was 10 months.

The current GOG study 204 compares the doublets *paclitaxel, topotecan, vinorelbine,* and *gemcitabine* in combination with *cisplatin,* and will determine which, if any is superior.

The two most important contemporary phase III studies have been carried out by the GOG. One compared *cisplatin* alone with *paclitaxel* and *cisplatin* and the other compared *cisplatin* alone with *topotecan* and *cisplatin.*

GOG 169 compared *cisplatin* and *paclitaxel* with *cisplatin* alone in 280 patients with stage IVB, recurrent, or persistent squamous cell carcinoma of the cervix (302). The patients were randomized to receive either *cisplatin* 50 mg/m^2 or *cisplatin* 50 mg/m^2 and *paclitaxel* 135 mg/m^2 every 3 weeks for six cycles, There were 234 patients eligible for response. Importantly, over 90% of all patients had prior radiation therapy. Objective responses occurred in 19% of patients receiving *cisplatin* (6% complete plus 13% partial), versus 36% (15% complete plus 21% partial) receiving *cisplatin* and *paclitaxel* (P = .002). The median progression-free survivals were 2.8 and 4.8 months, respectively, for *cisplatin* versus the combination (P <.001). There was no difference in median survival (8.8 months v 9.7 months). Grade 3 to 4 anemia and neutropenia were more common in the combination arm. The GOG concluded that the combination of *cisplatin* and *paclitaxel* was superior to *cisplatin* alone with respect to response rate and PFS with sustained quality of life.

Carboplatin and *paclitaxel* is a more attractive combination from the point of view of toxicity and ease of administration and although phase II studies have demonstrated that it is a very active regimen (303,304), this has not been confirmed in randomized trials.

GOG 179 demonstrated the superiority of *cisplatin* and *topotecan* over *cisplatin* alone in a study of 356 patients with stage IV, recurrent, or persistent cervical cancer (305). Patients were randomized to one of three treatment arms: single agent *cisplatin* 50 mg/m^2 every 3 weeks (n = 146), *topotecan* 0.75 mg/m^2 on days 1–3 plus *cisplatin* 50 mg/m^2 on day 1 every 3 weeks (n = 147), or *methotrexate* plus *vinblastine* plus *doxorubicin* plus *cisplatin* (MVAC) every four weeks.The MVAC arm was closed prematurely because of excessive toxicity. Nearly 80% of patients had received radiotherapy, and almost 60% had received *cisplatin*-based chemotherapy before randomization.

Objective responses were achieved in 39 of 147 patients (27%) on the combination, compared with 19 of 146 (13%) treated with single-agent *cisplatin* (p = 0.004). There were 14 complete responses observed with the combination (10%) compared with 4 (3%) with the single agent. Median progression-free survival for the combination was 4.6 months versus 2.9 months (p = 0.014), and median overall survival for the combination was 9.4 months versus 6.5 months (p = 0.017). Fifty seven percent of patients had been previously treated with *cisplatin* based chemoradiation. The median survival for patients who received no prior *cisplatin* was 15.4 months for the combination of *topotecan* and *cisplatin* compared to 7.9 months for those who had prior *cisplatin* chemoradiation. The probability of survival increased for both treatment groups the longer a patient was from prior *cisplatin* chemotherapy.

This is the only study to date that has reported an overall survival advantage with combination chemotherapy. The authors concluded that *topotecan* and *cisplatin* should be considered the standard of care for patients with advanced or recurrent cervical cancer. Quality of life scores were similar in the two arms of the study.

With increasing numbers of patients being treated with concurrent chemoradiotherapy with *cisplatin* as primary treatment, there is a need to develop new active non-*cisplatin* based combinations, as response rates to further *cisplatin*-based chemotherapy in these patients are much lower than in previously untreated patients. There have only been a few studies to evaluate non-*cisplatin* containing doublets in patients who have received *cisplatin* as part of their primary therapy and who have relapsed within 12 months. There are a number of possible agents that could be combined, and they include any of the active single agents discussed above. In a phase II study of **topotecan** and **paclitaxel** for recurrent, persistent, or metastatic cervical cancer, a New York group reported **7 responses (54%) among 13 evaluable patients** (1 complete, 6 partial) (3). Progression-free and overall survivals were 3.8 and 8.6 months, respectively.

The role of targeted therapies in cervical cancer is at present unknown, but there is a strong theoretical rationale to support such studies, and this is an area of active research. For example, EGFR-1 is highly expressed in primary and recurrent cervical tumors and drugs such as *cetuximab* may be of benefit (307). *Bevacuizimab* has shown activity in combination with *fluorouracil* in a small number of heavily pretreated patients and should also be investigated further (308). The GOG are investigating *cetuximab* and *cisplatin* (GOG 0076DD) as well as the activity of *erlotinib* (GOG 0277D) and *bevacizumab* (GOG 0277C) in patients with metastatic cervical cancer, and the results of these studies will influence the next generation of cervical cancer trials.

Ultimately, the approach to management and the choice of treatment is influenced by multiple factors. These include the age and performance status of the patient, the site of recurrence, the time to recurrence, the patient's symptoms, the number of metastatic sites, prior therapy including chemoradiation, and the pace of the disease. **Chemotherapy for metastatic cervical cancer is generally disappointing,** and, despite higher response rates with combination chemotherapy, the duration of response is relatively short in the majority of patients.

The objective of treatment is to palliate symptoms and improve quality of life. Ideally, eligible patients should be enrolled into clinical trials. However, in the absence of appropriate trials, **it is our practice to use platinum-based combinations such as *cisplatin* and *topotecan* or *carboplatin* and *paclitaxel* or *gemcitabine* in patients with a good performance status.** We would consider single agents such as *carboplatin* alone or weekly *cisplatin* in patients with a poorer performance status.

References

1. **Parkin DM, Bray F, Ferlay J, Pisani P.** Estimating the world cancer burden Globocan 2000, *Int J Cancer* 2001;94:153–156.
2. **Jemal A, Siegel R, Ward E, Hao Y, Xu J, Murray T, Thun MJ.** Cancer statistics, 2009. *CA Cancer J Clin* 2009;published online doi:10.3322/caac.20006.
3. **Walboomers JM, Jacobs MV, Manos MM.** Human papillomavirus is a necessary cause of invasive cervical cancer worldwide. *J Pathol* 1999;189:12–19.
4. **Schiffman M, Castle PE.** The promise of global cervical cancer prevention. *J Pathol* 2005;353:2101–2104.
5. **Trimble EL, Harlan LG, Clegg LX.** Untreated cervical cancer in the United States. *Gynecol Oncol* 2005;96:217–277.
6. **Pretorius R, Semrad N, Watring W, Fotherongham N.** Presentation of cervical cancer. *Gynecol Oncol* 1991;42:48–52.
7. **Sasieni PD, Cuzick J, Lynch-Farmery E, the National Co-ordinating Network for Cervical Screening Working Group.** Estimating the efficacy of screening by auditing smear histories of women with and without cervical cancer. *Br J Cancer* 1996;73:1001–1005.
8. **Burghardt E, Pickel H, Girardi F.** *Colposcopy and cervical pathology: textbook and atlas.* Stuttgart: Thieme, 1998:138–192.
9. **Quinn MA, Benedet JL, Odicino F, Maisonneuve P, Beller U, Creasman W, et al.** Carcinoma of the cervix uteri: annual report on the results of treatment in gynaecological cancer. *Int J Gynecol Obstet* 2006;95:S43–S103.
10. **Lagasse LD, Creasman WT, Shingleton HM, Blessing JA.** Results and complications of operative staging in cervical cancer: experience of the Gynecology Oncology Group. *Gynecol Oncol* 1980;9:90–98.
11. **La Polla JP, Schlaerth JB, Gaddis O, Morrow CP.** The influence of surgical staging on the evaluation and treatment of patients with cervical carcinoma. *Gynecol Oncol* 1986;24:194–199.
12. **Hacker NF, Berek JS.** Surgical staging of cervical cancer. In: **Surwit EA, Alberts DS, eds.** *Cervix cancer.* Boston: Martinus Nijhoff, 1987:43–47.
13. **Kim SH, Choi BI, Han JK, Kim HD, Lee HP, Kang SB, et al.** Preoperative staging of uterine cervical carcinoma: comparison of CT and MRI in 99 patients. *J Comput Assist Tomogr* 1993;17:633–640.
14. **Subak LL, Hricak H, Powell B, Azizi L, Stern JL.** Cervical carcinoma: computed tomography and magnetic resonance imaging for preoperative staging. *Obstet Gynecol* 1995;86:43–50.
15. **Narayan K, McKenzie A, Fisher R, Susil B, Jobling T, Bernshaw D.** Estimation of tumor volume in cervical cancer by magnetic resonance imaging. *Am J Clin Oncol* 2003;26:e163–168.
16. **Wagenaar HC, Trimbos JB, Postema S, Anastasopoulou A, van der Geest RJ, Reiber JHC, et al.** Tumor diameter and volume assessed by magnetic resonance imaging in the prediction of outcome for invasive cervical cancer. *Gynecol Oncol* 2001;82:474–482.
17. **Sahdev A, Sohaib SA, Wenaden AET, Shepherd JH, Rezrek RH.** The performance of magnetic resonance imaging in early cervical carcinoma: a long-term experience. *Int J Gynecol Cancer* 2007;17:629–36.
18. **Scheidler J, Hricak H, Yu KK, Subak L, Segal MR.** Radiological evaluation of lymph node metastases in patients with cervical cancer: a metaanalysis. *JAMA* 1997;278:1096–1101.
19. **Rose PG, Adler LP, Rodriguez M, Faulhaber PF, Abdul-Karim FW, Miraldi F.** Positron emission tomography for evaluating paraaortic nodal metastasis in locally advanced cervical cancer before surgical staging: a surgicopathological study. *J Clin Oncol* 1999;17:41–45.

20. Narayan K, Hicks RJ, Jobling T, Bernshaw D, McKenzie AF. A comparison of MRI and PET scanning in surgically staged locoregionally advanced cervical cancer: potential impact on treatment. *Int J Gynecol Cancer* 2001;11:263–271.

21. Grigsby PW, Siegel BA, Dehdashti F. Lymph node staging by positron emission tomography in patients with carcinoma of the cervix. *J Clin Oncol* 2001;19:3745–3749.

22. Narayan K, McKenzie AF, Hicks RJ, Fisher R, Bernshaw D, Bau S. Relation between FIGO stage, primary tumor volume, and presence of lymph node matastases in cervical cancer patients referred for radiotherapy. *Int J Gynecol Cancer* 2003;13:657–63.

23. Havrilesky LJ, Kulasingam SL, Matchar DB, Myers ER. FDG-PET for management of cervical and ovarian cancer. *Gynecol Oncol* 2005;97:183–191.

24. McDonald TW, Morley GW, Choo YL, Shields JJ, Cordoba RB, Naylor B. Fine needle aspiration of paraaortic and pelvic nodes showing lymphangiographic abnormalities. *Obstet Gynecol* 1983;61:383–388.

25. Ewing TL, Buchler DA, Hoogerland DL, Sonek MG, Wirtanen GW. Percutaneous lymph node aspiration in patients with gynecologic tumors. *Am J Obstet Gynecol* 1982;143:824–830.

26. Nelson JH Jr, Boyce J, Macasaet M, Lu T, Bohorquez JF, Nicastri AD, et al. Incidence, significance and follow-up of paraaortic lymph node metastases in late invasive carcinoma of the cervix. *Am J Obstet Gynecol* 1977;128:336–340.

27. Berman ML, Lagasse LD, Watring WG, Ballon SC, Schlesinger RE, Moore JG, et al. The operative evaluation of patients with cervical carcinoma by an extraperitoneal approach. *Obstet Gynecol* 1977;50:658–664.

28. Querleu D, Leblanc E, Castelain B. Laparoscopic pelvic lymphadenectomy in the staging of early carcinoma of the cervix. *Am J Obstet Gynecol* 1991;164:579–585.

29. Lai C-H, Huang K-G, Hong J-H, Lee C-L, Chou H-H, Chang T-C, et al. Randomized trial of surgical staging (extraperitoneal or laparoscopic) versus clinical staging in locally advanced cervical cancer. *Gynecol Oncol* 2003;89:160–167.

30. Gold MA, Tian C, Whitney CW, Rose PG, Lanciano R. Surgical versus radiographic determination of paraaortic lymph node metastases before chemoradiation for locally advanced cervical carcinoma. A Gynecologic Oncology Study. *Cancer* 2008;112:1954–1963.

31. Petereit DG, Hartenbach EM, Thomas GM. Paraaortic lymph node evaluation in cervical cancer: the impact of staging upon treatment decisions and outcome. *Int J Gynecol Cancer* 1998;8:353–364.

32. Plentyl AA, Friedman EA. *Lymphatic system of the female genitalia: the morphologic basis of oncologic diagnosis and therapy.* Philadelphia: WB Saunders, 1971.

33. Burke TW, Heller PB, Hoskins WJ, Weiser EB, Nash JD, Park PC. Evaluation of the scalene lymph nodes in primary and recurrent cervical carcinoma. *Gynecol Oncol* 1987;28:312–317.

34. Zander J, Baltzer J, Lobe KJ, Ober KG, Kaufman C. Carcinoma of the cervix: an attempt to individualize treatment. *Am J Obstet Gynecol* 1981;139:752–759.

35. Fuller AF, Elliott N, Kosloff C, Lewis JL Jr. Lymph node metastases from carcinoma of the cervix, stage IB and IIA: implications for prognosis and treatment. *Gynecol Oncol* 1982;13:165–174.

36. Timmer PR, Aalders JG, Bouma J. Radical surgery after preoperative intracavitary radiotherapy for stage IB and IIA carcinoma of the uterine cervix. *Gynecol Oncol* 1984;18:206–212.

37. Inoue T, Okamura M. Prognostic significance of parametrial extension in patients with cervical carcinoma stages IB, IIA, and IIB. *Cancer* 1984;54:1714–1719.

38. Creasman WT, Soper JT, Clarke-Pearson D. Radical hysterectomy as therapy for early carcinoma of the cervix. *Am J Obstet Gynecol* 1986;155:964–969.

39. Finan MA, De Cesare S, Fiorica JV, Chambers R, Hoffman MS, Kline RC, et al. Radical hysterectomy for stage IB1 vs IB2 carcinoma of the cervix: does the new staging system predict morbidity and survival? *Gynecol Oncol* 1996;62:139–147.

40. Artman LE, Hoskins WJ, Birro MC, Heller PB, Weiser EB, Barnhill DR, et al. Radical hysterectomy and pelvic lymphadenectomy for stage IB carcinoma of the cervix: 21 years experience. *Gynecol Oncol* 1987;28:8–13.

41. Monaghan JM, Ireland D, Mor-Yosef S, Pearson SE, Lopes A, Sinha DP. Role of centralization of surgery in stage IB carcinoma of the cervix: a review of 498 cases. *Gynecol Oncol* 1990;37:206–209.

42. Samlal RA, van der Velden J, Ten Kate FJW, Schilthuis MS, Hart AAM, Lammes FB. Surgical pathologic factors that predict recurrence in stage IB and IIA cervical carcinoma patients with negative pelvic nodes. *Cancer* 1997;80:1234–1240.

43. Delgado G, Chun B, Calgar H, Bepko F. Paraaortic lymphadenectomy in gynecologic malignancies confined to the pelvis. *Obstet Gynecol* 1977;50:418–423.

44. Piver MS, Barlow JJ. High dose irradiation to biopsy confirmed aortic node metastases from carcinoma of the uterine cervix. *Cancer* 1977;39:1243–1248.

45. Sudarsanam A, Charyulu K, Belinson J, Averette H, Goldberg M, Hintz B, et al. Influence of exploratory celiotomy on the management of carcinoma of the cervix. *Cancer* 1978;41:1049–1053.

46. Buchsbaum H. Extrapelvic lymph node metastases in cervical carcinoma. *Am J Obstet Gynecol* 1979;133:814–824.

47. Hughes RR, Brewington KC, Hanjani P, Photopulos G, Dick D, Votava C, et al. Extended field irradiation for cervical cancer based on surgical staging. *Gynecol Oncol* 1980;9:153–161.

48. Ballon SC, Berman ML, Lagasse LD, Petrilli ES, Castaldo TW. Survival after extraperitoneal pelvic and paraaortic lymphadenectomy and radiation therapy in cervical carcinoma. *Obstet Gynecol* 1981;57:90–95.

49. Welander CE, Pierce VK, Nori D, Hilaris BS, Kosloff C, Clark DCG, et al. Pretreatment laparotomy in carcinoma of the cervix. *Gynecol Oncol* 1981;12:336–347.

50. Berman ML, Keys H, Creasman WT, Di Saia P, Bundy B, Blessing J. Survival and patterns of recurrence in cervical cancer metastatic to periaortic lymph nodes: a Gynecologic Oncology Group study. *Gynecol Oncol* 1984;19:8–16.

51. Potish RA, Twiggs LB, Okagaki T, Prem KA, Adcock LL. Therapeutic implications of the natural history of advanced cervical cancer as defined by pretreatment surgical staging. *Cancer* 1985;56:956–960.

52. Dargent D, Martin X, Mathevet P. Laparoscopic assessment of sentinel lymph nodes in early cervical cancer. *Gynecol Oncol* 2000;79:411–415.

53. Levenback C, Coleman RL, Burke TW, Linn WM, Erdman W, Deavers M, et al. Lymphatic mapping and sentinel node identification in patients with cervical cancer undergoing radical hysterectomy and pelvic lymphadenectomy. *J Clin Oncol* 2002;20:688–693.

54. Rob L, Strnad P, Robova H, Charvat M, Pluta M, Shelgerova D, et al. Study of lymphatic mapping and sentinel node identification in early stage cervical cancer. *Gynecol Oncol* 2005;98:281–288.

55. Wydra D, Sawicki S, Wojtylak S, Bandurski T, Emerich J. Sentinel node identification in cervical cancer patients undergoing transperitoneal radical hysterectomy: a study of 100 cases. *Int J Gynecol Cancer* 2006;16:649–54.

56. Altgassen C, Hertel H, Brandstadt A, Kohler C, Durst M, Schneider A. AGO study group. Multicenter validation study of sentinel lymph node concept in cervical cancer:AGO Study Group. *J Clin Oncol* 2008;26:2943–51.

57. van Dam PA, Hauspy J, van der Hayden T, Sonnemans H, Spaepen A, Eggenstein G, et al. Intraoperative sentinel node identification with Technitium-99m-labelled nanocolloid in patients with cancer of the uterine cervix: a feasibility study. *Int J Gynecol Cancer* 2003;13:182–186.

58. Burghardt E, Girardi F. Local spread of cervical cancer. In: Burghardt E, ed. *Surgical gynecologic oncology.* New York: Thieme, 1993:203–212.

59. Shingleton HM, Orr JW. *Cancer of the cervix.* Philadelphia: JB Lippincott, 1995.

60. Sutton GP, Bundy BN, Delgado G, Sevin BU, Creasman WT, Major FJ, et al. Ovarian metastases in stage IB carcinoma of the cervix: a Gynecologic Oncology Group study. *Am J Obstet Gynecol* 1992;166:50–53.

61. Suprasert P, Srisomboon J, Kasamatsu T. Radical hysterectomy for stage IIB cervical cancer: a review. *Int J Gynecol Cancer* 2005;15:995–1001.

62. Kim JH, Kim HJ, Hong S, Wu HG, Ha SW. Post-hysterectomy radiotherapy for FIGO stage IB–IIB uterine cervical carcinoma. *Gynecol Oncol* 2005;96:407–414.

63. Hockel M, Horn L-C, Fritsch H. Association between the management compartment of uterovaginal organogenesis and local tumor spread in stage IB–IIB cervical cancer: a prospective study. *Lancet Oncol* 2005; 6:751–756.

64. **Mestwerdt G.** Die Fruhdiagnose des Kollumkarzinoms. *Zentralbl Gynakol* 1947;69:198–202.

65. **Creasman WT, Fetter BF, Clarke-Pearson DL, Kaufman L, Parker RT.** Management of stage IA carcinoma of the cervix. *Am J Obstet Gynecol* 1985;153:164–172.

66. **Van Nagell JR, Greenwell N, Powell DF, Donaldson ES, Hanson MB, Gay EC.** Microinvasive carcinoma of the cervix. *Am J Obstet Gynecol* 1983;145:981–991.

67. **Simon NL, Gore H, Shingleton HM, Soong SJ, Orr JW, Hatch KD.** Study of superficially invasive carcinoma of the cervix. *Obstet Gynecol* 1986;68:19–24.

68. **FIGO Cancer Committee.** Staging announcement. *Gynecol Oncol* 1986;25:383–385.

69. **Ostor AG.** Studies on 200 cases of early squamous cell carcinoma of the cervix. *Int J Gynecol Pathol* 1993;12:193–207.

70. **Ostor AG.** Pandora's box or Ariadne's thread? Definition and prognostic significance of microinvasion in the uterine cervix: squamous lesions. In: **Pathology annual,** part II. 1995:103–136.

71. **Elliott P, Coppleson M, Russell P, Liouros P, Carter J, Macleod C, et al.** Early invasive (FIGO stage IA) carcinoma of the cervix: a clinicopathologic study of 476 cases. *Int J Gynecol Cancer* 2000;10:42–52.

72. **Lee KBM, Lee JM, Park CY, Lee KB, Cho HY, Ha SY.** Lymph node metastases and lymphatic invasion in microinvasive squamous cell carcinoma of the uterine cervix. *Int J Gynecol Cancer* 2006;16:1184–1187.

73. **Roman LD, Felix JC, Muderspach LI, Agahjanian A, Qian D, Morrow CP.** Risk of residual invasive disease in women with microinvasive squamous cancer in a conization specimen. *Obstet Gynecol* 1997;90:759–764.

74. **Phongnarisorn C, Srisomboon J, Khumamornpong S, Siriaungkul S, Suprasert P, Charoenkwan K et al.** The risk of residual neoplasia in women with microinvasive squamous cell carcinoma and positive cone margins. *Int J Gynecol Cancer* 2006;16:655–659.

75. **Kolstad P.** Follow-up study of 232 patients with stage Ia1 and 411 patients with stage Ia2 squamous cell carcinoma of the cervix (microinvasive carcinoma). *Gynecol Oncol* 1989;33:265–272.

76. **Burghardt E, Girardi F, Lahousen M, Pickel H, Tamussino K.** Microinvasive carcinoma of the uterine cervix (FIGO stage IA). *Cancer* 1991;67:1037–1045.

77. **Van Nagell JR, Greenwell N, Powell DF, Donaldson ES, Hanson MB, Gay EC.** Microinvasive carcinoma of the cervix. *Am J Obstet Gynecol* 1983;145:981–989.

78. **Hasumi K, Sakamoto A, Sugano H.** Microinvasive carcinoma of the uterine cervix. *Cancer* 1980;45:928–931.

79. **Maiman MA, Fruchter RG, Di Maio TM, Boyce JG.** Superficially invasive squamous cell carcinoma of the cervix. *Obstet Gynecol* 1988;72:399–403.

80. **Buckley SL, Tritz DM, van Le L, Higgins R, Sevin B-U, Veland FR, et al.** Lymph node metastases and prognosis in patients with stage IA2 cervical cancer. *Gynecol Oncol* 1996;63:4–9.

81. **Creasman WT, Zaino R,T, Major FJ, Di Saia PJ, Hatch KD, Homesley HD.** Early invasive carcinoma of the cervix (3 to 5 mm invasion): risk factors and prognosis. A GOG study. *Am J Obstet Gynecol* 1998;178:62–65.

82. **Takeshima N, Yanoh K, Tabata T, Nagai K, Hirai Y, Hasumi K.** Assessment of the revised International Federation of Gynecology and Obstetrics staging for early invasive squamous cervical cancer. *Gynecol Oncol* 1999;74:165–169.

83. **Dargent D, Brun JL, Roy M, Remy I.** Pregnancies following radical trachelectomy for invasive cervical cancer. *Gynecol Oncol* 1994;52:105(abst).

84. **Covens A, Shaw P, Murphy J, De Petrillo D, Lickrish G, Laframboise S, et al.** Is radical trachelectomy a safe alternative to radical hysterectomy for patients with stage IA-B carcinoma of the cervix? *Cancer* 1999;86:2273–2279.

85. **Smith JR, Boyle DC, Corless DJ, Ungar L, Lawson AD, Del Priore G, et al.** Abdominal radical trachelectomy: a new surgical technique for the conservative management of cervical carcinoma. *BJOG* 1997;104:1196–1200.

86. **Rodriguez M, Guimares O, Rose PG.** Radical abdominal trachelectomy and pelvic lymphadenectomy with uterine conservation

and subsequent pregnancy in the treatment of early invasive cervical cancer. *Am J Obstet Gynecol* 2001;185:370–374.

87. **Alexander-Sefre F, Chee N, Spencer C, Menon U, Shepherd JH.** Surgical morbidity associated with radical trachelectomy and radical hysterectomy. *Gynecol Oncol* 2006;101:450–454.

88. **Peppercorn PD, Jeyarajah AR, Woolas R, Shepherd JH, Oram DH, Jacobs LI, et al.** Role of MR imaging in the selection of patients with early cervical carcinoma for fertility-preserving surgery: initial experience. *Radiology* 1999;212:395–399.

89. **Berek JS, Hacker NF, Fu Y-S, Sokale JR, Leuchter RC, Lagasse LD.** Adenocarcinoma of the uterine cervix: histologic variables associated with lymph node metastasis and survival. *Obstet Gynecol* 1985;65:46–52.

90. **Ostor A, Rome R, Quinn M.** Microinvasive adenocarcinoma of the cervix: a clinicopathologic study of 77 women. *Obstet Gynecol* 1997;89:88–93.

91. **Kaku T, Kamura T, Sakai K, Amada S, Kobayashi H, Shigematsu T, et al.** Early adenocarcinoma of the uterine cervix. *Gynecol Oncol* 1997;65:281–285.

92. **Teshima S, Shimosata Y, Kishi K, Kasamatsu T, Ohmi K, Uei Y.** Early stage adenocarcinoma of the cervix. *Cancer* 1985;56:167–172.

93. **Lee KR, Flynn CE.** Early invasive adenocarcinoma of the cervix: a histopathologic analysis of 40 cases with observations concerning histogenesis. *Cancer* 2000;89:1048–1055.

94. **Bisseling KCHM, Bekkers RLM, Rome RM, Quinn MA.** Treatment of microinvasive adenocarcinoma of the uterine cervix: a retrospective study and review of the literature. *Gynecol Oncol* 2007;107:424–430.

95. **Webb JC, Key CR, Qualls CR, Smith HO.** Population-based study of microinvasive adenocarcinoma of the uterine cervix. *Obstet Gynecol* 2001;97:701–706.

96. **Poynor EA, Marshall D, Sonoda Y, Slomovitz BM, Barakat RR, Soslow RA.** Clinicopathologic features of early adenocarcinoma of the cervix initially managed with cervical conization. *Gynecol Oncol* 2006; 103:960–965.

97. **Ostor AG.** Early invasive adenocarcinoma of the cervix. *Int J Gynecol Pathol* 2000;19:29–38.

98. **Poynor EA, Barakat RR, Hoskins WJ.** Management and follow-up of patients with adenocarcinoma *in situ* of the uterine cervix. *Gynecol Oncol* 1995;57:158–164.

99. **Landoni F, Maneo A, Colombo A, Placa F, Milani R, Perego P, et al.** Randomized study of radical surgery versus radiotherapy for stage IB–IIa cervical cancer. *Lancet* 1997;350:535–540.

100. **Eifel PJ, Moughan J, Erickson B, Iarocci T, Grant D,Owen J.** Patterns of radiotherapy practice for patients with carcinoma of the uterine cervix: a patterns of care study. *Int J Radiat Oncol Biol Phys* 2004;60:1144–1153.

101. **Lawton FG, Hacker NF.** Surgery for invasive gynecologic cancer in the elderly female population. *Obstet Gynecol* 1990;76:287–291.

102. **Brand AH, Bull CA, Cakir B.** Vaginal stenosis in patients treated with radiotherapy for carcinoma of the cervix. *Int J Gynecol Cancer* 2006; 16:288–293.

103. **Samlal RAK, van der Velden J, Schilthuis MS, Ten Kate FJW, Hart AAM, Lammes FB.** Influence of diagnostic conization on surgical morbidity and survival in patients undergoing radical hysterectomy for stage IB and IIA cervical carcinoma. *Eur J Gynaecol Oncol* 1997;18:478–481.

104. **Orr JW, Shingleton HM, Hatch KD, Mann WJ, Austin JM, Soong S.** Correlation of perioperative morbidity and conization to radical hysterectomy interval. *Obstet Gynecol* 1982;59:726–731.

105. **Piver M, Rutledge F, Smith J.** Five classes of extended hysterectomy for women with cervical cancer. *Obstet Gynecol* 1974;44:265–272.

106. **Wertheim E.** The extended abdominal operation for carcinoma uteri (based on 500 operative cases). *Am J Obstet* 1912;66:169–174.

107. **Meigs J.** Carcinoma of the cervix: the Wertheim operation. *Surg Gynecol Obstet* 1944;78:195–199.

108. **Querleu D, Morrow CP.** Classification of radical hysterectomy. *Lancet Oncol* 2008;9:297–303.

109. **Hockel M.** Laterally extended endopelvic resection: surgical treatment of infrailiac pelvic wall recurrences of gynecologic malignancies. *Am J Obstet Gynecol* 1999;180:306–312.

110. **Hacker NF, Wain GV, Nicklin JL.** Resection of bulky positive lymph nodes in patients with cervical cancer. *Int J Gynecol Cancer* 1995;5:250–256.

111. Fujii S, Tanakura K, Matsumura N, Higuchi T, Yura S, Mandai M et al. Anatomic identification and functional outcomes of the nerve sparing Okabayashi radical hysterectomy. *Gynecol Oncol* 2007;107:4–13.

112. Trimbos JB, Maas CP, Derviter MC, Peters AAW, Kenter GG. A nerve-sparing radical hysterectomy: guidelines and feasibility in Western patients. *Int J Gynecol Cancer* 2001;11:180–186.

113. Jensen JK, Lucci JA, Di Saia PJ, Manetta A, Berman ML. To drain or not to drain: a retrospective study of closed-suction drainage following radical hysterectomy with pelvic lymphadenectomy. *Gynecol Oncol* 1993;51:46–49.

114. Pikaat DP, Holloway RW, Ahmad S, Finkler NJ, Bigsby GE, Ortiz BH, et al. Clinico-pathologic morbidity analysis of types 2 and 3 abdominal radical hysterectomy for cervical cancer. *Gynecol Oncol* 2007;107:205–210.

115. Samlal RAK, van der Velden J, Ketting BW, Gonzalez DG, Ten Kate FJW, Hart AAM, et al. Disease-free interval and recurrence pattern after the Okabayashi variant of Wertheim's radical hysterectomy for stage IB and IIA cervical carcinoma. *Int J Gynecol Cancer* 1996;6:120–127.

116. Sivanesaratnam V, Sen DK, Jayalakshmi P, Ong G. Radical hysterectomy and pelvic lymphadenectomy for early invasive cancer of the cervix: 14 years experience. *Int J Gynecol Cancer* 1993;3:231–238.

117. Krishnan CS, Grant PT, Robertson G, Hacker NF. Lymphatic ascites following lymphadenectomy for gynecological cancer. *Int J Gynecol Cancer* 2001; 11:392–396.

118. Covens A, Rosen B, Gibbons A, Osborne R, Murphy J, DePetrillo A, et al. Differences in the morbidity of radical hysterectomy between gynecological oncologists. *Gynecol Oncol* 1993;51:39–45.

119. Lee RB, Park RC. Bladder dysfunction following radical hysterectomy. *Gynecol Oncol* 1981;11:304–308.

120. Bergmark K, Avall-Lundqvist E, Dickman PW, Henningsohn L, Steineck G. Vaginal function and sexuality in women with a history of cervical cancer. *N Engl J Med* 1999;340:1383–1389.

121. Grumann M, Robertson R, Hacker NF, Sommer G. Sexual functioning in patients following radical hysterectomy for stage IB cancer of the cervix. *Int J Gynecol Cancer* 2001;11:372–380.

122. Frumovitz M, Sun CC, Schover LR, Munsell MF, Jhingran A, Wharton JT et al. Quality of life and sexual functioning in cervical cancer survivors. *J Clin Oncol* 2005;23:7428–7436.

123. Greenwald HP, McCorkle R. Sexuality and sexual function in long-term survivors of cervical cancer. *J Women's Health* 2008;17:955–963.

124. Sakamoto S, Takazawa K. An improved radical hysterectomy with fewer urological complications and with no loss of therapeutic results for cervical cancer. *Baillieres Clin Obstet Gynaecol* 1999;2:953–962.

125. Yabuki Y, Asamoto A, Hoshiba T, Nishimoto H, Nishikawa Y, Nakajima T. Radical hysterectomy: an anatomic evaluation of parametrial dissection. *Gynecol Oncol* 2000;77:155–163.

126. Possover M, Stober S, Phaul K, Schneider A. Identification and preservation of the motoric innervation of the bladder in radical hysterectomy type III. *Gynecol Oncol* 2000;79:154–157.

127. Raspagliesi F, Ditto A, Fontanelli R, Zanaboni F, Solima E, Spatti G et al. Type II versus type III nerve-sparing radical hysterectomy: comparison of lower urinary tract dysfunctions. *Gynecol Oncol* 2006;102:256–262.

128. Todo Y, Kuwabara M, Watari H, Ebina Y, Takeda M, Kudo M et al. Urodynamic study on postsurgical bladder function in cervical cancer treated with systematic nerve-sparing radical hysterectomy. *Int J Gynecol Cancer* 2006;16:369–375.

129. Yalla SV, Andriole GL. Vesicourethral dysfunction following pelvic visceral ablative surgery. *J Urol* 1984;132:503–509.

130. Levin RJ. The physiology of female sexual function in women. *Clin Obstet Gynecol* 1980;7:213–252.

131. Landoni F, Maneo A, Cormio G, Perego P, Milani R, Caruso O, et al. Class II versus class III radical hysterectomy in stage IB–IIA cervical cancer: a prospective randomized study. *Gynecol Oncol* 2001;80:3–12.

132. Stegman M, Louwen M, van der Velden J, ten Kate FJW, den Bakker MA, Burger CW, et al. The incidence of parametrial tumor involvement in select patients with early cervix cancer is too low to justify parametrectomy. *Gynecol Oncol* 2007;105:475–480.

133. Wright JD, Grigsby PW, Brooks R, Powell MA, Gibb RK, Gao F et al. Utility of parametrectomy for early stage cervical cancer treated with radical hysterectomy. *Cancer* 2007;110:1281–1286.

134. Ryan M, Stainton C, Slaytor EK, Jaconelli C, Watts S, Mackenzie P. Aetiology and prevalence of lower limb lymphoedema following treatment for gynaecological cancer. *Aust N Z J Obstet Gynaecol* 2003;143:148–151.

135. Eifel PJ, Morris M, Wharton TJ, Oswald MJ. The influence of tumor size and morphology on the outcome of patients with FIGO stage IB squamous cell carcinoma of the uterine cervix. *Int J Radiat Oncol Biol Phys* 1994;29:9–16.

136. Perez CA, Grigsby PW, Chao KSC, Mutch D, Lockett MA. Tumor size, irradiation dose, and long term outcome of carcinoma of the cervix. *Int J Radiat Oncol Biol Phys* 1998;41:307–317.

137. Tan LT, Zahra M. Long term survival and late toxicity after chemoradiotherapy for cervical cancer–the Addenbrooke's Experience. *Clin Oncol* 2008;20:358–364.

138. Perez CA, Grigsby PW, Camel HM, Galakatos AE, Mutch D, Lockett MA. Irradiation alone or combined with surgery in stage IB, IIA and IIB carcinoma of the uterine cervix: update of a nonrandomized comparison. *Int J Radiat Oncol Biol Phys* 1995;31:706–716.

139. Montana GS, Fowler WC, Varia MA, Walton LA, Mack Y. Analysis of results of radiation therapy for stage IB carcinoma of the cervix. *Cancer* 1987;60:2195–2200.

140. Rose PG, Bundy B, Watkins EB, Thigpen T, Deppe G, Maiman MA, et al. Concurrent *cisplatin*-based radiotherapy and chemotherapy for locally advanced cervical cancer. *N Engl J Med* 1999;340:1144–1153.

141. Durrance FY, Fletcher GH, Rutledge FN. Analysis of central recurrent disease in stages I and II squamous cell carcinomas of the cervix on intact uterus. *Am J Roentgenol Rad Ther Nuclear Med* 1969;106:831–838.

142. Keys HM, Bundy BN, Stehman FB, Okagaki T, Gallup DG, Burnett AF, et al. for the Gynecology Oncology Group. Radiation therapy with and without extrafascial hysterectomy for bulky stage IB cervical carcinoma: a randomized trial of the Gynecologic Oncology Group. *Gynecol Oncol* 2003;89:343–353.

143. Keys HM, Bundy BN, Stehman FB, Muderspach LI, Chafe EW, Suggs CL, et al. *Cisplatin*, radiation, and adjuvant hysterectomy compared with radiation and adjuvant hysterectomy for bulky stage IB cervical carcinoma. *N Engl J Med* 1999;340:1154–1161.

144. Sardi J, Sananes C, Giaroli A, Bayo J, Gomez Rueda N, Vighi S, et al. Results of a prospective randomized trial with neoadjuvant chemotherapy in stage IB, bulky, squamous carcinoma of the cervix. *Gynecol Oncol* 1993;49:156–165.

145. Stewart LA, Stewart LA, Tierney JF. Neoadjuvant chemotherapy and surgery versus standard radiotherapy for locally advanced cervix cancer: a metaanalysis using individual patient data from randomized controlled trials. *Int J Gynecol Cancer* 2002;15:579(abst).

146. Neoadjuvant chemotherapy for cervical cancer metaanalysis collaboration. Neoadjuvant chemotherapy for locally advanced cervical cancer: a systematic review and metaanalysis of individual patient data from 21 randomized trials. *Euro J Cancer* 2003;39:2470–2486.

147. Ikushima H, Takegawa Y, Osaki K, Furutani S, Yamashita K, Kawanaka T et al. Radiation therapy for cervical cancer in the elderly. *Gynecol Oncol* 2007;107:339–343.

148. Mitchell PA, Waggoner S, Rotmensch J, Mundt AJ. Cervical cancer in the elderly treated with radiation therapy. *Gynecol Oncol* 1998;71:291–298.

149. Hacker NF. Clinical and operative staging of cervical cancer. *Baillieres Clin Obstet Gynecol* 1988;2:747–759.

150. Cosin JA, Fowler JM, Chen MD, Paley PJ, Carson LF, Twiggs LB. Pretreatment surgical staging of patients with cervical carcinoma: the case for lymph node debulking. *Cancer* 1998;82:2241–2248.

151. Allen HH, Nisker JA, Anderson RJ. Primary surgical treatment in one hundred ninety-five cases of stage IB carcinoma of the cervix. *Am J Obstet Gynecol* 1982;143:581–584.

152. Inoue T, Chihara T, Morita K. The prognostic significance of the size of the largest nodes in metastatic carcinoma from the uterine cervix. *Gynecol Oncol* 1984;19:187–193.

153. Bloss JD, Berman ML, Mukhererjee J, Manetta A, Emma D, Ramsanghani NS, et al. Bulky stage IB cervical carcinoma

managed by primary radical hysterectomy followed by tailored radiotherapy. *Gynecol Oncol* 1992;47:21–27.

154. **Boronow RC.** The bulky 6cm barrel-shaped lesion of the cervix: primary surgery and postoperative chemoradiation. *Gynecol Oncol* 2000;78:313–317.

155. **Rutledge TL, Kamelle S, Tillmanns TD, Cohn DE, Wright JD, Radar JS, et al.** A comparison of stage IB1 vs IB2 cervical cancers treated with radical hysterectomy: is size the real difference? *Gynecol Oncol* 2002;84:522(abst).

156. **Havrilesky LJ, Leath CA, Huh W, Calingaert B, Bentley RC, Soper JT, et al.** Radical hysterectomy and pelvic lymphadenectomy for stage IB2 cervical cancer. *Gynecol Oncol* 2004;93:429–434.

157. **Yessaian A, Magistris A, Burger RA, Monk BJ.** Radical hysterectomy followed by tailored postoperative therapy in the treatment of stage IB2 cervical cancer: feasibility and indications for adjuvant therapy. *Gynecol Oncol* 2004;94:61–66.

158. **Rocconi RP, Estes JM, Leath CA 3rd, Kilgore LC, Huh WK, Straughn JM Jr.** Management strategies for stage IB2 cervical cancer: a cost effectiveness analysis. *Gynecol Oncol* 2005;97:387–394.

159. **Langley I, Moore DW, Tarnasky J, Roberts P.** Radical hysterectomy and pelvic node dissection. *Gynecol Oncol* 1980;9:37–42.

160. **Benedet JL, Turko M, Boyes DA, Nickerson KG, Bienkowska BT.** Radical hysterectomy in the treatment of cervical cancer. *Am J Obstet Gynecol* 1980;137:254–260.

161. **Kenter GG, Ansink AG, Heintz APM, Aartsen EJ, Delamarre JF, Hart AA.** Carcinoma of the uterine cervix stage IB and IIA: results of surgical treatment: complications, recurrence and survival. *Eur J Surg Oncol* 1989;15:55–60.

162. **Lee Y-N, Wang KL, Lin CH, Liu C-H, Wang K-G, Lan CC, et al.** Radical hysterectomy with pelvic lymph node dissection for treatment of cervical cancer: a clinical review of 954 cases. *Gynecol Oncol* 1989;32:135–142.

163. **Monaghan JM, Ireland D, Shlomo MY, Pearson SE, Lopes A, Sinha DP.** Role of centralization of surgery in stage IB carcinoma of the cervix: a review of 498 cases. *Gynecol Oncol* 1990;37:206–209.

164. **Ayhan A, Tuncer ZS.** Radical hysterectomy with lymphadenectomy for treatment of early stage cervical cancer: clinical experience of 278 cases. *J Surg Oncol* 1991;47:175–177.

165. **Averette HE, Nguyen HN, Donato DM, Penalver MA, Sevin B-U, Estape R, et al.** Radical hysterectomy for invasive cervical cancer: a 25-year prospective experience with the Miami technique. *Cancer* 1993;71:1422–1437.

166. **Kim SM, Choi HS, Byun JS.** Overall 5-year survival rate and prognostic factors in patients with stage IB and IIA cervical cancer treated by radical hysterectomy and pelvic lymph node dissection. *Int J Gynecol Cancer* 2000;10:305–312.

167. **Noguchi H, Shiozawa I, Sakai Y, Yamazaki T, Fukuta T.** Pelvic lymph node metastases in uterine cervical cancer. *Gynecol Oncol* 1987;27:150–155.

168. **Inoue T, Morita K.** The prognostic significance of number of positive nodes in cervical carcinoma stage IB, IIA, and IIB. *Cancer* 1990;65:1923–1928.

169. **Tsai C-S, Lai C-H, Wang C-C, Chang JT, Chang T-C, Tseng C-J, et al.** The prognostic factors for patients with early cervical cancer treated by radical hysterectomy and postoperative radiotherapy. *Gynecol Oncol* 1999;75:328–333.

170. **Delgado G, Bundy B, Zaino R, Sevin B-U, Creasman WT, Major F.** Prospective surgical-pathological study of disease-free interval in patients with stage IB squamous cell carcinoma of the cervix: a Gynecologic Oncology Group study. *Gynecol Oncol* 1990;38:352–357.

171. **Rubin SC, Brookland R, Mikuta JJ, Mangan C, Sutton G, Danoff B.** Paraaortic nodal metastases in early cervical carcinoma: long term survival following extended field radiotherapy. *Gynecol Oncol* 1984;18:213–217.

172. **Roman LD, Felix JC, Muderspach LI, Varkey T, Burnett AF, Qian D, et al.** Influence of quantity of lymph-vascular space invasion on the risk of nodal metastases in women with early-stage squamous cancer of the cervix. *Gynecol Oncol* 1998;68:220–225.

173. **Chernofsky MR, Felix JC, Muderspach LI, Morrow CP, Ye W, Groshen SG, et al.** Influence of quantity of lymph vascular space invasion on time to recurrence in women with early-stage squamous cancer of the cervix. *Gynecol Oncol* 2006;100:288–293.

174. **Burghardt E, Baltzer J, Tulusan AH, Haas J.** Results of surgical treatment of 1028 cervical cancers studied with volumetry. *Cancer* 1992;70:648–655.

175. **Zreik TG, Chambers JT, Chambers SK.** Parametrial involvement, regardless of nodal status: a poor prognostic factor for cervical cancer. *Obstet Gynecol* 1996;87:741–746.

176. **Uno T, Ho H, Isobe K, Kaneyasu Y, Tanaka N, Mitsuhashi A et al.** Post operative pelvic radiotherapy for cervical cancer patients with positive parametrial invasion. *Gynecol Oncol* 2005;96:335–340.

177. **van Nagell JR Jr, Powell DE, Gallion HH, Elliott DG, Donaldson ES, Carpenter AE, et al.** Small cell carcinoma of the uterine cervix. *Cancer* 1988;62:1586–1593.

178. **Eifel PJ, Burke TW, Morris M, Smith TL.** Adenocarcinoma as an independent risk factor for disease recurrence in patients with stage IB cervical cancer. *Gynecol Oncol* 1995;59:38–44.

179. **Samlal RAK, van der Velden J, Ten Kate FJW, Schilthuis MS, Hart AAM, Lammes FB.** Surgical pathologic factors that predict recurrence in stage IB and IIA cervical carcinoma patients with negative pelvic lymph nodes. *Cancer* 1997;80:1234–1240.

180. **Shingleton HM, Bell MC, Fremgen A, Chmiel JS, Russell AH, Jones WB, et al.** Is there really a difference in survival of women with squamous cell carcinoma, adenocarcinoma and adenosquamous cell carcinoma of the cervix? *Cancer* 1995;76:1948–1955.

181. **Adcock LL, Potish RA, Julian TM, Ogagaki T, Prem KA, Twiggs LB, et al.** Carcinoma of the cervix, FIGO stage IB: treatment failures. *Gynecol Oncol* 1984;18:218–225.

182. **Gallup DG, Harper RH, Stock RJ.** Poor prognosis in patients with adenosquamous cell carcinoma of the cervix. *Obstet Gynecol* 1985;65:416–422.

183. **Yazigi R, Sandstad J, Munoz AK, Choi DJ, Nguyen PD, Risser R.** Adenosquamous carcinoma of the cervix: prognosis in stage IB. *Obstet Gynecol* 1990;75:1012–1015.

184. **Dos Reis R, Frumovitz M, Milam MR, Capp E, Sun CC, Coleman RL, Ramirez PT.** Adenosquamous carcinoma versus adenocarcinoma in early-stage cervical cancer patients undergoing radical hysterectomy: an outcome analysis. *Gynecol Oncol* 2007;107:458–463.

185. **Farley JH, Hickey KW, Carlson JW, Rose GS, Kost ER, Harrison TA.** Adenosquamous histology predicts a poor outcome for patients with advanced-stage, but not early-stage cervical carcinoma. *Cancer* 2003;97:2196–2202.

186. **Duk JM, Groenier KH, de Bruijn HWA, Hollema H, ten Hoor KA, van der Zee AGJ, et al.** Pretreatment serum squamous cell carcinoma antigen: a newly identified prognostic factor in early stage cervical carcinoma. *J Clin Oncol* 1996;14:111–118.

187. **Ogino I, Nakayama H, Kitamura T, Okamotos N, Inoue T.** The curative role of radiotherapy in patiets with isolated paraaortic node recurrence from cervical cancer and the value of squamous cell carcinoma antigen for early detection. *Int J Gynecol Cancer* 2005;15:630–638.

188. **Rose BR, Thompson CH, Simpson JM, Jarrett CS, Elliott PM, Tattersall MHN, et al.** Human papillomavirus deoxyribonucleic acid as a prognostic indicator in early stage cervical cancer: a possible role for type 18. *Am J Obstet Gynecol* 1995;173:1461–1468.

189. **Lombard I, Vincent-Salomon A, Validire P, Zafrani B, de la Rochefordiere A, Clough K, et al.** Human papilloma genotype as a major determinant of the course of cervical cancer. *J Clin Oncol* 1998;16:2613–2619.

190. **Walker J, Bloss JD, Liao S-Y, Berman M, Bergen S, Wilczynski SP.** Human papilloma genotype as a prognostic indicator in carcinoma of the uterine cervix. *Obstet Gynecol* 1989;74:781–785.

191. **Obermair A, Warner C, Bilgi S, Speiser P, Kaider A, Reinthaller A, et al.** Tumor angiogenesis in stage IB cervical cancer: correlation of microvessel density with survival. *Am J Obstet Gynecol* 1998;178:314–319.

192. **Peters WA 3rd, Liu PY, Barrett RJ, Gordon W Jr, Stock R, Berek JS, et al.** *Cisplatin* and 5-FU plus radiation therapy are superior to radiation therapy as adjunctive in high- risk early-stage carcinoma of the cervix after radical hysterectomy and pelvic lymphadenectomy: report of a phase III intergroup study. *J Clin Oncol* 2000;18:1606–1613.

193. **Monk BJ, Wang J, Im S, Stock RJ, Peters WA III, Liu PY et al.** Rethinking the use of radiation and chemotherapy after radical hysterectomy: a clinical-pathologic analysis of a Gynecologic

Oncology Group/Southwest Oncology Group/Radiation Therapy Oncology Group trial. *Gynecol Oncol* 2005;96:721–728.

194. **Thomas GM, Dembo AJ.** Is there a role for adjuvant pelvic radiotherapy after radical hysterectomy in early stage cervical cancer? *Int J Gynecol Cancer* 1991;1:1–8.

195. **Sedlis A, Bundy BN, Rotman M, Lentz S, Muderspach LI, Zaino R.** A randomized trial of pelvic radiation therapy versus no further therapy in selected patients with stage IB carcinoma of the cervix after radical hysterectomy and pelvic lymphadenectomy: a Gynecologic Oncology Group study. *Gynecol Oncol* 1999;73: 177–183.

196. **Rotman M, Sedlis A, Piedmonte MR, Bundy B, Lentz SS, Muderspach LI, et al.** A phase III randomized trial of postoperative pelvic irradiation in stage IB cervical carcinoma with poor prognostic features: follow-up of a Gynecologic Oncology Group study. *Int J Radiat Oncol Biol Phys* 2006;65:169–176.

197. **Pieterse QD, Trimbos JBMZ, Dijkman A, Creutzberg CL, Gaarenstroom KN, Peters AAW, Kenter GG et al.** Postoperative radiation therapy improves prognosis in patients with adverse risk factors in localized, early-stage cervical cancer: a retrospective comparative study. *Int J Gynecol Cancer* 2006;16:1112–1118.

198. **Kridelka FJ, Berg DO, Neuman M, Edwards LS, Robertson G, Grant PT, et al.** Adjuvant small field pelvic radiation for patients with high-risk stage IB node negative cervical cancer after radical hysterectomy and pelvic lymph node dissection: a pilot study. *Cancer* 1999;86:2059–2065.

199. **Ohara K, Tsunoda H, Nishida M, Sugahara S, Hashimoto T, Shioyama Y, et al.** Use of small pelvic field instead of whole pelvic field in postoperative radiotherapy for node-negative, high-risk stage I and II cervical squamous carcinoma. *Int J Gynecol Cancer* 2003;13: 170–176.

200. **Ohara K, Tsunoda H, Satoh T, Oki A, Sugahara S, Yoshikawa H.** Use of the small pelvic field instead of the classic whole pelvic field in postoperative radiotherapy for cervical cancer: reduction of adverse events. *Int J Radiat Oncol Biol Phys* 2004;60:258–264.

201. **Takeshima N, Umayahara K, Fujiwara K, Hirai Y, Takizawa K, Hasumi K.** Treatment results of adjuvant chemotherapy after radical hysterectomy for intermediate and high-risk stage IB – IIA cervical cancer. *Gynecol Oncol* 2006;103:618–622.

202. **Thomas G, Dembo A, Ackerman I, Franssen E, Balogh J, Fyles A, et al.** A randomized trial of standard versus partially hyperfractionated radiation with or without concurrent *5-fluorouracil* in locally advanced cervical cancer. *Gynecol Oncol* 1998;69:137–145.

203. **Tierney JF, Stewart LA.** Neoadjuvant chemotherapy followed by radiotherapy for locally advanced cervix cancer: a metaanalysis using individual patient data from randomized controlled trials. *Int J Gynecol Cancer* 2002;12:576(abst).

204. **Stehman FB, Bundy BN, Thomas G, Keys HM, d'Ablaing G 3rd, Fowler WC Jr, et al.** *Hydroxyurea* versus *misonidazole* with radiation in cervical carcinoma: long term follow-up of a Gynecologic Oncology Group trial. *J Clin Oncol* 1993;11:1523–1528.

205. **Rose PG, Ali S, Watkins E, Thigpen JT, Deppe G, Clarke-Pearson DL, et al.** Long term follow-up of a randomized trial comparing concurrent single agent *cisplatin* or *cisplatin*-based combination chemotherapy for locally advanced cervical cancer: a Gynecologic Oncology Group Study. *J Clin Oncol* 2007;25:1–7.

206. **Morris M, Eifel PJ, Lu J, Grigsby PW, Levenback C, Stevens RE, et al.** Pelvic radiation with concurrent chemotherapy compared with pelvic and paraaortic radiation for high-risk cervical cancer. *N Engl J Med* 1999;340:1137–1143.

207. **Whitney CW, Sause W, Bundy BN, Malfetano JH, Hannigan EV, Fowler WC Jr, et al.** Randomized comparison of *fluorouracil* plus *cisplatin* vs *hydroxyurea* as an adjunct to radiation therapy in stage IIB–IVA carcinoma of the cervix with negative paraaortic nodes: a Gynecologic Oncology Group and Southwest Oncology Group study. *J Clin Oncol* 1999;17:1339–1348.

208. **Trimble EL, Harlan LC, Gius D, Stevens J, Schwartz SM.** Patterns of care for women with cervical cancer in the United States. *Cancer* 2008;113:743–749.

209. **Torres MA, Jhingran A, Thames HD, Levenback CF, Bodurka DC, Ramondetta LM, et al.** Comparison of treatment tolerance and outcomes in patients with cervical cancer treated with concurrent chemoradiotherapy in a prospective randomized trial or with standard treatment. *Int J Radiat Oncol Biol Phys* 2008;70:118–125.

210. **Clifford KS, Leung W, Grigsby PW, Mutch MD, Herzog T, Perez CA.** The clinical implications of hydronephrosis and the level of ureteral obstruction in stage IIIB cervical cancer. *Int J Radiat Oncol Biol Phys* 1998;40:1095–1100.

211. **Horan G, McArdle O, Martin J, Collins CD, Faul C.** Pelvic radiotherapy in patients with hydronephrosis in stage IIIB cancer of the cervix: renal effects and the optimnal timing of urinary diversion. *Gynecol Oncol* 2006;101:441–444.

212. **Piver MS, Barlow JJ, Krishnamsetty R.** Five-year survival (with no evidence of disease) in patients with biopsy confirmed aortic node metastases from cervical carcinoma. *Am J Obstet Gynecol* 1981; 139:575–580.

213. **Tewfik HH, Buchsbaum HJ, Lafourette HB.** Paraaortic lymph node irradiation in carcinoma of the cervix after exploratory laparotomy and biopsy-proven positive aortic nodes. *Int J Radiat Oncol Biol Phys* 1982;8:13–18.

214. **Vigliotti AP, Wen B-C, Hussey DH, Doornbos JF, Staples JJ, Jani SK, et al.** Extended field irradiation for carcinoma of the uterine cervix with positive periaortic nodes. *Int J Radiat Oncol Biol Phys* 1992;23:501–509.

215. **Boronow RC.** Should whole pelvic radiation therapy become past history? A case for the routine use of extended field therapy and multimodality therapy. *Gynecol Oncol* 1991;43:71–76.

216. **Rotman M, Choi K, Guze C, Marcial V, Hornback N, John M.** Prophylactic irradiation of the paraaortic lymph node chain in stage IIB and bulky stage IB carcinoma of the cervix: initial treatment results of RTOG 7920. *Int J Radiat Oncol Biol Phys* 1990; 19:513–521.

217. **Varia MA, Bundy BN, Deppe G, Mannel R, Averette HE, Rose PG.** Cervical carcinoma metastatic to paraaortic nodes: extended field radiation therapy with concomitant *5-fluorouracil* and *cisplatin* chemotherapy. A Gynecologic Oncology Group study. *Int J Radiat Oncol Biol Phys* 1998;4:1015–1023.

218. **Beriwal S, Gan GN, Heron DE, Selvaraj RN, Kim H, Lalonde R et al.** Early clinical outcome with concurrent chemotherapy and extended-field, intensity-modulated radiotherapy for cervical cancer. *Int J Radiat Oncol Biol Phys* 2007;68:166–171.

219. **Duyn A, van Eijkeran M, Kenter G, Zwinderman K, Ansink A.** Recurrent cervical cancer: detection and prognosis. *Acta Obstet Gynecol Scand* 2002;81:759–763.

220. **Chen N-J, Okuda H, Sekiba K.** Recurrent carcinoma of the vagina following Okabayashi's radical hysterectomy for cervical cancer. *Gynecol Oncol* 1985;20:10–16.

221. **Havrilesky LJ, Wong TZ, Secord AA, Berchuck A, Clarke-Pearson DL, Jones EL.** The role of PET scanning in the detection of recurrent cervical cancer. *Gynecol Oncol* 2003;90:186–190.

222. **Chung HH, Kim S-K, Kim TH, Lee S, Kang KW, Kim J-Y, et al.** Clinical impact of FDG-PET imaging in post-therapy surveillance of uterine cervical cancer: from diagnosis to prognosis. *Gynecol Oncol* 2006;103:165–170.

223. **Sakurai H, Suzuki Y, Nonaka T, Ishikawa H, Shioya M, Kiyohara H et al.** FDG-PET in the detectiuon of recurrence of uterine cervical carcinoma following radiation therapy – tumor volume and FDG uptake value. *Gynecol Oncol* 2006;100:601–607.

224. **Smith HO, Tiffany MF, Qualls CR, Key CR.** The rising incidence of adenocarcinoma relative to squamous cell carcinoma of the uterine cervix in the United States: a 24 year population-based study. *Gynecol Oncol* 2000;78:97–105.

225. **Bray F, Carstensen B, Møller H, Zappa M, Zakelj MP, Lawrence G et al.** Incidence trends of adenocarcinoma of the cervix in 13 European countries. *Cancer Epidemiol Biomarkers Prev* 2005;14: 2191–2199.

226. **Ursin G, Peters RK, Henderson BE, D'Ablaing G, Munroe KR, Pile MC.** Oral contraceptive use and adenocarcinoma of the cervix. *Lancet* 1994;344:1390–1394.

227. **Sasieni P, Adams J.** Changing rates of adenocarcinoma and adenosquamous carcinoma of the cervix in England. *Lancet* 2001;357: 1490–1493.

228. **Duggan MA, McGregor SE, Benoit JL, Inoue M, Natcon JG, Stuart GCE.** The human papilloma virus status of invasive cervical adenocarcinoma: a clinico-pathological and outcome analysis. *Hum Pathol* 1995;26:319–325.

229. **Harper DM, Franco EL, Wheeler C, Ferris DG, Jenkins D, Schuind A, et al.** Efficacy of a bivalent *L1* virus-like particle vaccine

in prevention of infection with human papilloma virus types 16 and 18 in young women: a randomized controlled trial. *Lancet* 2004;364:1757–1765.

230. **Mitchell H, Hocking J, Saville M.** Improvement in protection against adenocarcinoma of the cervix resulting from participation in cervical screening. *Cancer* 2003;99:336–341.

231. **Duk JM, De Bruijn HWA, Groenier KH, Fleuren GJ, Aalders JG.** Adenocarcinoma of the cervix. *Cancer* 1990;65:1830–1837.

232. **Nakanishi T, Ishikawa H, Suzuki Y, Inoue T, Nakamura S, Kuzuya K.** A comparison of prognoses of pathologic stage IB adenocarcinoma and squamous cell carcinoma of the uterine cervix. *Gynecol Oncol* 2000;79:289–293.

233. **Helm CW, Kinney WK, Keeney G, Lawrence WD, Frank TS, Gore H, et al.** A matched study of surgically treated stage IIB adenosquamous carcinoma and adenocarcinoma of the uterine cervix. *Int J Gynecol Cancer* 1993;3:245–249.

234. **Glucksman A, Cherry C.** Incidence, histology and response to radiation of mixed carcinomas (adenoacanthomas) of the uterine cervix. *Cancer* 1956;9:976–983.

235. **Maier RC, Norris HJ.** Glassy cell carcinoma of the cervix. *Obstet Gynecol* 1982;60:219–226.

236. **Tamimi HK, Ek M, Hesla J, Cain JM, Figge DC, Greer BE.** Glassy cell carcinoma of the cervix redefined. *Obstet Gynecol* 1988;71:837–841.

237. **Gray HJ, Garcia R, Tamimi HK, Koh W-J, Goff BA, Greer BE, et al.** Glassy cell carcinoma of the cervix revisited. *Gynecol Oncol* 2002;85:274–277.

238. **McKelvey JL, Goodlin RR.** Adenoma malignum of the cervix: a cancer of deceptively innocent histological pattern. *Cancer* 1963;16: 549–557.

239. **Silverberg SG, Hurt WG.** Minimal deviation adenocarcinoma ("adenoma malignum") of the cervix: a reappraisal. *Am J Obstet Gynecol* 1975;121:971–975.

240. **McGowan L, Young RH, Scully RE.** Peutz-Jeghers syndrome with "adenoma malignum" of the cervix: a report of two cases. *Gynecol Oncol* 1980;10:125–133.

241. **Hart WR.** Special types of adenocarcinomas of the uterine cervix. *Int J Gynecol Pathol* 2002;21:327–346.

242. **Hirai Y, Takeshima N, Haga A, Arai Y, Akiyama F, Hasumi K.** A clinicocytopathologic study of adenoma malignum of the cervix. *Gynecol Oncol* 1998;70:219–223.

243. **Gilks CB, Young RH, Aguirre P, De Lellis RA, Scully RE.** Adenoma malignum (minimal deviation adenocarcinoma) of the uterine cervix: a clinicopathological and immunohistochemical analysis of 26 cases. *Am J Surg Pathol* 1989;13:717–729.

244. **Musa AG, Hughes RR, Coleman SA.** Adenoid cystic carcinoma of the cervix: a report of 17 cases. *Gynecol Oncol* 1985;22:167–173.

245. **Berchuck A, Mullin TJ.** Cervical adenoid cystic carcinoma associated with ascites. *Gynecol Oncol* 1985;22:201–211.

246. **Prempree T, Villasanta U, Tang C-K.** Management of adenoid cystic carcinoma of the uterine cervix (cylindroma). *Cancer* 1980;46: 1631–1635.

247. **Ferry JA, Scully RE.** "Adenoid cystic" carcinoma and adenoid basal carcinoma of the uterine cervix: a study of 28 cases. *Am J Surg Pathol* 1988;12:134–140.

248. **Brainard JA, Hart WR.** Adenoid basal epithelioma of the uterine cervix. *Am J Surg Pathol* 1998;22:965–972.

249. **Herbst AL, Kurman RJ, Scully RE, Poskanzer DC.** Clear cell adenocarcinoma of the genital tract in young females. *N Engl J Med* 1972;287:1259–1264.

250. **Kaminski PF, Maier RC.** Clear cell adenocarcinoma of the cervix unrelated to *diethylstilbestrol* exposure. *Obstet Gynecol* 1983;62: 720–727.

251. **Reich O, Tamussino K, Lauhousen M, Pickel H, Haas J, Winter R.** Clear cell carcinoma of the uterine cervix: pathology and prognosis in surgically treated stage IB–IIB disease in women not exposed to *in utero diethylstilbestrol*. *Gynecol Oncol* 2000;76:331–335.

252. **Young RH, Scully RE.** Villoglandular papillary adenocarcinoma of the uterine cervix. *Cancer* 1989;63:1773–1779.

253. **Jones MW, Silverberg SG, Kurman RJ.** Well differentiated villoglandular adenocarcinoma of the uterine cervix: a clinicopathologic study of 24 cases. *Int J Gynecol Pathol* 1993;12:1–7.

254. **Kaku T, Kamura T, Shigematsu T, Sakai K, Nakanami W, Vehira K, et al.** Adenocarcinoma of the uterine cervix with predom-

inantly villoglandular papillary growth pattern. *Gynecol Oncol* 1997;64:147–152.

255. **Scully RE, Aguirre P, De Lellis RA.** Argyrophilia, serotonin, and peptide hormones in the female genital tract and its tumors. *Int J Gynecol Pathol* 1984;3:51–70.

256. **McCusker ME, Cote TR, Clegg LX, Tavassoli FJ.** Endocrine tumors of the uterine cervix: incidence, demographics, and survival with comparison to squamous cell carcinoma. *Gynecol Oncol* 2003; 88:333–339.

257. **Chen J, Macdonald K, Gaffey DK.** Incidence, mortality, and prognostic factors of small cell carcinoma of the cervix. *Obstet Gynecol* 2008;111:1394–1402.

258. **Chang T-C, Lai C-H, Tseng C-J, Hsueh S, Huang K-G, Chou H-H.** Prognostic factors in surgically treated small cell cervical carcinoma followed by adjuvant chemotherapy. *Cancer* 1998;83:712–718.

259. **Bermudez A, Vighi S, Garcia A, Sardi J.** Neuroendocrine cervical carcinoma: a diagnostic and therapeutic challenge. *Gynecol Oncol* 2001;82:32–39.

260. **Zhou C, Gilks CB, Hayes M, Clement PB.** Papillary serous carcinoma of the uterine cervix: a clinicopathologic study of 17 cases. *Am J Surg Path* 1998;22:113–120.

261. **Rotmensch J, Rosenshein NB, Woodruff JD.** Cervical sarcoma: a review. *Obstet Gynecol Surv* 1983;38:456–460.

262. **Daya DA, Scully RE.** Sarcoma botryoides of the uterine cervix in young women: a clinicopathological study of 13 cases. *Gynecol Oncol* 1988;29:290–304.

263. **Arndt CA, Donaldson SS, Anderson JR, Andrassy RJ, Laurie F, Link MP et al.** What constitutes optimal therapy for patients with rhabdomyosarcoma of the female genital tract? *Cancer* 2001;91: 2454–2468.

264. **Brand E, Berek JS, Nieberg RK, Hacker NF.** Rhabdomyosarcoma of the uterine cervix: sarcoma botryoides. *Cancer* 1987;60:1552–1560.

265. **Sharma NK, Sorosky JI, Bender D, Fletcher MS, Sood AK.** Malignant mixed müllerian tumor (MMMT) of the cervix. *Gynecol Oncol* 2005;97:442–445.

266. **Chorlton I, Karnei RF, King FM, Norris HJ.** Primary malignant reticuloendothelial disease involving the vagina, cervix and corpus uteri. *Obstet Gynecol* 1974;44:735–748.

267. **Harris NL, Scully RE.** Malignant lymphoma and granulocytic sarcoma of the uterus and vagina. *Cancer* 1984;52:2530–2545.

268. **Komaki R, Cox JD, Hansen RM, Gunn WG, Greenberg M.** Malignant lymphoma of the uterine cervix. *Cancer* 1984;54: 1699–1704.

269. **Perrin T, Farrant M, McCarthy K, Harper P, Wiltshaw E.** Lymphomas of the cervix and upper vagina: a report of five cases and a review of the literature. *Gynecol Oncol* 1992;44:87–95.

270. **Jennings RH, Barclay DL.** Verrucous carcinoma of the cervix. *Cancer* 1972;30:430–433.

271. **Crowther ME, Lowe DG, Shepherd JH.** Verrucous carcinoma of the female genital tract: a review. *Obstet Gynecol Surv* 1988;45: 263–280.

272. **Schwade JG, Wara WM, Dedo HH, Phillips TL.** Radiotherapy for verrucous carcinoma. *Radiology* 1976;120:677–683.

273. **Mordel N, Mor-Yosef S, Ben-Baruch N, Anteby SO.** Malignant melanoma of the uterine cervix: case report and review of the literature. *Gynecol Oncol* 1989;32:375–380.

274. **Santosa JT, Kucora PR, Ray J.** Primary malignant melanoma of the uterine cervix: two case reports and a century's review. *Obstet Gynecol Surv* 1990;45:733–744.

275. **Lemoine NR, Hall PA.** Epithelial tumors metastatic to the uterine cervix. *Cancer* 1986;57:2002–2005.

276. **Miller BE, Copeland LJ, Hamberger AD, Gershenson DM, Saul PB, Herson J, et al.** Carcinoma of the cervical stump. *Gynecol Oncol* 1984;18:100–108.

277. **Kinney WK, Egorshin EV, Ballard DJ, Podratz KC.** Long-term survival and sequelae after surgical management of invasive cervical carcinoma diagnosed at the time of simple hysterectomy. *Gynecol Oncol* 1992;44:24–27.

278. **Chapman JA, Mannel RS, Di Saia PJ, Walker JL, Di Saia ML.** Surgical treatment of unexpected invasive cervical cancer found at total hysterectomy. *Obstet Gynecol* 1992;80:931–934.

279. **Hopkins MP, Peters WA III, Andersen W, Morley GW.** Invasive cervical cancer treated initially by standard hysterectomy. *Gynecol Oncol* 1990;36:7–12.

280. **Choi DH, Huh SJ, Nam KH.** Radiation therapy results for patients undergoing inappropriate surgery in the presence of invasive cervical carcinoma. *Gynecol Oncol* 1997;65:506–511.

281. **Saibishkumar EP, Patel FD, Ghoshal S, Kumar V, Karunanidhi G, Sharma SC.** Results of salvage radiotherapy after inadequate surgery in invasive cervical carcinoma patients: a retrospective analysis. *Int J Radiat Oncol Biol Phys* 2005;63:828–833.

282. **Pisco JM, Martins JM, Correia MG.** Internal iliac artery embolization to control hemorrhage from pelvic neoplasms. *Radiology* 1989;172:337–343.

283. **Eifel PJ, Jhingran A, Brown J, Levenbach C, Thames H.** Time course and outcome of central recurrence after radiation therapy for carcinoma of the cervix. *Int J Gynecol Cancer* 2006;16:1106–1111.

284. **Grigsby PW.** Radiotherapy for pelvic recurrence after radical hysterectomy for cervical cancer. *Radiation Med* 2005;23:327–330.

285. **Thomas GM, Dembo AJ, Black B, Bean HA, Beale FA, Pringle JR.** Concurrent radiation and chemotherapy for carcinoma of the cervix recurrent after radical surgery. *Gynecol Oncol* 1987;27:254–260.

286. **Shiromizu K, Kasamatsu T, Takahashi M, Kikuchi A, Yoshinari T, Matsuzawa M.** A clinicopathological study of postoperative pulmonary metastases of uterine cervical carcinomas. *J Obstet Gynaecol Res* 1999;25:245–249.

287. **Rutledge S, Carey MS, Pritchard H, Allen HH, Kocha W, Kirk ME.** Conservative surgery for recurrent or persistent carcinoma of the cervix following irradiation: is exenteration always necessary? *Gynecol Oncol* 1994;52:353–359.

288. **Maneo A, Landoni F, Cormio G, Colombo A, Mangioni C.** Radical hysterectomy for recurrent or persistent cervical cancer following radiation therapy. *Int J Gynecol Cancer* 1999;9:295–301.

289. **Long HJ 3rd.** Management of metastatic cervical cancer: review of the literature. *J Clin Oncol* 2007 Jul 10;25:2966–2974. Review.

290. **Hogg R, Friedlander M.** Role of systemic chemotherapy in metastatic cervical cancer. *Expert Rev Anticancer Ther* 2003 Apr;3:234–240. Review.

291. **Vermorken JB.** The role of chemotherapy in squamous cell carcinoma of the uterine cervix: a review. *Int J Gynecol Cancer* 1993;3: 129–142.

292. **Cadron I, Van Gorp T, Amant F, Leunen K, Neven P, Vergote I.** Chemotherapy for recurrent cervical cancer. *Gynecol Oncol* 2007 Oct;107(1 Suppl 1):S113–118.

293. **Hirte HW, Strychowsky JE, Oliver T, Fung-Kee-Fung M, Elit L, Oza AM.** Chemotherapy for recurrent, metastatic, or persistent cervical cancer: a systematic review. *Int J Gynecol Cancer* 2007;17: 1194–1204.

294. **Bonomi P, Blessing JA, Stehman FB, Di Saia PJ, Walton L, Major FJ.** Randomized trial of three *cisplatin* dose schedules in squamous cell carcinoma of the cervix: a Gynecologic Oncology Group study. *J Clin Oncol* 1985;3:1079–1085.

295. **Khoury-Collado F, Bowes RJ, Jhamb N, Aghajanian C, Abu-Rustum NR.** Unexpected long-term survival without evidence of disease after salvage chemotherapy for recurrent metastatic cervical cancer: a case series. *Gynecol Oncol* 2007;105:823–825.

296. **Buxton EJ, Meanwell CA, Hilton C, Mould JJ, Spooner D, Chetiyawardana A, et al.** Combination *bleomycin, ifosfamide,* and *cisplatin* chemotherapy in cervical cancer. *J Natl Cancer Inst* 1989;81:359–361.

297. **Bloss JD, Blessing JA, Behrens BC, Mannel RS, Rader JS, Sood AK, et al.** Randomized trial of *cisplatin* and *ifosfamide* with or without *bleomycin* in squamous carcinoma of the cervix: a gynecologic oncology group study. *J Clin Oncol* 2002;20:1832–1837.

298. **Rose PG, Blessing JA, Gershensen DM, McGehee R.** *Paclitaxel* and *cisplatin* as first-line therapy in recurrent or advanced squamous cell carcinoma of the cervix: a Gynecologic Oncology Group study. *J Clin Oncol* 1999;17:2676–2680.

299. **Lorvidhaya V, Kamnerdsupaphon P, Chitapanarux I, Sukthomya V, Tonusin A.** *Cisplatin* and *gemcitabine* in patients with metastatic cervical cancer. *Gan To Kagaku Ryoho* 2004;31: 1057–1062.

300. **Morris M, Blessing JA, Monk BJ, McGehee R, Moore DH.** Phase II study of *cisplatin* and *vinorelbine* in squamous cell carcinoma of the cervix: a gynecologic oncology group study. *J Clin Oncol* 2004;22: 3340–3344.

301. **Fiorica J, Holloway R, Ndubisi B, Orr J, Grendys E, Boothby R, et al.** Phase II trial of *topotecan* and *cisplatin* in persistent or recurrent squamous and nonsquamous carcinomas of the cervix. *Gynecol Oncol* 2002;85:89–94.

302. **Moore DH, Blessing JA, McQuellon RP, Thaler HT, Cella D, Benda J, et al.** Phase III study of *cisplatin* with or without *paclitaxel* in stage IVB, recurrent, or persistent squamous cell carcinoma of the cervix: a gynecologic oncology group study. *J Clin Oncol* 2004;22: 3113–3119.

303. **Sit AS, Kelley JL, Gallion HH, Kunschner AJ, Edwards RP.** *Paclitaxel* and *carboplatin* for recurrent or persistent cancer of the cervix. *Cancer Invest* 2004;22:368–373.

304. **Moore KN, Herzog TJ, Lewin S, Giuntoli RL, Armstrong DK, Rocconi RP, et al.** A comparison of *cisplatin/paclitaxel* and *carboplatin/paclitaxel* in stage IVB, recurrent or persistent cervical cancer. *Gynecol Oncol* 2007;105:299–303.

305. **Long HJ 3rd, Bundy BN, Glendys ED, Benda J, McMeekin S, Sorosky J et al.** Randomized phase III trial of *cisplatin* with or without *topotecan* for carcinoma of the uterine cervix: A Gynecologic Oncology Group study. *J Clin Oncol* 2005;23:4626–4633.

306. **Tiersten AD, Sellack MJ, Hershman DL, Smith D, Resnik EE, Troxel AB, et al.** Phase II study of *topotecan* and *paclitaxel* for recurrent, persistent or metastatic cervical carcinoma. *Gynecol Oncol* 2004;92:635–638.

307. **Bellone S, Frera G, Landolfi G, Romani C, Bandiera E, Tognon G, et al.** Overexpression of epidermal growth factor type-1 receptor (EGF-R1) in cervical cancer: implications for *Cetuximab*-mediated therapy in recurrent/metastatic disease. *Gynecol Oncol* 2007;106: 513–520.

308. **Wright JD, Viviano D, Powell MA, Gibb RK, Mutch DG, Grigsby PW, et al.** *Bevacizumab* combination therapy in heavily pretreated, recurrent cervical cancer. *Gynecol Oncol* 2006;103:489–493.

10 Uterine Cancer

Neville F. Hacker
Michael Friedlander

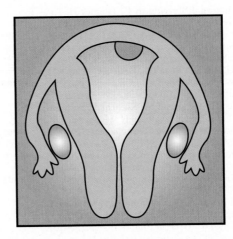

Endometrial carcinoma is the most common malignancy of the female genital tract in the Western world and the fourth most common cancer in women after breast, lung, and colorectum. Developing countries and Japan have incidence rates four to five times lower than Western industrialized nations, with the lowest rates being in India and south Asia (1).

In the United States, it is anticipated there will be 42,160 new cases and 7,780 deaths from the disease in 2009 (2). **Black women have a 40% lower risk of developing the disease but a 54% greater risk of dying from it, mainly because of late diagnosis** (3).

Two different clinicopathological subtypes of endometrial cancer are recognized: the estrogen-related (type I, endometrioid), and the non–estrogen-related (type II, nonendometrioid). Each subtype has specific genetic alterations, with endometrioid tumors showing microsatellite instability and mutations in *PTEN, PIK3CA, K-ras,* and *CTNNBI* (β-*catenin*), although nonendometrioid (predominantly serous and clear cell) tumors exhibit *p53* mutations and chromosomal instability (4).

Approximately 80% of newly diagnosed endometrial carcinomas in the Western world are endometrioid in type (4). **Any factor that increases exposure to unopposed estrogen (e.g., estrogen-replacement therapy, obesity, anovulatory cycles, estrogen-secreting tumors) increases the risk of these tumors, whereas factors that decrease exposure to estrogens or increase progesterone levels (e.g., oral contraceptives or smoking) tend to be protective** (1).

The average age of patients with endometrioid cancer is approximately 63 years, and 70% or so are confined to the corpus at the time of diagnosis. Their 5-year survival is approximately 83% (5). By contrast, the average age of patients with nonendometrioid cancer is 67 years, and at least half have already spread beyond the corpus at the time of diagnosis. Their 5-year survival is approximately 62% for clear cell carcinomas and 53% for papillary serous cancers (5).

Endometrial cancer may occasionally develop after radiation treatment for cervical cancer. In such cases, the majority are diagnosed at an advanced stage of disease and are high-risk histological subtypes. Their prognosis is poor but does not appear to be significantly worse when compared to patients with high-stage, high-grade sporadic cancers (6).

Screening of Asymptomatic Women

The ideal method for outpatient sampling of the endometrium has not yet been devised, and no blood test of sufficient sensitivity and specificity has been developed. Therefore, mass screening of the population is not practical. However, screening for endometrial

Table 10.1 Patients for Whom Screening for Endometrial Cancer Is Justified
1. Postmenopausal women on exogenous estrogens without *progestins*
2. Women from families with hereditary nonpolyposis colorectal cancer syndrome
3. Premenopausal women with anovulatory cycles, such as those with polycystic ovarian disease

carcinoma or its precursors is justified for certain high-risk people, including those shown in Table 10.1.

Only approximately 50% of women with endometrial cancer have malignant cells on a Papanicolaou (Pap) smear (7). However, compared with patients who have normal cervical cytologic findings, patients with suspicious or malignant cells are more likely to have deeper myometrial invasion, higher tumor grade, positive peritoneal cytologic findings, and a more advanced stage of disease (8).

The appearance of normal-appearing endometrial cells in cervical smears taken in the second half of the menstrual cycle or in postmenopausal women is controversial. Montz reported endometrial histology from 93 asymptomatic postmenopausal women receiving hormone-replacement therapy with normal endometrial cells on a Pap smear. Eighteen patients (19%) had abnormalities identified, including seven endometrial polyps, seven cases of simple hyperplasia (one with atypia), three cases of complex hyperplasia (one with atypia), and one endometrial carcinoma (9). A recent Dutch study of 29,144 asymptomatic postmenopausal women reported that **when normal endometrial cells were found in the cervical smear, the prevalence rate of (pre-) malignant uterine disease was significantly higher** (6.5%) as compared to smears without these cells (0.2%), resulting in a relative risk of 40.2 [95% confidence interval (CI) 9.4–172.2] (10). **If morphologically abnormal endometrial cells are present, then approximately 25% of women have endometrial carcinoma** (11).

Guidelines from the Bethesda system recommended that benign endometrial cells (BECs) should be reported in women age 40 and older. Beal et al. reported that BECs were rarely associated with significant endometrial pathology in asymptomatic premenopausal women and that these women may not need further evaluation (12). By contrast, Moroney et al., using liquid-based cytology, reported that 2.1% of asymptomatic premenopausal women with BECs had significant endometrial pathology (13).

The unsatisfactory results obtained with cervical cytology are the result of the indirect sampling of the endometrium, and several commercially available devices have been developed to allow direct sampling (e.g., Pipelle, Gyno Sampler, Vabra aspirator). A satisfactory endometrial biopsy specimen also may be obtained in the office with a small curette such as a Novak or Kevorkian (Fig. 10.1). All of these office techniques for endometrial sampling cause the patient some discomfort, and in approximately 8% of patients it is not possible to obtain a specimen because of a stenotic os. This failure rate increases to approximately 18% for women older than 70 years of age (14).

A metaanalysis reported that the Pipelle was the best device, with detection rates for endometrial cancer in postmenopausal and premenopausal women of 99.6% and 91%, respectively (15). The sensitivity for the detection of endometrial hyperplasia was 81%. The specificity for all devices was 98%.

In the 1990s, transvaginal ultrasonography, with or without color-flow imaging, was investigated as a screening technique. Mean thickness of the endometrial strip was measured as 3.4 ± 1.2 mm in women with atrophic endometrium, 9.7 ± 2.5 mm in women with hyperplasia, and 18.2 ± 6.2 mm in women with endometrial cancer (16). In a large, multiinstutional study of 1,168 women, all 114 women with endometrial cancer and 95% of the 112 women with endometrial hyperplasia had an endometrial thickness of 5 mm or more (17). **A metaanalysis reported that 4% of endometrial cancers would be missed using transvaginal ultrasonography for the investigation of postmenopausal bleeding, with a false positive rate as high as 50%** (18).

Tamoxifen increases the risk of endometrial cancer twofold to threefold (19) and produces a sonographically unique picture of an irregularly echogenic endometrium that is attributed to cystic glandular dilatation, stromal edema, and edema and hyperplasia of the adjacent

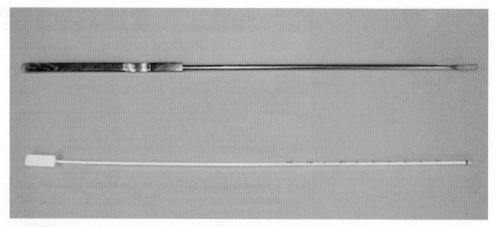

Figure 10.1   Devices used for sampling endometrium. Top, Metal curette, e.g., Kevorkian (pictured); Bottom, Flexible plastic endometrial sampler, e.g., Pipelle (Unimar), Endocell (pictured) (Wallach Surgical Devices, Inc.). From Hillard PJA. Benign Diseases of the Female Reproductive Tract. In: Berek JS, ed. *Berek & Novak's Gynecology.* 14th ed. Philadelphia: Lippincott Williams & Wilkins, 2007.

myometrium (20). Routine ultrasonic surveillance of asymptomatic women on *tamoxifen* is not useful because of its low specificity and positive predictive value. Canadian workers studied 304 women on *tamoxifen* as therapy for breast cancer. Even using an endometrial thickness cutoff of 9 mm, the positive predictive value for the detection of endometrial cancer was only 1.4% (21).

Patients taking *tamoxifen* should be informed of the increased risk of endometrial cancer and told to report any abnormal bleeding or spotting immediately. Any bleeding or spotting must be investigated by biopsy. A retrospective review of *tamoxifen* treated women who underwent dilatation and curettage found that uterine cancer was found only in those with vaginal bleeding (20).

Clinical Features

Symptoms

Endometrial carcinoma should be excluded in all patients shown in Table 10.2. **Ninety percent of patients with endometrial cancer will have abnormal vaginal bleeding**, most commonly postmenopausal bleeding, and the bleeding usually occurs early in the course of the disease. The usual causes of postmenopausal bleeding are shown in Table 10.3. **Intermenstrual bleeding or heavy prolonged bleeding in perimenopausal or anovulatory premenopausal women should arouse suspicion.**

The diagnosis may be delayed unnecessarily in these women because the bleeding is usually ascribed to "hormonal imbalance." A high index of suspicion also is needed to make an early diagnosis in women younger than 40 years of age.

Occasionally, vaginal bleeding does not occur because of cervical stenosis, particularly in thin, elderly, estrogen-deficient patients. In some patients with cervical stenosis, a hematometra develops, and a small percentage have a purulent vaginal discharge resulting from a pyometra.

Table 10.2 Patients in Whom a Diagnosis of Endometrial Cancer Should Be Excluded
1. All patients with postmenopausal bleeding
2. Postmenopausal women with a pyometra
3. Asymptomatic postmenopausal women with endometrial cells on a Papanicolaou smear, particularly if they are atypical
4. Perimenopausal patients with intermenstrual bleeding or increasingly heavy periods
5. Premenopausal patients with abnormal uterine bleeding, particularly if there is a history of anovulation

Table 10.3 Etiology of Postmenopausal Bleeding	
Factor	Approximate Percentage
Exogenous estrogens	30
Atrophic endometritis/vaginitis	30
Endometrial cancer	15
Endometrial or cervical polyps	10
Endometrial hyperplasia	5
Miscellaneous (e.g., cervical cancer, uterine sarcoma, urethral caruncle, trauma)	10

Reproduced from **Hacker NF, Moore JG, Gambone JC eds.** *Essentials of obstetrics and gynecology,* 4th ed. Philadelphia: Elsevier, 2004:479, with permission.

Signs

Physical examination commonly reveals an obese, hypertensive, postmenopausal woman, although approximately one-third of patients are not overweight. Abdominal examination is usually unremarkable except in advanced cases when ascites may be present and hepatic or omental metastases may be palpable. Occasionally, a hematometra appears as a large, smooth midline mass arising from the pelvis.

On pelvic examination, it is important to inspect and palpate the vulva, vagina, and cervix to exclude metastatic spread or other causes of abnormal vaginal bleeding. The uterus may be bulky, but often it is not significantly enlarged. Rectovaginal examination should be performed to evaluate the fallopian tubes, ovaries, and cul-de-sac. Endometrial carcinoma may metastasize to these sites or, alternatively, coexistent ovarian tumors such as a granulosa cell tumor, thecoma, or epithelial ovarian carcinoma may be noted.

Diagnosis

All patients suspected of having endometrial carcinoma should have an endocervical curettage and an office endometrial biopsy. A histologically positive endometrial biopsy allows the planning of definitive treatment.

Because there is a false negative rate of approximately 10%, a negative endometrial biopsy in a symptomatic patient must be followed by a fractional curettage under anesthesia. A diagnosis of endometrial hyperplasia on endometrial biopsy does not obviate the need for further investigation.

Hysteroscopy is often performed in conjunction with curettage and may identify some small bleeding polyps that would otherwise have been missed. There has been speculation that fluid hysteroscopy may facilitate the abdominal dissemination of malignant cells, but there is no evidence that it has any impact on the disease-free survival (22,23).

Fractional Curettage

While the patient is under anesthesia, careful bimanual rectovaginal examination is performed, a weighted speculum is placed in the vagina, and the cervix is grasped with a tenaculum. The endocervical canal is curetted before cervical dilatation, and the tissue placed in a specially labeled container. The uterus then is sounded, the cervix dilated, and the endometrium systematically curetted. The tissue is placed in a separate container so that the histopathologic status of the endocervix and endometrium can be determined separately.

Preoperative Investigations

Routine preoperative investigations for early stage endometrial carcinoma are shown in Table 10.4. If a fractional curettage has not been performed, then an endocervical curettage should be performed to evaluate the endocervix.

Nonroutine tests are sometimes indicated, particularly for more advanced cases or high-risk histologies on curettage. A colonoscopy should be performed if there is occult blood in the stool or a recent change in bowel habits because concomitant colon cancer occasionally occurs, particularly if there is a family history of bowel cancer. A **pelvic and abdominal computed**

Table 10.4 Routine Preoperative Investigations for Early Stage Endometrial Carcinoma
Full blood count
Serum creatinine and electrolytes
Liver function tests
Blood sugar
Urinalysis
CT scan of chest, pelvis, and abdomen, particularly for high-risk histologies

tomographic (CT) scan may be helpful to determine the extent of metastatic disease in the following circumstances:

1. abnormal liver function test results
2. clinical hepatomegaly
3. palpable upper abdominal mass
4. palpable extrauterine pelvic disease
5. clinical ascites
6. grade 3 endometrioid or nonendometrioid carcinomas

However, it has limited usefulness in determining the depth of myometrial invasion or the presence of nodal disease (24,25). **Magnetic resonance imaging (MRI)** was evaluated as a tool for preoperative staging in a National Cancer Institute cooperative study (26). Eighty-eight patients from five participating hospitals were entered in the study. For evaluating the depth of myometrial invasion, the overall accuracy was 66%, but the imaging was considered adequate for the evaluation of paraaortic lymph nodes in only 8% of the cases. Subsequent studies have shown an 83.3% accuracy (100 of 120 cases) for differentiating deep from superficial myometrial invasion (27) and a positive predictive value of 89.8% for the detection of cervical involvement (28). Hence, **MRI may help differentiate between low- and high-risk patients.**

Positron emission tomography (PET) has only recently been evaluated for the preoperative assessment of patients with endometrial cancer. Although its sensitivity for the detection of extrauterine lesions (excluding retroperitoneal nodes) was somewhat superior to CT or MRI (83.3% vs. 66.7%), its utility is limited by its inability to identify lymph nodes less than 1 cm in diameter (29).

Elevated CA125 levels have been demonstrated to correlate with **advanced stage of disease** and positive lymph node status (30).

Staging

In 1988, the Cancer Committee of the International Federation of Gynecology and Obstetrics (FIGO) replaced the old clinical staging system (Table 10.5) **with a surgical staging system for endometrial cancer** (Table 10.6). **For updated FIGO surgical staging tables (2008), see table 10.6A on page 666.** Previously, the disease was staged clinically, based on examination under anesthesia, sounding the uterus, and a limited number pf preoperative investigations. **The change was mainly in response to the Gynecologic Oncology Group (GOG) studies, which demonstrated the high incidence of lymph node metastases in high-risk cases** (31,32).

As increasing experience with the surgical staging of endometrial cancer has been reported, it seems apparent that **there is no need to perform systematic lymphadenectomy in low-risk cases** (grade 1 or 2 endometrioid tumors confined to the inner half of the myometrium) (33). These patients require only removal of palpably suspicious nodes.

For high-risk cases (grade 3, serous or clear cell histologies, stages IC or II disease), a systematic pelvic lymphadenectomy should be performed, with at least removal of any clinically suspicious paraaortic lymph nodes (33).

Spread Patterns

Endometrial carcinoma spreads by the following routes:

1. direct extension to adjacent structures

Table 10.5 1971 FIGO Clinical Staging for Endometrial Carcinoma	
Stage 0	Carcinoma *in situ*
Stage I	The carcinoma is confined to the corpus.
Stage IA	The length of the uterine cavity is 8 cm or less.
Stage IB	The length of the uterine cavity is more than 8 cm.
Stage I cases should be subgrouped with regard to the histologic grade of the adenocarcinoma as follows:	
Grade 1	Highly differentiated adenomatous carcinoma
Grade 2	Moderately differentiated adenomatous carcinoma with partly solid areas
Grade 3	Predominantly solid or entirely undifferentiated carcinoma
Stage II	The carcinoma has involved the corpus and the cervix but has not extended outside the uterus.
Stage III	The carcinoma has extended outside the uterus but not outside the true pelvis.
Stage IV	The carcinoma has extended outside the true pelvis or has obviously involved the mucosa of the bladder or rectum. A bullous edema as such does not permit a case to be allocated to stage IV.
Stage IVA	Spread of the growth to adjacent organs.
Stage IVB	Spread to distant organs.

FIGO, International Federation of Gynecology and Obstetrics.

2. transtubal passage of exfoliated cells
3. lymphatic dissemination
4. hematogenous dissemination

Direct Extension   Direct extension is the most common route of spread, and it results in penetration of the myometrium and eventually the serosa of the uterus. The cervix and fallopian tubes and ultimately the vagina and parametrium may be invaded. Tumors arising in the upper corpus may involve the tube or serosa before involving the cervix, whereas tumors arising from the lower segment of the uterus involve the cervix early. The exact anatomic route by which endometrial cancer involves the cervix has not been clearly defined, but it probably involves a combination of contiguous surface spread, invasion of deep tissue planes, and lymphatic dissemination (34).

Transtubal Dissemination   The presence of malignant cells in peritoneal washings and the development of widespread intraabdominal metastases in some patients with early stage endometrial cancer strongly suggest that cells may be exfoliated from the primary tumor and transported to the peritoneal cavity by retrograde flow along the fallopian tubes.

Lymphatic Dissemination   Lymphatic dissemination is clearly responsible for spread to pelvic and paraaortic lymph nodes. **Although lymphatic channels pass directly from the fundus to the paraaortic nodes through the infundibulopelvic ligament, it is rare to find positive paraaortic nodes in the absence of positive pelvic nodes.** However, it is quite common to find microscopic metastases in both pelvic and paraaortic nodes, suggesting simultaneous spread to pelvic and paraaortic nodes in some patients. This is in contrast to cervical cancer, where paraaortic nodal metastases are always secondary to pelvic nodal metastases.

It seems likely that vaginal metastases also result from lymph-vascular spread. They commonly occur in the absence of cervical involvement, excluding direct spread as the mechanism, and may occur despite preoperative sterilization of the uterus with intracavitary radiation, excluding implantation of cells at the time of surgery as the mechanism (35). In a study of 632 patients with stage I endometrial cancer managed with hysterectomy at the Mayo Clinic between 1984 and 1996, Mariani and colleagues reported that **grade 3 histology and lymphovascular invasion were significant predictors of vaginal relapse,** whereas depth of myometrial invasion was not (36).

Table 10.6 1988 FIGO Surgical Staging for Endometrial Carcinoma	
Stage IA G123	Tumor limited to endometrium
Stage IB G123	Invasion to less than one-half the myometrium
Stage IC G123	Invasion to more than one-half the myometrium
Stage HA G123	Endocervical glandular involvement only
Stage IIB G123	Cervical stromal invasion
Stage IIIA G123	Tumor invades serosa and/or adnexa, and/or positive peritoneal cytology
Stage IIIB G123	Vaginal metastases
Stage IIIC G123	Metastases to pelvic and/or paraaortic lymph nodes
Stage IVA G123	Tumor invasion of bladder and/or bowel mucosa
Stage IVB G123	Distant metastases including intraabdominal and/or inguinal lymph nodes

Histopathology—degree of differentiation:

Cases of carcinoma of the corpus should be classified (or graded) according to the degree of histologic differentiation, as follows:

G_1 = 5% or less of a nonsquamous or nonmorular solid growth pattern

G_2 = 6% to 50% of a nonsquamous or nonmorular solid growth pattern

G_3 = more than 50% of a nonsquamous or nonmorular solid growth pattern

Notes on pathological grading:

1. Notable nuclear atypia, inappropriate for the architectural grade, raises the grade of a grade 1 or a grade 2 tumor by 1.

2. In serous adenocarcinomas, clear cell adenocarcinomas, and squamous cell carcinomas, nuclear grading takes precedence.

3. Adenocarcinomas with squamous differentiation are graded according to the nuclear grade of the glandular component.

Rules related to staging:

1. Because corpus cancer is now staged surgically, procedures previously used for determination of stages are no longer applicable, such as the findings from fractional dilatation and curettage to differentiate between stage I and stage II.

2. It is appreciated that there may be a small number of patients with corpus cancer who will be treated primarily with radiation therapy. If that is the case, the clinical staging adopted by FIGO in 1971 would still apply, but designation of that staging system should be noted.

3. Ideally, width of the myometrium should be measured along with the width of tumor invasion.

For updated Carcinoma of the Endometrium staging table 10.6A on page 666.

FIGO, International Federation of Gynecology and Obstetrics.

Reproduced from **International Federation of Gynecology and Obstetrics.** Annual report on the results of treatment in gynecologic cancer. *Int J Gynecol Obstet* 1989;28:189–190, with permission.

Hematogenous Spread   Hematogenous spread most commonly results in lung metastases, but liver, brain, bone, and other sites are involved less commonly.

Prognostic Variables

Although stage of disease is the most significant prognostic variable, a number of factors have been shown to correlate with outcome in patients with the same stage of disease. These prognostic variables are summarized in Table 10.8. Knowledge of them is essential if appropriate treatment programs are to be devised.

Table 10.7 Carcinoma of the Endometrium: Distribution by Surgical Stage for Patients Treated in 1999 to 2001

Stage	No.	Percent
I	6,260	71.1
II	1,071	12.1
III	1,190	13.5
IV	280	3.3
Total	8,807	100.0

Modified from the **26th Annual Report on the Results of Treatment in Gynecological Cancer** (5).

Age

Age appears to be an independent prognostic variable. The GOG reported 5-year relative survival rates of 96.3% for 28 patients no older than 40 years of age, 87.3% for 261 patients 51 to 60 years, 78% for 312 patients 61 to 70 years, 70.7% for 119 patients 71 to 80 years, and 53.6% for 23 patients older than 80 ($p = 0.001$) (37). All patients had clinical stage I or occult stage II disease. Using proportional hazards modeling of relative survival time, and taking 45 years of age as the arbitrary reference point, the relative risks for death from disease were as follows: 2.0 at 55 years, 3.4 at 65 years, and 4.7 at 75 years of age.

A study of 51,471 patients from the Surveillance, Epidemiology, and End Results (SEER) data base of the National Cancer Institute in the United States demonstrated that patients 40 years and younger had an overall survival advantage compared with women older than 40 years, independent of other clinicopathological prognosticators (38).

Japanese workers have reported menopausal status to be an independent prognostic variable for early endometrial cancer but not for patients with advanced disease (39).

Histologic Type

A retrospective review of 388 patients treated at the Mayo Clinic recorded an uncommon histologic subtype in 52 patients (13%). There were 20 adenosquamous, 14 serous papillary, 11 clear cell, and 7 undifferentiated carcinomas (40). In contrast to the 92% survival rate among patients with endometrioid carcinoma, the overall survival rate for these patients was only 33%. **At the time of surgical staging, 62% of the patients with an unfavorable histologic subtype had extrauterine spread of disease.**

Zaino et al. (41) investigated the prognostic significance of squamous differentiation in 456 patients with typical adenocarcinomas and 175 women with areas of squamous differentiation who had been entered into a GOG clinicopathologic study of stage I and II disease. They reported that the biologic behavior of these tumors reflected the histologic grade and depth of invasion of the glandular component. Although prognostically valuable information was provided by dividing these tumors into adenoacanthomas and adenosquamous carcinomas, more information was gained when they were stratified by the histologic grade of the glandular component. **Zaino et al.** (41) **recommended that the terms** *adenoacanthoma* **and** *adenosquamous carcinoma* **be replaced by the simple term** *adenocarcinoma with squamous differentiation.*

Papillary serous carcinomas have a poor prognosis even in the absence of deep myometrial invasion or lymph node metastasis (4,42–45). They disseminate widely, with a particular predilection for recurrence in the upper abdomen (46,47). The mechanisms that have been proposed to explain the characteristic intraabdominal dissemination of these tumors include transtubal spread, vascular-lymphatic invasion, and multifocal disease. Sherman et al. (42) made the interesting observation that "intraepithelial serous carcinoma" was present in the endocervix in 22% of their cases, in the fallopian tube in 5%, on the surface of the ovary in 10%, and on peritoneal surfaces or omentum in 25%. **Serous papillary elements are often admixed with endometrioid carcinomas, but a serous component of 25% will portend a poor prognosis** (42).

Table 10.8 Prognostic Variables in Endometrial Cancer Other than FIGO Stage
Age
Histologic type
Histologic grade
Nuclear grade
Myometrial invasion
Vascular space invasion
Tumor size
Peritoneal cytology
Hormone receptor status
DNA ploidy and other biological markers
Type of therapy (surgery vs. radiation)

FIGO, International Federation of Gynecology and Obstetrics.

In contrast to the slow, estrogen-driven pathway leading to the biologically more indolent endometrioid carcinoma, a rapid, *p53*-driven pathway appears to lead to the aggressive serous (4,45) and clear cell carcinomas (4).

Clear cell carcinomas represent fewer than 5% of endometrial carcinomas, although clear cell elements are commonly present in papillary serous tumors (42). **Vascular space invasion is more common in these lesions** (46). In a review of 181 patients with clear cell endometrial carcinoma treated between 1970 and 1992, Abeler et al. (47) reported 5- and 10-year actuarial disease-free survival rates of 43% and 39%, respectively. Two-thirds of the relapses were outside the pelvis, most frequently in the upper abdomen, liver, and lungs.

SEER data from 1988 to 2001 were used to compare uterine papillary serous ($n = 1,473$), clear cell ($n = 391$), and grade 3 endometrioid carcinomas ($n = 2,316$) (44). Serous and clear cell carcinomas occurred in older patients, and were diagnosed at a more advanced stage. They represented 10%, 3%, and 15% of endometrial cancer, respectively, but accounted for 39%, 8%, and 27% of cancer deaths.

When papillary serous or clear cell carcinomas are limited to the curettings, with no adverse features in the hysterectomy specimen, prognosis may not be impaired (48).

Squamous cell carcinomas of the endometrium are rare. In a review of the literature, Abeler and Kjorstad (49) estimated that the survival rate for patients with clinical stage I disease was 36%.

Histologic Grade and Myometrial Invasion

There is a strong correlation between histologic grade, myometrial invasion, and prognosis. The GOG reported the surgicopathologic features of 621 patients with stage I endometrial carcinoma (32). The frequency of positive pelvic and paraaortic nodal metastases in relation to histologic grade and depth of myometrial invasion is shown in Tables 10.9 and 10.10. When grade 1 carcinomas were confined to the inner third of the myometrium, the incidence of positive pelvic nodes was less than 3%, whereas when grade 3 lesions involved the outer third, the incidence of positive pelvic nodes was 34%. For aortic nodes, the corresponding figures were less than 1% and 23%, respectively.

Local recurrence at the vaginal vault can usually be prevented by prophylactic vault brachytherapy, but the risk of distant metastases in relation to histologic grade and myometrial invasion is shown in Table 10.11 (50).

Vascular Space Invasion

Vascular space invasion appears to be an independent risk factor for recurrence and for death from endometrial carcinoma of all histologic types (36,51–53). Aalders et al. (51) reported recurrences and deaths in 26.7% of patients with stage I disease who had vascular space invasion compared with 9.1% of those without vessel invasion ($p = 0.01$). Abeler et al.

Table 10.9 Grade, Depth of Invasion, and Pelvic Nodal Metastasis of Endometrial Carcinoma

Depth of Myometrial Invasion	Histologic Grade		
	G_1 (n = 180)	G_2 (n = 288)	G_3 (n = 153)
Endometrium only (n = 86)	0/44 (0%)	1/31 (3%)	0/11 (0%)
Inner third (n = 281)	3/96 (3%)	7/131 (5%)	5/54 (9%)
Middle third (n = 115)	0/22 (0%)	6/69 (9%)	1/24 (4%)
Outer third (n = 139)	2/18 (11%)	11/57 (19%)	22/64 (34%)

Reproduced from **Creasman WT, Morrow CP, Bundy BN, Homesley HD, Graham JE, Heller PB.** Surgical pathologic spread patterns of endometrial cancer: a Gynecologic Oncology Group study. *Cancer* 1987; 60:2035–2041, with permission.

Table 10.10 Grade, Depth of Invasion, and Aortic Nodal Metastasis of Endometrial Carcinoma

Depth of Myometrial Invasion	Histologic Grade		
	G_1 (n = 180)	G_2 (n = 288)	G_3 (n = 153)
Endometrium only (n = 86)	0/44 (0%)	1/31 (3%)	0/11 (0%)
Inner third (n = 281)	1/96 (1%)	5/131 (4%)	2/54 (4%)
Middle third (n = 115)	1/22 (5%)	0/69 (0%)	0/24 (0%)
Outer third (n = 139)	1/18 (6%)	8/57 (14%)	15/64 (23%)

Reproduced from **Creasman WT, Morrow CP, Bundy BN, Homesley HD, Graham JE, Heller PB.** Surgical pathologic spread patterns of endometrial cancer: a Gynecologic Oncology Group study. *Cancer* 1987;60:2035–2041, with permission.

reviewed 1,974 cases of endometrial carcinoma from the Norwegian Radium Hospital and reported an 83.5% 5-year survival rate for patients without demonstrable vascular invasion compared with 64.5% for those in whom invasion was present (52). A Japanese study reported that lymph-vascular space invasion and the number of positive paraaortic lymph nodes were independent prognostic factors for patients with stage IIIC endometrial cancer (54).

The overall incidence of lymph-vascular invasion in stage I endometrial carcinoma is approximately 15%, although it increases with increasing myometrial invasion and decreasing tumor differentiation. Hanson et al. (55) reported vascular space invasion in 5% of patients with invasion limited to the inner one-third of the myometrium compared with 70% of those with invasion to the outer one-third. Similarly, it was present in 2% of grade 1 carcinomas and 42% of grade 3 lesions. Ambros and Kurman (56), using multivariate analysis, reported that only depth of myometrial invasion, DNA ploidy, and vascular-invasion–associated changes correlated significantly with survival for patients with stage I endometrioid adenocarcinomas. Vascular invasion–associated changes were defined as vascular invasion by tumor, or the presence of myometrial perivascular lymphocytic infiltrates, or both. In the GOG study, vascular space invasion carried a relative risk of death of 1.5 (37).

Peritoneal Cytologic Results

The significance of a positive peritoneal cytologic result is controversial (57). The incidence of positive cytologic findings in stage I disease is shown in Table 10.12. **Positive washings are most common in patients with grade 3 histologic type, metastases to the adnexae, deep myometrial invasion, or positive pelvic or paraaortic nodes** (32,57–62).

The GOG study reported by Morrow et al. (63) analyzed 697 patients with information on peritoneal cytologic results and adequate follow-up. Disease recurred in 25 of 86 patients (29.1%) with positive washings, compared with 64 of 611 patients (10.5%) with negative washings. The authors noted, however, that 17 of the 25 recurrences were outside the peritoneal cavity. **The GOG estimated that the relative risk of death for patients with positive cytologic washings was increased threefold** (37).

Table 10.11 Clinical Stage I Endometrial Carcinoma: Distant Metastases versus Histologic Grade and Myometrial Invasiona			
Variable	*Number*	*Metastases*	*Percent*
Histologic grade			
Grade 1	93	2	2.2
Grade 2	88	9	10.2
Grade 3	41	16	39.0
Myometrial invasion			
None	92	4	4.3
Inner third	80	8	10.0
Middle third	17	2	11.8
Outer third	33	13	39.4

aGynecologic Oncology Group data.

Reproduced from **DiSaia PJ, Creasman WT, Boronow RC, Blessing. JA.** Risk factors and recurrent patterns in stage I endometrial cancer. *Am J Obstet Gynecol* 1985;151:1009–1015, with permission.

In a review of the literature concerning patients with clinical stage I endometrial cancer, Milosevic et al. (64) reported positive peritoneal cytology in 8.3%, 12.1%, and 15.9% of patients with grades 1, 2, and 3 histologic types, respectively. Superficial and deep myometrial invasion were associated with positive washings in 7.6% and 17.2% of the cases, respectively. They concluded that the poor prognosis associated with malignant washings was largely a reflection of other adverse prognostic factors.

Kadar et al. (62) studied 269 patients with clinical stage I and stage II endometrial cancer and reported that if the disease was confined to the uterus, then positive peritoneal cytologic results did not influence survival. If the disease had spread to the adnexa, lymph nodes, or peritoneum, then positive peritoneal cytologic findings decreased the survival rate from 73% to 13% at 5 years, but all recurrences were at distant sites. Others have also reported no prognostic significance when the disease was confined to the uterus (65-68). Grimshaw et al. reported that 70% of patients with endometrial cancer and positive peritoneal cytology had extrauterine disease at the time of surgery, and the prognosis for these patients was impaired (66). Contrary findings were reported from Duke University, where Havrilesky et al. showed that positive cytology was an independent poor prognostic factor for patients with stages I to IIIA disease (69). Saga et al. from Japan also found positive peritoneal cytology to be an independent poor prognostic factor after reviewing 307 surgically staged patients with disease confined to the uterus (70).

Takeshima et al. (61) studied 534 patients with endometrial cancer to assess the prognostic significance of positive peritoneal washings. They concluded that they were not an independent negative prognostic indicator but potentiated other prognostic indicators. **They felt**

Table 10.12 Incidence of Positive Peritoneal Cytology in Clinical Stage I Endometrial Carcinoma			
Author	*Cases*	*Positive Cytology*	*Percent*
Creasman et al. 1987 (32)	621	76	12.2
Harouny et al. 1988 (58)	276	47	17.0
Hirai et al. 1989 (59)	173	25	14.4
Lurain et al. 1989 (60)	157	30	19.1
Takeshima et al. 2001 (61)	534	119	22.3
Total	1,761	297	16.7

that patients with positive peritoneal cytology in the absence of other adverse prognostic factors did not warrant upstaging.

These same workers placed a tube in the abdomen to allow peritoneal irrigation in 50 patients with early stage endometrial cancer and positive peritoneal smears detected at surgery (65). Washings were obtained via the tube 7 and 14 days postoperatively. Persistence of positive peritoneal cytology was observed in only five of 50 patients (10%), and four of these patients had adnexal metastases completely resected. They concluded that malignant cells found in the peritoneal cavity generally have a low malignant potential and that only malignant cells from special cases, such as patients with adnexal metastases, may be capable of independent growth.

Hormone Receptor Status

In general, mean estrogen receptor (ER) and progesterone receptor (PR) levels are inversely proportional to histologic grade (71–74). However, **ER and PR content have been shown to be independent prognostic indicators for endometrial cancer; that is, patients whose tumors are positive for one or both receptors have longer survival than patients whose carcinoma lacks the corresponding receptors** (71–73,75). Liao et al. (72) reported that, even for patients with lymph node metastases, the prognosis was significantly improved if the tumor was receptor positive. PR appears to be a stronger predictor of survival than ER and, at least for the ER, the absolute level of the receptors may be important: The higher the level, the better the prognosis (76).

Nuclear Grade

Nuclear grade is a significant prognostic indicator (76). Christopherson et al. (77) found nuclear grading to be a more accurate prognosticator than histologic grade.

The FIGO grading system takes into account the nuclear grade of the tumor, and "nuclear atypia" inappropriate for the architectural grade raises the grade by 1. However, there is great variability in the literature regarding the criteria for nuclear grading, and intraobserver and interobserver reproducibility of nuclear grading are poor (78).

Tumor Size

In an analysis of 142 patients with clinical stage I endometrial carcinoma, Schink et al. (79) reported tumor size as an independent prognostic factor. Lymph node metastases occurred in 4% of the patients with tumors no more than 2 cm in diameter, 15% with tumors greater than 2 cm in diameter, and 35% with tumors involving the entire uterine cavity. The incidence of nodal metastases in relation to tumor size and depth of invasion is shown in Table 10.13.

DNA Ploidy and Other Biologic Markers

Approximately one-fourth of patients with endometrial carcinomas have aneuploid tumors, which is a low incidence compared with many other solid tumors, including ovarian and cervical carcinomas. However, patients with aneuploid tumors are at significantly increased risk of early recurrence and death from disease (56,80,81).

In a prospective study of 174 patients, Susini et al. reported a 10-year survival probability of 53.2% for patients with DNA aneuploid tumors, compared with 91.0% for patients with DNA diploid tumors. By multivariate analysis, DNA aneuploid type was the strongest independent predictor of poor outcome, followed by age and stage (81). **The GOG estimated the relative risk to be 4.1 for disease-related death for patients with aneuploid tumors** (82).

A number of genetic mutations have also been shown to have prognostic significance in endometrial cancer. Greek workers reported that **loss of *beta-catenin* expression** was a strong, independent predictor of a poor prognosis, whereas **loss of *PTEN*** was associated with a worse

Table 10.13 Incidence of Lymph Node Metastasis in Endometrial Cancer by Tumor Size and Depth of Myometrial Invasion

Depth of Invasion	Tumor Size		
	≤2 cm Diameter (%)	>2 cm Diameter (%)	Entire Surface (%)
None	0/17 (0)	0/8 (0)	0/0 (0)
<1/2	0/27 (0)	5/41 (12)	2/9 (22)
≥1/2	2/9 (22)	6/23 (26)	4/8 (50)

Reproduced from **Schink JC, Lurain JR, Wallemark CB, Chmiel JS.** Tumor size in endometrial cancer: a prognostic factor for lymph node metastasis. *Obstet Gynecol* 1987;70:216–219, with permission.

Table 10.14 Clinical Stage II Carcinoma of the Endometrium: Comparison of Treatment Methods

	No. of Patients	Distant Metastases (%)	Pelvic Recurrence (%)	5-Year Survival Rate (%)
Radiation and surgery	90	13.3	8.9	78
Radiation alone	26	11.5	34.6	48

Reproduced from **Grigsby PW, Perez CA, Camel HM, Galakatos AE.** Stage II carcinoma of the endometrium: results of therapy and prognostic factors. *Int J Radiat Oncol Biol Phys* 1985;11:1915–1921, with permission.

prognosis for patients with early stage disease (83). The *p53* mutation correlated with increased stage, lymph node metastases, and nonendometrioid histology in univariate analysis but was not an independent prognostic factor in multivariate analysis (83). **Increasing expression of matrix metalloproteinases** (MMPs) (84), **nuclear *bcl-2* expression** (85), and **Ki-67 expression** (86) also have prognostic significance. The clinical implications of these biologic markers are not yet clear.

Method of Treatment

In contrast to cervical cancer, patients with endometrial cancer treated with hysterectomy alone or hysterectomy and radiation do significantly better than those treated with radiation alone This appears to be related to the inability of radiation therapy effectively to eliminate disease in the myometrium (87,88). Grigsby et al. (87) reported on 116 patients with stage II endometrial carcinoma. Ninety were treated with combined radiation and surgery, whereas 26 received radiation alone. The results of treatment are shown in Table 10.14.

Endometrial Hyperplasia

Classic teaching has been that endometrial hyperplasias represent a continuum of morphologic severity; the most severe form, termed *atypical adenomatous hyperplasia* or *carcinoma in situ,* was considered the immediate precursor of endometrial carcinoma (89,90). Since the mid-1980s, this continuum concept has been challenged. Independent studies by Kurman et al. (91) and Ferenczy et al. (92) have suggested the following:

1. **Endometrial hyperplasia and endometrial neoplasia are two biologically different diseases.**

2. **The only important distinguishing feature is the presence or absence of cytologic atypia.**

Ferenczy et al. (92) suggested that the term **endometrial hyperplasia** be used for any degree of glandular proliferation devoid of cytologic atypia and the term **endometrial intraepithelial neoplasia for lesions with cytologic atypia.** Using similar criteria in a long-term follow-up study of 170 patients with endometrial hyperplasia, Kurman et al. (91) reported a 1.6% risk of progression to carcinoma in patients devoid of cytologic atypia, compared with a 23% risk in patients with cytologic atypia.

Subsequently, Ferenczy and Gelfand (93) reported 85 menopausal women with endometrial hyperplasia. Sixty-five patients had no cytologic atypia, and 84% of this group responded to *medroxyprogesterone acetate* (MPA). Four (6%) had recurrent hyperplasia after discontinuing the MPA, and none developed carcinoma, with a mean follow-up of 7 years. By contrast, 20 patients had cytologic atypia, and only 50% responded to MPA. Recurrent hyperplasia developed in five (25%), and adenocarcinoma in five (25%). The World Health Organization (WHO) classification of endometrial hyperplasia is shown in Table 10.15

Although the studies of Kurman and Ferenczy are important, **the reproducibility of the diagnosis has been questioned.** In a GOG study, a panel of three expert gynecologic pathologists reviewed outside slides from 306 patients referred with a diagnosis of atypical endometrial hyperplasia. The majority panel diagnosis was adenocarcinoma in 29%, cycling endometrium in 7%, and nonatypical hyperplasia in 18% of cases (94). Interobserver variation was also common.

Hysterectomy slides from the same GOG study were reviewed by the study pathologists, and 289 hysterectomy specimens were available for review (95). Concurrent endometrial carcinoma

Table 10.15 World Health Organization Classification of Endometrial Hyperplasia
Hyperplasia
Simple
Complex (adenomatous)
Atypical hyperplasia
Simple
Complex (atypical adenomatous)

Reproduced from **Scully RE, Bonfiglio TA, Kurman RJ, Silverberg SG, Wilkinson EJ.** Uterine corpus. In: *Histological typing of female genital tract tumors.* New York: Springer-Verlag, 1994:13–31.

was present in 42.6% (123 of 289 specimens). Of these, 30.9% (38 of 123 specimens) had myometrial invasion, and 10.6% (13 of 123 specimens) had invasion to the outer half of the myometrium. Even when the study panel consensus diagnosis was less than atypical endometrial hyperplasia, 14 of 74 women (18.9%) still had carcinoma in the hysterectomy specimen.

Treatment

Most women with endometrial hyperplasia respond to *progestin* therapy. Patients who do not respond are at a significantly increased risk of progressing to invasive cancer and should be advised to have a hysterectomy. Patients who are unlikely to respond can be identified on the basis of cytologic atypia. A suggested scheme of management is outlined in Figure 10.2.

Ferenczy and Gelgand reported on 85 women with endometrial hyperplasia treated with *medroxyprogesterone* (93). The 65 patients who had no cytologic atypia received 10 mg daily for 14 days per month, whereas the 20 patients with cytologic atypia received 20 mg daily. Both groups had endometrial sampling every 3 months. In the group without cytologic atypia, 14% had persistence of their hyperplasia, but none progressed to carcinoma. **Of the 20 patients with cytologic atypia, 50% had persistence of their hyperplasia, and 25% developed frank carcinoma at a mean of 5.5 years after initiation of hormonal therapy.**

The type of *progestin* used does not appear to be important, the optimal dosage has not been investigated, and the regimens advocated are essentially arbitrary (96). High doses of *progestins* are often better tolerated than low doses. The main side effects are weight gain, edema, thrombophlebitis, and occasionally hypertension. The incidence of venous thrombosis and embolism may also be slightly increased.

Other approaches to hormonal therapy include *levonorgestrel*-releasing intrauterine devices (97), the use of *danazol* in a dose of 400 mg daily for 3 months (98), and the combined use of gonadotropin-releasing hormone (GnRH) analogues and *progestins* (99).

Treatment of Endometrial Cancer

The cornerstone of treatment for endometrial cancer is total abdominal hysterectomy and bilateral salpingo-oophorectomy, and this operation should be performed in all cases whenever feasible. In addition, many patients require some type of adjuvant radiation therapy to help prevent vaginal vault recurrence and to sterilize disease in lymph nodes. It is difficult to document that radiation actually improves survival rates, but both the GOG study (100) and the postoperative radiation therapy in endometrial carcinoma (PORTEC) trial (101) of surgery versus surgery plus adjuvant pelvic radiation for patients with intermediate to high-risk stage I endometrial cancer showed an improved disease-free survival rate for the radiation-treated group. Neither trial showed an improvement in overall survival because of the ability to salvage most pelvic recurrences in the surgery-only arm with radiation therapy. There may be a survival benefit for patients with high-grade, deeply invasive tumors, but currently there are no prospective data to demonstrate this (102).

With the increasing emphasis on surgicopathologic staging, a more individualized approach to adjuvant radiation is now possible.

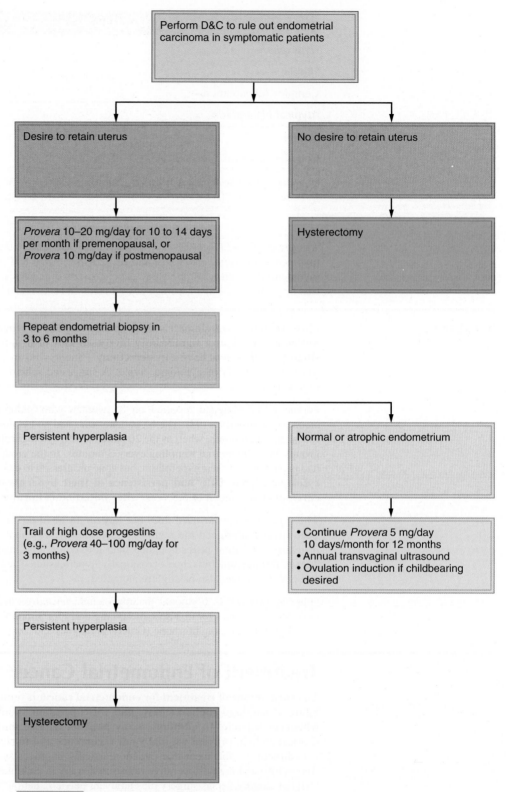

Figure 10.2   **Management of endometrial hyperplasia.**

Microscopic cervical involvement (positive endocervical curettage) is often designated (unofficially) as stage II occult disease. For practical purposes, if the cervix is not hard or expanded, such patients can be managed in the same way as patients with stage I disease.

Stage I and Stage II Occult

Operative Technique

A recommended treatment plan is shown in Fig. 10.3.

The initial approach for all medically fit patients should be total abdominal hysterectomy and bilateral salpingo-oophorectomy. Removal of a vaginal cuff is not necessary. The adnexa should be removed because they may be the site of microscopic metastases. In addition, patients with endometrial carcinoma are at increased risk for ovarian cancer. Such tumors sometimes occur concurrently (103). Surgical staging, including lymphadenectomy, should be performed in those patients listed in Table 10.16 The use of laparoscopically assisted vaginal hysterectomy is addressed in Chapter 21.

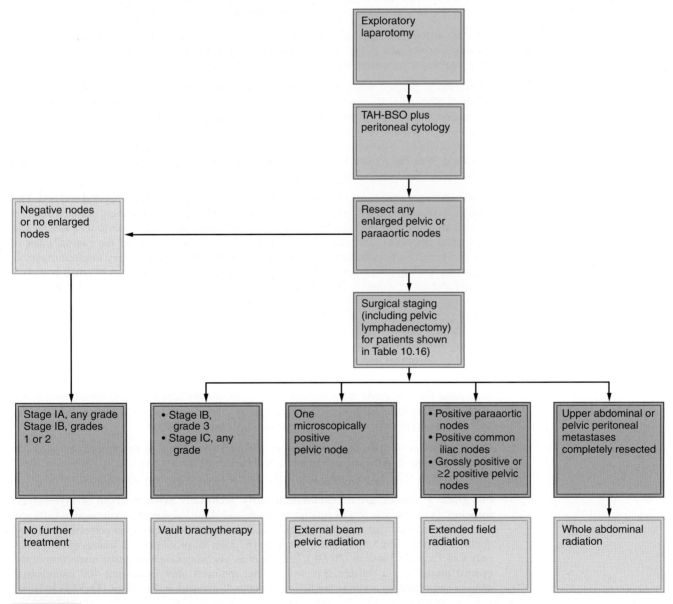

Figure 10.3 **Management of patients with stage I and occult stage II endometrial carcinoma.** TAH, total abdominal hysterectomy; BSO, bilateral salpingo-oophorectomy.

Table 10.16 Endometrial Carcinoma Stages I and Occult II: Patients Requiring Surgical Staging
1. Patients with grade 3 lesions
2. Patients with grade 2 tumors >2 cm in diameter
3. Patients with clear cell or papillary serous carcinomas
4. Patients with greater than 50% of myometrial invasion
5. Patients with cervical extension

The laparotomy is best performed through a lower midline abdominal incision, particularly in the obese patient. This incision allows easy access to the upper abdomen, including the omentum and paraaortic lymph nodes. A Pfannenstiel incision is commonly used for patients with grade 1 or 2 tumors and a normally sized uterus **An alternative approach is to use a transverse, muscle-dividing incision (e.g., the Maylard or Cherney),** as discussed in Chapter 20. This incision also gives reasonable access to the upper abdomen.

After the abdomen is opened, peritoneal washings are taken with 50 dL normal saline solution. Thorough exploration of the abdomen and pelvis is performed, with particular attention to the liver, diaphragm, omentum, and paraaortic nodes. Any suspicious lesions are excised or biopsied.

The uterus is grasped with clamps that encompass the round and ovarian ligaments and the fallopian tube. After the round ligaments are divided, the incision is carried anteriorly around the vesicouterine fold of peritoneum and posteriorly parallel and lateral to the infundibulopelvic ligaments. With a narrow Deaver retractor in the retroperitoneum providing gentle traction cephalad in the direction of the common iliac vessels, the iliac vessels and ureter are displayed. With the retroperitoneum displayed, the pelvic lymph nodes can be visualized and palpated, and any enlarged nodes can be removed.

With each ureter under direct vision, the infundibulopelvic ligaments are divided and tied. The bladder is dissected off the front of the cervix, and then the uterine vessels are skeletonized and divided at the level of the isthmus. Straight Kocher clamps are used to secure the cardinal and uterosacral ligaments. The uterus, tubes, and ovaries are removed, and the vaginal vault is closed. The pelvic peritoneum is not closed, and it usually is not necessary to place drains in the pelvis. The sigmoid colon is placed in the pelvis to help exclude loops of small bowel. A vertical abdominal wound is best closed with a continuous Smead-Jones type of internal retention suture, using a long-acting, absorbable suture such as Maxon or PDS.

Surgical Staging

The decision to undertake surgical staging is usually based on the histopathology from the uterine curettings, the gross findings on opening the uterus on the operating table, and possibly a frozen section of the resected uterus.

A relatively poor correlation has been reported between the grade of cancer on curettings or biopsy and the final grade in the resected uterus, presumably because of a sampling error in the diagnostic procedure. The poorest correlation is for grade 1 tumors, where 20% to 40% may be upgraded after evaluation of the hysterectomy specimen (104,105).

Our practice is to open the specimen on the operating table to determine the need for surgical staging in patients with grade 1 or 2 tumors (Figs. 10.4 and 10.5). All patients with grade 3 tumors (Fig. 10.6), serous papillary, or clear cell carcinomas are surgically staged.

For grade 1 tumors, gross examination fairly accurately predicts depth of myometrial invasion. In an analysis of 113 patients with surgical stage I endometrial carcinoma, Goff and Rice (106) reported that macroscopic examination of the fresh specimen correctly predicted depth of invasion in 55 of 63 grade 1 lesions (87.3%), 24 of 37 grade 2 lesions (64.9%), but only 4 of 13 grade 3 lesions (30.8%). Franchi et al. also concluded that gross inspection of the opened uterus was a reliable and inexpensive approach after evaluating 403 endometrial cancers and noting an accurate prediction of depth of invasion in 344 cases (85.3%) (107).

Tumor diameter should also be taken into account when determining the need for surgical staging, and we use this particularly for grade 2 lesions. Schink et al. (79) reported a 22%

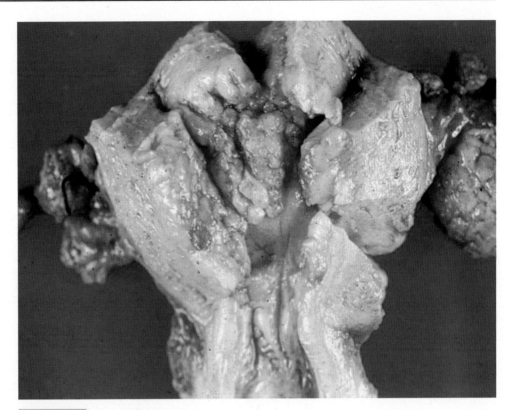

Figure 10.4   **A small fundal grade 1 endometrial carcinoma.** This patient does not require surgical staging.

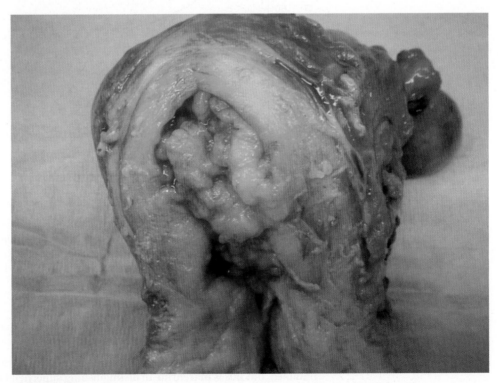

Figure 10.5   **A grade 2 endometrial carcinoma occupying most of the corpus.** A patient such as this should undergo surgical staging.

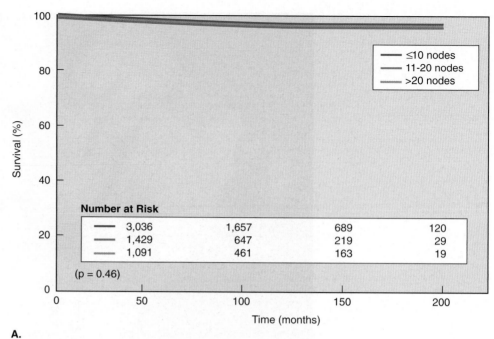

A.

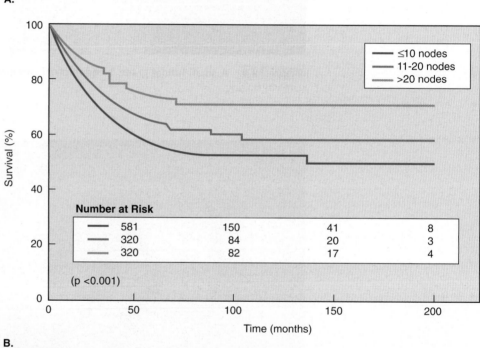

B.

Figure 10.6   **Survival for patients with (A) low-risk endometrial cancer and (B) high-risk endometrial cancer versus extent of lymphadenectomy.** Reproduced with permission from **Chan J et al.** Therapeutic role of lymph node resection in endometrioid corpus cancer: A study of 12,333 patients. *Cancer* 2006; 107:1823–1828.

incidence of lymph node metastases for grade 2 tumors greater than 2 cm in diameter (7 of 32). None of 19 grade 2 tumors less than 2 cm in diameter had nodal metastases.

If doubt exists regarding the need for surgical staging, intraoperative frozen section can be obtained, but this is inaccurate in distinguishing superficial from deep myometrial invasion in 5% to 10% of cases (106–108). If the final histopathology is worse than was anticipated intraoperatively, the prognosis will not be impaired if external-beam pelvic radiation is given on the basis of histologic grade and depth of myometrial invasion, as long as any enlarged pelvic or paraaortic nodes have been resected as part of the standard management for all patients.

Pelvic Lymphadenectomy

No preoperative scan is able to detect micrometastases in lymph nodes, so if accurate surgical staging is to be obtained, then full pelvic lymphadenectomy should be performed on all patients who meet the criteria in Table 10.16. Sampling will only lead to inaccurate information (109).

In an analysis of 11,443 patients registered on the SEER data base between 1990 and 2001, Chan et al. reported that the removal of 21 to 25 lymph nodes significantly increased the probability of detecting at least one positive lymph node in endometrioid uterine cancer (110). Lutman et al. also reported that the pelvic lymph node count was an important prognostic variable for patients with FIGO stages I and II endometrial carcinoma and high-risk histology (111). On the other hand, in an analysis of 5,556 patients with low-risk endometrioid endometrial carcinoma from the SEER data base, Chan et al. were unable to find any survival advantage regardless of the extent of the lymphadenectomy (33) (Figure 10.6).

The dissection should include removal of common iliac nodes and of the fat pad overlying the distal inferior vena cava. If full pelvic lymphadenectomy is considered inadvisable because of the patient's general medical condition, which is uncommon, then resection of any enlarged pelvic nodes should be performed.

Management of Paraaortic Lymph Nodes

Although some authors recommend systematic paraaortic lymphadenectomy on all high-risk patients (112) or in patients with two or more positive pelvic lymph nodes (113), this is major surgery for a group of patients who are usually elderly and obese. An extensive paraaortic lymphadenectomy significantly increases operating time and blood loss and also increases postoperative morbidity, particularly lower limb lymphedema. The latter occurs in 20% of patients in our experience (114).

Lymphedema is a lifelong affliction, which is often complicated by recurrent episodes of cellulitis. To avoid progressive deterioration of the condition, regular massage and use of surgical stockings are essential, and both become progressively more burdensome, particularly for elderly patients. In our opinion, primary prevention of lymphedema by selective use of pelvic lymphadenectomy and avoidance of systematic paraaortic lymphadenectomy is highly desirable.

The GOG data (63) suggested that **patients with positive paraaortic nodes were likely to have:**

1. **grossly positive pelvic nodes,**
2. **grossly positive adnexae, or**
3. **grade 2 or 3 lesions with outer-third myometrial invasion.**

Nomura et al. retrospectively reviewed 841 patients with endometrial cancer who underwent their initial surgery at Keio University Hospital in Japan (115). In a multivariate analysis, the clinicopathologic factor most strongly related to paraaortic nodal metastasis was pelvic lymph node metastasis. Among 155 patients who underwent systematic pelvic and paraaortic lymphadenectomy, **96.2% (101 of 105 cases) had negative paraaortic nodes when the pelvic nodes were negative.** However, when the pelvic nodes were positive, 48% (24 of 50 cases) also had positive paraaortic nodes. These findings are consistent with those from the Mayo Clinic (112).

Omental Biopsy

In addition to the lymphadenectomy, **an omental biopsy is also performed as part of the surgical staging** because occult omental metastases may occur, particularly in patients with grade 3 tumors or deeply invasive lesions (116). The omentum should be carefully inspected, along with all peritoneal surfaces, and any suspicious lesions excised. If the omentum appears normal, then a generous biopsy (e.g., 5 × 5 cm) should be taken.

Our current approach is to resect any enlarged paraaortic nodes and give extended-field radiation to all patients with any grossly positive pelvic nodes or more than one microscopically positive pelvic node.

Sentinel Node Biopsy

Sentinel node identification has been investigated in a number of solid tumors, the hypothesis being that if one or more sentinel nodes are negative, the remainder of the regional nodes will be negative, so complete lymphadenectomy can be avoided (117). Lymphatic mapping is performed by infecting tracers around the tumor and identifying the draining node(s). Usually, a blue dye and a radioactive tracer are used, and the best results are

Table 10.17 Sentinel Lymph Node Involvement in Endometrial Cancer				
Author	*Number*	*Injection Site*	*Mean Number of Nodes*	*Detection Rate (%)*
Pelosi 2002 (118)	11	Cervix	1.5	100
Barranger 2004 (119)	17	Cervix	2.6	93
Lelievre 2004 (120)	12	Cervix	2.0	92
Niikura 2004 (121)	28	Tumor	3.1	82
Maccauro 2005 (122)	26	Tumor	3.0	100
Delaloye 2007 (123)	60	Tumor	3.7	82
Lopes 2007 (124)	40	Fundus	2.0	77.5
Frumovitz 2007 (125)	18	Fundus	1.7	45

achieved when both techniques are used together. Technetium-99 is the most commonly used radioactive substance because of its short half-life (6 hours).

Three approaches have been used for sentinel node identification in endometrial cancer: (i) injection into the cervix, (ii) injection around the tumor via a hysteroscope, and (iii) injection into the subserosal myometrium at the fundus.

Results of some preliminary studies are shown in Table 10.17. **Injection around the tumor would seem the most logical approach, but data are scant, and studies are still addressing feasibility and standardization of technique.** Although detection of at least one sentinel node is reported to occur in as many as 100% of cases, bilateral pelvic sentinel node detection and paraaortic sentinel node detection both occur in less than 50% of cases. **Sentinel node identification is still entirely experimental for endometrial cancer.**

Role of Lymphadenectomy

Pelvic lymphadenectomy, with or without paraaortic lymphadenectomy, plays an important role in the surgical staging of endometrial cancer and thus **provides more accurate prognostic information. The therapeutic role of lymphadenectomy is less well understood, but its ability to modify adjuvant therapy is being increasingly accepted.**

The therapeutic value of pelvic lymph node dissection was investigated by Kilgore et al. from Birmingham, Alabama, who reported on 649 surgically managed patients with adenocarcinoma of the endometrium (126). Two hundred twelve patients had multiple-site pelvic node sampling (mean number of nodes 11), 205 had limited-site sampling (mean number of nodes 4), and 208 had no node sampling. The decision regarding lymph node sampling was surgeon dependent, and prognostic features—including tumor grade, depth of invasion, adnexal metastasis, cervical involvement, and positive cytologic findings—were equally distributed among the three groups. All patients had adjuvant radiation therapy based on traditional prognostic factors. With a mean follow-up of 3 years, patients undergoing multiple-site pelvic node sampling had a significantly better overall survival ($p = 0.0002$) as well as a better survival for both low-risk and high-risk groups (low-risk, $p = 0.026$; high-risk, $p = 0.0006$).

The authors concluded that their results strongly suggested a therapeutic benefit to lymphadenectomy, but confirmation of this must await randomized studies. **If there is a therapeutic benefit, it must surely be related to the resection of bulky, positive nodes, which are unlikely to be sterilized with external-beam radiation therapy.**

A randomized trial to evaluate the therapeutic effects of lymphadenectomy was conducted by the U.K. Medical Research Council's ASTEC study. The results were published recently (127). No therapeutic benefit was found. However, the number of lymph nodes resected was insufficient to show a benefit in at least one third of patients, paraaortic node dissection was not required, and subsequent radiation was not tailored to the nodal status, so it is difficult to draw any definitive conclusions.

The feasibility of using the results of pelvic lymphadenectomy to modify adjuvant radiation therapy has been addressed in several nonrandomized trials and will be discussed under adjuvant radiation.

Vaginal Hysterectomy

In selected patients with marked obesity and medical problems that place them at high risk for abdominal operations, vaginal hysterectomy should be considered.

Peters et al. (128) reported a 94% survival rate among 56 patients with stage I endometrial carcinoma who underwent vaginal hysterectomy. Seventy-five percent had grade 1 lesions, and 32 patients received adjuvant radiation, mainly brachytherapy.

Japanese workers reported on 171 patients aged 70 years and older, 128 (75%) of whom were treated with vaginal hysterectomy and 43 of whom underwent abdominal hysterectomy (129) The 10-year disease-specific survival rates were 83% and 84%, respectively (p = ns). Patients in the vaginal hysterectomy group had significantly shorter operating times, less blood loss, and shorter postoperative stays. Severe complications occurred in 5.4% of the vaginal and 7.0% of the abdominal procedures. Perioperative mortality was zero after vaginal hysterectomy and 2.3% after abdominal hysterectomy. The researchers concluded that vaginal hysterectomy should be considered the elective approach for the treatment of elderly patients with endometrial cancer.

Laparoscopically assisted vaginal hysterectomy is increasingly being used for the management of endometrial cancer, particularly in obese patients. Use of the laparoscope facilitates removal of the adnexae and the pelvic lymph nodes.

Adjuvant Radiation

The use of adjuvant radiation is decreasing for patients with endometrial cancer. For high-risk patients, surgical staging has allowed the therapy to be better tailored to the needs of the individual patient. The options for postoperative radiation are as follows:

1. observation
2. vault brachytherapy
3. external pelvic irradiation
4. extended-field irradiation
5. whole-abdominal irradiation (WAR)

Observation

Patients with stage IA or IB, grade 1 or 2 tumors have an excellent prognosis, and no adjuvant radiation is necessary for this group. Canadian workers reported 227 such patients who were followed without radiation, and the 5-year relapse-free survival rate was 95% (130). Elliot et al. (131) from Australia treated 308 patients with grade 1 or 2 lesions confined to the inner third of the myometrium with hysterectomy alone. There were ten vaginal recurrences (3.2%), eight at the vault, and one each in the middle and lower third. The Danish Endometrial Cancer Group (DEMCA) prospectively followed 641 patients with grade 1 and 2 tumors with no more than 50% myometrial invasion (stages IA and IB) who were treated by total abdominal hysterectomy and bilateral salpingo-oophorectomy without adjuvant radiation (132). With follow-up of 68 to 92 months, the disease-free survival rate was 93% (596 of 641). Fanning and colleagues compared surgery and adjuvant radiation with surgery alone for patients with stage I, grade 2 adenocarcinomas of favorable histologic subtype and less than one-third myometrial invasion (133). The 5-year survival rate for surgery and radiation was 94% (128 of 136), and the recurrence rate was 2.2% (3 of 136). The 5-year survival rate for the surgery-alone group was 98% (51 of 52), and the recurrence rate was 1.9% (1 of 52).

If patients are treated without adjuvant therapy, then they must be followed carefully so that vault recurrences can be diagnosed early or when they are eminently curable (132–135). The diagnosis of recurrence is sometimes first suspected when adenocarcinoma cells are seen on a routine vault smear.

Vaginal Brachytherapy

Vaginal brachytherapy significantly reduces the incidence of vault recurrence. With high dose-rate therapy, treatment can be accomplished as an outpatient, and the morbidity is low. A recent study from the University of Virginia reported that compared to observation, postoperative brachytherapy improved survival at a cost of $65,900 per survivor (136).

Several reported studies have demonstrated low recurrence rates at the vaginal vault and pelvic sidewall using vault brachytherapy without external pelvic radiation after pelvic lymphadenectomy

Table 10.18 Vault Brachytherapy for Stage I or Occult Stage II Endometrial Cancer after Pelvic Lymphadenectomy

Author	Number	Dose	Fractions	Follow-Up	Recurrence Vault	Recurrence Sidewall
COSA-NZ-UK 1996 (137)	207	LDR 60 Gy to surface	1	3–10 years	2	7
Orr et al. 1997 (138)	310	LDR 60 Gy to surface	1	Up to 10 yrs.	0	0
Mohan et al. 1998 (139)	159	LDR 20 Gy at 10 mm HDR 21 Gy	1 3	96 months median	0	1
Ng et al. 2000 (140)	77	LDR 60 Gy to surface HDR 36 Gy to mucosa	1 6	45 months median	2*	1
Fanning 2001 (141)	66	LDR 40 Gy at 0.5 cm HDR 21 Gy at 0.5 cm	1 3	4.4 years mean	0	0
Seago et al. 2001 (142)	23	HDR 21 Gy at 0.5 cm	3	25 months median	0	0
Horrowitz et al. 2002 (143)	143	HDR 21 Gy	3	65 months median	1	2
Jolly et al. 2005 (144)	50	HDR 30 Gy	6	38 months median	2	1
Solhjem et al. 2005 (145)	100	HDR 21 Gy	3	23 months median	0	0
Total	1,135				7 (0.6%)	12 (1.1%)

*Five recurrences in lower 2/3 of vagina

with negative nodes. Table 10.18 reveals an incidence of vault recurrence of 0.6% and an incidence of pelvic sidewall recurrence of 1.1% following this approach in 1,135 mainly high-risk patients with stage I and stage II occult disease. **Data from the Mayo Clinic would suggest that high-dose-rate brachytherapy should also be considered in low-risk cases with extensive vascular space invasion** (36).

The exact place of vaginal brachytherapy alone must await randomized, controlled trials. If lymph node sampling only has been performed, then it may be safer to use external pelvic radiation because of the increased risk of pelvic sidewall recurrence.

External Pelvic Irradiation

With an increasing number of patients in cancer centers having pelvic lymphadenectomy as part of their primary surgery, the indications for external pelvic irradiation are decreasing. **Patients with negative pelvic nodes generally receive vault brachytherapy alone, whereas patients with bulky positive pelvic nodes or more than one microscopically positive pelvic node are better treated with pelvic and paraaortic radiation.** External pelvic radiation is a reasonable option for high-risk patients who have not undergone surgical staging but have a negative pelvic and abdominal CT scan and a normal serum CA125 titer.

The GOG reported results of a randomized study of adjuvant pelvic radiation after complete surgical staging for patients with intermediate-risk endometrial carcinoma (100). Eligible patients had surgical stages IB, IC, IIA (occult), or IIB (occult) disease and were randomized to receive either no additional therapy or 5,040 centiGray of external pelvic radiation therapy. There were 390 eligible patients in the study, and median follow-up was 56 months.

The 2-year progression-free survival rate was significantly higher in the group receiving adjuvant radiation (96% vs. 88%; p 0.004). **However, overall survival rates were not significantly different** because there were more pelvic or vaginal recurrences in the no-treatment arm (17 vs. 3), and these were often effectively treated with second-line therapy.

A European randomized trial (the PORTEC study) of surgery and postoperative external pelvic radiation (46 Gy) **versus surgery alone for patients with stage I endometrial cancer was published in 2000** (101). Eligible patients were those with stage IC, grade 1; stage IB or IC, grade 2; or stage IB, grade 3 disease. Patients with serous papillary or clear cell carcinoma were also eligible. Surgery consisted of total abdominal hysterectomy and bilateral salpingo-oophorectomy without lymphadenectomy. A total of 715 patients from 19 radiation oncology centers were randomized.

Actuarial 5-year overall survival rates were similar in the two groups: 81% (radiotherapy) and 85% (controls) ($p = 0.31$). Endometrial-cancer–related death rates were 9% in the radiotherapy group and 6% in the control group ($p = 0.37$). Treatment-related complications occurred in 25% of the radiotherapy patients and in 6% of the controls ($p = 0.0001$). Grade 3–4 complications were seen in eight patients, of which seven were in the radiotherapy group (2%). **Two-year survival after vaginal recurrence was 79% in contrast to 21% after pelvic recurrence or distant metastases.** Survival after relapse was significantly better ($p = 0.02$) for patients in the control group. After multivariate analysis, investigators concluded that postoperative radiotherapy was not indicated in patients with stage I endometrial cancer younger than 60 years and in patients with grade 2 tumors with superficial invasion.

A subsequent 10-year follow-up of the PORTEC trial revealed that the 10-year locoregional relapse rates were 5% after radiation and 14% for controls ($p <0.0001$), and the 10-year overall survival rates were 66% and 73%, respectively ($p = 0.09$) (146). Endometrial-cancer–related death rates were 11% (RT) and 9% (controls) ($p = 0.47$). **The researchers concluded that radiotherapy was indicated for patients who were unstaged surgically but had high-risk features because of the significant locoregional control benefit.**

To clarify the effect of postoperative external-beam pelvic radiotherapy in patients with early endometrial cancer, Johnson and Cornes from the United Kingdom performed a metaanalysis of data from five randomized trials. Pelvic lymphadenectomy was performed in only two of the five trials. The authors concluded that adjuvant external-beam pelvic radiation should not be used for low (IA or IB, grade 1) or intermediate risk (IB, grade 2) cancer but was associated with a 10% survival advantage for high-risk (stage IC, grade 3) disease (147).

External irradiation appears to be as effective as vaginal brachytherapy for sterilizing micrometastases at the vaginal vault; thus, there seems to be no reason to give both external and vault irradiation after surgery because morbidity will be significantly increased. Weiss and colleagues treated 61 women with stage IC endometrial cancer with postoperative pelvic radiation without vaginal brachytherapy. No patient developed a vaginal recurrence (148).

Indications for external pelvic radiation are shown in Table 10.19

Extended-Field Radiation

Risk factors for pelvic lymph node metastases portend a lower but significant risk of paraaortic metastases, and failure rates of 15% to 20% in the paraaortic area have been reported for patients receiving pelvic radiation only (149). Approximately 50% of patients with positive pelvic nodes will have positive paraaortic nodes (115). **Paraaortic lymph node metastases are associated with an increasing number of pelvic lymph node metastases and with bilateral pelvic nodal involvement** (150).

Using what is now considered relatively unsophisticated radiation techniques and a dose between 45 and 50 Gy, **approximately 40% of patients with positive paraaortic nodes may achieve long-term disease-free survival with extended-field radiation therapy** (151). Mariani et al. reported that none of 11 patients with positive paraaortic nodes failed in the paraaortic area after adequate lymphadenectomy (defined as removal of five or more paraaortic nodes) and extended-field radiation (112).

Our current indications for extended-field radiation are shown in Table 10.20.

Table 10.19 Indications for External Pelvic Radiation in Patients with Stages I and II Occult Endometrial Cancer
1. Patients with 1 microscopically positive pelvic node after surgical staging.
2. Patients with high-risk features who have undergone TAH-BSO without surgical staging, and who have a negative pelvic and abdominal CT scan and a normal serum CA125 level.

Table 10.20 Indications for Extended-Field Radiation Therapy in Patients with Endometrial Cancer

1. Biopsy-proven paraaortic nodal metastasis

2. Grossly positive pelvic nodes

3. 2 or more positive pelvic nodes

Whole-Abdominal Radiation

Whole-abdominal radiation has been used for many years in selected patients with omental, adnexal, or peritoneal metastases that have been completely resected, but the GOG recently reported a randomized phase III trial of WAR versus chemotherapy in patients with stage III or IV endometrial carcinoma having a maximum of 2 cm of postoperative residual disease. There were 396 assessable patients. Irradiation dosage was 30 Gray (Gy) in 20 fractions, with a 15-Gy boost. Chemotherapy consisted of *doxorubicin* 60 mg/m^2 and *cisplatin* 50 mg/m^2 every 3 weeks for seven cycles, followed by one cycle of *cisplatin* (152).

The study showed a significant improvement in 2-year disease-free survival for the chemotherapy arm, 58% versus 46% ($p < 0.01$). At 60 months, and adjusting for stage, 55% of chemotherapy patients were predicted to be alive compared to 42% of patients receiving radiation. Chemotherapy was also more toxic and probably contributed to the deaths of eight patients (4%) compared to five (2%) on the radiation arm. In the chemotherapy arm, distant failure was reduced from 18% to 10%, but there was no difference in pelvic or abdominal failure rates in the two arms.

In a nonrandomized study of 180 patients with surgically staged III and IV endometrial cancer treated with WAR with pelvic, plus or minus paraaortic boost, the GOG reported 3-year recurrence-free survival rates of 29% for endometrial and 27% for serous and clear cell carcinomas, respectively (153). No patient with gross residual disease survived. Severe toxicity included bone marrow depression in 12.6%, gastrointestinal toxicity in 15%, and hepatic toxicity in 2.2% of patients.

The group at Duke University reported on 356 patients with advanced stage endometrial cancer. Postoperatively, whole-abdominal radiation alone was used in 48% ($n = 171$), chemotherapy alone in 29% ($n = 102$), and chemotherapy plus radiation in 23% ($n = 83$) of patients. After adjusting for age, grade stage, and debulking status, there was a significant survival benefit for combined therapy compared to either modality used alone (154).

A retrospective view of 86 patients from the University of Minnesota with peritoneal spread of endometrial carcinoma reported a recurrence rate of only 16% for patients with stage IIIA disease and only one peritoneal site of spread after treatment with WAR (155). Six percent of patients required surgical intervention for small-bowel obstruction.

Martinez and colleagues reported 10-year survival data on a nonrandomized, prospective trial of whole-abdominal radiation with a pelvic boost in patients with stages I to III endometrial cancer who were considered at high risk for intraabdominopelvic recurrence (156). There were 132 patients treated between 1981 and 2001, including 89 (68%) with stage III disease and 58 (45%) with serous papillary or clear cell histology. The 5- and 10-year cause-specific survival for patients with serous papillary or clear cell tumors was 80% and 74%, respectively. Chronic grade 3 or 4 gastrointestinal toxicity was seen in 14% of patients, and 2% developed grade 3 renal toxicity.

The above **studies suggest an advantage to combining radiation with chemotherapy in patients with advanced-stage endometrial cancer,** but we would still consider using whole-abdominal radiation in the circumstances shown in Table 10.21.

Table 10.21 Indications for Whole-Abdominal Radiation in Patients with Endometrial Cancer

1. Patients with endometrioid, serous papillary, or clear cell carcinomas and omental, adnexal, or peritoneal metastases that have been completely excised

2. Patients with serous papillary or clear cell carcinomas with positive peritoneal washings

Adjuvant *Progestins*

Although the role of *progestins* in the management of patients with advanced and recurrent endometrial cancer has been established, they have not been shown to be of value in an adjuvant setting (157–160). In a randomized study of 1,148 patients with clinical stage I or II endometrial cancer at the Norwegian Radium Hospital, death resulting from intercurrent disease, particularly cardiovascular disease, was actually more common in the *progesterone*-treated group ($p = 0.04$) (159). In 461 high-risk patients, a tendency toward fewer cancer-related deaths and a better disease-free survival rate in the treatment group was observed, but crude survival was unchanged. It was concluded that further studies were needed in high-risk patients but that the evidence suggested that prophylactic *progestin* therapy was not likely to be a cost-effective approach for patients with endometrial cancer unless the patient had a high-risk, receptor-positive tumor.

An Australian, New Zealand, and United Kingdom trial of 1,012 patients with high-risk disease showed more relapses in the control group, but no difference in survival (160). Patients received *medroxyprogesterone acetate* 200 mg twice daily for at least 3 years or until recurrence. Steroid receptor status had no influence on outcome in either arm.

Adjuvant Chemotherapy

The value of adjuvant systemic therapy in patients with high-risk early stage endometrial cancer is still controversial.

Four randomized trials have been conducted that evaluated the efficacy of chemotherapy in the adjuvant setting. The oldest trial (GOG 34), using single-agent *doxorubicin,* did not show any benefit in a study of 192 patients with clinical stage I or II (occult) disease who had one or more risk factors for recurrence after surgical staging (161). Maggi et al. conducted a randomized controlled trial in 345 high-risk endometrial cancer patients comparing 5 cycles of *cisplatin, doxorubicin,* and *cyclophosphamide* with external pelvic radiation. In a multivariate analysis, the researchers reported no difference between therapies in terms of progression-free or overall survival (162).

A Japanese multicenter randomized trial compared whole-pelvic irradiation (WPI) with three or more cycles of *cyclophosphamide, doxorubicin,* and *cisplatin* (CAP) chemotherapy in 385 evaluable patients with stages IC to IIIC endometrioid adenocarcinoma ("intermediate risk"; 60% stage IC, 15% grade 3) (163). At a median follow-up of 5 years, there were no significant differences in progression-free (WPI 83.5%.5 vs. CAP 81.8%) or overall survival (85.3% vs. 86.7%). In a subgroup analysis of "high to intermediate risk" cases [stage IC >70 yrs; stage IC grade 3; stage II or stage IIIA (cytology), $n = 120$], a survival benefit for CAP was suggested (163).

Hogberg et al. presented the results of a European trial of radiation alone *versus* adjuvant chemotherapy before or after radiation in 382 patients with stage I, II, IIIA (positive peritoneal cytology only), or IIIC disease who had high-risk factors for recurrence (one or more of deep myometrial invasion, nondiploid DNA, or serous, clear cell, grade 3, anaplastic histology) (164). Chemotherapy was not standardized and could be *doxorubicin* and *platinum* (AP); *paclitaxel, doxorubicin,* and *platinum* (TAP); *paclitaxel* and *platinum* (TP); or *paclitaxel, cisplatin,* and *epirubicin.* The study suggested an improvement in progression-free survival with chemotherapy (7% improvement at 5 years, $p = 0.03$), but survival data were too early to draw any conclusions (164).

These data reinforce the need for adequately powered trials with a single adjuvant chemotherapy treatment in endometrial cancer. Increased pelvic relapse rates have been reported when using adjuvant chemotherapy alone in patients with high-risk or advanced stage disease. The recently opened PORTEC 3 study is a phase III randomized trial comparing chemoradiation and adjuvant chemotherapy with pelvic radiation in patients with high-risk endometrial cancer, and it should establish the role, if any, of concurrent chemoradiation and adjuvant chemotherapy.

Clinical Stage II

When both the cervix and the endometrium are clinically involved with adenocarcinoma, it may be difficult to distinguish between a stage IB adenocarcinoma of the cervix and a stage II endometrial carcinoma. Histopathologic evaluation is not helpful in the differentiation of these two conditions, and the diagnosis must be based on clinical and epidemiologic features. The obese, elderly woman with a bulky uterus is more likely to have endometrial cancer, whereas the younger woman with a bulky cervix and a normal corpus is more likely to have cervical cancer.

The lack of randomized, prospective studies precludes dogmatic statements about the optimal mode of therapy, but modern management favors primary surgery, with adjuvant radiation tailored to the surgical findings.

A large retrospective Italian study reported on 203 patients who underwent primary surgery for stage II endometrial cancer (165). Simple hysterectomy was performed in 135 patients (66%) and radical hysterectomy in 68 (34%). Adjuvant radiation was given to 66 of 111 patients (59%) with stage IIA disease and to 67 of 92 patients (73%) with stage IIB. Survival rates were 79% in the simple hysterectomy group and 94% in the radical hysterectomy group at 5 years, and 74% and 94% at 10 years, respectively ($p = 0.05$). Although adjuvant radiation reduced locoregional recurrence, there was no significant difference in survival.

Surveillance, Epidemiology, and End Results data were used in the United States to determine whether primary treatment with simple or radical hysterectomy, with or without adjuvant radiation, altered disease-related survival for patients with FIGO stage II endometrial cancer (166). Cases diagnosed between 1988 and 1994 were analyzed, and included 555 patients (60%) undergoing simple hysterectomy and 377 patients (40%) undergoing radical hysterectomy. The 5-year cumulative survival rates for patients who received surgery alone was 84.4% with simple hysterectomy and 93% with radical hysterectomy ($p = 0.05$). There was no significant survival difference for adjuvant radiation versus no radiation in either arm. **The researchers concluded that radical hysterectomy was associated with better survival when compared with simple hysterectomy for FIGO stage II corpus adenocarcinoma.**

A multicenter study from the United States evaluated 162 patients with surgical stage II endometrial cancer (167). An extrafascial hysterectomy was performed in 75% of patients and a radical hysterectomy in 25%. At least ten nodes were removed in more than 90% of cases. **A significantly better 5-year disease-free survival was seen in patients undergoing radical hysterectomy** (94%) compared with extrafascial hysterectomy (76%) ($p = 0.05$). **Adjuvant radiation did not improve survival.**

Our current approach to patients with stage II endometrial carcinoma is to perform primary surgery and surgical staging, provided the patient is medically fit.

The surgery is as follows:

1. modified (type II) radical hysterectomy
2. bilateral salpingo-oophorectomy
3. peritoneal washings for cytologic study
4. pelvic lymphadenectomy to the aortic bifurcation
5. resection of grossly enlarged paraaortic nodes
6. omental biopsy
7. biopsy of any suspicious peritoneal nodules

Postoperatively, adjuvant radiation is individualized. If lymph nodes are negative, then no adjuvant radiation is given. Patients with one nodal micrometastases in the pelvis receive external pelvic radiation, whereas those with multiple positive pelvic nodes or grossly positive pelvic nodes are given extended-field, external-beam therapy. Patients with upper abdominal disease have cytoreductive surgery.

Surgical Stage IIIA

Patients with stage IIIA endometrial cancer include those with positive peritoneal washings, those with tumor involving the uterine serosa, and those with disease involving the tubes or ovaries. All macroscopic disease can be removed in these patients. Patients with endometrioid histology and positive washings only have a favorable prognosis, with or without adjuvant therapy (168). Adjuvant chemotherapy with or without pelvic radiation is appropriate when the disease involves the adnexae or uterine serosa.

Surgical Stage IIIB

The only study specifically of patients with surgical FIGO stage IIIB endometrial cancer was reported by Nicklin and Petersen in 2000 (169). Isolated vaginal metastases are very uncommon, and only 14 patients (0.7%) could be identified out of 1,940 patients with endometrial cancer treated at the Queensland Centre for Gynaecological Cancer from January 1982 to December

1996. None of the 14 patients in the study had pelvic or paraaortic lymph node dissection, so many may have been upstaged to IIIC had this been done. **Survival was similar to patients with stage IIIC disease,** and the authors concluded that a case could be made to abolish this substage and include these patients with those currently classified as having stage IIIC disease.

Surgical Stage IVA

Endometrial cancer extending only into the bladder or rectal mucosa is very uncommon. In the latest FIGO annual report, only 49 of 7,990 patients (0.6%) with endometrial cancer had stage IVA disease (5). Treatment must be individualized but would require some type of modified pelvic exenteration, with or without pelvic radiation or chemotherapy.

Surgical Stage IVB

Stage IVB endometrial carcinoma is uncommon, and results of therapy are in general poor. However, an occasional patient is seen with a well-differentiated adenocarcinoma that has metastasized because of prolonged patient or physician delay or because cervical stenosis has prevented the appearance of abnormal bleeding. Such tumors usually contain ER and PR, and prolonged survival may occur with *progestin* therapy before or after total abdominal hysterectomy, bilateral salpingo-oophorectomy, and possibly radiation therapy.

In a series of 83 patients reported by Aalders et al. (170) from the Norwegian Radium Hospital, the lung was the main site of extrapelvic spread, with 36% of patients having lung metastases. **Treatment of stage IV disease must be individualized but usually involves a combination of surgery, radiation therapy, or chemotherapy.**

There may be a role for cytoreductive surgery, although data are limited to small, retrospective studies. The largest series, from workers in Baltimore, reported results from 65 patients with stage IVB endometrial cancer. Optimal cytoreduction, defined as residual tumor 1 cm diameter, was accomplished in 36 patients (55.4%), whereas 29 patients (44.6%) underwent suboptimal resection (171). Median survival was 34 months in the optimal group compared with 11 months in the suboptimal group ($p = 0.0001$). Patients with no macroscopic residual disease had a median survival of 40.6 months. Similar results have been reported from the Netherlands in a smaller series (172).

In making a decision to undertake primary surgery in a patient with advanced endometrial cancer, both the location and the extent of metastatic disease must be taken in account. In the study by Goff and colleagues, factors that influenced a decision not to undertake cytoreductive surgery included the presence of lung metastases, bladder invasion, clinical involvement of the pelvic sidewall, bone metastases, and liver metastases (173).

A major objective of therapy should be to try to achieve local disease control in the pelvis and to palliate bleeding, discharge, pain, and fistula formation.

Hormonal therapy and chemotherapy for patients with advanced and recurrent endometrial cancer is discussed later in the chapter.

Special Clinical Circumstances

Endometrial Cancer Diagnosed after Hysterectomy

This situation is best avoided by the appropriate investigation of any abnormal vaginal bleeding preoperatively and by routinely opening the excised uterus in the operating room so that the adnexae can be removed and appropriate staging performed if unsuspected endometrial cancer is discovered.

When the diagnosis is made during the postoperative period, the following investigations are recommended:

1. a PET or CT scan of the chest, pelvis, and abdomen
2. a serum CA125 measurement

If the CA125 level is elevated or if the PET or CT scan reveals lymphadenopathy or other evidence of metastatic disease, then laparotomy is usually indicated.

If all investigations are negative, then our approach is as follows.

1. Grade 1 or 2 endometrioid lesions with less than one-half myometrial invasion: no further treatment, although laparoscopic prophylactic oophorectomy is advisable

because of the risk of subsequent ovarian cancer. This is particularly important if there is any family history of breast, ovarian, or colon cancer (Lynch II syndrome).

2. All other lesions: further laparotomy with removal of adnexae, surgical staging, and appropriate postoperative radiation.

Synchronous Primary Tumors in the Endometrium and Ovary

This uncommon circumstance occurs much more commonly in young women (174). In at least half of the cases, both endometrial and ovarian tumors are of the endometrioid type, and distinguishing between primary and metastatic lesions may be difficult.

Israeli workers reported that 62% of cases with simultaneous tumors of the endometrium and ovary could be differentiated from metastatic tumors by distinct immunohistochemical expression of ER and PR ($p = 0.0006$), and 32% could be differentiated by distinct immunostaining for *bcl-2* ($p = 0.03$) (175).

The Gynecologic Oncology Group reported 74 cases, 23 (31%) of whom had microscopic spread of tumor in the pelvis or abdomen (103). Sixty-four patients (86%) had endometrioid tumors in both sites, and endometriosis was found in the ovary in 23 patients (31%). Patients with tumor confined to the uterus and ovary had a 10% probability of recurrence within 5 years, compared with a 27% probability for those with metastatic disease ($p = 0.006$). Similarly, patients with no more than grade I disease at either site had an 8% probability of recurrence within 5 years, compared with a 22% probability for those with a higher grade in either the ovary or the endometrium ($p = 0.05$).

Treatment should be determined on the premise that each represents a primary lesion and many require surgery only without adjuvant chemotherapy or radiation (176).

Endometrial Carcinomas in Young Women

Approximately 5% of endometrial cancers occur in women aged 40 years or younger. The majority are associated with a history of chronic anovulation and are usually well-differentiated tumors. A minority occur in association with the hereditary nonpolyposis colorectal cancer syndrome in which case a more variable histologic spectrum occurs (177). **Adenocarcinomas of the endometrium occasionally occur in very young women (30 years of age or younger), usually in association with the polycystic ovarian syndrome. Approximately 90% of the lesions are well differentiated and limited to the endometrium** (178).

Fertility preservation is often a concern for these young women, and several small series have reported **regression of the carcinoma in approximately 80% of cases with a variety of progestins** (179–183). An MRI is desirable pretreatment to exclude significant myometrial invasion, and **the tumors should have grade 1 histology and be PR positive.** In spite of successful conservative management, only some 40% of these patients will carry a successful pregnancy.

A 3-month trial of *megestrol acetate* orally 160 to 320 mg/day or *medroxyprogesterone acetate* 200 to 500 mg/day is the usual approach. Using *megestrol acetate*, Gotlieb and colleagues reported a complete response in all 13 patients treated, within a mean period of 3.5 months. Six patients (46%) recurred 19 to 358 months later, four of whom responded to a second course of *progestins* (179). Taiwanese workers reported complete remission in eight of nine patients (89%) using a combination of ***megestrol acetate*** and ***tamoxifen*** (180). One patient failed to respond but achieved complete remission after a change from *tamoxifen* to a gonadotropin-releasing hormone analogue. Four (50%) of the responders later developed recurrent endometrial cancer.

Adequate imaging of the ovaries is important before any decision is made regarding conservative management. In our review of 254 patients with endometrial cancer at the Royal Hospital for Women in Sydney, synchronous ovarian malignancies were found in five of 17 patients (29.4%) younger than 45 years of age compared with 11 of 237 patients (4.6%) older than 45 ($p < 0.001$). Three other younger patients (17.7%) had secondary ovarian involvement (174). In a series of 102 women aged 24 to 45 years who underwent hysterectomy for endometrial cancer in Los Angeles, 26 (25%) were found to have a coexisting epithelial ovarian tumor; 23 were classified as synchronous primaries, and three were metastases (184).

In the combined series (179–183), **approximately 40% of patients who initially respond will recur.** Therefore, **it is reasonable to recommend hysterectomy once childbearing has been completed to avoid the need for ongoing hormonal manipulation and surveillance with transvaginal ultrasonography.** Given the significant incidence of ovarian involvement

(174,184) and the efficacy of modern hormonal therapy, there seems **little justification for ovarian preservation, unless for psychological reasons.**

Endometrial Carcinoma after Endometrial Ablation

With increasing use of endometrial ablation as an alternative to hysterectomy for some women with dysfunctional uterine bleeding unresponsive to hormonal therapy, there have been several reports of the subsequent development of endometrial cancer.

Valle and Baggish (185) reviewed eight case reports and cautioned about the need for proper patient selection. They recommended that all patients should have a preablation biopsy showing a normal endometrium and that patients with persistent hyperplasia unresponsive to hormonal therapy should be recommended for hysterectomy. They also suggested that if endometrial ablation is performed in high-risk patients because of medical contraindications to laparotomy, then vigorous follow-up, including periodic ultrasonography and endometrial sampling, is required. Hysteroscopy with biopsies of the endometrium should be done if bleeding occurs.

Follow-Up

Follow-up after management of endometrial cancer should be negotiated with the patient, but our own policy is to alternate visits with the referring gynecologist. Visits are scheduled every 3 months for the first year, every 4 months for the second year, and every 6 months until 5 years. **Approximately 10% of recurrences occur beyond 5 years** (186), so patients should be told to report early with any abnormal bleeding or other symptoms.

Surveillance gives valuable psychological support to patients and allows accurate collection of data. At each visit, a relevant history should be taken, and any suspicious symptoms investigated appropriately. We do not perform any routine radiological studies, but **a vault smear is important to perform on all women who have not had adjuvant radiation.** Bristow and colleagues reported that routine vaginal cytology detected an asymptomatic isolated vault recurrence in only two of 377 patients (0.5%), and that it was not cost effective (187). However, most of their patients had received postoperative radiation and would not benefit from early detection of vault recurrence.

Recurrent Endometrial Cancer

According to figures reported in the *26th Annual Report on the Results of Treatment in Gynecological Cancer,* approximately 22% of patients treated for endometrial cancer die within 5 years (5) (Table 10.17).

Serum CA125 levels are usually elevated in patients with recurrent disease, particularly if the recurrence is intraperitoneal (188). Pastner et al. (189) reported that none of six patients with an isolated vaginal recurrence had elevated levels, but false positive values may occur in the presence of severe radiation injury of the bowel.

The large series of 379 patients with recurrent disease reported by Aalders et al. (186) from the Norwegian Radium Hospital provides some important information, although management protocols have changed somewhat since that report (190). Local recurrence was found in 50% of the patients, distant metastases in 29%, and simultaneous local and distant metastases in 21%. The median time from primary treatment to detection of recurrence was 14 months for patients with local recurrence and 19 months for those with distant metastases. **Thirty-four percent of all recurrences were detected within 1 year and 76% within 3 years of primary treatment.** At the time of diagnosis, 32% of all patients were free of symptoms, and the diagnosis was made on routine physical or radiologic examination. For patients with local recurrence, 36% were free of symptoms, 37% had vaginal bleeding, and 16% had pelvic pain.

Isolated Vaginal Recurrence

Isolated vaginal metastases are the most amenable to therapy with curative intent. Before undertaking treatment for an apparent localized recurrence, a PET or CT scan should be obtained to exclude systematic spread.

In the Danish endometrial cancer study in which low-risk patients were followed without radiation, 17 vaginal recurrences were reported, and 15 of these **(88.2%) were salvaged with radiation therapy.** By contrast, none of seven pelvic recurrences was salvaged (132).

A multiinstitutional study in the United States identified 69 patients with surgical stage I endometrial cancer who were treated without adjuvant radiation and developed an isolated vaginal recurrence (135). Of these, ten (15%) were diagnosed initially with stage IA disease. Histologically, 22 patients (32%) had grade 1 disease, 26 (38%) had grade 2, and 21 (30%) had grade 3. **Radiation therapy salvaged 81% of the patients,** although 18% died from a subsequent recurrence.

A five-year disease-free survival of 68% for 50 patients was reported from St. Louis with a low rate of complications. Median time to recurrence was 25 months (range 4 to 179 months) (190). On multivariate analysis, age, histologic grade, and size of recurrence were significant predictors of overall survival. All patients who had grade 3 disease were dead by 3.6 years from the time of recurrence.

High-dose-rate brachytherapy usually combined with external-beam therapy, has been reported in a series of 22 patients from Canada (191). After a median follow-up of 32 months, all patients had locoregional control. One developed a distant metastasis and died from disease.

For bulky lesions (>4 cm diameter), surgical resection before radiation may improve local control. Laparotomy has the advantage of allowing a thorough exploration of the pelvis and abdomen to exclude other metastatic foci.

If the patient has had prior pelvic radiation, exploratory laparotomy with a view to some type of pelvic exenteration, offers the only possibility for cure.

Systematic Recurrence: Role of Surgery

Surgery—usually combined with radiation, chemotherapy, or hormonal therapy—may play a role in selected patients with recurrent endometrial cancer, particularly if all residual disease can be resected.

A study of 35 patients undergoing salvage cytoreductive surgery at Johns Hopkins Medical Center reported complete cytoreduction in 23 patients (66%) (192). These patients had a median survival of 39 months compared to 13.5 months for patients with gross residual disease. **On multivariate analysis, salvage surgery and residual disease status were significant and independent predictors of postrecurrence survival.** Similar conclusions were drawn from a smaller series of patients from Memorial Sloan-Kettering Cancer Center (193).

Patients with a long disease-free interval (>2 years) and an isolated recurrence at any site (e.g., lungs, liver, or lymph nodes) should be considered for surgical resection as long as the patient is medically fit and the surgery is technically feasible.

Role of Hormonal Therapy

Progestational agents have been used successfully as treatment for patients with advanced or recurrent endometrial cancer. Although parenteral administration has been used, oral administration is equally effective (194,195).

The Gynecologic Oncology Group randomized 299 patients with advanced or recurrent endometrial cancer to receive either 200 mg per day or 1,000 mg per day of oral *medroxyprogesterone acetate* (196). Among 145 patients receiving the low-dose regimen, there were 25 complete (17%) and 11 partial (8%) responses, for an overall response rate of 25%. For the 154 patients receiving the high-dose regimen, there were 14 complete (9%) and 10 partial (6%) responses, for an overall response rate of 15%. Median survival durations were 11.1 months and 7.0 months, respectively, for the low-dose and high-dose regimens.

The GOG concluded that 200 mg per day of MPA was a reasonable initial approach to the treatment of advanced or recurrent endometrial cancer, particularly for patients whose tumors were well differentiated or PR positive. Patients with poorly differentiated or PR negative tumors had only an 8% to 9% response rate (196).

If an objective response is obtained, then the progestogen should be continued indefinitely. Some responses may be sustained for several years. Side effects from *progestins* are usually minor and include weight gain, edema, thrombophlebitis, headache, and occasionally hypertension. There is an increased risk of thromboembolism.

The nonsteroidal antiestrogen *tamoxifen* has also been used to treat patients with recurrent endometrial cancer. It is a first-generation selective estrogen response modulator (SERM) and inhibits the binding of estradiol to uterine ER, presumably blocking the proliferative stimulus of circulating estrogens. **Responses are usually seen in patients who have previously responded to *progestins,*** but an occasional response may occur in a patient who is unresponsive to them (197,198). *Tamoxifen* may be administered orally in a dose of 10 to 20 mg twice daily and continued for as long as the disease is responding. In a review of the literature, Moore et al. (199) reported a pooled response rate of 22% for single-agent *tamoxifen.*

The third-generation SERM *arzoxifene* has been evaluated in 29 patients with advanced or recurrent endometrial cancer (200). The drug was administered orally in a dose of 20 mg per day, and toxicity was minimal. There were nine responses (31%) and a median duration of response of 13.9 months, the longest reported in a phase II trial of this patient population. *Arzoxifene* **warrants further evaluation for patients with advanced and recurrent endometrial cancer.**

Role of Cytotoxic Chemotherapy

Cytotoxic chemotherapy for endometrial cancer is given with palliative intent, and responses are generally of short duration. Many women with endometrial cancer are elderly and have other comorbidities such as obesity, diabetes mellitus, and cardiovascular disease. They may have had pelvic radiation, which can limit hematological reserve. All of these factors have to be taken into consideration when making treatment recommendations, but **chemotherapy should be considered in patients with a good performance status.**

The most active drugs are the *platinum* agents, *taxanes*, and *anthracyclines*. Response rates are in the order of 30%, but the duration of response is usually only measured in months (201–204).

The response to second-line therapy is generally poor. The best response rates are with *taxanes*, and the GOG has reported *paclitaxel* to have a 35% response rate in previously untreated women (205) and a 27% response rate in previously treated patients. In the latter group, the median duration of response was 4.2 months, and the median overall survival was 10.3 months. *Topotectan* was also studied as a second-line agent by the GOG, but the response rate was only 9% (206).

There have been a number of randomized trials of combination versus single agent chemotherapy, and there have two recent systematic reviews of chemotherapy for metastatic endometrial cancer. Both concluded that **combination chemotherapy with *doxorubicin* and *cisplatin* resulted in higher response rates than *doxorubicin* alone** (207,208). The combination was associated with response rates in the order of 40% with progression-free survivals of 5 to 7 months. The addition of *paclitaxel* to either of the above regimens resulted in a higher response rate (57% versus 37%) and a small survival advantage. However, the toxicity is excessive, and there have been a number of treatment-related deaths (209).

The combination of *carboplatin* and *paclitaxel* has been evaluated in a nonrandomzed setting, and response rates as high as 67%, with 29% complete responses, have been reported. Toxicity is acceptable, the median progression-free survival has been as high as 14 months, and overall survival has been approximately 26 months (210,211). **This regimen is commonly used in the community to treat patients with metastatic endometrial cancer.** The GOG is comparing *carboplatin* and *paclitaxel* with *paclitaxel, doxorubicin,* and *cisplatin* (TAP), and the results of this study will be important for the further development of chemotherapy for endometrial cancer.

Recently, the GOG reported the results of a randomized, phase III trial of whole-abdominal radiation versus *doxorubicin–cisplatin* in advanced endometrial cancer (152). To be eligible, the maximum size of residual disease had to be 2 cm diameter, and there were 388 evaluable patients. There was a significantly better progression-free and overall survival in the chemotherapy arm, but approximately 55% of all patients recurred.

Newer targeted treatments are also being investigated, including *sorafenib* and *bevacizumab,* as well as *traztusumab* in HER-2 amplified tumors (15% to 30% of serous and high-grade endometrial cancers have evidence of amplification). One of the most active new agents (*temsirolimus*) is directed against the mammalian target of rapamycin (mTOR), and a response rate of 26% has been reported in chemonaive patients (212).

Uterine papillary serous carcinomas are histologically similar to ovarian serous tumors, but the reported response rate to *cisplatin*-containing combination chemotherapy has been inconsistent, with some studies suggesting a lower response (213). However, there are data to suggest high response rates to *carboplatin* or *cisplatin* and *paclitaxel*. Rodriguez et al. (214) reported a complete response in three of 13 patients (23%) and a partial response in eight of 13 (62%) to various *platinum* combinations, including *cisplatin* or *paclitaxel* in three patients. Median duration of response was 7.5 months (range 1 to 30 months).

Our experience at the Royal Hospital for Women would justify further study of *platinum*-based chemotherapy in patients with serous endometrial carcinomas (215). All six patients with stages I or II disease given adjuvant *platinum*-based chemotherapy were tumor free with a mean follow-up of 31.6 months (range 12 to 68 months) and four of 12 (33%) with stages III to IV disease remained tumor free with a mean follow-up of 22.5 months.

There have been a number of similar retrospective phase II reports (216–218). Kelly et al. studied 75 patients with stage I serous carcinomas and reported that *platinum*-based chemotherapy improved both disease-free and overall survival (216). They concluded that patients with stage IA disease could be observed but recommended concomitant *platinum*-based chemotherapy and vaginal vault radiation for all other patients with stage I disease.

The impact of adjuvant chemotherapy in patients with uterine serous papillary carcinomas should be clarified by the PORTEC 3 study, which is in progress.

Hormone-Replacement Therapy

Particularly for younger women, hormone-replacement therapy is an important issue after treatment for endometrial cancer. **Patients with stage I disease have a good prognosis, and protection against osteoporosis and quality of life issues are important.** Although it has been frequently stated that estrogen-replacement therapy is contraindicated in patients who have had endometrial cancer, Creasman et al. (219) have challenged this concept. In a nonrandomized study, they reported no deleterious effect from estrogen given to 47 patients with stage I endometrial cancer compared with 174 patients with similar risk factors who did not receive estrogen. In fact, the estrogen group experienced a significantly longer disease-free survival.

Our practice is to offer patients daily conjugated estrogens (*Premarin*) 0.625 mg or *tibilone* (*Livial*).

Prognosis

Although individual institutions may report superior results, the most comprehensive survival data are provided in the *Annual Report on the Results of Treatment in Gynecological Cancer*. Survival by FIGO surgical stage for the years 1999 through 2001 are shown in Table 10.22. Survival by histological grade is shown in Table 10.23. The significance of histologic grade is highlighted by the fact that **patients with stage II, grade 1 and 2 tumors have a better prognosis than patients with stage I, grade 3 lesions.**

Survival in relation to grade and depth of myometrial invasion for stage I disease is shown in Table 10.24, and the poor prognosis associated with papillary serous and clear cell carcinomas is shown in Table 10.25.

Table 10.22 Carcinoma of the Corpus Uteri: Patients Treated from 1999 to 2001; Survival Rates by FIGO Surgical Stage ($n = 7,990$)

Strata	Patients	Overall Survival (%)		
		1-Year	3-Year	5-Year
IA	1,054	98.2	95.3	90.8
IB	2,833	98.7	94.6	91.1
IC	1,426	97.5	89.7	85.4
IIA	430	95.2	89.0	83.3
IIB	543	93.5	80.3	74.2
IIIA	612	89.0	73.3	66.2
IIIB	80	73.5	56.7	49.9
IIIC	356	89.9	66.3	57.3
IVA	49	63.4	34.4	25.5
IVB	206	59.5	29.0	20.1

Modified from the **26th Annual Report on the Results of Treatment in Gynecological Cancer** (5).

Table 10.23 Carcinoma of the Corpus Uteri: Patients Treated from 1999 to 2001; Survival Rates for Surgical Stages I and II by Histologic Grade

| | Overall 5-Year Survival Rates (%) | | | |
| | Stage I | | Stage II | |
Grade	No.	Percent	No.	Percent
1	2,373	92.9	267	86.0
2	2,014	89.9	444	82.1
3	708	78.9	208	66.0

Modified from *the 26th Annual Report on the Results of Treatment in Gynecological Cancer* (5).

Table 10.24 Carcinoma of the Corpus Uteri: Patients Treated from 1999 to 2001; Survival Rates in Stage I by Surgical Stage and Grade of Differentiation ($n = 5,095$)

| | | Overall Survival Rates (%) | | |
Strata	Patients	1-Year	3-Year	5-Year
IA G_1	627	98.9	97.7	93.4
IB G_1	1,113	99.2	94.9	91.6
IC G_1	441	98.6	93.9	90.6
IA G_2	253	98.8	95.0	91.3
IB G_2	1,305	98.8	96.2	93.4
IC G_2	648	98.0	90.7	86.3
IA G_3	107	94.2	83.5	79.5
IB G_3	328	97.2	88.1	82.0
IC G_3	273	95.5	80.0	74.9

Modified from *the 26th Annual Report on the Results of Treatment in Gynecological Cancer* (5).

Table 10.25 Carcinoma of the Corpus Uteri: Patients Treated from 1999 to 2001; Survival Rates by Histologic Type ($n = 8,033$)

Histologic Type	No.	5-Year Survival Rate (%)
Endometrioid	6,735	83.2
Adenosquamous	338	80.6
Mucinous	80	77.0
Clear cell	173	62.5
Papillary serous	323	52.6
Squamous	25	68.9

Modified from *the 26th Annual Report on the Results of Treatment in Gynecological Cancer* (5).

Uterine Sarcomas

Uterine sarcomas are rare mesodermal tumors that account for approximately 3% of uterine cancers (220). They are a heterogeneous group of tumors, and thus individual experience with each lesion is limited. **The main lesions are leiomyosarcomas, carcinosarcomas, and endometrial stromal sarcomas,** the first two tumors having a higher incidence in black women in the United States (221). Treatment protocols are not standardized, and there are few controlled studies evaluating different therapeutic approaches. Most subgroups behave in an aggressive manner and have a poor prognosis, with high rates of local recurrence and distant metastases (222).

Pelvic radiation is thought to predispose to the subsequent development of uterine sarcomas (223). Zelmanowicz et al. (224) reported that endometrial carcinomas and malignant mixed müllerian tumors have a similar risk factor profile, which is compatible with the hypothesis that the pathogenesis of these two tumors is similar.

Criteria for the histopathological classification of sarcomas has been changing, and such lesions should be reviewed by an expert gynecologic pathologist. **Much less emphasis is placed on mitotic counts than was previously the case.**

Classification

Mesodermal derivatives from which sarcomas may arise include uterine smooth muscle, endometrial stroma, and blood and lymphatic vessel walls. Uterine sarcomas can be divided basically into two types:

1. **pure,** in which only malignant mesodermal elements are present (e.g., leiomyosarcoma and endometrial stromal sarcomas)

2. **mixed,** in which malignant mesodermal and malignant epithelial elements are present (e.g., carcinosarcoma)

They also may be subdivided into **homologous** and **heterologous** tumors, depending on whether the malignant mesodermal elements are normally present in the uterus. Malignant smooth muscle and stroma represent homologous elements, whereas malignant striated muscle and cartilage represent heterologous elements.

Staging

There is a new FIGO staging system for Uterine Sarcomas (Table 10.26) on page 667. More accurate prognostic information is obtained by surgical staging, particularly for carcinosarcomas.

Smooth Muscle Tumors

Leiomyosarcomas, which must be distinguished from the cellular leiomyomas and atypical leiomyomas (see Chapter 5), occur most commonly in the 45- to 55-year age group and account for approximately 30% of uterine sarcomas. In the SEER study of 1,396 patients, the median age of the patients was 52 years (225).

Leiomyosarcomas usually arise *de novo* **from uterine smooth muscle, although rarely they may arise in a preexisting leiomyoma.** A subset of myomas with a deletion of a specific portion of chromosome 1 has both a specific cellular morphology and a genetic-transcription profile similar to those of leiomyosarcomas. Thus **cytogenetics may** help identify these exceptions to the rule, and **allow prediction of malignant progression** (226). A review of 1,432 patients undergoing hysterectomy for presumed fibroids at the University of Southern California revealed leiomyosarcoma in the hysterectomy specimens in ten patients (0.7%). The incidence increased steadily from the fourth to the seventh decades of life (0.2%, 0.9%, 1.4%, and 1.7%, respectively) (227).

Most leiomyosarcomas are accompanied by pain, a sensation of pressure, abnormal uterine bleeding, or a lower abdominal mass. **Rapid enlargement of a fibroid is a possible sign of malignancy.** A few patients may have signs of metastatic disease such as a persistent cough, back pain, or ascites. On physical examination, it is impossible to distinguish leiomyosarcomas from large leiomyomas or from other uterine sarcomas. Pap smears are unrewarding, and uterine curettings are diagnostic for only the 10% to 20% of tumors that are submucosal (228). Diagnosis usually is not made before surgery.

Intravenous leiomyomatosis is a rare, relatively benign uterine smooth muscle tumor in which much of the tumor is present in (and may arise from) veins (229). It may extend as rubbery cords beyond the uterus into the parametrium or occasionally into the vena cava. Some patients may survive for prolonged periods in spite of incomplete resection of diseased tissue. High levels of ER and PR are present in some tumors, and regression may occur after menopause.

Leiomyomatosis peritonealis disseminata is a condition in which numerous nodules of histologically benign smooth muscle are present on peritoneal surfaces (230). It is frequently associated with a term pregnancy or with the use of oral contraceptives, and regression may occur after termination of pregnancy.

Benign metastasizing leiomyoma is a rare disorder characterized by a histologically benign smooth muscle tumor that originates in the uterus and spreads elsewhere, usually to the lungs. Controversy exists regarding whether lung lesions represent metastases of a benign uterine primary tumor or synchronous or metachronous development of an independent lung lesion. Optimal therapy is also unclear, but surgical resection and hormonal therapy are generally recommended (231).

Surgical Treatment

The only treatment of any proven curative value for the frankly malignant leiomyosarcomas is surgical excision. This typically involves total abdominal hysterectomy and bilateral salpingo-oophorectomy, although in young patients it is reasonable to preserve the ovaries, particularly if the tumor has arisen in a fibroid (232).

Lissoni et al. (233) reported eight young patients with a diagnosis of leiomyosarcoma after **myomectomy** who were followed conservatively. All were nulliparous, and all had no evidence of disease on ultrasonography, hysteroscopy, chest radiography, and pelvic and abdominal CT scan or MRI. The mean mitotic count of the leiomyosarcomas was 6 per 10 high-power field (HPF), with a range of 5 to 33. With a median follow-up of 42 months, three live births were recorded, but one patient recurred and died.

For **leiomyosarcomas** the GOG study of 59 patients reported positive lymph nodes in only 3.5% of patients, positive washings in only 5.3%, and adnexal involvement in only 3.4% (233). For 71 patients with leiomyosarcoma confined to the uterus and/or cervix, the Memorial Sloan-Kettering group reported ovarian metastases in two patients (2.8%) and lymph node metastases in none. Three of 37 patients (8.1%) with gross extrauterine disease had positive nodes, and all were clinically suspicious (234). Wu et al. reported no pelvic or paraaortic lymph node involvement in 21 patients who underwent complete surgical staging (235). The SEER study reported lymph node metastases in 23 of 348 patients (6.6%) who underwent lymphadenectomy, but performance of a lymphadenectomy was not associated with improved survival (224), because most lymph node metastases are found in patients with advanced disease.

Spread of leiomyosarcomas is mainly hematogenous, so surgical staging appears to be of less importance for these tumors.

A possible role for **secondary cytoreduction** for leiomyosarcomas was reported from the Johns Hopkins Medical Center. In a recent review of 128 patients with recurrent uterine leiomyosarcoma, researchers reported prolonged survival **in a select group who had a prolonged progression-free survival and an isolated site of recurrent disease amenable to complete resection.** Neither chemotherapy nor radiation therapy was beneficial (237).

Chemotherapy

A large study of 1,042 patients with uterine sarcomas recorded in the Cancer Registry of Norway from 1956 to 1992 reported no change in the 5-year survival rate after the introduction of chemotherapy into the treatment protocols (238).

The most active drugs include *doxorubicin, cisplatin, ifosfamide, paclitaxel, docetaxel,* and *gemcitabine.* Unfortunately, most responses are partial and of short duration.

In the GOG trials, leiomyosarcomas had a 25% (7 of 28) overall response rate to *doxorubicin* (239). *Liposomal doxorubicin (Doxil)* showed no advantage over historical results with *doxorubicin* (240). There was a 17.2% (6 of 35) partial response rate to *ifosfamide* (241) and a 3% (1 of 33) partial response rate to *cisplatin* (242). For *paclitaxel,* there were three complete responses (9%) whereas eight patients (24%) had stable disease for at least two courses of treatment (243). The combination of *gemcitabine* plus *docetaxel* demonstrated activity in patients with metastatic leiomyosarcomas, the GOG reporting objective responses in 15 of 42 patients (35.8%) overall. The complete response rate was 4.8%, and the partial response rate was 31%, with an additional 11 patients (26.2%) having stable disease (244).

The combination of *docetaxel* and *gemcitabine* has also been reported to be active as second-line therapy for patients with metastatic leiomyosarcoma. In a study of 48 patients, 90% of whom had progressed following *doxorubicin*-based chemotherapy, Hensley et al. reported a complete response in three patients (8.8%) and a partial response in 15 patients (44.1%) for an overall response of 53% (95% CI 35% to 70%) (245). An additional seven patients (20.6%) had stable disease. Fifty percent of patients who were treated previously with *doxorubicin* had a response. The median time to progression was 5.6 months.

Because of the propensity for early hematogenous spread, adjuvant chemotherapy after hysterectomy to eliminate micrometastases is an attractive concept. However, in a randomized GOG study of *doxorubicin* after total abdominal hysterectomy and bilateral salpingo-oophorectomy for stage I or II uterine sarcoma, neither survival nor progression-free interval was prolonged by the adjuvant chemotherapy (246).

A study of 27 patients from the Massachusetts General Hospital also reported that use of adjuvant chemotherapy after optimal surgery did not decrease the rate of recurrence for patients with leiomyosarcomas (247). Future studies should evaluate the use of *docetaxel* and *gemcitabine*.

Radiation Therapy

Postoperative external-beam pelvic radiation is of no proven benefit in terms of survival, although it has generally been thought to improve tumor control in the pelvis (248). However, **the recent randomized clinical trial of adjuvant external pelvic radiation versus observation for patients with nonmetastatic leiomyosarcomas revealed no benefit even in terms of local control** (249).

Summation of Management of Leiomyosarcomas

The only proven benefit for patients with leiomyosarcomas is total abdominal hysterectomy. Ovaries should normally be removed in postmenopausal women. Surgical staging appears to be of no value, and neither does adjuvant chemotherapy. These patients should be entered onto clinical trials of new therapeutic agents, particularly *docetaxel* and *gemcitabine*. Pelvic radiation appears to offer no benefits in terms of local control or survival.

Endometrial Stromal Tumors

Endometrial stromal tumors are divided into two major categories: **benign endometrial stromal nodules** and **endometrial stromal sarcomas.** The division of endometrial stromal sarcomas into low-grade and high-grade categories has fallen out of favor, and **the term *endometrial stromal sarcoma* is now considered best restricted to neoplasms that were formally referred to as "low-grade" endometrial stromal sarcomas (250). High-grade tumors** without recognizable evidence of a definite endometrial stromal phenotype are **now termed *endometrial sarcomas* (251) or *undifferentiated uterine sarcomas*.** Mitotic counts are no longer used to differentiate high-grade from low-grade lesions. **Endometrial stromal sarcomas constitute 15% to 25% of uterine sarcomas (252).**

Most patients are in the age range of 42 to 53 years. More than half the patients are premenopausal, and young women and girls may be affected. Abnormal vaginal bleeding is the most common presenting symptom, and abdominal pain and uterine enlargement may occur (253). **Although they may be intramural, most endometrial stromal sarcomas involve the endometrium, and uterine curettage usually leads to diagnosis.**

Endometrial stromal sarcomas have infiltrating margins and demonstrate venous and lymphatic invasion. Although their behavior is relatively indolent, late recurrences and distant metastases may occur (252,253). **The most frequent sites of recurrence for patients with stage I disease are the pelvis and abdomen** (252,253). Prolonged survival and even cure are not uncommon after surgical resection of recurrent or metastatic lesions.

Undiffentiated uterine sarcomas behave aggressively compared with endometrial stromal sarcomas. In the original series reported by Evans, six of the seven patients died of disease between 10 and 34 months after diagnosis (251).

Surgical Treatment

Total abdominal hysterectomy and bilateral salpingo-oophorectomy, with radical cytoreductive surgery for extrauterine involvement, has been the standard recommendation for endometrial stromal sarcomas (254).

Preservation of the ovaries may be an option for premenopausal women with stage I disease. In a multiinstitutional case-control study, Li et al. reported no differences in progression-free or overall survival when 12 premenopausal patients who did not undergo bilateral salpingo-oophorectomy were matched with 24 controls (255). Twenty-two available tumors demonstrated positivity for both estrogen and progesterone receptors.

There are limited data available on the incidence of lymph node metastases in endometrial stromal sarcomas. Goff et al. reported five low-grade and five high-grade endometrial stromal tumors, seven of which had lymph node sampling. None of the seven had positive nodes (256). Ayhan et al. reported eight cases of endometrial stromal sarcoma (two low-grade and six high-grade). Four had lymph node sampling, and none had lymph node metastases (257). Riopel et al. reported positive nodes in five of 15 patients (33%) with low-grade endometrial stromal sarcomas. In two of the five patients, nodal metastases were found years later at the time of recurrence; of the three patients who had lymph node metastases at their initial presentation, two had gross extrauterine involvement (258).

Patients with a late recurrence of an endometrial stromal sarcoma benefit from aggressive cytoreductive surgery to remove all macroscopic disease if possible.

Chemotherapy or Hormonal Therapy

Endometrial stromal sarcomas usually contain estrogen and progesterone receptors (255), and patients with advanced and recurrent disease respond well to *progestins* **or aromatase inhibitors such as** *letrozole* (259). Chu et al. reported eight patients with recurrent endometrial stromal sarcoma who were treated with *progestin* therapy. Complete responses were seen in four patients (50%), and three others (38%) had stable disease. There are many anecdotal case reports of hormonal therapy, and the responses can be very durable. There are no data to support prophylactic hormonal therapy (260)

Patients with a previous history of low-grade endometrial stromal sarcoma should not receive estrogens or *tamoxifen* (259) because there may be stimulation of growth, although the estrogen and progesterone of normally functioning ovaries does not seem to be a problem (255,260).

There are limited data on the role of systemic chemotherapy in women with endometrial stromal sarcoma. However, chemotherapy could be considered in selected patients who progress on hormonal therapy as well as those with metastatic undifferentiated endometrial sarcomas. There are anecdotal case reports of response to a variety of agents, and similar drugs to those used in carcinosarcomas would be a reasonable option. A recent report from China suggested that a **combination of** *ifosfamide, epirubicin,* and *cisplatin* **had activity in patients with undifferentiated endometrial sarcomas** (261).

Radiation Therapy

Radiation therapy is not appropriate for endometrial stromal sarcomas. It may decrease pelvic recurrence without improving survival for patients with endometrial sarcomas.

Summation of Management for Endometrial Stromal Tumors

Patients with endometrial stromal sarcomas should undergo total abdominal hysterectomy, bilateral salpingo-oophorectomy, and resection of any extrauterine disease. Preservation of ovaries is an option for premenopausal patients with stage I disease. Patients with advanced disease respond well to *progestins* or aromatase inhibitors. **Late recurrences are not infrequent, and aggressive secondary cytoreduction to remove all macroscopic disease may result in long-term survival.**

Patients with undifferentiated uterine sarcomas should undergo total abdominal hysterectomy and bilateral salpingo-oophorectomy. Pelvic radiation will decrease pelvic recurrence without improving survival.

Carcinosarcomas

Malignant mixed mesodermal tumors (MMMTs) or carcinosarcomas usually occur in an older age group, most patients being postmenopausal (234). The frankly malignant variants grow rapidly and usually are accompanied by postmenopausal bleeding, pelvic pain, a palpable lower abdominal mass, or symptoms of metastatic disease. **Most patients have an enlarged uterus, and the tumor protrudes through the cervical os like a polyp in approximately half the patients** (220). Uterine curettage usually detects malignant tissue in the uterus, although determination of the exact nature of the tumor may require histologic examination of the entire specimen.

There is now convincing evidence that most, but not all, uterine carcinosarcomas are monoclonal tumors and really metaplastic carcinomas (262). The behavior of these tumors is similar to that of high-grade endometrioid adenocarcinomas. Metastases are usually from the carcinomatous element, and the sarcomatous element is believed to be derived as a result of dedifferentiation of the carcinomatous component (263). Heterologous differentiation, including rhabdomyosarcomotous differentiation, is not uncommon in MMMTs, and occasionally pure heterologous sarcomas have been reported (264).

Surgery

Carcinosarcomas should undergo surgical staging in the same manner as high-grade endometrial carcinomas. The Gynecologic Oncology Group reported a clinicopathologic study of 301 carcinosarcomas in 1993 (234). Adnexal metastases were present in 12% of patients, lymph node metastases in 18%, and positive peritoneal washings in 21%. No omental biopsies were taken.

A Californian study of 62 patients with carcinosarcoma apparently confined to the uterus reported occult metastases in 38 patients (61%) (265). Adnexal metastases were present in 23% of patients, positive pelvic nodes in 31%, positive paraaortic nodes in 6%, omental involvement in 13%, and positive peritoneal washings in 29%.

Our experience in Sydney suggests that very good survival rates can be obtained in patients with carcinosarcomas if they are subjected to surgical staging, postoperative radiation based on the surgical findings, and adjuvant chemotherapy with *cisplatin* and *epirubicin* (266). In a study of 38 patients with disease clinically confined to the uterus, 9 patients (24%) were upstaged to III or IV. Positive lymph nodes were present in 13%, adnexal metastases in 11%, and omental metastases in 8%.

Chemotherapy

There are a number of active agents, including *cisplatin, carboplatin, anthracyclines, ifosfamide,* and *paclitaxel.* As these are relatively uncommon tumors, the studies have generally been small and patient accrual has been slow. For *cisplatin* (50 mg/m^2 every 3 weeks), the GOG reported a complete response rate of 8% and a partial response rate of 11% among 63 patients with advanced or recurrent mixed mesodermal tumors who had received no previous chemotherapy (242).

***Ifosfamide* is also an active agent for mixed mesodermal sarcomas,** the GOG demonstrating nine responses among 28 patients (31.2%) (267). A small improvement in progression-free survival was noted with the addition of *cisplatin* to *ifosfamide* in a phase III GOG trial, but the added toxicity may not justify use of this combination (268).

The GOG also evaluated *paclitaxel* in 44 patients with carcinosarcoma of the uterus. Four patients (9.1%) had a complete response, and four (9.1%) had a partial response (269).

More recently, the GOG reported the results of a randomized study comparing ***ifosfamide* alone versus *ifosfamide* and *paclitaxel*** in 179 patients with advanced uterine carcinosarcomas (270). They reported a response rate of 29% with *ifosfamide* alone and 45% with the combination. The odds of response stratified by performance status were 2.21 times greater for the combination arm ($p = 0.017$). The median progression-free and overall survivals for *ifosfamide* compared with *ifosfamide* and *paclitaxel* were 3.6 versus 5.8 months and 8.4 versus 13.5 months, respectively.

Adjuvant Chemotherapy for Early Stage Disease

In a nonrandomized study, Peters et al. (271) reported 17 patients with high-risk clinical stage I uterine stromal sarcomas or mixed mesodermal tumors who were treated with six cycles of *cisplatin* 100 mg/m^2 and *doxorubicin* 40 to 60 mg/m^2 every 3 to 4 weeks. Fourteen of the patients had invasion to the outer third of the myometrium, seven had documented lymph node metastases, and five had positive peritoneal washings. With a median follow-up of 34 months, there were only four recurrences, giving a projected 5-year survival rate of 75%.

This experience is similar to our own data from the Royal Hospital for Women (266) with *cisplatin* and *epirubicin,* together with tailored radiation based on the surgical findings.

The GOG reported an overall 5-year survival of 62% for 65 patients with completely resected clinical stage I or II disease treated with adjuvant *ifosfamide* and *cisplatin.* No postoperative radiation was given, and the authors commented that pelvic relapse remained problematic (272).

Wolfson et al. recently reported the results of a relatively large randomized clinical trial comparing whole-abdominal radiation with three cycles of *cisplatin, ifosfamide,* and *mesna* (CIM) in 201 patients with stages I to IV uterine carcinosarcomas (273). The estimated crude probability of recurring within 5 years was 58% for WAR and 52% for CIM. Adjusting for stage and age, the recurrence rate was 29% lower for patients receiving CIM. They concluded that the results of the trial favored chemotherapy although the differences were small.

Radiation

Several nonrandomized studies have suggested that **radiotherapy reduces local recurrence** (274–276). In a report of 300 patients treated at the M.D. Anderson Hospital between 1954 and 1998, Callister et al. reported that radiotherapy reduced the risk of local recurrence from 48% to 28% and prolonged the time to distant relapse but did not improve overall survival (276). **The recent EORTC randomized study of stages I and II uterine sarcomas confirmed that external pelvic radiation decreases pelvic relapse but does not improve overall survival for carcinosarcomas** (249). There were 91 patients with carcinosarcomas in the study.

Based on the limited available data, our current approach is to treat patients with negative nodes with vault brachytherapy. We give whole-pelvic radiation to patients who have had no lymph node dissection or who have one positive pelvic node and give extended-field radiation to patients with multiple positive pelvic nodes or positive paraaortic nodes.

Summation of Management of Carcinosarcomas

Current evidence would suggest that carcinosarcomas of the uterus should undergo full surgical staging and resection of any gross metastatic disease. Postoperative radiation should be tailored to the operative findings. Adjuvant chemotherapy with either *cisplatin* and *epirubicin* or an *ifosfamide*-based combination **may be beneficial** based on small phase II studies, but confirmation requires a randomized phase III trial.

Prognosis

The frankly malignant uterine sarcomas usually have a poor prognosis. Surgical stage is the most important prognostic variable, with younger age (less than 50 years) also significant in a Japanese multiinstitutional study (277).

In the Mayo study of 208 patients with leiomyosarcoma (232), the median disease-specific survival for 130 patients with stage I disease was 7.8 years, whereas it was 3.7 years for 13 patients with stage II disease, 2.3 years for 18 patients with stage III, and 1.3 years for 41 patients with stage IV. Thirty-three patients with a tumor <5 cm diameter had a median survival of more than 30 years, whereas 128 patients with tumors larger than 5 cm diameter had a median survival of 3.5 years. The significance of tumor size confirmed the findings from a large Nordic study (278). Adjuvant chemotherapy or radiation therapy did not seem to be of any benefit (232). **If the leiomyosarcoma arises in a benign fibroid, the prognosis appears to be better** (228).

A recent analysis of 1,396 leiomyosarcomas identified from the SEER database from 1988 to 2003 reported 5-year disease specific survivals of 75.8%, 60.1%, 44.9%, and 28.7% for stages I, II, III, and IV, respectively (224). Independent prognostic factors on multivariate analysis were age, race, stage, grade, and primary surgery. Oophorectomy or lymphadenectomy had no impact on survival.

For 301 mixed mesodermal tumors, the GOG reported a recurrence rate of 53% (homologous 44%; heterologous 63%) (234). Factors significantly related to progression-free interval by univariate analysis were adnexal spread, lymph node metastases, tumor size, vascular space invasion, depth of myometrial invasion, positive peritoneal washings, histologic grade, and cell type. **On multivariate analysis, the significant prognostic factors were adnexal spread, lymph node metastases, cell type, and cell grade.**

Better survivals have been reported in smaller studies, including our own, following surgical staging, tailored radiation, and adjuvant chemotherapy (266,271). A randomized trial to determine the role of adjuvant chemotherapy after surgical staging and tailored postoperative radiation would be justified.

Endometrial stromal nodules are benign but can usually only be distinguished from endometrial stromal sarcomas after hysterectomy. For younger women wishing to preserve fertility, a combination of diagnostic imaging and hysteroscopy may be useful in monitoring the growth of the lesion, and local excision has been successful in occasional cases (279).

Endometrial stromal sarcomas are relatively indolent tumors with a tendency to very late recurrence, one-third to one-half of patients recurring as many as 30 years after treatment (253,260).

Chang et al. (253) reported that for endometrial stromal sarcomas, stage and mitotic index were both independent predictors of overall and disease-free survival, but when only stage I patients were considered, mitotic index disappeared from the Cox model. These authors placed most high-grade sarcomas into the undifferentiated sarcoma category on the basis of anaplastic cells that had mitotic indices in excess of 20 per 10 HPF.

Endometrial sarcomas are highly aggressive tumors with a very poor prognosis (251). Li et al. reported a recurrence rate of 24% (9 of 37) for stage I endometrial stromal sarcomas compared to 73% (8 of 11) for endometrial sarcomas (261).

References

1. **Parazzini F, LaVecchia C, Bocciolone L, Franceschi S.** The epidemiology of endometrial cancer. *Gynecol Oncol* 1991;41:1–16.
2. **Jemal A, Siegel R, Murray T, Hao Y, Xu J, Murray T, et al.** Cancer statistics, 2009. *CA Cancer J Clin* 2009; published online. doi:10.3322/caac.20006.
3. **Madison T, Schottenfeld D, Baker V.** Cancer of the corpus uteri in white and black women in Michigan, 1985–1994. *Cancer* 1998;83:1546–1554.
4. **Prat J, Gallardo A, Cuatrecasas M, Catasus L.** Endometrial carcinoma: pathology and genetics. *Pathology* 2007;39:1–7.
5. **Creasman WT, Odicino F, Mausinneuve P, Quinn MA, Beller U, Benedet JL et al.** Carcinoma of the corpus uteri. FIGO Annual Report, Vol 26. *Int J Gynaecol Obstet* 2006;95(suppl 1):S105–S143.
6. **Pothuri B, Ramondetta L, Winton A, Alektiar K, Eifel PJ, Deavers MT, et al.** Radiation-associated endometrial cancers are prognostically unfavorable tumors: A clinicopathologic comparison with 527 sporadic endometrial cancers. *Gynecol Oncol* 2006;103:948–951.
7. **Gusberg SB, Milano C.** Detection of endometrial carcinoma and its precursors. *Cancer* 1981;47:1173–1179.
8. **DuBeshter B, Warshal DP, Angel C, Dvoretsky PM, Lin JY, Raubertas RF.** Endometrial carcinoma: the relevance of cervical cytology. *Obstet Gynecol* 1991;77:458–462.
9. **Montz FJ.** Significance of "normal" endometrial cells in cervical cytology from asymptomatic postmenopausal women receiving hormone replacement therapy. *Gynecol Oncol* 2001;81:33–39.
10. **Siebers AG, Verbeck ALM, Massuger LF, Grefte JMM, Bulten J.** Normal appearing endometrial cells in cervical smears of asymptomatic postmenopausal women have predictive value of significant endometrial pathology. *Int J Gynecol Cancer* 2006;16:1069–1074.
11. **Zucker PK, Kasdon EJ, Feldstein ML.** The validity of Pap smear parameters as predictors of endometrial pathology in menopausal women. *Cancer* 1985;56:2256–2263.
12. **Beal HN, Stone J, Beckman MJ, McAsey ME** Endometrial cells identified in cervical cytology in women > 40 years of age: criteria for appropriate endometrial evaluation. *Am J Obstet Gynecol* 2007;196:568.e1–5; discussion 568.e5–6.
13. **Moroney JW, Zahn CM, Heaton RB, Crothers B, Kendall BS, Elkas JC** Normal endometrial cells in liquid-based cervical cytology specimens in women aged 40 or older. *Gynecol Oncol* 2007;105: 672–676.
14. **Koss LG, Schreiber K, Oberlander SG, Moukhtar M, Levine HS, Moussouris HF.** Screening of asymptomatic women for endometrial cancer. *Obstet Gynecol* 1981;57:681–691.
15. **Dijkhuizen FPH, Mol BWJ, Brolmann HAM, Heintz APM.** The accuracy of endometrial sampling in the diagnosis of patients with endometrial carcinoma and hyperplasia. *Cancer* 2000;89: 1765–1772.
16. **Granberg S, Wikland M, Karlsson B.** Endometrial thickness as measured by endovaginal ultrasonography for identifying endometrial abnormality. *Am J Obstet Gynecol* 1991;164:47–52.
17. **Karlsson B, Granberg S, Wikland M, Ylöstalo P, Torvid K, Marsal K, et al.** Transvaginal ultrasonography of the endometrium in women with postmenopausal bleeding: a Nordic multicenter study. *Am J Obstet Gynecol* 1995;172:1488–1494.
18. **Tabor A, Watt HC, Wald NJ.** Endometrial thickness as a test for endometrial cancer in women with postmenopausal vaginal bleeding. *Obstet Gynecol* 2002;99:663–670.
19. **Fisher B, Constantino JP, Redmond CK, Fisher ER, Wickerham DL, Cronin WM.** Endometrial cancer in *tamoxifen*-treated breast cancer patients: findings from the National Surgical Adjuvant Breast and Bowel Project B-14. *J Natl Cancer Inst* 1994;86:527–537.
20. **Assikis VJ, Neven P, Jordan VC, Vergote I.** A realistic clinical perspective on *tamoxifen* and endometrial carcinogenesis. *Eur J Cancer* 1996;32A:1464–1476.
21. **Fung MFK, Reid A, Faught W, Le T, Chenier C, Verma S, et al.** Prospective longitudinal study of ultrasound screening for endometrial abnormalities in women with breast cancer receiving *tamoxifen*. *Gynecol Oncol* 2003;91:154–159.
22. **Gücer F, Tamussino K, Reich O, Moser F, Arikan G, Winter R.** Two-year follow-up of patients with endometrial carcinoma after preoperative fluid hysteroscopy. *Int J Gynecol Cancer* 1998;8:476–480.
23. **Obermair O, Geramou M, Gücer F, Denison U, Graf AH, Kapshammer E.** Impact of hysteroscopy on disease-free survival in clinically stage I endometrial cancer patients. *Int J Gynecol Cancer* 2000;10:275–279.
24. **Connor JP, Andrews JI, Anderson B, Buller RE.** Computed tomography in endometrial carcinoma. *Obstet Gynecol* 2000;95:692–696.
25. **Zerbe MJ, Bristow R, Grumbine FC, Montz FJ.** Inability of preoperative computed tomography scans to accurately detect the extent of myometrial invasion and extracorporal spread in endometrial cancer. *Gynecol Oncol* 2000;78:67–70.
26. **Hricak H, Rubinstein LV, Gherman GM, Karstaedt N.** MR imaging evaluation of endometrial carcinoma: results of an NCI cooperative study. *Radiology* 1991;179:829–834.
27. **Chung HH, Kang S-B, Cho JY, Kim JW, Park N-H, Song Y-S, et al.** Accuracy of MR imaging for the prediction of myometrial invasion of endometrial carcinoma. *Gynecol Oncol* 2007;104:654–659.
28. **Nagar H, Dodds S, McClelland HR, Price J, McCluggage WG, Grey A** The diagnostic accuracy of magnetic resonance imaging in detecting cervical involvement in endometrial cancer. *Gynecol Oncol* 2006;103:431–434.
29. **Suzuki R, Miyagi E, Takahashi N, Sukegawa A, Suzuki A, Koike I, et al.** Validity of positron emission tomography using fluro-2-deoxyglucose for the preoperative evaluation of endometrial cancer. *Int J Gynecol Cancer* 2007;17:890–896.
30. **Jhang H, Chuang L, Visintainer P, Ramaswamy G.** CA125 levels in the preoperative assessment of advanced stage uterine cancer. *Am J Obstet Gynecol* 2003;188:1195–1197.
31. **Boronow RC, Morrow CP, Creasman WT, DiSaia PJ, Silverberg SG, Miller A, et al.** Surgical staging in endometrial cancer: clinico-pathologic findings of a prospective study. *Obstet Gynecol* 1984;63:825–832.
32. **Creasman WT, Morrow CP, Bundy BN, Homesley HD, Graham JE, Heller PB.** Surgical pathologic spread patterns of endometrial cancer. *Cancer* 1987;60:2035–2041.
33. **Chan JK, Cheung MK, Huh WK, Osann K, Husain A, Teng N, et al.** Therapeutic role of lymph node resection in endometrioid corpus cancer. *Cancer* 2006;107:1823–1830.
34. **Bigelow B, Vekshtein V, Demopoulos RI.** Endometrial carcinoma, stage II: route and extent of spread to the cervix. *Obstet Gynecol* 1983;62:363–366.
35. **Truskett ID, Constable WC.** Management of carcinoma of the corpus uteri. *Am J Obstet Gynecol* 1968;101:689–694.
36. **Mariani A, Dowdy SC, Keeney GL, Haddock MG, Lesnick TG, Podratz KC** Predictors of vaginal relapse in stage I endometrial cancer. *Gynecol Oncol* 2005;97:820–827.
37. **Zaino RJ, Kurman RJ, Diana KL, Morrow CP.** Prognostic models to predict outcome for women with endometrial adenocarcinoma. *Cancer* 1996;77:1115–1121.
38. **Lee NK, Cheung MK, Shin JY, Husain A, Teng NN, Berek JS, et al.** Prognostic factors for uterine cancer in reproductive-aged women. *Obstet Gynecol* 2007;109:655–662.

39. Nakanishi T, Ishikawa H, Suzuki Y, Inove T, Nakamura S, Kuzuya K. Association between menopausal state and prognosis of endometrial cancer. *Int J Gynecol Cancer* 2001;11:483–487.

40. Wilson TD, Podratz KC, Gaffey TA, Malkasian GD, O'Brien PC, Naessens JM. Evaluation of unfavourable histologic subtypes in endometrial adenocarcinoma. *Am J Obstet Gynecol* 1990;162:418–426.

41. Zaino RJ, Kurman R, Herbold D, Gliedman J, Bundy BN, Voet R, et al. The significance of squamous differentiation in endometrial carcinoma. *Cancer* 1991;68:2293–2302.

42. Sherman ME, Bitterman P, Rosenshein NB, Delgado G, Kurman RJ. Uterine serous carcinoma. *Am J Surg Pathol* 1992;16:600–610.

43. Sakuragi N, Hareyama H, Todo Y, Yamada H, Yamamoto R, Fujino T. Prognostic significance of serous and clear cell adenocarcinoma in surgically staged endometrial carcinoma. *Acta Obstet Gynecol Scand* 2000;79:311–316.

44. Hamilton CA, Cheung MK, Osann K, Chen L, Teng NN, Longacre TA, et al. Uterine papillary serous and clear cell carcinomas predict for poorer survival compared to grade 3 endometrioid corpus cancers. *Brit J Cancer* 2006;94:642–646.

45. Sherman ME, Bur ME, Kurman RJ. *P53* in endometrial carcinoma and its putative precursors: evidence for diverse pathways for tumorigenesis. *Hum Pathol* 1995;26:1268–1274.

46. Christopherson WM, Alberhasky RG, Connelly PJ. Carcinoma of the endometrium: I. a clinicopathologic study of clear cell carcinoma and secretory carcinoma. *Cancer* 1982;49:1511–1516.

47. Abeler VM, Vergote IB, Kjorstad KE, Trope CG. Clear cell carcinoma of the endometrium. *Cancer* 1996;78:1740–1747.

48. Aquino-Parsons C, Lim P, Wong F, Mildenberger M. Papillary serous and clear cell carcinoma limited to endometrial curettings in FIGO stage Ia and Ib endometrial adenocarcinoma: treatment implications. *Gynecol Oncol* 1998;71:83–86.

49. Abeler VM, Kjorstad KE. Endometrial squamous cell carcinoma: report of three cases and review of the literature. *Gynecol Oncol* 1990;36:321–325.

50. DiSaia PJ, Creasman WT, Boronow RC, Blessing JA. Risk factors and recurrent patterns in stage I endometrial cancer. *Am J Obstet Gynecol* 1985;151:1009–1015.

51. Aalders J, Abeler V, Kolstad P, Onsrud M. Postoperative external irradiation and prognostic parameters in stage I endometrial carcinoma. *Obstet Gynecol* 1980;56:419–424.

52. Abeler VM, Kjorstad KE, Berle E. Carcinoma of the endometrium in Norway: a histopathological and prognostic survey of a total population. *Int J Gynecol Cancer* 1992;2:9–22.

53. Cohn D, Horowitz N, Mutch D, Kim S, Manolitsas T, Fowler J. Should the presence of lymphvascular space involvement be used to assign patients to adjuvant therapy following hysterectomy for unstaged endometrial cancer? *Gynecol Oncol* 2002;87:249–252.

54. Watari H, Todo Y, Takeda M, Ebina Y, Yamamoto R, Sakuragi N. Lymph-vascular space invasion and number of positive paraaortic node groups predict survival in node positive patients with endometrial cancer. *Gynecol Oncol* 2005;96:651–657.

55. Hanson MB, van Nagell JR Jr, Powell DE, Donaldson ES, Gallion H, Merhige M, et al. The prognostic significance of lymphvascular space invasion in stage I endometrial cancer. *Cancer* 1985;55:1753–1757.

56. Ambros RA, Kurman RJ. Identification of patients with stage I uterine endometrioid adenocarcinoma at high risk of recurrence by DNA ploidy, myometrial invasion, and vascular invasion. *Gynecol Oncol* 1992;45:235–240.

57. Lurain JR. The significance of positive peritoneal cytology in endometrial cancer. *Gynecol Oncol* 1992;46:143–147.

58. Harouny VR, Sutton GP, Clark SA, Geisler HE, Stehman FB, Ehrlich CE. The importance of peritoneal cytology in endometrial carcinoma. *Obstet Gynecol* 1988;72:394–398.

59. Hirai Y, Fujimoto I, Yamauchi K, Hasumi K, Masubuchi K, Sano Y. Peritoneal fluid cytology and prognosis in patients with endometrial carcinoma. *Obstet Gynecol* 1989;73:335–338.

60. Lurain JR, Rumsey NK, Schink JC, Wallemark CB, Chmiel JS. Prognostic significance of positive peritoneal cytology in clinical stage I adenocarcinoma of the endometrium. *Obstet Gynecol* 1989;74:175–179.

61. Takeshima N, Nishida H, Tabata T, Hirai Y, Hasumi K. Positive peritoneal cytology in endometrial cancer: enhancement of other prognostic indicators. *Gynecol Oncol* 2001;82:470–473.

62. Kadar N, Homesley HD, Malfetano JH. Positive peritoneal cytology is an adverse factor in endometrial carcinoma only if there is other evidence of extrauterine disease. *Gynecol Oncol* 1992;46:145–150.

63. Morrow CP, Bundy BN, Kurman RJ, Creasman WT, Heller P, Homesley HD, et al. Relationship between surgical-pathologic risk factors and outcome in clinical stage I and II carcinoma of the endometrium: a Gynecologic Oncology Group study. *Gynecol Oncol* 1991;40:55–65.

64. Milosevic MF, Dembo AJ, Thomas GM. The clinical significance of malignant peritoneal cytology in stage I endometrial carcinoma. *Int J Gynecol Cancer* 1992;2:225–235.

65. Hirai Y, Takeshima N, Kato T, Hasumi K. Malignant potential of positive peritoneal cytology in endometrial cancer. *Obstet Gynecol* 2001;97:725–728.

66. Grimshaw RN, Tupper WC, Fraser RC, Tompkins MG, Jeffrey JF. Prognostic value of peritoneal cytology in endometrial cancer. *Gynecol Oncol* 1990;36:97–100.

67. Kasamatsu T, Onda T, Katsumata N, Sawada H, Yamada T, Tsunematsu R, et al. Prognostic significance of positive peritoneal cytology in endometrial carcinoma confined to the uterus. *Brit J Cancer* 2003;88:245–250.

68. Tebeu P-M, Popowski Y, Verkooijen HM, Bouchardy C, Ludicke F, Usel M, et al. Positive peritoneal cytology in early-stage endometrial cancer does not influence prognosis. *Brit J Cancer* 2004;91:720–724.

69. Havrilesky LJ, Cragan JM, Calingaert B, Alvarez Secord A, Valea FA, Clarke-Pearson DL, et al. The prognostic significance of positive peritoneal cytology and adnexal/serosal metastasis in stage IIIA endometrial cancer. *Gynecol Oncol* 2007;104:401–405.

70. Saga Y, Imai M, Jobo T, Kuramoto H, Takahashi K, Konno R, et al. Is peritoneal cytology a prognostic factor of endometrial cancer confined to the uterus. *Gynecol Oncol* 2006;103:277–280.

71. Ehrlich CE, Young PCM, Stehman FB, Sutton GP, Alford WM. Steroid receptors and clinical outcome in patients with adenocarcinoma of the endometrium. *Am J Obstet Gynecol* 1988;158:796–807.

72. Liao BS, Twiggs LB, Leung BS, Yu WCY, Potish RA, Prem KA. Cytoplasmic estrogen and progesterone receptors as prognostic parameters in primary endometrial carcinoma. *Obstet Gynecol* 1986;67:463–467.

73. Creasman WT, Soper JT, McCarty KS Jr, McCarty KS Sr, Hinshaw W, Clarke-Pearson DL. Influence of cytoplasmic steroid receptor content on prognosis of early stage endometrial carcinoma. *Am J Obstet Gynecol* 1985;151:922–932.

74. Zaino RJ, Satyaswaroop PG, Mortel R. The relationship of histologic and histochemical parameters to progesterone receptor status in endometrial adenocarcinomas. *Gynecol Oncol* 1983;16:196–208.

75. Palmer DC, Muir IM, Alexander AI, Cauchi M, Bennett RC, Quinn MA. The prognostic importance of steroid receptors in endometrial carcinoma. *Obstet Gynecol* 1988;72:388–393.

76. Geisinger KR, Homesley HD, Morgan TM, Kute TE, Marshall RB. Endometrial adenocarcinoma: a multiparameter clinicopathologic analysis including DNA profile and the sex steroid hormone receptors. *Cancer* 1986;58:1518–1525.

77. Christopherson WM, Connelly PJ, Alberhasky RC. Carcinoma of the endometrium: V. an analysis of prognosticators in patients with favorable subtypes and stage I disease. *Cancer* 1983;51:1705–1710.

78. Nielson AL, Thomsen HK, Nyholm HCJ. Evaluation of the reproducibility of the revised 1988 International Federation of Gynecology and Obstetrics grading system of endometrial cancers with special emphasis on nuclear grading. *Cancer* 1991;68:2303–2309.

79. Schink JC, Lurain JR, Wallemark CB, Chmiel JS. Tumor size in endometrial cancer: a prognostic factor for lymph node metastasis. *Obstet Gynecol* 1987;70:216–219.

80. Larson DM, Berg R, Shaw G, Krawisz BR. Prognostic significance of DNA ploidy in endometrial cancer. *Gynecol Oncol* 1999;74:356–360.

81. Susini T, Amunni G, Molino C, Carriero C, Rapi S, Branconi F, et al. Ten-year results of a prospective study on the prognostic role of ploidy in endometrial carcinoma. *Cancer* 2007;109:882–890.

82. Zaino RJ, Davis ATL, Ohlsson-Wilhelm BM, Brunetto VL. DNA content is an independent prognostic indicator in endometrial adenocarcinoma. *Int J Gynecol Pathol* 1998;17:312–319.

83. Athanassiadou P, Athanassiades P, Grapsa D, Gonida M, Athanassiadou AM, Stamati PN, et al. The prognostic value of *PTEN, p53,* and *beta-catenin* in endometrial carcinoma: a prospective immunocytochemical study. *Int J Gynecol Cancer* 2007;17:697–704.

84. Di Nezza LA, Misajon A, Zhang J, Jobling T, Quinn MA, Ostör AG, et al. Presence of active gelatinases in endometrial carcinoma and correlation of matrix metalloproteinase expression with increasing tumor grade and invasion. *Cancer* 2002;94:1466–1475.

85. Sakuragi N, Ohkouchi T, Hareyama H, Ikeda K, Watari H, Fujimoto M, et al. Bcl-2 expression and prognosis of patients with endometrial carcinoma. *Int J Cancer* 1998;79:153–158.

86. Salvesen H, Iversen OE, Akslen LA. Prognostic significance of angiogenesis and Ki-67, *p53,* and p21 expression: a population-based endometrial carcinoma study. *J Clin Oncol* 1999;17:1382–1390.

87. Grigsby PW, Perez CA, Camel HM, Galakatos AE. Stage II carcinoma of the endometrium: results of therapy and prognostic factors. *Int J Radiat Oncol Biol Phys* 1985;11:1915–1921.

88. Nahhas WA, Whitney CW, Stryker JA, Curry SL, Chung CK, Mortel R. Stage II endometrial carcinoma. *Gynecol Oncol* 1980; 10:303–311.

89. Gusberg SB, Kaplan AL. Precursors of corpus cancer: IV. adenomatous hyperplasia as stage 0 carcinoma of the endometrium. *Am J Obstet Gynecol* 1963;87:662–668.

90. Vellios F. Endometrial hyperplasias, precursors of endometrial carcinoma. *Pathol Annu* 1972;7:201–229.

91. Kurman RJ, Kaminski PF, Norris HJ. The behavior of endometrial hyperplasia: a long-term study of "untreated" hyperplasia in 170 patients. *Cancer* 1985;56:403–412.

92. Ferenczy A, Gelfand MM, Tzipris F. The cytodynamics of endometrial hyperplasia and carcinoma: a review. *Ann Pathol* 1983; 3:189–201.

93. Ferenczy A, Gelfand M. The biologic significance of cytologic atypia in *progestin*-treated endometrial hyperplasia. *Am J Obstet Gynecol* 1989;160:126–131.

94. Zaino RJ, Kauderer J, Trimble CL, Silverberg SG, Curtin JP, Lim PC, et al. Reproducibility of the diagnosis of atypical hyperplasia. A GOG study. *Cancer* 2006;106:804–811.

95. Trimble CL, Kauderer J, Zaino R, Silverberg S, Lim PC, Burke JJ 2nd, et al. Concurrent endometrial carcinoma in women with a biopsy diagnosis of atypical endometrial hyperplasia. A GOG study. *Cancer* 2006;106:812–819.

96. Marsden DE, Hacker NF. The classification, diagnosis and management of endometrial hyperplasia. *Reviews in Gynecol Practice* 2003;3:89–97.

97. Vereide AB, Kaino T, Sager G, Arnes M, Orbo A. Effect of *levonorgestrel* IUD and oral *medroxyprogesterone acetate* on glandular and stromal progesterone receptors (PRA and PRB) and estrogen receptors (ER-alpha and ER- beta) in human endometrial hyperplasia. *Gynecol Oncol,* 2006; 101:214–223.

98. Soh E, Sato K. Clinical effects of *danazol* on endometrial hyperplasia in menopausal and postmenopausal women. *Cancer* 1990;66: 983–988.

99. Perez-Medina T, Bajo J, Falgueira G, Haya J, Ortega P. Atypical hyperplasia treatment with *progestins* and gonadotropin releasing hormone analogues: long term follow up. *Gynecol Oncol* 1999;73: 299–304.

100. Keys HM, Roberts JA, Brunetto VL, Zaino R, Spirtos NM, Bloss JD, et al. A phase III randomized trial of surgery with or without adjunctive external pelvic radiation therapy in intermediate risk endometrial adenocarcinoma: a Gynecologic Oncology Group study. *Gynecol Oncol* 2004;92:744–751.

101. Creutzberg CL, van Putten WLJ, Koper PCM, Lybeert MLM, Jobsen JJ, Wárlám-Rodenhuis CC, et al. for the PORTEC Study Group. *Lancet* 2000;355:1404–1411.

102. Look K. Stage I–II endometrial adenocarcinoma-evolution of therapeutic paradigms: the role of surgery and adjuvant radiation. *Int J Gynecol Cancer* 2002;12:237–249.

103. Zaino R, Whitney C, Brady MF, DeGeest K, Burger RA, Buller RE. Simultaneously detected endometrial and ovarian carcinomas—a prospective clinicopathologic study of 74 cases: a Gynecologic Oncology Group study. *Gynecol Oncol* 2001;83:355–362.

104. Obermair A, Geramou M, Gücer F, Denison U, Kapshammer E, Medl M, et al. Endometrial cancer: accuracy of the finding of a well differentiated tumor at dilatation and curettage compared to the findings at subsequent hysterectomy. *Int J Gynecol Cancer* 1999;9: 383–386.

105. Petersen RW, Quinlivan JA, Casper GR, Nicklin JL. Endometrial adenocarcinoma–presenting pathology is a poor guide to surgical management. *Aust N Z J Obstet Gynaecol* 2000;40:191–194.

106. Goff BA, Rice LW. Assessment of depth of myometrial invasion in endometrial adenocarcinoma. *Gynecol Oncol* 1990;38:46–48.

107. Franchi M, Ghezzi F, Melpignano M, Cherchi PL, Scarabelli C, Apolloni C, Zanaboni F. Clinical value of intraoperative gross examination in endometrial cancer. *Gynecol Oncol* 2000;76:357–361.

108. Fanning J, Tsukada Y, Piver MS. Intraoperative frozen section diagnosis of depth of myometrial invasion in endometrial adenocarcinoma. *Gynecol Oncol* 1990;37:47–50.

109. Boronow RC. Endometrial cancer and lymph node sampling: short on science and common sense, long on cost and hazard. *J Pelvic Surg* 2001;7:187–190.

110. Chan JK, Urban R, Cheung MK, Shin JY, Husain A, Teng NN, et al. Lymphadenectomy in endometrioid uterine cancer staging. How many nodes are enough? A study of 11,443 patients. *Cancer* 2007;109:2454–2460.

111. Lutman CV, Havrilesky LJ, Cragun JM, Secord AA, Calingaert B, Berchuck A, et al. Pelvic lymph node count is an important prognostic variable for FIGO stage I and II endometrial carcinoma with high-risk histology. *Gynecol Oncol* 2006;102:92–97.

112. Mariani A, Dowdy SC, Cliby WA, Haddock MG, Keeney GL, Lesnick TG, et al. Efficacy of systematic lymphadenectomy and adjuvant radiotherapy in node-positive endometrial cancer patients. *Gynecol Oncol* 2006;10:200–208.

113. Fujimoto T, Nanjyo H, Nakamura A, Yokoyama Y, Takano T, Shoji T, et al. Paraaortic lymphadenectomy may improve disease-related survival in patients with multipositive pelvic lymph node stage IIIC endometrial cancer. *Gynecol Oncol* 2007;107:253–259.

114. Ryan M, Stainton C, Slaytor EK, Jaconelli C, Watts S, Mackenzie P. Aetiology and prevalence of lower limb lymphoedema following treatment for gynaecological cancer. *Aust N Z J Obstet Gynaecol* 2003;143:148–151.

115. Nomura H, Aoki D, Suzuki N, Susumu N, Suzuki A, Tamada Y, et al. Analysis of clinicopathologic factors predicting paraaortic lymph node metastasis in endometrial cancer. *Int J Gynecol Cancer* 2006;16:799–804.

116. Saygili U, Kavaz S, Altunyurt S, Uslu T, Koyuncuoglu M, Erten O. Omentectomy, peritoneal biopsy and appendectomy in patients with clinical stage I endometrial carcinoma. *Int J Gynecol Cancer* 2001; 11:471–474.

117. Morton DL, Wen DR, Wong JH, Economou JS, Cagk LA, Storm FR et al. Technical details of intraoperative lymphatic mapping for early stage melanoma. *Arch Surg* 1992;127:392–399.

118. Pelosi E, Arena V, Baudino B, Bello M, Gargiulo T, Giusti M, et al. Preliminary study of sentinel node identification using 99mTc colloid and blue dye in patients. *Tumori* 2002;88:S9–S10.

119. Barranger E, Cortez A, Grahek D, Callard P, Uzan S, Darai E. Laparoscopic sentinel node procedure using a combination of patent blue and radiocolloid in women with endometrial cancer. *Annals Surg Onc* 2004;11:334–349.

120. Lelièvre L, Camatte S, Le Frere-Belda MA, Kerrou K, Froissart M, Taurelle R, et al. Sentinel lymph node biopsy in cervical and endometrial cancers: a feasibility study. *Bull Cancer* 2004;91:379–384. French.

121. Niikura H, Okamura C, Utsunomiya H, Yoshinaga K, Akahira J, Ito K, et al. Sentinel lymph node detection in patients with endometrial cancer. *Gynecol Oncol* 2004;92:660–674.

122. Maccauro M, Lucignani G, Aliberti G, Villano C, Castellani MR, Solima E, et al. Sentinel lymph node detection following the hysteroscopic peritumoural injection of 99mTc-labelled albumen nanocolloid in endometrial cancer. *European J of Nuclear Medicine and Molecular Imaging* 2005;32:569–574.

123. Delaloye JF, Pampallona S, Chardonnens E, Fiche M, Lehr HA, De Grandi P, et al. Intraoperative lymphatic mapping and sentinel node biopsy using hysteroscopy in patients with endometrial cancer. *Gynecol Oncol* 2007;106:89–93.

124. Lopes LAF, Nicolau SM, Baracat FF, Baracat EC, Goncalves WJ, Santos HVB. Sentinel lymph node in endometrial cancer. *Int J Gynecol Cancer* 2007;17:1113–1117.

125. Frumovitz M, Bodurka DC, Broaddus RR, Coleman RL, Sood AK, Gershenson DM, et al. Lymphatic mapping and sentinel node biopsy in women with high-risk endometrial cancer. *Gynecol Oncol* 2007;104:100–103.

126. Kilgore LC, Partridge EE, Alvarez RD, Austin JM, Shingleton HM, Noojin F 3rd, et al. Adenocarcinoma of the endometrium: survival comparisons of patients with and without pelvic node sampling. *Gynecol Oncol* 1995;56:29–33.

127. The writing committee on behalf of the ASTEC study group. Efficacy of systematic pelvic lymphadenectomy in endometrial cancer (MRC ASTEC trial): a randomized study Lancet 2009;373:125–36.

128. Peters WA 3rd, Andersen WA, Thornton N Jr, Morley GW. The selective use of vaginal hysterectomy in the management of adenocarcinoma of the endometrium. *Am J Obstet Gynecol* 1983;146:285–289.

129. Susini T, Massi G, Amunni G, Carriero C, Marchionni M, Toddei G, et al. Vaginal hysterectomy and abdominal hysterectomy for treatment of endometrial cancer in the elderly. *Gynecol Oncol* 2005;96:362–367.

130. Carey MS, O'Connell GJ, Johanson CR, Goodyear MD, Murphy KJ, Daya DM, et al. Good outcome associated with a standardized treatment protocol using selective postoperative radiation in patients with clinical stage I adenocarcinoma of the endometrium. *Gynecol Oncol* 1995;57:138–144.

131. Elliot P, Green D, Coats A, Krieger M, Russell P, Coppleson M, et al. The efficacy of postoperative vaginal irradiation in preventing vaginal recurrence in endometrial cancer. *Int J Gynecol Cancer* 1994;4:84–93.

132. Poulsen HK, Jacobsen M, Bertelsen K, Andersen JE, Ahrons S, Bock J, et al. Adjuvant radiation therapy is not necessary in the management of endometrial carcinoma stage I, low-risk cases. *Int J Gynecol Cancer* 1996;6:38–43.

133. Fanning J, Evans MC, Peters AJ, Samuel M, Harmon ER, Bates JS. Adjuvant radiotherapy for stage I, grade 2 endometrial adenocarcinoma and adenoacanthoma with limited myometrial invasion. *Obstet Gynecol* 1987;70:920–922.

134. Ackerman I, Malone S, Thomas G, Franssen E, Balogh J, Dembo A. Endometrial carcinoma: relative effectiveness of adjuvant radiation vs therapy reserved for relapse. *Gynecol Oncol* 1996;60:177–183.

135. Huh WK, Straughn JM Jr, Mariani A, Podratz KC, Havrilesky LJ, Alvarez-Secord A, et al. Salvage of isolated vaginal recurrences in women with surgical stage I endometrial cancer: a multiinstitutional experience. *Int J Gynecol Cancer* 2007;17:886–889.

136. Lachance JA, Stukenborg GJ, Schneider BF, Rice LW, Jazaeri AA. A cost-effective analysis of adjuvant therapies for the treatment of stage I endometrial adenocarcinoma. *Gynecol Oncol* 2008:108:77–83.

137. COSA-NZ-UK Endometrial Cancer Study Groups. Pelvic lymphadenectomy in high-risk endometrial cancer. *Int J Gynecol Cancer* 1996;6:102–107.

138. Orr JW, Holimon JL, Orr PF. Stage I corpus cancer: is teletherapy necessary. *Am J Obstet Gynecol* 1997;176:777–789.

139. Mohan DS, Samuels MA, Selim MA, Shalodi AD, Ellis RJ, Samuels JR, et al. Long-term outcomes of therapeutic pelvic lymphadenectomy for stage I endometrial adenocarcinoma. *Gynecol Oncol* 1998;70:165–171.

140. Ng TY, Perrin LC, Nicklin JL, Cheuk R, Crandon AJ. Local recurrence in high-risk node-negative stage I endometrial carcinoma treated with postoperative vaginal vault brachytherapy. *Gynecol Oncol* 2000;79:490–494.

141. Fanning J. Long term survival of intermediate risk endometrial cancer (stage IG3, IC, II) treated with full lymphadenectomy and brachytherapy without teletherapy. *Gynecol Oncol* 2001;82:371–374.

142. Seago DP, Raman A, Lele S. Potential benefit of lymphadenectomy for the treatment of node-negative locally advanced uterine cancers. *Gynecol Oncol* 2001;83: 282–285.

143. Horowitz NS, Peters WA, Smith MR, Drescher CW, Atwood M, Mate TP. Adjuvant high dose rate vaginal brachytherapy as treatment of stage I and II endometrial cancer. *Obstet Gynecol* 2002;99:235–240.

144. Jolly S, Vargas C, Kumar T, Weiner S, Brabbins D, Chen P, et al. Vaginal brachytherapy alone: an alternative to adjuvant whole pelvis radiation for early stage endometrial cancer. *Gynecol Oncol* 2005;97:887–892.

145. Solhjem MC, Petersen IA, Haddock MG. Vaginal brachytherapy alone is sufficient adjuvant treatment of surgical stage I endometrial cancer. *Int J Radiation Oncol Biol Phys* 2005;62:1379–84.

146. Scholten AN, van Putten WLJ, Beerman H, Smit VTH, Koper PCM, Lybeert MLM, et al. Postoperative radiotherapy for stage I endometrial carcinoma: long term outcome of the randomized PORTEC trial with central pathology review. *Int J Radiation Oncol Biol Phys* 2005;63:834–838.

147. Johnson N, Cornes P. Survival and recurrent disease after postoperative radiotherapy for early endometrial cancer: systematic review and metaanalysis. *Brit J Obstet Gynaecol* 2007;114:1313–1320.

148. Weiss MF, Connell PP, Waggoner S, Rotmensch J, Mundt AJ. External pelvic radiation therapy in stage IC endometrial carcinoma. *Obstet Gynecol* 1999;93:599–602.

149. Komaki R, Cox JD, Hartz A, Wilson JF, Greenberg M. Influence of preoperative irradiation on failures of endometrial carcinoma with high risk of lymph node metastases. *Am J Clin Oncol* 1984;7:661–668.

150. McMeekin DS, Lashbrook D, Gold M, Scribner DR, Kamelle S, Tillmanns TD, et al. Nodal distribution and its significance in FIGO stage IIIC endometrial cancer. *Gynecol Oncol* 2001;82:375–379.

151. Aalders JG, Thomas G Endometrial cancer—revisiting the importance of pelvic and paraaortic lymph nodes. *Gynecol Oncol* 2007;104:222–231.

152. Randall ME, Filiaci VL, Muss H, Spirtos NM, Manuel RS, Fowley J, et al. for the Gynecologic Oncology Group Study. Randomized phase III trial of whole-abdominal irradiation versus *doxorubicin* and *cisplatin* chemotherapy in advanced endometrial carcinoma: a Gynecologic Oncology Group Study *J Clin Oncol* 2006;24:36–44.

153. Sutton G, Axelrod JH, Bundy BN, Roy T, Homesley H, Malfetano JH, et al. Whole-abdominal radiotherapy in the adjuvant treatment of patients with stage III and IV endometrial cancer: a Gynecologic Oncology Group Study. *Gynecol Oncol* 2005;97:755–763.

154. Alvarez Secord A, Havrilesky LJ, Bae-Jump V, Chin J, Calingaert B, Bland A, et al. The role of multimodality chemotherapy and radiation in women with advanced stage endometrial cancer. *Gynecol Oncol* 2007;107:285–291.

155. Dusenbery KE, Potish RA, Gold DG, Boente MP. Utility and limitations of abdominal radiotherapy in the management of endometrial carcinomas. *Gynecol Oncol* 2005;96:635–642.

156. Martinez AA, Weiner S, Podratz K, Armin A-R, Stromberg JS, Stanhope R, et al. Improved outcome at 10 years for serous papillary/clear cell or high-risk endometrial cancer patients treated by adjuvant high-dose whole-abdominal pelvic irradiation. *Gynecol Oncol* 2003;90:537–546.

157. MacDonald RR, Thorogood J, Mason MK. A randomized trial of progestogens in the primary treatment of endometrial carcinoma. *BJOG* 1988;95:166–174.

158. Hirsch M, Lilford RJ, Jarvis GJ. Adjuvant progestogen therapy for the treatment of endometrial cancer: review and metaanalysis of published, randomized controlled trials. *Eur J Obstet Gynecol Reprod Biol* 1996;65:201–207.

159. Vergote I, Kjorstad K, Abeler V, Kolstad P. A randomized trial of adjuvant protestogen in early endometrial cancer. *Cancer* 1989;64:1011–1016.

160. COSA-NZ-UK Endometrial Cancer Study Groups. Adjuvant *medroxyprogesterone acetate* in high-risk endometrial cancer. *Int J Gynecol Cancer* 1998;8:387–391.

161. Thigpen T, Vance RB, Balducci L, Blessing J. Chemotherapy in the management of advanced or recurrent cervical and endometrial carcinoma. *Cancer* 1981;48(2 supp l):658–665.

162. Maggi R, Lissoni A, Spina F, Melpignano M, Zola P, Favalli G, et al. Adjuvant chemotherapy vs radiotherapy in high-risk endometrial carcinoma: results of a randomized trial. *Br J Cancer* 2006;95:266–71.

163. Sasumu N, Sagae S, Udagawa Y, Niwa K, Kuramoto H, Satoh S, et al. Randomized phase III trial of pelvic radiotherapy versus *cisplatin*-based combined chemotherapy in patients with intermediate

and high-risk endometrial cancer: a Japanese Gynecologic Oncology Group study. *Gynecol Oncol* 2008;108:226–233.

164. Hogberg T, Rosenberg P, Kristensen G, de Oliveira CF, de Pont Christensen R, Sorbe B, et al. A randomized phase III study on adjuvant treatment with radiation (RT) ± chemotherapy (CT) in early-stage high-risk endometrial cancer (NSGO-EC-9501/EORTC 55991). *J Clin Oncol* 2007;25(18S):5503.

165. Sartori E, Gadducci A, Landoni F, Lissoni A, Maggino T, Zola P, et al. Clinical behavior of 203 stage II endometrial cancer cases: the impact of primary surgical approach and of adjuvant radiation therapy. *Int J Gynecol Cancer* 2001;11:430–437.

166. Cornelison TL, Trimble EL, Kosary CL. SEER data, corpus uteri cancer: treatment trends versus survival for FIGO stage II, 1988–1994. *Gynecol Oncol* 1999;74:350–355.

167. Cohn DE, Woeste EM, Cacchio S, Zanagnolo VL, Havrilesky LJ, Mariani A, et al. Clinical and pathologic correlates in surgical stage II endometrial carcinoma. *Obstet Gynecol* 2007;109:1062–1067.

168. Slomovitz BM, Ramondetta LM, Lee CM, Oh JC, Eifel PJ, Jhingran A, et al. Heterogeneity of stage IIIA endometrial carcinomas: implications for adjuvant therapy. *Int J Gynecol Cancer* 2005; 15:510–516.

169. Nicklin JL, Petersen RW. Stage 3B adenocarcinoma of the endometriom: a clinicopathologic study. *Gynecol Oncol* 2000;78: 203–207.

170. Aalders J, Abeler V, Kolstad P. Stage IV endometrial carcinoma: a clinical and histopathological study of 83 patients. *Gynecol Oncol* 1984;17:75–84.

171. Bristow RE, Zerbe MJ, Rosenshein NB, Grumbine FC, Montz FJ. Stage IVB endometrial carcinoma: the role of cytoreductive surgery and determinants of survival. *Gynecol Oncol* 2000;78:85–91.

172. Van Wijk FH, Huikeshoven FJ, Abdulkadir L, Ewing PC, Burger CW. Stage III and IV endometrial cancer: a 20 year review of patients. *Int J Gynecol Cancer* 2006;16:1648–1655.

173. Goff BA, Goodman A, Muntz HG, Fuller AF Jr, Nikrui N, Rice LW. Surgical stage IV endometrial carcinoma: a study of 47 cases. *Gynecol Oncol* 1994;52:237–240.

174. Gitsch G, Hanzal E, Jensen D, Hacker NF. Endometrial cancer in premenopausal women 45 years and younger. *Obstet Gynecol* 1995; 85:504–508.

175. Halperin R, Zehavi S, Hadas E, Habler L, Bukovsky I, Schneider D. Simultaneous carcinoma of the endometrium and ovary vs endometrial carcinoma with ovarian metastases: a clinical and immunohistochemical determination. *Int J Gynecol Cancer* 2003;13: 32–37.

176. Farias-Eisner R, Nieberg RK, Berek JS. Synchronous primary neoplasms of the female reproductive tract. *Gynecol Oncol* 1989; 33:335–339.

177. Broaddus RR, Lynch HT, Chen L-M, Daniels MS, Conrad P, Munsell MF, et al. Pathologic features of endometrial carcinoma associated with HNPCC. A comparison with sporadic endometrial carcinoma. *Cancer* 2006;106:87–94.

178. Farhi DC, Nosanchuk J, Silberberg SG. Endometrial adenocarcinoma in women under 25 years of age. *Obstet Gynecol* 1986;68: 741–745.

179. Gotlieb WH, Beiner ME, Shalmon B, Korach Y, Segal Y, Zmira N, et al. Outcome of fertility-sparing treatment with *progestins* in young patients with endometrial cancer. *Obstet Gynecol* 2003;102: 718–725.

180. Wang C-B, Wang C-J, Huang H-J, Hsueh S, Chou H-H, Soong Y-K, et al. Fertility-preserving treatment in young patients with endometrial adenocarcinoma. *Cancer* 2002;94:2192–2198.

181. Yamazawa K, Hirai M, Fujito A, Nishi H, Terauchi F, Ishikura H, et al. Fertility-preserving treatment with *progestin* and pathological criteria to predict responses in young women with endometrial cancer. *Hum Reprod* 2007;22:1953–1958.

182. Niwa K, Tagami K, Lian Z, Onogi K, Mori H, Tamaya T. Outcome of fertility-preserving treatment in young women with endometrial carcinomas *BJOG* 2005;112:317–320.

183. Oda T, Yoshida M, Kimura M, Kinoshita K. Clinicopathologic study of uterine endometrial carcinoma in young women aged 40 years and younger. *Int J Gynecol Cancer* 2005;15:657–662.

184. Walsh C, Holschneider C, Hoang Y, Tieu K, Karlan B, Cass I. Coexisting ovarian malignancy in young women with endometrial cancer. *Obstet Gynecol* 2005;106:693–699.

185. Valle RF, Baggish MS. Endometrial carcinoma after endometrial ablation: high-risk factors predicting its occurrence. *Am J Obstet Gynecol* 1998;179:569–572.

186. Aalders J, Abeler V, Kolstad P. Recurrent adenocarcinoma of the endometrium: a clinical and histopathological study of 379 patients. *Gynecol Oncol* 1984;17:85–103.

187. Bristow RE, Purinton SC, Santillan A, Dias-Montes TP, Gardner GJ, Giuntoli RL 2nd. Cost effectiveness of routine vaginal cytology for endometrial cancer surveillance. *Gynecol Oncol* 2006;103: 709–713.

188. Duk JM, Aalders JG, Fleuren GJ, de Bruijn HW. CA125: a useful marker in endometrial carcinoma. *Am J Obstet Gynecol* 1986;155: 1092–1102.

189. Pastner B, Orr JW, Mann WJ. Use of serum CA125 measurement in post-treatment surveillance of early-stage endometrial carcinoma. *Am J Obstet Gynecol* 1990;162:427–429.

190. Lin LL, Grigsby PW, Powell MA, Mutch DG Definitive radiotherapy in the management of isolated vaginal recurrences of endometrial cancer. *Int J Radiation Oncol Biol Phys* 2005;63: 500–504.

191. Petignat P, Jolicoeur M, Alobaid A, Drouin P, Gauthier P, Provencher D, et al. Salvage treatment with high-dose-rate brachytherapy for isolated vaginal endometrial cancer recurrence. *Gynecol Oncol* 2006;101:445–449.

192. Bristow RE, Santillan A, Zahurak ML, Gardner GJ, Giuntoli RL 2nd, Armstrong DK. Salvage cytoreductive surgery for recurrent endometrial cancer. *Gynecol Oncol* 2006;103:281–287.

193. Awtrey CS, Cadungog MG, Leitao MM, Alektiar KM, Aghajanian C, Hummer AJ, et al. Surgical resection of recurrent endometrial cancer. *Gynecol Oncol* 2006;102:480–488.

194. Kauppila A. *Progestin* therapy of endometrial, breast and ovarian carcinoma. *Acta Obstet Gynecol Scand* 1984;63:441–447.

195. Piver MS, Barlow JJ, Lurain JR, Blumenson LE. *Medroxyprogesterone acetate* (Depo-Provera) vs *hydroxyprogesterone caproate* (Delalutin) in women with metastatic endometrial adenocarcinoma. *Cancer* 1980;45:268–272.

196. Thigpen JT, Brady MF, Alvarez RD, Adelson MD, Homesley HD, Manetta A, et al. Oral *medroxyprogesterone acetate* in the treatment of advanced or recurrent endometrial carcinoma: a dose-response study by the Gynecologic Oncology Group. *J Clin Oncol* 1999;17: 1736–1744.

197. Swenerton KD. Treatment of advanced endometrial adenocarcinoma with *tamoxifen*. *Cancer Treat Rep* 1980;64:805–810.

198. Bonte J, Ide P, Billiet G, Wynants P. *Tamoxifen* as a possible chemotherapeutic agent in endometrial adenocarcinoma. *Gynecol Oncol* 1981;11:140–161.

199. Moore TD, Phillips PH, Nerenstone SR, Cheson BD. Systemic treatment of advanced and recurrent endometrial carcinoma: current status and future directions. *J Clin Oncol* 1991;9:1071–1088.

200. McMeekin DS, Gordon A, Fowler J, Melemed A, Buller R, Burke T, et al. A phase II trial of *arzoxifene*, a selective estrogen response modulator, in patients with recurrent or advanced endometrial cancer. *Gynecol Oncol* 2003; 90: 64–69.

201. Thigpen JT, Buchsbaum HJ, Mangan C, Blessing JA. Phase II trial of *Adriamycin* in the treatment of advanced or recurrent endometrial carcinoma: a Gynecologic Oncology Group study. *Cancer Treat Rep* 1979;63:21–27.

202. Cohen CJ, Bruckner HW, Deppe G, Blessing JA, Homesley H, Lee JH, et al. Multidrug treatment of advanced and recurrent endometrial carcinoma: a Gynecologic Oncology Group study. *Obstet Gynecol* 1984;63:719–726.

203. Thigpen T, Blessing J, Homesley H, Malfetano J, DiSaia P, Yordan E. Phase III trial of *doxorubicin* ± *cisplatin* in advanced or recurrent endometrial carcinoma: a Gynecologic Oncology Group (GOG) Study. *Proc Am Soc Clin Onc* 1993;12:261(abst).

204. Ball HG, Blessing JA, Lentz SS, Mutch DG. A phase II trial of Taxol in advanced or recurrent adenocarcinoma of the endometrium: a Gynecologic Oncology Group study. *Gynecol Oncol* 1995;56: 120(abst).

205. Lincoln S, Blessing JA, Lee RB, Rocereto TF. Activity of *paclitaxel* as second-line chemotherapy in endometrial carcinoma: a Gynecologic Oncology Group study. *Gynecol Oncol* 2003;88:277–281.

206. Miller DS, Blessing JA, Lentz SS, Waggoner SE. A phase II trial of *topotecan* in patients with advanced, persistent, or recurrent

endometrial carcinoma: a Gynecologic Oncology Group study. *Gynecol Oncol* 2002;87:247–251.

207. **Carey MS, Gawlik C, Fung-Kee-Fung M, Chambers A, Oliver T.** Cancer Care Ontario Practice Guidelines Initiative. Gynecology Cancer Disease Site Group. Systematic review of systemic therapy for advanced or recurrent endometrial cancer. *Gynecol Oncol* 2006;101:158–167.

208. **Humber CE, Tierney JF, Symonds RP, Collingwood M, Kirwan J, Williams C, et al.** Chemotherapy for advanced, recurrent or metastatic endometrial cancer: a systematic review of the Cochrane collaboration. *Ann Oncol* 2007;18:409–420.

209. **Fleming GF, Brunetto VL, Cella D, Look KY, Reid GC, Munkarah AR, et al.** Phase III trial of *doxorubicin* plus *cisplatin* with or without *paclitaxel* plus filgrastim in advanced endometrial carcinoma: a Gynecologic Oncology Group Study. *J Clin Oncol* 2004;22:2159–2166.

210. **Sorbe B, Andersson H, Boman K, Rosenberg P, Kalling M.** Treatment of primary advanced and recurrent endometrial carcinoma with a combination of *carboplatin* and *paclitaxel*—long-term follow-up. *Int J Gynecol Cancer* 2008;18:803–808.

211. **Hoskins PJ, Swenerton KD, Pike JA, Wong F, Lim P, Acquino-Parsons C, et al.** *Paclitaxel* and *carboplatin* alone or with irradiation, in advanced or recurrent endometrial cancer: a phase II study *J Clin Oncol* 2001;19:4048–4053.

212. **Fleming GF.** Systemic chemotherapy for uterine carcinoma: metastatic and adjuvant. *J Clin Oncol* 2007;25:2983–2990.

213. **Levenback C, Burke TW, Silva E, Morris M, Gershenson DM, Kavanagh JJ, et al.** Uterine papillary serous carcinoma (UPSC) treated with *cisplatin, doxorubicin,* and *cyclophosphamide* (PAC). *Gynecol Oncol* 1992;46:317–321.

214. **Rodriguez M, Abdul-Karim F, Nelson B, Sommers R, Ali R, Rose PG.** *Platinum* based chemotherapy is an active compound in advanced and recurrent papillary serous carcinoma of the endometrium. *Gynecol Oncol* 1998;68:135(abst).

215. **Gitsch G, Friedlander ML, Wain GV, Hacker NF.** Uterine papillary serous carcinoma. *Cancer* 1995;75:2239–2243.

216. **Kelly MG, O'Malley DM, Hui P, McAlpine J, Yu H, Rutherford TJ, et al.** Improved survival in surgical stage I patients with uterine papillary serous carcinoma (UPSC) treated with adjuvant *platinum*-based chemotherapy. *Gynecol Oncol* 2005;98:353–359.

217. **Vaidya AP, Littell R, Krasner C, Duska LR.** Tretment of uterine papillary serous carcinoma with *platinum*-based chemotherapy and *paclitaxel*. *Int J Gynecol Cancer* 2006;16(suppl 1):267–272.

218. **Dietrich CS 3rd, Modesitt SC, DePriest PD, Ueland FR, Wilder J, Reedy MB, et al.** The efficiency of adjuvant *platinum*-based chemotherapy in stage I uterine papillary serous carconoma (UPSC). *Gynecol Oncol* 2005;99:557–563.

219. **Creasman WT, Henderson D, Hinshaw W, Clarke-Pearson DL.** Estrogen replacement therapy in the patient treated for endometrial cancer. *Obstet Gynecol* 1986;67:326–330.

220. **Zaloudek CJ, Norris HJ.** Mesenchymal tumors of the uterus. In: **Fengolio C, Wolff M, eds.** *Progress in surgical pathology,* vol. 3. New York: Masson, 1981:1–35.

221. **Brooks SE, Zhan M, Cote T, Baquet CR.** Surveillance, Epidemiology and End Results analysis of 2677 cases of uterine sarcoma 1989–1999. *Gynecol Oncol* 2004;93:204–208.

222. **Kelly K-LJ, Craighead PS** Characteristics and management of uterine sarcoma patients treated at the Tom Baker Cancer Center. *Int J Gynecol Cancer* 2005;15:132–139.

223. **Norris HJ, Taylor HB.** Postirradiation sarcomas of the uterus. *Obstet Gynecol* 1965;26:689–693.

224. **Zelmanowicz A, Hildesheim A, Sherman ME, Sturgeon SR, Kurman RJ, Barrett RJ, et al.** Evidence for a common etiology for endometrial carcinomas and malignant mixed mŸllerian tumors. *Gynecol Oncol* 1998;69:253–257.

225. **Kapp DS, Shin JY, Chan JK.** Prognostic factors and survival in 1396 patients with uterine leiomyosarcomas. Emphasis on impact of lymphadenectomy and oophorectomy. *Cancer* 2008;112:820–830.

226. **Stewart EA, Morton CC** The genetics of uterine leiomyonta. What clinicians need to know. *Obstet Gynecol* 2006;107:917–921.

227. **Leibsohn S, d'Ablaing G, Mishell DR, Schlaerth JB.** Leiomyosarcoma in a series of hysterectomies performed for presumed uterine leiomyomas. *Am J Obstet Gynecol* 1990;162:968–976.

228. **Dinh TV, Woodruff JD.** Leiomyosarcoma of the uterus. *Am J Obstet Gynecol* 1982;144:817–823.

229. **Norris HJ, Parmley T.** Mesenchymal tumors of the uterus: V. intravenous leiomyomatosis: a clinical and pathologic study of 14 cases. *Cancer* 1975;36:2164–2170.

230. **Goldberg MF, Hurt WG, Frable WJ.** Leiomyomatosis peritonealis disseminata: report of a case and review of the literature. *Obstet Gynecol* 1977;49:465–468.

231. **Wentling GK, Serin B-U, Geiger XJ, Bridges MD.** Bening metastasing leiomyoma responsive to megestrol: a case report and review of the literature. *Int J Gynecol Cancer* 2005;15:1213–1217.

232. **Giuntoli RL 2nd, Metzinger DS, DiMarco CS, Cha SS, Sloan JA, Keeney GL, et al.** Retrospective review of 208 patients with leiomyosarcoma of the uterus: prognostic indicators, surgical management, and adjuvant therapy. *Gynecol Oncol* 2003;89:460–469.

233. **Lissoni A, Cormio G, Bonazzi C, Perego P, Lomonico S, Gabriele A, Bratina G.** Fertility-sparing surgery in uterine leiomyosarcoma. *Gynecol Oncol* 1998;70:348–350.

234. **Major FJ, Blessing JA, Silverberg SG, Morrow CP, Creasman WT, Currie JL, et al.** Prognostic factors in early-stage uterine sarcoma. *Cancer* 1993;71:1702–1709.

235. **Barakat R, Leitao M, Sonoda Y, Brennan MF, Barakat RR, Chi DS.** Incidence of lymph node and ovarian metastasis in leiomyosarcoma of the uterus. *Gynecol Oncol*;91:209–212.

236. **Wu T-I, Chang T-C, Hsueh S, Hsu K-H, Chou H-H, Huang H-J, et al.** Prognostic factors and impact of adjuvant chemotherapy for uterine leiomyosarcoma. *Gynecol Oncol* 2006;100:166–172.

237. **Giuntoli RL II, Garrett-Mayer E, Bristow RE, Gostout BS.** Secondary cytoreduction in the management of recurrent uterine leiomyosarcoma. *Gynecol Oncol* 2007;106:82–88.

238. **Nordal RR, Thoresen SO.** Uterine sarcomas in Norway 1956–1992: incidence, survival and mortality. *Eur J Cancer* 1997;33:907–911.

239. **Omura GA, Major FJ, Blessing JA, Sedlacek TV, Thigpen JT, Creasman WT, et al.** A randomized study of *Adriamycin* with and without dimethyl triazenoimidazole carboxamide in advanced uterine sarcomas. *Cancer* 1983;52:626–632.

240. **Sutton G, Blessing J, Hanjani P, Kramer P.** Phase II evaluation of *liposomal doxorubicin* (*Doxil*) in recurrent or advanced leiomyosarcoma of the uterus. A GOG study. *Gynecol Oncol* 2005;96:749–752.

241. **Sutton GP, Blessing JA, Barrett RJ, McGehee R.** Phase II trial of *ifosfamide* and *mesna* in leiomyosarcoma of the uterus: a Gynecologic Oncology Group study. *Am J Obstet Gynecol* 1992;166:556–559.

242. **Thigpen JT, Blessing JA, Beecham J, Homesley H, Yordan E.** Phase II trial of *cisplatin* as first-line chemotherapy in patients with advanced or recurrent uterine sarcomas: a Gynecologic Oncology Group study. *J Clin Oncol* 1991;9:1962–1966.

243. **Sutton G, Blessing JA, Ball H.** Phase II trial of *paclitaxel* in leiomyosarcoma of the uterus: a Gynecologic Oncology Group study. *Gynecol Oncol* 1999;74:346–349.

244. **Hensley ML, Blessing JA, Mannel R.** Fixed-dose rate *gemcitabine* plus *docetaxel* as first-line therapy for metastatic uterine leiomyosarcoma: a Gynecologic Oncology Group (GOG) phase II trial. *Gynecol Oncol* 2008;109:329–334.

245. **Hensley ML, Blessing JA, DeGeest K, Abulafia O, Rose PG, Homesley HD.** Fixed-dose rate *gemcitabine* and *docetaxel* as second-line therapy for metastatic uterine leiomyosarcoma: A Gynecologic Oncology Group Phase II study. *Gynecol Oncol* 2008;109:323–328.

246. **Omura GA, Blessing JA, Major E, Silverberg S.** A randomized trial of *Adriamycin* versus no adjuvant chemotherapy in stage I and II uterine sarcomas. *J Clin Oncol* 1985;9:1240–1245.

247. **Dinh TA, Oliva EA, Fuller AF, Lee H, Goodman A.** The treatment of uterine leiomyosarcomas: results from a 10-year experience (1990–1999) at the Massachusetts General Hospital. *Gynecol Oncol* 2004;92:648–652.

248. **Knocke TH, Kucera H, Dotfler D, Pokrajac B, Potter R.** Results of post-operative radiotherapy in the treatment of sarcoma of the corpus uteri. *Cancer* 1998;83:1972–1979.

249. **Reed NS, Mangioni C, Malmström H, Scarfone G, Poveda A, Pecorelli S, et al.** Phase III randomized study to evaluate the role of adjuvant pelvic radiotherapy in the treatment of uterine sarcomas stages I and II: An European Organization for Research and

Treatment of Cancer, Gynaecological Cancer Group Study. *Eur J Cancer* 2008;44:808–818.

250. **Clement PB, Young RH.** Mesenchymal and mixed epithelial-mesenchymal tumors of the uterine corpus and cervix. In: **Clement PB, Young RH,** eds. *Atlas of gynecologic surgical pathology.* Philadelphia: WB Saunders, 2000:177–210.

251. **Evans HL.** Endometrial stromal sarcoma and poorly differentiated endometrial sarcoma. *Cancer* 1982;50:2170–2182.

252. **DeFusco PA, Gaffey TA, Malkasian GD, Long HJ, Cha SS.** Endometrial stromal sarcoma: review of Mayo Clinic experience, 1945–1980. *Gynecol Oncol* 1989;35:8–14.

253. **Chang KL, Crabtree GS, Lim-Tan SK, Kempson RL, Hendrickson MR.** Primary uterine endometrial stromal neoplasms. *Am J Surg Pathol* 1990;14:415–438.

254. **Blank SV, Mikuta JJ.** Low grade stromal sarcoma: confusion and clarification. *Postgrduate Obstet Gynecol* 2001;21:1–4.

255. **Li AJ, Giuntoli RL 2nd, Drake R, Byan SY, Rojas F, Barbuto D, et al.** Ovarian preservation in stage I low-grade endometrial stromal sarcomas. *Obstet Gynecol* 2005;106:1304–1308.

256. **Goff BA, Rice LW, Fleischhacker D, Muritz HG, Falkenberry SS, Nikrui N, et al.** Uterine leiomyosarcoma and endometrial stromal sarcoma: lymph node metastases and sites of recurrence. *Gynecol Oncol* 1993;50:105–109.

257. **Ayhan A, Tuncer ZS, Tanir M, Yuce K, Ayhan A.** Uterine sarcoma:the Hacettepe Hospital experience of 88 consecutive patients. *Eur J Gynecol Oncol* 1997;18:146–148.

258. **Riopel J, Plante M, Renaud MC, Ray M, Têtu B.** Lymph node metastases in low-grade endometrial stromal sarcoma. *Gynecol Oncol* 2005;96:402–406.

259. **Pink D, Linder T, Mrozek A, Kretzschmar A, Thuss-Patience PC, Dorken B, et al.** Harm or benefit of hormonal treatment in metastatic low-grade endometrial stromal sarcoma. Simple Center experience with 10 cases and review of the literature. *Gynecol Oncol* 2006;101:464–469.

260. **Chu MC, Mor G, Lim C, Zheng W, Parkash V, Schwartz PE.** Low grade endometrial stromal sarcoma: hormonal aspects. *Gynecol Oncol* 2003;90:170–176.

261. **Li N, Wu L-Y, Zhang H-T, An J-S, Li X-G, Ma S-K.** Treatment options in stage I endometrial stromal sarcoma: a retrospective analysis of 53 cases. *Gynecol Oncol* 2008;108:306–311.

262. **McCluggage WG.** Malignant leiphasic uterine tumors, carcinosarcomas or metaplastic carcinoma? *J Clin Pathol* 2002;55:321–325.

263. **McCluggage WG.** Uterine carcinosarcomas (malignant mixed müllerian tumors) are metaplastic carcinomas *Int J Gynecol Cancer* 2002;12:687–690.

264. **Reynolds EA, Logani S, Moller K, Horowitz IR.** Embryonal rhabdomyosarcoma of the uterus in a post menopausal woman. Case report and review of the literature. *Gynecol Oncol* 2006;103:736–739.

265. **Yamada SD, Burger RA, Brewster WR, Anton D, Kohler MF, Monk BJ.** Pathologic variables and adjuvant therapy as predictors of recurrence and survival for patients with surgically evaluated carcinosarcoma of the uterus. *Cancer* 2000;88:2782–2786.

266. **Manolitsas TP, Wain GV, Williams KE, Friedlander MF, Hacker NF.** Multimodality therapy for patients with clinical stage I and II

malignant mixed müllerian tumors of the uterus. *Cancer* 2001;91:1437–1443.

267. **Sutton G, Blessing JA, Rosenshein N, Photopulos G, DiSaia PJ.** Phase II trial of *ifosfamide* and *mesna* in mixed mesodermal tumors of the uterus (a Gynecologic Oncology Group study). *Am J Obstet Gynecol* 1989;161:309–312.

268. **Sutton G, Brunetto VL, Kilgore L, Soper JT, McGehee R, Olt G, et al.** A phase III trial of *ifosphamide* with or without *cisplatin* in carcinosarcoma of the uterus: a Gynecologic Oncology Group study. *Gynecol Oncol* 2000;79:147–153.

269. **Curtin JP, Blessing JA, Soper JT, De Geest K.** *Paclitaxel* in the treatment of carcinosarcoma of the uterus: a Gynecologic Oncology Group study. *Gynecol Oncol* 2001;83:268–270.

270. **Homesley HD, Filiaci V, Markman M, Bitterman P, Eaton L, Kilgore LC, et al.** for the Gynecologic Oncology Group. Phase III trial of *ifosfamide* with or without *paclitaxel* in advanced uterine carcinosarcoma: a Gynecologic Oncology Group study. *J Clin Oncol* 2007;25:526–531.

271. **Peters WA III, Rivkin SE, Smith MR, Tesh DE.** *Cisplatin* and *Adriamycin* combination chemotherapy for uterine stromal sarcomas and mixed mesodermal tumors. *Gynecol Oncol* 1989;34:323–327.

272. **Sutton G, Kauderer J, Carson LF, Lentz SS, Whitney CW, Gallion H.** Adjuvant *ifosfamide* and *cisplatin* in patients with completely resected stage I or II carcinosarcomas (mixed mesodermal tumors) of the uterus: a Gynecology Oncology Group study. *Gynecol Oncol* 2005;96:630–634.

273. **Wolfson AH, Brady MF, Rocereto T, Mannel RS, Lee YC, Futoran RJ, et al.** A Gynecologic Oncology Group randomized phase III trial of whole-abdominal irradiation (WAI) vs *cisplatin-ifosfamide* and *mesna* (CIM) as post-surgical therapy in stage I–IV carcinosarcoma (CS) of the uterus. *Gynecol Oncol* 2007;107:177–185.

274. **Molpus KL, Redlin-Frazier S, Reed G, Burnett LS, Jones HW 3rd.** Postoperative pelvic irradiation in early stage uterine mixed müllerian tumors. *Eur J Gynecol Oncol* 1998;19:541–546.

275. **Sartori E, Bazzorini L, Gadducci A.** Carcinosarcoma of the uterus: A clinicopathological multicenter CTF study. *Gynecol Oncol* 1997;67:70–75.

276. **Callister M, Ramondetta LM, Jhingran A, Burke TW, Eifel PJ** Malignant mixed müllerian tumors of the uterus: analysis of patterns of failure, prognostic factors and treatment outcomes. *Int J Radiat Oncol Biol Phys* 2004;58:786–796.

277. **Kokawa K, Nishiyama K, Ikeuchi M, Ihara Y, Akamatsu N, Enomoto T, et al.** Clinical outcomes of uterine sarcomas: results from 14 years worth of experience in the Kinki district in Japan (1990–2003). *Int J Gynecol Cancer* 2006;16:1358–1363.

278. **Nordal RR, Kristensen GB, Kaern J, Stenwig AE, Pettersen EO, Trope CG.** The prognostic significance of stage, tumor size, cellular atypia and DNA ploidy in uterine leiomyosarcoma. *Acta Oncol* 1995;34:797–802.

279. **Schilder JM, Hurd WW, Roth LM.** Hormonal therapy of an endometrioid stromal nodule followed by local excision. *Obstet Gynecol* 1999;93:805–809.

11 Epithelial Ovarian, Fallopian Tube, and Peritoneal Cancer

Jonathan S. Berek
Michael Friedlander
Neville F. Hacker

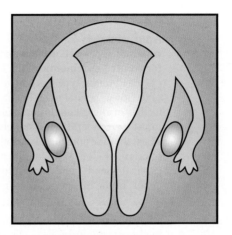

Epithelial ovarian cancer has the highest fatality-to-case ratio of all the gynecologic malignancies because more than two-thirds of patients have advanced disease at diagnosis (1). It presents a major surgical challenge, requires intensive and often complex therapies, and is extremely demanding of the patient's psychological and physical energy. **Serous carcinomas, which are the most common, are now believed to be related etiologically to fallopian tube and peritoneal cancer** (2–7).

There are more than 21,550 new cases of ovarian cancer annually in the United States, and more than 14,600 women can be expected to succumb to their illness (1). It is the fifth most common cancer in women in the United States after cancers of the lung, breast, colon, and uterus. It accounts for 4% of all female cancers and 31% of cancers of the female genital tract. Ovarian cancer is the fourth most common cause of death from malignancy in women.

A woman's risk at birth of having ovarian cancer some time in her lifetime is nearly 1.5%, and the risk of dying from ovarian cancer is almost 1% (2). Five-year survival from ovarian cancer of all stages and histologies has improved significantly in the United States from 37% in 1975–77 to 45% in 1996–2003 ($p < .05$) (1). The death rate per 100,000 has decreased by 8% from 9.51 in 1991 to 8.75 in 2004.

Classification

Approximately 90% of ovarian cancers are derived from cells of the coelomic epithelium or *modified mesothelium* (2). The cells are a product of the primitive mesoderm, which can undergo metaplasia. Neoplastic transformation can occur when the cells are genetically predisposed to oncogenesis or exposed to an oncogenic agent.

Epithelial ovarian cancers are thought to arise from a single layer of cells that covers the ovary or that lines cysts immediately beneath the ovarian surface. These cells are generally quiescent but proliferate following ovulation to repair the defect created by rupture of a follicle. Our understanding of the molecular pathogenesis of ovarian cancer is rapidly increasing. It is now recognized that **there are at least two different molecular pathways that lead to the** development of ovarian cancers and that these result in tumors that have quite distinct biological behaviors and probably different cells of origin (3). **There are those tumors (so-called type I tumors) that arise from ovarian surface epithelium and müllerian inclusions,** either from endosalpingiosis or invagination of the ovarian surface epithelium during repair of ovulation or implantation of cells from endometrium. This process typically **involves a relatively slow and multistep pathway** and **accounts for many early stage cancers such as endometrioid, clear cell, mucinous, and low-grade serous cancers.** In contrast, **the more common high-grade serous cancers (type II) have a phenotype that resembles the fallopian tube mucosa, and they commonly have p53 mutations.** These tumors **appear to develop rapidly** and are almost always at an advanced stage at presentation (3).

Pathology

Invasive Cancer

Approximately 75% to 80% of epithelial cancers are of the serous histologic type. Less common types are mucinous (10%), endometrioid (10%), clear cell, Brenner, and undifferentiated carcinomas, each of the latter three representing less than 1% of epithelial lesions (2). Each tumor type has a histologic pattern that reproduces the epithelial features of a section of the lower genital tract. For example, the serous or papillary pattern has an appearance similar to that of the glandular epithelium lining the fallopian tube, and it has been **proposed that many serous epithelial cancers may originate in the distal fallopian tubal epithelium.** Thus, these lesions involve both the ovaries and tubes, making it difficult to ascertain the site of origin (4–7) (see discussion below). **Mucinous tumors** contain cells that resemble the endocervical glands, and the **endometrioid tumors** resemble the endometrium. More specific details of the histology are discussed in Chapter 5.

Borderline Tumors

worry about GI obstruction w/ borderline tumors.

An important group of tumors to distinguish is the tumor of low malignant potential, also called the **borderline tumor** (8–11). Borderline tumors tend to remain confined to the ovary for long periods of time, occur predominantly in premenopausal women, and are associated with a very good prognosis. **They are encountered most frequently between the ages of 30 and 50 years,** whereas invasive carcinomas are found more commonly between the ages of 50 and 70 years (2).

Although uncommon, metastatic implants may occur with borderline tumors. Such implants have been divided into noninvasive and invasive forms. The latter group has a higher likelihood of developing progressive, proliferative disease in the peritoneal cavity, which can lead to intestinal obstruction and death (9–11).

Peritoneal Carcinoma

The primary malignant transformation of the peritoneum has been called **peritoneal carcinoma** or **primary peritoneal papillary serous carcinoma. This has the appearance of a "müllerian" carcinoma and simulates ovarian cancer clinically.** In such cases, there may be microscopic or small macroscopic cancer on the surface of the ovary and extensive disease in the upper abdomen, particularly in the omentum. Peritoneal carcinoma also explains how "ovarian cancer" can arise in a patient whose ovaries were surgically removed many years earlier (12–14).

Clinical Features

The peak incidence of invasive epithelial ovarian cancer is 56 to 60 years (2,15). The age-specific incidence of this disease rises precipitously from 20 to 80 years of age and subsequently declines (16). The average patient age of those with borderline tumors is approximately 46 years (2,8). Eighty percent to 90% of ovarian cancers, including borderline forms, occur after the age of 40 years, whereas 30% to 40% of malignancies occur after the age of 65.

The chance that a primary epithelial tumor will be of borderline or invasive malignancy in a patient younger than age 40 years is approximately 1 in 10, but after that age it rises to 1 in 3 (2). Less than 1% of epithelial ovarian cancers occur before the age of 20, two-thirds of ovarian malignancies in such patients being germ cell tumors (2,16). **Approximately 30% of ovarian neoplasms in postmenopausal women are malignant, whereas only about 7% of ovarian epithelial tumors in premenopausal patients are frankly malignant** (2).

Etiology

Ovarian cancer has been associated with low parity and infertility (17). Although there has been a variety of epidemiologic variables correlated with ovarian cancer—such as increased risk with talc use, galactose consumption, and decreased risk with tubal ligation (see Chapter 7)—none has been so strongly correlated as prior reproductive history and duration of the reproductive career (17,18). **Early menarche and late menopause increase the risk of ovarian cancer** (18). These factors and the relationship of parity and infertility to the risk of ovarian cancer have led to the hypothesis that suppression of ovulation may be an important factor. Theoretically, the surface epithelium undergoes repetitive disruption and repair. It is thought that this process might lead to a higher probability of spontaneous mutations that can unmask germ-line mutations or otherwise lead to the oncogenic phenotype (see Chapter 1).

Some serous ovarian cancers may actually arise in the fallopian tube (4–7), **a situation that may have been obscured by an overly rigid definition of fallopian tube cancer.** Molecular and genetic evidence supports this etiology, as well as the finding of very early histologic alterations in the tubal epithelium that appear to be precursor lesions in serous carcinomas (3).

In a cohort study of more than 1.1 million Norwegian women, a positive association was found between body mass index (BMI), height, and risk of ovarian cancer, particularly of the endometrioid type in women younger than 60 years (19). Women who had a very high BMI and were clinically obese in adolescence and childhood had a relative risk of 1.56 of developing ovarian cancer compared with women with a medium BMI.

There has been considerable controversy as to whether fertility-enhancing drugs increase the risk of ovarian cancer. In a metaanalysis of eight case-control studies of fertility drugs and ovarian cancer (20), there were 5,207 women with cancer compared with 7,705 controls. The relative risk (RR) of fertility drug exposure for ovarian cancer was 0.97—that is, the use of the drugs was not associated with an increased risk. However, in the same cohort, **nulliparity** (compared with multiparity >4) **carried a RR of 2.42, and infertility** *per se* **for 5 years or longer** (compared with < 1 year) **carried a RR of 2.7.** These results support the hypothesis that **the higher risk in these women is related to infertility, independent of fertility drug use.**

Most case-control and cohort studies have failed to link hormone-replacement therapy to an increased risk of epithelial ovarian cancer (21). A large cohort study has reopened controversy regarding this issue (22). Among 44,241 postmenopausal women in the Breast Cancer Detection Demonstration Project, 329 developed ovarian cancer. **Women who had received estrogen-replacement therapy only for more than 10 years without progestin were at increased risk of developing ovarian cancer.** By 20 years, the relative risk was 3.2-fold.

The incidence of ovarian cancer varies in different geographic locations throughout the world. **Western countries, including the United States and the United Kingdom, have an incidence of ovarian cancer that is three to seven times greater than in Japan, where epithelial ovarian tumors are considered rare** (2). In Asia, the incidence of germ cell tumors of the ovary appears to be somewhat higher than in the West. Japanese immigrants to the United States exhibit a significant increase in the incidence of epithelial ovarian cancer, the rate eventually approaching that of white U.S. women. The incidence of epithelial tumors is about 1.5 times greater in whites than in blacks (1).

Prevention

As parity is inversely related to the risk of ovarian cancer, having at least one child is protective of the disease, with a risk reduction of 0.3 to 0.4. **The oral contraceptive reduces the risk of epithelial ovarian cancer** (17). **Women who use the oral contraceptive for 5 or more years reduce their relative risk to 0.5—that is, there is a 50% reduction in the likelihood of developing ovarian cancer.** Women who have had two children and have used the oral contraceptive for 5 or more years have a relative risk of ovarian cancer as low as 0.3, or a 70% reduction (23). **Therefore, the oral contraceptive pill is the only documented method of chemoprevention for ovarian cancer, and it should be recommended to women for this purpose.** When counseling patients regarding birth control options, this important benefit of the oral contraceptive should be emphasized. This is also important for women with a strong family history of ovarian cancer.

Fenretinide, a retinoid, was thought to be a chemoprophylactic agent for ovarian cancer (24). However, in a prospective, randomized, placebo-controlled trial, there was no difference in the incidence or survival from ovarian cancer after 5 years (25). The Gynecology Oncology Group (GOG) initiated a confirmatory trial, but it was closed because of poor accrual.

Because some serous epithelial tumors might arise in the fallopian tube and because there is a higher rate of tubal carcinoma in women with *BRCA1* and *BRCA2* mutations, it is essential that risk-reducing prophylactic surgery include the removal of both ovaries and both fallopian tubes. The performance of a prophylactic salpingo-oophorectomy will significantly reduce, but not eliminate, the risk of ovarian and fallopian tube cancer (13,14) because the entire peritoneum is potentially at risk. **Peritoneal carcinomas can occur even after prophylactic oophorectomy.** Because the ovaries provide protection from cardiovascular and orthopedic diseases, prophylactic oophorectomy should not be routinely performed in premenopausal women at low risk for ovarian cancer.

*[handwritten margin notes: prophylactic BSO! ; PROSE study; we may use HRT in these pts *]*

Screening

There is no proven effective method of screening for ovarian cancer. Given the false positive results for both <u>CA125</u> and transvaginal ultrasonography, particularly in premenopausal women, these tests are not cost-effective and should not be used routinely to screen for ovarian cancer. In the future, new markers or technologies may improve the specificity of screening, but proof of this will require large prospective studies (27–41). Screening in women who have a familial risk may have a better yield, but additional studies are necessary.

Routine annual pelvic examinations are disappointing for the early detection of ovarian cancer (26). **Screening with transabdominal and transvaginal ultrasonography has been encouraging** (27–29), but specificity has been limited. However, recent advances in transvaginal ultrasonography (30–33) have allowed a very high (>95%) sensitivity for the detection of early stage ovarian cancer, although this test alone might require as many as 10–15 laparotomies per ovarian cancer detected (34). Transvaginal color-flow Doppler to assess the vascularity of the ovarian vessels has been shown to be a useful adjunct to ultrasonography (31–33), but it has not been shown to be useful in screening.

CA125 has been shown to contribute to the early diagnosis of epithelial ovarian cancer (34–41). CA125 has been cloned, and although the function of the molecule is unclear, the elucidation of the MUC16 gene and its control may enhance the understanding of this important marker in ovarian cancer (42–44). Binding of MUC16 to mesothelin appears to mediate cell adhesion and facilitates peritoneal metastasis in animal models (45–47). Regarding the sensitivity of the test, CA125 can detect 50% of patients with stage I disease and 60% with stage II (28). Data suggest that the specificity of CA125 is improved when the test is combined with transvaginal ultrasonography (35) or when the CA125 levels are followed over time (41–51). In this manner, the risk of ovarian cancer (ROC) algorithm might help to improve the efficacy of screening (51).

Altered levels of more than 50 biomarkers have been reported in the serum or urine of ovarian cancer patients. **A number of novel markers for ovarian cancer have been identified in recent years, including mesothelin,** a 110-kd fragment of EGFR (sEGFR), **lysophosphatidic acid, HE4, prostasin, osteopontin, and human kallikreins 6 and 10** (52–58). **Multiplex assays** can measure more than 50 biomarkers with a few hundred microliters of serum (59). Using the multiplex technology, a combination of CA125, HE4, sEGFR, and soluble vCAM-1 has distinguished 90% of stage I ovarian cancer patients from 98% of healthy controls.

Use of **surface-enhanced laser desorption and ionization (SELDI)** with subsequent resolution by mass spectroscopy has demonstrated a pattern of low molecular weight moieties that has been reported to distinguish sera from ovarian cancer patients from those of healthy individuals with 100% sensitivity and 95% specificity (60). Prospective replication of these results and determination of sensitivity for stage I disease should be available in the near future. **Methodological issues have been raised regarding these data** (61). SELDI may also identify a limited number of protein peaks that could be assayed by more conventional techniques (62).

Another approach is the measurement of plasma DNA levels and allelic imbalance by a technique known as **digital single-nucleotide polymorphism analysis.** In a study by Chang and colleagues (63), this analysis had an 87% positive correlation (13 of 15) in stages I and II and a 95% correlation (37 of 39) in patients with stages III and IV disease.

A complete discussion of screening is presented in Chapter 7.

Genetic Risk for Epithelial Ovarian Cancer

Ovarian cancers appear to arise from a single clone—that is, they are monoclonal—and thus are initiated from a single mutation (see Chapter 1) (64). Conversely, there is evidence that peritoneal carcinomas may have a multifocal origin (65).

Hereditary Ovarian Cancer

The risk of ovarian cancer is higher than that of the general population in women with certain family histories (66–80). Although **most epithelial ovarian cancer is sporadic, as many as 10% to 14% of women with epithelial ovarian cancer have a germ-line mutation in *BRCA1* or *BRCA2*** (67,79,80). Further discussion of germ-line mutations and their biology is presented in Chapter 1.

BRCA1 and *BRCA2*

Most hereditary ovarian cancer results from mutations in the *BRCA1* gene, which is located on chromosome 17 (66), **with a small proportion associated with mutations in *BRCA2*, which is located on chromosome 13** (41). Although these appear to be responsible for most hereditary ovarian cancers, it is likely that there are other, as yet undiscovered, genes that also predispose to ovarian or breast cancer or both (75).

In the past, it had been thought that there were two distinct syndromes associated with a genetic risk: site-specific hereditary ovarian cancer and hereditary breast or ovarian cancer syndrome. However, it is now accepted that these groups essentially represent a continuum of mutations of *BRCA1* and *BRCA2* with different degrees of penetrance within a given family (43,51). There are other less common genetic causes of ovarian cancer, and **there is a higher risk of ovarian and endometrial cancer in women with the Lynch II syndrome, which is also known as the *hereditary nonpolyposis colorectal cancer syndrome* (HNPCC syndrome)** (76).

The mutations are autosomal dominant, and thus a complete family history and pedigree analysis, including both maternal and paternal sides of the family, must be carefully evaluated (70). There are numerous distinct mutations that have been identified on each of these genes, and the mutations have different degrees of penetrance, which may account for the preponderance of either breast cancer, ovarian cancer, or both, in any given family. **Based on analysis of women who have a mutation in the *BRCA1* gene and are from high-risk families, the lifetime risk of ovarian cancer may be as high as 28% to 44%, and the risk has been calculated to be as high as 27% for those women with a *BRCA2* mutation** (67,68,74). **In women with a *BRCA1* or *BRCA2* mutation, the risk of ovarian and breast cancer may be as high as 54% and 82%, respectively** (78).

Hereditary ovarian cancers generally occur in women approximately 10 years younger than those with nonhereditary tumors (67,78). As the median age of epithelial ovarian cancer is in the mid- to late 50s, a woman with a first- or second-degree relative who had premenopausal ovarian cancer may have a higher probability of carrying an affected gene.

Breast and ovarian cancer may exist in a family in which there is a combination of epithelial ovarian and breast cancers, affecting a mixture of first- and second-degree relatives. Women with this syndrome tend to have their breast cancers at a very young age, and the breast cancers may be bilateral. If two first-degree relatives are affected, this pedigree is consistent with an autosomal dominant mode of inheritance (66,71).

Founder Effect

There is a higher carrier rate of *BRCA1* and *BRCA2* mutations in women of Ashkenazi Jewish descent, Icelandic women, and in other ethnic groups (72,73,75). There have been three specific mutations that are carried by the Ashkenazi population: 185delAG and 5382insC on *BRCA1*, and 6174delT on *BRCA2*. **The total carrier rate of at least one of these mutations for a patient of Ashkenazi Jewish descent is 1 in 40 or 2.5%, which is considerably higher than the general white population.** The increased risk is a result of the *founder effect*—that is, a higher rate of mutations that have occurred within a defined geographic area.

Pedigree Analysis

The risk of ovarian cancer depends on the number of first- or second-degree relatives with a history of epithelial ovarian carcinoma or breast cancer, and on the age of onset. The

degree of risk is difficult to determine precisely unless a full pedigree analysis is performed, and all patients should be referred to a familial cancer service for genetic counseling.

Risch et al. (79) found that **the hereditary proportion of invasive ovarian tumors was approximately 13% and was as high as 18% in the large subgroup of serous ovarian cancers.** This was independent of family history. Similar findings have been reported in a smaller study from Poland (80). If confirmed in other population-based studies, this will have major implications on genetic testing and argues for consideration of genetic testing in most patients with high-grade serous cancers irrespective of the pedigree and family history.

Lynch II Syndrome or HNPCC Syndrome

HNPCC syndrome, which includes multiple adenocarcinomas, **involves a combination of familial colon cancer** (known as the Lynch I syndrome); a high rate of ovarian, endometrial, and breast cancers; and other malignancies of the gastrointestinal and genitourinary systems (76). The mutations that have been associated with this syndrome are *MSH2, MLH1, PMS1,* and *PMS2.* The risk that a woman who is a member of one of these families will develop epithelial ovarian cancer depends on the frequency of this disease in first- and second-degree relatives, although these women appear to have at least three times the relative risk of the general population. A full pedigree analysis of such families should be performed by a geneticist to more accurately determine the risk.

Management of Women at High Risk for Ovarian Cancer

The management of a woman with a strong family history of epithelial ovarian cancer must be individualized and depends on her age, her reproductive plans, and the level of risk. A thorough pedigree analysis is important. A geneticist should evaluate the family pedigree for at least three generations. Decisions about management are best made after careful study of the pedigree and, whenever possible, verification of the histologic diagnosis of the family members' ovarian cancer as well as the age of onset and other tumors in the family.

The value of testing for *BRCA1* and *BRCA2* has been clearly established, and guidelines for testing now exist (70,77,78). The importance of genetic counseling cannot be overemphasized because the decision is complex. The American Society of Clinical Oncologists has offered guidelines that emphasize careful evaluation by geneticists, careful maintenance of medical records, and a clear understanding in a genetic screening clinic of how to counsel and manage these patients. There remain concerns of how the information will be used, the impact on insurability, how the results will be interpreted, and how the information will be used within a specific family—for example, to counsel children.

Although there are some conflicting data, the behavior of breast cancers arising in women with germ-line mutations in *BRCA1* or *BRCA2* appears to be comparable to that of sporadic tumors (69). **Women with breast cancer who carry these mutations, however, are at a greatly increased risk of ovarian cancer as well as of a second breast cancer. The lifetime risk of ovarian cancer is 54% for women who have a *BRCA1* mutation and 23% for those with a *BRCA2* mutation; for the two groups together, there is an 82% lifetime risk of breast cancer** (78).

Although recommended by the National Institutes of Health Consensus Conference on Ovarian Cancer (81), **the value of screening with transvaginal ultrasonography, CA125 levels, or other procedures has not been clearly established in women at high risk.** Bourne et al. (49) have shown that this approach can detect tumors about 10 times more often than in the general population, and thus they recommend screening in high-risk women. However, **the findings of two prospective studies of annual transvaginal ultrasonography and CA125 screening** in 888 *BRCA1* and *BRCA2* mutation carriers in the Netherlands and 279 mutation carriers in the United Kingdom are not encouraging and **suggest a very limited benefit, if any, of screening even in high-risk women** (82,83).

Despite annual gynecological screening, Hermsen et al. (82) reported that a high proportion of ovarian cancers in *BRCA1* and *BRCA2* carriers were interval cancers, and the majority of all cancers diagnosed were at an advanced stage. Similar findings were reported by Woodward (83). **Therefore, it is unlikely that annual screening will reduce mortality from ovarian cancer in *BRCA1* and *BRCA2* mutation carriers** (82,84).

This important question has also been addressed in GOG 199, a study of screening with annual transvaginal ultrasonography and CA125 ROCA compared to prophylactic bilateral salpingo-oophorectomy. Study accrual is complete as of November 2006 with 2,605 participants enrolled: 1,030 (40%) in the surgical cohort and 1,575 (60%) in the screening cohort. Five years of prospective follow-up ends in November 2011 (85).

Data derived from a multiinstitutional consortium of genetic screening centers indicate that the use of the oral contraceptive pill is associated with a lower risk of development of ovarian cancer in women who have a mutation in either *BRCA1* or *BRCA2* (86). In women who had taken the oral contraceptive pill for 5 or more years, the relative risk of ovarian cancer was 0.4, or a 60% reduction in the incidence of the disease. Another study, however, failed to confirm this finding (87). Tubal ligation may also decrease the risk of ovarian cancer in patients with *BRCA1* (but not *BRCA2*) mutations, but the protective effect is not nearly as strong as oophorectomy (88).

The value of prophylactic oophorectomy in these patients has been documented (89–94). Women at high risk for ovarian cancer who undergo prophylactic oophorectomy have a risk of harboring occult neoplasia: In one series of 98 such operations, three patients (3.1%) had a low-stage ovarian malignancy (90). **The protection against ovarian cancer is very high: the performance of a prophylactic salpingo-oophorectomy reduces the risk of *BRCA*-related gynecologic cancer by 96%** (92). Although the risk of ovarian cancer is diminished, there remains a small risk of subsequently developing a peritoneal carcinoma, a tumor that may also have a higher predisposition in women who have mutations in the *BRCA1* and *BRCA2* genes. In these series, the risk of development of peritoneal carcinoma was 0.8% and 1%, respectively (90,91). **Prophylactic salpingo-oophorectomy in premenopausal women reduced the risk of developing subsequent breast cancer by 50% to 80%** (90,91).

The role of hysterectomy is more controversial. Although most studies show no increase in the rate of uterine and cervical tumors, there are some reports of an increased risk of papillary serous tumors of the endometrium (95). Women on *tamoxifen* are at higher risk for benign endometrial lesions (e.g., polyps) and endometrial cancer. Therefore, **it is reasonable to consider the performance of a prophylactic hysterectomy in conjunction with salpingo-oophorectomy,** and this decision should be individualized.

Grann and associates reported the application of Markov modeling—that is, quality-adjusted survival estimate analysis—in a simulated cohort of 30-year-old women who tested positive for *BRCA1* or *BRCA2* mutations (96). The analysis predicted that a 30 year-old woman could prolong her survival beyond that associated with surveillance alone by 1.8 years with *tamoxifen,* 2.6 years with prophylactic salpingo-oophorectomy, 4.6 years with both *tamoxifen* and prophylactic salpingo-oophorectomy, 3.5 years with prophylactic mastectomy, and 4.9 years with both prophylactic surgeries. **Quality-adjusted survival** was estimated to be prolonged by 2.8 years for *tamoxifen,* 4.4 years with prophylactic salpingo-oophorectomy, 6.3 years for *tamoxifen* and prophylactic salpingo-oophorectomy, 2.6 years with mastectomy, and 2.6 years with both operations.

The survival of women who have a *BRCA1* or *BRCA2* mutation and develop ovarian cancer is longer than that for those who do not have a mutation. In one study, the median survival for mutation carriers was 53.4 months compared with 37.8 months for those with sporadic ovarian cancer from the same institution (97). These findings have recently been confirmed in a population-based-study from Israel in which Chetrit et al. reported that, among Ashkenazi women with ovarian cancer, those with *BRCA1* and *BRCA2* mutations had an improved long-term survival (38% vs. 24% at 5 years). This may result from distinct clinical behavior or from a better response to chemotherapy (98).

Recommendations

Current recommendations for management of women with high risk for ovarian cancers are summarized below (77,78,81,86–96):

1. **Women who appear to be at high risk for ovarian and or breast cancer should undergo genetic counseling; if there is a probability of 10% or greater of having a *BRCA* mutation, they should be offered genetic testing for *BRCA1* and *BRCA2*.**

2. **Women who wish to preserve their reproductive capacity or delay prophylactic surgery can undergo periodic screening by transvaginal ultrasonography every 6 months,** although the efficacy of this approach is not clearly established.

3. **Oral contraceptives should be recommended** to young women before a planned family.

4. **Women who do not wish to maintain their fertility or who have completed their family should be recommended to undergo prophylactic bilateral salpingo-oophorectomy. The majority of *BRCA1*-related ovarian cancers occur in women after the age of 40, and *BRCA2* ovarian cancers are more likely in postmenopausal women. The risk of ovarian cancer under the age of 40 is very low.** The potential risk should be clearly documented and preferably established by *BRCA1* and *BRCA2* testing, preoperatively. These women should be counseled that this operation does not offer absolute protection, because peritoneal carcinomas may occasionally occur (90,91). The concurrent performance of a prophylactic hysterectomy is acceptable, and the option should be discussed with these patients.

5. **In women who have a strong family history of breast or ovarian cancer, annual mammographic and MRI screening should be performed commencing at age 30 years or younger if there are family members with documented very early onset breast cancer.**

6. **Women with a documented HNPCC syndrome should be treated as above; in addition, they should undergo periodic screening mammography, colonoscopy, and endometrial biopsy** (76).

Symptoms

The majority of women with epithelial ovarian cancer have vague and nonspecific pelvic, abdominal, and menstrual symptoms (99–103). Goff et al. (104) recently developed an **ovarian cancer symptom index** and reported that symptoms associated with ovarian cancer were pelvic or abdominal pain, urinary frequency or urgency, increased abdominal size or bloating, and difficulty eating or feeling full. These symptoms were particularly suspicious when they were present for less than 1 year and lasted longer than 12 days a month. The index had a sensitivity of 56.7% for early ovarian cancer and 79.5% for advanced stage disease.

A study from the Royal Hospital for Women in Sydney compared 100 patients with early stage epithelial ovarian cancer with 100 patients with advanced stage disease. **Ninety percent of women with early disease and 100% with advanced disease reported at least one symptom.** With early disease, abdominal pain was reported by 51% and abdominal swelling by 32%; with advanced disease, abdominal swelling was reported by 62% and abdominal pain by 40%. **Seventy percent of patients with early disease and 69% of those with advanced disease reported symptoms of less than 3 months duration.** Patients with tumors less than 5 cm in diameter were three times more likely to have advanced disease. Patients with grade I tumors were 40 times more likely to have early stage disease when compared to patients with grade 3 tumors (105). **These findings were confirmed in a population-based study from Australia in which there did not appear to be a significant difference in the duration of symptoms or the nature of symptoms in patients with early as opposed to advanced stage disease** (106).

These two studies reinforce the concept that early and late-stage ovarian cancer are biologically different entities and argue against the widely held misconception that ovarian cancer is diagnosed at an early stage because the symptoms are recognized earlier than in patients with more advanced disease (84,105,106,107).

Signs

The most important sign is the presence of a pelvic mass on physical examination. A solid, irregular, fixed pelvic mass is highly suggestive of an ovarian malignancy. If, in addition, an upper abdominal mass or ascites is present, then the diagnosis of ovarian cancer is almost certain. Because the patient usually reports abdominal symptoms, she may not be subjected to a pelvic examination, and the presence of a tumor may be missed. Pleural effusions commonly occur in association with ascites and very occasionally in the absence of ascites in patients with advanced disease.

Diagnosis

The diagnosis of an ovarian cancer requires an exploratory laparotomy. The preoperative evaluation of the patient with an adnexal mass is outlined in Fig. 11.1.

Ultrasonographic signs of malignancy include an adnexal pelvic mass with areas of complexity such as irregular borders; multiple echogenic patterns within the mass; and dense, multiple,

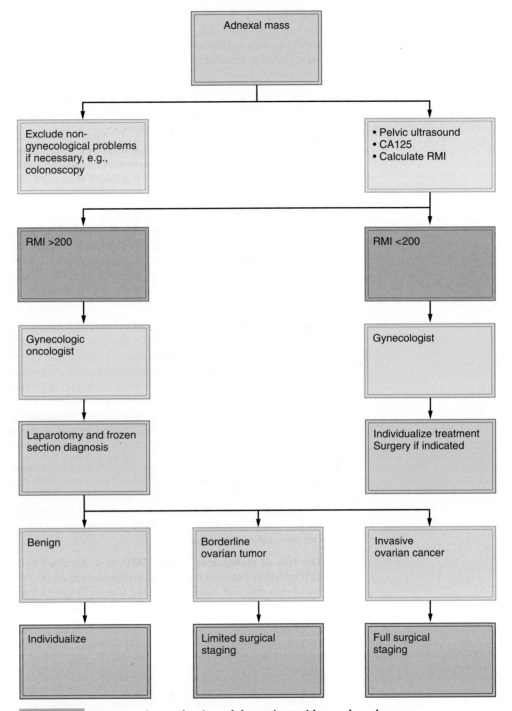

Figure 11.1 Preoperative evaluation of the patient with an adnexal mass.

irregular septae. Bilateral tumors are more likely to be malignant, although the individual characteristics of the lesions are of greater significance. **Transvaginal ultrasonography may have a somewhat better resolution than transabdominal ultrasonography for adnexal neoplasms** (27–30). Doppler color-flow imaging may enhance the specificity of ultrasonography for demonstrating findings consistent with malignancy (31–33).

The size of the lesion is of importance. If a complex cystic mass is more than 8 to 10 cm in diameter, then the probability is high that the lesion is neoplastic, unless the patient has been taking *clomiphene citrate* or other agents to induce ovulation (100). **In the premenopausal patient, a period of observation is reasonable, provided the adnexal mass is not clinically** suspicious (i.e., it is mobile, mostly cystic, unilateral, and of regular contour). Generally, an interval of no more than 2 months is allowed for observation. If the lesion is not neoplastic, it should remain stable or regress, as measured by pelvic examination and pelvic ultrasonography. If a mass increases in size or complexity, then it must be presumed to be neoplastic and removed surgically.

In postmenopausal women with unilocular cysts measuring 8 to 10 cm or less and normal serial CA125 levels, expectant management is acceptable, and this approach may decrease the number of surgical interventions (108–110).

Premenopausal patients whose lesions are clinically suspicious (i.e., large, predominantly solid, relatively fixed, or irregularly shaped) should undergo laparotomy, as should postmenopausal patients with complex adnexal masses of any size.

Before the planned exploration, the patient should undergo routine hematologic and biochemical assessments. A preoperative evaluation in a patient older than 40 years undergoing laparotomy should include a radiograph of the chest. An abdominal and pelvic computed tomographic (CT) or magnetic resonance imaging (MRI) scan is of no value in patients with a definite pelvic mass (111–115). Patients with ascites and no pelvic mass should have a CT or MRI scan to look particularly for liver or pancreatic tumors (112). The value of positron-emission tomography (PET) scans is being evaluated but may contribute to the specificity of the CT scan findings (114).

The preoperative evaluation should exclude other primary cancers metastatic to the ovary. A **colonoscopy** is indicated in selected patients with symptoms and signs suspicious for colon cancer. This would include any patient who has evidence of frank or occult blood in the stool or gives a recent history of diarrhea or constipation. A **gastroscopy** is indicated if there are upper gastrointestinal symptoms such as nausea, vomiting, or hematemesis (116). **Bilateral mammography** is indicated if there is any breast mass, because occasionally breast cancer metastatic to the ovaries can simulate primary ovarian cancer. **Patients who have irregular menses or postmenopausal bleeding should have an endometrial biopsy and an endocervical curettage** to exclude the presence of uterine or endocervical cancer metastatic to the ovary.

Differential Diagnosis   Ovarian epithelial cancers must be differentiated from benign neoplasms and functional cysts of the ovaries (117–119). A variety of benign conditions of the reproductive tract—such as pelvic inflammatory disease, endometriosis, and pedunculated uterine leiomyomata—can simulate ovarian cancer. Nongynecologic causes of a pelvic tumor, such as an inflammatory or neoplastic colonic mass, must be excluded (100). A pelvic kidney can simulate ovarian cancer.

The **risk of malignancy index** (RMI), first described by Jacobs in 1990, is one method of differentiating between benign and malignant masses (117). Utilization of this index may facilitate better triage of suspicious pelvic masses to gynecologic oncologists. **The RMI incorporates the menopausal status, an ultrasonic score, and the serum CA125 level.**

In an analysis of 204 consecutive patients with an ovarian mass at the Royal Hospital for Women in Sydney, an RMI of <200 correctly identified 83 of 108 (77%) benign ovarian masses (118). An RMI of >200 correctly identified 11 of 19 (58%) borderline ovarian tumors and 70 of 77 (91%) invasive ovarian cancers. An RMI of >200 had a sensitivity of 84%, specificity of 77%, positive predictive value of 76%, and a negative predictive value of 85% for the detection of both borderline and invasive ovarian tumors (118).

Patterns of Spread

Ovarian epithelial cancers spread primarily by exfoliation of cells into the peritoneal cavity, by lymphatic dissemination, and by hematogenous spread.

Transcoelomic   The most common and earliest mode of dissemination is by exfoliation of cells that implant along the surfaces of the peritoneal cavity. The cells tend to follow the circulatory path of the peritoneal fluid. The fluid tends to move with the forces of respiration from the pelvis, up the paracolic gutters, especially on the right, along the intestinal mesenteries, to the right hemidiaphragm. Therefore, metastases are typically seen on the posterior cul-de-sac, paracolic gutters, right hemidiaphragm, liver capsule, the peritoneal surfaces of the intestines and their mesenteries, and the omentum. The disease seldom invades the intestinal lumen but progressively agglutinates loops of bowel, leading to a functional intestinal obstruction. This condition is known as **carcinomatous ileus.**

Lymphatic   Lymphatic dissemination to the pelvic and paraaortic lymph nodes is common, particularly in advanced-stage disease (120–123). Spreading through the lymphatic channels of the diaphragm and through the retroperitoneal lymph nodes can lead to dissemination above the diaphragm, especially to the supraclavicular lymph nodes (120).

Burghardt et al. performed systematic pelvic and paraaortic lymphadenectomy on 123 patients (122) and reported that 78% of patients with stage III disease have metastases to the pelvic lymph nodes. In another series (123), the rate of positive paraaortic lymph nodes was 18% in stage I, 20% in stage II, 42% in stage III, and 67% in stage IV.

Hematogenous   Hematogenous dissemination at the time of diagnosis is uncommon, with spread to vital organ parenchyma, such as the lungs and liver, in only some 2% to 3% of patients. Most patients with disease above the diaphragm at the time of presentation have a right pleural effusion. Systemic metastases are seen more frequently in patients who have survived for some years. Dauplat et al. from UCLA (124) reported that **distant metastasis consistent with stage IV disease ultimately occurred in 38% of the patients whose disease was originally intraperitoneal.** Sites of hematogenous spread and their median survivals were as follows:

- parenchymal lung metastasis in 7.1%, median survival 9 months
- subcutaneous nodules in 3.5%, 12 months
- malignant pericardial effusion in 2.4%, 2.3 months
- central nervous system in 2%, 1.3 months
- bone metastases in 1.6%, 4 months

Significant risk factors for distant metastases were malignant ascites, peritoneal carcinomatosis, large metastatic disease within the abdomen, and retroperitoneal lymph node involvement at the time of initial surgery.

Prognostic Factors

The outcome of patients after treatment can be evaluated in the context of prognostic factors, which can be grouped into pathologic, biologic, and clinical factors.

Pathologic Factors

The morphology and histologic pattern, including the architecture and grade of the lesion, are important prognostic variables (125–130). **In general, stage for stage, histologic type is not of prognostic significance, with the exception of clear cell carcinomas,** which are associated with a worse prognosis than the other histologic types (128,129).

Histologic grade, as determined either by the pattern of differentiation or by the extent of cellular anaplasia and the proportion of undifferentiated cells, seems to be of prognostic significance (129,131). However, studies of the reproducibility of grading ovarian cancers have shown a high degree of intraobserver and interobserver variation (130). **Because there is significant heterogeneity of tumors and observational bias, the value of histologic grade as an independent prognostic factor has not been clearly established.** Baak et al. (131) have presented a standard grading system based on morphometric analysis, and the system appears to correlate with prognosis, especially in its ability to distinguish low-grade or borderline patterns from other tumors.

Biologic Factors

Several biologic factors have been correlated with prognosis in epithelial ovarian cancer (132–164). Using flow cytometry, Friedlander et al. (133) showed that ovarian cancers were commonly aneuploid. Furthermore, they and others showed that there was a high correlation between FIGO* stage and ploidy; that is, low-stage cancers tend to be diploid and high-stage tumors tend to be aneuploid (132–139) (Fig. 11.2). **Patients with diploid tumors have a significantly longer median survival than those with aneuploid tumors:** 5 years versus 1 year, respectively (134). Multivariate analyses have demonstrated that **ploidy is an independent prognostic variable** and one of the most significant predictors of survival (135).

*International Federation of Gynecology and Obstetrics

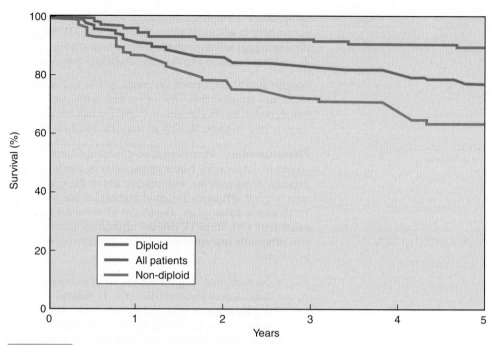

Figure 11.2   **Survival of patients with stage I epithelial ovarian cancer based on ploidy evaluation.** (From **Tropé C, Kaern J, Vergote I.** Adjuvant therapy for early-stage epithelial ovarian cancer. In: **Gershenson DM, McGuire WP, eds.** *Ovarian cancer: controversies in management.* New York: Churchill Livingstone, 1998:41–63, with permission.)

More than 100 protooncogenes have been identified, and studies have focused on the amplification or expression of these genetic loci and their relationship to the development and progression of ovarian cancer (140–155). For example, Slamon et al. (142) reported that 30% of epithelial ovarian tumors expressed HER2/*neu* oncogene and that this group had a poorer prognosis, especially those patients with more than five copies of the gene. Berchuck et al. (143) reported a similar incidence (32%) of HER2/*neu* expression. In their series, patients whose tumors expressed the gene had a poorer median survival (15.7 months versus 32.8 months). Others have not substantiated this finding (144), and a review of the literature by Leary et al. (145) revealed an overall incidence of HER2/*neu* expression of only 11%.

Additional prognostic variables include *p53, bcl-2, K-ras,* Ki67, interleukin 6, *PTEN*, lysophospholipids, and platelet-derived growth factor (150–160). Further discussion of these molecular variables is presented in Chapter 1.

The *in vitro* **clonogenic assay** has been studied in ovarian cancer. A significant inverse correlation has been reported between clonogenic growth *in vitro* and survival (161–164). Multivariate analysis has found that clonogenic growth in a semisolid culture medium is a significant independent variable (163). The use of an "**extreme drug resistance assay**" has been suggested as a possible means of directing therapy by defining platinum-sensitive and resistant tumors *in vitro* but, the assay does not independently predict or alter the outcome in either a primary or recurrent disease setting (164).

Clinical Factors

In addition to stage, the extent of residual disease after primary surgery, the volume of ascites, patient age, and performance status are all independent prognostic variables (165–174). Among patients with stage I disease, Dembo et al. (165) showed, in a multivariate analysis, that tumor grade and "dense adherence" to the pelvic peritoneum had a significant adverse impact on prognosis, whereas intraoperative tumor spillage or rupture did not. A subsequent study by Sjövall et al. confirmed these findings (166). A multivariate analysis of these and several other studies was performed by Vergote et al. (168), who reported that poor prognostic variables for early stage disease were the tumor grade, capsular penetrance, surfaces excrescences, and malignant ascites, but not iatrogenic rupture.

Initial Surgery for Ovarian Cancer

Staging

Ovarian epithelial malignancies are staged according to the International Federation of Gynecology and Obstetrics (FIGO) system, and the staging system of 1988 is presented in Table 11.1 and in Fig. 11.3. The TNM staging is correlated with the FIGO stage in Fig 11.3. The FIGO staging is based on findings at surgical exploration. A preoperative evaluation should exclude the presence of extraperitoneal metastases. **The 2008 FIGO staging for Ovarian epithelial malignancies remains unchanged.**

A thorough surgical staging should be performed because subsequent treatment will be determined by the stage of disease. In patients in whom exploratory laparotomy does not reveal any macroscopic evidence of disease on inspection and palpation of the entire intraabdominal space, a careful search for microscopic spread must be undertaken.

In earlier series in which patients did not undergo careful surgical staging, the overall 5-year survival for patients with apparent stage I epithelial ovarian cancer was only approximately 60% (175). Since then, survival rates of 90% to 100% have been reported for patients who have been properly staged and found to have stage IA or IB disease (175–179).

Table 11.1 FIGO Staging for Primary Carcinoma of the Ovary	
Stage I	Growth limited to the ovaries.
Stage IA	Growth limited to one ovary; no ascites containing malignant cells. No tumor on the external surface; capsule intact.
Stage IB	Growth limited to both ovaries; no ascites containing malignant cells. No tumor on the external surfaces; capsules intact.
Stage IC[a]	Tumor either stage IA or IB but with tumor on the surface of one or both ovaries; or with capsule ruptured; or with ascites present containing malignant cells or with positive peritoneal washings.
Stage II	Growth involving one or both ovaries with pelvic extension.
Stage IIA	Extension or metastases to the uterus or tubes.
Stage IIB	Extension to other pelvic tissues.
Stage IIC[a]	Tumor either stage IIA or IIB but with tumor on the surface of one or both ovaries; or with capsule(s) ruptured; or with ascites present containing malignant cells or with positive peritoneal washings.
Stage III	Tumor involving one or both ovaries with peritoneal implants outside the pelvis or positive retroperitoneal or inguinal nodes. Superficial liver metastasis equals stage III. Tumor is limited to the true pelvis but with histologically proven malignant extension to small bowel or omentum.
Stage IIIA	Tumor grossly limited to the true pelvis with negative nodes but with histologically confirmed microscopic seeding of abdominal peritoneal surfaces.
Stage IIIB	Tumor of one or both ovaries with histologically confirmed implants of abdominal peritoneal surfaces, none exceeding 2 cm in diameter. Nodes negative.
Stage IIIC	Abdominal implants >2 cm in diameter or positive retroperitoneal or inguinal nodes.
Stage IV	Growth involving one or both ovaries with distant metastasis. If pleural effusion is present, there must be positive cytologic test results to allot a case to stage IV. Parenchymal liver metastasis equals stage IV.

FIGO Annual Report, Vol 26, *Int J Gynecol Obstet* 2006;105:3–4.

These categories are based on findings at clinical examination or surgical exploration. The histologic characteristics are to be considered in the staging, as are results of cytologic testing as far as effusions are concerned. It is desirable that a biopsy be performed on suspect areas outside the pelvis.

[a]To evaluate the impact on prognosis of the different criteria for allotting cases to stage IC or IIC, it would be of value to know if rupture of the capsule was (a) spontaneous or (b) caused by the surgeon, and if the source of malignant cells detected was (a) peritoneal washings or (b) ascites.

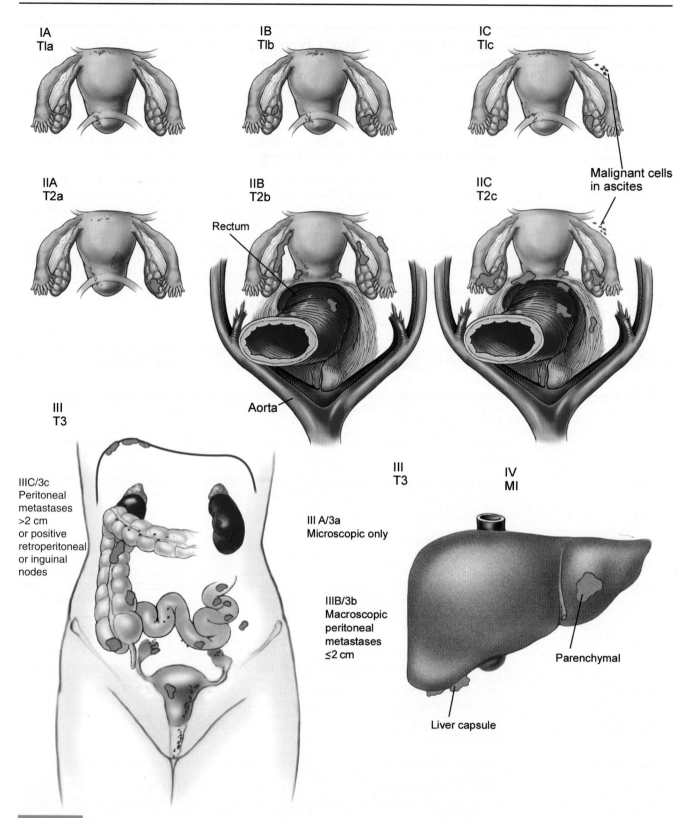

Figure 11.3   Staging ovarian cancer (FIGO and TNM). (From **Heintz APM, Odicino F, Maisonneuve P, Quinn MA, Benedet JL, Creasman WT, et al.** Carcinoma of the ovary. In **Pecorelli S, ed.** Twenty-Sixth Annual Report on the Results of Treatment in Gynaecological Cancer. *Int J Gynecol Oncol* 2006;95(suppl 1):S161–S192, with permission.)

Technique for Surgical Staging

In patients whose preoperative evaluation suggests a probable ovarian malignancy, a midline or paramedian abdominal incision is recommended to allow adequate access to the upper abdomen. When a malignancy is unexpectedly discovered in a patient who has a lower transverse incision, the rectus muscles can be either divided or detached from the symphysis pubis to allow better access to the upper abdomen (see Chapter 20). If this is not sufficient, the incision can be extended on one side to create a "J" incision.

The ovarian tumor should be removed intact, if possible, and a frozen histologic section obtained. If ovarian malignancy is present and the tumor is apparently confined to the ovaries or the pelvis, then thorough surgical staging should be carried out. This involves the following steps:

1. **Any free fluid, especially in the pelvic cul-de-sac, should be submitted for cytologic evaluation.**

2. **If no free fluid is present, then peritoneal "washings" should be performed by instilling and recovering 50 to 100 dl of saline from the pelvic cul-de-sac, each paracolic gutter, and from beneath each hemidiaphragm.** Obtaining the specimens from under the diaphragms can be facilitated with the use of a red rubber catheter attached to the end of a bulb syringe.

3. **A systematic exploration of all the intraabdominal surfaces and viscera is performed.** This should proceed in a clockwise fashion from the cecum cephalad along the paracolic gutter and the ascending colon to the right kidney, the liver and gallbladder, the right hemidiaphragm, the entrance to the lesser sac at the paraaortic area, across the transverse colon to the left hemidiaphragm, and down the left gutter and the descending colon to the rectosigmoid colon. The small intestine and its mesentery from the ligament of Treitz to the cecum should be inspected.

4. **Any suspicious areas or adhesions on the peritoneal surfaces should be biopsied.** If there is no evidence of disease, then multiple intraperitoneal biopsies should be performed. The peritoneum of the pelvic cul-de-sac, both paracolic gutters, the peritoneum over the bladder, and the intestinal mesenteries should be biopsied.

5. **The diaphragm should be sampled either by biopsy or by scraping with a tongue depressor and making a cytologic smear** (180). Biopsies of any irregularities on the surface of the diaphragm can be facilitated by use of the laparoscope and the associated biopsy instrument.

6. **The omentum should be resected from the transverse colon, a procedure called an *infracolic omentectomy*.** The procedure is initiated on the underside of the greater omentum, where the peritoneum is incised just a few millimeters away from the transverse colon. The branches of the gastroepiploic vessels are clamped, ligated, and divided, along with all the small branching vessels that feed the infracolic omentum. If the gastrocolic ligament is palpably normal, it does not need to be resected.

7. **The retroperitoneal spaces should be dissected and explored to evaluate the pelvic lymph nodes.** The pelvic retroperitoneal dissection is performed by incising the peritoneum over the psoas muscles. This may be done on the ipsilateral side only for unilateral tumors. Any enlarged lymph nodes should be resected and submitted for frozen section. If no metastases are present, then a formal pelvic lymphadenectomy should be performed.

8. **The paraaortic area should be explored.** A vertical incision should be made cephalad in the paracolic gutter and an oblique incision across the posterior parietal peritoneum from the right iliac fossa to the ligament of Treitz. The right colon can then be mobilized and the paraaortic lymph nodes exposed. Any enlarged nodes should be removed and at least the nodes caudal to the inferior mesenteric artery resected (181).

Results

As many as three in ten patients whose tumor appears confined to the pelvis have occult metastatic disease in the upper abdomen or the retroperitoneal lymph nodes. At surgical staging, metastases in apparent low-stage epithelial ovarian cancer are found in the diaphragm in approximately 7% of patients, in paraaortic lymph nodes in 15%, pelvic nodes in 6%, omentum in 9%, and peritoneal cytology in 26% (121,175–178).

The importance of careful initial surgical staging is emphasized by the findings of a cooperative national study (175) in which 100 patients with apparent stage I and II disease who were referred for subsequent therapy underwent additional surgical staging. In this series, 28% of the patients initially thought to have stage I disease were "upstaged," as were 43% of those thought to have stage II disease. A total of 31% of the patients were upstaged as a result of additional surgery, and 77% were reclassified as having stage III disease. **Histologic grade was a significant predictor of occult metastasis**; that is, 16% of the patients with grade 1 lesions were upstaged, compared with 34% with grade 2 and 46% with grade 3 disease.

After a comprehensive staging laparotomy, only a minority of women will have local disease (FIGO stage I). Of the 21,650 women diagnosed yearly with epithelial ovarian cancer in the United States, nearly 4,000 have disease confined to the ovaries (1,182). The prognosis for these patients depends on the clinical–pathologic features, as outlined below. Because of this emphasis on the importance of surgical staging, the rate of lymph node sampling has increased in the United States, with a study showing that for women with stage I and II disease, the percentage having lymph nodes sampled increased from 38% to 59% from 1991 to 1996 (183).

Early Stage Ovarian Cancer

The primary treatment for stage I epithelial ovarian cancer is surgical—that is, a total abdominal hysterectomy, bilateral salpingo-oophorectomy, and surgical staging (175,184). In certain circumstances, a unilateral oophorectomy may be permitted, as discussed below. Based on the prognostic variables outlined above (126,135,165–170,172,173,184), early stage epithelial ovarian cancer can be subdivided into low-risk and high-risk disease (Table 11.2).

Borderline Tumors

The principal treatment of borderline ovarian tumors is surgical resection of the primary tumor (3,185–192). There are no data to suggest that either adjuvant chemotherapy or radiation therapy improves survival (193–195). After a frozen section has determined that the histology is borderline, premenopausal patients who desire preservation of ovarian function may be managed with a "conservative" operation—that is, a unilateral oophorectomy (3,186,188). In a study of patients who underwent unilateral ovarian cystectomy only for apparent stage I borderline serous tumors, Lim-Tan et al. (187) found that this conservative operation was also safe; only 8% of the patients having recurrences 2 to 18 years later, all with curable disease confined to the ovaries. Recurrence was associated with "positive margins" of the removed ovarian cyst.

In a retrospective series of 339 patients by Zaetta et al. (191), seven (2%) progressed to invasive carcinoma, five serous and two mucinous. **Although the recurrence rate after fertility-sparing surgery was 18.5% versus 4.6% after nonfertility-sparing surgery, all but one woman with recurrence of borderline tumor or progression to carcinoma was cured.** The disease-free survival was 99.6% for stage I, 95.8% for stage II, and 89% for stage III. Thus, hormonal function and fertility can be maintained in the majority of patients with borderline tumors. In patients in whom an oophorectomy or cystectomy has been performed and a borderline tumor is later documented in the permanent pathology, no additional staging surgery is necessary, but the patient should be monitored with transvaginal ultrasonography.

Table 11.2 Prognostic Variables in Early Stage Epithelial Ovarian Cancer	
Low-Risk	*High-Risk*
Low-grade	High-grade
Non–clear cell histologic type	Clear cell histologic type
Intact capsule	Tumor growth through capsule
No surface excrescences	Surface excrescences
No ascites	Ascites
Negative peritoneal cytologic findings	Malignant cells in fluid
Unruptured or intraoperative rupture	Preoperative rupture
No dense adherence	Dense adherence
Diploid tumor	Aneuploid tumor

Fertility Preservation in Early Stage Ovarian Cancer

In patients who have undergone a thorough staging laparotomy and in whom there is no evidence of spread beyond the ovary, the uterus and contralateral ovary can be retained in women who wish to preserve fertility (196,197). In a study by Park et al. (197), 59 women with stages IA–IC underwent fertility-sparing surgery, and there were no recurrences in women whose disease was grade 1 or 2. Women with grade 3 or higher stage disease had a significantly higher recurrence rate and lower survival. Women who undergo fertility-sparing surgery for low-stage, low-grade epithelial ovarian cancer should be followed carefully with routine transvaginal ultrasonography and determination of serum CA125 levels. Generally, the other ovary and the uterus should be removed at the completion of childbearing (see treatment section below).

Advanced-Stage Ovarian Cancer

The surgical management of all patients with advanced-stage disease is approached in a similar manner, with modifications made for the overall status and general health of the patient, as well as the extent of residual disease present at the time treatment is initiated. A treatment scheme is outlined in Fig. 11.4.

If the patient is medically stable, she should undergo an initial exploratory procedure with removal of as much disease as possible (199–216). The operation to remove the primary tumor as well as the associated metastatic disease is referred to as *debulking* or *cytoreductive surgery*. Most patients subsequently receive combination intravenous chemotherapy with an empiric number of cycles, six to eight. In some patients with completely resected disease, intraperitoneal chemotherapy may be considered. In selected patients who are not candidates for initial cytoreductive surgery, neoadjuvant chemotherapy may be given for a few cycles before surgery, as discussed below. Second-look laparotomy has not been shown to improve outcomes. It is best limited to investigational protocols (198).

The preoperative assessment of resectability is limited. Using a cutoff of 500 IU, CA125 levels have been suggested as a means of predicting the probability of an optimal resection (211,214), but others have shown that these determinations have low predictive value (215). **CT , MR, and CT-PET scans have been used to try to predict suboptimal resection (216–219).** In a series by Dowdy et al. (216), the presence of diffuse peritoneal thickening and ascites on CT scan was associated with a 32% optimal debulking, as opposed 71% in the group that did not have these findings, with a positive predictive value of 68%. **However, in a larger multiinstititonal validation study, the accuracy of CT (218) in predicting suboptimal cytoreduction dropped to as low as 34% in some cohorts.** CT-PET was also found to have limited positive predictive value (219).

Vergote and colleagues from Belgium reported the use of open laparoscopy in 173 patients with a pelvic mass, an omental "cake," or large volume ascites to exclude other primary tumors and to determine resectability. Seventy-one of the patients (41%) developed a port site metastasis (220).

In our experience, it is virtually always possible to remove the primary tumor (if necessary, with an *en bloc* resection of the rectosigmoid colon) and the omental cake, so the major reason for recommending neoadjuvant chemotherapy is to improve the medical fitness of the patient.

Cytoreductive Surgery

Patients with advanced-stage epithelial ovarian cancer documented at initial exploratory laparotomy should undergo cytoreductive surgery (199–216). The operation typically includes the performance of a total abdominal hysterectomy and bilateral salpingo-oophorectomy, along with a complete omentectomy and resection of any metastatic lesions from the peritoneal surfaces or from the intestines. The pelvic tumor often directly involves the rectosigmoid colon, the terminal ileum, and the cecum (Fig. 11.5). In a minority of patients, most or all of the disease is confined to the pelvic viscera and the omentum so that removal of these organs will result in extirpation of all gross tumor, a situation that is associated with a reasonable chance of prolonged progression-free survival.

Theoretic Rationale

The rationale for cytoreductive surgery relates to general theoretic considerations (207,221,222): **(i) the physiologic benefits of tumor excision and (ii) the improved tumor perfusion and increased growth fraction,** both of which increase the likelihood of response to chemotherapy or radiation therapy.

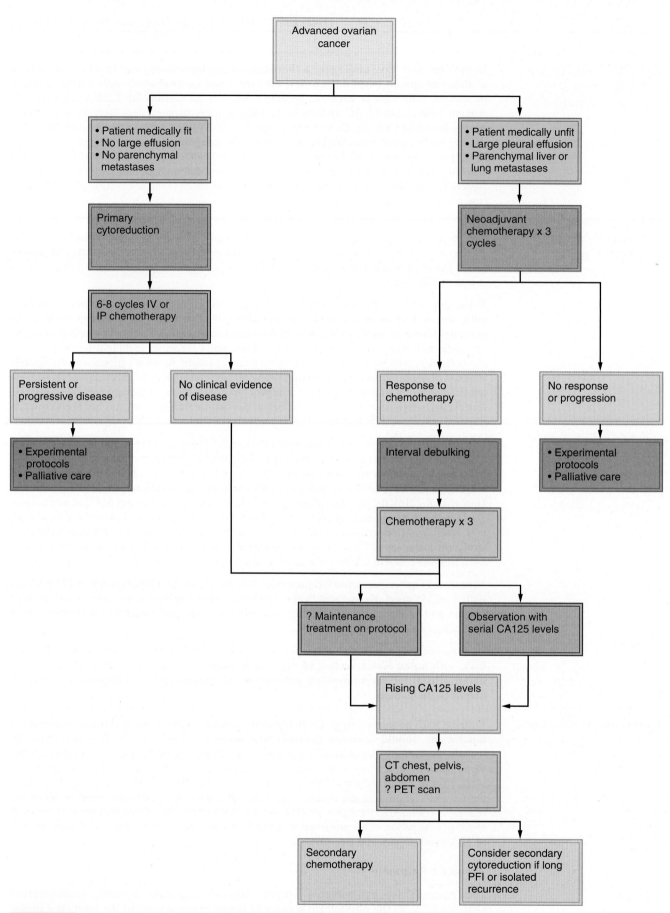

Figure 11.4 **Treatment scheme for patients with advanced-stage epithelial ovarian cancer.** PFI, progression-free interval

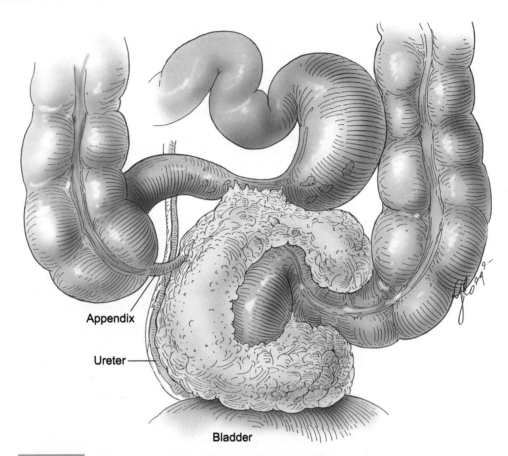

Appendix

Ureter

Bladder

Figure 11.5   **Extensive ovarian carcinoma involving the bladder, rectosigmoid, and ileocecal area.** (From **Heintz APM, Berek JS.** Cytoreductive surgery for ovarian carcinoma. In: **Piver MS, ed.** *Ovarian malignancies.* Edinburgh: Churchill Livingstone, 1987:134, with permission.)

Physiologic Benefits   Ascites may be sometimes reasonably well controlled after removal of the primary tumor and a large omental cake. Also, removal of the omental cake often alleviates the nausea and early satiety that many patients experience. Removal of intestinal metastases may restore adequate intestinal function and lead to an improvement in the overall nutritional status of the patient, thereby facilitating the patient's ability to tolerate subsequent chemotherapy.

Tumor Perfusion and Cellular Kinetics   A large, bulky tumor may contain areas that are poorly vascularized, and such areas will be exposed to suboptimal concentrations of chemotherapeutic agents. Similarly, these areas are poorly oxygenated, so radiation therapy, which requires adequate oxygenation to achieve maximal cell kill, will be less effective. Thus, surgical removal of these bulky tumors may eliminate areas that are most likely to be relatively resistant to treatment.

In addition, larger tumor masses tend to be composed of a higher proportion of cells that are either nondividing or in the "resting" phase (i.e., G_0 cells, which are essentially resistant to the therapy). A low-growth fraction is characteristic of bulky tumor masses, and cytoreductive surgery can result in smaller residual masses with a relatively higher growth fraction.

The fractional cell kill hypothesis of Skipper (221) postulates that a constant proportion of the tumor cells are destroyed with each treatment. This theory suggests that a given dose of a drug will kill a constant fraction of cells as long as the growth fraction and phenotype are the same. Therefore, a treatment that reduces a population of tumor cells from 10^9 to 10^4 cells also would reduce a population of 10^5 cells to a single cell. If the absolute number of tumor cells is lower at the initiation of treatment, then fewer cycles of therapy should be necessary to eradicate the cancer, provided that the cells are not inherently resistant to the therapy.

The larger the initial tumor burden, the longer the necessary exposure to the drug and, therefore, the greater the chance of developing acquired drug resistance. However, because the spontaneous mutation rate of tumors is an inherent property of the malignancy, the likelihood of developing phenotypic drug resistance also increases as the size of the tumor increases. **The chance of developing a clone of cells resistant to a specific agent is related to both the tumor size and its mutation frequency** (221,222). This is one of the inherent problems with cytoreductive surgery for large tumor masses: Phenotypic drug resistance may have already developed before any surgical intervention.

Goals of Cytoreductive Surgery

The principal goal of cytoreductive surgery is the removal of all of the primary cancer and, if possible, all metastatic disease. If resection of all metastases is not feasible, then the goal is to reduce the tumor burden by resection of all individual tumors to an "optimal" status. Griffiths (199) initially proposed that all metastatic nodules should be reduced to ≤1.5 cm in maximum diameter and showed that survival was significantly longer in such patients.

Subsequently, Hacker and Berek (201,204–207) showed that patients whose largest residual lesions were ≤5 mm had a superior survival, and this was substantiated by Hoskins et al. presenting the data of the Gynecologic Oncology Group (203). The median survival of patients in this category was 40 months, compared with 18 months for patients whose lesions were ≤1.5 cm and 6 months for patients with nodules >1.5 cm (Fig. 11.6). Clearly, **those patients whose disease has been completely resected have the best prognosis, and approximately 60% of patients in this category will be free of disease at 5 years** (Fig. 11.7).

The resectability of the metastatic tumor is usually determined by the location of the disease. Optimal cytoreduction is difficult to achieve in the presence of extensive disease on the diaphragm, in the parenchyma of the liver, along the base of the small-bowel mesentery, in the lesser omentum, or in the porta hepatis (212).

The ability of cytoreductive surgery to influence survival is limited by the extent of metastases before cytoreduction, possibly because of the higher likelihood of phenotypically resistant clones of cells in large metastatic masses (201,204). Patients whose metastatic tumor is very large (i.e., >10 cm before cytoreductive surgery) have a shorter survival than those with smaller areas of disease (134) (Fig. 11.8). Extensive carcinomatosis, the presence of ascites, and poor tumor grade, even with lesions that measure <5 mm, are also poor prognostic factors (204–207,212).

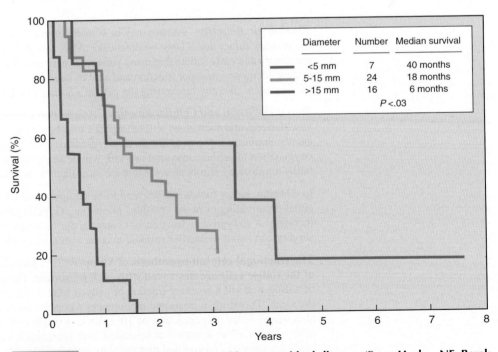

Diameter	Number	Median survival
<5 mm	7	40 months
5-15 mm	24	18 months
>15 mm	16	6 months

P <.03

Figure 11.6   **Survival versus diameter of largest residual disease.** (From **Hacker NF, Berek JS, Lagasse LD, Nieberg RK, Elashoff RM.** Primary cytoreductive surgery for epithelial ovarian cancer. *Obstet Gynecol* 1983;61:413–420, with permission from the American College of Obstetricians and Gynecologists.)

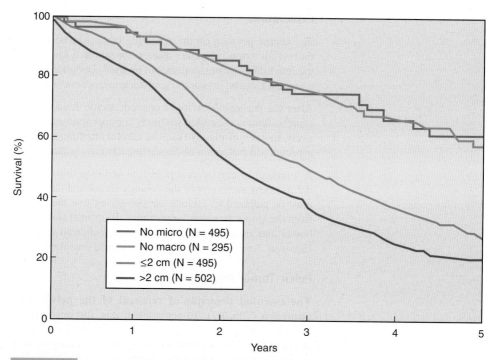

Figure 11.7   **Survival of patients with stage IIIC epithelial ovarian cancer based on the maximum size of the residual tumor after exploratory laparotomy and tumor resection.** (From **Heintz APM, Odicino F, Maisonneuve P, Quinn MA, Benedet JL, Creasman WT, et al.** Carcinoma of the ovary. In: **Pecorelli S, ed.** Twenty-Sixth Annual Report on the Results of Treatment in Gynaecological Cancer. *Int J Gynecol Oncol* 2006;95(suppl 1):S161–S192, with permission.)

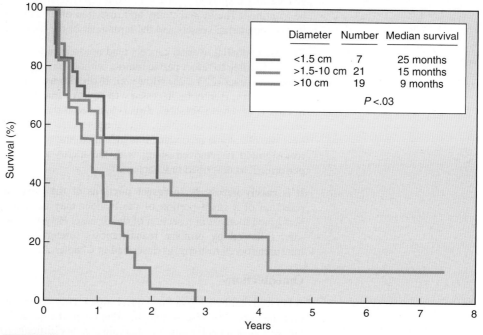

Figure 11.8   **Survival versus diameter of largest metastatic disease before cytoreduction.** (From **Hacker NF, Berek JS, Lagasse LD, Nieberg RK, Elashoff RM.** Primary cytoreductive surgery for epithelial ovarian cancer. *Obstet Gynecol* 1983;61:413–420, with permission from the American College of Obstetricians and Gynecologists.)

Exploration

The supine position on the operating table may be sufficient for most patients. However, for those with extensive pelvic disease for whom a low resection of the colon may be necessary, the low lithotomy position should be used. Debulking operations should be performed through a vertical incision in order to gain adequate access to the upper abdomen as well as to the pelvis.

After the peritoneal cavity is opened, ascitic fluid, if present, should be evacuated. In some centers, fluid is submitted routinely for appropriate *in vitro* studies, particularly the clonogenic assay. In cases of massive ascites, careful attention must be given to hemodynamic monitoring, especially in patients with borderline cardiovascular function.

A thorough inspection and palpation of the peritoneal cavity and retroperitoneum are carried out to assess the extent of the primary tumor and the metastatic disease. All abdominal viscera must be palpated to exclude the possibility that the ovarian disease is metastatic, particularly from the stomach, colon, or pancreas. If optimal status is not considered achievable, extensive bowel and urologic resections are not indicated except to overcome a bowel obstruction. However, removal of the primary tumor and omental cake is usually both feasible and desirable.

Pelvic Tumor Resection

The essential principle of removal of the pelvic tumor is to use the retroperitoneal approach (206,207). To accomplish this, the retroperitoneum is entered laterally, along the surface of the psoas muscles, which avoids the iliac vessels and the ureters. The procedure is initiated by division of the round ligaments bilaterally if the uterus is present. The peritoneal incision is extended cephalad, lateral to the ovarian vessels within the *infundibulopelvic ligament* and caudally toward the bladder. With careful dissection, the retroperitoneal space is explored, and the ureter and pelvic vessels are identified. The pararectal and paravesicle spaces are identified and developed as described in Chapter 9.

The peritoneum overlying the bladder is dissected to connect the peritoneal incisions anteriorly. The vesicouterine plane is identified, and, with careful sharp dissection, the bladder is mobilized from the anterior surface of the cervix. The ovarian vessels are isolated, doubly ligated, and divided.

The hysterectomy, which is often not a "simple" operation, is performed. The ureters need to be carefully displayed in order to avoid injury. During this procedure, the uterine vessels can be identified. The hysterectomy and resection of the contiguous tumor are completed by ligation of the uterine vessels and the remainder of the tissues within the cardinal ligaments.

Because epithelial ovarian cancers tend not to invade the lumina of the colon or bladder, it is usually feasible to resect pelvic tumors without having to resect portions of the lower colon or the urinary tract (223–226). However, **if the disease surrounds the rectosigmoid colon and its mesentery, it may be necessary to remove that portion of the colon to clear the pelvic disease** (Fig. 11.9) (223,224). This is justified if the patient will be left with "optimal" disease at the end of the cytoreduction. After the pararectal space is identified in such patients, the proximal site of colonic involvement is identified, the colon and its mesentery are divided, and the rectosigmoid is removed along with the uterus *en bloc*. A reanastomosis of the colon is performed, as described in Chapter 20.

It is rarely necessary to resect portions of the lower urinary tract (225). Occasionally, resection of a small portion of the bladder may be required. If so, a cystotomy should be performed to assist in resection of the disease. Rarely, partial ureteric resection may be necessary, followed by primary reanastomosis (ureteroureterostomy), ureteroneocystostomy, or transureteroureterostomy, as described in Chapter 20.

Omentectomy

Advanced epithelial ovarian cancer often completely replaces the omentum, forming an omental cake. This disease may be adherent to the parietal peritoneum of the anterior abdominal wall, making entry into the abdominal cavity difficult. After freeing the omentum from any adhesions to parietal peritoneum, adherent loops of small intestine are freed by sharp dissection. The omentum is then lifted and pulled gently in the cranial direction, exposing the attachment of the infracolic omentum to the transverse colon. The peritoneum is incised to open the appropriate plane, which is developed by sharp dissection along the serosa of the transverse

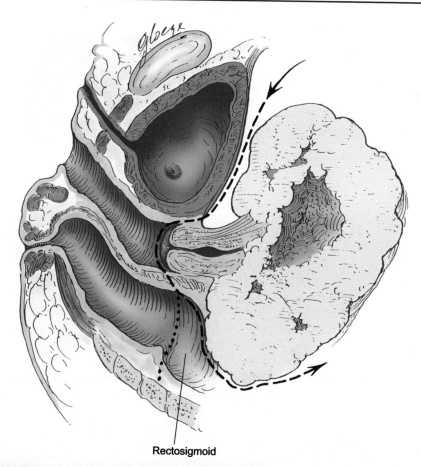

Rectosigmoid

Figure 11.9   **Resection of the pelvic tumor may include removal of the uterus, tubes, and ovaries, as well as portions of the lower intestinal tract.** The arrows represent the plane of resection.

colon. Small vessels are ligated with hemoclips. The omentum is then separated from the greater curvature of the stomach by ligation of the right and left gastroepiploic arteries and ligation of the short gastric arteries (Fig. 11.10).

The disease in the gastrocolic ligament can extend to the hilus of the spleen and splenic flexure of the colon on the left and to the capsule of the liver and the hepatic flexure of the colon on the right. Usually, the disease does not invade the parenchyma of the liver or spleen, and a plane can be found between the tumor and these organs. However, **it will occasionally be necessary to perform splenectomy to remove all the omental disease** (213,226,227) (Fig. 11.11). Diaphragm stripping and diaphragm resection have been used to optimally resect upper abdominal disease in selected cases (213).

Intestinal Resection

The disease may involve focal areas of the small or large intestine, and resection should be performed if it would permit the removal of all or most of the abdominal metastases. Apart from the rectosigmoid colon, the most frequent sites of intestinal metastasis are the terminal ileum, the cecum, and the transverse colon. Resection of one or more of these segments of bowel may be necessary (223–226).

Resection of Other Metastases

Other large masses of tumor that are located on the parietal peritoneum should be removed, particularly if they are isolated masses, and their removal will permit optimal cytoreduction. Resection of extensive disease from the surfaces of the diaphragm is generally neither practical nor feasible, although solitary metastases may be resected, the diaphragm sutured, and a

465

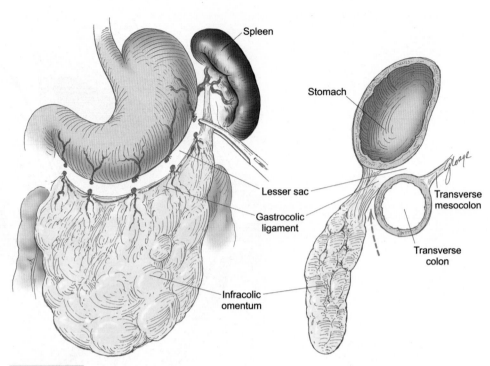

Figure 11.10   Separation of the omentum from stomach and transverse colon. (From **Heintz APM, Berek JS.** Cytoreductive surgery for ovarian carcinoma. In: **Piver MS, ed.** *Ovarian malignancies.* Edinburgh: Churchill Livingstone, 1987:134, with permission.)

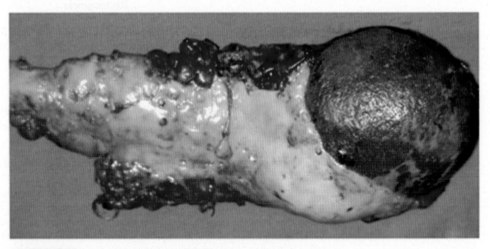

Figure 11.11   Omental "cake" densely adherent to the spleen.

chest tube placed if necessary for a few days (228). The use of the Cavitron Ultrasonic Surgical Aspirator (CUSA), the argon beam laser, and the loop electrosurgical device may help facilitate resection of small tumor nodules, especially those on flat surfaces (229–231).

Resection of Pelvic and Paraaortic Lymph Nodes

The performance of a pelvic and paraaortic lymphadenectomy in patients with stage IIIC–IV disease has been reported to prolong survival (123), but an international randomized study failed to confirm this (232). **Patients who were optimally cytoreduced in the peritoneal cavity were randomized between systematic pelvic and paraaortic lymphadenectomy versus resection of bulky nodes only.** There were 216 evaluable patients in the systematic lymphadenectomy arm and 211 in the nodal debulking arm of the study. Patients in each group were well matched for clinical characteristics such as stage of disease, grade of tumor, and residual disease status. Although there was a 6-month improvement in progression-free survival, **there was no difference in 5-year overall survival** [48.5% versus 47% respectively; 95% confidence interval (CI)—8.4% to 10.6%].

Du Bois and colleagues analyzed three phase III German trials to try to retrospectively determine the role of lymphadenectomy (233). There were a total of 3,336 patients, of whom 1,059 (32%) had no macroscopic residual intraperitoneal disease. Retroperitoneal lymphadenectomy was performed in 757 of the 1,059 patients (72%), and there was a significant survival advantage for the group having the lymphadenectomy (66% vs. 55%; $p = 0.003$). No advantage could be demonstrated if there was any macroscopic residual disease. **The authors concluded that a randomized controlled trial was warranted to address the question of systematic pelvic and paraaortic lymph node dissection versus nodal debulking in patients with no intraperitoneal residual disease.**

Feasibility and Outcome

An analysis of the retrospective data available suggests that these operations are feasible in 70% to 90% of patients when performed by gynecologic oncologists (205,207,210,213). Major morbidity is in the range of 5% and operative mortality in the range of 1% (182,187). Intestinal resection in these patients does not appear to increase the overall morbidity of the operation (205,207).

Some have questioned the ability of cytoreductive surgery to improve the overall outcome of patients with ovarian cancer (234). Concern has been expressed that these operations are excessively morbid and that modern chemotherapies are sufficient. No randomized prospective study has ever been performed to define the value of primary cytoreductive surgery. However, all retrospective studies indicate that the diameter of **the largest residual tumor nodule before the initiation of chemotherapy is significantly related to progression-free survival in patients with advanced ovarian cancer.** In addition, quality of life is likely to be significantly enhanced by removal of bulky tumor masses from the pelvis and upper abdomen.

In a metaanalysis of 81 studies of women who underwent cytoreductive surgery for advanced ovarian cancer, Bristow and colleagues (235) **documented that the extent of debulking correlated with incremental benefits in survival–that is, the greater the percentage of tumor reduction, the longer the survival. Each 10% increase in cytoreduction equated to a 5.5% increase in median survival. Women whose cytoreduction was greater than 75% of their tumor burden had a median survival of 33.9 months compared with 22.7 months for women whose tumors were cytoreduced to less than 75%.** ($p < 0.001$).

Patients with stage IV disease can benefit from optimal cytoreduction (208,236). In selected cases, resection of isolated hepatic metastasis to <1 cm results in an optimal resection of disease (236).

A prospective randomized study of "interval" cytoreductive surgery was carried out by the European Organization for the Research and Treatment of Cancer (EORTC). Interval surgery was performed after three cycles of platinum-combination chemotherapy in patients whose primary attempt at cytoreduction was suboptimal. Patients in the surgical arm of the study demonstrated a survival benefit when compared with those who did not undergo interval debulking (237). Most of these patients had not had an aggressive attempt to debulk their tumor at their initial surgery. In a 10-year follow-up analysis, the risk of mortality was reduced by more than 40% in the group that was randomized to the debulking arm of the study (238). Therefore, **the performance of a debulking operation as early as possible in the course of the patient's treatment should be considered the standard of care** (239).

A prospective phase III study of interval cytoreductive surgery was conducted by the GOG (240), but the study design was different because **the patients entered on the trial had already undergone a maximal attempt at tumor resection at their initial surgery.** The randomized findings showed no difference between the group of patients who had an additional attempt at debulking after three cycles of chemotherapy compared with those who did not. The median survival of the 216 women who underwent interval cytoreduction was 32 months compared with 33 months for the 209 women who did not undergo surgical cytoreduction.

There is evidence that the survival of women with advanced ovarian cancer is improved when the surgeon is specifically trained to perform cytoreductive surgery (241) and when there is centralization of care (242). Therefore, **whenever feasible, patients with advanced ovarian malignancy should be referred to a subspecialty unit for primary surgery, and every effort should be made to attain as complete a cytoreduction as possible.**

Treatment with Chemotherapy and Radiation

Early Stage Low-Risk Ovarian Cancer

Guthrie et al. (184) studied the outcome of 656 patients with early stage epithelial ovarian cancer. No untreated patients who had stage IA, grade 1 cancer died of their disease; thus, adjuvant radiation and chemotherapy were unnecessary. Furthermore, the Gynecologic Oncology Group carried out a prospective, randomized trial of observation versus *melphalan* for patients with stages IA and IB, grades 1 and 2 disease. **Five-year survival for each group was 94% and 96%, respectively, confirming that no further adjuvant treatment is needed for such patients.**

Early Stage High-Risk Ovarian Cancer

In patients whose disease is high risk—for example, more poorly differentiated or in whom there are malignant cells either in ascitic fluid or in peritoneal washings—additional therapy is indicated. Treatment options include chemotherapy or whole-abdominal radiation (186–206). Some comparisons of these modalities have been made and are summarized below.

Chemotherapy

Chemotherapy for patients with early stage high-risk epithelial ovarian cancer can be either single agent or multiagent (243–249). Some researchers have questioned the wisdom of overly aggressive chemotherapy in women with early stage disease, suggesting that the evidence for a durable impact on survival is marginal (250,251). Furthermore, **the possibility of leukemia with *alkylating agents* and platinum** make the administration of adjuvant therapy risky unless there is a significant benefit (244,245).

Cisplatin, carboplatin, cyclophosphamide, **and** *paclitaxel* **are all active as single agents against epithelial ovarian cancer** and have been administered either alone or in various combinations in the adjuvant setting. There were some early series in which *cisplatin* or *cyclophosphamide* or both (PC) were used to treat patients with stage I disease (252–260). In a GOG trial of three cycles of *cisplatin* and *cyclophosphamide* versus intraperitoneal ^{32}P in patients with stages IB and IC disease, the progression-free survival of women receiving the platinum-based chemotherapy was 31% higher than that of those receiving the radiocolloid (254). Similar results were reported from a multicenter trial performed in Italy by the Gruppo Italiano Collaborativo Oncologica Ginecologica for progression-free survival, although there was no overall survival advantage (259). *Carboplatin* can be substituted for *cisplatin* in the therapy of these patients (260) because it is much better tolerated, has fewer side effects, and appears to have similar efficacy.

Two large, parallel, randomized phase III clinical trials have been recently reported on women with early stage disease: the **International Collaborative Ovarian Neoplasm Trial 1 (ICON1)** and the **Adjuvant Chemotherapy Trial in Ovarian Neoplasia (ACTION)** (260,261).

In the ICON1 trial, 477 patients from 84 centers in Europe were entered. Patients of all stages were eligible for the trial if, in the opinion of the investigator, it was unclear whether adjuvant therapy would be of benefit. Most patients were said to have stages I and IIA disease, but optimal **surgical staging was not required,** so it is likely an unquantified number of these women had stage III disease. Adjuvant platinum-based chemotherapy was given to 241 patients, and no adjuvant chemotherapy was given to 236 patients. **The 5-year survival was 73% in the group that received adjuvant chemotherapy compared with 62% in the control group** [hazard ratio (HR) = 0.65, $p = 0.01$] (261).

In the ACTION trial, 440 patients from 40 European centers were randomized; 224 patients received adjuvant platinum-based chemotherapy, and 224 patients did not (260). Patients with stages I and IIA, grades 2 and 3 were eligible. Only **one-third of the total group was optimally staged** (151 patients). **In the observation arm, optimal staging was associated with a better survival** (HR = 2.31, $p = 0.03$); **in the nonoptimally staged patients, adjuvant**

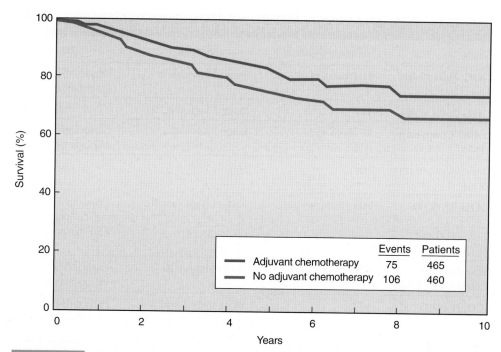

Figure 11.12 **Overall survival in patients with early-stage ovarian carcinoma** (The ICON1/ ACTION Trials). Adjuvant *cisplatin-* or *carboplatin-*based single agent or combination chemotherapy (*n* = 465 patients) (blue line) versus no adjuvant chemotherapy (*n* = 460 patients) (purple line) until clinical progression. The hazard ratio is 0.67 (95% CI = 0.50 to 0.90, *p* = 0.008 using log-rank test) in favor of chemotherapy. Five-year survivals were 82% for the adjuvant chemotherapy group versus 74% for those who do not receive adjuvant chemotherapy (221). These data should be interpreted with caution because most of the patients were not completely staged, and the benefit of treatment appears to be only in patients who did not have a complete staging laparotomy. (From **Trimbos JB, Parmar M, Guthrie D, Swart AM, Vergote I, Bolls G, et al.** International Collaborative Ovarian Neoplasm Trial 1 and Adjuvant Chemotherapy in Ovarian Neoplasm Trial: two parallel randomized phase III trials of adjuvant chemotherapy in patients with early-stage ovarian carcinoma. *J Natl Cancer Inst* 2003;95:105–112, with permission.)

chemotherapy was associated with an improvement in survival (HR = 1.78, *p* = 0.009). **In optimally staged patients, no benefit of adjuvant chemotherapy was seen.** Therefore, in the ACTION trial, the benefit from adjuvant chemotherapy was limited to the patients with nonoptimal staging, suggesting that patients might only benefit if they had a higher likelihood of occult microscopic dissemination.

When the data from the two trials were combined and analyzed (262), a total of 465 patients were randomized to receive platinum-based adjuvant chemotherapy and 460 to observation until disease progression (Fig. 11.12). After a median follow-up of more than 4 years, the overall survival was 82% in the chemotherapy arm and 74% in the observation arm (HR = 0.67, *p* = 0.001). Recurrence-free survival was also better in the chemotherapy arm: 76% versus 65% (HR = 0.64, *p* = 0.001). The results of this analysis must be interpreted with caution because most of the patients did not undergo thorough surgical staging, but **the findings suggest that platinum-based chemotherapy should be given to patients who have not been optimally staged.**

The GOG reported the results of a randomized study of three cycles versus six cycles of *carboplatin* **and** *paclitaxel* in 457 patients with early stage ovarian cancer (231). An unexpectedly large number of patients (126, or approximately 28%) had incomplete or inadequately documented surgical staging. The recurrence rate was 24% lower (HR = 0.76, CI = 0.5–1.13, *p* = 0.18) for six versus three cycles, but this was not statistically significant. The estimated probability of recurrence at 5 years was 20.1% for six cycles and 25.4% for three cycles. They **concluded that three cycles of adjuvant** *carboplatin* **and** *paclitaxel* **was a reasonable option for women with high-risk early stage ovarian cancer.**

Table 11.3 Randomized Trials in Stage I Epithelial Ovarian Cancer (Since 1995)				
Study	*Patients (Author)*	*Stages*	*Treatment*	*Best Arm*
GOG 7601 (248)	81 (Young et al.)	Stage I low risk	Observation vs. *melphalan*	No difference
GOG 7602 (248)	141	Stage I high risk, II	^{32}P vs. *melphalan*	No difference
Italian Cooperative (255)	47 (Bolis et al.)	Stage I low risk	Observation vs. *cisplatin* $\times$ 6	No difference
Italian Cooperative (255)	104	Stage I high risk	^{32}P vs. *cisplatin* $\times$ 6	*Cisplatin* 79% vs. 69% 5-yr survival
GOG 95 (254)	205 (Young et al.)	Stage I high risk, II	*Cisplatin* 75 mg/m^2; *cyclophosphamide* 750 mg/m^2 vs. ^{32}P	*Cisplatin, cyclophosphamide* 77% vs. 66% 5-yr survival
Scandinavian Cooperative (258)	134 (Tropé et al.)	Stage I high risk	*Carboplatin* AUC $\times$ vs. observation	No difference
ICON1 (261)	477	Most stage I and II, optimal staging not required	Platinum-based vs. observation	73% (chemotherapy) vs. 62% (observation) 5-yr survival
ACTION (260)	448 (Trimbos et al.)	Stage I high risk, IIA, one-third staged	Platinum-based vs. observation	Improved survival in optimally staged patients only
ICON1–ACTION (262)	925 (Trimbos et al.)	Combined analysis		82% (chemotherapy) vs. 72% (observation) 5-yr survival
GOG 157 (263)	421	Stage I high risk/II	*Paclitaxel* 175 mg/m^2; *carboplatin* AUC 7.5 3 vs. 6 cycles	3 cycles equivalent to 6 cycles of chemotherapy
GOG 175	Accruing	Stage I high risk/II	*Paclitaxel* 175 mg/m^2; *carboplatin* AUC 6 followed by observation vs. *paclitaxel* 40 mg/m^2 weekly $\times$ 26 weeks	

GOG, Gynecologic Oncology Group; AUC, area under the curve.

The current GOG trial includes patients with high-risk stage I and II disease and **offers three cycles of *carboplatin* and *paclitaxel* followed by a randomization to either observation versus 26 weeks of weekly low-dose (40 mg/m^2) *paclitaxel*.** High-risk stage I is defined as stages IA or IB, grade 3, stage IC, or clear cell carcinomas.

A summary of randomized phase III trials reported since 1995 for the treatment of patients with low-stage disease is presented in Table 11.3 (247,248,252,260,262).

Radiation Therapy

There are two general approaches to the treatment of low-stage epithelial ovarian cancer with radiation: intraperitoneal radiocolloids and whole-abdominal radiation therapy. In one retrospective study of ^{32}P, the 5-year survival was 85% (215). In a series of patients with stage I disease treated with whole-abdominal radiation (246), the 5-year relapse-free survival rate was 78%, but many of these patients had high-risk variables (e.g., poor histologic grade).

A prospective trial was conducted by the GOG of patients with stage IB, grade 3, stage IC, or stage II with no residual disease. Twelve cycles of *melphalan* were compared with intraperitoneal ^{32}P, and there was no difference in survival (248). However, in a multicenter Italian trial (182), a randomized comparison of six cycles of *cisplatin* as a single agent versus ^{32}P showed an 84% disease-free survival with *cisplatin* and 61% with ^{32}P ($p <0.01$). Furthermore, the GOG protocol that randomized *cisplatin* and *cyclophosphamide* versus ^{32}P showed that the platinum-based chemotherapy was superior (254). Therefore, **although ^{32}P produces results similar to single-agent *melphalan*, platinum-based chemotherapy is preferable** (Table 11.3). Pelvic radiation alone is not as effective as *melphalan* in these patients and should not be used in ovarian cancer (243).

Recommendation for Adjuvant Treatment of Early Stage Ovarian Cancer

Low-Risk Early Stage Disease

No adjuvant chemotherapy is recommended for these patients.

High-Risk Early Stage Disease

1. **Patients with high-risk stage I epithelial ovarian cancer should be given adjuvant chemotherapy. The type depends on the patient's overall health and presence of medical comorbidities.**

2. **Treatment with *carboplatin* and *paclitaxel* chemotherapy for three to six cycles is used in most patients, although single-agent *carboplatin* may be preferable for frailer women.**

Advanced-Stage Ovarian Cancer

Chemotherapy

Systemic chemotherapy is the standard treatment for metastatic epithelial ovarian cancer (264–288). After the introduction of *cisplatin* in the latter half of the 1970s, platinum-based combination chemotherapy has become the most frequently used treatment regimen in the United States (240). *Paclitaxel* became available in the 1980s, and this drug was incorporated into ovarian combination chemotherapy in the 1990s (264–271). Comparative trials of *paclitaxel, cisplatin,* and *carboplatin* are summarized below (Table 11.4).

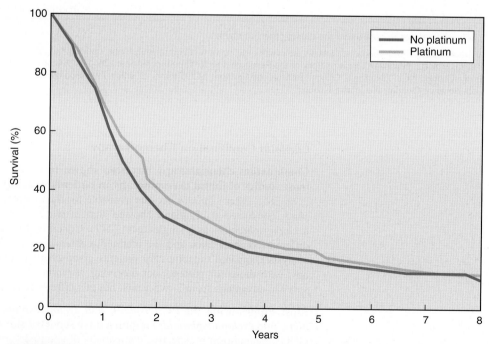

Figure 11.13 Survival of patients with advanced-stage ovarian cancer: a metaanalysis of multiple trials comparing *cisplatin*-containing combination chemotherapy with regimens without *cisplatin*. (From **Advanced Ovarian Cancer Trialists Group.** Chemotherapy in advanced ovarian cancer: an overview of randomized clinical trials. *BMJ* 1991;303:884, with permission.)

Table 11.4 Randomized Trials Involving Platinum and Taxanes in Patients with Advanced-Stage Epithelial Ovarian Cancer

Group Protocol	Ref. Update	Year	Author	Status	Drugs/Doses/(hrs)[a]	Best
GOG 111	(272)	1996	McQuire et al.	Subopt	Paclitaxel 135 (3); cisplatin 75 vs. cyclophosphamide 750; cisplatin 75	Paclitaxel, cisplatin
OV 10 EORTC, NOCOVA, NCIC	(273)	1998	Piccart et al.	Opt, subopt	Paclitaxel 175; cisplatin 75 vs. cyclophosphamide 750; cisplatin 75	Paclitaxel, cisplatin
GOG 132	(274)	2000	Muggia et al.	Subopt	Cisplatin 100 vs. paclitaxel 200 (24) vs. cisplatin 75; paclitaxel 135 (24)	Paclitaxel, cisplatin
GOG 158	(288)	2003	Ozols et al.	Opt	Carboplatin 7.5; paclitaxel 175(3) vs. cisplatin 75; paclitaxel 135 (24)	Paclitaxel, carboplatin
SCOT-ROC	(292)	1999	Vasey et al.	Opt, subopt	Docetaxel; cisplatin vs. paclitaxel; cisplatin	Docetaxel, carboplatin
ICON 3	(290)	2002	ICON3 collaborators	Opt, subopt	Carboplatin; paclitaxel vs. carboplatin vs. cisplatin; cyclophosphamide; doxorubicin	Carboplatin
GOG 182, ICON 5	(294)	2004	Completed	Opt, subopt	Paclitaxel; carboplatin × 8 vs. paclitaxel; carboplatin; gemcitabine × 8 vs. paclitaxel; carboplatin; liposomal doxorubicin × 8 vs. carboplatin; topotecan × 4 followed by paclitaxel; carboplatin × 4 vs. carboplatin; gemcitabine × 4 followed by paclitaxel; carboplatin × 4	Carboplatin[a], paclitaxel

[a]Carboplatin doses in area under the curve; others in mg/m^2.

IV, intravenous; IP, intraperitoneal; AUC, area under the curve (Calvert formula); opt, optimal; subopt, suboptimal; GOG, Gynecologic Oncology Group; EORTC, European Organization for the Research and Treatment of Cancer; OV 10, Ovarian Protocol; NOCOVA, Nordic Ovarian Cancer Study Group; NCIC, National Cancer Institute of Canada; SCOT-ROC, Scottish Gynaecological Cancer Trials Group; ICON, International Collaborative Ovarian Neoplasm Group.

Cisplatin Combination Chemotherapy

Combination chemotherapy has been shown to be superior to single-agent therapy in most studies of initial chemotherapy in patients with advanced epithelial ovarian cancer (272–285). After *cisplatin* became available for the treatment of ovarian cancer, a prospective study conducted in England showed that *cisplatin* was better than an *alkylating agent, cyclophosphamide,* as a single agent (277). Concurrently, *cisplatin* was tested in a variety of different combinations, and the platinum-containing regimens were superior (278). A meta-analysis compared outcomes for patients given *cisplatin*-containing combination chemotherapy, with those for patients not receiving *cisplatin* (275). The *cisplatin* group had a slight survival advantage from 2 to 5 years, but this difference disappeared by 8 years (Fig 11.13).

Most studies using the PC (*cisplatin* and *cyclophosphamide*) or PAC (*cisplatin, doxorubicin,* and *cyclophosphamide*) regimen have reported similar survival rates (279–284). The GOG's randomized prospective comparison of equitoxic doses of PAC versus PC showed no benefit to the inclusion of *doxorubicin* in the combination (280). Although a metaanalysis of the combined data from four trials showed a 7% survival advantage at 6 years for those patients treated with the *doxorubicin*-containing regimen (284), the survival curves converged at 8 years.

Paclitaxel

The next major advance in the treatment of advanced-stage disease was the incorporation of *paclitaxel* **into the chemotherapeutic regimens.** A series of randomized, prospective clinical trials with *paclitaxel*-containing arms have defined the current recommended treatment protocol in advanced epithelial ovarian cancer (272–274,288). These studies are listed in Table 11.4.

Paclitaxel **was shown to be a very active agent in ovarian cancer** (264–270). The overall response rate of *paclitaxel* in phase II trials was 36% in previously treated patients (268), which is a higher rate than was seen for *cisplatin* when it was first tested.

Reporting the Gynecologic Oncology Group data (Protocol 111), McGuire et al. showed that **the combination of** *cisplatin* **(75 mg/m^2) and** *paclitaxel* **(135 mg/m^2) was superior to** *cisplatin* **(75 mg/m^2) and** *cyclophosphamide* **(600 mg/m^2), each given for six cycles** (272). In suboptimally resected patients, the *paclitaxel*-containing arm produced a 36% reduction in mortality (Fig 11.14). These data were verified in a trial conducted jointly by the European Organization for the Research and Treatment of Cancer, the Nordic Ovarian Cancer Study Group (NOCOVA), and the National Cancer Institute of Canada (NCIC), in which patients with both optimal and suboptimal disease were treated (273). In this study, the *paclitaxel*-containing arm produced a significant improvement in both progression-free interval and overall survival in both optimal and suboptimal groups (Fig 11.15). **Based on these two studies,** *paclitaxel* **should be included in the primary treatment of all women with advanced-stage epithelial ovarian cancer unless precluded by toxicity.**

A three-arm comparison of *paclitaxel* (T) versus *cisplatin* (P) versus PT in suboptimal stage III and IV patients (protocol 132) showed equivalency in the three groups, but crossover from one drug to the other was permitted (274). The study essentially showed that the combination regimen was better tolerated than the sequential administration of the agents in suboptimally resected patients.

Carboplatin

The second-generation platinum analogue, *carboplatin*, was introduced and developed to have less toxicity than its parent compound, *cisplatin*. **Fewer gastrointestinal side effects, especially nausea and vomiting, are observed with** *carboplatin*, **and there is less nephrotoxicity, neurotoxicity, and ototoxicity** (285,286). *Carboplatin* is associated with a higher degree of myelosuppression than *cisplatin*.

The initial studies showed that *carboplatin* and *cisplatin* had approximately a 4:1 equivalency ratio. Thus, a standard single-agent dose of approximately 400 mg/m^2 *carboplatin* was used in most phase II trials. **The optimal way to dose** *carboplatin* **is by using the area under the curve (AUC) and the glomerular filtration rate according to the Calvert formula** (287), as discussed in Chapter 4. **The target AUC is 5 to 7 for previously untreated patients with ovarian cancer.** A platelet nadir of approximately 50,000/dL is a suitable target (287).

Carboplatin and Paclitaxel

Two randomized, prospective clinical studies have compared the combination of *paclitaxel* **and** *carboplatin* **with** *paclitaxel* **and** *cisplatin* **(288,289) (Table 11.4). In both studies, the efficacy and survivals were similar, but the toxicity was more acceptable for the** *carboplatin*-**containing regimen.**

In the first trial, GOG Protocol 158, the randomization was *carboplatin* AUC 7.5 and *paclitaxel* 175 mg/m^2 over 3 hours versus *cisplatin* 75 mg/m^2 and *paclitaxel* 135 mg/m^2 over 24 hours (288). The progression-free survival of the *carboplatin*-containing arm was 20.7 months versus 19.4 months for the control arm (Fig. 11.16). The overall survival was 57.4 months for the *carboplatin* arm versus 48.7 months for control arm. The relative risk of progression for the *carboplatin* plus *paclitaxel* group was 0.88, and the RR of death was 0.84. **The gastrointestinal and neurotoxicity of the** *carboplatin* **arm were appreciably lower than in the** *cisplatin* **arm.**

A similar result was obtained in a large randomized trial in Germany (289) in which the dose of *carboplatin* was AUC = 6, and *paclitaxel* was 185 mg/m^2 over 3 hours compared with the same dose of *paclitaxel* and *cisplatin* 75 mg/m^2. The overall survival was 44.1 months for the *carboplatin*-containing arm versus 43.3 months for the control arm. **Thus, the preferred regimen in patients with advanced stage disease is the** *paclitaxel* **plus** *carboplatin* **combination.**

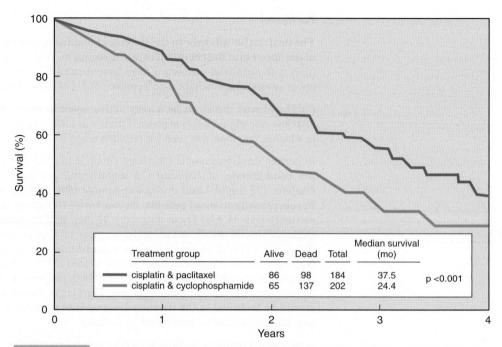

Figure 11.14 Survival of patients with suboptimal stage III and IV epithelial ovarian cancer treated with *paclitaxel* and *cisplatin* versus *cyclophosphamide* and *cisplatin:* a Gynecologic Oncology Group study (Protocol 111). (From **McGuire WP, Hoskins W, Brady MF, Kucera PR, Partridge EE, Look KY, et al.** *Cyclophosphamide* and *cisplatin* compared with *paclitaxel* and *cisplatin* in patients with stage III and stage IV ovarian cancer. *N Engl J Med* 1996;334:1–6, with permission.)

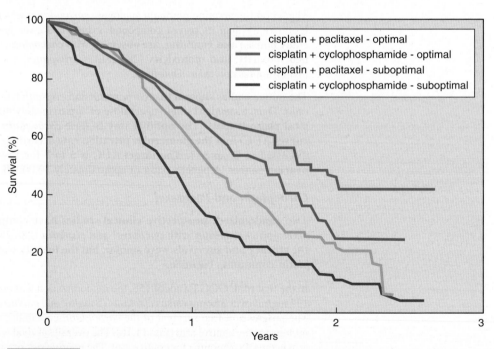

Figure 11.15 Survival of patients with stage III and IV epithelial ovarian cancer treated with *paclitaxel* and *cisplatin* or *cyclophosphamide* and *cisplatin:* results of a European cooperative group trials study. Survival by treatment, and survival by treatment group (optimal vs. suboptimal). [From **Stuart G, Bertelsen K, Mangioni C, Tropé C, James K, Kaye S, et al.** Updated analysis shows a highly significant improved survival for *cisplatin-paclitaxel* as first line treatment of advanced stage epithelial ovarian cancer: mature results of the EORTC-GCCG, NOCOVA, NCIC CTG and Scottish Intergroup Trial. *Proc Am Soc Clin Oncol* 1998;34: 1394(abst), with permission.]

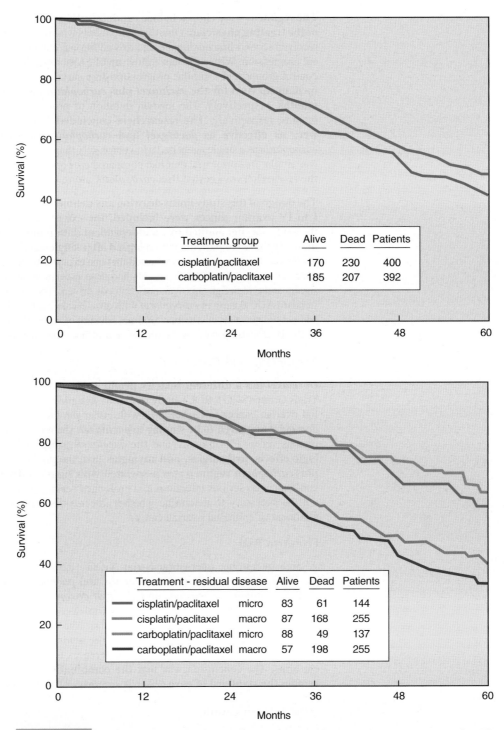

Figure 11.16   Survival of patients with stage III epithelial ovarian cancer treated with *carboplatin* and *paclitaxel* versus *cisplatin* and *paclitaxel:* a Gynecologic Oncology Group study (Protocol 158) **Top:** Survival by treatment. **Bottom:** Survival by treatment group (microscopic vs. macroscopic) [From **Ozols RF, Bundy BN, Greer BE, Fowler JM, Clarke-Pearson D, Burger RA, et al.** Phase III trial of *carboplatin* and *paclitaxel* compared with *cisplatin* and *paclitaxel* in patients with optimally resected stage III ovarian cancer: a Gynecologic Oncology Group study. *J Clin Oncol* 2003;21:3194–3200, with permission.]

The **International Collaborative Ovarian Neoplasm 3 (ICON3) trial** was a study of **2,074 women with all stages of ovarian cancer, including 20% who had stage I or II disease** (290). The combination of *carboplatin* plus *paclitaxel* was compared with two *nonpaclitaxel* regimens, *carboplatin* (**70%**) or *cyclophosphamide, doxorubicin,* and *cisplatin* (CAP) (**30%**).

The regimens were chosen before randomization and were based on the clinical preference of the treating physician. One-third of patients who received *carboplatin* or CAP subsequently received second-line *paclitaxel,* and this additional chemotherapy was often given before clinical progression. With a median follow-up of 51 months, the *carboplatin* plus *paclitaxel* and the control groups had a similar progression-free survival (0.93) and overall survival (0.98). **The median survival for the *paclitaxel* plus *carboplatin* and control groups was 36.1 and 35.4 months, respectively.** The median duration of progression-free survival was 17.3 and 16.1 months, respectively. **The researchers concluded that single-agent *carboplatin* and CAP were as effective as *paclitaxel* and *carboplatin* for first-line chemotherapy.** Because *carboplatin* as a single agent had a lower toxicity than the other regimens and the median survival was similar in a prior trial that had compared *carboplatin* and CAP as first-line treatment (291), **the researchers suggested that *carboplatin* alone was the preferred therapy.**

The design of this study limits drawing any definitive conclusions. Patients with FIGO stages I to IV ovarian cancer were included, the extent of primary surgery was variable, and the study was not audited by an independent data-monitoring committee. Furthermore, the majority (85%) of patients who relapsed after single-agent *carboplatin* subsequently received *paclitaxel.* The investigators suggested that one explanation for the favorable outcome with *carboplatin* alone was that 30% of patients had dose escalation based on their nadir counts not falling significantly, although this was not protocol driven. They have commenced a study comparing standard AUC dosing of *carboplatin* with dose escalation based on nadir counts, and this will help address the question of whether "optimal" dosing of *carboplatin* makes a difference. **The findings of the ICON study were not conclusive and have not altered the standard of care.**

Carboplatin and *Docetaxel*

Docetaxel* has a different toxicity profile to *paclitaxel. The Scottish Gynaecological Cancer Trials Group (SCOT-ROC) study randomly assigned 1,077 women with stages IC to IV epithelial ovarian cancer to *carboplatin* with either *paclitaxel* or *docetaxel* (292). **The efficacy of *docetaxel* appeared to be similar to *paclitaxel:*** the median progression-free survival was 15.1 months versus 15.4 months, and **the *docetaxel* group had less extremity weakness, neurologic effects, arthralgias, and myalgias** than the *paclitaxel* group. However, **the *docetaxel* plus *carboplatin* regimen was associated with significantly more myelosuppression** and its consequences: serious infections and prolonged severe neutropenia. Therefore, additional study will be necessary to determine whether *docetaxel* should supplant *paclitaxel* in the primary treatment of epithelial ovarian cancer.

Five-Arm Trial

A large intergroup, international trial (GOG 182/SWOG 182/ICON5/ANZGOG) compared the standard **combination of *carboplatin* and *paclitaxel* with these drugs in combination with *gemcitabine, topotecan,* or *liposomal doxorubicin* in sequential doublets or triplets** (292,293).This was the largest randomized trial ever carried out in women with advanced ovarian cancer and recruited more than 4000 patients. The results have been presented, and **there was no apparent difference between any of the arms in terms of progression-free survival or median survival** although there were differences in the side effects experienced in the different arms. The conclusion was that **the combination of *carboplatin* and *paclitaxel* should remain the standard of care** (294). A summary of these trials is presented in Table 11.4.

Dose Intensification

Intravenous Chemotherapy   The issue of dose intensification of *cisplatin* was examined in a prospective trial conducted by the GOG (295). In this study, **243 patients with suboptimal ovarian cancer were randomized to receive 50 mg/m² or 100 mg/m² *cisplatin* plus 500 mg/m² *cyclophosphamide.* There was no difference in response rates in those patients with measurable disease,** and the overall survival times were identical. There was greater toxicity associated with the high-dose regimen. A Scottish group reported that patients who received 100 mg/m² *cisplatin* plus 750 mg/m² *cyclophosphamide* had a significantly longer median survival compared with those receiving 50 mg/m² *cisplatin* plus the same dose of *cyclophosphamide* (296). The overall median survival time was 114 weeks in the high-dose group and 69 weeks in the low-dose group ($p = 0.0008$), but this difference disappeared with longer follow-up (297). **Therefore, the doubling of the dose of *cisplatin* does not improve the survival of these patients.**

Dose escalations of *paclitaxel* and *carboplatin* require granulocyte colony-stimulating factor (G-CSF) because of the combined myelosuppressive effects, but there is no evidence to support a role for a more intensive course of either agent (270,298).

Intraperitoneal Chemotherapy   A randomized, prospective trial in 546 evaluable patients of intraperitoneal *cisplatin* versus intravenous *cisplatin* (100 mg/m^2), each given with 750 mg/m^2 *cyclophosphamide,* was performed jointly by the Southwest Oncology Group (SWOG) and the GOG in patients with advanced ovarian cancer following optimal cytoreduction (residual nodules <2 cm diameter) (299). **The intraperitoneal *cisplatin* arm had a somewhat longer overall median survival than the intravenous arm, 49 versus 41 months** ($p = 0.03$). **In the patients with minimal residual disease (<0.5 cm maximum residual diameter), who would be expected to derive the most benefit, there was no difference between the two treatments, 51 versus 46 months** ($p = 0.08$) (Table 11.5).

In a follow-up trial of 532 patients (GOG Protocol 114), the dose-intense arm was initiated by giving a moderately high dose of *carboplatin* (dose AUC $= 9$) for two induction cycles followed by intraperitoneal *cisplatin* 100 mg/m^2 and intravenous *paclitaxel* 135 mg/m^2 over 24 hours versus intravenous *cisplatin* 75 mg/m^2 and intravenous *paclitaxel* 135 mg/m^2 (300). In the dose-intense arm, progression-free median survival was 27.6 months compared with 22.5 months for the control arm ($p = 0.02$). However, there was no difference in overall survival (52.9 months versus 47.6 months, $p = 0.056$). Thus, **it is unclear if dose intensification with intraperitoneal *cisplatin* has a long-term impact on the survival of these patients.** A phase II trial of intravenous *paclitaxel* plus intraperitoneal *cisplatin* and *paclitaxel* was well tolerated and associated with a 2-year survival of 91% (302).

A randomized prospective GOG study compared intraperitoneal *cisplatin* and *paclitaxel* with intravenous *cisplatin* and *paclitaxel* (301). Four hundred and twenty-nine patients were randomly assigned, and 415 were eligible. The median progression-free survival was 23.8 months in the IP arm versus 18.3 months in the IV arm ($p = 0.05$). The median overall survival was 65.6 months in the IP group and 49.7 months in the IV group ($p = 0.03$) (Fig. 11.17). Ninety percent of patients in the IV arm received the six planned cycles of therapy, whereas **only 42% of patients received the assigned 6 cycles of IP therapy with the remainder switching to IV therapy.** The reasons for discontinuing were primarily for catheter-related problems, but there were also significantly more side effects in the IP group, with more patients experiencing severe fatigue, pain, hematological toxicity, nausea, and vomiting as well as metabolic and neurotoxicity. It is likely that with more training, appropriate dose modifications, and better antiemetics, the toxicity can be reduced.

The results of this study, together with the previous studies, led to an NCI clinical announcement recommending that women with optimally debulked stage III ovarian cancer be considered for IP chemotherapy. There has been a Cochrane Review as well as a separate metaanalysis that concluded that IP chemotherapy was associated with better outcomes than intravenous chemotherapy (304,305). The metaanalysis included six randomized trials with a total of 1,716 ovarian cancer patients. The pooled HR for progression-free survival of IP *cisplatin* as compared to IV treatment regimens was 0.792 (95% CI: 0.688–0.912, $p = 0.001$), and the pooled hazard ratio for overall survival was 0.799 (95% CI: 0.702–0.910, $p = 0.0007$). The authors concluded that these findings strongly supported the incorporation of an IP *cisplatin* regimen in the first-line treatment of stage III optimally debulked ovarian cancer (304).

Similar conclusions were reached in the **Cochrane review.** The reviewers concluded that their analysis established that **IP chemotherapy was associated with an increased overall survival and progression-free survival in patients with optimally debulked stage III ovarian cancer.** However, they also commented on the **potential for catheter-related complications and increased toxicity** with IP therapy and concluded that the optimal dose, timing, and mechanism of administration should be addressed in the next phase of clinical trials (305).

The role of IP chemotherapy is still contentious, with some researchers arguing that the trials to date were not pure tests of IP therapy and were flawed. In addition, concerns have been raised about the technical difficulties and increased toxicity of IP therapy (306).

Neoadjuvant Chemotherapy

Some authors have suggested that for patients with advanced disease, chemotherapy may be given before cytoreductive surgery. A series performed at Yale by Schwartz et al. (307) suggested

Group Protocol	Ref.	Year	Author	Status	Drugs/Doses/(hrs)	Best Arm
Table 11.5 Randomized Trials of IV Versus IP Chemotherapy in Patients with Advanced Epithelial Ovarian Cancer						
GOG 104	(299)	1996	Alberts et al.	Optimal	IP *cisplatin;* IV *cyclophosphamide* vs. IV *cisplatin;* IV *cyclophosphamide*	IP *cisplatin;* IV *cyclophosphamide*[a] 49 vs. 41 mos (*p* = 0.03)
GOG 114	(300)	2001	Markman et al.	Optimal	IV *carboplatin* AUC = 9 IP *cisplatin* 100; IV *paclitaxel* 135 (24) vs. IV *cisplatin* 75; IV *paclitaxel* 135 (24)	IP *cisplatin;* IV *carboplatin;* IV *paclitaxel*[b] 52.9 vs. 47.6 mos (*p* = 0.056)
GOG 172	(301)	2006	Armstrong et al.	Optimal	IV *paclitaxel* 135 (24); IP *cisplatin* 100-day 2; IP *paclitaxel* 60-day 8 vs. IV *paclitaxel* 135 (24); IV *cisplatin* 75	IP *cisplatin,* IV *paclitaxel* and IP *paclitaxel* 65.6 vs. 49.7 mos i (*p* = 0.03)

[a]Median survival longer in IP arm, not in minimal residual (<0.5 mm) group.

[b]Progression-free survival longer in IP arm, no difference in overall survival.

AUC; area under the curve.

that the survival of patients treated with *neoadjuvant* chemotherapy was comparable to that of patients historically treated with primary cytoreductive surgery in the same institution.

Neoadjuvant chemotherapy might be appropriate in selected patients who are at high risk for operative morbidity or mortality [e.g., those with significant cardiac disease (308,309) or those with large pleural effusions], but primary cytoreductive surgery should be considered the standard of care for most patients. Bristow et al. (310) recently reported the results of a systemic overview of neoadjuvant chemotherapy and concluded that **neoadjuvant chemotherapy represented a viable alternative strategy for the limited number of patients felt to be**

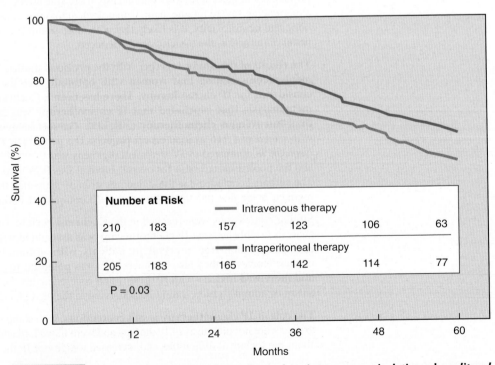

Figure 11.17   Overall survival after intraperitoneal vs. intravenous *cisplatin* and *paclitaxel* chemotherapy. (From **Armstrong DK, Bundy B, Wenzel L, Huang HQ, Baergen R, Lele S, et al.** Intraperitoneal *cisplatin* and *paclitaxel* in ovarian cancer. *N Eng J Med* 2006:354:34–43, with permission.)

Table 11.6 Combination Chemotherapy for Advanced Epithelial Ovarian Cancer: Recommended Regimens

Drugs	Dose	Administration (hr)	Interval	No. of Treatments
Standard Regimens				
Paclitaxel	175 mg/m^2	3	Every 3 weeks	6–8 cycles
Carboplatin	AUC = 5–6			
Paclitaxel	135 mg/m^2	3	Every 3 weeks	6–8 cycles
Cisplatin	75 mg/m^2			
Alternative Drugs[a] (Can be given with platinum)				
Topotecan	1.0–1.25 mg/m^2		Daily × 3–5 days	
	4.0 mg/m^2		Every 3 weeks, or weekly	
Gemcitabine	800–1,000 mg/m^2		Every 3 weeks	
Doxorubicin, liposomal	40–50 mg/m^2		Every 4 weeks	

AUC, area under the curve dose by Calvert formula (287).

[a]Drugs that can be substituted for *paclitaxel* if hypersensitivity to that drug occurs.

optimally unresectable by an experienced ovarian cancer surgical team; however, currently available data suggest that the survival outcome achievable with initial chemotherapy may be inferior to successful primary cytoreductive surgery.

The EORTC has completed a large randomized trial of surgery followed by six cycles of *carboplatin* and *paclitaxel* versus three cycles of chemotherapy followed by surgical debulking and a further three cycles of chemotherapy. As these data become available, the results will help address the potential role of neoadjuvant chemotherapy.

Chemotherapy and Molecular Targeted Therapies

Inhibition of angiogenesis with drugs such as ***bevacizumab*** has demonstrated activity and benefit in women with recurrent ovarian cancer; in view of this, there are two large randomized trials investigating the impact, if any, of the addition of *bevacizumab* to standard *carboplatin* and *paclitaxel* in patients with advanced ovarian cancer. There is evidence in other tumor types such as breast cancer, colon cancer, and lung cancer that the addition of *bevacizumab* to chemotherapy increases response rates and progression-free survival and also survival in some studies (311–313).

GOG 218 is a phase III, three-arm randomized, double-blind, placebo-controlled trial. Patients in **arm 1** will receive **six cycles of *carboplatin* and *paclitaxel* and placebo** starting with the second cycle and continuing for ten additional cycles after the completion of chemotherapy. Patients in **arm 2** will receive **six cycles of *carboplatin* and *paclitaxel* plus *bevacizumab*** starting with cycle 2 and administered with chemotherapy **followed by ten cycles of placebo,** and in **arm 3** patients will **receive *bevacizumab* to start with cycle 2 of *carboplatin* and *paclitaxel* and then ten additional cycles of *bevacizumzab* after the completion of chemotherapy.** This study is designed to investigate the benefit of *bevacizumab* in combination with chemotherapy as well as for maintenance. The *bevacizumab* is administered at a dose of 15mg/kg and starts with the second cycle of chemotherapy to decrease the risk of gastrointestinal perforation, which has been a rare complication of this agent in the setting of its use in colorectal cancer. **The ICON7 study is similar but is a two-arm study of *carboplatin* and *paclitaxel* plus or minus *bevacizumab*** 7.5 mg/kg administered every 3 weeks with chemotherapy and then as maintenance therapy. The results of these studies will be available in several years.

Chemotherapeutic Recommendations for Patients with Advanced Ovarian Cancer

For first-line chemotherapy of advanced epithelial ovarian cancer, we recommend the following (Table 11.6).

1. **Combination chemotherapy with *carboplatin* and *paclitaxel* for six to eight cycles.** The recommended doses and schedule are *carboplatin* (starting dose AUC = 5–6) and *paclitaxel* (175 mg/m^2) given over 3 hours every 3 weeks.

2. **Consideration should be given to intraperitoneal chemotherapy with *cisplatin* and *paclitaxel* in selected patients with stage III ovarian cancer who have been optimally debulked.**

3. **Consider participation in a clinical trial** if the patient is eligible and gives signed informed consent.

4. **In frail patients who may not tolerate the combination, single-agent *carboplatin* (AUC = 5–6) can be given.**

5. **In those who have a hypersensitivity to *paclitaxel*, an alternative drug can be substituted—for example, *docetaxel*, *topotecan*, *gemcitabine*, or *liposomal doxorubicin*.**

6. **In patients who cannot tolerate intravenous chemotherapy, an oral agent can be substituted—for example, an oral *alkylating agent* or oral *etoposide*.**

Consolidation and Maintenance of Complete Clinical Response to First-Line Chemotherapy

Because as many as 80% of women with advanced-stage disease who completely respond to their first-line chemotherapy will ultimately relapse, several trials have been conducted that administer a drug to these patients immediately following their primary treatment in an effort to decrease the relapse rate.

Paclitaxel

In a study conducted by the GOG and SWOG, 277 women with advanced ovarian cancer who had a complete clinical response to first-line chemotherapy were randomized to receive 3 or 12 cycles of additional single-agent *paclitaxel* (175 or 135 mg/m^2 every 28 days) (314). Patients were excluded if they had developed grade 2 or 3 neurotoxicity during their initial chemotherapy. Because of cumulative toxicity, the mean number of actual cycles of *paclitaxel* received by the group assigned to receive 12 cycles was 9. The treatment-related grade 2 to 3 neuropathy was more common with longer treatment, 24% versus 14% of patients, respectively. **The study was closed after a median follow-up of only 8.5 months, and an interim analysis showed a significant 7-month prolongation in median progression-free survival (28 versus 21 months) with 9 versus 3 months of consolidation *paclitaxel*. However, there was no difference in median overall survival.** The rate of disease progression increased significantly after maintenance therapy was discontinued, which suggested that long-term survival would not be likely to be improved. Furthermore, it is unlikely that a survival benefit will be seen with longer follow-up because patients assigned to three cycles were given the option of receiving an additional nine courses of *paclitaxel* after the study was discontinued (315).

Topotecan

Four additional courses of *topotecan* were administered to patients following six cycles of *carboplatin* and *paclitaxel* in two randomized trials, one conducted in Italy (316) and the other in Germany (317). In the larger trial conducted in Germany, 1,059 evaluable patients were randomly assigned to six cycles of *paclitaxel* (175 mg/m^2 over 3 hours) and *carboplatin* (AUC 5) with (537 patients) or without (522 patients) four additional cycles of *topotecan* (1.25 mg/m^2 IV days 1 to 5 every 3 weeks) (316). In the Italian trial, 273 women were randomly assigned to receive four additional cycles (137 patients) of *topotecan* at a dose of 1 mg/m^2 on days 1 to 5 every 3 weeks or no further chemotherapy (136 patients) (316). There were **no significant differences in either progression-free or overall survival in patients who received four to six cycles of maintenance *topotecan*.**

Cisplatin

In a randomized clinical trial of intraperitoneal *cisplatin* for consolidation versus observation, there was no difference in survival between the treatment arms (316).

Summary

The clinical benefit of consolidation and maintenance chemotherapy seems doubtful. Patients and their physicians may consider prolonged single-agent *paclitaxel* an option, but it should not be considered the standard of care.

Administration of Chemotherapy and Amelioration of Toxicity

Paclitaxel   **The principal concern of combining *paclitaxel* and *carboplatin* is the potential for enhanced bone marrow toxicity.** In general, shorter infusions of *paclitaxel* (e.g., 3 hours) tend to reduce the likelihood of bone marrow depression when combining the drug with *carboplatin* (270), although in practice this is not usually a problem. **Conversely, when *paclitaxel* is combined with *cisplatin*, the principal concern is the potentiation of neurotoxicity.** This toxicity can be minimized by using a lower dose of *paclitaxel* administered over a longer period of time (e.g., 135 mg/m^2 over 24 hours).

Carboplatin   **The renal and gastrointestinal toxicities of *carboplatin* are modest compared with *cisplatin;* thus, patients do not require prehydration, and outpatient administration is standard practice.** *Carboplatin* does tend to have more bone marrow toxicity than *cisplatin.* **Growth factors such as G-CSF have facilitated the administration of drug combinations that have neutropenia as a dose-limiting toxicity,** although they are not commonly required with *carboplatin* and *paclitaxel.* The use of growth factors is discussed more fully in Chapter 2.

There are some data to suggest that ***amifostine*** can reduce *carboplatin and paclitaxel*-induced neurotoxicity (319). In a phase III randomized trial of 187 women, the incidence of grade 3–4 neutropenia was lower in the arm with *amifostine* (31.3% vs. 37.9%; $p = 0.03$), as was the incidence of severe mucositis (4.7% vs. 15.4%, respectively; $p <0.0001$). *Amifostine* appeared to be protective against neurotoxicity (grade 3–4 neurotoxicity, 3.7% vs. 7.2%; $p = 0.02$). In a similar study, De Vos et al. (320) found that *amifostine* had only minor albeit statistically significant benefit in decreasing neurotoxicity, without preventing *paclitaxel* plus *carboplatin*-induced bone marrow toxicity. The drug has not found widespread use.

Cisplatin   *Cisplatin* combination chemotherapy is given every 3 to 4 weeks by intravenous infusion over 1 to 1.5 hours. ***Cisplatin* requires appropriate hydration and can be administered on either an inpatient or outpatient basis.** Hydration is administered with intravenous one-half normal saline at a rate of 300 to 500 dL per hour for 2 to 4 hours until the urinary output is greater than 100 dl per hour. When the urinary output is satisfactory, the *cisplatin* is infused in normal saline and the intravenous fluid rate is decreased to 150 to 200 dl per hour for 6 hours and then discontinued if the patient is stable.

The principal toxicities of this regimen are renal, gastrointestinal, hematologic, and neurologic. The renal and neurologic toxicities generally limit the duration of treatment to six cycles.

The acute and delayed gastrointestinal toxicity of *cisplatin* (i.e., nausea and vomiting) can be minimized with appropriate antiemetics, including a 5HT3 antagonist together with *dexamethasone* and *aprepitant*, an NK1 receptor blocker. All three published guidelines recommend this approach to prevent acute nausea and vomiting, and they also recommend *dexamethasone* and *aprepitant* to reduce delayed nausea and vomiting (321–323). For example, the ASCO guidelines recommend a 5HT3 antagonist (e.g., *ondansetron* 8 mg IV, *palonsetron* 0.25 mg, or one other 5HT3 antagonist) as well as *dexamethasone* 12 mg orally and *aprepitant* 125 mg orally prior to *cisplatin* followed by *dexamethasone* 8 mg daily from days 2 to 4 and *aprepitant* 80 mg orally on days 2 and 3 as appropriate antiemetic cover (323).

Radiation Therapy

An alternative to first-line combination chemotherapy for selected patients with metastatic ovarian cancer is the use of whole-abdominal radiation therapy. This approach is not used in the United States, but it was standard treatment in some institutions in Canada for patients with no residual macroscopic tumor in the upper abdomen (246). It has been compared with oral *chlorambucil* and appears to be superior (246), but it has not been tested against combination chemotherapy. A trial of three cycles of high-dose *cisplatin* and *cyclophosphamide* "induction" chemotherapy followed by whole-abdominal radiation therapy to "consolidate" the initial response has been reported (324). No apparent benefit could be shown by adding whole-abdominal radiation after chemotherapy in patients with optimal disease.

Hormonal Therapy

There is no evidence that hormonal therapy alone is appropriate primary therapy for advanced ovarian cancer (325).

Immunotherapy

There is some interest in the use of biologic response modifiers in ovarian cancer, and in a trial of ***gamma interferon*** (*γ-interferon*) **with *cisplatin* and *cyclophosphamide*, there appeared to be a benefit to the addition of the *interferon* (326). A trial of *carboplatin* and *paclitaxel* with or without *γ-interferon*** concluded that there were more adverse events with *γ-interferon* and no survival benefits in women with advanced ovarian cancer (327).

Trials of monoclonal antibodies directed toward ovarian cancer-associated antigens have been conducted (328–334). Women who were in clinical remission following platinum and *taxane* chemotherapy were studied in a randomized, prospective trial of maintenance *OvaRex*, a monoclonal antibody directed toward CA125, and no progression-free survival benefit was seen (330–331). Studies with monoclonal antibodies directed at human milk fat globulin (HMFG) tumor-associated antigens for consolidation have shown no survival benefit (331); however, there was an improved control of intraperitoneal disease, which was offset by increased extraperitoneal disease (331). *Herceptin,* an humanized antibody directed toward the extracellular protein produced when the HER2/*neu* oncogene is overexpressed, has been used extensively in breast cancer, where it has been shown to improve the response rate to chemotherapy in selected patients with HER2 amplified breast cancer. **A trial of** *herceptin* **antibody in HER-2/***neu* **overexpressing ovarian cancers has been conducted by the GOG, and the response rate was low: 9.7%** (334). The rationale for the use of these agents in ovarian cancer is discussed in Chapter 2.

Treatment Assessment

Many patients who undergo optimal cytoreductive surgery and subsequent chemotherapy for epithelial ovarian cancer will have no evidence of disease at the completion of treatment. The *second-look operation* was previously considered to be standard practice, but is now seldom performed (335–343).

Tumor Markers

Elevated CA125 levels are useful in predicting the presence of disease, but normal levels are an insensitive determinant of the absence of disease. In a prospective study (347), the positive predictive value was shown to be 100%—that is, if the level of CA125 was >35 U/dL, disease was always detectable in patients at second-look laparotomy. The predictive value of a negative test was only 56%—that is, if the level was <35 U/dL, disease was present in 44% of the patients. **A review of the literature suggests that an elevated CA125 level predicts persistent disease at second-look in 97% of the cases** (36).

Serum CA125 levels can be used during chemotherapy to follow those patients whose level was elevated at the initiation of treatment (36,347). The change in level generally correlates with response. Those patients with persistently elevated levels after three cycles of treatment most likely have resistant clones. **Rising levels on treatment almost invariably indicate treatment failure. A retrospective study determined that a doubling of the CA125 level from its nadir in those patients with a persistently elevated level accurately predicts disease progression** (348).

The Gynecologic Cancer Intergroup (GCIG) developed a standard definition for CA125 level progression, which is now widely used in clinical trials. **Patients with elevated CA125 levels pretreatment who normalize their levels must demonstrate CA125 levels greater than or equal to twice the upper limit of normal on two occasions at least 1 week apart. Patients with elevated CA125 levels pretreatment, which never normalize, must show evidence of CA125 levels greater than or equal to twice the nadir value on two occasions at least 1 week apart** (349). However, a trial of 527 patients, randomized to early treatment of relapse based on CA 125 level alone versus delay treatment commencing when clinical symptomatic recurrence appear, showed no survival benefits from early treatment based on raised serum marker levels alone (350).

Radiologic Assessment

In patients with stage I to III epithelial ovarian cancer, radiologic tests have generally been of limited value in determining the presence of subclinical disease. Ascites can be readily detected, but **even quite large omental metastases can be missed on CT scan** (112,351,352). If liver enzymes are abnormal, then the liver can be evaluated with a CT scan or ultrasonography. CT-scan–directed fine-needle aspiration cytology will indicate tumor persistence if positive, but a negative result is not definitive. The false negative rate of a CT scan is approximately 45% (351).

Positron-emission tomography with or without CT imaging may help in the detection of relapse, but there appears to be a higher false positive rate with PET compared with CT (113–115). A review concluded that PET had a sensitivity of 90% and a specificity of 85% for the detection of recurrent ovarian cancer and that it appeared to be particularly useful for the diagnosis of recurrent disease when CA125 levels were rising and conventional imaging was inconclusive or negative (113). Technologic advances have led to combined [18]fluorodeoxyglucose ([18]FDG)-PET–computed tomographic that provide contemporaneous [18]FDG-PET and CT images. **The role of [18]FDG-PET–CT for the detection of recurrent ovarian cancer is promising,** and this technique may be especially useful for the selection of patients with late recurrent disease who may benefit from secondary cytoreductive surgery (353–355). **MRI can be used as an alternative to CT in patients with allergies to the contrast medium** (115).

Second-Look Operations

A second-look operation is one performed on a patient who has no clinical evidence of disease after a prescribed course of chemotherapy in order to determine the response to therapy.

Second-Look Laparotomy	**The technique for a second-look laparotomy is essentially identical to that for a staging laparotomy. Areas of previously documented tumor are the most important areas to biopsy** because they are most likely to give a positive result. Any adhesions or surface irregularities should be sampled. In addition, biopsy specimens should be taken from the pelvic sidewalls, the pelvic cul-de-sac, the bladder, the paracolic gutters, the residual omentum, and the diaphragm. At least a pelvic and paraaortic lymph node sampling should be performed in those patients whose nodal tissues have not been previously removed.

Approximately 30% of patients with no evidence of macroscopic disease will have microscopic metastases (335). Also, in many patients with microscopic disease, macroscopic disease will be detected in only the occasional biopsy or cytologic specimen. Therefore, a large number of specimens (20–30) should be obtained to minimize the false negative rate of the operation. **In selected patients in whom gross residual tumor is discovered at second-look surgery, resection of isolated masses may be performed.** The removal of all macroscopic areas of disease might facilitate response to salvage therapies (356,357), as well as permitting the collection of tissue for *in vitro* analyses.

Second-look laparotomy has not been shown to influence patient survival, although the information obtained at second-look correlates with subsequent outcome and survival (336–339,342,343). Patients who have no histologic evidence of disease have a significantly longer survival than those in whom microscopic or macroscopic disease is documented. **The operation should be performed selectively—for example, in patients receiving therapy in a setting where second-line therapies are undergoing clinical trials.**

The likelihood that a patient will have a recurrence after a negative second-look laparotomy ranges from 30% to 60% at 5 years (339–342). The majority of recurrences after a negative second-look laparotomy are in patients with poorly differentiated cancers (342). Patients whose tumors are initially stage I and II have negative second-look laparotomy rates of 85% to 95% and 70% to 80%, respectively. In patients with optimally resected stage III disease treated with the platinum and *paclitaxel* regimen, the negative second-look rate is approximately 45% to 50% (256).

Second-Look Laparoscopy	Second-look laparoscopy may be useful for patients on experimental treatment protocols. The advantage of laparoscopy is that it is a less invasive operation; the disadvantage is that visibility may be limited by the frequent presence of intraperitoneal adhesions (344–346). **The development of newer techniques for retroperitoneal lymph node dissection has potentially increased the utility of the endoscopic approach to second-look.**

Secondary Therapy

Secondary Cytoreduction	**Secondary cytoreduction maybe defined as an attempt at cytoreductive surgery at some stage following completion of first-line chemotherapy** (356). Patients with progressive disease on chemotherapy are not suitable candidates for secondary cytoreduction, but patients who are clinically free of disease and undergo second-look laparotomy may benefit if all macroscopic residual disease can be resected (357). Patients with recurrent disease are sometimes candidates for surgical excision of their disease. **Tumor resection under these circumstances should be restricted to those who have a disease-free interval of at least 12, but preferably 24 months, or those in whom all macroscopic disease can be resected,** regardless of the disease-free interval (358,360,361).

Chemotherapy for Recurrent Ovarian Cancer	The majority of women who relapse will be offered further chemotherapy with the likelihood of benefit related in part to the initial response and the duration of response. **The goals of treatment include improving disease-related symptoms, maintaining or improving quality of life, delaying time to progression, and possibly prolonging survival, particularly in women with platinum-sensitive recurrences.**

Many active chemotherapeutic agents (platinum, *paclitaxel*, *topotecan*, *liposomal doxorubicin*, *docetaxel*, *gemcitabine*, and *etoposide*) as well as targeted agents (*bevacizumab*) are

Table 11.7 Second-Line Chemotherapy in Recurrent or Persistent Epithelial Ovarian Cancer

Drugs Used in Platinum- and Taxane-Sensitive Disease

Response Rates 20%–40%

Cisplatin

Carboplatin

Paclitaxel (Taxol)

Docetaxel (Taxotere)

Drugs Used in Platinum- and Taxane-Resistant and Refractory Disease

Response Rates 10%–25%

Topotecan (Hycamtin)

Etoposide (oral) (VP-16)

Liposomal doxorubicin (Doxil)

Gemcitabine (Gemzar)

Hexamethylmelamine (Altretamine)

available, and the choice of treatment is based on many factors including likelihood of benefit, potential toxicity, and patient convenience (367,368). **Women who relapse later than 6 months after primary chemotherapy are classified as** *platinum-sensitive* and usually receive further platinum-based chemotherapy, with response rates ranging from 27% to 65% and a median survival of 12 to 24 months (369,370). **Patients who relapse within 6 months of completing first-line chemotherapy are classified as** *platinum-resistant* and have a median survival of 6 to 9 months and a 10% to 30% likelihood of responding to chemotherapy. **Patients who progress while on treatment are classified as having** *platinum-refractory disease.* Objective response rates to chemotherapy in patients with platinum-refractory ovarian cancer are less than 20% (368).

Patients with platinum-refractory and platinum-resistant ovarian cancer are commonly treated with chemotherapy and may have a number of lines of therapy depending on response, performance status, patient request, and doctor recommendations. A study comparing *topotecan* with *liposomal doxorubicin* demonstrated the **low response rates and poor prognosis for women with platinum-resistant ovarian cancer** (371). In a subset analysis of platinum-resistant patients, the median time to progression ranged from 9.1 to 13.6 weeks for *topotecan* and *liposomal doxorubicin,* respectively. The median survival was 35.6 weeks for *pegylated liposomal doxorubicin* (PLD) and 41.3 weeks for *topotecan* ($p = 0.455$). Objective response rates were recorded in 6.5% of patients who received *topotecan* and in 12.3% of those who received PLD ($p = 0.118$). It is not known whether the treatment improved symptom control or quality of life because this was not specifically addressed.

The potential adverse effects associated with chemotherapy should not be underestimated and have been well documented in trials involving women with recurrent ovarian cancer. The three most commonly used drugs are *paclitaxel, topotecan,* and *liposomal doxorubicin.* The reported adverse effects associated with **paclitaxel** included **alopecia** in 62% to 100% of patients, **neurotoxicity** (any grade) in 5% to 42%, and **severe leukopenia** in 4% to 24%. **Topotecan** is associated with **myelosuppression** in 49% to 76% of patients, which is significantly greater than with *liposomal doxorubicin* or *paclitaxel.* **Liposomal doxorubicin** is associated with **palmar–plantar erythrodysesthesia** of any grade in more than 50% of patients, and it is severe in 23%. In addition, severe stomatitis has been reported in as many as 10% of patients (368). A large international study that is evaluating the impact of chemotherapy on quality of life and symptom improvement in patients with platinum-resistant or platinum-refractory ovarian cancer is currently underway.

Second-Line Chemotherapy

The response rates for second-line chemotherapies are in the range of 10% to >40% for most drugs tested by the oral or intravenous route and depend on many factors. The most important predictors of response are response to first-line chemotherapy and the treatment-free interval (370–434) (Table 11.7).

Platinum-Sensitive Disease

Some studies suggest that **a combination of platinum plus** *paclitaxel* **may be better** in some patients for second-line therapy than platinum alone (376,377). In a study of 25 women who relapsed 6 months or longer after first-line *carboplatin* and *paclitaxel*, retreatment with the same combination had a response rate of 91% and a median progression-free survival of more than 9 months (377). Other studies suggest that single-agent therapy (*cisplatin* or *carboplatin*) should be considered the standard of care for platinum-sensitive disease (378,379).

In most studies, there is a lack of survival advantage and greater toxicity with multiagent compared with single-agent regimens. However, the combination of *carboplatin* and *paclitaxel* is relatively well tolerated and has been shown to have a higher response rate and to be associated with a longer survival than *carboplatin* alone (379,380).

The use of combination platinum plus *paclitaxel* **chemotherapy versus a single-agent platinum has been tested in two multinational randomized phase III trials** (381) and a randomized phase II study (382). In a report (381) of the ICON4 and AGO-OVAR-2.2 trials, 802 women with platinum-sensitive ovarian cancer who relapsed after being treatment free for at least 6 to 12 months were randomized to platinum-based chemotherapy (72% *carboplatin*, or *cisplatin* alone; 17% CAP; 4% *carboplatin* plus *cisplatin;* and 3% *cisplatin* plus *doxorubicin*) or *paclitaxel* plus platinum-based chemotherapy (80% *paclitaxel* plus *carboplatin;* 10% *paclitaxel* plus *cisplatin;* 5% *paclitaxel* plus both *carboplatin* and *cisplatin;* and 4% *paclitaxel* alone). The AGO-OVAR-2.2 trial did not accrue its planned number of patients. **In both trials, a significant proportion of the patients had not received** *paclitaxel* **as part of their initial chemotherapeutic regimen. Combining the trials for analysis, there was a significant survival advantage for the** *paclitaxel*-**containing therapy** (HR = 0.82), with a median follow-up of 42 months. **The absolute 2-year survival advantage was 7% (57% vs. 50%), and there was a 5-month improvement in median survival (29 vs. 24 months).** Progression-free survival was better with the *paclitaxel* regimen (HR = 0.76); there was a 10% difference in 1-year progression-free survival (50% vs. 40%) and a 3-month prolongation in median progression-free survival (13 vs. 10 months). The toxicities were comparable, except there was a significantly higher incidence of neurologic toxicity and alopecia in the *paclitaxel* group, whereas myelosuppression was significantly greater with the non–*paclitaxel*-containing regimens. **These data support the slight advantage of a second-line regimen containing both** *paclitaxel* **and a platinum agent in patients who have not received** *paclitaxel* **in their primary chemotherapeutic regimen.**

Two randomized trials have compared *carboplatin* alone to *carboplatin* and *gemcitabine* or *liposomal doxorubicin* (435,436). There was a higher response rate with the combination therapy and a longer progression-free survival, but the studies were not powered to look at overall survival. **In the GCIG study comparing** *carboplatin* **and** *gemcitabine* **with** *carboplatin* **alone, the response rate was 47.2% for the combination and 30.9% for** *carboplatin*, **with the progression-free survival being 8.6 months and 5.8 months, respectively** (435). A SWOG study of *carboplatin* versus *carboplatin* and *liposomal doxorubicin* was closed early because of poor accrual, but with 61 patients recruited the response rate was 67% for the combination and 32% for *carboplatin*. The progression-free survival was 12 months versus 8 months; intriguingly, the overall survival was 26 months compared to 18 months ($p = 0.02$) (436). A phase II study from France confirmed the high response rate of 67% with *carboplatin* and *liposomal doxorubicin* in patients with platinum-sensitive recurrent ovarian cancer. **A large GCIG study (CALYPSO) comparing** *carboplatin* **and** *liposomal doxorubicin* **with** *carboplatin* **and** *paclitaxel* **has completed recruitment,** and the results are expected in the next 18 months (437).

Platinum-Resistant and Refractory Disease

In *cisplatin*-**refractory patients—that is, those progressing on treatment—response rates to second-line** *carboplatin* **are less than 10%** (375). The management of women who are platinum-resistant (i.e., progressing within 6 months of completion of chemotherapy) is difficult, and *noncrossresistant agents* are usually selected, but there does not appear to be one best treatment. Single-agent therapy is typically used because combination regimens are associated with more toxicity without any apparent additional benefit. **Response rates of 48% to 64%**

have been reported with dose-dense weekly *carboplatin* (AUC = 4) and *paclitaxel* (90 mg/m²), and this deserves further study (438). **There are a variety of active drugs; the most frequently used are *paclitaxel, docetaxel, topotecan, liposomal doxorubicin, gemcitabine,* oral *etoposide, tamoxifen,* and *bevacizumab*.** Other active agents include *vinorelbine* and *ifosfamide* and newer drugs such as *trabectidin*.

The poor results achieved with chemotherapy in this population of patients are well demonstrated by a recent trial in which 195 patients with platinum-resistant ovarian cancer were randomized to receive either *liposomal doxorubicin* or *gemcitabine*. In the *gemcitabine* and PLD groups, median progression-free survival was 3.6 versus 3.1 months, median overall survival was 12.7 versus 13.5 months, and overall response rate was 6.1% versus 8.3%. In the subset of patients with measurable disease, overall response rate was 9.2% versus 11.7%, respectively. None of the efficacy end points showed a statistically significant difference between treatment groups. The *liposomal doxorubicin* group experienced significantly more hand–foot syndrome and mucositis, whereas the *gemcitabine* group experienced significantly more constipation, nausea and vomiting, fatigue, and neutropenia (439).

Some researchers have attempted to treat patients with non-platinum drugs to prolong the *platinum-free interval,* hoping that their use will allow the tumor to become platinum-sensitive during the interval use of non-cross-resistant agents. The rationale for this approach was that the platinum-free interval was equivalent to the treatment-free interval; before the availability of other active drugs, these two terms were synonymous. However, **there are no data to support the hypothesis that the interposition of another drug can produce an increased platinum sensitivity as a result of a longer interval since the last platinum treatment.**

Taxanes

Single-agent *paclitaxel* shows objective responses in 20% to 30% of patients in phase II trials of women with platinum-resistant ovarian cancer (380,383–388). The main toxicities are asthenia and peripheral neuropathy. A dose of 135 to 175 mg/m² every 3 weeks, either as a 3-hour or 24-hour infusion, may be considered standard because a randomized trial showed similar response rates for both regimes (384). Three-hour infusions produce more neurotoxicity but less myelosuppression. Higher doses of *paclitaxel* (250 mg/m² vs. 175 mg/m² per dose) using hematopoietic growth factor support can result in higher response rates but with significantly more toxicity and no survival benefit (386).

Weekly *paclitaxel* is active, and the toxicity, especially myelosuppression, is less than with the 3-week regimens. In a study of 53 women with platinum-resistant ovarian cancer, weekly *paclitaxel* (80 mg/m² over 1 hour) had an objective response of 25% in patients with measurable disease, and 27% of patients without measurable disease had a 75% decline in serum CA125 levels (386).

Docetaxel also has some activity in these patients (389–391). The GOG studied 60 women with platinum-resistant ovarian or primary peritoneal cancer (391). Although there was a 22% objective response rate, the median response duration was only 2.5 months, and therapy was complicated by severe neutropenia in three-quarters of the patients.

Topotecan

***Topotecan* is an active second-line treatment for patients with platinum-sensitive and platinum-resistant disease** (392–407). In a study of 139 women receiving *topotecan* 1.5 mg/m² daily for 5 days, response rates were 19% and 13% in patients with platinum-sensitive and platinum-resistant disease, respectively (392). **The predominant toxicity of *topotecan* is hematologic, especially neutropenia.** With the 5-day dosing schedule, 70% to 80% of patients have severe neutropenia, and 25% have febrile neutropenia with or without infection (359,360). In some studies, regimens of 5 days produce better response rates than regimens of shorter duration (392–402), but in others, reducing the dose to 1.0 mg/m²/day for 3 days is associated with similar response rates but lower toxicity (403,404). In a study of 31 patients, one-half of whom were platinum refractory (405), *topotecan* 2 mg/m²/day for 3 days every 21 days had a 32% response rate. Continuous infusion *topotecan* (0.4 mg/m²/day for 14–21 days) had a 27% to 35% objective response rate in platinum-refractory patients (398,399). **Weekly *topotecan* administered at a dose of 4 mg/m²/week for 3 weeks with a week off every month**

produced a response rate similar to the 5-day regimen with considerably less toxicity. Therefore, this is now considered the regimen of choice for this agent (407).

Oral *topotecan,* not currently available in the United States, **results in similar response rates with less hematologic toxicity** (401). The intravenous and oral formulations of *topotecan* were compared in a randomized trial of 266 women as a third-line regimen after an initial platinum-based regimen (406). Compared with intravenous *topotecan* (1.5 mg/m^2 daily for 5 days every 3 weeks), oral *topotecan* (2.3 mg/m^2/day for 5 days every 3 weeks) produced a similar response rate (13% vs. 20%), less severe myelosuppression, and only a slightly shorter median survival (51 vs. 58 weeks).

Liposomal Doxorubicin

Liposomal doxorubicin (*Doxil* in the United States and *Caelyx* in Europe) has activity in platinum- and *taxane*-refractory disease (371,408,409). **The predominant severe toxicity of liposomal doxorubicin is the hand–foot syndrome, also known as palmar–plantar erythrodysesthesia or acral erythema. This morbidity is observed in 20% of patients who receive 50 mg/m^2 every 4 weeks** (408). *Liposomal doxorubicin* tends to produce a low rate of both neurologic toxicity and alopecia. In a study of 89 patients with platinum-refractory disease, including 82 *paclitaxel*-resistant patients, *liposomal doxorubicin* (50 mg/m^2 every 3 weeks) produced a response in 17% (one complete and 14 partial responses) (409). In another study, an objective response of 26% was reported, although there were no responses in women who progressed during first-line therapy (408).

There have been two randomized trials comparing *liposomal doxorubicin* with either *topotecan* or *paclitaxel*. In a study of 237 women who relapsed after receiving one platinum-containing regimen, 117 of whom (49.4%) had platinum-refractory disease (371), *liposomal doxorubicin* 50 mg/m^2 over 1 hour every 4 weeks **was compared with *topotecan*** 1.5 mg/m^2/day for 5 days every 3 weeks. **The two treatments had a similar overall response rate (20% vs. 17%), time to progression (22 vs. 20 weeks), and median overall survival (66 vs. 56 weeks).** The myelotoxicity was significantly lower in the *liposomal doxorubicin*–treated patients than with those receiving *topotecan*. **In a second study comparing *liposomal doxorubicin* with single-agent *paclitaxel* in 214 platinum-treated patients who had not received prior *taxanes* (410), the overall response rates for *liposomal doxorubicin* and *paclitaxel* were 18% versus 22%, respectively, and median survival durations were 46 and 56 weeks, respectively.** Neither was significantly different. In practice, most patients are treated with a starting dose of 40mg/m^2 of *liposomal doxorubicin* every 4 weeks because of the toxicity associated with the higher dose and the need to commonly dose reduce when 50mg/m^2 is used.

Gemcitabine

Gemcitabine has been associated with response rates of 20% to 50% with, 6% in patients who are platinum-resistant (413–417). **The principal toxicities are myelosuppression and gastrointestinal.** The drug has been used in doublet combinations with *cisplatin* or *carboplatin* with acceptable responses and toxicities and in the triplet combination with *carboplatin* and *paclitaxel* (415).

Oral *Etoposide*

The most common toxicities with oral *etoposide* are myelosuppression and gastrointestinal: Grade 4 neutropenia is observed in approximately one-fourth of patients, and 10% to 15% have severe nausea and vomiting (418–420). Although an initial study of intravenous *etoposide* reported an objective response rate of only 8% among 24 patients (418), a subsequent study of oral *etoposide* given for a prolonged treatment (50 mg/m^2 daily for 21 days every 4 weeks) had a 27% response rate in 41 women with platinum-resistant disease, three of whom had durable complete responses (419). In 25 patients with platinum- and *taxane*-resistant disease, eight objective responses (32%) were reported. **Oral *etoposide* should be considered one of the principal drugs to be used in patients with *paclitaxel*- and platinum-resistant disease.**

Other Chemotherapeutic Agents

Other active oral agents associated with response rates of 20% to 25% include ***hexamethamelamine*** (418–422), ***capecitabine*** (424), ***ifosfamide*** with ***mesna*** (425), and ***trabectedin*** (440).

Hormonal Therapy

Tamoxifen has been associated with response rates of 15% to 20% in well-differentiated carcinomas of the ovary (426–430). The gonadotropin-agonist *leuprolide acetate (Lupron)* has been shown to produce a response rate of 10% in one series (431). Trials combining *tamoxifen* and *leuprolide acetate*, and *tamoxifen* and combination chemotherapy are being conducted (432). Aromatase inhibitors (e.g., *letrozole, anastrozole*, and *exemestane*, which have been shown to have activity in metastatic breast cancer) are being studied in relapsed ovarian cancer (433). One principal advantage of this class of agents is the very low toxicity (434).

Targeted Therapies

A new era of cancer treatment is being entered in which knowledge of molecular pathways within normal and malignant cells has led to the development of agents with specific molecular targets. The greatest success to date in ovarian cancer has been in targeting angiogenesis, in particular VEGF, which has been found to play a major role in the biology of epithelial ovarian cancer (441). There are three main approaches to targeting angiogenesis: The first is to target VEGF itself, the second to target the VEGF receptor, and the third to inhibit tyrosine kinase activation and downstream signaling with small molecules that work at the intracellular level.

Bevacizumab is the first targeted agent to show significant single-agent activity in ovarian cancer. It is a humanized monoclonal antibody that targets angiogenesis by binding to VEGF-A, thereby blocking the interaction of VEGF with its receptor. There have been a number of phase II studies reported using *bevacizumab* in patients with platinum-sensitive and platinum-resistant ovarian cancer, with response rates ranging from 16% to 22% in both platinum-sensitive and platinum-refractory patients (442,443). Furthermore, as many as 40% of patients have had stabilization of disease for at least 6 months.

A study of 70 patients with recurrent ovarian cancer using low-dose metronomic chemotherapy with 50 mg of *cyclophosphamide* daily and *bevacizumab* 10 mg/kg intravenously every 2 weeks showed significant activity (444). The primary end point was progression-free survival at 6 months. The probability of being alive and progression free at 6 months was 56%. A partial response was achieved in 17 patients (24%). Median times to progression and survival were 7.2 and 16.9 months, respectively. The side effects of *bevacizumab* are now well recognized and include hypertension, fatigue, proteinuria, and gastrointestinal perforation or fistula. Uncommonly, vascular thrombosis and CNS ischemia, pulmonary hypertension, bleeding, and wound healing complications may occur. The most common side effect is hypertension. This is grade 3 in 7% of patients and is usually readily treatable, whereas the most concerning side effect is bowel perforation. The study by Cannistra was stopped after recruiting 44 patients because of an 11% incidence of perforation of the bowel (441–444).

It has been suggested that the complication of bowel perforation can be avoided by careful screening of patients. Simpkins et al. (445) limited *bevacizumab* treatment to patients without clinical symptoms of bowel obstruction, evidence of rectosigmoid involvement on pelvic examination, or bowel involvement on CT scan. Their study included 25 patients with platinum-resistant ovarian cancer, and all had been heavily pretreated. They observed a response rate of 28% and had no bowel perforations or any other grade 3 or 4 toxicity (445). This highlights the importance of patient selection and also suggests that as clinicians become more experienced with these agents, there should be less toxicity.

VEGF-Trap functions as a soluble decoy receptor, soaking up a ligand before it can interact with its receptor. It is also currently being evaluated in phase II trials in patients with recurrent ovarian cancer. There are also a number of other oral agents that target angiogenesis through tyrosine kinase inhibition that are currently in clinical trial (446).

Dose-Intense Second-Line Chemotherapy

In patients with minimal residual (≤5 mm) or microscopic disease confined to the peritoneal cavity, intraperitoneal chemotherapy or immunotherapy has been used (447–464). Cytotoxic chemotherapeutic agents such as *cisplatin, paclitaxel, 5-fluorouracil (5-FU), etoposide* (VP-16), and *mitoxantrone*, have been used as single agents in patients with persistent epithelial ovarian cancer (447–452), and complete responses have been seen in patients who start their treatment with minimal residual disease. The surgically documented response rates reported with this approach are approximately 20% to 40% for carefully selected patients, and the complete response rate is 10% to 20%. Although it has been suggested that this approach produces a significant subsequent improvement in survival (455), there are no prospective phase III data that demonstrate this, and the patients so treated tend to be those with a more favorable prognosis regardless of subsequent therapy.

Of historical interest is intraperitoneal immunotherapy with *alpha interferon* (α-*interferon*), γ-*interferon,* tumor necrosis factor, and *interleukin 2,* which were shown to have some activity in patients with minimal residual disease (456–463) (see Chapter 2). The response rate for the intraperitoneal cytokines, α-*interferon* and γ-*interferon,* is the same as that for the cytotoxic agents: approximately 28% to 50% (456–458,461,463). The combination of *cisplatin* and α-*interferon* produced a surgically documented 50% complete response rate, which was greater than that produced by either single agent alone (458). However, because *interferons* are not FDA approved for use in ovarian cancer, they are no longer used.

Second-line intraperitoneal treatment is not suitable for most patients because they often have extensive intraperitoneal adhesions or extraperitoneal disease. **Therefore, second-line intraperitoneal chemotherapy and immunotherapy should be considered experimental.**

High-Dose Chemotherapy and Autologous Bone Marrow Transplantation   The use of high-dose chemotherapy and either autologous bone marrow transplantation or peripheral stem cell protection has been tested in patients with advanced ovarian cancer (465–467). **In one trial of high-dose *carboplatin* with autologous bone marrow transplantation, 7 of the 11 patients with extensive refractory disease had an objective response**. The maximum tolerated dose of high-dose *carboplatin* was 2 g/m^2 (465).

A phase III randomized trial of 57 patients treated with high-dose chemotherapy (***cyclophosphamide* 6,000 mg/m^2 and *carboplatin* 1,600 mg/m^2**) **with peripheral blood stem cell support as consolidation** versus 53 patients treated with **conventional dose maintenance** (*cyclophosphamide* 600 mg/m^2 and *carboplatin* 300 mg/m^2) has been reported (467). Only 43 of the 57 women (75%) completed the high-dose therapy, while 48 of 53 (92%) completed the standard dose regimen. **There was no statistically significant difference in progression-free and overall survival between the two groups of patients.**

A prospective randomized clinical trial of a combination, very high-dose chemotherapy supported with autologous bone marrow transplantation versus standard-dose chemotherapy with *paclitaxel* and *carboplatin* was initiated by the Gynecologic Oncology Group, but the trial was discontinued because of poor accrual.

A European study of high-dose chemotherapy was recently reported (468). One hundred forty-nine patients with untreated ovarian cancer were randomly assigned after debulking surgery to receive standard combination chemotherapy or sequential high-dose treatment with two cycles of *cyclophosphamide* and *paclitaxel* followed by three cycles of high-dose *carboplatin* and *paclitaxel* with stem cell support. High-dose *melphalan* was added to the final cycle**. After a median follow-up of 38 months, the progression-free survival was 20.5 months in the standard arm and 29.6 months in the high-dose arm.** The median overall survival was 62.8 months in the standard arm and 54.4 months in the high-dose arm. This is the first randomized trial comparing sequential high-dose with standard-dose chemotherapy in first-line treatment of patients with advanced ovarian cancer, and **no statistically significant difference in progression-free survival or overall survival was observed**. The investigators concluded that high-dose chemotherapy does not appear to be superior to conventional-dose chemotherapy.

Whole-Abdominal Radiation

Whole-abdominal radiation therapy given as a second-line treatment has been shown to be potentially effective in a small subset of selected patients with microscopic disease, but it is associated with a relatively high morbidity. The principal problem associated with this approach is the development of acute and chronic intestinal morbidity. **As many as 30% of patients treated with this approach develop intestinal obstruction, and this may** necessitate potentially morbid exploratory surgery (469). Because there are many new chemotherapeutic agents available for the treatment of relapsed ovarian cancer, most centers have stopped using second-line whole-abdominal radiation therapy.

Intestinal Obstruction

Patients with epithelial ovarian cancer often develop intestinal obstruction, either at the time of initial diagnosis or, more frequently, in association with recurrent disease (470–478). **Obstruction may be related to a mechanical blockage or to carcinomatous ileus.** Correction of the intestinal blockage can be accomplished in most patients whose obstruction appears at the time of initial diagnosis. However, the decision to perform an exploratory procedure to palliate intestinal obstruction in patients with recurrent disease is more difficult. In patients whose life expectancy is very short (e.g., less than 2 months), surgical relief of the obstruction is not indicated (470). **In those whose projected life span is longer, features that predict a reasonable likelihood of correcting the obstruction include young age, good nutritional status, and the absence of rapidly accumulating ascites.**

For most patients with recurrent ovarian cancer who present with intestinal obstruction, initial management should include radiographic documentation of the obstruction, hydration, correction of any electrolyte disturbances, and parenteral alimentation (471–475). In many patients, the obstruction may be alleviated by this conservative approach. A preoperative upper gastrointestinal series and a barium enema will define possible sites of obstruction.

If exploratory surgery is deemed appropriate, the type of operation to be performed will depend on (i) the site and (ii) the number of obstructions. **Multiple sites of obstruction are not uncommon in patients with recurrent epithelial ovarian cancer.** More than one-half of the patients have small-bowel obstruction, one-third have colonic obstruction, and one-sixth have both (474–476). If the obstruction is principally contained in one area of the bowel (e.g., the terminal ileum), then this area can either be resected or bypassed, depending on what can be accomplished safely. **Intestinal bypass is generally less morbid than resection;** in patients with progressive cancer, the survival time after these two operations is the same (474–476).

If multiple obstructions are present, then resection of several segments of intestine is usually not indicated, and intestinal bypass or colostomy should be performed. A gastrostomy may occasionally be useful in this circumstance (476), and this can usually be placed percutaneously (477).

Surgery for bowel obstruction in patients with ovarian cancer carries an operative mortality of approximately 10% and a major complication rate of some 30% (470–476). The need for multiple reanastomoses and preceding radiation therapy increase the morbidity, which consists primarily of sepsis and enterocutaneous fistulae. The median survival ranges from 3 to 12 months, although approximately 20% of such patients survive longer than 12 months (471).

Survival

There is a trend toward improved survival for ovarian cancer (1,447). **FIGO has reported a statistically significant improvement in survival for all stages from 29.8% for the interval 1976 to 1978 to 49.7% for the interval 1999 to 2001** (479). In the United States, the 5-year survival for all stages combined increased from 37% in 1975–1977 to 45% in 1996–2003 (1). The death rate decreased from 9.51 per 100,000 to 8.75 per 100,000 from 1991 to 2003, an 8% decline (1).

The 5-year survival rate for carefully staged patients with stage IA disease is 89.6%, whereas it is 86.1% for stage IB and 83.4% for stage IC (479). The 5-year survival for stage II disease is 70.7%, 65.5%, and 71.4% for stages IIA, IIB, and IIC, respectively. For stage IIIA, 5-year survival is 46.7%, whereas it is 41.5% for stage IIIB, 32.5% for stage IIIC, and 18.6% for stage IV (479). The proportion in each stage at the time of diagnosis is shown in Fig. 11.18, and the survival by substage is presented in Fig. 11.19.

The 5-year survival of patients with stage III disease with microscopic residual disease only at the start of treatment is 63.5% compared with 32.9% for those with optimal residual disease (≤2 cm), and 24.8% for those with suboptimal residual disease (>2 cm) (279) (Fig. 11.19).

Including patients at all stages, patients younger than 50 years of age have a 5-year survival rate of approximately 40%, compared with some 15% for patients older than 50 (279). Patients whose Karnofsky's index (KI) is low (<70) have a significantly shorter survival than those with a KI >70 (169,174).

Regarding patients with invasive cancer, for stages I and II disease, the 5-year survival rate for grade 1 epithelial ovarian cancer is approximately 90.3%, compared with approximately 79.7% for grade 2 and 75% for grade 3 (479) (Fig. 11.20). Examining stages III and IV patients, the 5-year survivals for grades 1, 2, and 3 are 57.2%, 31%, and 28.5%, respectively (479) (Fig. 11.21).

Survival of patients with borderline tumors is excellent, with stage I lesions having a 98% 10-year survival (8,10,185,192,479). When all stages of borderline tumors are included, the 5-year survival rate is 87% (479) (Fig. 11.22).

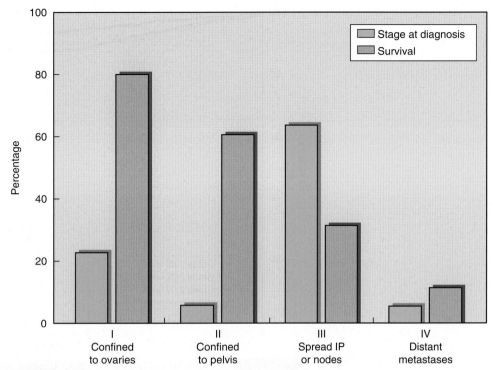

Figure 11.18   **Survival of patients with epithelial ovarian cancer by stage.** The percentage of patients diagnosed at a particular stage is shown next to the 5-year survival by stage. (Data from **Heintz APM, Odicino F, Maisonneuve P, Quinn MA, Benedet JL, Creasman WT, et al.** Carcinoma of the ovary. In: **Pecorelli S, ed.** Twenty-Sixth Annual Report on the Results of Treatment in Gynaecological Cancer. *Int J Gynecol Oncol* 2006;95(suppl 1):S161–S192, with permission.)

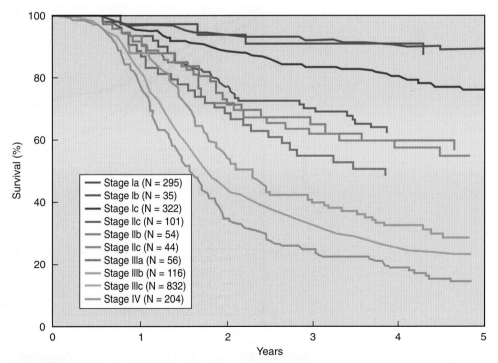

Figure 11.19   **Survival of patients with epithelial ovarian cancer by substage.** (From **Heintz APM, Odicino F, Maisonneuve P, Quinn MA, Benedet JL, Creasman WT, et al.** Carcinoma of the ovary. In: **Pecorelli S, ed.** Twenty-Sixth Annual Report on the Results of Treatment in Gynaecological Cancer. *Int J Gynecol Oncol* 2006;95(suppl 1):S161–S192, with permission.)

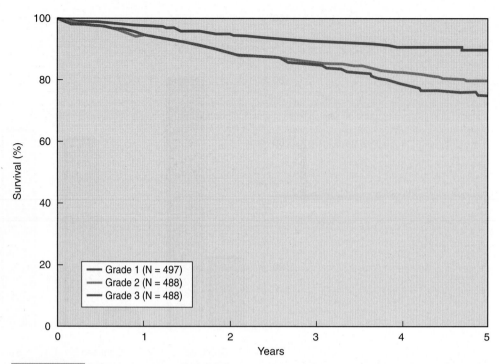

Figure 11.20   **Survival of patients with FIGO stages I and II epithelial ovarian cancer by grade of the tumor.** (From **Heintz APM, Odicino F, Maisonneuve P, Quinn MA, Benedet JL, Creasman WT, et al.** Carcinoma of the ovary. In: **Pecorelli S, ed.** Twenty-Sixth Annual Report on the Results of Treatment in Gynaecological Cancer. *Int J Gynecol Oncol* 2006;95(suppl 1): S161–S192, with permission.)

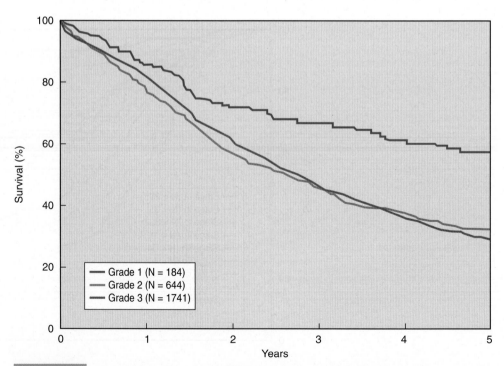

Figure 11.21   **Survival of patients with FIGO stages III and IV epithelial ovarian cancer by grade of the tumor.** (From **Heintz APM, Odicino F, Maisonneuve P, Quinn MA, Benedet JL, Creasman WT, et al.** Carcinoma of the ovary. In: **Pecorelli S, ed.** Twenty-Sixth Annual Report on the Results of Treatment in Gynaecological Cancer. *Int J Gynecol Oncol* 2006;95(suppl 1):S161–S192, with permission.)

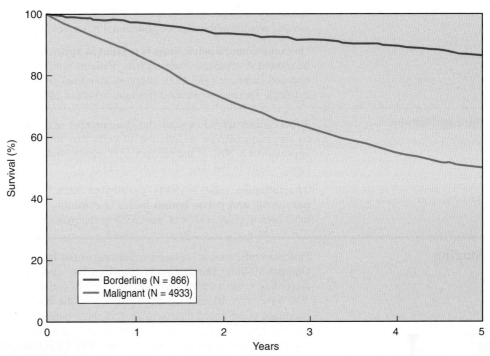

Figure 11.22 **Survival of patients with borderline versus invasive epithelial ovarian cancer.** (From **Heintz APM, Odicino F, Maisonneuve P, Quinn MA, Benedet JL, Creasman WT, et al.** Carcinoma of the ovary. In: **Pecorelli S, ed.** Twenty-Sixth Annual Report on the Results of Treatment in Gynaecological Cancer. *Int J Gynecol Oncol* 2006;95(suppl 1):S161–S192, with permission.)

Fallopian Tube Cancer

Carcinoma of the fallopian tube currently accounts for 0.3% of all cancers of the female genital tract (99,480–485). Molecular and genetic data suggest that many serous ovarian cancers arise in the distal fallopian tube (2). The definitions of ovarian and fallopian tube malignancies may need to be revised as the distinction between these two entities is reassessed.

In histologic features and clinical behavior, fallopian tube carcinoma is similar to ovarian cancer; thus, the management is essentially the same. Almost all fallopian tube cancers are of "epithelial" origin, most frequently of serous histology. Rarely, sarcomas have also been reported. The fallopian tubes are frequently involved secondarily from other primary sites, most often the ovaries, endometrium, gastrointestinal tract, or breast (99). They may be secondarily involved in primary peritoneal cancer.

Clinical Features

Tubal cancers are seen most frequently in the fifth and sixth decades, with a mean age of 55 to 60 years (99,480–484). **Women who have germ-line mutations in *BRCA1* and *BRCA2* are at substantially higher risk of developing fallopian tube carcinoma; therefore, prophylactic surgery in these women should include a complete removal of both fallopian tubes along with the ovaries** (90,486).

Symptoms and Signs

The classic triad of symptoms and signs associated with fallopian tube cancer is (i) a **prominent watery vaginal discharge**—that is, *hydrops tubae profluens;* (ii) **pelvic pain**; and (iii) **a pelvic mass.** However, this triad is noted in fewer than 15% of patients (90).

Either vaginal discharge or bleeding is the most common symptom reported and is documented in more than 50% of patients (302,482). Lower abdominal or pelvic pressure and pain also are noted in many patients. However, the presentation may be rather vague and nonspecific. In perimenopausal and postmenopausal women with an unexplained or persistent vaginal discharge, even in the absence of bleeding, the clinician should be concerned about the

493

possibility of an occult tubal cancer. Fallopian tube cancer is often found incidentally in asymptomatic women at the time of abdominal hysterectomy and bilateral salpingo-oophorectomy.

On examination, **a pelvic mass is present in approximately 60% of patients**, and ascites may be present if advanced disease exists. Patients with tubal carcinoma will have a negative dilation and curettage (483,487), although abnormal or adenocarcinomatous cells may be seen in cytologic specimens obtained from the cervix in 10% of patients.

Spread Pattern

Tubal cancers spread in much the same manner as epithelial ovarian malignancies, principally by the transcoelomic exfoliation of cells that implant throughout the peritoneal cavity. In approximately 80% of the patients with advanced disease, metastases are confined to the peritoneal cavity at the time of diagnosis (482).

The fallopian tube is richly permeated with lymphatic channels, and spread to the paraaortic and pelvic lymph nodes is common. Metastases to the paraaortic lymph nodes have been documented in at least 33% of the patients with all stages of disease (482).

Staging

Fallopian tube cancer is staged according to the International Federation of Gynecology and Obstetrics (480). The staging is based on the surgical findings at laparotomy (Table 11.8). According to this system, approximately 29% of patients have stage I disease, 23% have stage II, 39% have stage III, and 7% have stage IV at the time of diagnosis (480). A somewhat lower incidence of advanced disease is seen in these patients than in patients with epithelial ovarian carcinomas, which may result from many advanced-staged fallopian tube cancers being designated ovarian or peritoneal cancers. **The 2008 FIGO staging for carcinoma of the fallopian tube is unchanged.**

Table 11.8 FIGO Staging for Carcinoma of the Fallopian Tube	
Stage 0	Carcinoma *in situ* (limited to tubal mucosa).
Stage I	Growth is limited to the fallopian tubes.
Stage IA	Growth is limited to one tube with extension into the submucosa[c] or muscularis but not penetrating the serosal surface; no ascites.
Stage IB	Growth is limited to both tubes with extension into the submucosa[c] or muscularis but not penetrating the serosal surface; no ascites.
Stage IC	Tumor either stage IA or IB but with tumor extension through or onto the tubal serosa; or with ascites present containing malignant cells or with positive peritoneal washings.
Stage II	Growth involving one or both fallopian tubes with pelvic extension.
Stage IIA	Extension or metastasis to the uterus or ovaries.
Stage IIB	Extension to other pelvic tissues.
Stage IIC	Tumor either stage IIA or IIB but with tumor extension through or onto the tubal serosa; or with ascites present containing malignant cells or with positive peritoneal washings.
Stage III	Tumor involves one or both fallopian tubes with peritoneal implants outside of the pelvis or positive retroperitoneal or inguinal nodes. Superficial liver metastases equals stage III. Tumor appears limited to the true pelvis but with histologically proven malignant extension to the small bowel or omentum.
Stage IIIA	Tumor is grossly limited to the true pelvis with negative nodes but with histologically confirmed microscopic seeding of abdominal peritoneal surfaces.
Stage IIIB	Tumor involving one or both tubes with histologically confirmed implants of abdominal peritoneal surfaces, none exceeding 2 cm in diameter. Lymph nodes are negative.
Stage IIIC	Abdominal implants greater than 2 cm in diameter or positive retroperitoneal or inguinal nodes.
Stage IV	Growth involving one or both fallopian tubes with distant metastases. If pleural effusion is present, there must be positive cytology to be stage IV. Parenchymal liver metastases equals stage IV.

FIGO Annual Report, Vol 26, *Int J Gynecol Obstet* 2006;105:3–4.

Treatment

The treatment of this disease is identical to that of epithelial ovarian cancer.

Surgery

Patients with tubal carcinoma should undergo total abdominal hysterectomy and bilateral salpingo-oophorectomy (99,484,488–493). **If there is no evidence of gross tumor spread, a staging operation is performed.** The retroperitoneal lymph nodes should be adequately evaluated, and peritoneal cytologic studies and biopsies should be performed, along with an infracolic omentectomy.

In patients with metastatic disease, an effort should be made to remove as much tumor bulk as possible. Extrapolation from the experience with epithelial ovarian cancer suggests that the best outcome should be achieved in patients in whom all macroscopic disease can be resected (459).

Chemotherapy

As with epithelial ovarian cancer, the most active agents are platinum and the taxanes. *Cisplatin* or *carboplatin* plus *paclitaxel* **has response and survival outcomes that are similar to that for epithelial ovarian cancer** (99,489–493). **Therefore, the same treatments used for epithelial ovarian cancer should be used in patients with epithelial tubal malignancies** (490,493).

A variety of other chemotherapeutic agents that are effective against ovarian cancer appear to be active in fallopian tube carcinomas as well. These agents include *docetaxel, etoposide, topotecan, gemcitabine,* and *liposomally encapsulated doxorubicin* (494–498).

Data on well-staged lesions are scarce, so it is unclear whether patients with disease confined to the fallopian tube (i.e., a stage IA, grade 1 or 2 carcinoma) benefit from adjuvant therapy.

Radiation

The role of radiation in the management of the disease remains unclear because patients have not been treated in any consistent manner and the small numbers treated preclude any meaningful conclusions (485,499–501). In advanced stage disease, chemotherapy appears to be more effective (501). Whole-abdominal radiation has been used in patients with no evidence of gross disease in the abdomen (i.e., completely resected disease or microscopic metastases only) but was ineffective (499). As with epithelial ovarian cancer, there may be a role in properly selected patients.

Prognosis

The overall 5-year survival for patients with epithelial tubal carcinomas is 56% (480). This number is higher than for patients with ovarian cancer and reflects the somewhat higher proportion of patients with early stage disease. The reported 5-year survival rate for patients with stage I disease is 81%, 67% for stage II disease, 41% for stage III disease, and 33% for stage IV (480).

Tubal Sarcomas

Tubal sarcomas, mostly malignant mixed mesodermal tumors, have been described but are rare (502). Leiomyosarcomas have been reported (503). They occur mainly in the sixth decade and are typically advanced at the time of diagnosis (2). An attempt should be made to resect all gross disease, and platinum-based combination chemotherapy should be given (502). These lesions need to be distinguished from extragastrointestinal stromal tumors, which are treated with *imatinib* (467). Survival of patients with primary tubal sarcomas is generally poor, and most die of their disease within 2 years (2).

References

1. **Jemal A, Siegel R, Murray T, Hao Y, Xu J, Murray T, et al.** Cancer statistics, 2009. *CA Cancer J Clin* 2009; published online. doi:10.3322/caac.20006.
2. **Scully RE, Young RH, Clement PB.** Tumors of the ovary, maldeveloped gonads, fallopian tube, and broad ligament. In: *Atlas of tumor pathology*, 3rd Series, Fascicle 23. Washington, DC: Armed Forces Institute of Pathology, 1998:1–168.
3. **Kurman RJ, Shih IeM.** Pathogenesis of ovarian cancer: lessons from morphology and molecular biology and their clinical implications. *Int J Gynecol Pathol* 2008;27:151–160.
4. **Kindelberger DW, Lee Y, Miron A, Hirsch MS, Feltmate C, Medeiros F, et al.** Intraepithelial carcinoma of the fimbria and pelvic serous carcinoma: Evidence for a causal relationship. *Am J Surg Pathol* 2007;31:161–169.
5. **Callahan MJ, Crum CP, Medeiros F, Kindelberger DW, Elvin JA, Garber JE, et al.** Primary fallopian tube malignancies in *BRCA*-positive women undergoing surgery for ovarian cancer risk reduction. *J Clin Oncol* 2007;25:3985–3990.
6. **Carlson JW, Miron A, Jarboe EA, Parast MM, Hirsch MS, Lee Y, et al.** Serous tubal intraepithelial carcinoma: its potential role in primary peritoneal serous carcinoma and serous cancer prevention. *J Clin Oncol* 2008; 26:4160–4165.

7. **Levanon K, Crum C, Drapkin R.** New insights into the pathogenesis of serous ovarian cancer and its clinical impact. *J Clin Oncol* 2008:26:5284–93.

8. **Barnhill DR, Kurman RJ, Brady MF, Omura GA, Yordan E, Given FT, et al.** Preliminary analysis of the behavior of stage I ovarian serous tumors of low malignant potential: a Gynecologic Oncology Group study. *J Clin Oncol* 1995;13:2752–2756.

9. **Seidman JD, Kurman RJ.** Subclassification of serous borderline tumors of the ovary into benign and malignant types: a clinicopathologic study of 65 advanced stage cases. *Am J Surg Pathol* 1996;20:1331–1345.

10. **Seidman JD, Kurman RJ.** Pathology of ovarian carcinoma. *Hematol Oncol Clin North Am* 2003;17:909–925.

11. **Bell DA, Weinstock MA, Scully RE.** Peritoneal implants of ovarian serous borderline tumors: histologic features and prognosis. *Cancer* 1988;62:2212–2222.

12. **Fowler JM, Nieberg RK, Schooler TA, Berek JS.** Peritoneal adenocarcinoma (serous) of müllerian type: a subgroup of women presenting with peritoneal carcinomatosis. *Int J Gynecol Cancer* 1994;4:43–51.

13. **Tobacman JK, Greene MH, Tucker MA, Costa J, Kase R, Frameni JF Jr.** Intraabdominal carcinomatosis after prophylactic oophorectomy in ovarian cancer-prone families. *Lancet* 1982;2:795–797.

14. **Piver MS, Jishi MF, Tsukada Y, Nava G.** Primary peritoneal carcinoma after prophylactic oophorectomy in women with a family history of ovarian cancer: a report of the Gilda Radner Familial Ovarian Cancer Registry. *Cancer* 1993;71:2751–2755.

15. **Heintz APM, Odicino F, Maisonneuve P, Beller U, Benedet JL, Creasman W, et al.** Carcinoma of the ovary. *Int J Gynecol Obstet* 2003;83(suppl 1):135–166.

16. **Koonings PP, Campbell K, Mishell DR Jr, Grimes DA.** Relative frequency of primary ovarian neoplasms: a 10-year review. *Obstet Gynecol* 1989;74:921–926.

17. **Negri E, Franceschi S, Tzonou A, Booth M, La Vecchia C, Parazzini F, et al.** Pooled analysis of three European case-control studies of epithelial ovarian cancer: I. Reproductive factors and risk of epithelial ovarian cancer. *Int J Cancer* 1991;49:50–56.

18. **Franceschi S, La Vecchia C, Booth M, Tzonou A, Negri E, Parazzini F, et al.** Pooled analysis of three European case-control studies of epithelial ovarian cancer: II. Age at menarche and menopause. *Int J Cancer* 1991;49:57–60.

19. **Engeland A, Tretli S, Bjorge T.** Height, body mass index, and ovarian cancer: a follow-up of 1.1 million Norwegian women. *J Natl Cancer Inst* 2003;95:1244–1248.

20. **Ness RB, Cramer DW, Goodman MT, Kjaer SK, Mallin K, Mosgaard BJ, et al.** Infertility, fertility drugs, and ovarian cancer: a pooled analysis of case-control studies. *Am J Epidemiol* 2002;155:217–224.

21. **Sit AS, Modugno F, Weissfeld JL, Berga SL, Ness RB.** Hormone replacement therapy and formulations and risk of epithelial ovarian carcinoma. *Gynecol Oncol* 2002;86:118–123.

22. **Lacey JV Jr, Mink PJ, Lubin JH, Sherman ME, Troisi R, Hartge P, et al.** Menopausal hormone replacement therapy and risk of ovarian cancer. *J Am Med Assoc* 2002;288:334–341.

23. **Franceschi, S, Parazzini F, Negri E, Booth M, La Vecchia C, Beral V, et al.** Pooled analysis of three European case-control studies of epithelial ovarian cancer: III. Oral contraceptive use. *Int J Cancer* 1991;49:61–65.

24. **De Palo G, Vceronesi U, Camerini T, Formelli F, Mascotti G, Boni C, et al.** Can *fenretinide* protect women against ovarian cancer? *J Natl Cancer Inst* 1995;87:146–147.

25. **De Palo G, Mariani L, Camerini T, Marubini E, Formelli F, Pasini B, et al.** Effect of *fenretinide* on ovarian carcinoma occurrence. *Gynecol Oncol* 2002;86:24–27.

26. **Rulin MC, Preston AL.** Adnexal masses in postmenopausal women. *Obstet Gynecol* 1987;70:578–581.

27. **Campbell S, Royston P, Bhan V, Whitehead MI, Collins WP.** Novel screening strategies for early ovarian cancer by transabdominal ultrasonography. *BJOG* 1990;97:304–311.

28. **van Nagell JR Jr, Higgins RV, Donaldson ES, Gallion HH, Powell DE, Pavlik EJ, et al.** Transvaginal sonography as a screening method for ovarian cancer: a report of the first 1,000 cases screened. *Cancer* 1990;65:573–577.

29. **van Nagell JR Jr, Gallion HH, Pavlik EJ, DePriest PD.** Ovarian cancer screening. *Cancer* 1995;76:2086–2091.

30. **van Nagell JR Jr, DePriest PD, Reedy MB, Gallion HH, Ueland FR, Pavlik EJ, et al.** The efficacy of transvaginal sonographic screening in asymptomatic women at risk for ovarian cancer. *Gynecol Oncol* 2000;77:350–356.

31. **Ueland FR, DePriest PD, Pavlik EJ, Kryscio RJ, van Nagell JR Jr.** Preoperative differentiation of malignant from benign ovarian tumors: the efficacy of morphology indexing and Doppler flow sonography. *Gynecol Oncol* 2003;91:46–50.

32. **Cohen LS, Escobar PF, Scharm C, Glimco B, Fishman DA.** Three-dimensional power Doppler ultrasound improves the diagnostic accuracy for ovarian cancer prediction. *Gynecol Oncol* 2001;82:40–48.

33. **Kurjak A, Kupesic S, Sparac V, Prka M, Bekavac I.** The detection of stage I ovarian cancer by three-dimensional sonography and power Doppler. *Gynecol Oncol* 2003;90:258–264.

34. **Jacobs I, Oram D, Fairbanks J, Turner J, Frost C, Grudzinskas JG.** A risk of malignancy index incorporating CA125, ultrasound and menopausal status for the accurate preoperative diagnosis of ovarian cancer. *BJOG* 1990;97:922–929.

35. **Jacobs I, Davies AP, Bridges J, Stabile I, Fay T, Lower A, et al.** Prevalence screening for ovarian cancer in postmenopausal women by CA125 measurements and ultrasonography. *BMJ* 1993;306:1030–1034.

36. **Rustin GJS, van der Burg MEL, Berek JS.** Tumor markers. *Ann Oncol* 1993;4:S71–S77.

37. **Jacobs IJ, Skates S, Davies AP, Woolas RP, Jeyerajah A, Weidemann P, et al.** Risk of diagnosis of ovarian cancer after raised serum CA125 concentration: a prospective cohort study. *BMJ* 1996;313:1355–1358.

38. **Einhorn N, Sjövall K, Knapp RC, Hall P, Scully RE, Bast RC Jr, et al.** A prospective evaluation of serum CA125 levels for early detection of ovarian cancer. *Obstet Gynecol* 1992;80:14–18.

39. **Jacobs IJ, Oram DH, Bast RC Jr.** Strategies for improving the specificity of screening for ovarian cancer with tumor-associated antigens CA125, CA15-3, and TAG 72.3. *Obstet Gynecol* 1992;80:396–399.

40. **Berek JS, Bast RC Jr.** Ovarian cancer screening: the use of serial complementary tumor markers to improve sensitivity and specificity for early detection. *Cancer* 1995;76:2092–2096.

41. **Skates SJ, Xu FJ, Yu YH, Sjövall K, Einhorn N, Chang Y, et al.** Towards an optimal algorithm for ovarian cancer screening with longitudinal tumour markers. *Cancer* 1995;76:2004–2010.

42. **Yin BW, Lloyd KO.** Molecular cloning of the CA125 ovarian cancer antigen: identification of a new mucin, MUC16. *J Biol Chem* 2001;27:371–375.

43. **Lloyd KO, Yin BW, Kudryashov V.** Isolation and characterization of ovarian cancer antigen CA125 using a new monoclonal antibody (VK-8): identification as a mucin-type molecule. *Int J Cancer* 1997;71:842–850.

44. **O'Brien TJ, Beard JB, Underwood LJ, Dennis RA, Santin AD, York L.** The CA125 gene: an extracellular superstructure dominated by repeat sequences. *Tumour Biol* 2001;22:345–347.

45. **Gubbels JA, Belisle J, Onda M, Rancourt C, Migneault M, Ho M, et al.** Mesothelin-MUC16 binding is a high affinity, N-glycan dependent interaction that facilitates peritoneal metastasis of ovarian tumors. *Mol Cancer* 2006;5:50.

46. **Maeda T, Inoue M, Koshiba S, Yabuki T, Aoki M, Nunokawa E, et al.** Solution structure of the SEA domain from the murine homologue of ovarian cancer antigen CA125 (MUC16). *J Biol Chem* 2004;279:13174–13182.

47. **Rump A, Morikawa Y, Tanaka M, Minami S, Umesaki N, Takeuchi M, et al.** Binding of ovarian cancer antigen CA125/MUC16 to mesothelin mediates cell adhesion. *J Biol Chem* 2004;279:9190–9198.

48. **Jacobs IJ, Skates SJ, MacDonald N, Menon U, Rosenthal AN, Davies AP, et al.** Screening for ovarian cancer: a pilot randomised controlled trial. *Lancet* 1999;353:1207–1210.

49. **Bourne TH, Campbell S, Reynolds KM, Whitehead MI, Hampson J, Royston P, et al.** Screening for early familial ovarian cancer with transvaginal ultrasonography and colour blood flow imaging. *BMJ* 1993;306:1025–1029.

50. European Randomised Trial of Ovarian Cancer Screening (protocol). Department of Environmental and Preventive Medicine, Wolfson

Institute of Preventive Medicine, Barts and The London, Queen Mary's School of Medicine and Dentistry, London, United Kingdom, 1999.

51. **Skates SJ, Menon U, MacDonald N, Rosenthal AN, Oram DH, Knapp RC, et al.** Calculation of the risk of ovarian cancer from serial CA-125 values for preclinical detection in postmenopausal women. *J Clin Oncol* 2003;21(suppl 10):206–210.

52. **Scholler N, Fu N, Yang Y, Ye Z, Goodman GE, Hellström KE, et al.** Soluble member(s) of the mesothelin/megakaryocyte potentiating factor family are detectable in sera from patients with ovarian carcinoma. *Proc Natl Acad Sci U S A* 1999;96:11531–11536.

53. **Baron AT, Lafky JM, Boardman CH, Balasubramanian S, Suman VJ, Podratz KC, et al.** Serum sErbB1 and epidermal growth factor levels as tumor biomarkers in women with stage III or IV epithelial ovarian cancer. *Cancer Epidemiol Biomarkers* 1999; 8:129–137.

54. **Schummer M, Ng WV, Bumgarner RE, Nelson PS, Schummer B, Bednarski DW, et al.** Comparative hybridization of an array of 21,500 ovarian cDNAs for the discovery of genes overexpressed in ovarian carcinomas. *Gene* 1999;238:375–385.

55. **Mok SC, Chao J, Skates S, Wong K, Yiu GK, Muto MG, et al.** Prostasin, a potential serum marker for ovarian cancer: identification through microarray technology. *J Natl Cancer Inst* 2001;93: 1458–1464.

56. **Kim JH, Skates SJ, Uede T, Wong KK, Schorge JO, Feltmate CM, et al.** Osteopontin as a potential diagnostic for ovarian cancer. *JAMA* 2002;282:1671–1679.

57. **Diamandis EP, Yousef GM, Soosaipillai AR, Bunting P.** Human kallikrein 6 (zyme/protease M/neurosin): a new serum biomarker of ovarian carcinoma. *Clin Biochem* 2000;33:579–583.

58. **Luo LY, Bunting P, Scorilas A, Diamandis EP.** Human kallikrein 10: a novel tumor marker for ovarian carcinoma? *Clin Chim Acta* 2001;306:111–118.

59. **Gorelik E, Landsittel DP, Morangonni AM, Modugno F, Velikokhatnaya L, Winans MT, et al.** Multiplexed immunobead-based cytokine profiling for early detection of ovarian cancer. *Epidemiol Biomarkers Prev* 2005;14:981–987.

60. **Petricoin EF, Ardekani AM, Hitt BA, Levine PJ, Fusaro VA, Steinberg SM, et al.** Use of proteomic patterns in serum to identify ovarian cancer. *Lancet* 2002;359:572–577.

61. **Zhang Z, Barnhill SD, Baggerly KA, Morris JS, Coombes KR.** Reproducibility of SELDI-TOF protein patterns in serum: comparing datasets from different experiments. *Bioinformatics* 2004;20:777–785.

62. **Zhang Z, Bast RC Jr, Yu Y, Li J, Sokoll LJ, Rai AJ, et al.** Three biomarkers identified from serum proteomic analysis for the detection of early stage ovarian cancer. *Cancer Res* 2004; 64:5882–5890.

63. **Chang HW, Lee SM, Goodman SN, Singer G, Cho SK, Sokoll LJ, et al.** Assessment of plasma DNA levels, allelic imbalance, and CA125 as diagnostic tests for cancer. *J Natl Cancer Inst* 2002;94: 1697–1703.

64. **Mok CH, Tsao SW, Knapp RC, Fishbaugh PM, Lau CC.** Unifocal origin of advanced human epithelial ovarian cancers. *Cancer Res* 1992;52:5119–5122.

65. **Muto MG, Welch WR, Mok SC, Bandera CA, Fishbaugh PM, Tsao SW, et al.** Evidence for a multifocal origin of papillary serous carcinoma of the peritoneum. *Cancer Res* 1995;55:490–492.

66. **Easton DF, Ford D, Bishop DT.** Breast and ovarian cancer incidence in *BRCA1*-mutation carriers. Breast Cancer Linkage Consortium. *Am J Hum Genet* 1995;56:265–271.

67. **Whittemore AS, Gong G, Itnyre J.** Prevalence and contribution of *BRCA1* mutations in breast cancer and ovarian cancer: results from three U.S. population-based case-control studies of ovarian cancer. *Am J Hum Genet* 1997;60:496–504.

68. **Frank TS, Manley SA, Olopade OI, Cummings S, Garber JE, Bernhardt B, et al.** Sequence analysis of *BRCA1* and *BRCA2*: correlation of mutations with family history and ovarian cancer risk. *J Clin Oncol* 1998;16:2417–2425.

69. **Johannsson OT, Ranstam J, Borg A, Olsson H.** Survival of *BRCA1* breast and ovarian cancer patients: a population-based study from southern Sweden. *J Clin Oncol* 1998;16:397–404.

70. **Burke W, Daly M, Garber J, Botkin J, Kahn MJ, Lynch P, et al.** Recommendations for follow-up care of individuals with an inherited predisposition to cancer. II. *BRCA1* and *BRCA2*. Cancer Genetics Studies Consortium. *JAMA* 1997;277:997–1003.

71. **Berchuck A, Cirisano F, Lancaster JM, Schildkraut JM, Wiseman RW, Marks JR.** Role of *BRCA1* mutation screening in the management of familial ovarian cancer. *Am J Obstet Gynecol* 1996;175:738–746.

72. **Struewing JP, Hartge P, Wacholder S, Baker SM, Berlin M, McAdams M, et al.** The risk of cancer associated with specific mutations of *BRCA1* and *BRCA2* among Ashkenazi Jews. *N Engl J Med* 1997;336:1401–1408.

73. **Beller U, Halle D, Catane R, Kaufman B, Hornreich G, Levy-Lahad E.** High frequency of *BRCA1* and *BRCA2* germline mutations in Ashkenazi Jewish ovarian cancer patients, regardless of family history. *Gynecol Oncol* 1997;67:123–126.

74. **Lerman C, Narod S, Schulman K, Hughes C, Gomez-Caminero A, Bonney G, et al.** *BRCA1* testing in families with hereditary breast-ovarian cancer: a prospective study of patient decision making and outcomes. *JAMA* 1996;275:1885–1892.

75. **Ponder B.** Genetic testing for cancer risk. *Science* 1997;278: 1050–1058.

76. **Lynch HT, Cavalieri RJ, Lynch JF, Casey MJ.** Gynecologic cancer clues to Lynch syndrome II diagnosis: a family report. *Gynecol Oncol* 1992;44:198–203.

77. **American Society of Clinical Oncology.** Statement of the American Society of Clinical Oncology: genetic testing for cancer susceptibility. *J Clin Oncol* 1996;14:1730–1736.

78. **King MC, Marks JH, Mandell JB for the New York Breast Cancer Study Group.** Breast and ovarian cancer risks due to inherited mutations in *BRCA1* and *BRCA2*. *Science* 2003;302:643–646.

79. **Risch HA, McLaughlin JR, Cole DE, Rosen B, Bradley L, Fan I, et al.** Population *BRCA1* and *BRCA2* mutation frequencies and cancer penetrances: a kin-cohort study in Ontario, Canada. *J Natl Cancer Inst* 2006;98:1694–1706.

80. **Brozek I, Ochman K, Debniak J, Morzuch L, Ratajska M, Stepnowska M, et al.** High frequency of *BRCA1/2* germline mutations in consecutive ovarian cancer patients in Poland. *Gynecol Oncol* 2008;108:433–437.

81. **NIH Consensus Development Panel on Ovarian Cancer.** Ovarian cancer: screening, treatment and follow-up. *JAMA* 1995;273: 491–497.

82. **Hermsen BB, Olivier RI, Verheijen RH, van Beurden M, de Hullu JA, Massuger LF, et al.** No efficacy of annual gynaecological screening in *BRCA1/2* mutation carriers; an observational follow-up study. *Br J Cancer* 2007;96:1335–1342.

83. **Woodward ER, Sleightholme HV, Considine AM, Williamson S, McHugo JM, Cruger DG.** Annual surveillance by CA125 and transvaginal ultrasound for ovarian cancer in both high-risk and population risk women is ineffective. *BJOG* 2007;114:1500–1509.

84. **Hogg R, Friedlander M.** Biology of epithelial ovarian cancer: implications for screening women at high genetic risk. *J Clin Oncol* 2004;22:1315–1327.

85. **Greene MH, Piedmonte M, Alberts D, Gail M, Hensley M, Miner Z, et al.** Prospective study of risk-reducing salpingo-oophorectomy and longitudinal CA-125 screening among women at increased genetic risk of ovarian cancer: design and baseline characteristics: a Gynecologic Oncology Group study. *Cancer Epidemiol Biomarkers Prev* 2008;17:594–604.

86. **Narod SA, Risch H, Moslehi R, Dorum A, Neuhausen S, Olsson H, et al.** Oral contraceptives and the risk of hereditary ovarian cancer. Hereditary Ovarian Cancer Clinical Study Group. *N Engl J Med* 1998;339:424–428.

87. **Modan B, Hartge P, Hirsh-Yechezkel G, Chetrit A, Lubin F, Beller U, et al.** Parity, oral contraceptives, and the risk of ovarian cancer among carriers and noncarriers of a *BRCA1* or *BRCA2* mutation. *N Engl J Med* 2001;345:235–240.

88. **Narod SA, Sun P, Ghadirian P, Lynch H, Isaacs C, Garber J, et al.** Tubal ligation and risk of ovarian cancer in carriers of *BRCA1* or *BRCA2* mutations: a case-control study. *Lancet* 2001;357:1467–1470.

89. **Averette HE, Nguyen HN.** The role of prophylactic oophorectomy in cancer prevention. *Gynecol Oncol* 1994;55:S38–S41.

90. **Kauff ND, Satagopan JM, Robson ME, Scheuer L, Hensley M, Hudis CA, et al.** Risk-reducing salpingo-oophorectomy in women with a *BRCA1* or *BRCA2* mutation. *N Engl J Med* 2002;346: 1609–1615.

91. **Rebbeck TR, Lynch HT, Neuhausen SL, Narod SA, Van't Veer L, Garber JE, et al. for the Prevention and Observation of Surgical**

End Points Study Group. Prophylactic oophorectomy in carriers of *BRCA1* or *BRCA2* mutations. *N Engl J Med* 2002;346:1616–1622.

92. **Haber D.** Prophylactic oophorectomy to reduce the risk of ovarian and breast cancer in carriers of *BRCA* mutations. *N Engl J Med* 2002;346:1660–1661.

93. **Rebbeck TR, Levin AM, Eisen A, Snyder C, Watson P, Cannon-Albright L, et al.** Breast cancer risk after bilateral prophylactic oophorectomy in *BRCA1* mutation carriers. *J Natl Cancer Inst* 1999;91:1475–1479.

94. **Schrag D, Kuntz KM, Garber JE, Weeks JC.** Decision analysis-effects of prophylactic mastectomy and oophorectomy on life expectancy among women with *BRCA1* and *BRCA2* mutations. *N Engl J Med* 1997;336:1465–1471 [erratum, *N Engl J Med* 1997;337: 434].

95. **Lavie O, Hornreich G, Ben-Arie A.** *BRCA* germline mutations in Jewish women with uterine papillary carcinoma. *Gynecol Oncol* 2004;92:521–524.

96. **Grann VR, Jacobson JS, Thomason D, Hershman D, Heitjan DF, Neugut AI.** Effect of prevention strategies on survival and quality-adjusted survival of women with *BRCA1/2* mutations: an updated decision analysis. *J Clin Oncol* 2002;20:2520–2529.

97. **Ben David Y, Chetrit A, Hirsh-Yechezkel G, Friedman E, Beck BD, Beller U, et al.** Effect of *BRCA* mutations on the length of survival in epithelial ovarian tumors. *J Clin Oncol* 2002;20:463–466.

98. **Chetrit A, Hirsh-Yechezkel G, Ben-David Y, Lubin F, Friedman E, Sadetzki S.** Effect of *BRCA1/2* mutations on long-term survival of patients with invasive ovarian cancer: the national Israeli study of ovarian cancer. *J Clin Oncol* 2008;26:20–25.

99. **Chen LM, Berek JS.** Ovarian and fallopian tubes. In: **Haskell CM, ed.** *Cancer treatment.* 5th ed. Philadelphia: WB Saunders, 2000: 900–932.

100. **Berek JS, Bast RC.** Ovarian cancer. In: **Kufe DW, Pollock RE, Weichselbaum RR, Bast RC, Gansler TS, Holland JF, Frei E.** *Cancer medicine,* 6th ed. Hamilton, ON: BC Decker, 2004: 1831–1861.

101. **Goff BA, Masndel L, Muntz HG, Melancon CH.** Ovarian carcinoma diagnosis. *Cancer* 2000;89:2068–2075.

102. **Olson SH, Mignone L, Nakraseive C, Caputo TA.** Symptoms of ovarian cancer. *Obstet Gynecol* 2001;98:212–217.

103. **Vine MF, Calingaert B, Berchuck A, Schildkraut JM.** Characterization of prediagnostic symptoms among primary epithelial ovarian cancer cases and controls. *Gynecol Oncol* 2003;90:75–82.

104. **Goff BA, Mandel LS, Drescher CW, Urban N, Gough S, Schurman KM, et al.** Development of an ovarian cancer symptom index: possibilities for earlier detection. *Cancer* 2007;109:221–227.

105. **Lataifeh I, Marsden DE, Robertson G, Gebski V, Hacker NF.** Presenting symptoms of epithelial ovarian cancer. *Aust NZ J Obstet Gynaecol* 2005;45:211–214.

106. **Olsen CM, Cnossen J, Green AC, Webb PM.** Comparison of symptoms and presentation of women with benign, low malignant potential and invasive ovarian tumors. *Eur J Gynaecol Oncol* 2007; 28:376–380.

107. **Barber HK, Grober EA.** The PMPO syndrome (postmenopausal palpable ovary syndrome). *Obstet Gynecol* 1971;138:921–923.

108. **Nardo LG, Kroon ND, Reginald PW.** Persistent unilocular ovarian cysts in a general population of postmenopausal women: is there a place for expectant management? *Obstet Gynecol* 2003;102: 589–593.

109. **Modesitt SC, Pavlik EJ, Ueland FR, DePriest PD, Kryscio RJ, van Nagell JR Jr.** Risk of malignancy in unilocular ovarian cystic tumors less than 10 centimeters in diameter. *Obstet Gynecol* 2003; 102:594–599.

110. **Roman LD.** Small cystic pelvic masses in older women: is surgical removal necessary? *Gynecol Oncol* 1998;69:1–2.

111. **Bristow RE, Duska LR, Lambrou NC, Fishman EK, O'Neill MJ, Trimble EL, et al.** A model for predicting surgical outcome in patients with advanced ovarian carcinoma using computed tomography. *Cancer* 2000;89:1532–1540.

112. **Togashi K.** Ovarian cancer: the clinical role of US, CT, and MRI. *Eur Radiol* 2003;13(suppl 4):S87–104.

113. **Makhija S, Howden N, Edwards R, Kelley J, Townsend DW, Meltzer CC.** Positron emission tomography/computed tomography imaging for the detection of recurrent ovarian and fallopian tube carcinoma: a retrospective review. *Gynecol Oncol* 2002;85:53–58.

114. **Kurokawa T, Yoshida Y, Kawahara K, Tsuchida T, Fujibayashi Y, Yonekura Y, et al.** Whole-body PET with FDG is useful for following up an ovarian cancer patient with only rising CA-125 levels within the normal range. *Ann Nucl Med* 2002;16:491–493.

115. **Jung SE, Lee JM, Rha SE, Byun JY, Jung JI, Hahn ST.** CT and MR imaging of ovarian tumors with emphasis on differential diagnosis. *Radiographics* 2002;22:1305–1325.

116. **Hacker NF, Berek JS, Lagasse LD.** Gastrointestinal operations in gynecologic oncology. In: **Knapp RE, Berkowitz RS, eds.** *Gynecologic oncology,* 2nd ed. New York: McGraw-Hill, 1993: 361–375.

117. **Jacobs I, Oram D, Fairbanks J, Turner J, Frost C, Grudzinskas JG.** A risk of malignancy index incorporating CA125, ultrasound and menopausal status in the preoperative diagnosis of ovarian cancer. *Brit J Obstet Gynaecol* 1990;97:922–929.

118. **Chia YN, Marsden DE, Robertson G, Hacker NF.** Triage of ovarian masses. *Aust NZ Obstet Gynaecol* 2008;48:322–328.

119. **Malkasian GD, Knapp RC, Lavin PT, Zurawski VR, Podratz KC, Stanhope CR, et al.** Preoperative evaluation of serum CA125 levels in premenopausal and postmenopausal patients with pelvic masses: discrimination of benign from malignant disease. *Am J Obstet Gynecol* 1988;159:341–346.

120. **Plentl AM, Friedman EA.** *Lymphatic system of the female genitalia.* Philadelphia: WB Saunders, 1971.

121. **Chen SS, Lee L.** Incidence of paraaortic and pelvic lymph node metastasis in epithelial ovarian cancer. *Gynecol Oncol* 1983;16: 95–100.

122. **Burghardt E, Pickel H, Lahousen M, Stettner H.** Pelvic lymphadenectomy in operative treatment of ovarian cancer. *Am J Obstet Gynecol* 1986;155:315–319.

123. **Scarbelli C, Gallo A, Zarrelli A, Visentin C, Campagnutta E.** Systematic pelvic and para-aortic lymphadenectomy during cytoreductive surgery in advanced ovarian cancer: potential benefit on survival. *Gynecol Oncol* 1995;56:328–337.

124. **Dauplat J, Hacker NF, Neiberg RK, Berek JS, Rose TP, Sagae S.** Distant metastasis in epithelial ovarian carcinoma. *Cancer* 1987;60:1561–1566.

125. **Krag KJ, Canellos GP, Griffiths CT, Knapp RC, Parker LM, Welch WR, et al.** Predictive factors for long term survival in patients with advanced ovarian cancer. *Gynecol Oncol* 1989;34:88–93.

126. **Haapasalo H, Collan Y, Atkin NB.** Major prognostic factors in ovarian carcinomas. *Int J Gynecol Cancer* 1991;1:155–162.

127. **Haapasalo H, Collan Y, Seppa A, Gidland AL, Atkin NB, Pesonen E.** Prognostic value of ovarian carcinoma grading methods: a method comparison study. *Histopathology* 1990;16:1–7.

128. **Silverberg SG.** Prognostic significance of pathologic features of ovarian carcinoma. *Curr Top Pathol* 1989;78:85–109.

129. **Ludescher C, Weger AR, Lindholm J, Oefner D, Hausmaninger H, Reitsamer R, et al.** Prognostic significance of tumor cell morphometry, histopathology, and clinical parameters in advanced ovarian carcinoma. *Int J Gynecol Pathol* 1990;9:343–351.

130. **Henson DE.** The histologic grading of neoplasms. *Arch Pathol Lab Med* 1988;112:1091–1096.

131. **Baak JP, Chan KK, Stolk JG, Kenemans P.** Prognostic factors in borderline and invasive ovarian tumours of the common epithelial type. *Pathol Res Pract* 1987;182:755–774.

132. **Gajewski WH, Fuller AF Jr, Pastel-Ley C, Flotte TJ, Bell DA.** Prognostic significance of DNA content in epithelial ovarian cancer. *Gynecol Oncol* 1994;53:5–12.

133. **Friedlander ML, Hedley DW, Swanson C, Russell P.** Prediction of long term survivals by flow cyto-metric analysis of cellular DNA content in patients with advanced ovarian cancer. *J Clin Oncol* 1988;6:282–290.

134. **Rice LW, Mark SD, Berkowitz RS, Goff BA, Lage JM.** Clinicopathologic variables, operative characteristics, and DNA ploidy in predicting outcome in epithelial ovarian carcinoma. *Obstet Gynecol* 1995;86:379–385.

135. **Vergote IB, Kaern J, Abeler VM, Petterson EO, De Vos LN, Tropé CG.** Analysis of prognostic factors in stage I epithelial ovarian cancer. Importance of degree of differentiation and deoxyribonucleic acid ploidy in predicting relapse. *Am J Obstet Gynecol* 1993;169:40–52.

136. **Fox H.** Clinical value of a new technique of gynecologic tumor assessment. *Int J Gynecol Cancer* 1997;7:337–349.

137. Khoo SK, Hurst T, Kearsley J, Dickie G, Free K, Parsons PG, et al. Prognostic significance of tumour ploidy in patients with advanced ovarian carcinoma. *Gynecol Oncol* 1990;39:284–288.

138. Reles AE, Conway G, Schellerschmidt I, Schmider A, Unger M, Freidman W, et al. Prognostic significance of DNA content and S-phase fraction in epithelial ovarian carcinomas analyzed by image cytometry. *Gynecol Oncol* 1998;71:3–13.

139. Kaern J, Tropé CG, Kristensen GB, Pettersen EO. Flow cytometric DNA ploidy and S-phase heterogeneity in advanced ovarian carcinoma. *Cancer* 1994;73:1870–1877.

140. Berek JS, Martinez-Maza O. Molecular and biological factors in the pathogenesis of ovarian cancer. *J Reprod Med* 1994;39:241–248.

141. Berek JS, Martinez-Maza O, Hamilton T, Tropé C, Kaern J, Baak J, et al. Molecular and biological factors in the pathogenesis of ovarian cancer. *Ann Oncol* 1993;4:S3–S16.

142. Slamon DJ, Godolphin W, Jones LA, Holt JA, Wong SG, Keith DE, et al. Studies of the HER-2/*neu* protooncogene in human breast and ovarian cancer. *Science* 1989;244:707–712.

143. Berchuck A, Kamel A, Whitaker R, Kerns B, Olt G, Kinney R, et al. Overexpression of HER-2/*neu* is associated with poor survival in advanced epithelial ovarian cancer. *Cancer Res* 1990;50:4087–4091.

144. Rubin SC, Finstad CL, Wong GY, Almadrones L, Plante M, Lloyd KO. Prognostic significance of HER-2/*neu* expression in advanced epithelial ovarian cancer: a multivariate analysis. *Am J Obstet Gynecol* 1993;168:162–169.

145. Leary JA, Edwards BG, Houghton CRS. Amplification of HER-2/*neu* oncogene in human ovarian cancer. *Int J Gynecol Oncol* 1993;2:291–294.

146. Meden H, Marx D, Rath W, Kron M, Fattahi-Meibodi A, Hinney B, et al. Overexpression of the oncogene c-erb B2 in primary ovarian cancer: evaluation of the prognostic value in a Cox proportional hazards multiple regression. *Int J Gynecol Pathol* 1994;13:45–53.

147. Makar AP, Holm R, Kristensen GB, Neskland JM, Tropé CG. The expression of c-erb-B-2 (her-2/*neu*) oncogene in invasive ovarian malignancies. *Int J Gynecol Cancer* 1994;4:194–199.

148. Rubin SC, Finstad CL, Federici MG, Scheiner L, Lloyd KO, Hoskins WJ. Prevalence and significance of her-2/*neu* expression in early epithelial ovarian cancer. *Cancer* 1994;73:1456–1459.

149. Singleton TP, Perrone T, Oakley G, Niehans GA, Carson L, Cha SS. Activation of c-erb-B-2 and prognosis in ovarian carcinoma. Comparison with histologic type, grade, and stage. *Cancer* 1994;73:1460–1466.

150. Hutson R, Ramsdale J, Wells M. p53 protein expression in putative precursor lesions of epithelial ovarian cancer. *Histopathology* 1995;27:367–371.

151. Gotlieb WH, Watson JM, Rezai BA, Johnson MT, Martinez-Maza O, Berek JS. Cytokine-induced modulation of tumor suppressor gene expression in ovarian cancer cells: upregulation of *p53* gene expression and induction of apoptosis by tumor necrosis factor-α. *Am J Obstet Gynecol* 1994;170:1121–1128.

152. Kohler MF, Kerns BJ, Humphrey PA, Marks JR, Bast RC Jr, Berchuck A. Mutation and overexpression of p53 in early-stage ovarian cancer. *Obstet Gynecol* 1993;81:643–650.

153. Skomedal H, Kristensen G, Abeler V, Borresen AL, Tropé C, Holm R. *TP53* protein accumulation and gene mutation in relation to overexpression of *MDM2* protein in ovarian borderline tumors and stage I carcinoma. *J Pathol* 1997;181:158–165.

154. Henriksen R, Strang P, Backstom T, Wilander E, Tribukait B, Oberg K. Ki-67 immunostaining and DNA flow cytometry as prognostic factors in epithelial ovarian cancers. *Anticancer Res* 1994;14:603–608.

155. Mok SC, Bell DA, Knapp RC, Fishbaugh PM, Welch WR, Muto MG, et al. Mutation of K-*ras* protooncogene in human ovarian epithelial tumors of borderline malignancy. *Cancer Res* 1993;53:1489–1492.

156. Henriksen R, Funa K, Wilander E, Backstom T, Ridderheim M, Oberg K. Expression and prognostic significance of platelet-derived growth factor and its receptors in epithelial ovarian neoplasms. *Cancer Res* 1993;53:4550–4554.

157. Mills GB, Lu Y, Fang X, Wang H, Eder A, Mao M, et al. The role of genetic abnormalities of *PTEN* and the phosphatidylinositol 3-kinase pathway in breast and ovarian tumorigenesis, prognosis, and therapy. *Semin Oncol* 2001;28:125–141.

158. Liu J, Yang G, Thompson-Lanza JA, Glassman A, Hayes K, Patterson A, et al. A genetically defined model for human ovarian cancer. *Cancer Res* 2004;64:1655–1663.

159. Yu YH, Xu FJ, Peng H, Fang X, Zhao S, Li Y, et al. NOEY2 (ARHI), an imprinted putative tumor suppressor gene in ovarian and breast carcinomas. *Proc Natl Acad Sci U S A* 1999;96:214–219.

160. Mills GB, Eder A, Fang X, Hasegawa Y, Mao M, Lu Y, et al. Critical role of lysophospholipids in the pathophysiology, diagnosis and management of ovarian cancer. *Cancer Treat Res* 2002;107:259–283.

161. Dittrich C, Dittrich E, Sevelda P, Hudec M, Salzer H, Grunt T, Eliason J. Clonogenic growth *in vitro*: an independent biologic prognostic factor in ovarian carcinoma. *J Clin Oncol* 1991;9:381–388.

162. Sevin BU, Perras JP, Averette HE, Donato DM, Penalver M. Chemosensitivity testing in ovarian cancer. *Cancer* 1993;71:1613–1620.

163. Federico M, Alberts DS, Garcia DJ, Emerson J, Fanta P, Liu R, et al. *In vitro* drug testing of ovarian cancer using the human tumor colony-forming assay: comparison of in vitro response and clinical outcome. *Gynecol Oncol* 1994;55:S156–S163.

164. Karam A, Wang Chiang, Fung E, Nossov V, Karlan BY. Influence of residual disease and extreme drug resistance assays on outcome on patients with epithelial ovarian cancer. *J Clin Oncol* 2009;27:15s(abst5504).

165. Dembo AJ, Davy M, Stenwig AE, Berle EJ, Bush RS, Kjorstad K. Prognostic factors in patients with stage I epithelial ovarian cancer. *Obstet Gynecol* 1990;75:263–273.

166. Sjövall K, Nilsson B, Einhorn N. Different types of rupture of the tumour capsule and the impact on survival in early ovarian cancer. *Int J Gynecol Cancer* 1994;4:333–336.

167. Sevelda P, Dittich C, Salzer H. Prognostic value of the rupture of the capsule in stage I epithelial ovarian carcinoma. *Gynecol Oncol* 1989;35:321–322.

168. Vergote I, De Brabanter J, Fyles A, Bertelsen K, Einhorn N, Sevelda P, et al. Prognostic importance of degree of differentiation and cyst rupture in stage I invasive epithelial ovarian carcinoma. *Lancet* 2001;357:176–182.

169. Voest EE, van Houwelingen JC, Neijt JP. A meta-analysis of prognostic factors in advanced ovarian cancer with median survival and overall survival measured with log (relative risk) as main objectives. *Eur J Cancer Clin Oncol* 1989;25:711–720.

170. van Houwelingen JC, ten Bokkel Huinink WW, van der Burg ATM, van Oosterom AT, Neijt JP. Predictability of the survival of patients with ovarian cancer. *J Clin Oncol* 1989;7:769–773.

171. Berek JS, Bertlesen K, du Bois A, Brady MF, Carmichael J, Eisenhauer EA, et al. Advanced epithelial ovarian cancer: 1998 consensus statement. *Ann Oncol* 1999;10(suppl 1):87–92.

172. Sharp F, Blackett AD, Berek JS, Bast RC Jr. Conclusions and recommendations from the Helene Harris Memorial Trust sixth biennial international forum on ovarian cancer. *Int J Gynecol Cancer* 1997;7:416–424.

173. Balkwill F, Bast RC, Berek JS, Chenevix-Trench G, Gore M, Hamilton T, et al. Current research and treatment for epithelial ovarian cancer: a position paper from the Helene Harris Memorial Trust. *Eur J Cancer* 2003;39:1818–1827.

174. Omura GA, Brady MF, Homesley HD, Yordan E, Major FJ, Buchsbaum HJ, et al. Long-term follow-up and prognostic factor analysis in advanced ovarian carcinoma: the Gynecologic Oncology Group experience. *J Clin Oncol* 1991;9:1138–1150.

175. Young RC, Decker DG, Wharton JT, Piver MS, Sindelar WF, Edwards BK, et al. Staging laparotomy in early ovarian cancer. *JAMA* 1983;250:3072–3076.

176. Yoshimura S, Scully RE, Bell DA, Taft PD. Correlation of ascitic fluid cytology with histologic findings before and after treatment of ovarian cancer. *Am J Obstet Gynecol* 1984;148:716–721.

177. Benedetti-Panici P, Greggi S, Maneschi F, Scambia G, Amoroso M, Rabitti C, et al. Anatomical and pathological study of retroperitoneal nodes in epithelial ovarian cancer. *Gynecol Oncol* 1993;51:150–154.

178. Zanetta G, Rota S, Chiari S, Bonazzi C, Bratina G, Torri V, et al. The accuracy of staging: an important prognostic determinator in stage I ovarian carcinoma. *Ann Oncol* 1998;9:1097–1101.

179. Schueler JA, Cornelisse CJ, Hermans J, Trimbos JB, van der Burg MEL, Fleuran GJ. Prognostic factors in well-differentiated early-stage epithelial ovarian cancer. *Cancer* 1993;71:787–795.

180. **Eltabbakh GH, Mount SL.** Comparison of diaphragmatic wash and scrape specimens in staging of women with ovarian cancer. *Gynecol Oncol* 2001;81:461–465.

181. **Benedetti-Panici P, Scambia G, Baiocchi G, Greggi S, Mancuso S.** Technique and feasibility of radical para-aortic and pelvic lymphadenectomy for gynecologic malignancies: a prospective study. *Int J Gynecol Cancer* 1991;1:133–140.

182. **Green JA.** Early ovarian cancer—time for a rethink on stage? *Gynecol Oncol* 2003;90:235–237.

183. **Harlan LC, Clegg LX, Trimble EL.** Trends in surgery and chemotherapy for women diagnosed with ovarian cancer in the United States. *J Clin Oncol* 2003;21:3488–3494.

184. **Guthrie D, Davy MLJ, Phillips PR.** Study of 656 patients with "early" ovarian cancer. *Gynecol Oncol* 1984;17:363–369.

185. **Gershenson DM.** Clinical management potential tumours of low malignancy. *Best Pract Res Clin Obstet Gynaecol* 2002;16:513–527.

186. **Kurman RJ, Trimble CL.** The behavior of serous tumors of low malignant potential: are they ever malignant? *Int J Gynecol Pathol* 1993;12:120–127.

187. **Lim-Tan SK, Cajigas HE, Scully RE.** Ovarian cystectomy for serous borderline tumors: a follow-up study of 35 cases. *Obstet Gynecol* 1988;72:775–781.

188. **Rose PG, Rubin RB, Nelson BE, Hunter RE, Reale FR.** Accuracy of frozen section (intraoperative consultation) diagnosis of ovarian tumors. *Am J Obstet Gynecol* 1994;171:823–826.

189. **Tropé C, Kaern J, Vergote IB, Kristensen G, Abeler V.** Are borderline tumors of the ovary overtreated both surgically and systemically? A review of four prospective randomized trials including 253 patients with borderline tumors. *Gynecol Oncol* 1993;51: 236–243.

190. **Kaern J, Tropé CG, Abeler VM.** A retrospective study of 370 borderline tumors of the ovary treated at the Norwegian Radium Hospital from 1979 to 1982: a review of clinicopathologic features and treatment modalities. *Cancer* 1993;71:1810–1820.

191. **Zaetta G, Rota S, Chiari S, Bonazzi C, Bratina G, Mangioni C.** Behavior of borderline tumors with particular interest to persistence, recurrence, and progression to invasive carcinoma: a prospective study. *J Clin Oncol* 2001;19:2658–2664.

192. **Trimble CL, Korsary C, Trimble EL.** Long-term survival and patterns of care in women with ovarian tumors of low malignant potential. *Gynecol Oncol* 2002;86:34–37.

193. **Sutton GP, Bundy GN, Omura GA, Yordan EL, Beecham JB, Bonfoglio T.** Stage III ovarian tumors of low malignant potential treated with *cisplatin* combination therapy: a Gynecologic Oncology Group study. *Gynecol Oncol* 1991;41:230–233.

194. **Barakat RR, Benjamin IB, Lewis JL Jr, Saigo PE, Curtin JP, Hoskins WJ.** Platinum-based chemotherapy for advanced-stage serous ovarian tumors of low malignant potential. *Gynecol Oncol* 1995;59:390–393.

195. **Ronnett BM, Kurman RJ, Shmookler BM, Jablonski KS, Kass ME, Sugarbaker PH.** Pseudomyxoma peritonei in women: a clinicopathologic analysis of 30 cases with emphasis on site of origin, prognosis, and relationship to ovarian mucinous tumors of low malignant potential. *Hum Pathol* 1995;26:509–524.

196. **Gershenson DM.** Fertility-sparing surgery for malignancies in women. *J Natl Cancer Inst Monogr* 2005;34:43–47.

197. **Park JY, Kim DY, Suh DS, Kim JH, Kim YM, Kim YT, et al.** Outcomes of fertility-sparing surgery for invasive epithelial ovarian cancer: oncologic safety and reproductive outcomes. *Gynecol Oncol* 2008;110:345–353.

198. **Greer BE, Bundy BN, Ozols RF, Fowler JM, Clarke-Pearson D, Burger RA, et al.** Implications of second-look laparotomy in the context of optimally resected stage III ovarian cancer: a nonrandomized comparison using an explanatory analysis: a Gynecologic Oncology Group study. *Gynecol Oncol* 2005;99:71–79.

199. **Griffiths CT.** Surgical resection of tumor bulk in the primary treatment of ovarian carcinoma. *J Natl Cancer Inst Monogr* 1975;42: 101–104.

200. **Heintz APM, Berek JS.** Cytoreductive surgery in ovarian cancer. In: **Piver MS, ed.** *Ovarian cancer.* Edinburgh: Churchill Livingstone, 1987;129–143.

201. **Hacker NF, Berek JS, Lagasse LD, Nieberg RK, Elashoff RM.** Primary cytoreductive surgery for epithelial ovarian cancer. *Obstet Gynecol* 1983;61:413–420.

202. **Hoskins WJ, Bundy BN, Thigpen JT, Omura GA.** The influence of cytoreductive surgery on recurrence-free interval and survival in small volume stage III epithelial ovarian cancer: a Gynecologic Oncology Group study. *Gynecol Oncol* 1992;47:159–166.

203. **Hoskins WJ, McGuire WP, Brady MF, Homesley HD, Creasman WT, Berman M, et al.** The effect of diameter of largest residual disease on survival after primary cytoreductive surgery in patients with suboptimal residual epithelial ovarian carcinoma. *Am J Obstet Gynecol* 1994;170:974–979.

204. **Farias-Eisner R, Teng F, Oliveira M, Leuchter R, Karlan B, Lagasse LD, Berek JS.** The influence of tumor grade, distribution and extent of carcinomatosis in minimal residual epithelial ovarian cancer after optimal primary cytoreductive surgery. *Gynecol Oncol* 1994;55:108–110.

205. **Berek JS.** Complete debulking of advanced ovarian cancer. *Cancer J* 1996;2:134–135.

206. **Farias-Eisner R, Kim YB, Berek JS.** Surgical management of ovarian cancer. *Semin Surg Oncol* 1994;10:268–275.

207. **Hacker NF.** Cytoreduction for advanced ovarian cancer in perspective. *Int J Gynecol Cancer* 1996;6:159–160.

208. **Bristow R, Montz FJ, Lagasse LD, Leuchter RS, Karlan BY.** Survival impact of surgical cytoreduction in stage IV epithelial ovarian cancer. *Gynecol Oncol* 1999;72:278–287.

209. **Hunter RW, Alexander NDE, Soutter WP.** Meta-analysis of surgery in advanced ovarian carcinoma: Is maximum cytoreductive surgery an independent determinant of prognosis? *Am J Obstet Gynecol* 1992;166:504–511.

210. **Eisenkop SM, Spirtos NM, Friedman RL, Lin WC, Pisani AL, Perticucci S.** Relative influences of tumor volume before surgery and the cytoreductive outcome on survival for patients with advanced ovarian cancer: a prospective study. *Gynecol Oncol* 2003; 90:390–396.

211. **Brockbank EC, Ind TE, Barton DP, Shepherd JH, Gore ME, A'Hern R, et al.** Preoperative predictors of suboptimal primary surgical cytoreduction in women with clinical evidence of advanced primary epithelial ovarian cancer. *Int J Gynecol Cancer* 2004;14: 42–50.

212. **Crawford SC, Vasey PA, Paul J, Hay A, Davis JA, Kaye SB.** Does aggressive surgery only benefit patients with less advanced ovarian cancer? Results from an international comparison within the SCOTROC-1 Trial. *J Clin Oncol* 2005;23:8802–8811.

213. **Eisenkop SM, Spirtos NM, Lin WC.** Splenectomy in the context of primary cytoreductive operations for advanced ovarian cancer. *Gynecol Oncol* 2006;100:344–348.

214. **de Jong D, Eijkemans MJ, Lie Fong S, Gerestein CG, Kooi GS, Baalbergen A, et al.** Preoperative predictors for residual tumor after surgery in patients with ovarian carcinoma. *Oncology* 2007;72: 293–301.

215. **Memarzadeh S, Lee SB, Berek JS, Farias-Eisner R.** CA125 levels are a weak predictor of optimal cytoreductive surgery in patients with advanced epithelial ovarian cancer. *Int J Gynecol Cancer* 2003; 13:120–124.

216. **Dowdy SC, Mullany SA, Brandt KR, Huppert BJ, Cliby WA.** The utility of computed tomography scans in predicting suboptimal cytoreductive surgery in women with advanced ovarian cancer. *Cancer* 2004;101:346–352.

217. **Oayyum A, Coakley FV, Westphalen AC, Hricak H, Okuno WT, Powell B.** Role of CT and MR imaging in predicting optimal cytoreduction of newly diagnosed primary epithelial ovarian cancer. *Gynecol Oncol* 2005;96:301–306.

218. **Axtell AE, Lee MH, Bristow RE, Dowdy SC, Cliby WA, Raman S, et al.** Multi-institutional reciprocal validation study of computed tomography predictors of suboptimal primary cytoredcution in patients with advanced ovarian cancer. *J Clin Oncol* 2007;25: 384–389.

219. **Risum S, Høgdall C, Loft A, Berthelsen AK, Høgdall E, Nedergaard L, et al.** Prediction of suboptimal primary ovarian cancer with combined positron emission tomography/computed tomography: a prospective study. *Gynecol Oncol* 2008;108: 265–270.

220. **Vergote I, Marquette S, Amant F, Berteloot P, Neven P.** Port-site metastases after open laparoscopy: a study in 173 patients with advanced ovarian cancer. *Int J Gynecol Cancer* 2005;15:776–779.

221. **Skipper HE.** Adjuvant chemotherapy. *Cancer* 1978;41:936–940.

222. **Goldie JH, Coldman AJ.** A mathematic model for relating the drug sensitivity of tumors to their spontaneous mutation rate. *Cancer Treat Rep* 1979;63:1727–1733.

223. **Berek JS, Hacker NF, Lagasse LD.** Rectosigmoid colectomy and reanastomosis to facilitate resection of primary and recurrent gynecologic cancer. *Obstet Gynecol* 1984;64:715–720.

224. **Bridges JE, Leung Y, Hammond IG, McCartney AJ.** En bloc resection of epithelial ovarian tumors with concomitant rectosigmoid colectomy: the KEMH experience. *Int J Gynecol Cancer* 1993;3:199–202.

225. **Berek JS, Hacker NF, Lagasse LD, Leuchter RS.** Lower urinary tract resection as part of cytoreductive surgery for ovarian cancer. *Gynecol Oncol* 1982;13:87–92.

226. **Heintz AM, Hacker NF, Berek JS, Rose T, Munoz AK, Lagasse LD.** Cytoreductive surgery in ovarian carcinoma: feasibility and morbidity. *Obstet Gynecol* 1986;67:783–788.

227. **Montz FJ, Schlaerth J, Berek JS.** Resection of diaphragmatic peritoneum and muscle: role in cytore-ductive surgery for ovarian carcinoma. *Gynecol Oncol* 1989;35:338–340.

228. **Nicklin JL, Copeland LJ, O'Toole RV, Lewandowski GS, Vaccarello L, Havenar LP.** Splenectomy as part of cytoreductive surgery for ovarian carcinoma. *Gynecol Oncol* 1995;58:244–247.

229. **Brand E, Pearlman N.** Electrosurgical debulking of ovarian cancer: a new technique using the argon beam coagulator. *Gynecol Oncol* 1990;39:115–118.

230. **Deppe G, Malviya VK, Boike G, Malone JM Jr.** Use of Cavitron surgical aspirator for debulking of diaphragmatic metastases in patients with advanced carcinoma of the ovaries. *Surg Gynecol Obstet* 1989;168:455–456.

231. **Fanning J, Hilgers R.** Loop electrosurgical excision procedure for intensified cytoreduction of ovarian cancer. *Gynecol Oncol* 1995;57:188–190.

232. **Panici PB, Maggioni A, Hacker NF, Landoni F, Ackermann S, Campagnutta E, et al.** Systematic aortic and pelvic lymphadenectomy versus resection of bulky nodes only in optimally debulked advanced ovarian cancer: a randomized clinical trial. *J Nat Cancer Inst* 2005;97:560–566.

233. **du Bois A, Reuss A, Harter A, Meier W, Wagner U, Sehouli J, et al.** The role of lymphadenectomy in advanced epithelial ovarian cancer in patients with macroscopically complete resection of intraperitoneal disease. *Int J Gyn Cancer* 2006;16(suppl 3):601.

234. **Venesmaa P, Ylikorkala O.** Morbidity and mortality associated with primary and repeat operations for ovarian cancer. *Obstet Gynecol* 1992;79:168–172.

235. **Bristow RE, Tomacruz RS, Armstrong DK, Trimble EL, Montz FJ.** Survival effect of maximal cytore-ductive surgery for advanced ovarian carcinoma during the platinum era: a meta-analysis. *J Clin Oncol* 2002;20:1248–1259.

236. **Naik R, Nordin A, Cross PA, Hemming D, de Barros Lopes A, et al.** Optimal cytoreductive surgery is an independent prognostic indicator in stage IV epithelial ovarian cancer with hepatic metastases. *Gynecol Oncol* 2000;78:171–175.

237. **van der Burg MEL, van Lent M, Buyse M, Kobierska A, Columbo N, Favalli G, et al.** The effect of debulking surgery after induction chemotherapy on the prognosis in advanced epithelial ovarian cancer. *N Engl J Med* 1995;332:629–634.

238. **van der Burg MEL, Vergote I.** The role of interval debulking surgery in ovarian cancer. *Curr Oncol Rep* 2003;5:473–481.

239. **Berek JS.** Interval debulking of ovarian cancer—an interim measure. *N Engl J Med* 1995;332:675–677.

240. **Rose PG, Nerenstone S, Brady MF, Clarke-Pearson D, Olt G, Rubin SC, et al.** Secondary surgical cytoreduction for advanced ovarian carcinoma. *N Engl J Med* 2004;351:2544–2546.

241. **Junor EJ, Hole DJ, McNulty L, Mason M, Young J.** Specialist gynecologists and survival outcome in ovarian cancer: a Scottish National Study of 1966 patients. *BJOG* 1999;106:1130–1136.

242. **Tingulstad S, Skjeldestad FE, Hagen B.** The effect of centralization of primary surgery on survival in ovarian cancer patients. *Obstet Gynecol* 2003;102:499–505.

243. **Hreshchyshyn MM, Park RC, Blessing JA, Norris HJ, Levy D, Lagasse LD, et al.** The role of adjuvant therapy in stage I ovarian cancer. *Am J Obstet Gynecol* 1980;138:139–145.

244. **Greene MH, Boice JD, Greer BE, Blessing JA, Dembo AJ.** Acute nonlymphocytic leukemia after therapy with *alkylating agents* for ovarian cancer: a study of the five randomized clinical trials. *N Engl J Med* 1982;307:1416–1421.

245. **Travis LB, Holowaty EJ, Bergfeldt K, Lynch CF, Kohler BA, Wiklund T, et al.** Risk of leukemia after platinum-based chemotherapy for ovarian cancer. *N Engl J Med* 1999;340:351–357.

246. **Thomas GM.** Radiotherapy in early ovarian cancer. *Gynecol Oncol* 1994;55:S73–S79.

247. **Sell A, Bertlesen K, Andersen JE, Streyer I, Panduro J.** Randomized study of whole-abdomen irradiation versus pelvic irradiation plus *cyclophosphamide* in treatment of early ovarian cancer. *Gynecol Oncol* 1990;37:367–373.

248. **Young RC, Walton LA, Ellenberg SS, Homesley HD, Wilbanks GD, Decker DG, et al.** Adjuvant therapy in stage I and stage II epithelial ovarian cancer: results of two prospective randomized trials. *N Engl J Med* 1990;322:1021–1027.

249. **Berek JS.** Adjuvant therapy for early-stage ovarian cancer. *N Engl J Med* 1990;322:1076–1078.

250. **Ahmed FY, Wiltshaw E, Hern RP, Shepard J, Blake P, Fisher C, et al.** Natural history and prognosis of untreated stage I epithelial ovarian carcinoma. *J Clin Oncol* 1996;14:2968–2975.

251. **Finn CB, Luesley DM, Buxton EJ, Blackledge GR, Kelly K, Dunn JA, et al.** Is stage I epithelial ovarian cancer overtreated both surgically and systemically? Results of a five-year cancer registry review. *BJOG* 1992;99:54–58.

252. **Vergote I, Vergote-De Vos LN, Abeler V, Aas M, Lindegaard M, Kjoerstad KE, et al.** Randomized trial comparing *cisplatin* with radioactive phosphorus or whole abdominal irradiation as adjuvant treatment of ovarian cancer. *Cancer* 1992;69:741–749.

253. **Rubin SC, Wong GY, Curtin JP, Barakat RR, Hakes TB, Hoskins WJ.** Platinum based chemotherapy of high risk stage I epithelial ovarian cancer following comprehensive surgical staging. *Obstet Gynecol* 1993;82:143–147.

254. **Young RC, Brady MF, Nieberg RK, Long HJ, Mayer AR, Lentz SS, et al.** Adjuvant treatment for early ovarian cancer: a randomized phase III trial of intraperitoneal 32P or intravenous *cyclophosphamide* and *cisplatin*: a Gynecologic Oncology Group study. *J Clin Oncol* 2003;21:4350–4355.

255. **Bolis G, Colombo N, Pecorelli S, Torri V, Marsoni S, Bonazzi C, et al.** Adjuvant treatment for early epithelial ovarian cancer: results of two randomized clinical trials comparing *cisplatin* to no further treatment or chromic phosphate (32P). *Ann Oncol* 1995;6:887–893.

256. **Colombo N, Maggioni A, Bocciolone L, Rota S, Cantu MG, Mangioni C.** Multimodality therapy of early-stage (FIGO I-II) ovarian cancer: review of surgical management and postoperative adjuvant treatment. *Int J Gynecol Cancer* 1996;6:13–17.

257. **Vermorken JB, Pecorelli S.** Clinical trials in patients with epithelial ovarian cancer: past, present and future. *Eur J Surg Oncol* 1996;22:455–466.

258. **Tropé C, Kaern J, Hogberg T, Abeler V, Hagen B, Kristensen G, et al.** Randomized study on adjuvant chemotherapy in stage I high-risk ovarian cancer with evaluation of DNA-ploidy as prognostic instrument. *Ann Oncol* 200;11:281–288.

259. **Gadducci A, Sartori E, Maggino T, Zola P, Landoni F, Stegh ER, et al.** Analysis of failure in patients with stage I ovarian cancer: an Italian multicenter study. *Int J Gynecol Cancer* 1997;7:445–450.

260. **Trimbos JB, Vergote I, Bolis G, Vermorken JB, Mangioni C, Madronal C, et al.** Impact of adjuvant chemotherapy and surgical staging in early-stage ovarian carcinoma: European Organisation for Research and Treatment of Cancer-Adjuvant Chemotherapy in Ovarian Neoplasm Trial. *J Natl Cancer Inst* 2003;95:113–125.

261. **International Collaborative Ovarian Neoplasm (ICON1) Collaborators.** International collaborative ovarian neoplasm trial 1: a randomized trial of adjuvant chemotherapy in women with early-stage ovarian cancer. *J Natl Cancer Inst* 2003;95:125–132.

262. **Trimbos JB, Parmar M, Vergote I, Guthrie D, Bolis G, Columbo N, et al.** International Collaborative Ovarian Neoplasm Trial 1 and Adjuvant Chemotherapy in Ovarian Neoplasm Trial: two parallel randomized phase III trials of adjuvant chemotherapy in patients with early-stage ovarian carcinoma. *J Natl Cancer Inst* 2003;95:105–112.

263. **Bell J, Brady MF, Young RC, Lage J, Walker JL, Look KY, et al. for the Gynecologic Oncology Group.** Randomized phase III trial of three versus six cycles of adjuvant *carboplatin* and *paclitaxel* in

early stage epithelial ovarian carcinoma: a Gynecologic Oncology Group study. *Gynecol Oncol* 2006;102:432–439.

264. **McGuire WP, Rowinski EK, Rosensheim NE, Grumbine FC, Ettinger DS, Armstrong DK, et al.** *Taxol:* a unique antineoplastic agent with significant activity in advanced ovarian epithelial neoplasms. *Ann Intern Med* 1989;111:273–279.

265. **Rowinsky EK, Czaenave LA, Donehower RC.** *Taxol:* a novel investigational antimicrotubule agent. *J Natl Cancer Inst* 1990;82: 1247–1259.

266. **Sarosy G, Kohn E, Stone DA, Rothenberg M, Jacob J, Adamo DO, et al.** Phase I study of *Taxol* and granulocyte colony-stimulating factor in patients with refractory ovarian cancer. *J Clin Oncol* 1992;10:1165–1170.

267. **Einzig AI, Wiernik PH, Sasloff J, Runowicz CD, Goldberg GL.** Phase II study and long-term follow-up of patients treated with *Taxol* for advanced ovarian adenocarcinoma. *J Clin Oncol* 1992;10: 1748–1753.

268. **Trimble EL, Adams JD, Vena D, Hawkins MJ, Friedman MA, Fisherman JS, et al.** *Paclitaxel* for platinum-refractory ovarian cancer: results from the first 1,000 patients registered to National Cancer Institute Treatment Referral Center 9103. *J Clin Oncol* 1993; 11:2405–2410.

269. **Thigpen JT, Blessing JA, Ball H, Hummel SJ, Barrett RJ.** Phase II trial of *paclitaxel* in patients with progressive ovarian carcinoma after platinum-based chemotherapy: a Gynecologic Oncology Group study. *J Clin Oncol* 1994;12:1748–1753.

270. **Eisenhauer EA, ten Bokkel Huinink WW, Swenerton KD, Gianni L, Myles J, van der Burg MEL, et al.** European-Canadian randomized trial of *paclitaxel* in relapsed ovarian cancer: high-dose versus low-dose and long versus short infusion. *J Clin Oncol* 1994; 12:2654–2666.

271. **Bookman MA, McGuire WP, Kilpatrick D, Keenan E, Hogan WM, Johnson SW, et al.** *Carboplatin* and *paclitaxel* in ovarian carcinoma: a phase I study of the Gynecologic Oncology Group. *J Clin Oncol* 1996;14:1895–1902.

272. **McGuire WP, Hoskins WJ, Brady MF, Kucera PR, Partridge EE, Look KY, et al.** *Cyclophosphamide* and *cisplatin* compared with *paclitaxel* and *cisplatin* in patients with stage III and stage IV ovarian cancer. *N Engl J Med* 1996;334:1–6.

273. **Piccart MJ, Bertelsen K, Stuart G, Cassidy J, Mangioni C, Simonsen E, et al.** Long-term follow-up confirms a survival advantage of the *paclitaxel-cisplatin* regimen over the *cyclophosphamide-cisplatin* combination in advanced ovarian cancer. *Int J Gynecol Cancer* 2003;13(suppl 2):144–148.

274. **Muggia FM, Braly PS, Brady MF, Sutton G, Niemann TH, Lentz SL, et al.** Phase III randomized study of *cisplatin* versus *paclitaxel* versus *cisplatin* and *paclitaxel* in patients with suboptimal stage III or IV ovarian cancer: a gynecologic oncology group study. *J Clin Oncol* 2000;18:106–115.

275. **Advanced Ovarian Cancer Trialists Group.** Chemotherapy in advanced ovarian cancer: an overview of randomized clinical trials. *BMJ* 1991;303:884–891.

276. **Young RC, Chabner BA, Hubbard SP, Fisher RI, Anderson T, Simon RM, et al.** Advanced ovarian adenocarcinoma: a prospective clinical trial of *melphalan* (L-PAM) versus combination chemotherapy. *N Engl J Med* 1978;299:1261–1266.

277. **Lambert HE, Berry RI.** High dose *cisplatin* compared with high dose *cyclophosphamide* in the management of advanced epithelial ovarian cancer (FIGO Stages III and IV): report from the North Thames Cooperative Group. *BMJ* 1985;290:889–893.

278. **Neijt JP, ten Bokkel Huinink WW, van der Burg ME, Hamerlynck JV, van Lent M, van Houwelingen JC, et al.** Randomized trial comparing two combination chemotherapy regions (Hexa-CAF vs. CHAP-5) in advanced ovarian carcinoma. *Lancet* 1984;2:594–600.

279. **Neijt JP, ten Bokkel Huinink WW, van der Burg MEL, van Oosteron AT, Willemse PH, Heintz AP, et al.** Randomized trial comparing two combination chemotherapy regimens (CHAP-5 versus CP) in advanced ovarian carcinoma: a randomized trial of the Netherlands joint study group for ovarian cancer. *J Clin Oncol* 1987;5:1157–1168.

280. **Omura G, Bundy B, Berek JS, Curry S, Delgado G, Mortel R.** Randomized trial of *cyclophosphamide* plus *cisplatin* with or

without *doxorubicin* in ovarian carcinoma: a Gynecologic Oncology Group study. *J Clin Oncol* 1989;7:457–465.

281. **Bertelsen K, Jakobsen A, Andersen JE, Ahrons S, Pedersen PH, Kiaer H, et al.** A randomized study of *cyclophosphamide* and *cisplatin* with or without *doxorubicin* in advanced ovarian cancer. *Gynecol Oncol* 1987;28:161–169.

282. **Conte PF, Bruzzone M, Chiara S, Sertoli MR, Daga MG, Rubagotti A, et al.** A randomized trial comparing *cisplatin* plus *cyclophosphamide* versus *cisplatin*, *doxorubicin* and *cyclophosphamide* in advanced ovarian cancer. *J Clin Oncol* 1986;4:965–971.

283. **Gruppo Interegionale Cooperativo Oncologico Ginecologia.** Randomized comparison of *cisplatin* with *cyclophosphamide/cisplatin* with *cyclophosphamide/doxorubicin/cisplatin* in advanced ovarian cancer. *Lancet* 1987;2:353–359.

284. **Ovarian Cancer Meta-Analysis Project.** *Cyclophosphamide* plus *cisplatin* versus *cyclophosphamide*, *doxorubicin*, and *cisplatin* chemotherapy of ovarian carcinoma: a meta-analysis. *J Clin Oncol* 1991;9:1668–1674.

285. **Swenerton K, Jeffrey J, Stuart G, Roy M, Krepart G, Carmichael J, et al.** *Cisplatin-cyclophosphamide* versus *carboplatin-cyclophosphamide* in advanced ovarian cancer: a randomized phase III study of the National Cancer Institute of Canada Clinical Trials Group. *J Clin Oncol* 1992;10:718–726.

286. **Alberts DS, Green S, Hannigan EV, O'Toole R, Stock-Novack D, Anderson P, et al.** Improved therapeutic index of *carboplatin* plus *cyclophosphamide* versus *cisplatin* plus *cyclophosphamide*: final report by the Southwest Oncology Group of a phase III randomized trial in stages III (suboptimal) and IV ovarian cancer. *J Clin Oncol* 1992;10:706–717.

287. **Calvert AH, Newell DR, Gumbrell LA, O'Reilly S, Burnell M, Boxall FE, et al.** *Carboplatin* dosage: prospective evaluation of a simple formula based on renal function. *J Clin Oncol* 1989;7:1748–1756.

288. **Ozols RF, Bundy BN, Greer B, Fowler JM, Clarke-Pearson D, Burger RA, et al.** Phase III trial of *carboplatin* and *paclitaxel* compared with *cisplatin* and *paclitaxel* in patients with optimally resected stage III ovarian cancer: a Gynecologic Oncology Group study. *J Clin Oncol* 2003;21:3194–3200.

289. **du Bois A, Lück HJ, Meier W, Adams HP, Möbus V, Costa SD, et al.** A randomized clinical trial of *cisplatin/paclitaxel* versus *carboplatin/paclitaxel* as first-line treatment of ovarian cancer. *J Natl Cancer Inst* 2003;95:1320–1330.

290. **The International Collaborative Ovarian Neoplasm (ICON) Group.** *Paclitaxel* plus *carboplatin* versus standard chemotherapy with either single agent *carboplatin* or *cyclophosphamide, doxorubicin,* and *cisplatin* in women with ovarian cancer: the ICON3 randomised trial. *Lancet* 2002;360:505–515.

291. **The ICON Collaborators.** International Collaborative Ovarian Neoplasm Study 2 (ICON2): randomised trial of single-agent *carboplatin* against three-drug combination of CAP (*cyclophosphamide, doxorubicin,* and *cisplatin*) in women with ovarian cancer. *Lancet* 1998;352:1571–1576.

292. **Vasey PA, Paul J, Birt A, Junor EJ, Reed NS, Symonds RP, et al.** *Docetaxel* and *cisplatin* in combination as first-line chemotherapy for advanced epithelial ovarian cancer. Scottish Gynaecological Cancer Trials Group. *J Clin Oncol* 1999;17:2069–2080.

293. **Copeland LJ, Bookman M, Trimble E, for the Gynecologic Oncology Group Protocol GOG 182–ICON5.** Clinical trials of newer regimens for treating ovarian cancer: the rationale for Gynecologic Oncology Group Protocol GOG 182-ICON5. *Gynecol Oncol* 2003;90:S1–S7.

294. **Bookman MA, Brady MF, McGuire WP, Harper PG, Alberts DS, Friedlander M, et al.** Evaluation of new platinum-based treatment regimens in advanced-stage ovarian cancer: a Phase III Trial of the Gynecologic Cancer Intergroup. *J Clin Oncol* 2009;27:1419–1425.

295. **McGuire WP, Hoskins WJ, Brady MS, Homesley HD, Creasman WT, Berman ML, et al.** An assessment of dose-intensive therapy in suboptimally debulked ovarian cancer: a Gynecologic Oncology Group study. *J Clin Oncol* 1995;13:1589–1599.

296. **Kaye SB, Lewis CR, Paul J, Duncan ID, Gordon HK, Kitchener HC, et al.** Randomized study of two doses of *cisplatin* with *cyclophosphamide* in epithelial ovarian cancer. *Lancet* 1992;340: 329–333.

297. Kaye SB, Paul J, Cassidy J, Lewis CR, Duncan ID, Gordon HK, et al. Mature results of a randomized trial of two doses of *cisplatin* for the treatment of ovarian cancer. *J Clin Oncol* 1996;14:2113–2119.

298. Reed E, Janik J, Bookman MA, Rothenberg M, Smith J, Young RC, et al. High-dose *carboplatin* and recombinant granulocyte-macrophage colony-stimulating factor in advanced-stage recurrent ovarian cancer. *J Clin Oncol* 1993;11:2118–2126.

299. Alberts DS, Liu PY, Hannigan EV, O'Toole R, Williams SD, Young JA, et al. Intraperitoneal *cisplatin* plus intravenous *cyclophosphamide* versus intravenous *cisplatin* plus intravenous *cyclophosphamide* for stage III ovarian cancer. *N Engl J Med* 1996; 335:1950–1955.

300. Markman M, Bundy BN, Alberts DS, Fowler JM, Clarke-Pearson DL, Carson LF, et al. Phase III trial of standard-dose intravenous *cisplatin* plus *paclitaxel* versus moderately high-dose intravenous *carboplatin* followed by intraperitoneal *paclitaxel* and intraperitoneal *cisplatin* in small-volume stage III ovarian cancer: an intergroup study of the Gynecologic Oncology Group, Southwestern Oncology Group, and the Eastern Cooperative Oncology Group. *J Clin Oncol* 2001;19:1001–1007.

301. Armstrong DK, Bundy B, Wenzel L, Huang HQ, Baergen R, Lele S, et al. Intraperitoneal *cisplatin* and *paclitaxel* in ovarian cancer. *N Eng J Med* 2006:354:34–43.

302. Rothenburg ML, Liu PY, Braly PS, Wilczynski SP, Hannigan EV, Wadler S, et al. Combined intraperitoneal and intravenous chemotherapy for women with optimally debulked ovarian cancer: results from an intergroup phase II trial. *J Clin Oncol* 2003;21: 1313–1319.

303. Alberts DS, Markman M, Armstrong D, Rothenberg ML, Muggia F, Howell SB. Intraperitoneal therapy for stage III ovarian cancer: a therapy whose time has come! *J Clin Oncol* 2002;20: 3944–3946.

304. Hess LM, Benham-Hutchins M, Herzog TJ, Hsu CH, Malone DC, Skrepnek GH, et al. A meta-analysis of the efficacy of intraperitoneal *cisplatin* for the front-line treatment of ovarian cancer. *Int J Gynecol Cancer* 2007;17:561–570.

305. Jaaback K, Johnson N. Intraperitoneal chemotherapy for the initial management of primary epithelial ovarian cancer. *Cochrane Database of Systematic Reviews* 2006, Issue 1. Art. No.: CD005340. DOI: 10.1002/14651858.CD005340.pub2.

306. Gore M, du Bois A, Vergote I. Intraperitoneal chemotherapy in ovarian cancer remains experimental. *J Clin Oncol* 2006;24: 4528–4530.

307. Schwartz PE, Rutherford TJ, Chambers JT, Kohorn EL Thiel RP. Neoadjuvant chemotherapy for advanced ovarian cancer: long-term survival. *Gynecol Oncol* 1999;72:93–99.

308. Shibata K, Kikkawa F, Mika M, Suzuki Y, Kajiyama H, Ino K, Mizutani S. Neoadjuvant chemotherapy for FIGO stage III or IV ovarian cancer: survival benefit and prognostic factors. *Int J Gynecol Cancer* 2003;13:587–592.

309. Chan YM, Ng TY, Ngan HY, Wong LC. Quality of life in women treated with neoadjuvant chemotherapy for advanced ovarian cancer: a prospective longitudinal study. *Gynecol Oncol* 2003;88:9–16.

310. Bristow RE, Eisenhauer EL, Santillan A, Chi DS. Delaying the primary surgical effort for advanced ovarian cancer: a systematic review of neoadjuvant chemotherapy and interval cytoreduction. *Gynecol Oncol* 2007;104:480–490.

311. Cohen MH, Gootenberg J, Keegan P, Pazdur R. FDA drug approval summary: *bevacizumab* (Avastin) plus *carboplatin* and *paclitaxel* as first-line treatment of advanced/metastatic recurrent nonsquamous non-small cell lung cancer. *Oncologist* 2007;12:713–718.

312. Miller K, Wang M, Gralow J, Dickler M, Cobleigh M, Perez EA, et al. *Paclitaxel* plus *bevacizumab* versus *paclitaxel* alone for metastatic breast cancer. *N Engl J Med* 2007;357:2666–2676.

313. Hurwitz H, Fehrenbacher L, Novotny W, Cartwright T, Hainsworth J, Heim W, et al. *Bevacizumab* plus *irinotecan*, *fluorouracil*, and *leucovorin* for metastatic colorectal cancer. *N Engl J Med* 2004;350:2335–2342.

314. Markman M, Liu PY, Wilczynski S, Monk B, Copeland LJ, Alvarez RD, et al. for the Southwest Oncology Group and Gynecologic Oncology Group. Phase III randomized trial of 12 versus 3 months of maintenance *paclitaxel* in patients with advanced ovarian cancer after complete response to platinum and *paclitaxel*-based chemotherapy: a Southwest Oncology Group and Gynecologic Oncology Group trial. *J Clin Oncol* 2003;21:2460–2465.

315. Ozols RF. Maintenance therapy in advanced ovarian cancer: progression-free survival and clinical benefit. *J Clin Oncol* 2003;21: 2451–2453.

316. De Placido S, Scambia G, DiVagno G, Naglieri E, Lombardi AV, Biamonte R, et al. *Topotecan* compared with no therapy after response to surgery and *carboplatin/paclitaxel* in patients with ovarian cancer: multicenter Italian trials in ovarian cancer (MITO-1) randomized study. *J Clin Oncol* 2004;22:2635–2642.

317. Pfisterer J, Weber B, Reuss A, Kimmig R, Du Bois A, Wagner U, et al. Randomized phase III trial of *topotecan* following *carboplatin* and *paclitaxel* in first-line treatment of advanced ovarian cancer: a gynecologic cancer intergroup trial of the AGO-OVAR and GINECO. *J Natl Cancer Inst* 2006;98:1024–1045.

318. Piccart MJ, Floquet A, Scarfone G, Willemse PH, Emerich J, Vergote I, et al. Intraperitoneal cis_platin versus no further treatment: 8-year results of EORTC 55875, a randomized phase III study in ovarian cancer patients with a pathologically complete remission after platinum-based intravenous chemotherapy. *Int J Gynecol Cancer* 2003;13(suppl 2):196–203.

319. Lorusso D, Ferrandina G, Greggi S, Gadducci A, Pignata S, Tateo S, et al.; Multicenter Italian Trials in Ovarian Cancer Investigators. Phase III multicenter randomized trial of *amifostine* as cytoprotectant in first-line chemotherapy in ovarian cancer patients. *Ann Oncol* 2003;14:1086–1093.

320. De Vos FY, Bos AM, Schaapveld M, de Swart CA, de Graaf H, van der Zee AG, et al. A randomized phase II study of *paclitaxel* with *carboplatin* +/– *amifostine* as first line treatment in advanced ovarian carcinoma. *Gynecol Oncol* 2005;97:60–67.

321. Jordan K, Sippel C, Schmoll HJ. Guidelines for antiemetic treatment of chemotherapy-induced nausea and vomiting: past, present, and future recommendations. *Oncologist* 2007;12:1143–1150.

322. Herrstedt J. Antiemetics: an update and the MASCC guidelines applied in clinical practice. *Nat Clin Pract Oncol* 2008;1:32–43.

323. American Society of Clinical Oncology, Kris MG, Hesketh PJ, Somerfield MR, Feyer P, Clark-Snow R, et al. American Society of Clinical Oncology guideline for antiemetics in oncology: update 2006. *J Clin Oncol* 2006;24:2932–2947.

324. Rothenberg ML, Ozols RF, Glatstein E, Steinberg SM, Reed E, Young RC. Dose-intensive induction therapy with *cyclophosphamide*, *cisplatin* and consolidative abdominal radiation in advanced stage epithelial cancer. *J Clin Oncol* 1992;10:727–734.

325. Rendina GM, Donadio C, Giovannini M. Steroid receptors and progestinic therapy in ovarian endometrioid carcinoma. *Eur J Gynaecol Oncol* 1982;3:241–246.

326. Windbichler G, Hausmaninger H, Stummvoll W, Graf AH, Kainz C, Lahodny J, et al. *Interferon-gamma* in the first-line therapy of ovarian cancer: a randomized phase III trial. *Br J Cancer* 2000;82:1138–1144.

327. Alberts DS, Marth C, Alvarez RD, Johnson G, Bidzinski M, Kardatzke DR, et al. GRACES Clinical Trial Consortium. Randomized phase 3 trial of *interferon gamma-1b* plus standard *carboplatin/paclitaxel* versus *carboplatin/paclitaxel* alone for first-line treatment of advanced ovarian and primary peritoneal carcinomas: results from a prospectively designed analysis of progression-free survival. *Gynecol Oncol* 2008;109:174–181.

328. Berek JS, Schultes BC, Nicodemus CF. Biologic and immunologic therapies for ovarian cancer. *J Clin Oncol* 2003;21:168S–174S.

329. Berek JS, Dorigo O, Schultes BC, Nicodemus CF. Immunological therapy for ovarian cancer. *Gynecol Oncol* 2003;88:S105–S109.

330. Berek JS, Taylor PT, Gordon A, Cunningham MJ, Finkler N, Orr J, et al. Randomized placebo-controlled study of *oregovomab* for consolidation of clinical remission in patients with advanced ovarian cancer. *J Clin Oncol* 2004;22:3507–3516.

331. Berek JS, Taylor P, McGuire W, Smith CT, Schultes B, Nicodemus C. Orogovamab maintenance therapy in advanced stage ovarian cancer: no impact on relapse-free survival. *J Clin Oncol* 2008;26:1–8.

332. Verheijen RH, Massuger LF, Benigno BB, Epenetos AA, Lopes A, Soper JT, et al. Phase III trial of intraperitoneal therapy with yttrium-90-labeled HMFG1 murine monoclonal antibody in patients with epithelial ovarian cancer after a surgically defined complete remission. *J Clin Oncol* 2006;24:571–578.

333. Oei AL, Verheijen RH, Seiden MV, Benigno BB, Lopes A, Soper JT, et al. Decreased intraperitoneal disease recurrence in epithelial ovarian cancer patients receiving intraperitoneal consolidation treatment with yttrium-90-labeled murine HMFG1 without improvement in overall survival. *Int J Cancer* 2007;120:2710–2714.

334. Bookman MA, Darcy KM, Clarke-Pearson D, Boothby RA, Horowitz IR. Evaluation of monoclonal humanized anti-HER2 antibody, *trastuzumab*, in patients with recurrent or refractory ovarian or primary peritoneal carcinoma with overexpression of HER2: a phase II trial of the Gynecologic Oncology Group. *J Clin Oncol* 2003;21: 283–290.

335. Berek JS, Hacker NF, Lagasse LD, Poth T, Resnick B, Nieberg RK. Second-look laparotomy in stage III epithelial ovarian cancer: clinical variables associated with disease status. *Obstet Gynecol* 1984;64:207–212.

336. Schwartz PE, Smith JP. Second-look operation in ovarian cancer. *Am J Obstet Gynecol* 1980;138:1124–1130.

337. Rubin SC, Jones WB, Curtin JP, Barakat RR, Hakes TB, Hoskins WJ. Second-look laparotomy in stage I ovarian cancer following comprehensive surgical staging. *Obstet Gynecol* 1993;82:139–142.

338. Podratz KC, Cliby WA. Second-look surgery in the management of epithelial ovarian carcinoma. *Gynecol Oncol* 1994;55:S128–S133.

339. Bolis G, Villa A, Guarnerio P, Ferraris C, Gavoni N, Giardina G, et al. Survival of women with advanced ovarian cancer and complete pathologic response at second-look laparotomy. *Cancer* 1996;77: 128–131.

340. Friedman JB, Weiss NS. Second thoughts about second-look laparotomy in advanced ovarian cancer. *N Engl J Med* 1990;322:1079–1082.

341. Berek JS. Second-look versus second-nature. *Gynecol Oncol* 1992;44:1–2.

342. Rubin SC, Hoskins WJ, Saigo PE, Chapman D, Hakes TB, Markman M, et al. Prognostic factors for recurrence following negative second-look laparotomy in ovarian cancer patients treated with platinum-based chemotherapy. *Gynecol Oncol* 1991;42:137–141.

343. Dowdy SC, Constantinou CL, Hartmann LC, Keeney GL, Suman VJ, Hillman DW, et al. Long-term follow-up of women with ovarian cancer after positive second-look laparotomy. *Gynecol Oncol* 2003;91:563–568.

344. Berek JS, Griffith CT, Leventhal JM. Laparoscopy for second-look evaluation in ovarian cancer. *Obstet Gynecol* 1981;58:192–198.

345. Berek JS, Hacker NF. Laparoscopy in the management of patients with ovarian carcinoma. In: DiSaia P, ed. *The treatment of ovarian cancer*. London: WB Saunders, 1983:213–222.

346. Lele S, Piver MS. Interval laparoscopy prior to second-look laparotomy in ovarian cancer. *Obstet Gynecol* 1986;68:345–347.

347. Berek JS, Knapp RC, Malkasian GD, Lavin PT, Whitney C, Niloff JM, et al. CA125 serum levels correlated with second-look operations among ovarian cancer patients. *Obstet Gynecol* 1986;67:685–698.

348. Rustin GJ, Marples M, Nelstrop AE, Mahmoudi M, Meyer T. Use of CA125 to define progression of ovarian cancer in patients with persistently elevated levels. *J Clin Oncol* 2001;19:4054–4057.

349. Rustin GJ, Timmers P, Nelstrop A, Shreeves G, Bentzen SM, Baron B, et al. Comparison of CA-125 and standard definitions of progression of ovarian cancer in the intergroup trial of *cisplatin* and *paclitaxel* versus *cisplatin* and *cyclophosphamide*. *J Clin Oncol* 2006;24:45–51.

350. Rustin GJ, van der Burg ME, On behalf of MRC and EORTC collaborators. A randomized trial in ovarian cancer (OC) of early treatment of relapse based on CA125 level alone versus delayed treatment based on conventional clinical indicators (MRC OV05/EORTC 55955 trials). *J Clin Oncol* 2009;27:18s(abst1).

351. De Rosa V, Mangioni di Stefano ML, Brunetti A, Caraco C, Graziano R, et al. Computed tomography and second-look surgery in ovarian cancer patients: correlation, actual role and limitations of CT scan. *Eur J Gynaecol Oncol* 1995;16:123–129.

352. Lund B, Jacobson K, Rasch L, Jensen F, Olesen K, Feldt-Rasmussen K. Correlation of abdominal ultrasound and computed tomography scans with second- or third-look laparotomy in patients with ovarian carcinoma. *Gynecol Oncol* 1990;37:279–283.

353. Gadducci A, Cosio S, Zola P, Landoni F, Maggino T, Sartori E. Diagnostic accuracy of FDG PET in the follow-up of platinum-sensitive epithelial ovarian carcinoma. *Eur J Nucl Med Mol Imaging* 2007;34:1396–1405.

354. Bristow RE, del Carmen MG, Pannu HK, Cohade C, Zahurak ML, Fishman EK, et al. Clinically occult recurrent ovarian cancer: a patient selection for secondary cytoreductive surgery using combined PET/CT. *Gynecol Oncol* 2003;90:519–528.

355. Bristow RE, Giuntoli RL 2nd, Pannu HK, Schulick RD, Fishman EK, Wahl RL. Combined PET/CT for detecting recurrent ovarian cancer limited to the retroperitoneal nodes. *Gynecol Oncol* 2005;99:294–300.

356. Berek JS, Hacker NF, Lagasse LD, Nieberg RK, Elashoff RM. Survival of patients following secondary cytoreductive surgery in ovarian cancer. *Obstet Gynecol* 1983;61:189–193.

357. Hoskins WJ, Rubin SC, Dulaney E, Chapman D, Almadrones L, Saigo P, et al. Influence of secondary cytoreduction at the time of second-look laparotomy on the survival of patients with epithelial ovarian carcinoma. *Gynecol Oncol* 1989;34:365–371.

358. Jänicke F, Hölscher M, Kuhn W, von Hugo R, Pache L, Siewert JR, et al. Radical surgical procedure improves survival time in patients with recurrent ovarian cancer. *Cancer* 1992;70:2129–2136.

359. Rubin SC, Benjamin I, Berek JS. Secondary cytoreductive surgery. In: Gershenson D, McGuire W, eds. *Ovarian cancer: controversies in management*. New York: Churchill Livingstone, 1998:101–113.

360. Tay EH, Grant PT, Gebski V, Hacker NF. Secondary cytoreductive surgery for recurrent epithelial ovarian cancer. *Obstet Gynecol* 2002;100:1359–1360.

361. Salani R, Santillan A, Zahurak ML, Giuntoli RL 2nd, Gardner GJ, Armstrong DK, et al. Secondary cytoreductive surgery for localized recurrent epithelial ovarian cancer: analysis of prognostic factors and survival outcome. *Cancer* 2007;109:685–691.

362. Rose PG. Surgery for recurrent ovarian cancer. *Semin Oncol* 2000;27:17–23.

363. Munkarah A, Levenback C, Wolf JK, Bodurka-Bevers D, Tortolero-Luna G, Morris RT, et al. Secondary cytoreductive surgery for localized intra-abdominal recurrences in epithelial ovarian cancer. *Gynecol Oncol* 2001;81:237–241.

364. Segna RA, Dottino PR, Mandeli JP, Konsker K, Cohen CJ. Secondary cytoreduction for ovarian cancer following *cisplatin* therapy. *J Clin Oncol* 1993;11:434–439.

365. Eisenkop SM, Friedman RL, Spirtos NM. The role of secondary cytoreductive surgery in the treatment of patients with recurrent epithelial ovarian carcinoma. *Cancer* 2000;88:144–153.

366. Scarabelli C, Gallo A, Carbone A. Secondary cytoreductive surgery for patients with recurrent epithelial ovarian carcinoma. *Gynecol Oncol* 2001;83:504–512.

367. Herzog TJ, Pothuri B. Ovarian cancer: a focus on management of recurrent disease. *Nat Clin Pract Oncol* 2006 3:604–611.

368. Fung-Kee-Fung M, Oliver T, Elit L, Oza A, Hirte HW, Bryson P. Optimal Chemotherapy treatment for women with recurrent ovarian cancer. *Curr Oncol* 2007;14:195–207.

369. Blackledge G, Lawton F, Redman C, Kelly K. Response of patients in phase II studies of chemotherapy in ovarian cancer: implications for patient treatment and the design of phase II trials. *Br J Cancer* 1989 59:650–653.

370. Markman M, Rothman R, Hakes T, Reichman B, Hoskins W, Rubin S, et al. Second-line platinum chemotherapy in patients with ovarian cancer previously treated with *cisplatin*. *J Clin Oncol* 1991;9:389–393.

371. Gordon AN, Fleagle JJ, Guthrie D, Parkin DE, Gore ME, Lacave AJ. Recurrent epithelial ovarian carcinoma: A randomized phase III study of *pegylated liposomal doxorubicin* versus *topotecan*. *J Clin Oncol* 2001;19:3312–3322.

372. Gershenson DM, Kavanagh JJ, Copeland LJ, Stringer CA, Morris M, Wharton JT. Retreatment of patients with recurrent epithelial ovarian cancer with *cisplatin*-based chemotherapy. *Obstet Gynecol* 1989;73:798–802.

373. Ozols RF, Ostchega Y, Curt G, Young RT. High dose *carboplatin* in refractory ovarian cancer patients. *J Clin Oncol* 1987;5:197–201.

374. Gore ME, Fryatt I, Wiltshaw E, Dawson T. Treatment of relapsed carcinoma of the ovary with *cisplatin* or *carboplatin* following initial treatment with these compounds. *Gynecol Oncol* 1990;36: 207–211.

375. Eisenhauer EA, Vermorken JB, van Glabbeke M. Predictors of response to subsequent chemotherapy in platinum pretreated ovarian cancer: a multivariate analysis of 704 patients. *Ann Oncol* 1997;8: 963–968.

376. **Rose PG, Fusco N, Fluellen L, Rodriguez M.** Second-line therapy with *paclitaxel* and *carboplatin* for recurrent disease following first-line therapy with *paclitaxel* and platinum in ovarian or peritoneal carcinoma. *J Clin Oncol* 1998;16:1494–1497.

377. **Gronlund B, Hogdall C, Hansen HH, Engelholm SA.** Results of reinduction therapy with *paclitaxel* and *carboplatin* in recurrent epithelial ovarian cancer. *Gynecol Oncol* 2001;83:128–134.

378. **Markman M.** Second-line therapy for potentially platinum-sensitive recurrent ovarian cancer: what is optimal treatment? *Gynecol Oncol* 2001;81:1–2.

379. **Cannistra SA.** Is there a "best" choice of second-line agent in the treatment of recurrent, potentially platinum-sensitive ovarian cancer? *J Clin Oncol* 2002;20:1158–1160.

380. **Havrilesky LJ, Tait DL, Sayer RA, Lancaster JM, Soper JT, Berchuck A, et al.** Weekly low-dose *carboplatin* and *paclitaxel* in the treatment of recurrent ovarian and peritoneal cancer. *Gynecol Oncol* 2003;88:51–57.

381. **Parmar MK, Ledermann JA, Colombo N, du Bois A, Delaloye JF, Kristensen GB, et al.** *Paclitaxel* plus platinum-based chemotherapy versus conventional platinum-based chemotherapy in women with relapsed ovarian cancer: the ICON4/AGO-OVAR-2.2 trial. *Lancet* 2003;361:2099–2106.

382. **Gonzalez-Martin AJ, Calvo E, Bover I, Rubio J, Arcusa A, Casado A, et al.** Randomized phase II study of *carboplatin* versus *paclitaxel* and *carboplatin* in platinum-sensitive recurrent advanced ovarian carcinoma: a GEICO (Grupo Espanol de Investigacion en Cancer de Ovario) study. *Ann Oncol* 2005;16:749–755.

383. **Greco FA, Hainsworth JD.** One-hour *paclitaxel* infusion schedules: a phase I/II comparative trial. *Semin Oncol* 1995;22:118–123.

384. **Chang AY, Boros L, Garrow G, Asbury R.** *Paclitaxel* by 3-hour infusion followed by 96-hour infusion on failure in patients with refractory malignant disease. *Semin Oncol* 1995;22:124–127.

385. **Kohn EC, Sarosy G, Bicher A, Link C, Christian M, Steinberg SM, et al.** Dose-intense *Taxol:* high response rate in patients with platinum-resistant recurrent ovarian cancer. *J Natl Cancer Inst* 1994;86:1748–1753.

386. **Omura GA, Brady MF, Look KY, Averette HE, Delmore JE, Long HJ, et al.** Phase III trial of *paclitaxel* at two dose levels, the higher dose accompanied by filgrastim at two dose levels in platinum-pretreated epithelial ovarian cancer: an intergroup study. *J Clin Oncol* 2003;21:2843–2848.

387. **Markman M, Hall J, Spitz D, Weiner S, Carson L, Van Le L, et al.** Phase II trial of weekly single-agent *paclitaxel* in platinum/ *paclitaxel*-refractory ovarian cancer. *J Clin Oncol* 2002;20:2365–2369.

388. **Ghamande S, Lele S, Marchetti D, Baker T, Odunsi K.** Weekly *paclitaxel* in patients with recurrent or persistent advanced ovarian cancer. *Int J Gynecol Cancer* 2003;13:142–147.

389. **Piccart MJ, Gore M, ten Bokkel Huinink W, Van Oosterom A, Verweij J, Wanders J, et al.** *Docetaxel*: an active new drug for treatment of advanced epithelial ovarian cancer. *J Natl Cancer Inst* 1995;87:676–681.

390. **Francis P, Schneider J, Hann L, Balmaceda C, Barakat R, Phillips M, et al.** Phase II trial of *docetaxel* in patients with platinum-refractory advanced ovarian cancer. *J Clin Oncol* 1994;12:2301–2308.

391. **Rose PG, Blessing, JA, Ball HG, Hoffman J, Warshal D, DeGeest K, et al.** A phase II study of *docetaxel* in *paclitaxel*-resistant ovarian and peritoneal carcinoma: a Gynecologic Oncology Group study. *Gynecol Oncol* 2003;88:130–135.

392. **Bookman MA, Malstrom H, Bolis G, Gordon A, Lissoni A, Krebs JB, et al.** *Topotecan* for the treatment of advanced epithelial ovarian cancer: an open-label phase II study in patients treated after prior chemotherapy that contained *cisplatin* or *carboplatin* and *paclitaxel*. *J Clin Oncol* 1998;16:3345–3352.

393. **ten Bokkel Huinink W, Gore M, Carmichael J, Gordon A, Malfetano J, Hudson I, et al.** *Topotecan* versus *paclitaxel* for the treatment of recurrent epithelial ovarian cancer. *J Clin Oncol* 1997;15:2183–2193.

394. **ten Bokkel Huinink W, Lane SR, Ross GA, for the International** *Topotecan* **Study Group.** Long-term survival in a phase III, randomised study of *topotecan* versus *paclitaxel* in advanced epithelial ovarian carcinoma. *Ann Oncol* 2004;15:100–103.

395. **Hoskins P, Eisenhauer E, Beare S, Roy M, Droin P, Stuart G, et al.** Randomized phase II study of two schedules of *topotecan* in

previously treated patients with ovarian cancer: a National Cancer Institute of Canada Clinical Trials Group study. *J Clin Oncol* 1998; 16:2233–2237.

396. **Markman M, Blessing JA, Alvarez RD, Hanjani P, Waggoner S, Hall K, et al.** Phase II evaluation of 24-h continuous infusion *topotecan* in recurrent, potentially platinum-sensitive ovarian cancer: a Gynecologic Oncology Group study. *Gynecol Oncol* 2000;77:112–115.

397. **Kudelka AP, Tresukosol D, Edwards CL, Freedman RS, Levenback C, Chantarawiroj P, et al.** Phase II study of intravenous *topotecan* as a 5-day infusion for refractory epithelial ovarian carcinoma. *J Clin Oncol* 1996;14:1552–1557.

398. **Hochster H, Wadler S, Runowicz C, Liebes L, Cohen H, Wallach R, et al.** Activity and pharmaco-dynamics of 21-day *topotecan* infusion in patients with ovarian cancer previously treated with platinum-based chemotherapy. New York Gynecologic Oncology Group. *J Clin Oncol* 1999;17:2553–2561.

399. **Elkas JC, Holschneider CH, Katz B, Li AJ, Louie R, McGonigle KF, et al.** The use of continuous infusion *topotecan* in persistent and recurrent ovarian cancer. *Int J Gynecol Cancer* 2003;13:138–141.

400. **Markman M, Kennedy A, Webster, K, Kulp B, Peterson G, Belinson J.** Phase 2 evaluation of *topotecan* administered on a 3-day schedule in the treatment of platinum- and *paclitaxel*-refractory ovarian cancer. *Gynecol Oncol* 2000;79:116–119.

401. **Clarke-Pearson DL, Van Le L, Iveson T, Whitney CW, Hanjani P, Kristensen G, et al.** Oral *topotecan* as single-agent second-line chemotherapy in patients with advanced ovarian cancer. *J Clin Oncol* 2001;19:3967–3975.

402. **McGuire WP, Blessing JA, Bookman MA, Lentz SS, Dunton CJ.** *Topotecan* has substantial antitumor activity as first-line salvage therapy in platinum-sensitive epithelial ovarian carcinoma: a Gynecologic Oncology Group Study. *J Clin Oncol* 2000;18:1062–1067.

403. **Rodriguez M, Rose PG.** Improved therapeutic index of lower dose *topotecan* chemotherapy in recurrent ovarian cancer. *Gynecol Oncol* 2001;83:257–262.

404. **Gronlund B, Hansen HH, Hogdall C, Engelholm SA.** Efficacy of low-dose *topotecan* in second-line treatment for patients with epithelial ovarian carcinoma. *Cancer* 2002;95:1656–1662.

405. **Brown JV, Peters WA, Rettenmaier MA, Graham CL, Smith MR, Drescher CW, et al.** Three-consecutive-day *topotecan* is an active regimen for recurrent epithelial ovarian cancer. *Gynecol Oncol* 2003;88:136–140.

406. **Gore M, Oza A, Rustin G, Malfetano J, Calvert H, Clarke-Pearson D, et al.** A randomised trial of oral versus intravenous *topotecan* in patients with relapsed epithelial ovarian cancer. *Eur J Cancer* 2002;38:57–63.

407. **Homesley HD, Hall DJ, Martin DA, Lewandowski GS, Vaccarello L, Nahhas WA, et al.** A dose-escalating study of weekly bolus *topotecan* in previously treated ovarian cancer patients. *Gynecol Oncol* 2001;83:394–399.

408. **Muggia F, Hainsworth J, Jeffers S, Miller P, Groshen S, Tan M, et al.** Phase II study of *liposomal doxorubicin* in refractory ovarian cancer: antitumor activity and toxicity modification by liposomal encapsulation. *J Clin Oncol* 1997;15:987–993.

409. **Gordon AN, Granai CO, Rose PG, Hainsworth J, Lopez A, Weissman C, et al.** Phase II study of *liposomal doxorubicin* in platinum- and *paclitaxel*-refractory epithelial ovarian cancer. *J Clin Oncol* 2000;18:3093–3100.

410. **Smith DH, Adams JR, Johnston SR, Gordon A, Drummond MF, Bennet CL.** A comparative economic analysis of *pegylated liposomal doxorubicin* versus *topotecan* in ovarian cancer in the USA and UK. *Ann Oncol* 2002;13:1590–1597.

411. **Gold MA, Walker JL, Berek JS, Hallum AV, Garcia DJ, Alberts DS.** *Amifostine* pretreatment for protection against *topotecan*-induced hematologic toxicity: results of a multicenter phase III trial in patients with advanced gynecologic malignancies. *Gynecol Oncol* 2003;90:325–330.

412. **Gore M, ten Bokkel Huinink W, Carmichael J, Gordon A, Davidson N, Coleman R, et al.** Clinical evidence for *topotecan*-*paclitaxel* non-cross-resistance in ovarian cancer. *J Clin Oncol* 2001;19:1893–1900.

413. **Shapiro JD, Millward MJ, Rischin D, Michael M, Walcher V, Francis PA, et al.** Activity of *gemcitabine* in patients with advanced

ovarian cancer: responses seen following platinum and *paclitaxel*. *Gynecol Oncol* 1996;63:89–93.

414. **Papadimitriou CA, Fountzilas G, Aravantinos G, Kalofonos C, Mouloupoulos LA, Briassoulis E, et al.** Second-line chemotherapy with *gemcitabine* and *carboplatin* in *paclitaxel*-pretreated, platinum-sensitive ovarian cancer patients: a Hellenic Cooperative Oncology Group Study. *Gynecol Oncol* 2004;92:152–159.

415. **Look KY, Bookman MA, Schol J, Herzog TJ, Rocereto T, Vinters J.** Phase I feasibility trial of *carboplatin, paclitaxel*, and *gemcitabine* in patients with previously untreated epithelial ovarian or primary peritoneal cancer: a Gynecologic Oncology Group study. *Gynecol Oncol* 2004;92:93–100.

416. **Belpomme D, Krakowski I, Beauduin M, Petit T, Canon JL, Janssens J, et al.** *Gemcitabine* combined with *cisplatin* as first-line treatment in patients with epithelial ovarian cancer: a phase II study. *Gynecol Oncol* 2003;91:32–38.

417. **Markman M, Webster K, Zanotti K, Kulp B, Peterson G, Belinson J.** Phase 2 trial of single-agent *gemcitabine* in platinum-*paclitaxel* refractory ovarian cancer. *Gynecol Oncol* 2003;90:593–596.

418. **Slayton RE, Creasman WT, Petty W, Bundy B, Blessing J.** Phase II trial of VP-16-213 in the treatment of advanced squamous cell carcinoma of the cervix and adenocarcinoma of the ovary: a Gynecologic Oncology Group Study. *Cancer Treat Rep* 1979;63:2089–2092.

419. **Hoskins PJ, Swenerton KD.** Oral *etoposide* is active against platinum-resistant epithelial ovarian cancer. *J Clin Oncol* 1994;12:60–63.

420. **Rose PG, Blessing JA, Mayer AR, Homesley HD.** Prolonged oral *etoposide* as second-line therapy for platinum-resistant and platinum-sensitive ovarian carcinoma: a Gynecologic Oncology Group study. *J Clin Oncol* 1998;16:405–410.

421. **Manetta A, MacNeill C, Lyter JA, Scheffler B, Podczaski ES, Larson JE, et al.** Hexam-ethylmelamine as a second-line agent in ovarian cancer. *Gynecol Oncol* 1990;36:93–96.

422. **Moore DH, Valea F, Crumpler LS, Fowler WC.** *Hexamethylmelamine* (*altretamine*) as second-line therapy for epithelial ovarian carcinoma. *Gynecol Oncol* 1993;51:109–112.

423. **Vasey PA, McMahon L, Paul J, Reed N, Kaye SB.** A phase II trial of *capecitabine* (*Xeloda*) in recurrent ovarian cancer. *Br J Cancer* 2003;89:1843–1848.

424. **Look KY, Muss HB, Blessing JA, Morris M.** A phase II trial of *5-fluorouracil* and high-dose *leucovorin* in recurrent ovarian carcinoma: a Gynecologic Oncology group study. *Am J Clin Oncol* 1995;18:19–22.

425. **Sorensen P, Pfeiffer P, Bertelsen K.** A phase II trial of ifosfamide/mesna as salvage therapy in patients with ovarian cancer refractory to or relapsing after prior platinum-containing chemotherapy. *Gynecol Oncol* 1995;56:75–78.

426. **Perez-Gracia JL, Carrasco EM.** *Tamoxifen* therapy for ovarian cancer in the adjuvant and advanced settings: systematic review of the literature and implications for future research. *Gynecol Oncol* 2002;84:201–209.

427. **Ansink AC, Williams CJ.** The role of *tamoxifen* in the management of ovarian cancer. *Gynecol Oncol* 2002;86:390.

428. **Williams CJ, Simera I.** *Tamoxifen* for relapse of ovarian cancer. *Cochrane Database of Systematic Reviews* 2001, Issue 1. Art. No.: CD001034. DOI: 10.1002/14651858.CD001034.

429. **Hatch KD, Beecham JB, Blessing JA, Creasman WT.** Responsiveness of patients with advanced ovarian carcinoma to *tamoxifen:* a Gynecologic Oncology Group study of second-line therapy in 105 patients. *Cancer* 1991;68:269–271.

430. **Van der Velden J, Gitsch G, Wain GV, Freidlander ML, Hacker NE.** *Tamoxifen* in patients with advanced epithelial ovarian cancer. *Int J Gynecol Cancer* 1995;5:301–305.

431. **Miller DS, Brady MF, Barrett RJ.** A phase II trial of leuprolide acetate in patients with advanced epithelial ovarian cancer. *J Clin Oncol* 1992;15:125–128.

432. **Lopez A, Tessadrelli A, Kudelka AP, Edwards CL, Freedman RS, Hord M, et al.** Combination therapy with leuprolide acetate and *tamoxifen* in refractory ovarian cancer. *Int J Gynecol Cancer* 1996;6:15–619.

433. **Smith IE, Dowsett M.** Aromatase inhibitors in breast cancer. *N Engl J Med* 2003;348:2431–2442.

434. **Le T, Leis A, Pahwa P, Wright K, Ali K, Reeder B, et al.** Quality of life evaluations in patients with ovarian cancer during chemotherapy treatment. *Gynecol Oncol* 2004;92:839–844.

435. **Pfisterer J, Plante M, Vergote I, du Bois A, Hirte H, Lacave AJ, et al., for AGO-OVAR; NCIC CTG; EORTC GCG.** *Gemcitabine* plus *carboplatin* compared with *carboplatin* in patients with platinum-sensitive recurrent ovarian cancer: an intergroup trial of the AGO-OVAR, the NCIC CTG, and the EORTC GCG. *J Clin Oncol* 2006;24:4699–4707.

436. **Alberts DS, Liu PY, Wilczynski SP, Clouser MC, Lopez AM, Michelin DP, et al., for the Southwest Oncology Group.** Randomized trial of *pegylated liposomal doxorubicin* (PLD) plus *carboplatin* versus *carboplatin* in platinum-sensitive (PS) patients with recurrent epithelial ovarian or peritoneal carcinoma after failure of initial platinum-based chemotherapy (Southwest Oncology Group Protocol S0200). *Gynecol Oncol* 2008;108:90–94.

437. **Ferrero JM, Weber B, Geay JF, Lepille D, Orfeuvre H, Combe M, et al.** Second-line chemotherapy with *pegylated liposomal doxorubicin* and *carboplatin* is highly effective in patients with advanced ovarian cancer in late relapse: a GINECO phase II trial. *Ann Oncol* 2007;18:263–268.

438. **van der Burg ME, van der Gaast A, Vergote I, Burger CW, van Doorn HC, de Wit R, et al.** What is the role of dose-dense therapy? *Int J Gynecol Cancer* 2005;15(suppl 3):233–240.

439. **Mutch DG, Orlando M, Goss T, Teneriello MG, Gordon AN, McMeekin SD, et al.** Randomized phase III trial of *gemcitabine* compared with *pegylated liposomal doxorubicin* in patients with platinum-resistant ovarian cancer. *J Clin Oncol* 2007;25:2811–2818.

440. **Krasner CN, McMeekin DS, Chan S, Braly PS, Renshaw FG, Kaye S, et al.** Phase II study of *trabectedin* single agent in patients with recurrent ovarian cancer previously treated with platinum-based regimens. *Br J Cancer* 2007 17;97:1618–1624.

441. **Martin L, Schilder R.** Novel approaches in advancing the treatment of epithelial ovarian cancer: the role of angiogenesis inhibition. *J Clin Oncol* 2007;25:2894–2901.

442. **Cannistra SA, Matulonis UA, Penson RT, Hambleton J, Dupont J, Mackey H, et al.** Phase II study of *bevacizumab* in patients with platinum-resistant ovarian cancer or peritoneal serous cancer. *J Clin Oncol* 2007;25:5180–5186.

443. **Burger RA, Sill MW, Monk BJ, Greer BE, Sorosky JI.** Phase II trial of *bevacizumab* in persistent or recurrent epithelial ovarian cancer or primary peritoneal cancer: a Gynecologic Oncology Group Study. *J Clin Oncol* 2007;25:5165–5171

444. **Garcia AA, Hirte H, Fleming G, Yang D, Tsao-Wei DD, Roman L, et al.** Phase II clinical trial of *bevacizumab* and low-dose metronomic oral *cyclophosphamide* in recurrent ovarian cancer: a trial of the California, Chicago, and Princess Margaret Hospital phase II consortia. *J Clin Oncol* 2008;26:76–82.

445. **Simpkins F, Belinson JL, Rose PG.** Avoiding *bevacizumab* related gastrointestinal toxicity for recurrent ovarian cancer by careful patient screening. *Gynecol Oncol* 2007;107:118–123.

446. **Ma WW, Jimeno A.** Strategies for suppressing angiogenesis in gynecological cancers. *Drugs Today (Barc)* 2007;43:259–273.

447. **Hacker NF, Berek JS, Pretorius G, Zuckerman J, Eisenkop S, Lagasse LD.** Intraperitoneal *cisplatinum* as salvage therapy in persistent epithelial ovarian cancer. *Obstet Gynecol* 1987;70:759–764.

448. **Braly PS, Berek JS, Blessing JA, Homesley HD, Averette H.** Intraperitoneal administration of *cisplatin* and *5-fluorouracil* in residual ovarian cancer: a phase II Gynecologic Oncology Group trial. *Gynecol Oncol* 1995;34:143–147.

449. **Francis P, Rowinsky E, Schneider J, Hakes T, Hoskins W, Markman M.** Phase I feasibility study and pharmacologic study of weekly intraperitoneal *Taxol:* a Gynecologic Oncology Group study. *J Clin Oncol* 1995;13:2961–2967.

450. **Feun LG, Blessing JA, Major FJ, DiSaia PJ, Alvarez RD, Berek JS.** A phase II study of intraperitoneal *cisplatin* and *thiotepa* in residual ovarian carcinoma: a Gynecologic Oncology Group study. *Gynecol Oncol* 1998;71:410–415.

451. **Markman M, Blessing JA, Major F, Manetta A.** Salvage intraperitoneal therapy of ovarian cancer employing *cisplatin* and *etoposide*: a Gynecologic Oncology Group study. *Gynecol Oncol* 1993;50:191–195.

452. **Kirmani S, Lucas WE, Kim S, Goel R, McVey L, Morris J, et al.** A phase II trial of intraperitoneal *cisplatin* and *etoposide* as salvage treatment for minimal residual ovarian carcinoma. *J Clin Oncol* 1991;9:649–657.

453. Markman M, Hakes T, Reichman B, Lewis JL Jr, Rubin S, Jones W, et al. Phase II trial of weekly or biweekly intraperitoneal mitox-antrone in epithelial ovarian cancer. *J Clin Oncol* 1991;9:978–982.

454. Markman M, Rowinsky E, Hakes T, Reichman B, Jones W, Lewis JL Jr, et al. Phase I trial of intraperitoneal *Taxol:* a Gynecologic Oncology Group study. *J Clin Oncol* 1992;10:1485–1491.

455. Howell SB, Zimm S, Markman M, Abramsoin IS, Cleary S, Lucas WE, et al. Long-term survival of advanced refractory ovarian carcinoma patients with small-volume disease treated with intraperitoneal chemotherapy. *J Clin Oncol* 1987;5:1607–1612.

456. Berek JS, Hacker NF, Lichtenstein A, Jung T, Spina C, Knox RM, et al. Intraperitoneal recombinant *alpha2 interferon* for salvage epithelial ovarian cancer immunotherapy in stage III: a Gynecologic Oncology Group study. *Cancer Res* 1985;45:4447–4453.

457. Willemse PHB, De Vries EGE, Mulder NH, Aalders JG, Bouma J, Sleijfer DT. Intraperitoneal human recombinant *interferon alpha-2b* in minimal residual ovarian cancer. *Eur J Cancer* 1990;26: 353–358.

458. Nardi M, Cognetti F, Pollera F, Giulia MD, Lombardi A, Atlante G, et al. Intraperitoneal *alpha-2-interferon* alternating with *cisplatin* as salvage therapy for minimal residual disease ovarian cancer: a phase II study. *J Clin Oncol* 1990;6:1036–1041.

459. Markman M, Berek JS, Blessing JA, McGuire WP, Bell J, Homesley HD. Characteristics of patients with small-volume residual ovarian cancer unresponsive to *cisplatin*-based IP chemotherapy: lessons learned from a Gynecologic Oncology Group phase II trial of IP *cisplatin* and recombinant α-*interferon*. *Gynecol Oncol* 1992; 45:3–8.

460. Berek JS, Markman M, Blessing JA, Kucera PR, Nelson BE, Anderson B, et al. Intraperitoneal α-*interferon* alternating with *cisplatin* in residual ovarian cancer: a phase II Gynecologic Oncology Group study. *Gynecol Oncol* 1999;74:48–52.

461. Berek JS, Markman M, Stonebraker B, Lentz S, Adelson MD, DeGeest K, et al. Intraperitoneal α-*interferon* in residual ovarian cancer: a phase II Gynecologic Oncology Group study. *Gynecol Oncol* 1999;75:10–14.

462. Bezwoda WR, Golombick T, Dansey R, Keeping J. Treatment of malignant ascites due to recurrent/refractory ovarian cancer: the use of *interferon-alpha* or *interferon-alpha* plus chemotherapy. *In vivo* and *in vitro* observations. *Eur J Cancer* 1991;27:1423–1429.

463. Pujade-Lauraine E, Guastalla JP, Colombo N, Franocois E, Fumoleau P, Monier A, et al. Intraperi-toneal administration of *interferon gamma*: an efficient adjuvant to chemotherapy of ovarian cancers. Apropos of a European study of 108 patients. *Bull Cancer* 1993;80:163–170.

464. Steis RG, Urba WJ, Vandermolen LA, Bookman MA, Smith JW II, Clark JW, et al. Intraperitoneal lymphokine-activated killer cell and interleukin 2 therapy for malignancies limited to the peritoneal cavity. *J Clin Oncol* 1990;10:1618–1629.

465. Broun ER, Belinson JL, Berek JS, McIntosh D, Hurd D, Ball H, et al. Salvage therapy for recurrent and refractory ovarian cancer with high-dose chemotherapy and autologous bone marrow support: a Gynecologic Oncology Group pilot study. *Gynecol Oncol* 1994;54: 142–146.

466. Stiff P, Bayer R, Camarda M, Tan S, Dolan J, Potkul R, et al. A phase II trial of high-dose mitox-antrone, *carboplatin* and *cyclophosphamide* with autologous bone marrow rescue for recurrent epithelial ovarian carcinoma: analysis of risk factors for clinical outcome. *Gynecol Oncol* 1995;57:278–285.

467. Cure H, Battista C, Guastalla JP, Fabbro M, Tubiana N, Bourgeois H, et al. Phase III randomized trial of high-dose chemotherapy (HDC) and peripheral blood stem cell (PBSC) support as consolidation in patients with advanced ovarian cancer: 5-year follow-up of a GINECO/FNCLCC/SFGM-TC Study. *Proc Am Soc Clin Oncol* 2004;23(abst 5006).

468. Möbus V, Wandt H, Frickhofen N, Bengala C, Champion K, Kimmig R, et al. Phase III trial of high-dose sequential chemotherapy with peripheral blood stem cell support compared with standard dose chemotherapy for first-line treatment of advanced ovarian cancer: intergroup trial of the AGO-Ovar/AIO and EBMT. *J Clin Oncol* 2007;25:4187–4193.

469. Hacker NF, Berek JS, Burnison CM, Heintz APM, Juillard GJF, Lagasse LD. Whole abdominal radiation as salvage therapy for epithelial ovarian cancer. *Obstet Gynecol* 1985;65:60–65.

470. Ripamonti C. Management of bowel obstruction in advanced cancer. *Curr Opin Oncol* 1994;6:351–357.

471. Feuer DJ, Broadley KE, Shepherd JH, Barton DP. Surgery for the resolution of symptoms in malignant bowel obstruction in advanced gynaecological and gastrointestinal cancer (Cochrane Review). *Cochrane Database of Systematic Reviews* 2000, Issue 3. Art. No.: CD002764. DOI: 10.1002/14651858.CD002764.

472. Ripamonti C, Bruera E. Palliative management of malignant bowel obstruction. *Int J Gynecol Cancer* 2002;12:135–143.

473. Coukos G, Rubin SC. Surgical management of epithelial ovarian cancer. *Oncology Spectrums* 2001;2:350–361.

474. Pothuri B, Vaidya A, Aghajanian C, Venkatraman E, Barakat RR, Chi DS. Palliative surgery for bowel obstruction in recurrent ovarian cancer: an updated series. *Gynecol Oncol* 2003;89:306–313.

475. Tamussino KF, Lim PC, Webb MJ, Lee RA, Lesnick TG. Gastrointestinal surgery in patients with ovarian cancer. *Gynecol Oncol* 2001;80:79–84.

476. Winter WE, McBroom JW, Carlson JW, Rose GS, Elkas JC. The utility of gastrojejunostomy in secondary cytoreduction and palliation of proximal intestinal obstruction in recurrent ovarian cancer. *Gynecol Oncol* 2003;91:261–264.

477. Jolicoeur L, Faught W. Managing bowel obstruction in ovarian cancer using a percutaneous endoscopic gastrostomy (PEG) tube. *Can Oncol Nurs J* 2003;13:212–219.

478. Campagnutta E, Cannizzaro R, Gallo A, Zarelli A, Valentini M, De Cicco M, et al. Palliative treatment of upper intestinal obstruction by gynecologic malignancy: the usefulness of percutaneous endoscopic gastrostomy. *Gynecol Oncol* 1996;62:103–105.

479. Heintz APM, Odicino F, Maisonneuve P, Quinn MA, Benedet JL, Creasman WT, et al. Carcinoma of the ovary. 26th Annual Report on the Results of Treatment in Gynaecological Cancer. *Internat J Gynecol Oncol* 2006;95(suppl 1):S161–S192.

480. Heintz APM, Odicino F, Maisonneuve P, Quinn MA, Benedet JL, Creasman WT, et al. Carcinoma of the fallopian tube. 26th Annual Report on the Results of Treatment in Gynaecological Cancer. *Internat J Gynecol Oncol* 2006;95(suppl 1):S145–S160.

481. Cormio G, Maneo A. Gabriele A, Rota SM, Lissone A, Zanatta G. Primary carcinoma of the fallopian tube: a retrospective analysis of 47 patients. *Ann Oncol* 1996;7:271–275.

482. Alvarado-Cabrero I, Young RH, Vamvakas EC, Scully RE. Carcinoma of the fallopian tube: a clinicopathological study of 105 cases with observations on staging and prognostic factors. *Gynecol Oncol* 1999;72:367–379.

483. Romagosa C, Tome A, Iglesias X, Cardesa A, Ordi J. Carcinoma of the fallopian tube presenting as acute pelvic inflammatory disease. *Gynecol Oncol* 2003;89:181–184.

484. Kosary C, Trimble EL. Treatment and survival for women with fallopian tube carcinoma: a population-based study. *Gynecol Oncol* 2002;86:190–191.

485. Hellström AC, Silfverswärd C, Nilsson B, Petterson F. Carcinoma of the fallopian tube: a clinical and histopathologic review. The Radiumhemmet series. *Int J Gynecol Cancer* 1994;4:395–407.

486. Levine DA, Argenta PA, Yee CJ, Marshall DS, Olvera N, Bogomolniy F, et al. Fallopian tube and primary peritoneal carcinomas associated with *BRCA* mutations. *Clin Oncol* 2003;21:4222–4227.

487. Mikami M, Tei C, Kurahashi T, Takehara K, Komiyama S, Suzuki A, et al. Preoperative diagnosis of fallopian tube cancer by imaging. *Abdom Imaging* 2003;28:743–747.

488. Barakat RR, Rubin SC, Saigo PE, Chapman D, Lewis JL, Jones WB, et al. *Cisplatin*-based combination chemotherapy in carcinoma of the fallopian tube. *Gynecol Oncol* 1991;42:156–160.

489. Cormio G. Experience at the Memorial Sloan-Kettering Cancer Center with *paclitaxel*-based combination chemotherapy following primary cytoreductive surgery in carcinoma of the fallopian tube. *Gynecol Oncol* 2002;84:185–186.

490. Baekelandt M, Nesbakken A, Kristensen GB, Trope CG, Abeler VM. Carcinoma of the fallopian tube. *Cancer* 2000;89:2076–2084.

491. Ajithkumar TV, Minimole AL, John MM, Ashokkumar OS. Primary fallopian tube carcinoma. *Obstet Gynecol Surv* 2005;60:247–252.

492. Clayton NL, Jaaback KS, Hirschowitz L. Primary fallopian tube carcinoma: the experience of a UK cancer centre and review of the literature. *J Obstet Gynaecol* 2005;25:694–702.

493. Moore KN, Moxley KM, Fader AN, Axtell AE, Rocconi RP, Abaid LN, et al. *Gynecol Oncol* 2007;107:398–403.

494. **Markman M, Zanotti K, Webster K, Peterson G, Kulp B, Belinson J.** Phase 2 trial of single agent *docetaxel* in platinum and *paclitaxel*-refractory ovarian cancer, fallopian tube cancer, and primary carcinoma of the peritoneum. *Gynecol Oncol* 2003;91: 573–576.

495. **Kuscu E, Oktem M, Haberal A, Erkanli S, Bilezikci B, Demirhan B.** Management of advanced-stage primary carcinoma of the fallopian tube: case report and literature review. *Eur J Gynaecol Oncol* 2003;24:557–560.

496. **Matulonis U, Campos S, Duska L, Fuller A, Berkowitz R, Gore S, et al.** A phase II trial of three sequential doublets for the treatment of advanced müllerian malignancies. *Gynecol Oncol* 2003;91: 293–298.

497. **Markman M, Glass T, Smith HO, Hatch KD, Weiss GR, Taylor SA, et al.** Phase II trial of single agent *carboplatin* followed by dose-intense *paclitaxel*, followed by maintenance *paclitaxel* therapy in stage IV ovarian, fallopian tube, and peritoneal cancers: a Southwest Oncology Group trial. *Gynecol Oncol* 2003;88:282–288.

498. **Rose PG, Rodriguez M, Walker J, Greer B, Fusco N, McGuire W.** A phase I trial of prolonged oral *etoposide* and *liposomal doxoru-* *bicin* in ovarian, peritoneal, and tubal carcinoma: a gynecologic oncology group study. *Gynecol Oncol* 2002;85:136–139.

499. **Kojs Z, Uranski K, Reinfuss M, Karolewski K, Klimek M, Pudelerk J, et al.** Whole abdominal external beam radiation in the treatment of primary carcinoma of the fallopian tube. *Gynecol Oncol* 1997;65:473–477.

500. **Wolfson AH, Tralins KS, Greven KM, Kim RY, Corn BW, Kuettel MR, et al.** Adenocarcinoma of the fallopian tube: results of a multi-institutional retrospective analysis of 72 patients. *Int J Radiat Oncol Biol Phys* 1998;40:71–76.

501. **Klein M, Rosen A, Lahousen M, Graf AH, Rainer A.** The relevance of adjuvant therapy in primary carcinoma of the fallopian tube stages I and II: irradiation vs. chemotherapy. *Int J Radiat Oncol Biol Phys* 2000;48:1427–1431.

502. **Topuz E, Eralp Y, Aydiner A, Saip P, Tas F, Yavuz E, et al.** The role of chemotherapy in malignant mixed müllerian tumors of the female genital tract. *Eur J Gynaecol Oncol* 2001;22:469–472.

503. **Mariani L, Quattrini M, Galati M, Dionisi B, Piperno G, Modafferi F, et al.** Primary leiomyosarcoma of the fallopian tube: a case report. *Eur J Gynaecol Oncol* 2005;26:333–335.

12

Germ Cell and Other Nonepithelial Ovarian Cancers

Jonathan S. Berek
Michael Friedlander
Neville F. Hacker

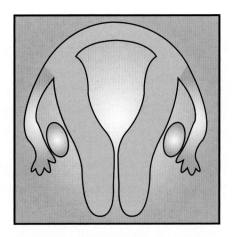

Compared with epithelial ovarian cancers, other malignant tumors of the female genital adnexal structures are uncommon. Nonepithelial ovarian cancers include malignancies of germ cell origin, sex-cord–stromal cell origin, metastatic carcinomas to the ovary, and a variety of extremely rare ovarian cancers (e.g., sarcomas, lipoid cell tumors).

Nonepithelial malignancies of the ovary account for approximately 10% of all ovarian cancers (1,2). Although there are many similarities in the presentation, evaluation, and management of these patients, these tumors also have unique qualities that require a special approach (1–5).

Germ Cell Malignancies

Germ cell tumors are derived from the primordial germ cells of the ovary. Their incidence is only about one-tenth the incidence of malignant germ cell tumors of the testis. Although they can arise in extragonadal sites such as the mediastinum and the retroperitoneum, the majority of germ cell tumors arise in the gonad from the undifferentiated germ cells. The variation in the site of these cancers is explained by the embryonic migration of the germ cells from the caudal part of the yolk sac to the dorsal mesentery before their incorporation into the sex cords of the developing gonads (1,2).

Germ cell tumors are a model of a curable cancer. The management of patients with ovarian germ cell tumors has largely been extrapolated from the experience of treating the more common testicular germ cell tumors. There have been many randomized trials for testicular germ cell tumors, which have provided a strong evidence base for treatment decision making (6,7). The outcome of patients with testicular germ cell tumors is better in experienced centers, and it is reasonable to suggest the same will be true for the less common ovarian counterparts. The cure rate is high, and currently efforts are being made to reduce toxicity without compromising survival. There are still a small number of patients who die from the disease, and studies are in progress to try to improve the outcome for this high-risk poor-prognostic subset (6,7).

In one of the largest reported series, which included 113 patients with advanced ovarian germ cell tumors treated with *cisplatin*-based chemotherapy, Murugaesu et al. (8) reported that **stage and elevated tumor markers were independent poor prognostic indicators.** These findings

Table 12.1 Histologic Typing of Ovarian Germ Cell Tumors

I. Primitive Germ Cell Tumors	III. Monodermal Teratoma and Somatic-Type Tumors Associated with Dermoid Cysts
Dysgerminoma	Thyroid tumor
Yolk sac tumor	Struma ovarii
Embryonal carcinoma	Benign
Polyembryoma	Malignant
Nongestational choriocarcinoma	Carcinoid
Mixed germ cell tumor	Neuroectodermal tumor
II. Biphasic or Triphasic Teratoma	Carcinoma
Immature teratoma	Melanocytic
Mature teratoma	Sarcoma
Solid	Sebaceous tumor
Cystic	Pituitary-type tumor
Dermoid cyst	Others
Fetiform teratoma (homunculus)	

Adapted from **Tavassoli FA, Devilee P, eds.** World Health Organization classification of tumours. *Pathology and genetics of tumours of the breast and female organs.* Lyon: France: IARC Press, 2003.

are important because they identify similar prognostic factors for ovarian germ cell tumors as has been described previously for testicular germ cell tumors. This is in accordance with the clinical observation that testicular and ovarian germ cell tumors behave similarly. This is relevant for the management of patients with ovarian germ cell tumors because it could help to identify patients who may require more intensive therapeutic strategies (8).

Classification

A histologic classification of ovarian germ cell tumors is presented in Table 12.1 (1). **Both α-fetoprotein (AFP) and human chorionic gonadotropin (hCG) are secreted by some germ cell malignancies;** therefore, the presence of circulating hormones can be clinically useful in the diagnosis of a pelvic mass and in monitoring the course of a patient after surgery. **Placental alkaline phosphatase (PLAP) and lactate dehydrogenase (LDH) are produced by as many as 95% of dysgerminomas,** and serial monitoring of serum LDH titers may be useful for monitoring the disease. PLAP is more useful as an immunohistochemical marker than as a serum marker. When the histologic and immunohistologic identification of these substances in tumors is correlated, a classification of germ cell tumors emerges (Fig. 12.1) (9).

In this scheme, **embryonal carcinoma,** which is a cancer composed of undifferentiated cells, **synthesizes both hCG and AFP,** and this lesion is the progenitor of several other germ cell tumors (4,9). More differentiated germ cell tumors—such as the endodermal sinus tumor, which secretes AFP, and choriocarcinoma, which secretes hCG—are derived from the extraembryonic tissues; the immature teratomas derived from the embryonic cells have lost the ability to secrete these substances. Elevated hCG levels are seen in 3% of dysgerminomas (1).

Epidemiology

Although 20% to 25% of all benign and malignant ovarian neoplasms are of germ cell origin, only some 3% of these tumors are malignant (1). Germ cell malignancies account for fewer than 5% of all ovarian cancers in Western countries. Germ cell malignancies represent as much as 15% of ovarian cancers in Asian and black societies, where epithelial ovarian cancers are much less common.

In the first two decades of life, almost 70% of ovarian tumors are of germ cell origin, and one-third of these are malignant (1,2). Germ cell tumors account for two-thirds of the ovarian malignancies in this age group. Germ cell cancers also are seen in the third decade, but thereafter they become quite rare.

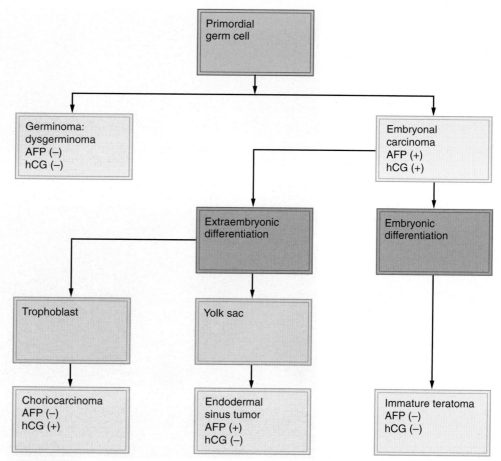

Figure 12.1   Relationship between examples of pure malignant germ cell tumors and their secreted marker substances.

Clinical Features

Symptoms

In contrast to the relatively slow-growing epithelial ovarian tumors, germ cell malignancies grow rapidly and often are characterized by subacute pelvic pain related to capsular distention, hemorrhage, or necrosis. The rapidly enlarging pelvic mass may produce pressure symptoms on the bladder or rectum, and menstrual irregularities also may occur in menarchal patients. Some young patients may misinterpret the early symptoms of a neoplasm as those of pregnancy, and this can lead to a delay in the diagnosis. Acute symptoms associated with torsion or rupture of the adnexa can develop. These symptoms may be confused with acute appendicitis. In more advanced cases, ascites may develop, and the patient can present with abdominal distention (3).

Signs

In patients with a palpable adnexal mass, the evaluation can proceed as outlined in Chapter 11. Some patients with germ cell tumors will be premenarchal and may require examination under anesthesia. If the lesions are principally solid or a combination of solid and cystic, as might be noted on an ultrasonographic evaluation, then a neoplasm is probable and a malignancy is possible (Fig. 12.2). The remainder of the physical examination should search for signs of ascites, pleural effusion, and organomegaly.

Diagnosis

Adnexal masses measuring 2 cm or more in premenarchal girls or complex masses 8 cm or more in premenopausal patients will usually require surgical exploration (Fig. 12.3). In young patients, blood tests should include serum hCG, AFP, and CA125 titers, a complete blood count, and liver function tests. A radiograph of the chest is important because germ cell tumors can metastasize to the lungs or mediastinum. **A karyotype should ideally be obtained preoperatively on all premenarchal girls because of the propensity of these tumors to**

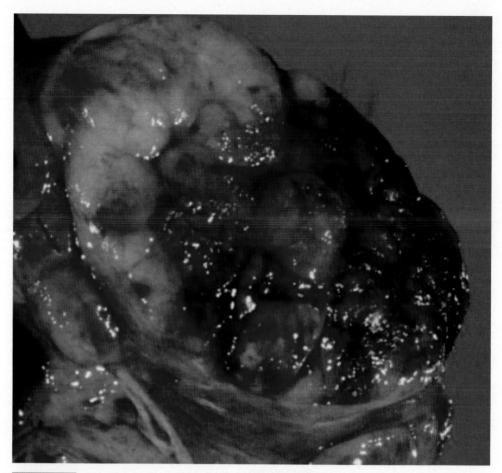

Figure 12.2   **Dysgerminoma of the ovary.** Note that the lesion is principally solid with some cystic areas and necrosis. From **Berek JS, Natarajan S.** Ovarian and fallopian tube cancer. In: **Berek JS, ed.** *Berek & Novak's Gynecology,* 14th ed. Philadelphia: Lippincott Williams & Wilkins, 2007.

arise in dysgenetic gonads, but this may not be practical (3,10). A preoperative computed tomographic (CT) scan or magnetic resonance imaging (MRI) may document the presence and extent of retroperitoneal lymphadenopathy or liver metastases, but unless there is very extensive metastatic disease, is unlikely to influence the decision to operate on the patient initially. If postmenarchal patients have predominantly cystic lesions up to 8 cm in diameter, they may undergo observation or a trial of hormonal suppression for two cycles (11).

Dysgerminoma

The dysgerminoma is the most common malignant germ cell tumor, accounting for approximately 30% to 40% of all ovarian cancers of germ cell origin (2,9). The tumors represent only 1% to 3% of all ovarian cancers, but they represent as many as 5% to 10% of ovarian cancers in patients younger than 20 years of age. Seventy-five percent of dysgerminomas occur between the ages of 10 and 30 years, 5% occur before the age of 10 years, and rarely after age 50 (1,4). Because these malignancies occur in young women, 20% to 30% of ovarian malignancies associated with pregnancy are dysgerminomas.

Approximately 5% of dysgerminomas are discovered in phenotypic females with abnormal gonads (1,10). This malignancy can be associated with patients who have pure gonadal dysgenesis (46XY, bilateral streak gonads), mixed gonadal dysgenesis (45X/46XY, unilateral streak gonad, contralateral testis), and the androgen insensitivity syndrome (46XY, testicular feminization). Therefore, in premenarchal patients with a pelvic mass, the karyotype should be determined (Fig 12.4).

In most patients with gonadal dysgenesis, dysgerminomas arise in a gonadoblastoma, which is a benign ovarian tumor composed of germ cells and sex-cord stroma. If gonadoblastomas

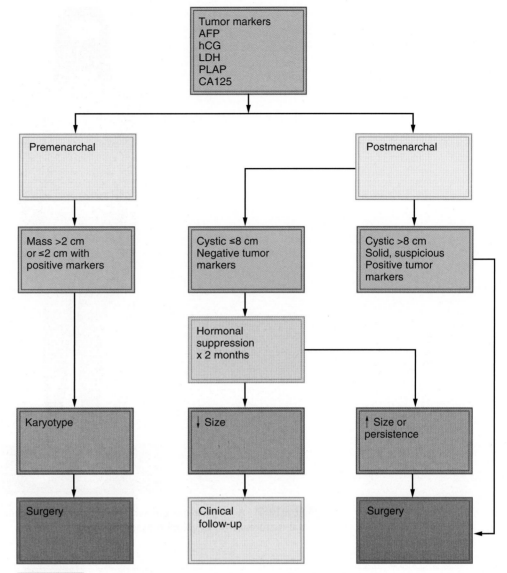

Figure 12.3   **Evaluation of a pelvic mass in young female patients.**

are left *in situ* in patients with gonadal dysgenesis, more than 50% will develop into ovarian malignancies (12).

Approximately 65% of dysgerminomas are stage I (i.e., confined to one or both ovaries) at diagnosis (1,3,5,13–16). **Approximately 85% to 90% of stage I tumors are confined to one ovary; 10% to 15% are bilateral. Dysgerminoma is the only germ cell malignancy that has this significant rate of bilaterality, other germ cell tumors being rarely bilateral.**

In patients whose contralateral ovary has been preserved, disease can develop in 5% to 10% of the retained gonads over the next 2 years (1). This figure includes those not given additional therapy, as well as patients with gonadal dysgenesis.

In the 25% of patients who present with metastatic disease, the tumor most commonly spreads via the lymphatics, particularly to the higher paraaortic nodes. It can also spread hematogenously, or by direct extension through the capsule of the ovary with exfoliation and dissemination of cells throughout the peritoneal surfaces. Metastases to the contralateral ovary may be present when there is no other evidence of spread. An uncommon site of metastatic disease is bone, and when metastasis to this site occurs, the lesions are seen principally in the lower vertebrae. Metastases to the lungs, liver, and brain are seen most often in patients with long-standing or recurrent disease. Metastasis to the mediastinum and supraclavicular lymph nodes is usually a late manifestation of disease (13,14).

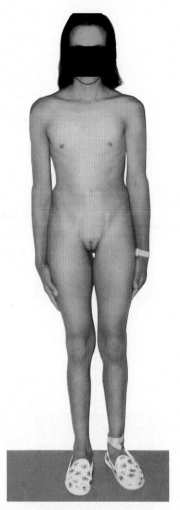

Figure 12.4   A 16-year-old girl with 46XY gonadal dysgenesis, showing lack of secondary sexual features, who developed dysgerminoma.

Treatment

The treatment of patients with early dysgerminoma is primarily surgical, including resection of the primary lesion and proper surgical staging. Chemotherapy or radiation or both is administered to patients with metastatic disease. Because the disease principally affects young women, special consideration must be given to the preservation of fertility whenever possible. An algorithm for the management of ovarian dysgerminoma is presented in Fig. 12.5.

Surgery

The minimum operation for ovarian dysgerminoma is unilateral oophorectomy (15,17). If there is a desire to preserve fertility, as is usually the case, then the contralateral ovary, fallopian tube, and uterus should be left *in situ,* even in the presence of metastatic disease because of the sensitivity of the tumor to chemotherapy. If fertility need not be preserved, then it may be appropriate to perform a total abdominal hysterectomy and bilateral salpingo-oophorectomy in patients with advanced disease (5), although this will be appropriate in only a small minority of patients. In patients whose karyotype contains a Y chromosome, both ovaries should be removed, although the uterus may be left *in situ* for possible future embryo transfer. Whereas cytoreductive surgery is of unproven value, bulky disease that can be readily resected (e.g., an omental cake) should be removed at the initial operation.

In patients in whom the neoplasm appears on inspection to be confined to the ovary, a careful staging operation should be undertaken to determine the presence of any occult metastatic disease. All peritoneal surfaces should be inspected and palpated, and any suspicious lesions should be biopsied. Unilateral pelvic lymphadenectomy and at least careful palpation and

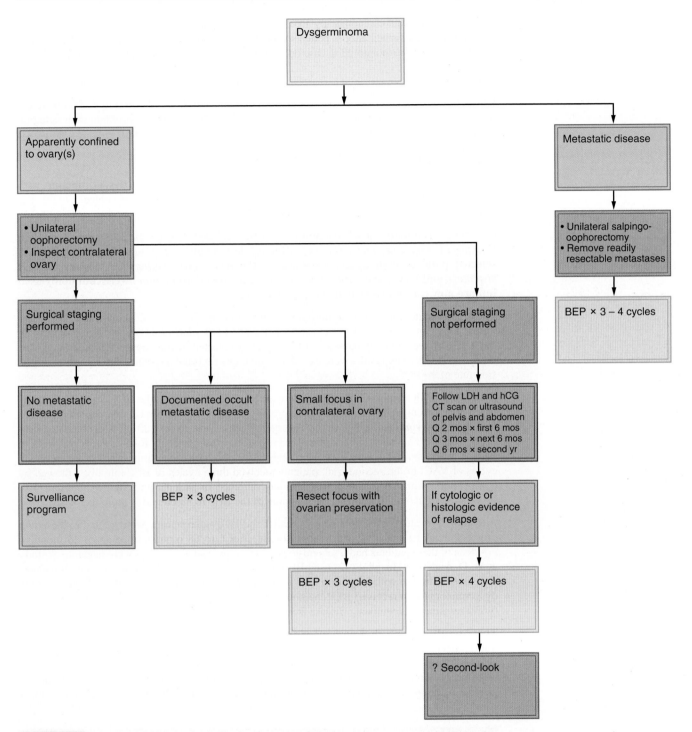

Figure 12.5   **Management of dysgerminoma of the ovary.** BEP = *bleomycin, etoposide,* and *cisplatin;* CT = computed tomogram.

excisional biopsy of enlarged paraaortic nodes are particularly important parts of the staging. These tumors often metastasize to the paraaortic nodes around the renal vessels. Dysgerminoma is the only germ cell tumor that tends to be bilateral, and not all of the bilateral lesions have obvious ovarian enlargement. Therefore careful inspection and palpation of the contralateral ovary and excisional biopsy of any suspicious lesion are desirable (5,15–17). If a small contralateral tumor is found, then it may be possible to resect it and preserve some normal ovary.

Many patients with a dysgerminoma will have a tumor that is apparently confined to one ovary and will be referred after unilateral salpingo-oophorectomy without surgical staging. The options for such patients are (i) repeat laparotomy for surgical staging, (ii) regular pelvic and abdominal CT scans, or (iii) adjuvant chemotherapy. Because these are rapidly growing tumors, our preference is to perform regular surveillance in patients with stage I tumors. Tumor markers (LDH, AFP, and β-hCG) should also be monitored in case occult mixed germ cell elements are present (Fig. 12.1).

Radiation

Dysgerminomas are very sensitive to radiation therapy, and doses of 2,500 to 3,500 centiGray may be curative, even for gross metastatic disease. Loss of fertility is a problem with radiation therapy, so radiation should rarely be used as first-line treatment (5,16).

Chemotherapy

There have been numerous reports of successful control of metastatic dysgerminomas with systemic chemotherapy, and this should be regarded as the treatment of choice (17–27). The obvious advantage is the preservation of fertility in most patients with chemotherapy (17,28–32).

The most frequently used chemotherapeutic regimen for germ cell tumors is BEP (*bleomycin, etoposide,*** and ***cisplatin***), although less-intensive regimens have been used in selected patients with dysgerminomas. In the past, VBP (***vinblastine, bleomycin,*** and ***cisplatin***), and VAC (***vincristine, actinomycin,*** and ***cyclophosphamide***) were commonly used but are now rarely prescribed** (17–22) (Table 12.2).

The Gynecologic Oncology Group (GOG) studied three cycles of EC: *etoposide* (120 mg/m^2 intravenously on days 1, 2, and 3 every 4 weeks) and *carboplatin* (400 mg/m^2 intravenously on day 1 every 4 weeks) in 39 patients with completely resected ovarian dysgerminoma, stages IB, IC, II, or III (25). The results were excellent, and GOG reported a sustained disease-free remission rate of 100%.

For patients with advanced, incompletely resected germ cell tumors, the GOG studied *cisplatin*-based chemotherapy on two consecutive protocols (18,19). In the first study, patients received four cycles of *vinblastine* (12 mg/m^2 every 3 weeks), *bleomycin* (20 units/m^2 intravenously every week for 12 weeks), and *cisplatin* (20 mg/m^2/day intravenously for 5 days every 3 weeks). Patients with persistent or progressive disease at second-look laparotomy were treated with six cycles of VAC. In the second trial, patients received three cycles of BEP initially, followed by consolidation with VAC, which was later discontinued in patients with dysgerminomas (19). VAC does not appear to improve the outcome of the BEP regimen and is no longer used.

A total of 20 evaluable patients with stages III and IV dysgerminoma were treated in these two protocols, and 19 are alive and free of disease after 6 to 68 months (median = 26 months). Fourteen of these patients had a second-look laparotomy, and all findings were negative. A study at M. D. Anderson Hospital (22) used BEP in 14 patients with residual disease, and all patients were free of disease with long-term follow-up. In another series of 26 patients with pure ovarian dysgerminoma who received BEP chemotherapy, 54% of whom had stage IIIC or IV disease, 25 (96%) remained continuously disease free following three to six cycles of therapy (27).

These results suggest that patients with advanced-stage, incompletely resected dysgerminoma have an excellent prognosis when treated with *cisplatin*-based combination chemotherapy (26–31). **The best regimen is three to four cycles of BEP based on the data from testis cancers** (32,33) depending on the extent of disease and the presence or absence of visceral metastases. These are uncommon tumors, and most of the principles of management

Table 12.2 Combination Chemotherapy for Germ Cell Tumors of the Ovary	
Regimen and Drugs	*Dose and Schedule*[a]
BEP	
Bleomycin	30,000 IU weekly for a total of 12 weeks
Etoposide	100 mg/m^2/day × 5 days every 3 weeks
Cisplatin	20 mg/m^2/day × 5 days every 3 weeks

[a]**Loehrer PJ, Johnson D, Elson P, Einhorn LH, Trump D.** Importance of *bleomycin* in favorable-prognosis disseminated germ cell tumors: an Eastern Cooperative Oncology Group trial. *J Clin Oncol* 1995;13: 470–476.

are extrapolated from seminomas, their counterparts in males. If *bleomycin* is contraindicated or omitted because of lung toxicity, then consideration should be given to four cycles of *cisplatin* and *etoposide.*

There is no need to perform a second-look laparotomy in patients with dysgerminomas (34–36). The role of surgery to resect residual masses following chemotherapy for dysgerminomas is not clear, and the vast majority of these patients will only have necrotic tissue and nonviable tumor. In general, these patients should be closely monitored with scans and tumor markers. **A positron emission tomography (PET) scan should be considered in patients who have bulky residual masses more than 4 weeks after chemotherapy.** A positive PET scan is a reliable predictor of residual seminoma in males with residual lesions >3cm (37), and the same may apply to females with dysgerminomas. If the PET is positive or if there is a suggestion of progressive disease on scans, then ideally there should be histological evaluation and confirmation of residual disease before embarking on salvage therapy.

Recurrent Disease	**Approximately 75% of recurrences occur within the first year after initial treatment** (1–4), **the most common sites being the peritoneal cavity and the retroperitoneal lymph nodes.** These patients should be treated with either radiation or chemotherapy, depending on their primary treatment. Patients with recurrent disease who have had no therapy other than surgery should be treated with chemotherapy. If previous chemotherapy with BEP has been given, then an alternative regimen such as **TIP** (*paclitaxel, ifosfamide,* and *cisplatin*) is a reasonable option based on the experience in testicular tumors (38).

These treatment decisions should be made in a multidisciplinary setting with the input of physicians experienced in the treatment of patients with germ cell tumors (Table 12.3).

Table 12.3 POMB-ACE Chemotherapy for Germ Cell Tumors of the Ovary	
POMB	
Day 1	*Vincristine* 1 mg/m^2 intravenously; *methotrexate* 300 mg/m^2 as a 12-h infusion
Day 2	*Bleomycin* 15 mg as a 24-h infusion: *folinic acid* rescue started at 24 h after the start of *methotrexate* in a dose of 15 mg every 12 h for 4 doses
Day 3	*Bleomycin* infusion 15 mg by 24-h infusion
Day 4	*Cisplatin* 120 mg/m^2 as a 12-h infusion, given together with hydration and 3 g *magnesium sulfate* supplementation
ACE	
Days 1–5	*Etoposide* (VP-16-213) 100 mg/m^2, days 1 to 5
Day 3, 4, 5	*Actinomycin D* 0.5 mg intravenously, days 3, 4, and 5
Day 5	*Cyclophosphamide* 500 mg/m^2 intravenously, day 5
OMB	
Day 1	*Vincristine* 1 mg/m^2 intravenously; *methotrexate* 300 mg/m^2 as a 12-h infusion
Day 2	*Bleomycin* 15 mg by 24-h infusion; *folinic acid* rescue started at 24 h after start of *methotrexate* in a dose of 15 mg every 12 h for 4 doses
Day 3	*Bleomycin* 15 mg by 24-h infusion

The sequence of treatment schedules is two courses of POMB followed by ACE. POMB is then alternated with ACE until patients are in biochemical remission as measured by human chorionic gonadotropin and α-fetoprotein, and placental alkaline phosphatase and lactate dehydrogenase. The usual number of courses of POMB is three to five. After biochemical remission, patients alternate ACE with OMB until remission has been maintained for approximately 12 weeks. The interval between courses of treatment is kept to the minimum (usually 9 to 11 days). If delays are caused by myelosuppression after courses of ACE, then the first two days of *etoposide* are omitted from subsequent courses of ACE.

Reproduced from **Newlands ES, Southall PJ, Paradinas FJ, Holden L.** Management of ovarian germ cell tumors. In: **Williams CJ, Krikorian JG, Green MR, Ragavan D, eds.** *Textbook of uncommon cancer.* New York: John Wiley & Sons, 1988:37–53, with permission.

Consideration should be given to the use of high-dose chemotherapy with peripheral stem cell support. A number of high dose regimens have been used in phase 2 studies, and the choice depends on the previous chemotherapy, the time to recurrence, and the residual toxicity from the previous therapy. Alternatively, radiation therapy may be given, but this has the major disadvantage of causing loss of fertility if pelvic and abdominal radiation is required. It will also compromise the ability to deliver further chemotherapy if unsuccessful.

Pregnancy

Because dysgerminomas tend to occur in young patients, they may coexist with pregnancy. When a stage IA cancer is found, the tumor can be removed intact and the pregnancy continued. In patients with more advanced disease, continuation of the pregnancy will depend on gestational age. Chemotherapy can be given in the second and third trimesters in the same dosages as given for the nonpregnant patient without apparent detriment to the fetus (28).

Prognosis

In patients whose initial disease is stage IA (i.e., a unilateral encapsulated dysgerminoma), unilateral oophorectomy alone results in a 5-year disease-free survival rate of greater than 95% (5,16). The features that have been associated with a higher tendency to recurrence include lesions larger than 10 to 15 cm in diameter, age younger than 20 years, and a microscopic pattern that includes numerous mitoses, anaplasia, and a medullary pattern (1,9).

Kumar et al. abstracted data on malignant ovarian germ cell tumors from the Surveillance, Epidemiology, and End Results (SEER) program from 1988 through 2004 (39). There were a total of 1,296 patients with dysgerminomas, immature teratomas, or mixed germ cell tumors, 613 (47.3%) of whom had lymphadenectomies. Lymph node metastases were present in 28% of dysgermanomas, 8% of immature teratomas, and 16% of mixed germ cell tumors ($p < 0.05$). The 5-year survival for patients with negative nodes was 95.7% compared to 82.8% for patients with positive nodes ($p < 0.001$). Multivariate analysis revealed the presence of lymph node involvement to be an independent predictor of poor survival.

Although surgery for advanced disease followed by pelvic and abdominal radiation resulted in the past in a 5-year survival rate of 63% to 83%, cure rates of 90% to 100% for this same group of patients are now being reported with the use of BEP or EC combination chemotherapy (18–31).

Immature Teratomas

Immature teratomas contain elements that resemble tissues derived from the embryo. Immature teratomatous elements may occur in combination with other germ cell tumors as mixed germ cell tumors. The pure immature teratoma accounts for fewer than 1% of all ovarian cancers, but it is the second most common germ cell malignancy. This lesion represents 10% to 20% of all ovarian malignancies seen in women younger than 20 years of age and 30% of the deaths from ovarian cancer in this age group (1). Approximately 50% of pure immature teratomas of the ovary occur between the ages of 10 and 20 years, and they rarely occur in postmenopausal women.

Semiquantification of the amount of neuroepithelium correlates with survival in ovarian immature teratomas and is the basis for the grading of these tumors (40–42). **Those with less than one lower-power field** (4) **of immature neuroepithelium on the slide with the greatest amount of such tissue (grade 1) have a survival of at least 95%, whereas greater amounts of immature neuroepithelium (grades 2 and 3) appear to have a lower overall survival (approximately 85%)** (42). This may not apply, however, to immature teratomas of the ovary in children because they appear to have a very good outcome with surgery alone, regardless of the degree of immaturity (43,44).

Some authorities have recommended a two-tier grading system and have recommended that immature teratomas be categorized as either low grade or high grade because of the significant inter- and intraobserver difficulty with a three-grade system (42). This is our current practice.

Immature ovarian teratomas are associated with gliomatosis peritonei, a favorable prognostic finding if composed of completely mature tissues. Recent reports using molecular methods have determined that these glial "implants" are not tumor derived but represent teratoma-induced metaplasia of pluripotential müllerian stem cells in the peritoneum (45,46).

Malignant transformation of a mature teratoma is a rare event. Squamous cell carcinoma is the most frequent subtype of malignancy in this setting, but adenocarcinomas, primary melanomas, and carcinoids also occur (see below) (24). The risk is reported to be between 0.5% and 2% of teratomas, usually in postmenopausal patients.

Diagnosis

The preoperative evaluation and differential diagnosis are the same as for patients with other germ cell tumors. Some of these lesions will contain calcifications similar to mature teratomas, and this can be detected by a radiograph of the abdomen or by ultrasonography. Rarely, they are associated with the production of steroid hormones and can be accompanied by sexual pseudoprecocity (4). Tumor markers are negative unless a mixed germ cell tumor is present.

Treatment

Surgery

In a premenopausal patient whose lesion appears confined to a single ovary, unilateral oophorectomy and surgical staging should be performed. In postmenopausal patients, a total abdominal hysterectomy and bilateral salpingo-oophorectomy may be performed. Contralateral involvement is rare, and routine resection or wedge biopsy of the contralateral ovary is unnecessary (2). Any lesions on the peritoneal surfaces should be sampled and submitted for histologic evaluation. The most frequent site of dissemination is the peritoneum and, much less commonly, the retroperitoneal lymph nodes. Blood-borne metastases to organ parenchyma such as the lungs, liver, or brain are uncommon. When present, they are usually seen in patients with late or recurrent disease and most often in tumors that are high grade (4).

It is unclear whether debulking of metastatic implants enhances the response to combination chemotherapy (47,48). Cure ultimately depends on the ability to deliver chemotherapy promptly. Any surgical resection that may be potentially morbid and therefore delay chemotherapy should be resisted, although surgical resection of any residual disease should be considered at the completion of chemotherapy.

Chemotherapy

Patients with stage IA, grade 1 tumors have an excellent prognosis, and no adjuvant therapy is required. In patients whose tumors are stage IA, grades 2 or 3, high grade, adjuvant chemotherapy has commonly been given although this has been questioned and excellent results have been also reported with close surveillance and only treating patients who have a recurrence (see below) (20–22,35,49–61).

The most frequently used combination chemotherapeutic regimen in the past has been VAC (55–57), but a GOG study reported a relapse-free survival rate in patients with incompletely resected disease of only 75% (57).

The approach over the last 20 years has been to incorporate *cisplatin* into the primary treatment of these tumors, and most of the experience has been with the VBP and BEP regimens.

The GOG has been prospectively studying three courses of BEP therapy in patients with completely resected stage I, II, and III ovarian germ cell tumors (24). Overall, the toxicity was acceptable, and 91 of 93 patients (97.8%) with nondysgerminomatous tumors were clinically free of disease. In nonrandomized studies, the BEP regimen is superior to the VAC regimen in the treatment of completely resected nondysgerminomatous germ cell tumors of the ovary. Some patients can progress rapidly postoperatively, and, in general, treatment should be initiated as soon as possible after surgery, preferably within 7 to 10 days.

The switch from VBP to BEP has been prompted by the experience in patients with testicular cancer, where the replacement of *vinblastine* with *etoposide* has been associated with a better therapeutic index (i.e., equivalent efficacy and lower morbidity), especially less neurologic and gastrointestinal toxicity. Furthermore, the use of *bleomycin* appears to be important in this group of patients. In a randomized study of three cycles of *etoposide* plus *cisplatin* with or without *bleomycin* (EP vs. BEP) in 166 patients with germ cell tumors of the testes, the BEP regimen had a relapse-free survival rate of 84% compared with 69% for the EP regimen ($p = 0.03$) (33).

***Cisplatin* is superior to *carboplatin* in metastatic germ cell tumors of the testis.** One hundred ninety-two patients with good prognosis germ cell tumors of the testes were entered into a study of four cycles of *etoposide* plus *cisplatin* (EP) versus 4 cycles of *etoposide* plus *carboplatin* (EC). There were three relapses with the EP regimen versus seven with the EC regimen (34). A German group randomized patients to (i) a BEP regimen of three cycles at standard doses given days 1–5 versus (ii) a CEB regimen of *carboplatin* (target AUC of 5 mg/dl × min) on

519

day 1), *etoposide* 120 mg/m² on days 1 to 3, and *bleomycin* 30 mg on days 1, 8, and 15 (62). Four cycles of CEB were given, with the omission of *bleomycin* in the fourth cycle so that the cumulative doses of *etoposide* and *bleomycin* in the two treatment arms were comparable. Fifty-four patients were entered on the trial; 29 were treated with PEB and 25 with CEB chemotherapy. More patients treated with CEB relapsed after therapy (32% versus 13%). Four patients (16%) treated with CEB died of disease progression in contrast to one patient (3%) after BEP therapy. The trial was terminated early after an interim analysis. The inferiority of *carboplatin* was confirmed in a larger randomized trial reported by Horwich et al. (63). In view of these results, **BEP is the preferred treatment regimen for patients with gross residual disease and has replaced the VAC regimen for patients with completely resected disease.**

Radiation

Radiation therapy is generally not used in the primary treatment of patients with immature teratomas. Furthermore, there is no evidence that the combination of chemotherapy and radiation has a higher rate of disease control than chemotherapy alone. Radiation should be reserved for patients with localized persistent disease after chemotherapy (5,35).

Second-Look Laparotomy

The need for a second-look operation for ovarian germ cell tumors has been questioned (36,37). It is not justified in patients who have received chemotherapy in an adjuvant setting (i.e., stage IA, grades 2 and 3) because these patients have an excellent prognosis. However, we continue to prefer second-look laparotomy in patients with residual disease at the completion of chemotherapy because these patients may have residual mature teratoma and are at risk of **growing teratoma syndrome,** a rare complication of immature teratomas (64,65). Furthermore, cancers can arise at a later date in residual mature teratoma, and it is important to resect any residual mass and exclude persistent disease because further chemotherapy may be indicated.

The principles of surgery are based on the much larger experience of surgery in males with residual masses following chemotherapy for germ cell tumors with a component of immature teratoma (66). Mathew et al. (67) reported their experience of laparotomy in assessing the nature of postchemotherapy residual masses in ovarian germ cell tumors. Sixty-eight patients completed combination chemotherapy with *cisplatin* regimens, of whom 35 had radiological residual masses. Twenty-nine of these 35 patients underwent laparotomy, and three patients (10.3%) had viable tumor, seven (24%) immature teratoma, three (10.3%) mature teratoma, and 16 (55.2%) necrosis or fibrosis only. None of the patients with a dysgerminoma or embryonal carcinoma and radiological residual mass of <5 cm had viable tumor present, whereas **all patients with primary tumors containing a component of teratoma had residual tumor,** strengthening the case for surgery in patients with immature teratoma and any residual mass (67). An enlarged contralateral ovary may contain a benign cyst or a mature cystic terotoma, and ovarian cystectomy should be performed (2,4).

Prognosis

The most important prognostic feature of the immature teratoma is the grade of the lesion (1,40). In addition, the stage of disease and the extent of tumor at the initiation of treatment also have an impact on curability. **Patients whose tumors have been incompletely resected before treatment have a significantly lower probability of 5-year survival than those whose lesions have been completely resected (i.e., 94% vs. 50%)** (4). Overall, the 5-year survival rate for patients with all stages of pure immature teratomas is 70% to 80%, and it is 90% to 95% for patients with surgical stage I lesions (35,40,49).

The degree or grade of immaturity generally predicts the metastatic potential and curability. The 5-year survival rates have been reported to be 82%, 62%, and 30% for patients with grades 1, 2, and 3, respectively (40). However, many of these patients were treated in an era before optimal chemotherapy was available, and these figures do not match current experience and more recently published data. For example, Lai et al. reported on the long-term outcome of 84 patients with ovarian germ cell tumors, including 29 immature teratomas, and the 5-year survival was 97.4% (68).

Occasionally, these tumors are associated with mature or low-grade glial elements that have implanted throughout the peritoneum. Such patients have a favorable long-term survival (4). However, mature glial elements can grow and mimic malignant disease and may need to be resected to relieve pressure on surrounding structures.

Endodermal Sinus Tumor

Endodermal sinus tumors (ESTs) have also been referred to as *yolk sac carcinomas* **because they are derived from the primitive yolk sac** (1). **These lesions are the third most frequent malignant germ cell tumor of the ovary.**

ESTs have a median age of 18 years (1–3,69,70). Approximately one-third of the patients are premenarchal at the time of initial presentation. Abdominal or pelvic pain is the most frequent presenting symptom, occurring in some 75% of patients, whereas an asymptomatic pelvic mass is documented in 10% of patients (3).

Most EST lesions secrete AFP and rarely may elaborate detectable alpha-1-antitrypsin (AAT). There is a good correlation between the extent of disease and the level of AFP, although discordance also has been observed. The serum level of these markers, particularly AFP, is useful in monitoring the patient's response to treatment (69–75).

Treatment

Surgery

The treatment of the EST consists of surgical exploration, unilateral salpingo-oophorectomy, and a frozen section for diagnosis. The addition of a hysterectomy and contralateral salpingo-oophorectomy does not alter outcome and is not indicated (4,72). Furthermore, with conservative surgery and adjuvant chemotherapy, fertility can be preserved as with other germ cell tumors (17). Any gross metastases should be resected if possible, but thorough surgical staging is not indicated because all patients need chemotherapy. At surgery, the tumors tend to be solid and large, ranging in size from 7 to 28 cm (median = 15 cm) in the GOG series. Bilaterality is not seen in these lesions, and the other ovary is involved with metastatic disease only when there are other metastases in the peritoneal cavity. Most patients have early stage disease: 71% stage I, 6% stage II, and 23% stage III (76).

Chemotherapy

All patients with endodermal sinus tumors are treated with either adjuvant or therapeutic chemotherapy. Before the routine use of combination chemotherapy for this disease, the 2-year survival rate was approximately 25%. After the introduction of the VAC regimen, this rate improved to 60% to 70%, indicating the chemosensitivity of the majority of these tumors (56,57). Currently, all patients are treated with *cisplatin*-based regimens such as BEP, which is considered the standard of care. The chance of cure now approaches 100% for early stage patients and at least 75% for more advanced-stage patients.

The optimal number of treatment cycles has not been established in ovarian germ cell tumors, but it is reasonable to extrapolate from the much larger experience in testicular germ cell tumors where three cycles of BEP is considered optimal for good prognosis, low-risk patients and four cycles for patients with intermediate to high-risk tumors (7). In patients for whom *bleomycin* **is omitted or discontinued because of toxicity, four cycles of** *cisplatin* **and** *etoposide* **are recommended.** An alternative approach is to use VIP (*etoposide, ifosfamide,* and *cisplatin*) in patients with more advanced disease in whom *bleomycin* is contraindicated. Four cycles of VIP are equivalent to four cycles of BEP, but it is more myelotoxic and generally requires growth-factor support (6,7).

A number of years ago, the group from the Charing Cross Hospital in London developed the **POMB-ACE* regimen for high-risk germ cell tumors of any histologic type** (75) (Table 12.3). Their results appear to be superior to BEP in patients with poor prognostic features. This protocol introduces seven drugs into the initial management, which is intended to minimize the chances of developing drug resistance. **This is particularly relevant for patients with massive metastatic disease.** We have tended to use the POMB-ACE regimen as primary therapy for such cases, as well as for patients with liver or brain metastases.

The POMB schedule is only moderately myelosuppressive, so the intervals between each course can be kept to a maximum of 14 days (usually 9 to 11 days), thereby minimizing the time for tumor regrowth between courses. When *bleomycin* is given by a 48-hour infusion, pulmonary toxicity is reduced. With a maximum of 9 years of follow-up, the Charing Cross group has seen no long-term side effects in patients treated with POMB-ACE. Children have

---

*POMB, *cisplatin, vincristine, methotrexate,* and *bleomycin*; ACE, *actinomycin D, cyclophosphamide,* and *etoposide.*

developed normally, menstruation has been physiologic, and several women have completed normal pregnancies. It is still not clear if POMB-ACE is superior to BEP, but it is unlikely that this will ever be addressed in a randomized trial.

Second-Look Laparotomy

The value of a second-look operation is not established in patients with EST. It is reasonable to omit surgery in patients whose AFP values return to normal and remain normal for the balance of their treatment (73,74). There have been reported cases in which the AFP titer has returned to normal in spite of persistent measurable disease; some of these cases have been mixed germ cell tumors (74).

Rare Germ Cell Tumors of the Ovary

Embryonal Carcinoma

Embryonal carcinoma of the ovary is an extremely rare tumor that is distinguished from a choriocarcinoma of the ovary by the absence of syncytiotrophoblastic and cytotrophoblastic cells. The patients are very young, their ages ranging between 4 and 28 years (median = 14 years) in two series (76). Older patients have been reported (77). Embryonal carcinomas may secrete estrogens, with the patient exhibiting symptoms and signs of precocious pseudopuberty or irregular bleeding (1). The presentation is otherwise similar to that of the endodermal sinus tumor. The primary lesions tend to be large, and approximately two-thirds are confined to one ovary at the time of presentation. These lesions frequently secrete AFP and hCG, which are useful for following the response to subsequent therapy (73).

The treatment of embryonal carcinomas is the same as for the EST (i.e., a unilateral oophorectomy followed by combination chemotherapy with BEP) (21,61,78).

Choriocarcinoma of the Ovary

Pure nongestational choriocarcinoma of the ovary is an extremely rare tumor. Histologically, it has the same appearance as gestational choriocarcinoma metastatic to the ovaries (79). The majority of patients with this cancer are younger than 20 years. The presence of hCG can be useful in monitoring the patient's response to treatment. In the presence of high hCG levels, isosexual precocity has been seen, occurring in approximately 50% of patients whose tumors appear before menarche (80).

There are only a few limited reports on the use of chemotherapy for these nongestational choriocarcinomas, but complete responses have been reported to the MAC regimen (*methotrexate, actinomycin D,* and *cyclophosphamide*) used in a manner described for gestational trophoblastic disease (79) (see Chapter 15). These tumors are so rare that no good data are available, but the options also include the BEP or POMB-ACE regimens. The prognosis for ovarian choriocarcinomas has been poor, with the majority of patients having metastases to organ parenchyma at the time of initial diagnosis.

Polyembryoma

Polyembryoma of the ovary is another extremely rare tumor, which is composed of "embryoid bodies." This tumor replicates the structures of early embryonic differentiation (i.e., the three somatic layers: endoderm, mesoderm, and ectoderm) (1,9). The lesion tends to occur in very young, premenarchal girls with signs of pseudopuberty, and AFP and hCG levels are elevated. **Women with polyembryomas that are surgically staged and confined to one ovary may be followed with serial tumor markers and diagnostic-imaging techniques to avoid cytotoxic chemotherapy. In patients who require chemotherapy, the BEP regimen is appropriate** (56).

Mixed Germ Cell Tumors

Mixed germ cell malignancies of the ovary contain two or more elements of the lesions described above. In one series (78), the most common component of a mixed malignancy was dysgerminoma, which occurred in 80%, followed by EST in 70%, immature teratoma in 53%, choriocarcinoma in 20%, and embryonal carcinoma in 16%. The most frequent combination was a dysgerminoma and an EST. The mixed lesions may secrete either AFP or hCG—or both or neither—depending on the components.

These lesions should be managed with combination chemotherapy, preferably BEP. The serum marker, if positive initially, may become negative during chemotherapy, but this may reflect regression of only a particular component of the mixed lesion. Therefore, **in these patients a second-look laparotomy may be indicated if there is residual disease following** chemotherapy, particularly if there was an immature teratomatous component in the original tumor.

The most important prognostic features are the size of the primary tumor and the relative amount of its most malignant component (78). In stage IA lesions smaller than 10 cm, survival is 100%. Tumors composed of less than one-third EST, choriocarcinoma, or grade 3 immature teratoma also have an excellent prognosis, but it is less favorable when these components compose the majority of the mixed lesions.

Surveillance for Stage I Ovarian Germ Cell Tumors	**Surveillance is a common approach to the management of young men with apparent stage I testicular germ cell tumors.** There is a large body of evidence to support this approach, as well as guidelines on what constitutes appropriate surveillance (6,7). **Although as many as 20% to 30% of patients will relapse, almost all will be cured with salvage chemotherapy with BEP,** and the potential adverse effects of chemotherapy can be avoided in most patients.

Although this is a very common approach to management of young men with stage I testicular germ cell tumors, it has not been widely adopted in females with ovarian germ cell tumors. However, **some data are now available to support surveillance in selected patients who have been surgically staged.** Cushing et al. reported a study of 44 pediatric patients with completely resected ovarian immature teratomas who were followed carefully for recurrence of disease with appropriate diagnostic imaging and serum tumor markers (81). Thirty-one patients (70.5%) had pure ovarian immature teratomas with a tumor grade of 1 ($n = 17$), 2 ($n = 12$), or 3 ($n = 2$). Thirteen patients (29.5%) had an ovarian immature teratoma plus microscopic foci of yolk sac tumor. The 4-year event-free and overall survival for the ovarian immature teratoma group and for the ovarian immature teratoma plus yolk sac tumor group was 97.7% (95% confidence interval, 84.9% to 99.7%) and 100%, respectively. The only yolk sac tumor relapse occurred in a child with ovarian immature teratoma and yolk sac tumor who was then treated and salvaged with chemotherapy (81).

The Charing Cross Group reported a study of 24 patients with stage IA ovarian germ cell tumors who were also enrolled in a surveillance program. The group consisted of nine patients (37.5%) with dysgerminoma, nine (37.5%) with pure immature teratoma, and six (25%) with endodermal sinus tumors (with or without immature teratoma). Treatment consisted of surgical resection without adjuvant chemotherapy, followed by a surveillance program of clinical, serologic, and radiologic review. A second-look operation was performed, and **all but one patient were alive and in remission after a median follow-up of 6.8 years.** The 5-year overall survival was 95%, and the 5-year disease-free survival was 68%. Eight patients required chemotherapy for recurrent disease or second primary ovarian germ cell tumor. This included three patients with grade II immature teratoma, three patients with dysgerminoma, and two patients with dysgerminoma who developed a contralateral dysgerminoma 4.5 and 5.2 years after their first tumor. All but one, who died of a pulmonary embolus, were successfully salvaged with chemotherapy (82).

More recently, the same group updated its experience and reported on the safety of the ongoing surveillance program of all stage IA female germ cell tumors (83). Thirty-seven patients (median age 26, range 14–48 years) with stage I disease were referred to Mount Vernon and Charing Cross Hospitals between 1981 and 2003. Patients underwent surgery and staging followed by intense surveillance, which included regular tumor markers and imaging. The median period of follow-up was 6 years. **Relapse rates for stage IA nondysgerminomatous tumors and dysgerminomas were 8 of 22 (36%) and 2 of 9 (22%), respectively.** In addition, one patient with mature teratoma and glial implants also relapsed. Ten of these 11 patients (91%) were successfully cured with platinum-based chemotherapy. Only one patient died from chemoresistant disease. **All relapses occurred within 13 months of initial surgery.** The overall disease-specific survival of malignant ovarian germ cell tumors was 94%.

More than 50% of patients who underwent fertility-sparing surgery went on to have successful pregnancies. They concluded that surveillance of all stage IA ovarian germ cell tumors is very safe, and that the outcome is comparable with testicular tumors. They questioned the need for potentially toxic adjuvant chemotherapy in patients with nondysgerminomas who have greater than 90% chance of being salvaged with chemotherapy if they relapse.

This strategy is appealing and is supported by a larger pediatric literature, but there is much less experience in adults. It deserves further study, but this will require international collaboration. If a surveillance program is to be instigated, it is essential that the protocols used by the Charing Cross group are closely adhered to and that patients understand that the data for adults are limited.

Late Effects of Treatment of Malignant Germ Cell Tumors of the Ovary

Although there are substantial data regarding late effects of *cisplatin*-based therapy in men with testicular cancer, much less information is available for women with ovarian germ cell tumors. **The toxicity of BEP chemotherapy** has been well documented and includes **significant pulmonary toxicity** in 5% of patients, with fatal lung toxicity in 1%; **acute myeloid leukemia or myelodysplastic syndrome** in 0.2% to 1% of patients; **neuropathy** in 20% to 30%; **Raynaud's phenomenon** in 20%; **tinnitus** in 24%; and **high-tone hearing loss** in as many as 70% of patients. In addition, late effects occur on **gonadal function,** there is an increased risk of **hypertension and cardiovascular disease,** and some degree of **renal impairment** occurs in 30% of patients (84,85). These side effects underscore the importance of limiting the number of cycles of chemotherapy and also highlight the need for these patients to be referred to clinicians with experience in managing germ cell tumors.

Gonadal Function

An important cause of infertility in patients with ovarian germ cell tumors is unnecessary bilateral salpingo-oophorectomy and hysterectomy. **Although temporary ovarian dysfunction or failure is common with platinum-based chemotherapy, most women will resume normal ovarian function, and childbearing is usually preserved** (10,16,17,28–32). In one representative series of 47 patients treated with combination chemotherapy for germ cell malignancies, 91.5% of patients resumed normal menstrual function, and there were 14 healthy live births and no birth defects (17). **Factors such as older age at initiation of chemotherapy, greater cumulative drug dose, and longer duration of therapy all have adverse effects on future gonadal function** (29).

A large study of reproductive and sexual function after platinum-based chemotherapy in ovarian germ cell tumor survivors was recently reported by the GOG, and 132 survivors were included in the study. Interestingly, and quite revealing, was the fact that only 71 (53.8%) had fertility-sparing surgery; of these, 87.3% were still having regular menstrual periods. Twenty-four survivors had 37 offspring after cancer treatment (86).

Secondary Malignancies

An important cause of late morbidity and mortality in patients receiving chemotherapy for germ cell tumors is the development of secondary tumors. *Etoposide* **in particular has been implicated in the development of treatment-related leukemias.**

The chance of developing treatment-related leukemia following *etoposide* **is dose related.** The incidence of leukemia is approximately 0.4% to 0.5% (representing a 30-fold increased likelihood) in patients receiving a cumulative *etoposide* dose of less than 2,000 mg/m^2 (87) compared with as much as 5% (representing a 336-fold increased likelihood) in those receiving more than 2,000 mg/m^2 (88). In a typical three- or four-cycle course of BEP, patients receive a cumulative *etoposide* dose of 1,500 or 2,000 mg/m^2, respectively.

Despite the risk of secondary leukemia, risk–benefit analyses have concluded that *etoposide*-**containing chemotherapy regimens are beneficial in advanced germ cell tumors;** one case of treatment-induced leukemia would be expected for every 20 additionally cured patients who receive BEP as compared with PVB (*cisplatin, vinblastine,* and *bleomycin*). The risk–benefit balance for low-risk disease or for high-dose *etoposide* in the salvage setting is less clear (88).

Sex-Cord–Stromal Tumors

Sex-cord–stromal tumors of the ovary account for approximately 5% to 8% of all ovarian malignancies (1–4,89–93). This group of ovarian neoplasms is derived from the sex cords and the ovarian stroma or mesenchyme. The tumors usually are composed of various combinations of elements, including the "female" cells (i.e., granulosa and theca cells) and "male" cells (i.e., Sertoli and Leydig cells), as well as morphologically indifferent cells. A classification of this group of tumors is presented in Table 12.4.

Table 12.4 Sex-Cord–Stromal Tumors
1. Granulosa-stromal cell tumors
A. Granulosa cell tumor
B. Tumors in thecoma–fibroma group
(1) Thecoma
(2) Fibroma
(3) Unclassified
2. Androblastomas; Sertoli-Leydig cell tumors
A. Well differentiated
(1) Sertoli cell tumor
(2) Sertoli-Leydig cell tumor
(3) Leydig cell tumor; hilus cell tumor
B. Moderately differentiated
C. Poorly differentiated (sarcomatoid)
D. With heterologous elements
3. Gynandroblastoma
4. Unclassified

Modified and reprinted from **Young RE, Scully RE.** Ovarian sex cord-stromal tumors: recent progress. *Int J Gynecol Pathol* 1980;1:153, with permission.

Granulosa–Stromal-Cell Tumors

Granulosa–stromal-cell tumors include granulosa cell tumors, thecomas, and fibromas. The granulosa cell tumor is a low-grade malignancy. Thecomas and fibromas are benign but rarely may have morphologic features of malignancy and then may be referred to as *fibrosarcomas.*

Granulosa cell tumors, which secrete estrogen, are seen in women of all ages. They are found in prepubertal girls in 5% of cases; the remainder are distributed throughout the reproductive and postmenopausal years (92–95). They are bilateral in only 2% of patients.

Of the rare prepubertal lesions, 75% are associated with sexual pseudoprecocity because of the estrogen secretion (93). In the reproductive age group, most patients have menstrual irregularities or secondary amenorrhea, and cystic hyperplasia of the endometrium is frequently present. In postmenopausal women, abnormal uterine bleeding is frequently the presenting symptom. Indeed, the estrogen secretion in these patients can be sufficient to stimulate the development of endometrial cancer. **Endometrial cancer occurs in association with granulosa cell tumors in at least 5% of cases, and 25% to 50% are associated with endometrial hyperplasia** (1,92–94). **Rarely, granulosa cell tumors may produce androgens and cause virilization.**

The other symptoms and signs of granulosa cell tumors are nonspecific and the same as most ovarian malignancies. Ascites is present in approximately 10% of cases, and rarely a pleural effusion is present (92,93). Granulosa tumors tend to be hemorrhagic; occasionally they rupture and produce a hemoperitoneum.

Granulosa cell tumors are usually stage I at diagnosis but may recur 5 to 30 years after initial diagnosis (91). The tumors may also spread hematogenously, and metastases can develop in the lungs, liver, and brain years after initial diagnosis. When they do recur, they can progress quite rapidly. Malignant thecomas are extremely rare, and their presentation, management, and outcome are similar to those of the granulosa cell tumors (95).

Diagnosis

Inhibin is secreted by granulosa cell tumors and is a useful marker for the disease (96–99). Inhibin is an ovarian product that decreases to nondetectable levels after menopause. However, certain ovarian cancers (mucinous epithelial ovarian carcinomas and granulosa cell tumors) produce inhibin, which may predate clinical disease (100–102). An elevated serum inhibin level in a premenopausal woman presenting with amenorrhea and infertility is suggestive of a granulosa cell tumor.

Müllerian inhibitory substance (MIS), which is produced by granulosa cells, is emerging as a potential marker for these tumors (99). An elevated MIS level appears to have high specificity, but the test is not clinically available except for research purposes. An elevated estradiol level is not a sensitive marker of this disease (101).

The histological diagnosis can be facilitated by staining for markers of ovarian granulosa cell tumors (e.g., inhibin, CD99, and MIS) (96,97). Antibodies against inhibin appear to be the most useful, but they are not specific. In one report, positive staining for inhibin was present in 94% of granulosa cell tumors and in 10% to 20% of ovarian endometrioid tumors and metastatic carcinomas to the ovary (99). The latter demonstrated significantly weaker staining.

Treatment

The treatment of granulosa cell tumors depends on the age of the patient and the extent of disease. For most patients, surgery alone is sufficient primary therapy, with radiation and chemotherapy reserved for the treatment of recurrent or metastatic disease (92–95).

Surgery

Because granulosa cell tumors are bilateral in only some 2% of patients, a unilateral salpingo-oophorectomy is appropriate therapy for stage IA tumors in children or in women of reproductive age (90). At the time of laparotomy, if a granulosa cell tumor is identified by frozen section, then a staging operation is performed, including an assessment of the contralateral ovary. If the opposite ovary appears enlarged, it should be biopsied. In perimenopausal and postmenopausal women for whom ovarian preservation is not important, a hysterectomy and bilateral salpingo-oophorectomy should be performed. **In premenopausal patients in whom the uterus is left *in situ*, a dilatation and curettage of the uterus should be performed because of the possibility of a coexistent adenocarcinoma of the endometrium** (92).

Radiation

There is no evidence to support the use of adjuvant radiation therapy for granulosa cell tumors, although pelvic radiation may help to palliate isolated pelvic recurrences (92). Radiation can induce clinical responses and occasional long-term remission in patients with persistent or recurrent granulosa cell tumors, particularly if the disease is surgically cytoreduced (102–104). In one review of 34 patients treated at one center for more than 40 years, 14 were treated with measurable disease (103). Three (21%) were alive without progression 10 to 21 years following treatment.

Chemotherapy

There is no evidence that adjuvant chemotherapy in patients with stage I disease will prevent recurrence.

Metastatic lesions and recurrences have been treated with a variety of different antineoplastic drugs. There has been no consistently effective regimen in these patients, although complete responses have been reported anecdotally in patients treated with the single agents *cyclophosphamide* and *melphalan,* as well as the combinations VAC, PAC (*cisplatin, doxorubicin, cyclophosphamide*), PVB, BEP (4,105–117), and, more recently, *carboplatin* and *paclitaxel* (102).

The rarity of these tumors has made it impossible to conduct well-designed randomized studies assessing the value of therapy for patients with stages II to IV disease. **In retrospective series, postoperative chemotherapy has been associated with a prolonged progression-free interval in women with stage III or IV disease** (107), but an overall survival benefit has not been shown (108). Despite the absence of data supporting a survival benefit, some experts recommend postoperative chemotherapy for women with completely resected stage II to IV disease because of the high risk of disease progression and the potential for long-term survival after platinum-based chemotherapy (102,109–112). Among the acceptable options are **BEP, EP, PAC,** and *carboplatin* and *paclitaxel* (102).

For patients with suboptimally cytoreduced disease, combinations of BEP have produced overall response rates of 58% to 83% (109,114). In one study, 14 of 38 patients (37%) with advanced disease undergoing second-look laparotomy following four courses of BEP had negative findings (109). With a median follow-up of 3 years, 11 of 16 patients (69%) with primary advanced disease and 21of 41 patients (51%) with recurrent disease were progression free. This regimen was associated with severe toxicity and two *bleomycin*-related deaths. **Carboplatin** and *etoposide* (115), **PVB** (92,116), and **PAC** (105,117) are other chemotherapeutic regimens with reported relatively high response rates.

There is a need to develop less-toxic and equally active regimens for this older group of patients. **Paclitaxel is an active agent, and the combination of platinum with a *taxane* has been reported to have a response rate of 60%,** which makes it a more viable alternative (118,119).

Recurrent Disease	**The median time to relapse is approximately 4 to 6 years after initial diagnosis** (91,112,113). There is no standard approach to the management of relapsed disease. A common site of recurrence is the pelvis, although the upper abdomen may be involved as well. Further surgery can be effective if the tumor is localized, but diffuse intraabdominal disease is difficult to treat. Chemotherapy or radiation may be useful in selected patients.

Approximately 30% of these tumors have estrogen receptors and 100% have progesterone receptors (120,121). The use of hormonal agents such as progestins or luteinizing hormone-releasing hormone (LHRH) agonists has been suggested as an option, but very limited data are available (101). Small clinical series and case reports have indicated that LHRH agonists had a 50% response rate in 13 patients (121–123), whereas four of five patients were reported to respond to a progestational agent (124). Freeman recently reported two patients with recurrent adult granulosa cell tumors who had received multiple treatment modalities, including chemotherapy, and had previously progressed on *leuprolide*. Both patients were treated with *anastrozole*. Inhibin B levels normalized, as did clinical findings. Both were maintained on treatment for 14 and 18 months, respectively (125). The numbers are too small to draw any conclusions, and it is likely that there has been significant publication bias, with more reports of responses to treatment.

Prognosis	The prognosis of granulosa cell tumor of the ovary depends on the surgical stage of disease at the time of diagnosis (91,93,102). **Most granulosa cell tumors have an indolent growth pattern and are confined to one ovary;** the cure rate for stage I disease is 75% to 92% (93,112). However, late recurrences are not uncommon (90,91,93). In one report of 37 women with stage I disease, survival rates at 5, 10, and 20 years were 94%, 82%, and 62%, respectively. The survival rates for stages II to IV at 5 and 10 years were 55% and 34%, respectively (102).

In adult tumors, cellular atypia, mitotic rate, and the absence of Call-Exner bodies are the only significant pathologic predictors of early recurrence (111). Neither an abnormal tumor karyotype nor *p53* overexpression appear to be prognostic (126). The DNA ploidy of the tumors has been correlated with survival. Holland and colleagues (106) reported DNA aneuploidy in 13 of 37 patients (35%) with primary granulosa cell tumors. **The presence of residual disease was found to be the most important predictor of progression-free survival, but DNA ploidy was an independent prognostic factor.** Patients with no residual disease and DNA diploid tumors had a 10-year progression-free survival of 96%.

Juvenile Granulosa Cell Tumors	Juvenile granulosa cell tumors of the ovary are rare and make up less than 5% of ovarian tumors in childhood and adolescence (115). Approximately 90% are diagnosed in stage I and have a favorable prognosis. The juvenile subtype behaves less aggressively than the adult type. Advanced-stage tumors have been successfully treated with platinum-based combination chemotherapy (e.g., BEP) (102).

Sertoli-Leydig Tumors	**Sertoli-Leydig tumors occur most frequently in the third and fourth decades, with 75% of the lesions seen in women younger than 40 years. These lesions account for less than 0.2% of ovarian cancers** (1). **Sertoli-Leydig cell tumors are most frequently low-grade malignancies, although occasionally a poorly differentiated variety may behave more aggressively.**

The tumors typically produce androgens, and clinical virilization is noted in 70% to 85% of patients (127,128). Signs of virilization include oligomenorrhea followed by amenorrhea, breast atrophy, acne, hirsutism, clitoromegaly, a deepening voice, and a receding hairline

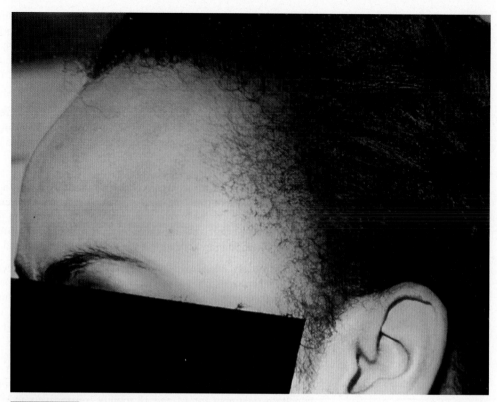

Figure 12.6 **A young woman with a Sertoli-Leydig cell tumor demonstrating temporal baldness.**

(Fig. 12.6). Measurement of plasma androgens may reveal elevated testosterone and androstenedione, with normal or slightly elevated dehydroepiandrosterone sulfate (1). Rarely, the Sertoli-Leydig tumor can be associated with manifestations of estrogenization (i.e., isosexual precocity, irregular or postmenopausal bleeding) (128).

Treatment

Because these low-grade lesions are bilateral in less than 1% of cases, the usual treatment is unilateral salpingo-oophorectomy and evaluation of the contralateral ovary in patients who are in their reproductive years (128). In older patients, hysterectomy and bilateral salpingo-oophorectomy are appropriate.

There are limited data regarding the utility of chemotherapy in patients with persistent disease, but responses in patients with measurable disease have been reported with *cisplatin* in combination with *doxorubicin* or *ifosfamide* or both (128) as well as the regimens mentioned above for granulosa cell tumors. Because of their rarity, most series have included them with granulosa cell tumors (110). Pelvic radiation can also be used for recurrent pelvic tumor but with limited responses.

Prognosis

The 5-year survival rate is 70% to 90%, and recurrences thereafter are uncommon (1,2,128). Poorly differentiated lesions compose the majority of fatalities.

Uncommon Ovarian Cancers

There are several varieties of malignant ovarian tumors, which together constitute only 0.1% of ovarian malignancies. These lesions include lipoid (or lipid) cell tumors, primary ovarian sarcomas, and small cell ovarian carcinomas.

Lipoid Cell Tumors

Lipoid cell tumors are thought to arise in adrenal cortical rests that reside in the vicinity of the ovary. More than 100 cases have been reported, and bilaterality has been noted in only a few (1). Most are associated with virilization and occasionally with obesity, hypertension, and glucose intolerance, reflecting glucocorticoid secretion. Rare cases of estrogen secretion and isosexual precocity have been reported.

The majority of these tumors have a benign or low-grade behavior, but approximately 20% develop metastatic lesions, most of which are initially larger than 8 cm in diameter. Metastases are usually in the peritoneal cavity but rarely occur at distant sites. The primary treatment is surgical extirpation of the primary lesion. There are no data regarding radiation or chemotherapy for this disease.

Sarcomas

Malignant mixed mesodermal sarcomas of the ovary are extremely rare (129–135). Most lesions are heterologous, and 80% occur in postmenopausal women. The presentation is similar to that of most ovarian malignancies. These lesions are biologically aggressive, and the majority of patients have evidence of metastases.

Such patients should be treated by cytoreductive surgery and postoperative platinum-containing combination chemotherapy (134,135). Silasi et al. recently reported their experience with 22 patients from Yale, all but two of whom presented with advanced-stage disease (136). The median survival for the entire cohort was 38 months. The median survival was 46 months for 18 optimally debulked (<1 cm) patients and 27 months for four suboptimally debulked (>1 cm) patients. Six patients were treated with optimal cytoreduction and adjuvant *cisplatin* and *ifosfamide*; they had a median progression-free interval of 13 months and median survival of 51 months. The combination of *carboplatin* and *paclitaxel* was administered to four patients following optimal cytoreduction; their median progression-free interval was 6 months, and median survival was 38 months. The difference in survival between the *cisplatin* and *ifosfamide* group and the *carboplatin* and *paclitaxel* group was not statistically significant ($p = 0.48$). **First-line *cisplatin* and *ifosfamide* or *carboplatin* and *paclitaxel* can achieve survival rates comparable to those observed in epithelial ovarian cancer.**

Leiser et al. reported the Memorial Sloan-Kettering experience with ***platinum*** and ***paclitaxel*** in 30 patients with carcinosarcomas of the ovary, and they also found it was very active (137). Twelve patients (40%) had a complete response, seven (23%) a partial response, two (7%) stable disease, and nine (30%) progression of disease. The median time to progression for responders was 12 months; with a median follow-up of 23 months, the median overall survival was 43 months for survivors. The 3- and 5-year survival rates were 53% and 30%, respectively.

Small Cell Carcinomas

This rare tumor occurs at an average age of 24 years (range 2 to 46 years) (138). The tumors are all bilateral. **Approximately two-thirds of the tumors are accompanied by paraneoplastic hypercalcemia.** This tumor accounts for one-half of all of the cases of hypercalcemia associated with ovarian tumors. Approximately 50% of the tumors have spread beyond the ovaries at the time of diagnosis (1,2).

Management consists of surgery followed by platinum-based chemotherapy or radiation therapy. In addition to the primary treatment of the disease, control of the hypercalcemia may require aggressive hydration, loop diuretics, and the use of bisphosphonates. There have been a number of recent reports on the treatment of patients with small cell carcinoma of the ovary. In a collaborative Gynecologic Cancer Intergroup study, data were collected for 17 patients treated in Australia, Canada, and Europe (139). The median follow-up was 13 months for all patients and 35.5 months for surviving patients. Ten patients had FIGO stage I tumors, six stage III tumors, and one stage unknown. All underwent surgical resection. Adjuvant platinum-based chemotherapy was given to all patients. Seven received adjuvant pelvic, whole-abdominal or extended-field radiation. The median survival for stage I tumors was not reached, whereas it was 6 months for stage III tumors. For the ten patients with stage I tumors, six received adjuvant radiotherapy, with five alive and disease-free; four received no adjuvant radiotherapy, with one alive and disease-free; and three have relapsed, with one alive and disease-free after resection. Of the seven patients with stage III or unknown stage tumors, all but one have died. Recurrences were most frequent in the pelvis and the abdomen. Patients receiving salvage treatment with chemotherapy and radiotherapy did poorly.

Although the optimal approach to management is not known, in view of these findings **we advocate a multimodality treatment approach including surgical resection of gross disease, chemotherapy with *carboplatin* and *paclitaxel* or *cisplatin* and *ifosfamide,* and the addition of radiotherapy either sequentially or concurrently.** Others have advocated high-dose chemotherapy with stem cell support and have reported a number of long-term survivors (140).

Metastatic Tumors

Approximately 5% to 6% of ovarian tumors are metastatic from other organs, most frequently from the female genital tract, the breast, or the gastrointestinal tract (141–155). The metastases may occur from direct extension of another pelvic neoplasm, by hematogenous spread, by lymphatic spread, or from transcoelomic dissemination, with surface implantation of tumors that spread in the peritoneal cavity.

Gynecologic

Nonovarian cancers of the genital tract can spread by direct extension or metastasize to the ovaries. Tubal carcinoma involves the ovaries secondarily in 13% of cases (1), usually by direct extension. Under some circumstances, it is difficult to know whether the tumor originates in the tube or in the ovary when both are involved. **Cervical cancer spreads to the ovary only in rare cases** (<1%), and most of these are of an advanced clinical stage or are adenocarcinomas. Although adenocarcinoma of the endometrium can spread and implant directly onto the surface of the ovaries in as many as 5% of cases, two synchronous primary tumors probably occur with greater frequency. In these cases, an endometrioid carcinoma of the ovary is usually associated with the adenocarcinoma of the endometrium (156).

Nongynecologic

The frequency of metastatic breast carcinoma to the ovaries varies according to the method of determination, but the phenomenon is common. In autopsy data of women who die of metastatic breast cancer, the ovaries are involved in 24% of cases, and 80% of the involvement is bilateral (141–147). Similarly, when ovaries are removed to palliate advanced breast cancer, approximately 20% to 30% of the cases reveal ovarian involvement, 60% bilaterally. The involvement of ovaries in early stage breast cancer appears to be considerably lower, but precise figures are not available. In almost all cases, either ovarian involvement is occult or a pelvic mass is discovered after other metastatic disease becomes apparent.

Krukenberg Tumor

The Krukenberg tumor, which can account for 30% to 40% of metastatic cancers to the ovaries, arises in the ovarian stroma and has characteristic mucin-filled, signet-ring cells (148,149). The primary tumor is most frequently the stomach (Fig. 12.7) but less commonly the colon, breast, or biliary tract. Rarely, the cervix or the bladder may be the primary site. Krukenberg tumors can account for approximately 2% of ovarian cancers at some institutions, and they are usually bilateral. The lesions are usually not discovered until the primary disease is advanced, and therefore most patients die of their disease within a year. In some cases, a primary tumor is never found.

Other Gastrointestinal

In other cases of metastasis from the gastrointestinal tract to the ovary, the tumor does not have the classic histologic appearance of a Krukenberg tumor; most of these are from the colon and, less commonly, the small intestine. One percent to 2% of women with intestinal carcinomas will develop metastases to the ovaries during the course of their disease (143,150,151). Before exploration for an adnexal tumor in a woman more than 40 years of age, a colonoscopy or gastroscopy is indicated to exclude a primary gastrointestinal carcinoma with metastases to the ovaries, if there are any gastrointestinal symptoms.

Metastatic colon cancer can mimic a mucinous cystadenocarcinoma of the ovary histologically, and the histological distinction between the two can be difficult (150–154). Lesions that arise in the appendix may be associated with ovarian metastasis and have frequently been confused with primary ovarian malignancies, especially when associated with pseudomyxoma peritonei (150,154) (see Chapters 5 and 11). Therefore, it is reasonable to consider the performance of prophylactic bilateral salpingo-oophorectomy at the time of surgery for women with colon cancer (155).

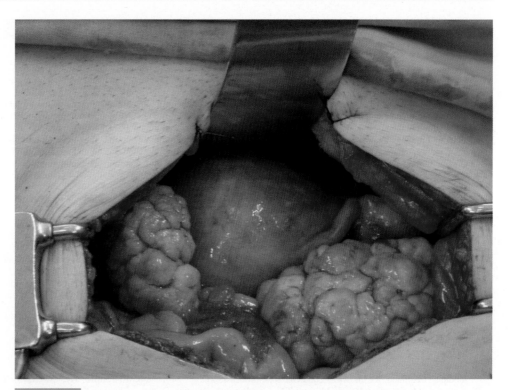

Figure 12.7   **Bilateral Krukenberg tumors from a primary stomach cancer.**

Melanoma

Rare cases of malignant melanoma metastatic to the ovaries have been reported (157). These must be distinguished from the rare case of a melanoma arising in an ovarian teratoma (158). In these circumstances, the melanomas are usually widely disseminated. Removal would be warranted for palliation of abdominal or pelvic pain, bleeding, or torsion.

Carcinoid

Metastatic carcinoid tumors are rare, representing fewer than 2% of metastatic lesions to the ovaries (159). Conversely, only some 2% of primary carcinoids have evidence of ovarian metastasis, and only 40% of these patients have the carcinoid syndrome at the time of discovery of the metastatic carcinoid (160). However, in perimenopausal and postmenopausal women explored for an intestinal carcinoid, it is reasonable to remove the ovaries to prevent subsequent ovarian metastasis. Furthermore, the discovery of an ovarian carcinoid should prompt a careful search for a primary intestinal lesion.

Lymphoma and Leukemia

Lymphomas and leukemia can involve the ovary. When they do, the involvement is usually bilateral (161–163). Approximately 5% of patients with Hodgkin's disease will have lymphomatous involvement of the ovaries, but this occurs typically with advanced-stage disease. With Burkitt's lymphoma, ovarian involvement is very common. Other types of lymphoma involve the ovaries much less frequently, and leukemic infiltration of the ovaries is uncommon.

Sometimes the ovaries can be the only apparent site of involvement of the abdominal or pelvic viscera with a lymphoma; if this circumstance is found, a careful surgical exploration may be necessary. An intraoperative consultation with a hematologist–oncologist should be obtained to determine the need for such procedures if frozen section of a solid ovarian mass reveals a lymphoma. In general, most lymphomas no longer require extensive surgical staging, although enlarged lymph nodes should generally be biopsied. In some cases of Hodgkin's disease, a more extensive evaluation may be necessary. Treatment involves that of the lymphoma or leukemia in general. Removal of a large ovarian mass may improve patient comfort and facilitate a response to subsequent radiation or chemotherapy (163).

References

1. **Scully RE, Young RH, Clement RB.** Tumors of the ovary, maldeveloped gonads, fallopian tube, and broad ligament. In: *Atlas of tumor pathology*: 3rd series, Fascicle 23. Washington, DC: Armed Forces Institute of Pathology, 1998:169–498.

2. **Chen LM, Berek JS.** Ovarian and fallopian tubes. In: **Haskell CM, ed.** *Cancer treatment,* 5th ed. Philadelphia: WB Saunders, 2000:900–932.

3. **Imai A, Furui T, Tamaya T.** Gynecologic tumors and symptoms in childhood and adolescence: 10-years' experience. *Int J Gynaecol Obstet* 1994;45:227–234.

4. **Gershenson DM.** Management of early ovarian cancer: germ cell and sex-cord stromal tumors. *Gynecol Oncol* 1994;55:S62–S72.

5. **Gershenson DM.** Update on malignant ovarian germ cell tumors. *Cancer* 1993;71:1581–1590.

6. **Krege S, Beyer J, Souchon R, Albers P, Albrecht W, Algaba F, et al.** European Consensus Conference on Diagnosis and Treatment of Germ Cell Cancer: A Report of the Second Meeting of the European Germ Cell Cancer Consensus group (EGCCCG): Part I. *Eur Urol* 2008 Mar;53:478–496.

7. **Krege S, Beyer J, Souchon R, Albers P, Albrecht W, Algaba F, et al.** European Consensus Conference on Diagnosis and Treatment of Germ Cell Cancer: A Report of the Second Meeting of the European Germ Cell Cancer Consensus Group (EGCCCG): Part II. *Eur Urol* 2008 Mar;53:497–513.

8. **Murugaesu N, Schmid P, Dancey G, Agarwal R, Holden L, McNeish I, et al.** Malignant ovarian germ cell tumors: identification of novel prognostic markers and long-term outcome after multimodality treatment. *J Clin Oncol* 2006 Oct 20;24:4862–4866.

9. **Kurman RJ, Scardino PT, Waldmann TA, Javadpour N, Norris HJ.** Malignant germ cell tumors of the ovary and testis: an immunohistologic study of 69 cases. *Ann Clin Lab Sci* 1979;9:462–466.

10. **Obata NH, Nakashima N, Kawai M, Nikkawa F, Mamba S, Tomoda Y.** Gonadoblastoma with dysgerminoma in one ovary and gonadoblastoma with dysgerminoma and yolk sac tumor in the contralateral ovary in a girl with 46XX karyotype. *Gynecol Oncol* 1995;58:124–128.

11. **Spanos WJ.** Preoperative hormonal therapy of cystic adnexal masses. *Am J Obstet Gynecol* 1973;116:551–556.

12. **Bremer GL, Land JA, Tiebosch A, Van Der Putten HW.** Five different histologic subtypes of germ cell malignancies in an XY female. *Gynecol Oncol* 1993;50:247–248.

13. **Mayordomo JI, Paz-Ares L, Rivera F, López-Brea M, López Martain E, Mendiola C, et al.** Ovarian and extragonadal malignant germ-cell tumors in females: a single-institution experience with 43 patients. *Ann Oncol* 1994;5:225–231.

14. **Piura B, Dgani R, Zalel Y, Nemet D, Yanai-Inbar I, Cohen Y, Glezerman M.** Malignant germ cell tumors of the ovary: a study of 20 cases. *J Surg Oncol* 1995;59:155–161.

15. **Gordon A, Lipton D, Woodruff JD.** Dysgerminoma: a review of 158 cases from the Emil Novak Ovarian Tumor Registry. *Obstet Gynecol* 1981;58:497–504.

16. **Thomas GM, Dembo AJ, Hacker NF, DePetrillo AD.** Current therapy for dysgerminoma of the ovary. *Obstet Gynecol* 1987;70:268–275.

17. **Low JJ, Perrin LC, Crandon AJ, Hacker NF.** Conservative surgery to preserve ovarian function in patients with malignant ovarian germ cell tumors: a review of 74 cases. *Cancer* 2000;89:391–398.

18. **Williams SD, Birch R, Einhorn LH, Irwin L, Greco FA, Loehrer PJ.** Treatment of disseminated germ cell tumors with *cisplatin, bleomycin* and either *vinblastine* or *etoposide*. *N Engl J Med* 1987;316:1435–1440.

19. **Williams SD, Blessing JA, Hatch K, Homesley HD.** Chemotherapy of advanced ovarian dysgerminoma: trials of the Gynecologic Oncology Group. *J Clin Oncol* 1991;9:1950–1955.

20. **Williams SD, Blessing JA, Moore DH, Homesley HD, Adcock L.** *Cisplatin, vinblastine,* and *bleomycin* in advanced and recurrent ovarian germ-cell tumors. *Ann Intern Med* 1989;111:22–27.

21. **Williams SD, Blessing JA, Liao S, Ball HJ 3rd, Hanjani P.** Adjuvant therapy of ovarian germ cell tumors with *cisplatin, etoposide,* and *bleomycin*: a trial of the Gynecologic Oncology Group. *J Clin Oncol* 1994;12:701–706.

22. **Gershenson DM, Morris M, Cangir A, Kavanagh JJ, Stringer CA, Edwards CL, et al.** Treatment of malignant germ cell tumors of the ovary with *bleomycin, etoposide,* and *cisplatin*. *J Clin Oncol* 1990;8:715–720.

23. **Bekaii-Saab T, Einhorn LH, Williams SD.** Late relapse of ovarian dysgerminoma: case report and literature review. *Gynecol Oncol* 1999;72:111–112.

24. **Kurtz JE, Jaeck D, Maloisel F, Jung GM, Chenard MP, Dufour P.** Combined modality treatment for malignant transformation of a benign ovarian teratoma. *Gynecol Oncol* 1999;73:319–321.

25. **Williams SD.** Ovarian germ cell tumors: an update. *Semin Oncol* 1998;25:407.

26. **Pawinski A, Favalli G, Ploch E, Sahmoud T, van Oosterom AT, Pecorelli S.** PVB chemotherapy in patients with recurrent or advanced dysgerminoma: a phase II study of the EORTC Gynaecological Cancer Cooperative Group. *Clin Oncol (R Coll Radiol)* 1998;10:301–305.

27. **Brewer M, Gershenson DM, Herzog CE, Mitchell MF, Silva EC, Wharton JT.** Outcome and reproductive function after chemotherapy for ovarian dysgerminoma. *J Clin Oncol* 1999;17:2670–2675.

28. **Gershenson DM.** Menstrual and reproductive function after treatment with combination chemotherapy for malignant ovarian germ cell tumors. *J Clin Oncol* 1988;6:270–275.

29. **Kanazawa K, Suzuki T, Sakumoto K.** Treatment of malignant ovarian germ cell tumors with preservation of fertility: reproductive performance after persistent remission. *Am J Clin Oncol* 2000;23:244–248.

30. **El-Lamie IK, Shehata NA, Abou-Loz SK, El-Lamie KI.** Conservative surgical management of malignant ovarian germ cell tumors: the experience of the Gynecologic Oncology Unit at Ain Shams University. *Eur J Gynaecol Oncol* 2000;21:605–609.

31. **Tangir J, Zelterman D, Ma W, Schwartz PE.** Reproductive function after conservative surgery and chemotherapy for malignant germ cell tumors of the ovary. *Obstet Gynecol* 2003;101:251–257.

32. **Loehrer PJ, Johnson D, Elson P, Einhorn LH, Trump D.** Importance of *bleomycin* in favorable-prognosis disseminated germ cell tumors: an Eastern Cooperative Oncology Group trial. *J Clin Oncol* 1995;13:470–476.

33. **Bajorin DF, Sarosdy MF, Pfister GD, Mazumdar M, Motzer RJ, Scher HI.** Randomized trial of *etoposide* and *cisplatin* versus *etoposide* and *carboplatin* in patients with good-risk germ cell tumors: a multi-institutional study. *J Clin Oncol* 1993;11:598–606.

34. **Schwartz PE, Chambers SK, Chambers JT, Kohorn E, McIntosh S.** Ovarian germ cell malignancies: the Yale University experience. *Gynecol Oncol* 1992;45:26–31.

35. **Williams SD, Blessing JA, DiSaia PJ, Major FJ, Ball HG 3rd, Liao SY.** Second-look laparotomy in ovarian germ cell tumors. *Gynecol Oncol* 1994;52:287–291.

36. **Culine S, Lhomme C, Michel G, Leclere J, Duvillard P, Droz JP.** Is there a role for second-look laparotomy in the management of malignant germ cell tumors of the ovary? Experience at Institute Gustave Roussy. *J Surg Oncol* 1996;62:40–45.

37. **De Santis M, Bokemeyer C, Becherer A, Stoiber F, Oechsle K, Kletter K, et al.** Predictive impact of 2-18fluoro-2-deoxy-D-glucose positron emission tomography for residual postchemotherapy masses in patients with bulky seminoma. *J Clin Oncol*. 2001;1:19:3740–3744.

38. **Motzer RJ, Sheinfeld J, Mazumdar M, Bains M, Mariani T, Bacik J, et al.** *Paclitaxel, ifosfamide,* and *cisplatin* second-line therapy for patients with relapsed testicular germ cell cancer. *J Clin Oncol* 2000;18:2413–8.

39. **Kumar S, Shah JP, Bryant CS, Imudia AN, Cote ML, Ali-fehmi R et al.** The prevalence and prognostic impact of lymph node metastases in malignant germ cell tumors of the ovary. *Gynecol Oncol* 2008;110:125–132.

40. **O'Conner DM, Norris HJ.** The influence of grade on the outcome of stage I ovarian immature (malignant) teratomas and the reproducibility of grading. *Int J Gynecol Pathol* 1994;13:283–289.

41. **Norris HJ, Zirkin HJ, Benson WL.** Immature (malignant) teratoma of the ovary: a clinical and pathologic study of 58 cases. *Cancer* 1976;37:2359–2372.

42. Ulbright, TM. Germ cell tumors of the gonads: a selective review emphasizing problems in differential diagnosis, newly appreciated, and controversial issues. A review. *Mod Pathol* 2005;18 Suppl 2:S61–S79.

43. Heifetz SA, Cushing B, Giller R, Shuster JJ, Stolar CJ, Vinocur CD, et al. Immature teratomas in children: pathologic considerations: a report from the combined Pediatric Oncology Group/Children's Cancer Group. *Am J Surg Pathol* 1998;22:1115–1124.

44. Marina NM, Cushing B, Giller R, Cohen L, Lauer SJ, Ablin A, et al. Complete surgical excision is effective treatment for children with immature teratomas with or without malignant elements: A Pediatric Oncology Group/Children's Cancer Group Intergroup Study. *J Clin Oncol* 1999; 17:2137–2143.

45. Ferguson AW, Katabuchi H, Ronnett BM, Cho KR. Glial implants in gliomatosis peritonei arise from normal tissue, not from the associated teratoma. *Am J Pathol* 2001 Jul;159:51–55.

46. Best DH, Butz GM, Moller K, Coleman WB, Thomas DB. Molecular analysis of an immature ovarian teratoma with gliomatosis peritonei and recurrence suggests genetic independence of multiple tumors. *Int J Oncol* 2004;25:17–25.

47. Dimopoulos MA, Papadopoulou M, Andreopoulou E, Papadimitriou C, Pavlidis N, Aravantinos G, et al. Favorable outcome of ovarian germ cell malignancies treated with *cisplatin* or *carboplatin*-based chemotherapy: a Hellenic Cooperative Oncology Group study. *Gynecol Oncol* 1998;70:70–74.

48. Bafna UD, Umadevi K, Kumaran C, Nagarathna DS, Shashikala P, Tanseem R. Germ cell tumors of the ovary: is there a role for aggressive cytoreductive surgery for nondysgerminomatous tumors? *Int J Gynecol Cancer* 2001;11:300–304.

49. De Palo G, Zambetli M, Pilotti S, Rottoli L, Spatti G, Fontanelli R, et al. Non-dysgerminomatous tumors of the ovary treated with *cisplatin, vinblastine,* and *bleomycin:* long-term results. *Gynecol Oncol* 1992;47:239–246.

50. Culine S, Kattan J, Lhomme C, Duvillard P, Michel G, Castaigne D, et al. A phase II study of high-dose *cisplatin, vinblastine, bleomycin,* and *etoposide* (PVeBV regimen) in malignant nondysgerminomatous germ-cell tumors of the ovary. *Gynecol Oncol* 1994;54:47–53.

51. Mann JR, Raafat F, Robinson K, Imeson J, Gornell P, Sokal M, et al. The United Kingdom Children's Cancer Study Group's second germ cell tumor study: *carboplatin, etoposide,* and *bleomycin* are effective treatment for children with malignant extracranial germ cell tumors, with acceptable toxicity. *J Clin Oncol* 2000;18: 3809–3818.

52. Segelov E, Campbell J, Ng M, Tattersall M, Rome R, Free K, et al. *Cisplatin*-based chemotherapy for ovarian germ cell malignancies: the Australian experience. *J Clin Oncol* 1994;12:378–384.

53. Marina NM, Cushing B, Giller R, Cohen L, Lauer SJ, Ablin A, et al. Complete surgical excision is effective treatment for children with immature teratomas with or without malignant elements: a Pediatric Oncology Group/Children's Cancer Group Intergroup Study. *J Clin Oncol* 1999;17:2137–2143.

54. Bonazzi C, Peccatori F, Colombo N, Lucchini V, Cantu MG, Mangioni C. Pure ovarian immature teratoma, a unique and curable disease: 10 years' experience of 32 prospectively treated patients. *Obstet Gynecol* 1994;84:598–604.

55. Cangir A, Smith J, van Eys J. Improved prognosis in children with ovarian cancers following modified VAC (*vincristine sulfate, dactinomycin,* and *cyclophosphamide*) chemotherapy. *Cancer* 1978;42: 1234–1238.

56. Chapman DC, Grover R, Schwartz PE. Conservative management of an ovarian polyembryoma. *Obstet Gynecol* 1994;83:879–882.

57. Slayton RE, Park RC, Silverberg SC, Shingleton H, Creasman WT, Blessing JA. *Vincristine, dactinomycin,* and *cyclophosphamide* in the treatment of malignant germ cell tumors of the ovary: a Gynecologic Oncology Group study (a final report). *Cancer* 1985;56:243–248.

58. Creasman WJ, Soper JT. Assessment of the contemporary management of germ cell malignancies of the ovary. *Am J Obstet Gynecol* 1985;153:828–834.

59. Taylor MH, DePetrillo AD, Turner AR. *Vinblastine, bleomycin,* and *cisplatin* in malignant germ cell tumors of the ovary. *Cancer* 1985;56:1341–1349.

60. Culine S, Lhomme C, Kattan J, Michel G, Duvillard P, Droz JP. *Cisplatin*-based chemotherapy in the management of germ cell tumors of the ovary: the Institute Gustave Roussy experience. *Gynecol Oncol* 1997;64:160–165.

61. Williams SD, Wong LC, Ngan HYS. Management of ovarian germ cell tumors. In: Gershenson DM, McGuire WP, eds. *Ovarian cancer.* New York: Churchill-Livingstone, 1998:399–415.

62. Bokemeyer C, Köhrmann O, Tischler J, Weissbach L, Räth U, Haupt A, et al. Schmoll HJA randomized trial of *cisplatin, etoposide,* and *bleomycin* (PEB) versus *carboplatin, etoposide,* and *bleomycin* (CEB) for patients with "good-risk" metastatic non-seminomatous germ cell tumors. *Ann Oncol* 1996;7:1015–1021.

63. Horwich A, Sleijfer DT, Fosså SD, Kaye SB, Oliver RT, Cullen MH, et al. Randomized trial of *bleomycin, etoposide,* and *cisplatin* compared with *bleomycin, etoposide,* and *carboplatin* in good-prognosis metastatic nonseminomatous germ cell cancer: a Multiinstitutional Medical Research Council/European Organization for Research and Treatment of Cancer Trial. *J Clin Oncol* 1997;15:1844–1852.

64. Hariprasad R, Kumar L, Janga D, Kumar S, Vijayaraghavan M. Growing teratoma syndrome of ovary. *Int J Clin Oncol* 2008;13:83–87.

65. Tangjitgamol S, Manusirivithaya S, Leelahakorn S, Thawaramara T, Suekwatana P, Sheanakul C. The growing teratoma syndrome: a case report and a review of the literature. *Int J Gynecol Cancer* 2006;16 Suppl 1:384–390.

66. Carver BS, Shayegan B, Serio A, Motzer RJ, Bosl GJ, Sheinfeld J. Long-term clinical outcome after postchemotherapy retroperitoneal lymph node dissection in men with residual teratoma. *J Clin Oncol* 2007;25:1033–1037.

67. Mathew GK, Singh SS, Swaminathan RG, Tenali SG. Laparotomy for post chemotherapy residue in ovarian germ cell tumors. *J Postgrad Med* 2006;52:262–265.

68. Lai CH, Chang TC, Hsueh S, Wu TI, Chao A, Chou HH, et al. Outcome and prognostic factors in ovarian germ cell malignancies. *Gynecol Oncol* 2005 Mar;96:784–791.

69. Talerman A. Germ cell tumors of the ovary. *Curr Opin Obstet Gynecol* 1997;9:44–47.

70. Kleiman GM, Young RH, Scully RE. Primary neuroectodermal tumors of the ovary: a report of 25 cases. *Am J Surg Pathol* 1993; 17:764–778.

71. Sasaki H, Furusata M, Teshima S, Kiyokawa T, Tada A, Aizawa S, et al. Prognostic significance of histopathological subtypes in stage I pure yolk sac tumour of the ovary. *Br J Cancer* 1994;69:529–536.

72. Fujita M, Inoue M, Tanizawa O, Miagawa J, Yamada T, Tani T. Retrospective review of 41 patients with endodermal sinus tumor of the ovary. *Int J Gynecol Cancer* 1993;3:329–335.

73. Kawai M, Kano T, Kikkawa F, Morikawa Y, Oguchi H, Nakashima N, et al. Seven tumor markers in benign and malignant germ cell tumors of the ovary. *Gynecol Oncol* 1992;45:248–253.

74. Abu-Rustum NR, Aghajanian C. Management of malignant germ cell tumors of the ovary. *Semin Oncol* 1998;25:235–242.

75. Newlands ES, Southall PJ, Paradinas FJ, Holden L. Management of ovarian germ cell tumours. In: Williams CJ, Krikorian JG, Green MR, Ragavan D, eds. *Textbook of uncommon cancer.* New York: John Wiley & Sons, 1988:37–53.

76. Ueda G, Abe Y, Yoshida M, Fujiwara T. Embryonal carcinoma of the ovary: a six-year survival. *Gynecol Oncol* 1990;31:287–292.

77. Kammerer-Doak D, Baurick K, Black W, Barbo DM, Smith HO. Endodermal sinus tumor and embryonal carcinoma of the ovary in a 53-year-old woman. *Gynecol Oncol* 1996;63:133–137.

78. Tay SK, Tan LK. Experience of a 2-day BEP regimen in postsurgical adjuvant chemotherapy of ovarian germ cell tumors. *Int J Gynecol Cancer* 2000;10:13–18.

79. Simosek T, Trak B, Thnoc M, Karaveli S, Uner M, Seonmez C. Primary pure choriocarcinoma of the ovary in reproductive ages: a case report. *Eur J Gynaecol Oncol* 1998;19:284–286.

80. Oliva E, Andrada E, Pezzica E, Prat J. Ovarian carcinomas with choriocarcinomatous differentiation. *Cancer* 1993;72:2441–2446.

81. Cushing B, Giller R, Ablin A, Cohen L, Cullen J, Hawkins E, et al. Surgical resection alone is effective treatment for ovarian immature teratoma in children and adolescents: a report of the Pediatric Oncology Group and the Children's Cancer Group. *Am J Obstet Gynecol* 1999;181:353–358.

82. Dark GG, Bower M, Newlands ES, Paradinas F, Rustin G. Surveillance policy for stage I ovarian germ cell tumors. *J Clin Oncol* 1997;15:620–624.

83. Patterson DM, Murugaesu N, Holden L, Seckl MJ, Rustin GJ. A review of the close surveillance policy for stage I female germ cell tumors of the ovary and other sites. *Int J Gynecol Cancer* 2008;18:43–50.

84. Efstathiou E, Logothetis CJ. Review of late complications of treatment and late relapse in testicular cancer. *J Natl Compr Canc Netw* 2006;4:1059–1070.

85. Chaudhary UB, Haldas JR. Long-term complications of chemotherapy for germ cell tumours. *Drugs* 2003;63:1565–1577.

86. Gershenson DM, Miller AM, Champion VL, Monahan PO, Zhao Q, Cella D, et al., for the Gynecologic Oncology Group. Reproductive and sexual function after platinum-based chemotherapy in long-term ovarian germ cell tumor survivors: a Gynecologic Oncology Group Study. *J Clin Oncol* 2007;25:2792–2797.

87. Schneider DT, Hilgenfeld E, Schwabe D, Behnisch W, Zoubek A, Wessalowski R, et al. Acute myelogenous leukemia after treatment for malignant germ cell tumors in children. *J Clin Oncol* 1999;17:3226–3233.

88. Kollmannsberger C, Beyer J, Droz JP, Harstrick A, Hartmann JT, Biron P, et al. Secondary leukemia following high cumulative doses of *etoposide* in patients treated for advanced germ cell tumors. *J Clin Oncol* 1998;16:3386–3391.

89. Young RE, Scully RE. Ovarian sex cord-stromal tumors: problems in differential diagnosis. *Ann Pathol* 1988;23:237–296.

90. Miller BE, Barron BA, Wan JY, Delmore JE, Silva EG, Gershenson DM. Prognostic factors in adult granulosa cell tumor of the ovary. *Cancer* 1997;79:1951–1955.

91. Malmström H, Högberg T, Risberg B, Simonsen E. Granulosa cell tumors of the ovary: prognostic factors and outcome. *Gynecol Oncol* 1994;52:50–55.

92. Segal R, DePetrillo AD, Thomas G. Clinical review of adult granulosa cell tumors of the ovary. *Gynecol Oncol* 1995;56:338–344.

93. Cronje HS, Niemand I, Barn, RH, Woodruff JD. Review of the granulosa–theca cell tumors from the Emil Novak ovarian tumor registry. *Am J Obstet Gynecol* 1999;180:323–328.

94. Aboud E. A review of granulosa cell tumours and thecomas of the ovary. *Arch Gynecol Obstet* 1997;259:161–165.

95. Young R, Clement PB, Scully RE. The ovary. In: Sternberg SS, ed. *Diagnostic surgical pathology.* New York: Raven Press, 1989:1687.

96. Lappohn RE, Burger HG, Bouma J, Bangah M, Krans M, de Bruijn HW. Inhibin as a marker for granulosa-cell tumors. *N Engl J Med* 1989;321:790–793.

97. Hildebrandt RH, Rouse RV, Longacre TA. Value of inhibin in the identification of granulosa cell tumors of the ovary. *Hum Pathol* 1997;28:1387–1395.

98. Richi M, Howard LN, Bratthauae GL, Tavassoli FA. Use of monoclonal antibody against human inhibin as a marker for sex-cord-stromal tumors of the ovary. *Am J Surg Pathol* 1997:21:583–589.

99. Matias-Guiu X, Pons C, Prat J. Müllerian inhibiting substance, alpha-inhibin, and CD99 expression in sex cord-stromal tumors and endometrioid ovarian carcinomas resembling sex cord-stromal tumors. *Hum Pathol* 1998;29:840–845.

100. McCluggage WG. Recent advances in immunohistochemistry in the diagnosis of ovarian neoplasms. *J Clin Pathol* 2000;53:327–334.

101. Rey RA, Lhomme C, Marcillac I, Lahlou N, Duvillard P, Josso N, et al. Antimüllerian hormone as a serum marker of granulosa cell tumors of the ovary: comparative study with serum alpha-inhibin and estradiol. *Am J Obstet Gynecol* 1996;174:958–965.

102. Schumer ST, Cannistra SA. Granulosa cell tumor of the ovary. *J Clin Oncol* 2003;21:1180–1189.

103. Wolf JK, Mullen J, Eifel PJ, Burke TW, Levenback C, Gershenson DM. Radiation treatment of advanced or recurrent granulosa cell tumor of the ovary. *Gynecol Oncol* 1999;73:35–41.

104. Savage P, Constenla D, Fisher C, Shepherd JH, Barton DP, Blake P, et al. Granulosa cell tumours of the ovary: demographics, survival and the management of advanced disease. *Clin Oncol (R Coll Radiol)* 1998;10:242–245.

105. Gershenson DM, Copeland IA, Kavanagh JJ, Stringer CA, Saul PB, Wharton JT. Treatment of metastatic stromal tumors of the ovary with *cisplatin, doxorubicin,* and *cyclophosphamide. Obstet Gynecol* 1987;5:765–769.

106. Holland DR, Le Riche J, Swenerton KD, Elit L, Spinelli J. Flow cytometric assessment of DNA ploidy is a useful prognostic factor for patients with granulosa cell ovarian tumors. *Int J Gynecol Cancer* 1991;1:227–232.

107. Uygun K, Aydiner A, Saip P, Kocak Z, Basaran M, Dincer M, et al. Clinical parameters and treatment results in recurrent granulosa cell tumor of the ovary. *Gynecol Oncol* 2003;88:400–403.

108. Al-Badawi IA, Brasher PM, Ghatage P, Nation JG, Schepansky A, Stuart GC. Postoperative chemotherapy in advanced ovarian granulosa cell tumors. *Int J Gynecol Cancer* 2002;12:119–123.

109. Homesley HD, Bundy BN, Hurteau JA, Roth LM. *Bleomycin, etoposide,* and *cisplatin* combination therapy of ovarian granulosa cell tumors and other stromal malignancies: a Gynecologic Oncology Group study. *Gynecol Oncol* 1999;72:131–137.

110. Colombo N, Sessa C, Landoni F, Sartori E, Pecorelli S, Mangioni C. *Cisplatin, vinblastine,* and *bleomycin* combination chemotherapy in metastatic granulosa cell tumor of the ovary. *Obstet Gynecol* 1986;67:265–268.

111. Zambetti M, Escobedo A, Pilotti S, De Palo G. *Cis-platinum/vinblastine/bleomycin* combination chemotherapy in advanced or recurrent granulosa cell tumors of the ovary. *Gynecol Oncol* 1990; 36:317–320.

112. Lauszus FF, Petersen,AC, Greisen J, Jakobsen A. Granulosa cell tumor of the ovary: a population-based study of 37 women with stage I disease. *Gynecol Oncol* 2001;81:456–460.

113. Miller BE, Barron BA, Wan JY, Delmore JE, Silva EG, Gershenson DM. Prognostic factors in adult granulosa cell tumor of the ovary. *Cancer* 1997;79:1951–1955.

114. Gershenson DM, Morris M, Burke TW, Levenback C, Matthews CM, Wharton JT. Treatment of poor-prognosis sex cord-stromal tumors of the ovary with the combination of *bleomycin, etoposide,* and *cisplatin. Obstet Gynecol* 1996;87:527–531.

115. Powell JL, Otis CN. Management of advanced juvenile granulosa cell tumor of the ovary. *Gynecol Oncol* 1997;64:282–284.

116. Pecorelli S, Wagenaar HC, Vergote IB, Curran D, Beex LV, Wiltshaw E, et al. *Cisplatin* (P), *vinblastine* (V), and *bleomycin* (B) combination chemotherapy in recurrent or advanced granulosa(-theca) cell tumours of the ovary. An EORTC Gynaecological Cancer Cooperative Group study. *Eur J Cancer* 1999;35:1331–1337.

117. Muntz HG, Goff BA, Fuller AF Jr. Recurrent ovarian granulosa cell tumor: role of combination chemotherapy with report of a long-term response to a *cyclophosphamide, doxorubicin,* and *cisplatin* regimen. *Eur J Gynaecol Oncol* 1990;11:263–268.

118. Tresukosol D, Kudelka AP, Edwards CL, Charnsangavej C, Narboni N, Kavanagh JJ. Recurrent ovarian granulosa cell tumor: a case report of a dramatic response to *Taxol. Int J Gynecol Cancer* 1995;5:156–159.

119. Brown J, Shvartsman HS, Deavers MT, Ramondetta LM, Burke TW, Munsell MF, et al. The activity of *taxanes* compared with *bleomycin, etoposide,* and *cisplatin* in the treatment of sex cord-stromal ovarian tumors. *Gynecol Oncol* 2005;97:489–496.

120. Hardy RD, Bell JG, Nicely CJ, Reid GC. Hormonal treatment of a recurrent granulosa cell tumor of the ovary: case report and review of the literature. *Gynecol Oncol* 2005;96:865–869.

121. Emons G, Schally AV. The use of luteinizing hormone releasing hormone agonists and antagonists in gynaecological cancers. *Hum Reprod* 1994;9:1364–1379.

122. Martikainen H, Penttinen J, Huhtaniemi I, Kauppila A. Gonadotropin-releasing hormone agonist analog therapy effective in ovarian granulosa cell malignancy. *Gynecol Oncol* 1989;35:406.

123. Fishman A, Kudelka. AP, Tresukosol D, Edwards CL, Freedman RS, Kaplan AL, et al. *Leuprolide acetate* for treating refractory or persistent ovarian granulosa cell tumor. *J Reprod Med* 1996;41:393–396.

124. Briasoulis E, Karavasilis V, Pavlidis N. Megestrol activity in recurrent adult type granulosa cell tumour of the ovary. *Ann Oncol* 1997;8:811–812.

125. Freeman SA, Modesitt SC. *Anastrozole* therapy in recurrent ovarian adult granulosa cell tumors: a report of 2 cases. *Gynecol Oncol* 2006 Nov;103:755–758.

126. Ala-Fossi SL, Maenpaa J, Aine R, Koivisto P, Koivisto AM, Punnonen R. Prognostic significance of *p53* expression in ovarian granulosa cell tumors. *Gynecol Oncol* 1997;66:475–479.

127. **Roth LM, Anderson MC, Govan AD, Langley FA, Gowing NF, Woodcock AS.** Sertoli-Leydig cell tumors: a clinicopathologic study of 34 cases. *Cancer* 1981;48:187–197.

128. **Tomlinson MW, Treadwell MC, Deppe G.** Platinum based chemotherapy to treat recurrent Sertoli-Leydig cell ovarian carcinoma during pregnancy. *Eur J Gynaecol Oncol* 1997;18:44–46.

129. **Le T, Krepart GV, Lotocki RJ, Heywood MS.** Malignant mixed mesodermal ovarian tumor treatment and prognosis: a 20-year experience. *Gynecol Oncol* 1997;65:237–240.

130. **Piura B, Rabinovich A, Yanai-Inbar I, Cohen Y, Glezerman M.** Primary sarcoma of the ovary: report of five cases and review of the literature. *Eur J Gynaecol Oncol* 1998;19:257–261.

131. **Topuz E, Eralp Y, Aydiner A, Saip P, Tas F, Yavuz E, et al.** The role of chemotherapy in malignant mixed müllerian tumors of the female genital tract. *Eur J Gynaecol Oncol* 2001;22:469–472.

132. **van Rijswijk RE, Tognon G, Burger CW, Baak JP, Kenemans P, Vermorken JB.** The effect of chemotherapy on the different components of advanced carcinosarcomas (malignant mixed mesodermal tumors) of the female genital tract. *Int J Gynecol Cancer* 1994;4:52–60.

133. **Berek JS, Hacker NF.** Sarcomas of the female genital tract. In: **Eilber FR, Morton DL, Sondak VK, Economou JS, eds.** *The soft tissue sarcomas.* Orlando, FL: Grune & Stratton, 1987:229–238.

134. **Barakat RR, Rubin SC, Wong G, Saigo PE, Markman M, Hoskins WJ.** Mixed mesodermal tumor of the ovary: analysis of prognostic factors in 31 cases. *Obstet Gynecol* 1992;80:660–664.

135. **Fowler JM, Nathan L, Nieberg RK, Berek JS.** Mixed mesodermal sarcoma of the ovary in a young patient. *Eur J Obstet Gynecol Reproduc Biol* 1996;65:249–253.

136. **Silasi DA, Illuzzi JL, Kelly MG, Rutherford TJ, Mor G, Azodi M, et al.** Carcinosarcoma of the ovary. *Int J Gynecol Cancer* 2008;18:22–29.

137. **Leiser AL, Chi DS, Ishill NM, Tew WP.** Carcinosarcoma of the ovary treated with platinum and taxane: the Memorial Sloan-Kettering Cancer Center experience. *Gynecol Oncol* 2007;105:657–661.

138. **Young RH, Oliva E, Scully RE.** Small cell sarcoma of the ovary, hypercalcemic type: a clinicopathological analysis of 150 cases. *Am J Surg Pathol* 1994;18:1102–1116.

139. **Harrison ML, Hoskins P, du Bois A, Quinn M, Rustin GJ, Ledermann JA, et al.** Small cell of the ovary, hypercalcemic type—analysis of combined experience and recommendation for management. A GCIG study. *Gynecol Oncol* 2006;100:233–238.

140. **Pautier P, Ribrag V, Duvillard P, Rey A, Elghissassi I, Sillet-Bach I, et al.** Results of a prospective dose-intensive regimen in 27 patients with small cell carcinoma of the ovary of the hypercalcemic type. *Ann Oncol* 2007;18:1985–1989.

141. **Petru E, Pickel H, Heydarfadai M, Lahousen M, Haas J, Schaider H, et al.** Non-genital cancers metastatic to the ovary. *Gynecol Oncol* 1992;44:83–86.

142. **Demopoulos RI, Touger L, Dubin N.** Secondary ovarian carcinoma: a clinical and pathological evaluation. *Int J Gynecol Pathol* 1987;6:166–175.

143. **Young RH, Scully RE.** Metastatic tumors in the ovary: a problem-oriented approach and review of the recent literature. *Semin Diagn Pathol* 1991;8:250–276.

144. **Moore RG, Chung M, Granai CO, Gajewski W, Steinhoff MM.** Incidence of metastasis to the ovaries from nongenital tract tumors. *Gynecol Oncol* 2004;93:87–91.

145. **Ayhan A, Tuncer ZS, Bukulmez O.** Malignant tumors metastatic to the ovaries. *J Surg Oncol* 1995;60:268–276.

146. **Curtin JP, Barakat RR, Hoskins WJ.** Ovarian disease in women with breast cancer. *Obstet Gynecol* 1994;84:449–452.

147. **Yada-Hashimoto N, Yamamoto T, Kamiura S, Seino H, Ohira H, Sawai K, et al.** Metastatic ovarian tumors: a review of 64 cases. *Gynecol Oncol* 2003;89:314–317.

148. **Kim HK, Heo DS, Bang YJ, Kim NK.** Prognostic factors of Krukenberg's tumor. *Gynecol Oncol* 2001;82:105–109.

149. **Yakushiji M, Tazaki T, Nishimura H, Kato T.** Krukenberg tumors of the ovary: a clinicopathologic analysis of 112 cases. *Acta Obstet Gynaecol Jpn* 1987;39:479–485.

150. **Misdraji J, Yantiss RK, Graeme-Cook FM, Balis UJ, Young RH.** Appendiceal mucinous neoplasms: a clinicopathologic analysis of 107 cases. *Am J Surg Pathol* 2003;27:1089–1103.

151. **Chou YY, Jeng YM, Kao HL, Chen T, Mao TL, Lin MC.** Differentiation of ovarian mucinous carci-noma and metastatic colorectal adenocarcinoma by immunostaining with beta-catenin. *Histopathology* 2003 ;43:151–156.

152. **Seidman JD, Kurman RJ, Ronnett BM.** Primary and metastatic mucinous adenocarcinomas in the ovaries: incidence in routine practice with a new approach to improve intraoperative diagnosis. *Am J Surg Pathol* 2003;27:985–993.

153. **Lee KR, Young RH.** The distinction between primary and metastatic mucinous carcinomas of the ovary: gross and histologic findings in 50 cases. *Am J Surg Pathol* 2003;27:281–292.

154. **McBroom JW, Parker MF, Krivak TC, Rose GS, Crothers B.** Primary appendiceal malignancy mimicking advanced stage ovarian carcinoma: a case series. *Gynecol Oncol* 2000;78:388–390.

155. **Schofield A, Pitt J, Biring G, Dawson PM.** Oophorectomy in primary colorectal cancer. *Ann R Coll Surg Engl* 2001;83:81–84.

156. **Ayhan A, Guvenal T, Coskun F, Basaran M, Salman MC.** Survival and prognostic factors in patients with synchronous ovarian and endometrial cancers and endometrial cancers metastatic to the ovaries. *Eur J Gynaecol Oncol* 2003;24:171–174.

157. **Young RH, Scully RE.** Malignant melanoma metastatic to the ovary: a clinicopathologic analysis of 20 cases. *Am J Surg Pathol* 1991;15:849–860.

158. **Davis GL.** Malignant melanoma arising in mature ovarian cystic teratoma (dermoid cyst): report of two cases and literature analysis. *Int J Gynecol Pathol* 1996;15:356–362.

159. **Motoyama T, Katayama Y, Watanabe H, Okazaki E, Shibuya H.** Functioning ovarian carcinoids induce severe constipation. *Cancer* 1991;70:513–518.

160. **Robbins ML, Sunshine TJ.** Metastatic carcinoid diagnosed at laparoscopic excision of pelvic endometriosis. *J Am Assoc Gynecol Laparosc* 2000;7:251–253.

161. **Fox H, Langley FA, Govan AD, Hill AS, Bennett MH.** Malignant lymphoma presenting as an ovarian tumour: a clinicopathological analysis of 34 cases. *BJOG* 1988;95:386–390.

162. **Monterroso V, Jaffe ES, Merino MJ, Medeiros LJ.** Malignant lymphomas involving the ovary: a clinicopathologic analysis of 39 cases. *Am J Surg Pathol* 1993;17:154–170.

163. **Azizoglu C, Altinok G, Uner A, Sokmensuer C, Kucukali T, Ayhan A.** Ovarian lymphomas: a clinicopathological analysis of 10 cases. *Arch Gynecol Obstet* 2001;265:91–93.

13 Vulvar Cancer

Neville F. Hacker

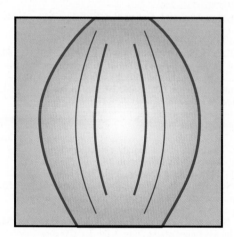

Vulvar cancer is uncommon, representing approximately 4% of malignancies of the female genital tract. There were estimated to be 3,580 new cases of vulvar cancer diagnosed in the United States in 2009 and 900 deaths (1). Squamous cell carcinomas account for approximately 90% of the cases, whereas melanomas, adenocarcinomas, basal cell carcinomas, and sarcomas are much less common.

There has been a significant increase in the incidence of vulvar intraepithelial neoplasia (VIN) and VIN-related cancer in young women in recent decades (2,3,4), and this relates to changing sexual behavior, human papilloma virus (HPV) infection, and cigarette smoking (5). Judson et al. reviewed 13,176 *in situ* and invasive vulvar carcinomas from the SEER database over a 28-year period (1973–2000); 57% of the cases were *in situ* (2). There was a 411% increase in the incidence of *in situ* carcinoma from 1973 to 2000, while the incidence of invasive carcinoma increased 20% during the same period. The incidence of *in situ* disease increased until the age of 40 to 49 years, and then decreased, whereas the invasive cancer risk increased with age, and increased more rapidly after age 50.

It may be anticipated that the recent implementation of prophylactic HPV vaccination in young females will ultimately result in a significant decrease in the incidence of HPV-related *in situ* and invasive vulvar cancer, particularly in younger women.

In the early part of the 20th century, patients commonly presented with advanced disease, and surgical techniques were poorly developed; thus, the 5-year survival rate for vulvar cancer was 20% to 25% (6,7). Basset (8), in France, was the first to suggest an *en bloc* dissection of the vulva, groin, and iliac lymph nodes, although he performed the operation only on cadavers. Taussig (9), in the United States, and Way (10), in Great Britain, pioneered the radical *en bloc* dissection for vulvar cancer and reported 5-year survival rates of 60% to 70%. Postoperative morbidity was high after these procedures, with wound breakdown, infection, and prolonged hospitalization the norm. For patients with disease involving the anus, rectum, or proximal urethra, pelvic exenteration was often combined with radical vulvectomy.

Since approximately 1980, there has been a paradigm shift in the approach to vulvar cancer (11). The most significant advances have included:

1. **Individualization of treatment** for all patients with invasive disease (12,13).
2. The introduction of **a multidisciplinary team approach** to management (11).
3. **Vulvar conservation** for patients with unifocal tumors and an otherwise normal vulva (12–16).

536

4. **Omission of the groin dissection for patients with T₁ tumors and no more than 1 mm of stroinal invasion** (12–13).

5. **Elimination of routine pelvic lymphadenectomy** (17–21).

6. **The use of separate groin incisions** for the groin dissection to improve wound healing (22).

7. **Omission of the contralateral groin dissection** in patients with lateral T₁ lesions and negative ipsilateral nodes (12,13,23).

8. **The use of preoperative radiation therapy** to obviate the need for exenteration in patients with advanced disease (24,25).

9. **The use of postoperative radiation to decrease the incidence of groin recurrence in patients with multiple positive groin nodes** (21).

Innovations that are currently being investigated include the **sentinel node procedure** to obviate the need for complete groin dissection in patients with early vulvar cancer (26-29) and **chemoradiation** for patients with advanced vulvar cancer (30-35). **Resection of bulky positive nodes** without complete groin dissection to decrease the risk of lymphedema prior to pelvic and groin radiation is another initiative aimed at decreasing morbidity without compromising survival (36).

This paradigm shift in the management philosophy of vulvar cancer has been well exemplified in retrospective reviews of the experience at the University of Miami (37) and the Mayo Clinic (38). Both centers reported a trend toward a more conservative approach, and both reported decreased postoperative morbidity, without compromised survival.

Etiology

No specific etiologic factor has been identified for vulvar cancer, and the relationship of the invasive disease to vulvar dystrophy and to vulvar intraepithelial neoplasia (VIN) is controversial. Chronic pruritus is usually an important antecedent phenomenon in patients with invasive vulvar cancer (39).

VIN has traditionally been considered to have a low malignant potential, with progression to invasive disease most likely in the elderly or immunosuppressed (40). **This concept has been challenged** by Jones et al. (41), who reported a series of 405 cases of VIN 2-3 seen between 1962 and 2003 in Auckland, New Zealand. Progression to malignant disease occurred in 10 of 16 (62.5%) untreated patients with persistent VIN. Progression occurred between 1.1 and 7.3 years (mean 3.9 years). Invasive vulvar, perianal, or urethral cancer occurred in 17 women (3.8%) after treatment (mean age 42 years). Nine (2%) of the cases represented treated failure, with a median treatment-to-invasion interval of 2.4 years, while eight (1.8%) represented new "field" carcinomas, with a median treatment-to-invasion interval of 13.5 years. **Spontaneous regression of VIN occurred in 47 women (11.6%). These women were young (mean age 24.6 years),** and the median interval to complete regression was 9.5 months.

Using data on 2,685 patients with invasive vulvar cancer from the National Cancer Institute's Surveillance Epidemiology and End Results program (SEER), Sturgeon et al. (42) reported **an increased risk of a subsequent cancer of 1.3 fold. Most of the second cancers were smoking related** (i.e., cancers of the lung, buccal cavity, pharynx, nasal cavity, and larynx) or related to infection with human papillomavirus (HPV; e.g., cervix, vagina, and anus).

The common association between cervical, vaginal, and vulvar cancer suggests a common pathogen, and the case-control study by Brinton et al. (43) found a significantly increased risk in association with multiple sexual partners, a history of genital warts, and smoking. **HPV DNA has been reported in 20% to 60% of patients with invasive vulvar cancer** (44). Hording et al. (45) reported HPV subtypes 16 or 33 in only 2 of 51 (4%) invasive keratinizing vulvar carcinomas, whereas one or the other was demonstrated in 12 of 17 (71%) invasive warty carcinomas and 10 of 10 (100%) invasive basaloid carcinomas. **The HPV-positive group has been characterized by a younger mean age, greater tobacco use, and the presence of VIN in association with the invasive component** (45–48).

These studies suggest two different etiologic types of vulvar cancer. **One type is seen mainly in younger patients, is related to HPV infection and smoking, and is commonly associated with basaloid or warty VIN. The more common type is seen mainly in elderly patients, is**

unrelated to smoking or HPV infection, and concurrent VIN is uncommon, but there is a high incidence of dystrophic lesions, including lichen sclerosus, adjacent to the tumor. If VIN is present, it is of the differentiated type, and is situated adjacent to the invasive cancer (49).

Other diseases known to be occasionally associated with vulvar cancer include syphilis and nonleutic granulomatous venereal disease, particularly lymphogranuloma venereum and granuloma inguinale (*Donovanosis*). Such diseases are not seen commonly in Western countries.

Noninvasive Disease

Nonneoplastic Epithelial Disorders

The most recent recommendation on classification of vulvar diseases from the International Society for the Study of Vulvar Disease (ISSVD) is shown in Table 13.1. **The new classification of squamous vulvar intraepithelial neoplasia (VIN) was introduced in 2004 (50). The term VIN 1 is no longer used, and VIN 2 and 3 are simply called VIN.** Diagnosis in all cases requires biopsy of suspicious lesions, which are best detected by careful inspection of the vulva in a bright light, aided if necessary by a magnifying glass.

The older classification of VIN 1, 2, and 3 was based on the degree of histologic abnormality. However, there is neither evidence that the VIN 1-3 morphologic spectrum reflects a biologic continuum, nor that VIN 1 is a cancer precursor (49,50). The high-grade VIN lesions (2 and 3) include 2 types: (i) **VIN usual type** (warty, basaloid, and mixed), which is HPV related in most cases. Invasive squamous cancer of the warty or basaloid type is associated with VIN, usual type, (ii) **VIN differentiated type,** which is seen particularly in older women with lichen sclerosus and/or squamous cell hyperplasia. **Neither VIN differentiated type nor associated keratinizing squamous cell carcinoma is HPV related.**

The malignant potential of these nonneoplastic epithelial disorders is low, particularly now that the lesions with atypia are classified as VIN. However, patients with lichen sclerosus and concomitant hyperplasia may be at particular risk. Rodke and colleagues (51) reported the development of vulvar carcinoma in 3 of 18 such cases (17%), postulating that the areas of hyperplasia were superimposed on a background of lichen sclerosus because of chronic irritation and trauma.

Table 13.1 Classification of Vulvar Diseases
Nonneoplastic epithelial disorders of skin and mucosa
Lichen sclerosus (as before)
Squamous hyperplasia, not otherwise specified (formerly "hyperplastic dystrophy without atypia")
Other dermatoses
Mixed nonneoplastic and neoplastic epithelial disorders
Intraepithelial neoplasia
Squamous intraepithelial neoplasia (formerly "dystrophies with atypia")
VIN, usual type
VIN differentiated type
Nonsquamous intraepithelial neoplasia
Paget's disease
Tumors of melanocytes, noninvasive
Invasive tumors
VIN, Vulvar intraepithelial neoplasia

From Committee on Terminology, International Society for the Study of Vulvar Disease. New nomenclature for vulvar disease. *J Reprod Med* 2005;50:807–810, with permission.

Table 13.2 Classification of Paget's Disease of the Vulva
1. *Primary Paget's disease of the vulva:*
a. **Intraepithelial Paget's disease**
b. **Intraepithelial Paget's disease with stromal invasion**
c. **As a manifestation of an underlying adenocarcinoma of a skin appendage or subcutaneous vulvar gland**
2. *Secondary Paget's disease of the vulva:*
a. **Secondary to an anorectal adenocarcinoma**
b. **Secondary to an urothelial carcinoma**
c. **As a manifestation of another noncutaneous adenocarcinoma (eg., endocervical, endometrial, ovarian)**

Modified from **Wilkinson RJ and Brown H.** *Human Pathology.* 2002;33:S49–S54.

Carli and colleagues from the Vulvar Clinic at the University of Florence, Italy, reported an association with lichen sclerosus in 32% of their cases of vulvar cancer that were not HPV related (52). They felt that the existence of accessory conditions necessary to promote the progression from lichen sclerosus to cancer remained to be established.

Scurry also supports an association between lichen sclerosus and vulvar cancer (53). He believes it contributes to a vicious cycle of itching and scratching which leads to superimposed lichen simplex chronicus, squamous cell hyperplasia, and ultimately carcinoma.

Vulvar Intraepithelial Neoplasia

The management of VIN is discussed in Chapter 8.

Paget's Disease of the Vulva

The original description of Paget's disease was of a breast lesion (Paget, 1874), in which the appearance of the nipple heralded an underlying carcinoma. Invasive carcinoma underlying Paget's disease of the vulvar is much less common.

Paget's disease of the vulva has been the subject of two recent classifications and that proposed by **Wilkinson and Brown** in 2002 is shown in Table 13.2 (54). In this classification, **Type 1 Paget's disease is of primary cutaneous origin,** and is divided into Type 1a, primary intraepithelial neoplasia; Type 1b, intraepithelial neoplasia with underlying invasion; and Type 1c, a manifestation of an underlying adenocarcinoma of a skin appendage or of vulvar glandular origin. **Type 2 Paget's disease is of noncutaneous origin.**

In the Kurman classification, Type 2 Paget's disease is a manifestation of an associated primary and/or rectal adenocarcinoma, and Type 3 is a manifestation of a urothelial neoplasm (55).

Type 1 Paget's Disease

In a review of Type 1 cases from the English literature, Niikura et al. reported on 565 cases of type 1 Paget's disease, including their own series of 22 cases (56). There were 425 patients (75%) with type 1a disease; 89 (16%) with type 1b; and 51 (9%) with type 1c. MacLean et al. reported that 6 of 76 patients (8%) on a British registry had an underlying carcinoma (type 1c) (57). In the British series, 14 patients (18.4%) had a systemic cancer. The primary was in the breast in six; bladder in three; and colorectum, cervix, uterus, and ovary in one each. One patient had a melanoma. Only four of these tumors were a synchronous cancer. Niikura et al. determined that if only synchronous neoplasms or those occurring within 12 months of the diagnosis were considered, only 8% of patients (44 of 534) with primary Paget's disease had a nonvulvar malignancy (56).

Fanning et al. reported on a combined series of 100 patients with Paget's disease of the vulva (58). Their median age was 70 years. There was a 12% prevalence of invasive vulvar Paget's disease, and a 4% prevalence of associated vulvar adenocarcinoma. Thirty-four percent of patients experienced a recurrence at a median of 3 years,

Clinical Features   The disease predominantly affects postmenopausal white women, and the presenting symptoms are usually pruritus and vulvar soreness. **The lesion has an eczematoid appearance macroscopically and usually begins on the hair-bearing portions of the vulva.** It may extend to involve the mons pubis, thighs, and buttocks. Extension to involve the mucosa of the rectum, vagina, or urinary tract also has been described (59). The more extensive lesions are usually raised and velvety in appearance and may weep persistently.

Investigations   **All patients with Paget's disease of the vulva should be screened for any associated malignancy.** These investigations should include mammography, computed tomography (CT) scan of the pelvis and abdomen, transvaginal ultrasonography, and cervical cytology. If the lesions involve the anus, colonoscopy should be undertaken, while if the urethra is involved, cystoscopy is indicated.

Treatment   The mainstay of treatment is wide superficial resection of the gross disease. **Underlying adenocarcinomas usually are clinically apparent, but this is not invariable. Paget cells may invade the underlying dermis, which should be removed for adequate histologic evaluation.** For this reason, laser therapy is unsatisfactory for primary Paget's disease. The surgical defect can usually be closed primarily, but sometimes a split thickness skin graft may be required to cover an extensive defect.

Unlike squamous cell carcinoma *in situ*, in which the histologic extent of disease usually correlates reasonably with the macroscopic lesion, Paget's disease usually extends well beyond the gross lesion (60). This results in frequent positive surgical margins. The group at Memorial Sloan-Kettering Cancer Center reported positive margins in 20 of 28 patients (71%) (61). Of the 20 patients with microscopically positive margins, 14 (70%) developed recurrent disease, while of the 8 patients with negative margins, 3 (38%) developed a recurrence. With a median follow-up of 49 months (range 3–186 months), there was no correlation between disease recurrence and margin status ($p = 0.20$).

Surgical margins may be checked with frozen sections (62), but these can be misleading when compared to the definitive histology (63). **Resection of the entire gross lesion will control symptoms and exclude invasive disease.**

The role of **radiotherapy** for vulvar Paget's cancer has been reviewed by Brown et al. (64). It **may be most useful when the disease involves the anus or urethra**, and surgery would involve diversion and stoma formation.

If an underlying invasive carcinoma is present, it should be treated in the same manner as a squamous vulvar cancer. This may require radical vulvectomy and at least an ipsilateral inguinofemoral lymphadenectomy. From their literature review, Niikura et al. reported positive nodes in 30% of patients (23 of 70) with types 1b or 1c Paget's disease of the vulva (56).

Lymph node metastases have been reported in patients with very superficially invasive tumors. Fine et al. reported a patient who had invasion no greater than 1 mm over a maximum length of 10 mm at her primary operation. Three weeks later, she was noted to have a palpable groin node, and at groin dissection, six positive groin nodes were resected from each groin (65). Ewing et al reported a positive sentinel node in a patient whose excised Paget's disease had scattered foci of superficial dermal invasion to a maximum depth of 0.7 mm (66).

Minimally invasive Paget's disease is rare, and in both cases the surgical margins were positive for intraepithelial disease. **It would seem prudent to at least monitor the groins carefully, preferably with ultrasound, if the nodes are not dissected in a patient with superficially invasive Paget's disease.**

The disease is characterized by local recurrences over many years (61,57). **Recurrent lesions are usually *in situ*, although 5 of 76 patients (6.7%) in the British registry showed progression to invasive disease** between 1 and 21 years after the initial diagnosis (57). The age at the time of diagnosis of the invasive recurrence ranged from 63 to 88 years (mean 76.2 years). Investigators at the Norwegian Radium Hospital have demonstrated that nondiploid tumors have an increased risk of recurrence regardless of surgical radicality (67). In general, recurrent lesions should be treated by further surgical resection, although laser therapy may occasionally be useful, particularly for perianal disease.

Invasive Vulvar Cancer

Squamous Cell Carcinoma

Squamous cell carcinoma of the vulva is predominantly a disease of postmenopausal women, with a mean age at diagnosis of approximately 65 years.

Clinical Features

Most patients present with a vulvar lump or mass, although there is often a long history of pruritus, usually associated with a vulvar dystrophy. Less common presenting symptoms include vulvar bleeding, discharge, or dysuria. Occasionally a large metastatic mass in the groin may be the initial presenting symptom, although this is much less common than in the past because women are now more likely to present with earlier-stage disease.

On physical examination, the lesion is usually raised and may be fleshy, ulcerated, leukoplakic, or warty in appearance. Warty lesions are often initially diagnosed as condylomata acuminata.

Most squamous carcinomas of the vulva occur on the labia majora, but the labia minora, clitoris, and perineum also may be primary sites. A recent study from one University Hospital in Germany reported that the tumor localization had changed significantly from the labia to the area between the clitoris and the urethra (3). Approximately 10% of the cases are too extensive to determine a site of origin, and approximately 5% of the cases are multifocal.

As part of the clinical assessment, the groin lymph nodes should be evaluated carefully and a complete pelvic examination performed. A Papanicolaou smear should be taken from the cervix, and **colposcopy of the cervix and vagina should be performed because of the common association with other squamous intraepithelial neoplasms of the lower genital tract.**

Diagnosis

Diagnosis requires a wedge or a Keyes biopsy specimen, which usually can be taken in the office under local anesthesia. The biopsy specimen must include some underlying dermis and connective tissue so that the pathologist can adequately evaluate the depth and nature of the stromal invasion. It is preferable to leave the primary lesion *in situ,* if possible, to allow the treating surgeon to fashion adequate surgical margins.

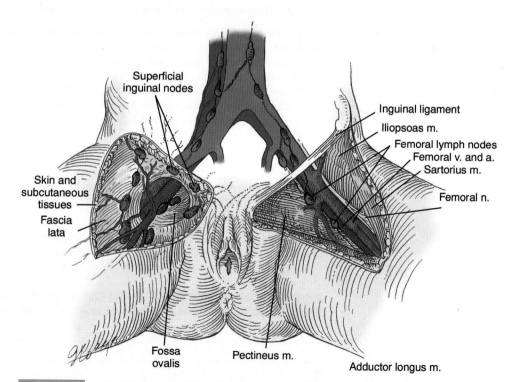

Figure 13.1   **Inguinal-femoral lymph nodes.** (Reproduced from **Hacker NF.** Vulvar cancer. In: **Hacker NF, Moore JG.** *Essentials of obstetrics and gynecology,* 5th ed. Philadelphia: Elsevier Saunders, 2008, with permission.)

Table 13.3 Incidence of Lymph Node Metastases in Operable Vulvar Cancer			
Author	*No. of Cases*	*Positive Nodes*	*Percent*
Rutledge *et al.*, 1970 (75)	110	40	36.4
Green, 1978 (76)	142	54	38.0
Krupp and Bohm, 1978 (77)	195	40	20.5
Benedet *et al.*, 1979 (78)	120	34	28.3
Curry *et al.*, 1980 (17)	191	57	29.8
Iversen *et al.*, 1980 (79)	268	86	32.1
Hacker *et al.*, 1983 (18)	113	31	27.4
Monaghan and Hammond, 1984 (19)	134	37	27.6
Rouzier *et al.*, 2002 (80)	180	54	30.0
Raspagliesi *et al.*, 2006 (81)	389	110	28.3
Bosquet *et al.*, 2007 (82)	320	108	33.8
Total	**2,162**	**651**	**30.1**

Physician delay is a common problem in the diagnosis of vulvar cancer, particularly if the lesion has a warty appearance. Although isolated condylomata do not require histologic confirmation for diagnosis, **any confluent warty lesion should be biopsied adequately before medical or ablative therapy is initiated.**

Routes of Spread

Vulvar cancer spreads by the following routes:

1. **Direct extension,** to involve adjacent structures such as the vagina, urethra, and anus.
2. **Lymphatic embolization** to regional lymph nodes.
3. **Hematogenous spread** to distant sites, including the lungs, liver, and bone.

Lymphatic metastases may occur early in the disease. Initially, spread is usually to the inguinal lymph nodes, which are located between Camper's fascia and the fascia lata. From these superficial groin nodes, the disease spreads to the femoral nodes, which are located medial to the femoral vein (Fig. 13.1). Cloquet's node, situated beneath the inguinal ligament, is the most cephalad of the femoral node group. **Metastases to the femoral nodes without involvement of the inguinal nodes have been reported** (68–71). In addition, Gordinier and colleagues reported groin recurrence in 9 of 104 patients (8.7%) treated by superficial inguinal lymphadenectomy at the M. D. Anderson Cancer Center (72). The median number of lymph nodes removed per groin was 7, and the median time to recurrence was 22 months.

From the inguinofemoral nodes, the cancer spreads to the pelvic nodes, particularly the external iliac group. **Although direct lymphatic pathways from the clitoris and Bartholin gland to the pelvic nodes have been described, these channels seem to be of minimal clinical significance** (17,73,74).

Since 1970, the overall incidence of lymph node metastases is reported to be approximately 30% (Table 13.3). The incidence in relation to clinical stage of disease is shown in Table 13.4, and that in relation to depth of invasion is shown in Table 13.5.

Table 13.4 Incidence of Lymph Node Metastases in Relation to Clinical Stage of Disease			
Stage	*No. of Cases*	*Positive Nodes*	*Percent*
I	140	15	10.7
II	145	38	26.2
III	137	88	64.2
IV	18	16	88.9

Data compiled from **Green,** 1978 (76); **Iversen *et al.*,** 1980 (79); and **Hacker *et al.*,** 1983 (18).

Table 13.5 Nodal Status in T_1 Squamous Cell Carcinoma of the Vulva Versus Depth of Stromal Invasion

Depth of Invasion	No.	Positive Nodes	Nodes
<1 mm	163	0	0
1.1–2 mm	145	11	7.6
2.1–3 mm	131	11	8.4
3.1–5 mm	101	27	26.7
>5 mm	38	13	34.2
Total	**578**	**62**	**10.7**

Data compiled from **Parker** *et al.*, 1975 (69); **Magrina** *et al.*, 1979 (83); **Iversen** *et al.*, 1981 (12); **Wilkinson** *et al.*, 1982 (84); **Hoffman** *et al.*, 1983 (85); **Hacker** *et al.*, 1984 (13); **Boice** *et al.*, 1984 (86); **Ross and Ehrmann**, 1987 (87); **Rowley** *et al.*, 1988 (88); **Struyk** *et al.*, 1989 (89).

Metastases to pelvic nodes are uncommon, the overall reported frequency being approximately 9%. Approximately 20% of patients with positive groin nodes have positive pelvic nodes (90). Pelvic nodal metastases are rare in the absence of clinically suspicious (N_2) groin nodes (18) and three or more positive groin nodes (17,18,79,82). Recent Mayo Clinic data suggested that in addition to having 3 or more positive groin nodes, all patients with positive pelvic nodes had a tumor with invasion >4 mm (82). **Systematic pelvic lymphadenectomy is no longer performed in the management of patients with vulvar cancer.**

Hematogenous spread usually occurs late in the course of vulvar cancer and is rare in the absence of lymph node metastases. Hematogenous spread is uncommon in patients with one or two positive groin nodes, but is more common in patients with three or more positive nodes (18).

Staging

A clinical staging system based on the TNM classification was adopted by the International Federation of Gynecology and Obstetrics (FIGO) in 1969 (Table 13.6). The staging was based on a clinical evaluation of the primary tumor and regional lymph nodes and a limited search for distant metastases.

Clinical evaluation of the groin lymph nodes is inaccurate in approximately 25% to 30% of the cases (10,19,91). Microscopic metastases may be present in nodes that are not clinically suspicious, and suspicious nodes may be enlarged because of inflammation only. **Compared with surgical staging of vulvar cancer, the percentage of error in clinical staging increases from 18% for stage I disease to 44% for stage IV disease** (92).

These factors led the Cancer Committee of FIGO to introduce a surgical staging for vulvar cancer in 1988. For updated FIGO surgical staging tables (2009) see pages 665–668. Various modifications have been made, with a subdivision of stage I in 1994. The current FIGO staging is shown in Table 13.7. Most available data are still based on the 1969 FIGO staging, which is appropriate because the new staging system requires further modification.

There are two major problems with the staging system as currently proposed. **First, patients with negative lymph nodes have a very good prognosis, regardless of the size of the primary tumor** (18,78,81,92), so the survival rate for both stages I and II should be better than 80%. **Second, survival depends on the number of positive lymph nodes** (17,18,92,93). **Therefore, stage III represents a very heterogeneous group of patients**, ranging from those with negative nodes and involvement of the distal urethra or vagina, who should have an excellent prognosis, to those with multiple positive groin nodes, who have a very poor prognosis. Rouzier et al. reported a cohort of 895 patients with FIGO Stage III vulvar cancer who had been registered with the SEER database from 1988 through 2004. The 5-year overall survival for patients with regional metastatic nodal disease (39%) was significantly worse than that of patients with locally advanced tumors but negative nodes (62%, p <0.0001) (94).

Treatment

After the pioneering work of Taussig (9) in the United States and Way (7,10) in Great Britain, *en bloc* **radical vulvectomy and bilateral dissection of the groin and pelvic nodes became the standard treatment for most patients with operable vulvar cancer.** If the disease involved the anus, rectovaginal septum, or proximal urethra, some type of pelvic exenteration was combined with this dissection.

Table 13.6 Clinical Staging of Carcinoma of the Vulva

FIGO Stage	TNM	Clinical Findings
Stage 0		Carcinoma *in situ* (e.g., VIN 3, noninvasive Paget's disease)
Stage I	$T_1N_0M_0$	Tumor confined to the vulva, 2 cm or less in largest diameter, and no suspect groin nodes
	$T_1N_1M_0$	
Stage II	$T_2N_0M_0$	Tumor confined to the vulva more than 2 cm in diameter, and no suspect groin nodes
	$T_2N_1M_0$	
Stage III	$T_3N_0M_0$	Tumor of any size with:
	$T_3N_1M_0$	1. Adjacent spread to the urethra and/or the vagina, the perineum, and the anus, and/or
	$T_3N_2M_0$	2. Clinically suspect lymph nodes in either groin
	$T_1N_2M_0$	
	$T_2N_2M_0$	
Stage IV	$T_xN_3M_0$	Tumor of any size:
	$T_4N_0M_0$	1. Infiltrating the bladder mucosa, or the rectal mucosa, or both,
	$T_4N_1M_0$	including the upper part of the urethral mucosa, and/or
	$T_4N_2M_0$	2. Fixed to the bone, and/or
	$T_xN_xM_{1a}$	3. Other distant metastases
	$T_xN_xM_{1b}$	

TNM Classification

T:	Primary Tumor	N:	Regional Lymph Nodes
T_1	Tumor confined to the vulva, ≤2 cm in largest diameter	N_0	No nodes palpable
T_2	Tumor confined to the vulva, >2 cm in diameter	N_1	Nodes palpable in either groin, not enlarged, mobile (not clinically suspect for neoplasm)
T_3	Tumor of any size with adjacent spread to the urethra and/or vagina and/or perineum and/or anus	N_2	Nodes palpable in either or both groins, enlarged, firm and mobile (clinically suspect for neoplasm)
T_4	Tumor of any size infiltrating the bladder mucosa and/or the rectal mucosa, or including the upper part of the urethral mucosa and/or fixed to the bone	N_3	Fixed or ulcerated nodes

		M:	Distant Metastases
		M_0	No clinical metastases
		M_1	Palpable deep pelvic lymph nodes
		M_{1b}	Other distant metastases

For updated Carcinoma of the Cervix Uteri staging table 13.7A on page 668.

FIGO, International Federation of Gynecology and Obstetrics; VIN, vulvar intraepithelial neoplasia; x, any T or N category.

Although the survival rate improved markedly with this aggressive surgical approach, **several factors have led to modifications of this "standard" treatment plan during the past 25 years.** These factors may be summarized as follows:

1. **The disease is occurring in younger women, who are presenting with smaller tumors.** Jones et al. (4) retrospectively reviewed two cohorts of women with squamous carcinoma of the vulva in New Zealand. Only 1 of 56 patients (1.8%) seen

Table 13.7 FIGO Staging for Vulvar Cancer (1994)

FIGO Stage	TNM	Clinical/Pathologic Findings
Stage 0	T_{is}	Carcinoma *in situ,* intraepithelial carcinoma
Stage I	$T_1N_0M_0$	Tumor ≤2 cm in greatest diameter, confined to the vulva or perineum; nodes are negative
IA	$T_1N_0M_0$	As above with stromal invasion ≤1.0 mm[a]
IB	$T_{1b}N_0M_0$	As above with stromal invasion >1 mm
Stage II	$T_2N_0M_0$	Tumor confined to the vulva and/or perineum, >2 cm in greatest dimension, nodes are negative
Stage III	$T_3N_0M_0$ $T_3N_1M_0$ $T_1N_1M_0$ $T_2N_1M_0$	Tumor of any size with: 1. Adjacent spread to the lower urethra and/or the vagina and/or the anus 2. Unilateral regional lymph node metastasis
Stage IVA	$T_1N_2M_0$ $T_2N_2M_0$ $T_3N_2M_0$ T_4, any N, M_0	Tumor invades any of the following: Upper urethra, bladder mucosa, rectal mucosa, pelvic bone, or bilateral regional node metastasis
Stage IVB	Any T, any N, M_1	Any distant metastasis including pelvic lymph nodes

TNM Classification

T:	Primary Tumor	N:	Regional Lymph Nodes
T_x	Primary tumor cannot be assessed		Regional lymph nodes are the femoral and inguinal nodes
T_0	No evidence of primary tumor	N_x	Regional lymph nodes cannot be assessed
T_{is}	Carcinoma *in situ* (preinvasive carcinoma)	N_0	No lymph node metastasis
T_1	Tumor confined to the vulva and/or perineum 2 cm or less in greatest dimension	N_1	Unilateral regional lymph node metastasis
T_2	Tumor confined to the vulva and/or perineum more than 2 cm in greatest dimension	N_2	Bilateral regional lymph node metastasis
T_3	Tumor involves any of the following: lower urethra, vagina, anus	M:	Distant Metastasis
T_4	Tumor involves any of the following: bladder mucosa, rectal mucosa, upper urethra, pelvic bone	M_x	Presence of distant metastasis cannot be assessed
		M_0	No distant metastasis
		M_1	Distant metastasis (pelvic lymph node metastasis is M1)

For updated 2008 FIGO staging of Carcinoma of the Vulva, see Table 13.7A, on page 668.

FIGO, International Federation of Gynecology and Obstetrics.

[a]The depth of invasion is defined as the measurement of the tumor from the epithelial–stromal junction of the adjacent most superficial dermal papilla to the deepest point of invasion.

between 1965 and 1974 was younger than 50 years, whereas 12 of 57 women (21%) seen between 1990 and 1994 were in the younger age group ($p = 0.001$). The younger women had significantly more basaloid or warty VIN associated with invasive carcinoma ($p = 0.001$), and cigarette smoking and multiple lower genital tract neoplasia were also more commonly seen ($p = 0.001$).

2. **There has been concern about the postoperative morbidity and associated long-term hospitalization common with the *en bloc* radical dissection.**

3. **There has been an increasing awareness of the psychosexual consequences of radical vulvectomy.**

Modern management of vulvar cancer requires an experienced, multidisciplinary team approach, which is available only in tertiary referral centers. The shortcomings of treatment in nonreferral units were highlighted in two community-based European studies.

In the British study, investigators retrospectively reviewed the records of 411 patients with squamous cell carcinoma who had been notified to the Central Intelligence Unit of the West Midlands during two 3-year periods; 1980 to 1982 and 1986 to 1988 (95). The women were treated at 35 different hospitals, 16 of which averaged 1 case or less per year.

Fifteen different operations were used, the most common of which were simple vulvectomy (35%) and radical vulvectomy with bilateral inguinal lymphadenectomy (34%). Hemivulvectomy was performed in only five patients (1.2%). Management of the lymph nodes was equally inappropriate. Only 190 of the 411 patients (46%) had a lymphadenectomy performed, and a unilateral dissection was performed in only 9 patients (2.1%).

Survival data for all FIGO stages compared unfavorably with the Gynecologic Oncology Group (GOG) data from tertiary units in the United States (92): 78% versus 98% for stage I disease; 53% versus 85% for stage II; 27% versus 74% for stage III; and 13% versus 31% for stage IV. **Omission of lymphadenectomy was the single most important prognostic factor, but treatment in a hospital with less than 20 cases in total was a poor prognostic factor in univariate analysis.**

A similar experience was reported from the Netherlands (96). As in the British study, older patients tended not to be referred to gynecologic oncology units, and 80% of patients in the community hospitals had omission of groin node dissection.

Management of Early Vulvar Cancer (T_1 or $T_2 N_0$ or N_1)

The modern approach to the management of patients with carcinoma confined to the vulva should be individualized (12,13,15,16,97–99). There is no "standard" operation applicable to every patient, and emphasis is on performing the most conservative operation consistent with cure of the disease.

In considering the appropriate operation, it is necessary to determine independently the appropriate management of:

1. **The primary lesion**
2. **The groin lymph nodes**

Before any surgery, all patients should have colposcopy of the cervix, vagina, and vulva because preinvasive (and rarely invasive) lesions may be present at other sites along the lower genital tract.

Management of the Primary Lesion

The two factors to take into account in determining the management of the primary tumor are:

1. **The condition of the remainder of the vulva**
2. **The patient's age**

Although radical vulvectomy has been regarded as the standard treatment for the primary vulvar lesion, this operation is associated with significant disturbances of sexual function and body image. DiSaia et al. (14) regarded psychosexual disturbance as the major long-term morbidity associated with the treatment of vulvar cancer. Andersen and Hacker (100) reported that, when compared with healthy adult women, sexual arousal was reduced to the eighth percentile and body image to the fourth percentile in women who had undergone vulvectomy.

Since the early 1980s, several investigators have advocated a radical local excision rather than a radical vulvectomy for the primary lesion in patients with T_1 and T_2 tumors (9–13,16,90,97,98,101,102). Regardless of whether a radical vulvectomy or a radical local excision is performed, the surgical margins adjacent to the tumor are the same, and **an analysis of the available literature indicates that the incidence of local invasive recurrence is low if the histopathologic margin is at least 8 mm** (Table 13.8). Allowing for 20% tissue shrinkage with formalin fixation, this translates to a surgical margin of at least 1 cm. De Hulla et al. reported that in 50% of patients, the histologic margins were 8 mm or less in spite of intentional macroscopic margins of 1 cm (102), but in the author's experience, this will happen only if the skin is placed under tension prior to making the incisions.

When vulvar cancer arises in the presence of VIN or some nonneoplastic epithelial disorder, treatment is influenced by the patient's age. Elderly patients who have often had many

Table 13.8 Invasive Vulvar Recurrence versus Histopathologic Resection Margins				
	Histologic Margins		Recurrence	
	≥8	<8	>8	<8
	No.	No.	No.	No.
Heaps et al., 1990 (104)	91	44	0	21
de Hulla et al., 2002 (102)	39	40	0	9
Chan et al., 2007 (103)	30	53	0	12
Tantipalakorn et al., 2009 (98)	92	24	6	7
Total	252	161	2.4%	49 (30.4%)

years of chronic itching are not usually disturbed by the prospect of a radical vulvectomy. In younger women, it is desirable to conserve as much of the vulva as possible; thus, radical local excision should be performed for the invasive disease, and the associated disease should be treated in the most appropriate manner. For example, topical steroids may be required for squamous hyperplasia or lichen sclerosus, whereas VIN should be treated by superficial local excision and primary closure or split thickness skin grafting.

Radical local excision is most appropriate for lesions on the lateral or posterior aspects of the vulva (Fig. 13.2), where preservation of the clitoris is feasible. For anterior lesions that involve the clitoris or are close to it, any type of surgical excision has psychosexual consequences, particularly in younger patients. Chan et al. identified 41 patients with squamous carcinoma of the anterior vulva not involving the clitoris (105). Thirteen patients (32%) had clitoral sparing modified radical vulvectomy and 28 (68%) had radical vulvectomy. The 13 patients who had clitoral sparing surgery included 8 with stage I, 2 with stage II, 2 with stage III, and 1 with stage IV disease. After a median follow-up of 59 months, none of the 13 patients having conservative surgery had locoregional failure.

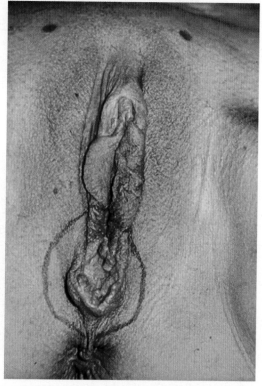

Figure 13.2   Small (T_1) vulvar carcinoma at the posterior fourchette.

In young patients with actual involvement of the clitoris or in whom surgical margins would be <5 mm, consideration should be given to treating the primary lesion with a small field of radiation therapy. Small vulvar lesions respond very well to approximately 5,000 cGy external radiation, and biopsy can be performed after therapy to confirm the absence of any residual disease (106).

Two recent papers have looked at a single institutional experience with T_1 and T_2 squamous cell carcinoma of the vulva (97,98).

In the study from Kentucky, 61 patients with a lateral T_1 lesion and 61 patients with a lateral T_2 lesion were seen from 1963 to 2003 (97). Radical vulvectomy was performed on 60 patients (49%) and radical hemivulvectomy on 62 (51%). Ipsilateral inguinal node metastases were present in 11% of patients (7 of 61) with a T_1 lesion, and 31% (19 of 61) of patients with a T_2 lesion. Disease-free survival of patients with T_1 and T_2 lesions was 98% and 93% respectively at 5 years. Local or distant recurrence was not more common in patients treated by radical vulvectomy or radical hemivulvectomy.

Our experience at the Royal Hospital for Women in Sydney with FIGO stages I and II vulvar cancer has recently been reported (98). There were 121 cases managed from 1987 through 2005, which represented 37.7% of the 339 patients with invasive vulvar cancer seen during this period. Radical local excision was performed in 116 patients (95.9%). Only 5 patients underwent radical vulvectomy, in all cases for tumor multifocality. With a median follow-up of 84 months, the overall survival at 5 years was 96.4%.

Technique for Radical Local Excision

Radical local excision implies a wide and deep excision of the primary tumor. The surgical margins should be at least 1 cm, and should be drawn using a marking pen with the vulva in its natural state. The incision should be carried down to the inferior fascia of the urogenital diaphragm, which is coplanar with the fascia lata and the fascia over the pubic symphysis. The surgical defect is closed in two layers. For perineal lesions, proximity to the anus may preclude adequate surgical margins, and consideration should be given to preoperative or postoperative radiation in such cases. For periurethral lesions, the distal half of the urethra may be resected without loss of continence. Figure 13.3 shows the satisfactory cosmetic result achieved in the treatment of the lesion shown in Fig. 13.2.

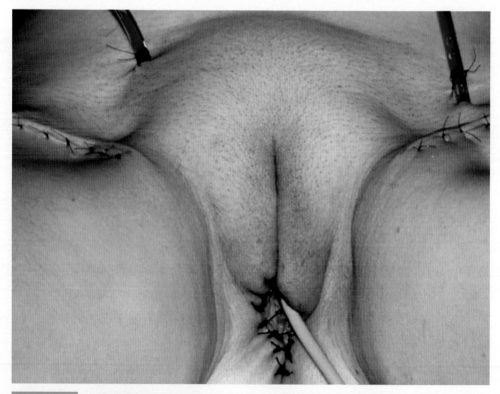

Figure 13.3 Satisfactory cosmetic result after radical local excision and bilateral groin dissection (for the small posterior vulvar carcinoma shown in Fig. 13.2).

Table 13.9 Death From Recurrence in an Undissected Groin		
Author	*Recurrence*	*Dead of Disease*
Rutledge *et al.*, 1970 (75)	4	3
Magrina *et al.*, 1979 (83)	4	3
Hoffman *et al.*, 1983 (85)	4	4
Hacker *et al.*, 1984 (13)	3	3
Monaghan and Hammond, 1984 (19)	4	4
Lingard *et al.*, 1992 (107)	7	7
Total	**26**	**24 (92%)**

Management of the Groin Lymph Nodes

Appropriate management of the regional lymph nodes is the single most important factor in decreasing the mortality from early vulvar cancer. With an increasing number of reports in the literature, two facts have become apparent:

1. **The only patients without significant risk of lymph node metastases are those with a T_1 tumor that invades the stroma to a depth no greater than 1 mm** (Table 13.5).

2. **Patients in whom recurrent disease develops in an undissected groin have a very high mortality rate** (Table 13.9).

All patients with a T_1 tumor with more than 1 mm of stromal invasion, and all patients with a T_2 tumor require inguinofemoral lymphadenectomy. A wedge or Keyes biopsy of the primary tumor should be obtained, and the depth of invasion determined. If it is less than 1 mm on the biopsy specimen, and the lesion is 2 cm or less in diameter, the entire lesion should be locally excised and analyzed histologically to determine the depth of invasion. If there is still no invasive focus deeper than 1 mm, groin dissection may be omitted. Although an occasional patient with a T_1 tumor and less than 1 mm of stromal invasion has had documented groin node metastases (108–110), the incidence is so low that it is of no practical significance.

If groin dissection is indicated in patients with early vulvar cancer, it should be a thorough inguinofemoral lymphadenectomy. The GOG reported six groin recurrences among 121 patients with T_1N_0 or N_1 tumors after a superficial (inguinal) dissection, even though the inguinal nodes were reported as negative (111). Whether all these recurrences were in the femoral nodes is unclear, but this large, multi-institutional study does indicate that modification of the groin dissection increases groin recurrences and, therefore, mortality.

From the accumulated experience now available in the literature, it is clear that **it is not necessary to perform a bilateral groin dissection if the primary lesion is unilateral and the ipsilateral nodes are negative** (Table 13.10). A recent series from the Mayo Clinic reported 48 positive groin nodes (29.4%) among 163 patients with a unilateral vulvar cancer. Only three patients (1.8%) had positive contralateral nodes with negative ipsilateral nodes and none had T_1 tumors. The only independent risk factor for bilateral nodal involvement was the total number of positive groin nodes, with an OR of 1.84 (CI: 1.30, 2.59). With each additional positive node, the possibility of having bilateral groin node involvement increased by 84%.

Lesions involving the anterior labia minora should have bilateral dissection because of the more frequent contralateral lymph flow from this region (114).

Measurement of Depth of Invasion

The Nomenclature Committee of the International Society of Gynecological Pathologists has recommended that depth of invasion should be measured from the most superficial dermal papilla adjacent to the tumor to the deepest focus of invasion. This method was originally proposed by Wilkinson et al. (84). Tumor thickness is also commonly measured (83,115), and Fu (116) estimated that the average difference between tumor thickness and depth of invasion as determined by the Wilkinson method was 0.3 mm.

Table 13.10 Incidence of Positive Contralateral Nodes in Patients With Lateral T₁ Squamous Cell Vulvar Carcinomas and Negative Ipsilateral Nodes			
Author	*Unilateral Lesions*	*Contralateral Nodes Positive*	*Percentage*
Wharton *et al.*, 1974 (112)	25	0	0
Parker *et al.*, 1975 (69)	41	0	0
Magrina *et al.*, 1979 (83)	77	2	2.6
Iversen *et al.*, 1981 (12)	112	0	0
Buscema *et al.*, 1981 (113)	38	0	0
Hoffman *et al.*, 1983 (85)[a]	70	0	0
Hacker *et al.*, 1984 (13)	60	0	0
Struyk *et al.*, 1989 (89)	53	0	0
De Simone *et al.*, 2007 (97)	61	0	0
Total	**537**	**2**	**0.37**

[a]Information not contained in reference but obtained from personal communication.

Technique for Groin Dissection

A linear incision is made along the medial four-fifths of a line drawn between the anterior superior iliac spine and the pubic tubercle. The incision is best made about 1 cm above the groin crease (Fig. 13.4). Studies of bipedal lymphangiograms have demonstrated that **there are no lymph nodes adjacent to the anterior superior iliac spine** (117). On the basis of embryological and anatomical studies, Micheletti et al. have proposed that the superficial circumflex iliac vessels could represent the lateral surgical landmark (118). The incision is carried through the subcutaneous tissues to the superficial fascia. The latter is incised and grasped with artery forceps to place it on traction, and the fatty tissue between it and the fascia lata is removed over

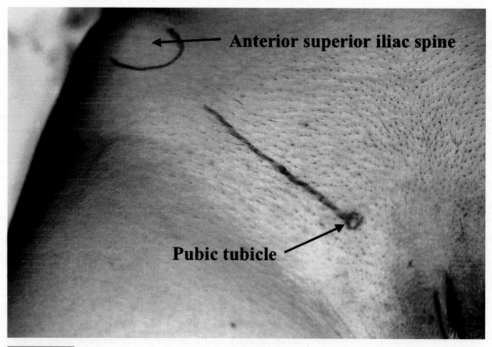

Figure 13.4   Skin incision for groin dissection through a separate incision. The incision is made along the medial four fifths of a line drawn between the anterior superior iliac spine and the pubic tubercle.

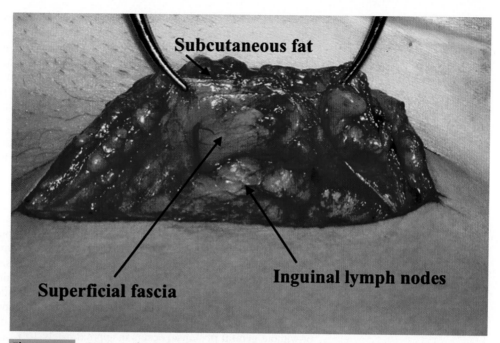

Figure 13.5   **Camper's fascia kept on traction with forceps while the underlying node-bearing fatty tissue is dissected out of the femoral triangle.** Note the preservation of the subcutaneous tissue above the superficial fascia. This ensures that skin necrosis will not occur.

the femoral triangle (Fig. 13.5). The dissection is carried 2 cm above the inguinal ligament to include all the inguinal nodes.

The saphenous vein is usually tied off at the apex of the femoral triangle and at its point of entry into the femoral vein. Some authors have suggested that saphenous vein sparing may decrease postoperative morbidity (119,120), although in a study of 64 patients, 31 of whom underwent saphenous sparing, Zhang et al. reported no difference in the incidence of postoperative fever, acute cellulitis, seroma, or lymphocyst formation (120). **To avoid skin necrosis, all subcutaneous tissue above the superficial fascia must be preserved.**

The fatty tissue containing the femoral lymph nodes is removed from within the fossa ovalis. **There are only one to three femoral lymph nodes, and they are always situated medial to the femoral vein in the opening of the fossa ovalis** (121). Hence, there is no need to remove the fascia lata lateral to the femoral vessels and no need to perform a sartorius muscle transposition. Cloquet's node is not consistently present but should be checked for by retraction of the inguinal ligament cephalad over the femoral canal. At the conclusion of the dissection, a suction drain is placed in the groin and the wound is closed in two layers.

Postoperative Management

In spite of the age and general medical condition of most patients with vulvar cancer, the surgery is usually remarkably well tolerated. However, a postoperative mortality rate of 1% to 2% can be expected, usually as a result of pulmonary embolism or myocardial infarction. Patients should be able to commence a low-residue diet on the first postoperative day. **Bed rest is advisable for 2 to 3 days to allow immobilization of the wounds to foster healing.** Pneumatic calf compression and subcutaneous heparin should be used to help prevent deep venous thrombosis, and active, non–weight-bearing leg movements are to be encouraged. Perineal swabs are given until the patient is fully mobilized, at which stage sitz baths or whirlpool therapy are helpful, followed by drying of the perineum with a hair dryer. Suction drainage of each groin is continued for approximately 7 to 10 days to help decrease the incidence of groin seromas. A Foley catheter is left in the bladder until the patient is ambulatory.

Early Postoperative Complications

The major immediate morbidity is related to the groin dissection. With the separate incision approach, and sparing of the subcutaneous fat in both the superior and inferior flap, the incidence of wound breakdown is now very low. **The most common problem is lymphocyst formation,** which occurs in about 40% of cases (122). These seem to have become more common since introduction of the practice of leaving the fascia lata over the muscles in the floor of the femoral triangle. If large, they are usually best managed by making a linear incision approximately 1 cm long to allow adequate drainage. Drainage must be maintained by placing a narrow gauze wick in the incision and changing it twice daily until the skin flaps seal to the underlying tissues. Early mobilization and long walks immediately after discharge from hospital seem to increase the incidence of lymphocysts.

Other early postoperative complications include cellulitis, **urinary tract infection, deep venous thrombosis, pulmonary embolism, myocardial infarction, hemorrhage, and, rarely, osteitis pubis.**

Late Complications

The major late complication is **chronic leg edema,** which has been reported in up to 69% of patients (93). In our experience at the Royal Hospital for Women, the incidence of lymphedema after groin dissection is 62% (123). In about 50% of patients, the onset of lymphedema occurs within 3 months, while about 85% experience the onset within 12 months (123). Lymphedema is significantly related to the occurrence of early complications (122), particularly cellulitis. **Recurrent lymphangitis** or cellulitis of the leg occurs in approximately 10% of patients and usually responds to *erythromycin* tablets or *flucloxacillin.* **Urinary stress incontinence,** with or without **genital prolapse,** occurs in approximately 10% of patients and may require corrective surgery. **Introital stenosis** can lead to dyspareunia and may require a vertical relaxing incision, which is sutured transversely. An uncommon late complication is **femoral hernia,** which can usually be prevented during surgery by closure of the femoral canal with a suture from the inguinal ligament to Cooper's ligament. **Pubic osteomyelitis** and **rectovaginal or rectoperineal fistulae** are rare late complications.

Management of a Patient With Positive Groin Nodes

Traditionally, patients with positive groin nodes had a pelvic lymphadenectomy, but in 1977, the GOG initiated a prospective trial in which patients with positive groin nodes were randomized to either ipsilateral pelvic node dissection or bilateral pelvic plus groin irradiation (21). Radiation therapy consisted of 4,500 to 5,000 cGy to the midplane of the pelvis at a rate of 180 to 200 cGy/day. The survival rate for the radiation group (68% at 2 years) was significantly better than that for the pelvic lymphadenectomy group (54% at 2 years; $p = 0.03$). The survival advantage was limited to patients with clinically evident groin nodes or more than one positive groin node. Groin recurrence occurred in 3 of 59 patients (5.1%) treated with radiation, compared with 13 of 55 (23.6%) treated with lymphadenectomy ($p = 0.02$). Four patients who received radiation had a pelvic recurrence, compared with one who had lymphadenectomy. **These data highlight the value of prophylactic groin irradiation in preventing groin recurrence in patients with multiple positive groin nodes.**

In the 1990s, several investigators demonstrated that the morphology of the positive groin nodes was also of prognostic significance, allowing further discrimination among patients with positive nodes. Origoni et al. (124) demonstrated that for patients with positive lymph nodes, there was a significant difference in survival, depending on the size of the involved nodes and the presence or absence of extracapsular spread. **Patients whose involved nodes were less than 5 mm in diameter had a 5-year survival rate of 90.9%, compared with 41.6% for nodes 5 to 15 mm in diameter and 20.6% for nodes larger than 15 mm diameter** ($p = 0.001$). Similarly, if nodal involvement remained intracapsular, the 5-year survival rate was 85.7%, compared with 25% if there was extracapsular spread ($p = 0.001$).

Similar results were obtained by the group at Gateshead, who reported that in a multivariate analysis, the only significant variables were FIGO stage (III, IVA, or IVB) and the presence or absence of extracapsular spread (125). Van der Velden et al. (126) demonstrated that **even for patients with one positive node, the presence of extracapsular spread decreased the survival rate from 88% (14 of 16 patients) to 44% (7 of 16 patients).** Raspagliesi et al. have recently reported a 10-year survival of 55% in lymph node positive patients with <50% of nodal replacements, compared to 34.3% in lymph node positive patients with >50% nodal replacement ($p < 0.01$) (81).

From the foregoing observations, our recommendations for the management of patients with positive groin nodes are as follows:

1. **Patients with one micrometastasis (metastatic deposit ≤5 mm diameter) should be observed.** The prognosis for this group of patients is excellent (18). Even if a unilateral groin dissection has been performed for a lateral lesion, there seems to be no indication for dissection of the other groin because contralateral lymph node involvement is likely only if there are multiple ipsilateral inguinal node metastases (21,82,127).

2. **Patients with three or more micrometastases, one macrometastasis (≥10 mm diameter), or any evidence of extracapsular spread should receive bilateral groin and pelvic radiation.**

3. **There are insufficent data on patients with two micrometastases to draw definitive conclusions.** If these patients are observed, which is our usual policy, it may be prudent to observe the contralateral groin with ultrasound for the first 6–12 months if it has not been dissected.

Lymphatic Mapping

The major morbidity associated with the modern management of vulvar cancer is chronic lymphedema, which occurs in about 60% of patients and is a lifelong affliction. Hence, there is significant interest in eliminating or modifying the groin dissection for patients with negative nodes.

Several noninvasive methods for detecting lymph node metastases from vulvar cancer have been disappointing, including positron emission tomography (128) and computerized tomographic scanning (129). Ultrasonic scanning, particularly when combined with fine needle aspiration cytology, shows more promise, but false negatives and false positives still occur (129,130).

For the past decade considerable investigation has been undertaken of the role of sentinel node identification in patients with vulvar cancer. This concept was initially introduced by Cabanas for the management of patients with penile cancer (131), and subsequently for the management of melanomas by Morton et al. (132). **The hypothesis is that if the sentinel node is negative, all other nodes will be negative, so the patient can be spared the morbidity of full groin dissection.**

The sentinel node (or nodes) is identified by the **injection of intradermal isosulfan blue dye** around the primary vulvar lesion, either alone or in combination with **intradermal radioactive ^{99m}Tc-labeled sulfur colloid** (26,28). After the injections, the node(s) is isolated in the groin by dissection and gamma counting.

In a review of the literature in 2001, Makar et al. reported successful identification of sentinel node(s) in 85 of 103 patients (82.5%) using the blue dye technique, and 128 of 128 patients (100%) using lymphoscintigraphy (29). **False-negative sentinel nodes have been reported** (132,133), **although the incidence appears to be low.** In the presence of palpably suspicious nodes, or nodes replaced by cancer, the incidence of false negatives is higher, presumably because metastatic disease obstructs flow to those nodes (134,135). **The incidence of false-negative sentinel nodes can be reduced by ultrastaging,** using either serial sectioning alone (136) or in combination with immunohistochemical staining for cytokeratin (137). Molpus et al. reported that 2 of 18 (11%) negative sentinel nodes had micrometastases (<0.2 mm) upon serial sectioning and immunohistochemical staining (138).

Results of a European multicenter observation study on sentinel node detection in vulvar cancer was recently reported by van der Zee et al. (26). Both radiotracer and blue dye were used, and eligible patients were those with T_1 or T_2 squamous cell carcinomas <4 cm diameter. If the sentinel node was negative at pathologic ultrastaging, groin dissection was omitted and the patient was observed clinically every 2 months for 2 years.

From March 2000 to June 2006, 403 assessable patients were recruited to the study, and they underwent 623 groin dissections. Metastatic sentinel nodes were found in 163 groins (26.2%). Routine pathologic examination detected 95 (58.3%) positive sentinel nodes and ultrastaging detected 68 (41.7%). **In eight of 276 patients in the observational study, groin recurrence was observed after a negative sentinel node procedure. The actuarial groin recurrence rate after 2 years was 3% (95%, CI 1%, to 6%).** All patients with a groin recurrence underwent bilateral inguinofemoral lymphadenectomy and adjuvant (chemo)radiation. **Six of the**

eight patients died of disease, while two remained disease-free at 6 and 50 months after recurrence. The median time to recurrence was 12 months (range 5–16 months). As expected, both short-term and long-term morbidity were significantly decreased.

While sentinel node biopsy is clearly superior to earlier attempts to decrease postoperative morbidity by selective omission (69,112) or modification (14) of the groin dissection, **the key issue really is to determine the false-negative rate of the procedure, not just from the best centers, but in the hands of the average operator.** The high mortality rate from recurrence in an undissected groin is vitally important to a patient undergoing this procedure, and **proper informed consent will be crucial.**

In this latter regard, a recent study by de Hulla et al. is important (139). They sent structured questionnaires both to patients who had been treated for vulvar cancer and to gynecologists. The response rate among patients was 91% (107 of 118), 40% of whom had experienced lower limb cellulitis and 49% of whom still experienced severe pain and/or lymphedema in the legs. Sixty percent of the patients preferred complete lymphadenectomy in preference to a 5% false-negative rate of the sentinel node procedure. Their preference was not related to age or the side effects they had experienced. The response among gynecologists was 80% (80 of 100), of whom 60% were willing to accept a 5% to 20% false-negative rate for the sentinel node procedure. The authors concluded that **although gynecologists may consider this a promising approach, the majority of vulvar cancer patients would not advise its introduction because they are not prepared to take any risk of missing a lymph node metastasis.**

Exactly similar sentiments have been expressed about the sentinel node procedure by women with breast cancer (140), even though most patients with breast cancer receive adjuvant treatment after surgery, and the nodal recurrence risk is much lower (0.1% to 0.3%) (141). A recent study from our own institution of 60 patients with vulvar cancer and clinically negative lymph nodes revealed similar findings. **Although 73% of these women reported lymphedema, 80% indicated they would choose complete lymphadenectomy rather than take a 5% risk of a false-negative sentinel node procedure** (142).

If the sentinel lymph node procedure is performed after proper informed consent, it is important to undertake complete inguinofemoral lymphadenectomy if a sentinel node is not detected. This is particularly likely to occur for lesions close to the midline, when bilateral groin dissection would normally be required (28,135).

In the author's opinion, an undissected groin should be followed with ultrasonography every 3 months for the first 12 months to allow early detection of any enlarging lymph nodes.

Advanced Disease

Vulvar cancer may be considered to be advanced on the basis of a T_3 or a T_4 primary tumor or the presence of bulky, positive groin nodes. Advanced vulvar cancer is uncommon in developed countries, and most data derive from single institutional experience or single-arm multiinstitutional reports.

Management should be individualized, and a multidisciplinary team approach is desirable. As with early stage disease, it is advantageous **to independently determine the most appropriate treatment for (i) the primary tumor and (ii) groin and pelvic lymph nodes.**

Management of the Groin and Pelvic Lymph Nodes

The author's preference is to initially determine the status of the groin and pelvic lymph nodes, using clinical examination and a CT scan of the groin, pelvis, and abdomen. Patients can then be triaged into 3 groups, as follows:

1. **Patients with no clinically or radiologically suspicious nodes.** These patients are treated by bilateral inguinofemoral lymphadenectomy, performed through separate groin incisions. If there are negative nodes or up to two micrometastases (<5 mm tumor deposits) without extracapsular spread, the groins are eliminated from any subsequent radiation fields. As with early stage disease, if there is one macrometastasis (>5 mm tumor deposit, 3 or more micrometastases, or extracapsular spread), pelvic and groin radiation is indicated.

2. **Patients with clinically or radiologically suspicious nodes.**

    i.   **All enlarged groin nodes are removed** through a separate incision approach and sent for frozen-section diagnosis. If metastatic disease is confirmed, full lymphadenectomy is not carried out.

    ii   **Any enlarged pelvic nodes seen on CT scan are removed** by an extraperitoneal approach.

    iii.   **Full pelvic and groin irradiation is given** as soon as the groin incisions are healed, which is usually approximately 2 weeks.

    iv.   **If the frozen section reveals no metastatic disease** in the removed nodes, **full groin dissection is performed.**

We have reported our experience with resection of bulky positive nodes rather than full groin dissection for patients with advanced vulvar cancer (36). Seventeen patients treated by nodal debulking in Australia were compared with 23 similar patients treated by full groin dissection at the Academic Medical Hospital in Amsterdam. Both groups of patients received groin and pelvic radiation post-operatively. **Both disease-specific survival and groin recurrence-free intervals were superior in the group having nodal debulking** although with the small numbers in both series, the differences were not statistically significant.

3. **Patients with fixed, unresectable groin nodes (Fig. 13.6).** These patients should be treated with primary groin and pelvic radiation, probably combined with chemotherapy. It may be appropriate to resect a residual groin mass following radiation if there is no other evidence of metastatic disease (143).

An algorithm for the management of patients with advanced vulvar cancer is shown in Fig. 13.7.

Management of the Primary Tumor

Surgery

If the tumor involves the distal vagina and/or urethral orifice, and can be resected without need for a stoma, primary surgical resection is the best option. Radical vulvectomy often will be

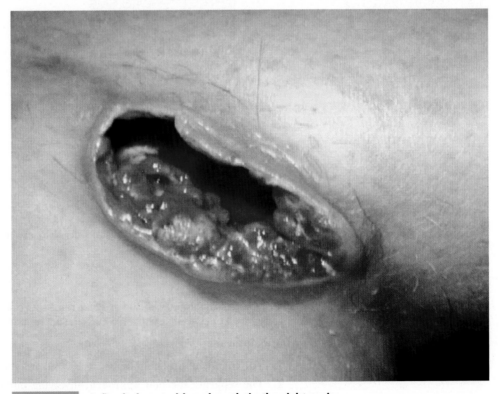

Figure 13.6   A fixed ulcerated lymph node in the right groin.

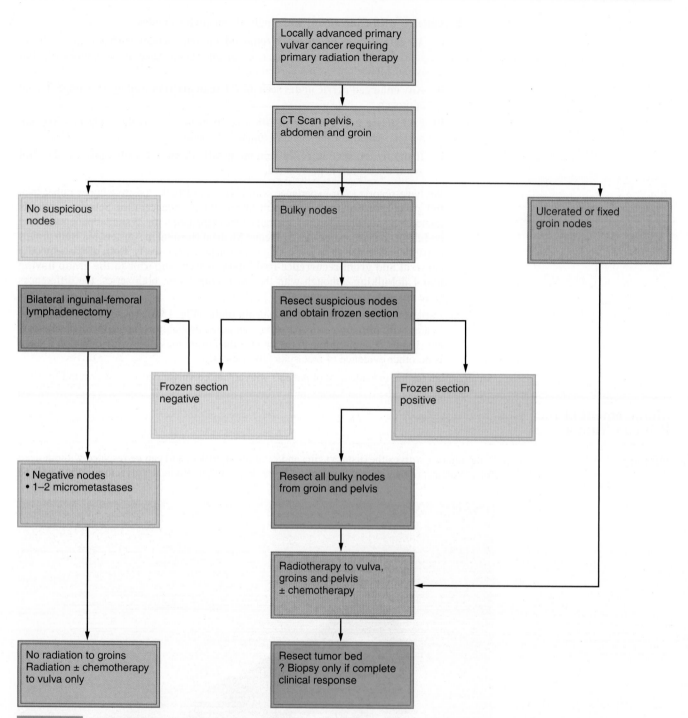

Figure 13.7 **Algorithm for the management of patients with locally advanced vulvar cancer, in whom surgical resection of the primary tumor would necessitate a stoma.**

required, although a modified radical vulvectomy to allow adequate clearance around the lesion while preserving some normal vulva may also be appropriate.

Two basic surgical approaches can be used:

1. **The *en bloc* approach** through a trapezoid or butterfly incision (91) (Fig. 13.8).
2. **The separate incision approach,** involving three separate incisions, one for the radical vulvectomy and one for each groin dissection (22).

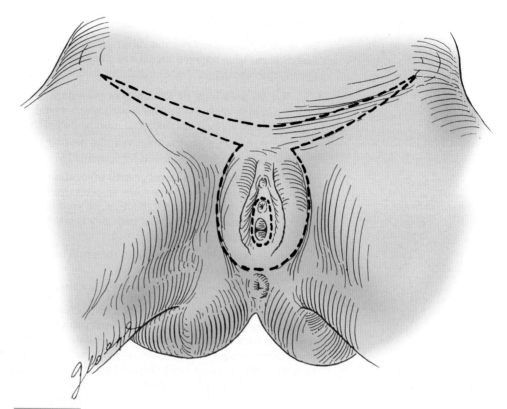

Figure 13.8   Incision used for *en bloc* radical vulvectomy and bilateral groin dissection.

Technique for *En Bloc* Radical Vulvectomy and Groin Dissection

The operation is usually performed with the patient in the low lithotomy position, and groin and vulvar dissections can proceed simultaneously with two teams of surgeons if appropriate. The skin incision has been significantly modified from the original Stanley Way technique to allow primary skin closure. The groin dissection is accomplished initially, with the abdominal incision carried down to the aponeurosis of the external oblique muscle, approximately 2 cm above the inguinal ligament. A skin flap is raised over the femoral triangle, with preservation of the subcutaneous fat above the superficial (Camper's) fascia. The technique for groin dissection has been described earlier.

The vulvar incision is carried posteriorly along each labiocrural fold, or within a 1-cm margin of the primary lesion. The technique for vulvectomy is described in the next section.

Technique for Radical Vulvectomy

If the radical vulvectomy is performed through a separate incision, the lateral incision is basically elliptical. Each lateral incision should commence on the mons pubis anteriorly and extend through the fat and superficial fascia to the fascia over the pubic symphysis. It is then easy to develop bluntly the plane immediately above the pubic symphysis and fascia lata. The skin incision is extended posteriorly along the labiocrural folds to the perianal area and carried down to the fascia lata. The medial incision is placed to clear the tumor with margins of at least 1 cm. If necessary, the distal half of the urethra may be resected without compromising continence. If the tumor is involving the urethra or the vagina, dissection around the tumor is facilitated by transection of the vulva, thereby improving exposure of the involved area.

The specimen includes the bulbocavernosus muscles and the vestibular bulb. Because of the vascularity, it is desirable to perform most of the dissection by diathermy after the initial skin incision. In addition, the vessels supplying the clitoris should be clamped and tied, as should the internal pudendal vessels posterolaterally.

Closure of Large Defects

It is usually possible to close the vulvar defect without tension. However, if a more extensive dissection has been required because of a large primary lesion, a number of options are available to repair the defect. These include the following:

1. **An area may be left open to granulate,** which it usually does over a period of 6 to 8 weeks (144). This is particularly useful around the urethra, where sutures can cause urethral deviation and misdirection of the urinary stream.

2. **Full-thickness skin flaps may be devised** (145,146). An example is the rhomboid flap, which is best suited for covering large defects of the posterior vulva (147).

3. **Unilateral or bilateral gracilis myocutaneous grafts** may be developed (Fig. 13.9). These are most useful when an extensive area from the mons pubis to the perianal area has been resected. Because the graft brings a new blood supply to the area, it is particularly applicable if the vulva is poorly vascularized from prior surgical resection or radiation (148).

4. **If extensive defects exist in the groin and vulva, the tensor fascia lata myocutaneous graft is applicable** (149).

The technique for these grafts is discussed in Chapter 20.

When the primary disease involves the anus, rectum, rectovaginal septum, or proximal urethra, **adequate surgical clearance of the primary tumor is possible only by pelvic exenteration combined with radical vulvectomy and bilateral groin dissection.** Such radical surgery is often inappropriate for these elderly patients, and even in suitable surgical candidates, psychological morbidity is high (100,150), and postoperative morbidity is significant. Nevertheless, a 5-year survival rate of approximately 50% can be expected with this approach (151,152). Surgery alone is rarely curative for patients with fixed or ulcerated (N_3) groin nodes.

Radiation Therapy

Boronow (24) was the first to suggest a combined radiosurgical approach as an alternative to pelvic exenteration for patients with advanced vulvar cancer. In his initial report, he recommended intracavitary radium, with or without external irradiation, to eliminate the internal genital disease, and subsequent surgery, usually radical vulvectomy and bilateral groin dissection, to treat the external genital disease.

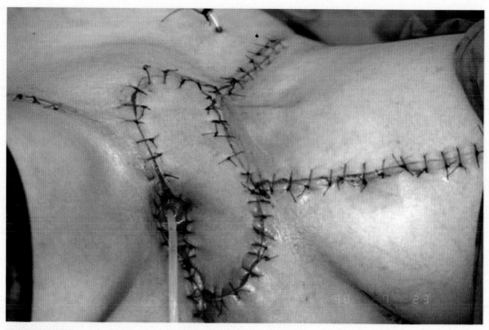

Figure 13.9   Unilateral gracilis myocutaneous graft used to cover a large lateral vulvar defect.

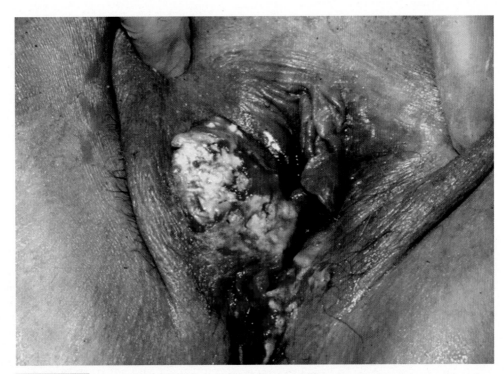

Figure 13.10   **Advanced squamous cell carcinoma of the vulva involving the anal canal.** A primary surgical approach would have necessitated radical vulvectomy, anoproctectomy, and permanent colostomy.

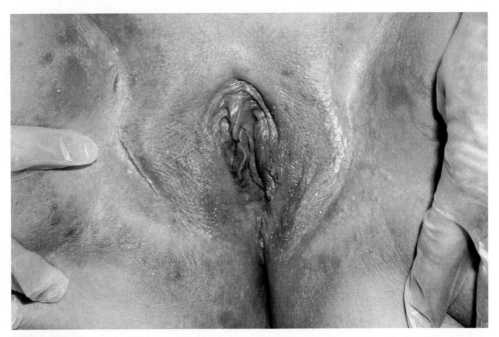

Figure 13.11   **Advanced vulvar cancer shown in Figure 13.10 after 50.4 cGy of external-beam radiation therapy.** Resection of the tumor bed showed microscopic residual disease. The radiation therapy prevented the need for a permanent stoma.

In 1984, Hacker et al. (25) reported the use of preoperative teletherapy in patients with advanced vulvar cancer; brachytherapy was reserved for patients with persistent disease that would otherwise necessitate exenteration (Figs. 13.10, 13.11). Rather than performing radical vulvectomy for all patients, **only the tumor bed was resected,** on the assumption that any microscopic foci originally present in the vulva would have been sterilized by the radiation.

In specimens from one-half of the patients, there was no residual disease. Long-term morbidity was low with the predominant use of teletherapy, and no patient developed a fistula. Two patients whose primary tumor was fixed to bone were long-term survivors (25).

In 1987, Boronow et al. (153) updated their experience with preoperative radiation for locally advanced vulvovaginal cancer, reporting 37 primary cases and 11 cases of recurrent disease. The 5-year survival rate for the primary cases was 75.6%, whereas the recurrent cases had a 5-year survival rate of 62.6%. Seventeen of 40 vulvectomy specimens (42.5%) contained no residual disease. Eight patients (16.7%) had a local recurrence, and five patients (10.4%) developed a fistula.

This second report had three major refinements: (i) the use of external-beam therapy for all cases, with more selective use of brachytherapy; (ii) more conservative vulvar surgery; and (iii) resection of bulky N_2 and N_3 nodes without full groin dissection to minimize lymphedema.

In 1989, Thomas et al. (154) reported on the use of radiation with concurrent infusional *5-fluorouracil (5-FU)*, with or without *mitomycin C* who received primary chemoradiation; six had an initial complete response in the vulva, but three of the six subsequently had a local recurrence.

Several subsequent studies have reported on the use of chemoradiation followed by wide excision of the tumor bed. Italian investigators reported 31 patients with locoregionally advanced vulvar cancer who were treated with a combination of *mitomycin C* and *5-FU* in combination with radiation to the vulva, groins, and pelvis (31). A total of 54 Gy was given, with a 2-week break after 36 Gy. The pathologic complete response rate was 36% in the vulva and 55% in the groin. The 5-year survival rate was 55% for patients treated for primary lesions and 57% for those with recurrent disease. A second similar Italian study of 58 patients reported a pathologic complete response rate of 31% in both the vulva and the groin (32).

The pathologic complete response rate in the vulva with these radiation doses is not greater than that seen with radiation alone, but the local acute toxicity is much greater with the addition of chemotherapy, invariably necessitating at least a 1-week break in therapy.

Cunningham et al. (34) used radiation therapy in combination with *cisplatin* (50 mg/m^2 on day 1) and *5-FU* (1,000 mg/m^2/24 hours × 96 hours) during the first and last weeks of therapy. Radiation doses to the vulva and groins ranged from 50 to 65 Gy. Nine of 14 patients (64%) had a complete clinical response, and surgical excision of the primary site was not performed in these 9 patients. Only one recurrence was noted with a mean follow-up of 36 months (range, 7 to 81 months).

Leiserowitz et al. (35) omitted groin dissection after preoperative chemoradiation with *5-FU,* with or without *cisplatin,* in 23 patients. No patient failed in the groins, but with a median radiation dose to the groins of only 36 Gy, it is difficult to believe that these results could be duplicated.

Beriwal et al. reported 18 patients having preoperative intensity-modulated radiotherapy and chemotherapy for locally advanced vulvar cancer (30). Fourteen patients had surgery performed with a pathological complete response in 9 patients (64%) and a partial response in 5 (36%).

With the experience now accrued, preoperative radiation, with or without concurrent chemotherapy, should be regarded as the treatment of first choice for patients with advanced vulvar cancer who would otherwise require some type of pelvic exenteration. Chemoradiation is associated with more acute and chronic toxicity, particularly if no break is given during therapy.

Role of Radiation

Radiation therapy, with or without the addition of concurrent chemotherapy, is playing an increasingly important role in the management of patients with vulvar cancer. The indications for radiation therapy in patients with this disease are still evolving. At present, radiation seems to be clearly indicated in the following situations:

1. **Before surgery, in patients with advanced disease** who would otherwise require pelvic exenteration.

2. **After surgery, to treat the pelvic lymph nodes and groins** in patients with more than two micrometastases, one macrometastasis, or extracapsular spread.

Bilateral groin and pelvic radiation is recommended (21) although workers in North England have suggested that unilateral groin and pelvic radiation may be appropriate for patients with unilaterally positive groin nodes. This recommendation (155) was based on experience with 20 patients, nine (45%) of whom recurred. None of the recurrences were in the contralateral (nonirradiated groin).

It has also been suggested that adjuvant radiation may benefit patients with a single positive node if a less extensive groin node dissection has been performed (156).

Possible roles for radiation therapy include the following:

1. **After surgery, to help prevent local recurrence** and improve survival **in patients with involved or close surgical margins** (<5 mm) (157–159), Faul et al. from Pittsburgh retrospectively reviewed 62 patients with invasive vulvar carcimoma who had either positive or close (<8 mm) margins of excision. Half the patients (31) were treated with adjuvant radiation to the vulva, and half were observed after surgery. Local recurrence occurred in 58% of the observed patients and 16% following adjuvant radiation (159).

2. **As primary therapy for patients with small primary tumors, particularly clitoral or periclitoral lesions** in young and middle-aged women, in whom surgical resection would have significant psychological consequences (106).

Groin irradiation has been proposed as an alternative to groin dissection in patients with N_0 lymph nodes. The GOG reported the results of a phase III trial in which patients with T_1, T_2, or T_3 tumors and N_0 or N_1 groin nodes were randomized between surgical resection (and postoperative irradiation for patients with positive groin nodes) and primary groin irradiation (160). Patients with N_1 nodes were allowed fine-needle aspiration cytologic analysis of the nodes and exclusion from the trial if findings were positive. The study was closed prematurely because 5 of 26 patients in the groin irradiation arm of the study had recurrences in the groin. Of 23 patients undergoing groin dissection, 5 showed groin node metastases, but no groin recurrences occurred after postoperative irradiation. The dose of radiation was 5,000 cGy given in daily 200-cGy fractions to a depth of 3 cm below the anterior skin surface.

Subsequently, Koh et al. (161) reviewed pretreatment CT scans of 50 patients with gynecologic cancer to determine the distance of each femoral vessel beneath the overlying skin surface. Femoral vessel depths in these patients ranged from 2.0 to 18.5 cm, with an average depth of 6.1 cm. It is apparent that many patients in the GOG study would have been underdosed because CT scanning was not used to define the target.

In 2002, van der Velden and Ansink published a **Cochrane review** of primary groin irradiation versus primary groin dissection for patients with early vulvar cancer (162). Only three studies *met* the minimum criteria for inclusion in the review, but **it was concluded that although groin irradiation is less morbid, it is associated with a higher risk of groin recurrence.** Large positive nodes, not likely to be controlled by radiation, may be quite inapparent clinically, even in relatively slim patients, so this finding is not surprising.

Recurrent Vulvar Cancer

Most recurrences from vulvar cancer occur on the vulva, but distant recurrences do occur, particularly in the presence of multiple lymph node metastases (18,163).

Rouzier et al. from France identified three patterns of local recurrence with very different prognoses: (i) primary tumor site recurrence (up to and including 2 cm from the vulvectomy scar); (ii) **remote vulvar recurrence** (>2 cm from the primary tumor site); and (iii) **skin bridge recurrence** (80). Their study included 215 patients, and the local relapse-free survival was 78.6% at 5 years. Patients with positive margins who did not receive radiotherapy and patients with greater than 1 mm stromal invasion who did not have a groin dissection were excluded from analysis.

Local recurrence at a site distant from the primary tumor (which could be considered a new primary lesion), **had a good prognosis,** 66.7% of patients surviving 3 years. **By contrast, survival after recurrence at the primary tumor site was poor,** only 15.4% of patients surviving 3 years. None of seven patients with a skin bridge recurrence was alive at 1 year.

Review of our own data from the Royal Hospital for Women in Sydney has confirmed that these three patterns of local recurrence are distinct entities (98). In our experience, **primary site recurrences** occurred at a median interval of 21 months, and were more commonly associated with surgical margins <8 mm. By contrast, **remote site vulvar recurrences** occurred at a median interval of 69 months, and were commonly associated with lichen sclerosus or VIN. In contrast to Rouzier, **our patients with both primary and remote site recurrence had an excellent prognosis.**

Local vulvar recurrences are usually amenable to further surgical resection (22,80,164). A variety of plastic surgical techniques may facilitate adequate surgical resection, particularly for larger recurrences. Myocutaneous grafts which may be used include the gluteus thigh flap, the rectus abdominus flap, the gracilis flap, and the tensor fascia lata flap (Fig. 13.12)(165).

Radiation therapy, particularly a combination of external-beam therapy plus interstitial needles, also has been used to treat vulvar recurrences. Hoffman et al. reported on 10 patients treated in this manner, and 9 were still alive with a mean follow-up of 28 months (166). However, 6 of the 10 had severe radionecrosis at a median of 8.5 months after radiation, and the authors concluded that although this treatment was highly effective, it was also highly morbid.

Regional and distant recurrences are difficult to manage (157). Radiation therapy may be used with surgery for groin recurrence, whereas chemotherapeutic agents that have activity against squamous carcinomas may be offered for distant metastases. The most active agents are *cisplatin, methotrexate, cyclophosphamide (Cytoxan), bleomycin,* and *mitomycin C,* but response rates are low and the duration of response is usually disappointing (167). Long-term survival is very uncommon with regional or distant recurrence (157).

Prognosis

With appropriate management, the prognosis for vulvar cancer is generally good, the overall 5-year survival rate in operable cases being approximately 70%. Survival

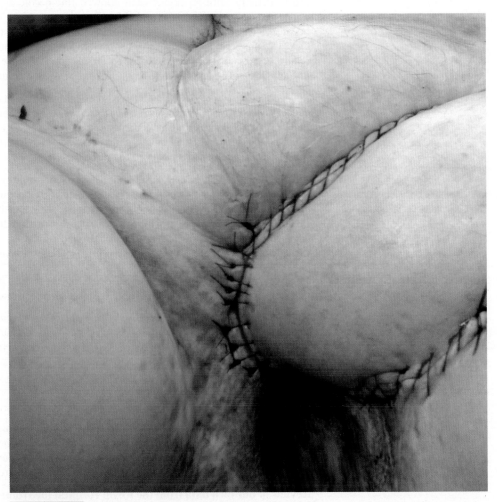

Figure 13.12 Tensor fascia lata myocutaneous graft used to cover the left groin following resection of a recurrence in an irradiated field.

Table 13.11 Five-Year Survival Rate Versus Stage for Patients Treated With Curative Intent

Clinical FIGO Stage	No.	Dead of Disease	Corrected 5-Year Survival (%)
I	376	36	90.4
II	310	71	77.1
III	238	116	51.3
IV	111	91	18.0
Total	**1,035**	**314**	**69.7**

FIGO, International Federation of Gynecology and Obstetrics.

Data compiled from **Rutledge et al.,** 1970 (75); **Boutselis,** 1972 (168); **Morley,** 1976 (91); **Japeze et al.,** 1977 (169); **Benedet et al.,** 1979 (78); **Hacker et al.,** 1983 (18); **Cavanagh et al.,** 1986 (170).

Table 13.12 Five-Year Survival Versus Lymph Node Status for Squamous Cell Carcinoma of the Vulva

Lymph node status	Patients	5-year survival (%)	Hazard ratio (95% CI)
Negative	302	80.7	Reference
1 positive	66	62.9	2.1 (1.2–3.4)
2 positive	43	30.4	6.0 (3.7–9.8)
3 positive	24	19.2	5.3 (3.0–9.5)
4+ positive	62	13.3	2.6 (1.9–3.7)

Modified from the 26th Annual Report on the Results of Treatment in Gynecological Cancer (168).

correlates with the FIGO clinical stage of disease (Table 13.11) and also with lymph node status. In the 26th FIGO annual report, **patients with negative lymph nodes had a 5-year survival rate of 80.7%, which fell to 13.3% for patients with 4 or more positive nodes (Table 13.12).**

The GOG staged 588 patients with vulvar cancer by the new surgical staging criteria and reported 5-year survival rates of 98%, 85%, 74%, and 31% for stages I, II, III, and IV, respectively (92).

The number of positive groin nodes is the single most important prognostic variable (18,20,21,93,171). Patients with one microscopically positive node have a good prognosis, regardless of the stage of disease (18,20), but patients with three or more positive nodes have a poor prognosis (18,103). Because the number of positive nodes correlates with the clinical status of the groin nodes (18), survival also correlates significantly with this variable. In the GOG study, patients with N_0 or N_1 nodes had a 2-year survival rate of 78%, compared with 52% for patients with N_2 nodes and 33% for patients with N_3 nodes ($p = 0.01$) (21). Extracapsular spread is a poor prognostic factor (124–126). **The survival rate for patients with positive pelvic nodes is approximately 11%** (90).

Workers at the Norwegian Radium Hospital evaluated DNA ploidy for its prognostic significance in 118 squamous cell carcinomas of the vulva (171). **The 5-year crude survival rate was 62% for the diploid and 23% for the aneuploid tumors** ($p < 0.001$). Aneuploid tumors without lymph node metastases had a 5-year cancer-related survival rate of 44%, compared with 58% for the diploid tumors with lymph node metastases. In a multivariate Cox regression analysis, **the most important independent prognostic parameters were:**

1. **Lymph node involvement** ($p < 0.0001$)
2. **Tumor ploidy** ($p < 0.0001$)
3. **Tumor size** ($p < 0.0039$)

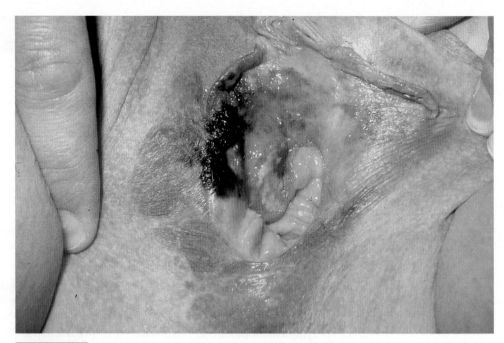

Figure 13.13   Melanoma of the vulva involving the right labium minus.

A more recent paper from the Norwegian Radiation Hospital evaluated the prognostic significance of aberrant expression of the cell cycle kinase inhibitors p16, p21, and p27 among 224 patients with squamous cell carcinoma of the vulva (173). A low level of p16 protein and a high level of p21 protein were associated with a shorter disease-related survival.

Dutch workers studied 75 patients age 80 years or older, 57 (76%) of whom had standard treatment (174). When preoperatively available parameters of all patients were assessed in relation to survival in the total group, Eastern Cooperative Oncology Group (ECOG) performance status was the only independent prognostic variable. When all clinical and histopathological variables were assessed in the subgroup that had standard treatment, both **ECOG performance status and extracapsular lymph node involvement were independent prognostic variables for overall survival. Age was not a significant prognostic variable.**

Melanoma

Vulvar melanomas are rare, although they are the second most common vulvar malignancy. Most arise *de novo* (175), but they may arise from a preexisting junctional nevus. **They occur predominantly in postmenopausal white women, most commonly on the labia minoris or the clitoris** (Fig. 13.13). The incidence of cutaneous melanomas worldwide is increasing significantly.

Most patients with a vulvar melanoma have no symptoms except for the presence of a pigmented lesion that may be enlarging. Some patients have itching or bleeding, and a few present with a groin mass. Amelanotic varieties occasionally occur. **Any pigmented lesion on the vulva should be excised or biopsied, unless it is known to have been present and unchanged for some years.**

There are three basic histologic types: (i) the **superficial spreading melanoma,** which tends to remain relatively superficial early in its development; (ii) **the mucosal lentiginous melanoma,** a flat freckle, which may become quite extensive but also tends to remain superficial; and (iii) the **nodular melanoma,** which is a raised lesion that penetrates deeply and may metastasize widely. A Swedish study of 219 cases reported that the mucosal lentiginous melanoma was the most frequent type (57%) (176).

Staging

The FIGO staging used for squamous lesions is not applicable for melanomas, because these lesions are usually much smaller and the prognosis is related to the depth of penetration rather than to the diameter of the lesion (177–179). The leveling system established

Table 13.13 Microstaging of Vulvar Melanomas		
Clark's Levels (180)	*Chung et al. (177)*	*Breslow (181)*
I Intraepithelial	Intraepithelial	<0.76 mm
II Into papillary dermis	≤1 mm from granular layer	0.76–1.50 mm
III Filling dermal papillae	1.1–2 mm from granular layer	1.51–2.25 mm
IV Into reticular dermis	>2 mm from granular layer	2.26–3.0 mm
V Into subcutaneous fat	Into subcutaneous fat	>3 mm

by Clark et al. (180) for cutaneous melanomas is less readily applicable to vulvar lesions because of the different skin morphology. Chung et al. (174) proposed a modified system that retained Clark's definitions for levels I and V but arbitrarily defined levels II, III, and IV, using measurements in millimeters. Breslow (181) measured the thickest portion of the melanoma from the surface of intact epithelium to the deepest point of invasion. A comparison of these systems is shown in Table 13.13.

A revised American Joint Committee on Cancer (AJCC) Staging System for cutaneous melanomas came into effect in 2002 to reflect the new prognostic factors that have been found to be important in predicting survival (182). These factors include primary tumor thickness (replacing level of invasion), ulceration, number of metastatic lymph nodes, micrometastatic disease based on the sentinel lymph node biopsy technique or elective node dissection, the site(s) of distant metastatic disease, and serum lactate dehydrogenase (LDH) levels.

Treatment

With better understanding of the prognostic significance of the microstage, some individualization of treatment has developed. **Lesions with less than 1 mm of invasion may be treated with radical local excision alone** (174,175). Traditionally, for more invasive lesions, *en bloc* radical vulvectomy and resection of regional groin nodes has been performed.

More conservative surgery for cutaneous melanomas commenced in the 1980s (183,184), and although vulvar melanomas seem to be biologically different and carry a much worse prognosis than cutaneous melanoma (185), this trend has been followed (186–189). In 1987, Davidson et al. reported on 32 patients with vulvar melanoma who underwent local excision ($n = 14$), simple vulvectomy ($n = 7$), or radical resection ($n = 11$) (184). No group had a superior survival, although the overall survival rate at 5 years was only 25%. Trimble et al. reported on 59 patients who underwent radical vulvectomy and 19 who underwent more conservative resections (188). Survival was not improved by the more radical approach, and they recommended radical local excision for the primary tumor, with groin dissection for tumors thicker than 1 mm. In 1994, the Gynecologic Oncology Group (GOG) conducted a prospective clinicopathologic study of 71 evaluable patients with melanoma of the vulva diagnosed between 1983 and 1990 (190). All patients were required to have a modified radical hemivulvectomy as minimal therapy. Seven of 37 patients (19%) having radical vulvectomy developed a local recurrence, compared with 3 of 34 (9%) having a hemivulvectomy.

The advisability of groin node dissection is controversial. **The Intergroup Surgical Melanoma Program conducted a prospective, multiinstitutional, randomized trial of elective lymph node dissection versus observation for intermediate thickness cutaneous melanomas** (1 to 4 mm) (191). There were 740 patients entered into the trial, and **elective lymph node dissection resulted in a significantly better 5-year survival rate for the 522 patients 60 years of age or younger** (88% vs. 81%; p <0.04), the 335 **patients with tumors 1 to 2 mm thick** (96% vs. 86%; p <0.02), the 403 **patients without tumor ulceration** (95% vs. 84%; p <0.01), and the 284 **patients with tumors 1 to 2 mm thick and no ulceration** (97% vs. 87%; p <0.005).

De Hulla et al. reported 9 patients with vulvar melanoma who underwent a **sentinel node procedure** (192). **Two of nine (22%) patients developed a groin recurrence after having negative sentinel nodes**, compared to 0 of 24 patients who were treated conventionally ($p = 0.06$). The authors postulated that the recurrences were due to in-transit metastases. In a study of 344 patients with cutaneous melanomas treated at the M.D. Anderson Hospital, 27 of 243 patients (11%) with a histologically negative sentinel node developed local, in transit, nodal, and/or distant metastases after a median follow-up of 35 months (193). Ten patients (4%) developed a nodal recurrence in the previously mapped basin, but ultrastaging demonstrated evidence of occult micrometastases in 80% of these 10 cases. The authors concluded that the data provided further support for sentinel node biopsy in patients with cutaneous melanomas.

As with sentinel nodes in squamous carcinoma of the vulva, sentinel node biopsy in patients with vulvar melanoma is a compromise operation, but in a well informed patient, in the hands of an experienced team, and with ultrastaging of the negative nodes, lymphatic mapping would seem to be significantly superior to no node dissection for patients with more than 1 mm of stromal invasion.

Pelvic node metastases do not occur in the absence of groin node metastases (194,195). In addition, the prognosis for patients with positive pelvic nodes is so poor that there appears to be no value in performing pelvic lymphadenectomy for this disease.

As melanomas commonly involve the clitoris and labia minora, the vaginourethral margin of resection is a common site of failure, and care should be taken to obtain an adequate "inner" resection margin. Podratz et al. (179) demonstrated a 10-year survival rate of 61% for lateral lesions, compared with 37% for medial lesions ($p < 0.027$).

The author's current policy is to perform a radical local excision with 1–2 cm margins for the primary lesion. In patients with more than 1 mm of stromal invasion, at least an ipsilateral inguinofemoral lymphadenectomy is performed. Sentinel node biopsy is reserved for the few patients who don't want to take the 50% to 60% risk of developing lymphedema.

Interferon alpha-2b (IFN-α-2b) **is the first agent to show significant value as an adjuvant for melanoma in a randomized controlled trial** (196). The Eastern Cooperative Oncology Group entered 287 patients onto an adjuvant trial of high-dose *IFN-α-2b* after surgery for deep primary (>4 mm) or regionally metastatic melanoma. With a median follow-up of 6.9 years, there was a significant prolongation of relapse-free and overall survival for the group receiving interferon. The proportion of patients who remained disease free also improved from 26% to 37%.

The results were confirmed in a larger intergroup trial that compared the efficacy of high-dose *interferon-α-2b* for 1 year with vaccination using GM2 conjugated to keyhole limpet hemocyanin (197). Eight hundred and eighty patients were randomized, and the trial was closed after interim analysis indicated inferiority of the vaccination compared with high-dose *interferon-α-2b*.

High-dose interferon regimens cause significant morbidity, but should be considered standard therapy for all high-risk melanoma patients expected to be able to tolerate the interferon (198). Immunotherapy for melanoma includes a number of different strategies with vaccines utilizing whole cell tumors, peptides, cytokine-mediated dendritic cells, DNA and RNA, and antibodies. Although initial clinical trials are promising, these approaches remain experimental (199).

Prognosis

The behavior of vulvar melanomas can be quite unpredictable, but the overall prognosis is poor. **The mean 5-year survival rate for reported cases of vulvar melanoma ranges from 21.7%** (175) **to 54%** (176). Patients with lesions invading to 1 mm or less have an excellent prognosis, but as depth of invasion increases, prognosis worsens. Chung et al. (177) reported a corrected 5-year survival rate of 100% for patients with level II lesions, 40% for level III or IV lesions, and 20% for level V lesions. Tumor volume has been reported to correlate with prognosis, with patients whose lesion has a volume less than 100 mm^3 having an excellent prognosis (195). DNA ploidy and angioinvasion have been shown to be independent prognostic factors for disease-free survival (200).

Bartholin Gland Carcinoma

Primary carcinoma of the Bartholin gland accounts for approximately 5% of vulvar malignancies. Because of its rarity, individual experience with the tumor is limited, and recommendations for management must be based on literature reviews (73,201).

The bilateral Bartholin glands are greater vestibular glands situated posterolaterally in the vulva. Their main duct is lined with stratified squamous epithelium, which changes to transitional epithelium as the terminal ducts are reached. Because tumors may arise from the gland or the duct, **a variety of histologic types may occur, including adenocarcinomas,** squamous carcinomas, and, rarely, transitional cell, adenosquamous, and adenoid cystic carcinomas. One case of small cell neuroendocrine cancer of the Bartholin gland has been reported (202).

Classification of a vulvar tumor as a Bartholin gland carcinoma has typically required that it fulfill criteria proposed by **Honan in 1897. These criteria are:**

1. **The tumor is in the correct anatomic position.**
2. **The tumor is located deep in the labium majus.**
3. **The overlying skin is intact.**
4. **There is some recognizable normal gland present.**

Strict adherence to these criteria results in underdiagnosis of some cases. Large tumors may ulcerate through the overlying skin and obliterate the residual normal gland. Although transition between normal and malignant tissue is the best criterion, some cases are diagnosed on the basis of their histologic characteristics and anatomic location.

Bartholin gland carcinomas are often misdiagnosed initially as a Bartholin cyst or abscess. A study from Tampa reported that 8 of 11 cases had initially been treated for an infectious process before referral (203). Hence, **delay of diagnosis is common, particularly in premenopausal patients.** Other differential diagnoses of any pararectovaginal neoplasm should include cloacogenic carcinoma and secondary neoplasm (201).

The **adenoid cystic variety** accounts for approximately 10% of Bartholin gland carcinomas (204,205). The largest series has been reported from the University of Michigan, where 11 cases were seen over a 58-year period (201). It is **a slow-growing tumor with a marked propensity for perineural and local invasion.** The perineural infiltration is quite characteristic and may account for the pruritus and burning sensation that many patients experience long before a palpable mass is evident (206).

Treatment

Although treatment has traditionally included radical vulvectomy and bilateral groin dissection, Copeland et al. (201) at the M. D. Anderson Hospital have reported good results with hemivulvectomy or radical local excision for the primary tumor. Because these lesions are deep in the vulva, extensive dissection is required in the ischiorectal fossa, and, this is facilitated by

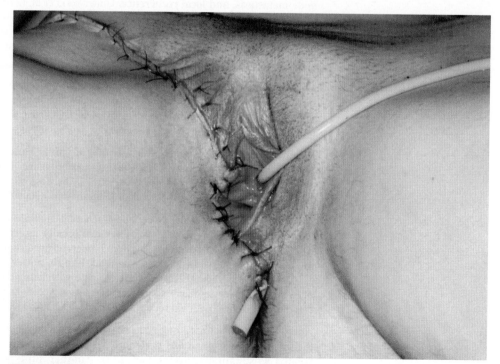

Figure 13.14   *En bloc* **resection of the right groin and right-posterior vulva for a Bartholin gland carcinoma.** Note the preservation of the clitoris and right anterior labium minus.

performing an *en bloc* resection of the primary lesion and the ipsilateral inguinofemoral lymph nodes (Fig. 13.14). **Postoperative radiation to the vulva decreased the likelihood of local recurrence** in Copeland's series from 27% (6 of 22) to 7% (1 of 14). If the ipsilateral groin nodes are positive, bilateral groin and pelvic radiation may be indicated, based on the same criteria as apply for squamous cell carcinomas.

Workers at the Massachusetts General Hospital reported 10 women with Bartholin's gland carcinoma who were treated with primary chemoradiation to the primary tumor and regional lymph nodes (207). There were four patients with stage I disease, one with stage II, three with stage III and two with stage IV. The 5-year survival was 66%, and the authors concluded that chemoradiation offered an effective alternative to surgery. Primary chemoradiation should certainly be used if the tumor is fixed to the inferior pubic ramus or involves adjacent structures, such as the anal sphincter or rectum, in order to avoid exenterative surgery.

Radical local excision, with or without ipsilateral inguinal-femoral lymphadenectomy, is also the treatment of choice for the primary lesion with adenoid cystic carcinomas, and adjuvant radiation is recommended for positive margins or perineural invasion.

Prognosis

Because of the deep location of the gland, cases tend to be more advanced than squamous carcinomas at the time of diagnosis, but stage for stage, the prognosis is similar.

Adenoid cystic tumors are less likely to metastasize to lymph nodes and carry a somewhat better prognosis. Late recurrences may occur in the lungs, liver, or bone, so 10- and 15-year survival rates are more appropriate when evaluating therapy (208). The slowly progressive nature of these tumors is reflected in the disparity between progression-free interval and survival curves (209).

Other Vulvar Adenocarcinomas

Adenocarcinomas of the vulva usually arise in a Bartholin gland or occur in association with Paget's disease. They **may rarely arise from the skin appendages, paraurethral glands, minor vestibular glands, aberrant breast tissue, endometriosis, or a misplaced cloacal remnant** (116).

A particularly aggressive type is the **adenosquamous carcinoma.** This tumor has a number of synonyms, including cylindroma, pseudoglandular squamous cell carcinoma, and adenoacanthoma of the sweat gland of Lever. **The tumor has a propensity for perineural invasion, early lymph node metastasis, and local recurrence.** Underwood et al. (210) reported a crude 5-year survival rate of 5.6% (1 of 18) for adenosquamous carcinoma of the vulva, compared with 62.3% (48 of 77) for patients with squamous cell carcinoma. Treatment should be by radical vulvectomy and bilateral groin dissection, and postoperative radiation may be appropriate.

Basal Cell Carcinoma

Basal cell carcinoma (BCC) is the most common human malignant neoplasm. As with melanomas, its incidence is strongly correlated with sun exposure, and the vast majority occurs in the head and neck region. Of 3,604 cases of BCC seen at the University of Florence, Italy, between 1995 and 2003, there were 63 cases (1.7%) arising on the vulva (211).

Basal cell carcinomas represent 2% to 4% of vulvar cancers. As with other basal cell carcinomas, vulvar lesions commonly appear as a "rodent ulcer" with rolled edges, although nodules and macules are other morphologic varieties. Most lesions are smaller than 2 cm in diameter and are usually situated on the anterior labia majora. Giant lesions occasionally occur (212).

Basal cell carcinomas usually affect postmenopausal white women, a Vancouver study reporting a mean age of 74 years (213). **They are locally aggressive, and radical local excision usually is adequate treatment.** They are moderately radiosensitive, so radiation may be useful in selected cases. **Metastasis to regional lymph nodes has been reported but is rare** (214,215), and there has been one reported case with hematogenous spread (212). The duration of symptoms prior to diagnosis is usually several years in patients with metastatic basal cell carcinomas (215). The local recurrence rate is 10% to 20% (215).

Approximately 3% to 5% of basal cell carcinomas contain a malignant squamous component, the so-called **basosquamous carcinoma. These lesions are more aggressive and should be treated as squamous carcinomas** (214). **Another subtype of basal cell carcinoma is the adenoid basal cell carcinoma,** which must be differentiated from the more aggressive adenoid cystic carcinoma arising in a Bartholin gland or the skin (215).

Verrucous Carcinoma

Verrucous carcinomas are most commonly found in the oral cavity, but may be found on any moist membrane composed of squamous epithelium (216). They are a distinct entity, with no association with human papillomavirus infection, and a peculiar distribution pattern of cytokeratins AE1 and AE3 on immunohistochemical staining (217).

Grossly, the tumors have a cauliflower-like appearance, and the diameter of reported lesions ranges from 1 to 15 cm (218). **Microscopically, they contain multiple papillary fronds that lack the central connective tissue core that characterizes condylomata acuminata.** The gross and microscopic features of a verrucous carcinoma are very similar to those of the **giant condyloma of Buschke-Loewenstein,** and they probably represent the same disease entity (116). Adequate biopsy from the base of the lesion is required to differentiate a verrucous carcinoma from a benign condyloma acuminatum or a squamous cell carcinoma with a verrucous growth pattern.

Clinically, verrucous carcinomas usually occur in postmenopausal women, and they are slowly growing but locally destructive lesions. Even bone may be invaded. Metastasis to regional lymph nodes is rare but has been reported (219).

Radical local excision is the basic treatment, although if there are palpably suspicious groin nodes, these should be evaluated with fine-needle aspiration cytologic testing or excisional biopsy. Usually, enlarged nodes are due to inflammatory hypertrophy (220). If the nodes contain metastases, radical local excision and at least an ipsilateral inguinofemoral lymphadenectomy are indicated.

Vulvar intraepithelial neoplasia or invasive squamous cell carcinoma may be seen in association with verrucous carcinoma. A Greek study of 17 cases diagnosed over a 12-year period reported coexistence of verrucous and squamous carcinoma of the vulva in 6 cases (35%) (221).

Radiation therapy is contraindicated because it may induce anaplastic transformation with subsequent regional and distant metastasis (222). Japaze et al. (220) reported a corrected 5-year survival rate of 94% for 17 patients treated with surgery alone, compared with 42% for 7 patients treated with surgery and radiation. If there is a recurrence, further surgical excision is the treatment of choice. This may occasionally necessitate some type of exenteration.

Vulvar Sarcomas

Sarcomas represent 1% to 2% of vulvar malignancies and comprise a heterogenous group of tumors. **Leiomyosarcomas** are the most common, and other histologic types include **fibrosarcomas, neurofibrosarcomas, liposarcomas, rhabdomyosarcomas, angiosarcomas, epithelioid sarcomas, and malignant schwannomas** (116). A recent paper from Johns Hopkins reported seven cases of vulvar sarcoma among 453 patients with vulvar malignancies seen from 1977 to 1997, an incidence of 1.5% (223).

The primary treatment is wide surgical excision (221). Adjuvant radiation may be helpful for high-grade tumors and locally recurrent low-grade lesions (222). **The overall survival rate is approximately 70%.** There were no recurrences in the series from Johns Hopkins (220), with follow-up ranging from 60 to 172 months. Only one of their patients had groin dissection.

Leiomyosarcomas usually appear as enlarging, often painful masses, usually in the labium majus. In a review of 32 smooth-muscle tumors of the vulva, in 1979, Tavassoli and Norris (226) reported that recurrence was associated with three main determinants: diameter greater than 5 cm, infiltrating margins, and five or more mitotic figures per 10 high-power fields. The absence of one, or even all, of these features did not guarantee that recurrence would not occur (226). A more recent study from the Massachusetts General Hospital suggested that a vulvar smooth muscle tumor should be considered a sarcoma when three or all of the following four features were present: (i) over 5 cm in greatest dimension; (ii) infiltrate margins; (iii) 5 mitoses/10 HPF; and (iv) moderate to severe cytologic atypia (227).

Lymphatic metastases are uncommon, and radical local excision is the usual treatment.

Epithelioid sarcomas characteristically develop in the soft tissues of the extremities of young adults but may rarely occur on the vulva. Ulbright et al. (228) described two cases and reviewed three other reports. They concluded that these tumors may mimic a Bartholin cyst, thus leading to inadequate initial treatment. They also suggested that vulvar epithelioid sarcomas behave more aggressively than their extragenital counterparts, with four of the five patients dying of metastatic disease.

Epithelioid sarcomas in general have a propensity for extensive local disease at presentation, local recurrence, lymph node metastasis, and distant metastasis (229,230). Treatment consists of radical excision of the tumor, and at least ipsilateral groin dissection. Systemic therapy is ineffective.

Rhabdomyosarcomas are the most common soft tissue sarcomas in childhood, and 20% involve the pelvis or genitourinary tract (231). Dramatic gains have been made in the treatment of these tumors since the late 1970s. Previously, **radical pelvic surgery was the standard approach, but results were poor. A multimodality approach has evolved, principally as a result of four successful protocols organized by the Intergroup Rhabdomyosarcoma Study Group (IRSG), and survival rates have improved significantly, with a corresponding decrease in morbidity (232).**

Arndt et al. summarized the results of these four protocols in 2001. There were 151 patients entered on the studies, and the vulva was the least common primary site, there being only 20 (13%) vulvar rhabdomyosarcomas. Only 5 (25%) of the patients were 15 years or older, and the histologic subtypes were enbryonal 8 (40%); botryoid 3 (15%); and alveolar/undifferentiated 9 (45%). All were managed with chemotherapy *(vincristine, dactinomycin ± cyclophosphamide ± doxorubicin)*, with or without radiation therapy. Wide local excision of the tumor, with or without inguinofemoral lymphadenectomy, was carried out before or after the chemotherapy.

Patients with local and/or regional rhabdomyosarcoma of the female genital tract have an excellent prognosis, with an estimated 5-year overall survival of 87% (232).

Lymphomas

The genital tract may be involved primarily by malignant lymphomas, but involvement more commonly is a manifestation of systemic disease. In the lower genital tract, the cervix is most commonly involved, followed by the vulva and the vagina (116). Most patients are in their third to sixth decade of life, and approximately three-fourths of the cases involve diffuse large cell or histiocytic non-Hodgkin's lymphomas. The remainder are nodular or Burkitt's lymphomas (233). **Treatment is by surgical excision followed by chemotherapy and/or radiation,** and the overall 5-year survival rate is approximately 70% (233).

Endodermal Sinus Tumor

There have been eight case reports of endodermal sinus tumor of the vulva. Three of the eight for whom data were available died of distant metastases (116,234). Most patients were young adults with a median age of 21 years, unlike vaginal yolk sac tumors, which usually occur in infants. Unlike their ovarian counterpart, they are not always associated with elevated serum alpha fetoprotein titers. Spread to lymph nodes occurs early, so wide excision of the primary tumor, ipsilateral groin dissection, and platinum based chemotherapy appears to be the most appropriate management (234).

Merkel Cell Carcinoma

Merkel cell carcinomas are **primary small cell carcinomas of the skin** that resemble oat cell carcinomas of the lung. They metastasize widely and have a very poor prognosis (235,236). They should be **locally excised and treated with *cisplatin*-based chemotherapy.**

Dermatofibrosarcoma Protuberans

This is a rare, low-grade cutaneous malignancy of the dermal connective tissue that occasionally involves the vulva. It has a marked tendency for local recurrence but a low risk of systemic spread (237,238). **Radical local excision should be sufficient treatment.**

Malignant Schwannoma

Five cases of malignant schwannoma in the vulvar region have been reported. The patients ranged in age from 25 to 45 years. Four of the five were free of tumor from 1 to 9 years after radical surgery, and the fifth patient died of multiple pulmonary metastases (116).

Secondary Vulvar Tumors

Eight percent of vulvar tumors are metastatic (116). **The most common primary site is the cervix, followed by the endometrium, kidney, and urethra.** Most patients in whom vulvar metastases develop have advanced primary tumors at presentation, and in approximately one-fourth of the patients, the primary lesion and the vulvar metastasis are diagnosed simultaneously (239).

References

1. **Jemal A, Siegel R, Ward E, Hao Y, Xu J, Murray T, et al.** Cancer statistics 2009. *CA Cancer J Clin* 2009;published online.doi:10.3322/caac.20006.

2. **Judson PL, Habermann EB, Baxter NN, Durham SB, Virnig BA.** Trends in the incidence of invasive and *in situ* vulvar carcinoma. *Obstet Gynecol* 2006;107:1018–1022.

3. **Hampl M, Deckers-Figiel S, Hampl JA, Rein D, Bender HG.** New aspects of vulvar cancer: changes in localization and age of onset. *Gynecol Oncol* 2008;109:340–345.

4. **Jones RW, Baranyai J, Stables S.** Trends in squamous cell carcinoma of the vulva: the influence of vulvar intraepithelial neoplasia. *Obstet Gynecol* 1997;90:448–452.

5. **Madeleine MM, Daling JR, Carter JJ, Wipf GC, Schwartz SM, McKnight B, et al.** Cofactors with human papillomarvirus in a population-based study of vulvar cancer. *J Natl Cancer Inst* 1997;89:1516–1523.

6. **Blair-Bell W, Datnow MM.** Primary malignant diseases of the vulva, with special reference to treatment by operation. *Journal of Obstetrics and Gynaecology of the British Empire* 1936;43:755–761.

7. **Way S.** The anatomy of the lymphatic drainage of the vulva and its influence on the radical operation for carcinoma. *Ann R Coll Surg Engl* 1948;3:187–197.

8. **Basset A.** Traitement chirurgical operatoire de l'epithelioma primitif du clitoris: indications—technique—results. *Revue de Chirurgie* 1912;46:546–552.

9. **Taussig FJ.** Cancer of the vulva: an analysis of 155 cases. *Am J Obstet Gynecol* 1940;40:764–770.

10. **Way S.** Carcinoma of the vulva. *Am J Obstet Gynecol* 1960;79:692–699.

11. **Hacker NF.** Radical resection of vulvar malignancies: a paradigm shift in surgical approaches. *Curr Opin Obstet Gynecol* 1999;11:61–64.

12. **Iversen T, Abeler V, Aalders J.** Individualized treatment of stage I carcinoma of the vulva. *Obstet Gynecol* 1981;57:85–89.

13. **Hacker NF, Berek JS, Lagasse LD, Nieberg RK, Leuchter RS.** Individualization of treatment for stage I squamous cell vulvar carcinoma. *Obstet Gynecol* 1984;63:155–162.

14. **DiSaia PJ, Creasman WT, Rich WM.** An alternative approach to early cancer of the vulva. *Am J Obstet Gynecol* 1979;133:825–831.

15. **Burke TW, Stringer CA, Gershenson DM, Edwards CL, Morris M, Wharton JT.** Radical wide excision and selective inguinal node dissection for squamous cell carcinoma of the vulva. *Gynecol Oncol* 1990;38:328–332.

16. **Burrell MO, Franklin EW III, Campion MJ, Crozier MA, Stacey DW.** The modified radical vulvectomy with groin dissection: an eight-year experience. *Am J Obstet Gynecol* 1988;159:715–722.

17. **Curry SL, Wharton JT, Rutledge F.** Positive lymph nodes in vulvar squamous carcinoma. *Gynecol Oncol* 1980;9:63–67.

18. **Hacker NF, Berek JS, Lagasse LD, Leuchter RS, Moore JG.** Management of regional lymph nodes and their prognostic influence in vulvar cancer. *Obstet Gynecol* 1983;61:408–412.

19. **Monaghan JM, Hammond IG.** Pelvic node dissection in the treatment of vulval carcinoma: is it necessary? *BJOG* 1984;91:270–274.

20. **Hoffman JS, Kumar NB, Morley GW.** Prognostic significance of groin lymph node metastases in squamous carcinoma of the vulva. *Obstet Gynecol* 1985;66:402–406.

21. **Homesley HD, Bundy BN, Sedlis A, Adcock L.** Radiation therapy versus pelvic node resection for carcinoma of the vulva with positive groin nodes. *Obstet Gynecol* 1986;68:733–738.

22. **Hacker NF, Leuchter RS, Berek JS, Castaldo TW, Lagasse LD.** Radical vulvectomy and bilateral inguinal lymphadenectomy through separate groin incisions. *Obstet Gynecol* 1981;58:574–579.

23. **Figge CD, Gaudenz R.** Invasive carcinoma of the vulva. *Am J Obstet Gynecol* 1974;119:382–387.

24. **Boronow RC.** Therapeutic alternative to primary exenteration for advanced vulvo-vaginal cancer. *Gynecol Oncol* 1973;1:223–229.

25. **Hacker NF, Berek JS, Juillard GJF, Lagasse LD.** Preoperative radiation therapy for locally advanced vulvar cancer. *Cancer* 1984;54:2056–2060.

26. **Van der Zee AGJ, Oonk MH, De Hulla JA, Ansink AC, Vergote I, Verheijen RH, et al.** Sentinel node dissection is safe in the treatment of early stage vulvar cancer. *J Clin Oncol* 2008;26:884–889.

27. **Hakim AA, Terada KY.** Sentinel node dissection in vulvar cancer. *Curr Treat Options Oncol* 2006;7:85–89.

28. **Hauspy J, Beiner M, Harley I, Ehrlich L, Rasty G, Covens A.** Sentinel lymph node in vulvar cancer. *Cancer* 2007;110:1015–1023.

29. **Makar APH, Scheistroen M, van den Weyngaert D, Trope CG.** Surgical management of stage I and II vulvar cancer: the role of sentinel node biopsy: review of literature. *Int J Gynecol Cancer* 2001;11:255–262.

30. **Beriwal S, Coon D, Heron DE, Kelly JL, Edwards RP, Sukumvanich P, et al.** Preoperative intensity-modulated radiotherapy and chemotherapy for locally advanced vulvar cancer. *Gynecol Oncol* 2008;109:291–295.

31. **Lupi G, Raspagliesi F, Zucali R, Fontanelli R, Paladini D, Kenda R, et al.** Combined preoperative chemoradiotherapy followed by radical surgery in locally advanced vulvar carcinoma. *Cancer* 1996;77:1472–1478.

32. **Landoni F, Maneo A, Zanetta G, Colombo A, Nava S, Placa F, et al.** Concurrent preoperative chemotherapy with 5-*fluorouracil* and *mitomycin-C* and radiotherapy (FUMIR) followed by limited surgery in locally advanced and recurrent vulvar carcinoma. *Gynecol Oncol* 1996;61:321–327.

33. **Landrum LM, Skaggs V, Gould N, Walker JL, McMeekin DS.** Comparison of outcome measures in patients with advanced squamous cell carcinoma of the vulva treated with surgery or primary chemoradiation. *Gynecol Oncol* 2008;108:584–590.

34. **Cunningham MJ, Goyer RP, Gibbons SK, Kredentser DC, Malfetano JH, Keys H.** Primary radiation, *cisplatin*, and 5-*fluorouracil* for advanced squamous cell carcinoma of the vulva. *Gynecol Oncol* 1997;66:258–261.

35. **Leiserowitz GS, Russell AH, Kinney WK, Smith LH, Taylor MH, Scudder SA.** Prophylactic chemoradiation of inguinal femoral lymph nodes in patients with locally extensive vulvar cancer. *Gynecol Oncol* 1997;66:509–514.

36. **Hyde SE, Valmadre S, Hacker NF, Schilthuis MS, van der Velden J.** Squamous cell carcinoma of the vulva with bulky positive groin nodes — nodal debulking versus full groin dissection prior to radiation therapy. *Int J Gynecol Cancer* 2007;17:154–158.

37. **Rodriguez M, Sevin B-U, Averette HE, Angioli R, Janicek M, Method M, et al.** Conservative trends in the surgical management of vulvar cancer: a University of Miami patient care evaluation study. *Int J Gynecol Cancer* 1997;7:151–157.

38. **Magrina JF, Gonzalez-Bosquet J, Weaver AL, Gaffey TA, Webb MJ, Podratz KC, et al.** Primary squamous cell cancer of the vulva: radical versus modified radical vulvar surgery. *Gynecol Oncol* 1998;71:116–121.

39. **Zacur H, Genandry R, Woodruff JD.** The patient-at-risk for development of vulvar cancer. *Gynecol Oncol* 1980;9:199–208.

40. **Buscema J, Woodruff JD, Parmley TH, Genadry R.** Carcinoma *in situ* of the vulva. *Obstet Gynecol* 1980;55:225–230.

41. **Jones RW, Rowan DM, Stewart AW.** Vulvar intraepithelial neoplasis. Aspects of the natural history and outcome in 405 women. *Obstet Gynecol* 2005;106:1319–1326.

42. **Sturgeon SR, Curtis RE, Johnson K, Ries L, Brinton LA.** Second primary cancers after vulvar and vaginal cancers. *Am J Obstet Gynecol* 1996;174:929–933.

43. **Brinton LA, Nasca PC, Mallin K, Baptiste MS, Wilbanks GW, Richart RM.** Case control study of cancer of the vulva. *Obstet Gynecol* 1990;75:859–866.

44. **Rusk D, Sutton GP, Look KY, Roman A.** Analysis of invasive squamous cell carcinoma of the vulva and vulvar intraepithelial neoplasia for the presence of human papillomavirus DNA. *Obstet Gynecol* 1991;77:918–922.

45. **Hording U, Junge J, Daugaard S, Lundvall F, Poulsen H, Bock J.** Vulvar squamous carcinoma and papillomaviruses: indications for two different etiologies. *Gynecol Oncol* 1994;52:241–246.

46. **Bloss JD, Liao SY, Wilczynski SP.** Clinical and histologic features of vulvar carcinomas analyzed for human papillomavirus status: evidence that squamous cell carcinoma of the vulva has more than one etiology. *Hum Pathol* 1991;22:711–718.

47. **Toki T, Kurman RJ, Park JS, Kessis T, Daniel RW, Shah KV.** Probable nonpapillomavirus etiology of squamous cell carcinoma of

the vulva in older women: a clinicopathologic study using *in situ* hybridization and polymerase chain reaction. *Int J Gynecol Pathol* 1991;10:107–125.

48. **Nuovo GJ, Delvenne P, MacConnel P, Chalas E, Neto C, Mann WJ.** Correlation of histology and detection of human papillomavirus DNA in vulvar cancers. *Gynecol Oncol* 1991;43:275–280.

49. **Scurry J, Campion M, Scurry B, Kim SN, Hacker NF.** Pathologic audit of 164 consecutive cases of vulvar intraepithelial neoplasia. *Int J Gynecol Path* 2006;25:176–181.

50. **Sideri M, Jones RW, Wilkinson EJ, Preti M, Heller DS, Scurry J.** Squamous vulvar intraepithelial neoplasia. 2004 modified terminology, ISSVD vulvar oncology subcommittee. *J Reprod Med* 2005; 50:807–810.

51. **Rodke G, Friedrich EG, Wilkinson EJ.** Malignant potential of mixed vulvar dystrophy (lichen sclerosis associated with squamous cell hyperplasia). *J Reprod Med* 1988;33:545–551.

52. **Carli P, De Magnis A, Mannone F, Botti E, Taddei G, Cattaneo A.** Vulvar carcinoma associated with lichen sclerosus: experience at the Florence, Italy, Vulvar Clinic. *J Reprod Med* 2003;48:313–318.

53. **Scurry J.** Does lichen sclerosus play a central role in the pathogenesis of human papilloma virus negative vulvar squamous cell carcinoma? The itch-scratch-lichen sclerosus hypothesis. *Int J Gynecol Cancer* 1999;9:89–97.

54. **Wilkinson EJ, Brown HM.** Vulvar Paget disease of urothelial origin: a report of three cases and a proposed classification of vulvar Paget disease. *Hum Pathol* 2002;33:549–554.

55. **Kurman RJ.** *Blaunstein's pathology of the female genital tract.* 5th ed. New York: Springer, 2002.

56. **Niikura H, Yoshida H, Ito K, Takano T, Watanabe H, Aiba S, et al.** Paget's disease of the vulva: a clinicopathologic study of type 1 cases treated at a single institution. *Int J Gynecol Cancer* 2006;16: 1212–1215.

57. **MacLean AB, Makwana M, Ellis PE, Cunningham F.** The management of Paget's disease of the vulva. *J Obstet Gynaecol* 2004; 24:124–128.

58. **Fanning J, Lambert L, Hale TM, Morris PC, Schuerch C.** Paget's disease of the vulva: prevalence of associated vulvar adenocarcinoma, invasive Paget's disease, and recurrence after surgical excision. *Am J Obstet Gynecol* 1999;180:24–27.

59. **Lee RA, Dahlin DC.** Paget's disease of the vulva with extension into the urethra, bladder, and ureters: a case report. *Am J Obstet Gynecol* 1981;140:834–836.

60. **Gunn RA, Gallager HS.** Vulvar Paget's disease: a topographic study. *Cancer* 1980;46:590–594.

61. **Black D, Tornos C, Soslow RA, Awtrey CS, Barakat RR, Chi DS.** The outcomes of patients with positive margins after excision for intraepithelial Paget's disease of the vulva. *Gynecol Oncol* 2007;104: 547–550.

62. **Stacy D, Burrell MO, Franklin EW III.** Extramammary Paget's disease of the vulva and anus: use of intraoperative frozen-section margins. *Am J Obstet Gynecol* 1986;155:519–522.

63. **Fishman DA, Chambers SK, Schwartz PE, Kohorn EI, Chambers JT.** Extramammary Paget's disease of the vulva. *Gynecol Oncol* 1995;56:266–270.

64. **Brown RSD, Lankester KJ, McCormack M, Power DA, Spittle MF.** Radiotherapy for perianal Paget's disease. *Clin Oncol* 2002;14:272–284.

65. **Fine BA, Fowler LJ, Valente PT, Gaudet T.** Minimally invasive Paget's disease of the vulva with extensive lymph node metastases. *Gynecol Oncol* 1995;57:262–265.

66. **Ewing T, Sawicki J, Ciaravino G, Rumore GJ.** Microinvasive Paget's disease. *Gynecol Oncol* 2004;95:755–758.

67. **Scheistroen M, Trope C, Kaern J, Petterson EO, Alfsen GC, Nesland JM.** DNA ploidy and expression of p53 and c-erbB-2 in extramammary Paget's disease of the vulva. *Gynecol Oncol* 1997;64:88–92.

68. **Hacker NF, Nieberg RK, Berek JS, Lagasse LD.** Superficially invasive vulvar cancer with nodal metastases. *Gynecol Oncol* 1983;15: 65–77.

69. **Parker RT, Duncan I, Rampone J, Creasman W.** Operative management of early invasive epidermoid carcinoma of the vulva. *Am J Obstet Gynecol* 1975;123:349–355.

70. **Chu J, Tamimi HK, Figge DC.** Femoral node metastases with negative superficial inguinal nodes in early vulvar cancer. *Am J Obstet Gynecol* 1981;140:337–341.

71. **Podczaski E, Sexton M, Kaminski P, Singapuri K, Sorosky J, Larson J, et al.** Recurrent carcinoma of the vulva after conservative treatment for "microinvasive" disease. *Gynecol Oncol* 1990;39: 65–68.

72. **Gordinier ME, Malpica A, Burke TW, Bodurka DC, Wolf JK, Jhingran A, et al.** Groin recurrence in patients with vulvar cancer with negative nodes on superficial inguinal lymphadenectomy. *Gynecol Oncol* 2003;90:625–628.

73. **Leuchter RS, Hacker NF, Voet RL, Berek JS, Townsend DE, Lagasse LD.** Primary carcinoma of the Bartholin gland: a report of 14 cases and a review of the literature. *Obstet Gynecol* 1982;60: 361–368.

74. **Piver MS, Xynos FP.** Pelvic lymphadenectomy in women with carcinoma of the clitoris. *Obstet Gynecol* 1977;49:592–598.

75. **Rutledge F, Smith JP, Franklin EW.** Carcinoma of the vulva. *Am J Obstet Gynecol* 1970;106:1117–1124.

76. **Green TH Jr.** Carcinoma of the vulva: a reassessment. *Obstet Gynecol* 1978;52:462–468.

77. **Krupp PJ, Bohm JW.** Lymph gland metastases in invasive squamous cell cancer of the vulva. *Am J Obstet Gynecol* 1978;130: 943–949.

78. **Benedet JL, Turko M, Fairey RN, Boyes DA.** Squamous carcinoma of the vulva: results of treatment, 1938 to 1976. *Am J Obstet Gynecol* 1979;134:201–206.

79. **Iversen T, Aalders JG, Christensen A, Kolstad P.** Squamous cell carcinoma of the vulva: a review of 424 patients, 1956–1974. *Gynecol Oncol* 1980;9:271–279.

80. **Rouzier R, Haddad B, Plantier F, Dubois P, Pelisse M, Paniel BJ.** Local relapse in patients treated for squamous cell vulvar carcinoma: incidence and prognostic values. *Obstet Gynecol* 2002;100: 1159–1167.

81. **Raspagliesi F, Hanozet F, Ditto A, Solima E, Zanaboni F, Vecchione F, et al.** Clinical and pathological prognostic factors in squamous cell carcinoma of the vulva. *Gynecol Oncol* 2006;102: 333–337.

82. **Bosquet JG, Magrina JF, Magtibay PM, Gaffey TA, Cha SS, Jones MB, et al.** Patterns of inguinal groin metastases in squamous cell carcinoma of the vulva. *Gynecol Oncol* 2007;105:742–746.

83. **Magrina JF, Webb MJ, Gaffey TA, Symmonds RE.** Stage I squamous cell cancer of the vulva. *Am J Obstet Gynecol* 1979;134: 453–457.

84. **Wilkinson EJ, Rico MJ, Pierson KK.** Microinvasive carcinoma of the vulva. *Int J Gynecol Pathol* 1982;1:29–35.

85. **Hoffman JS, Kumar NB, Morley GW.** Microinvasive squamous carcinoma of the vulva: search for a definition. *Obstet Gynecol* 1983;61:615–619.

86. **Boice CR, Seraj IM, Thrasher T, King A.** Microinvasive squamous carcinoma of the vulva: present status and reassessment. *Gynecol Oncol* 1984;18:71–77.

87. **Ross M, Ehrmann RL.** Histologic prognosticators in stage I squamous cell carcinoma of the vulva. *Obstet Gynecol* 1987;70:774–779.

88. **Rowley K, Gallion HH, Donaldson ES, Van Nagell JR, Higgins RV, Powell DE, et al.** Prognostic factors in early vulvar cancer. *Gynecol Oncol* 1988;31:43–49.

89. **Struyk APHB, Bouma JJ, van Lindert ACM.** Early stage cancer of the vulva: a pilot investigation on cancer of the vulva in gynecologic oncology centers in the Netherlands. *Proceedings of the International Gynecological Cancer Society* 1989;2:303(abst).

90. **van der Velden J, Hacker NF.** Update on vulvar carcinoma. In: **Rothenberg ML, ed.** *Gynecologic oncology: controversies and new developments.* Boston: Kluwer, 1994:101–119.

91. **Morley GW.** Infiltrative carcinoma of the vulva: results of surgical treatment. *Am J Obstet Gynecol* 1976;124:874–880.

92. **Homesley HD, Bundy BN, Sedlis A, Yordan E, Berek JS, Jahshan A, et al.** Assessment of current International Federation of Gynecology and Obstetrics staging of vulvar carcinoma relative to prognostic factors for survival (a Gynecologic Oncology Group study). *Am J Obstet Gynecol* 1991;164:997–1004.

93. **Podratz KC, Symmonds RE, Taylor WF, Williams TJ.** Carcinoma of the vulva: analysis of treatment and survival. *Obstet Gynecol* 1983; 61:63–74.

94. **Rouzier R, Preti M, Sideri M, Paniel B-J, Jones RW.** A suggested modification to FIGO stage III vulvar cancer. *Gynecol Oncol* 2008;110: 83–86.

95. **Rhodes CA, Cummings C, Shafi MI.** The management of squamous cell vulval cancer: a population-based retrospective study of 411 cases. *BJOG* 1998;105:200–205.

96. **van der Velden J, van Lindert ACM, Gimbrere CHF, Oosting H, Heintz APM.** Epidemiological data on vulvar cancer: comparison of hospital and population-based data. *Gynecol Oncol* 1996;62:379–383.

97. **De Simone CP, Van Ness JS, Cooper AL, Modesitt SC, De Priest PD, Veland FR, et al.** The treatment of lateral T1 and T2 squamous cell carcinomas of the vulva confined to the labium majus or minus. *Gynecol Oncol* 2007;104:390–395.

98. **Tantipalakorn C, Robertson G, Marsden DE, Gabski V, Hacker NF.** Outcome and Patterns of Recurrence for International Federation of Gynecology and Obstetrics (FIGO) Stages I and II squamous Cell Vulvar Cancer. *Obstet Gynecol* 2009;113:895–901.

99. **de Hulla JA, Oonk MHM, van der Zee AGJ.** Modern management of vulvar cancer. *Curr Opin Obstet Gynecol* 2004;16:65–72.

100. **Andersen BL, Hacker NF.** Psychological adjustment after vulvar surgery. *Obstet Gynecol* 1983;62:457–461.

101. **Farias-Eisner R, Cirisano F, Grouse D, Leuchter RS, Karlan BY, Lagasse LD, et al.** Conservative and individualized surgery for early squamous carcinoma of the vulva: the treatment of choice for stages I and II (T_{1-2}, N_{0-1}, M_0) disease. *Gynecol Oncol* 1994;53:55–58.

102. **de Hulla JA, Hollema H, Lolkema S, Boezen M, Boonstra H, Burger MPM, et al.** Vulvar carcinoma: the price of less radical surgery. *Cancer* 2002;95:2331–2338.

103. **Chan JK, Sugiyama V, Pham H, Gu M, Rutgers J, Osann K.** Margin distance and other clinico-pathologic prognostic factors in vulvar carcinoma: a multivariate analysis. *Gynecol Oncol* 2007;104:636–641.

104. **Heaps JM, Fu YS, Montz FJ, Hacker NF, Berek JS.** Surgical-pathologic variables predictive of local recurrence in squamous cell carcinoma of the vulva. *Gynecol Oncol* 1990;38:309–314.

105. **Chan JK, Sugiyama V, Tajalli TR, Pham H, Gu M, Rutgers J, et al.** Conservative clitoral preservation surgery in the treatment of vulvar squamous cell carcinoma. *Gynecol Oncol* 2004;95:152–156.

106. **Jones RW, Matthews JH.** Early clitoral carcinoma successfully treated by radiotherapy and bilateral inguinal lymphadenectomy. *Int J Gynecol Cancer* 1999;9:348–350.

107. **Lingard D, Free K, Wright RG, Battistutta D.** Invasive squamous cell carcinoma of the vulva: behaviour and results in the light of changing management regimes. *Aust N Z J Obstet Gynaecol* 1992;32:137–142.

108. **Atamdede F, Hoogerland D.** Regional lymph node recurrence following local excision for microinvasive vulvar carcinoma. *Gynecol Oncol* 1989;34:125–129.

109. **van der Velden J, Kooyman CD, van Lindert ACM, Heintz APM.** A stage 1A vulvar carcinoma with an inguinal lymph node recurrence after local excision: a case report and literature review. *Int J Gynecol Cancer* 1992;2:157–159.

110. **Vernooij F, Sie-Go DMDS, Heintz APM.** Lymph node recurrence following Stage IA vulvar cancer: two cases and a short overview of literature. *Int J Gynecol Cancer* 2007;17:517–535.

111. **Stehman FB, Bundy BN, Droretsky PM, Creasman WT.** Early stage I carcinoma of the vulva treated with ipsilateral superficial inguinal lymphadenectomy and modified radical hemivulvectomy: a prospective study of the Gynecologic Oncology Group. *Obstet Gynecol* 1992;79:490–495.

112. **Wharton JT, Gallager S, Rutledge RN.** Microinvasive carcinoma of the vulva. *Am J Obstet Gynecol* 1974;118:159–165.

113. **Buscema J, Stern JL, Woodruff JD.** Early invasive carcinoma of the vulva. *Am J Obstet Gynecol* 1981;140:563–568.

114. **Iversen T, Aas M.** Lymph drainage from the vulva. *Gynecol Oncol* 1983;16:179–189.

115. **Sedlis A, Homesley H, Bundy BN, Marshall R, Yordan E, Hacker NF, et al.** Positive groin lymph nodes in superficial squamous cell vulvar cancer. *Am J Obstet Gynecol* 1987;156:1159–1164.

116. **Fu YS.** Nonepithelial and metastatic tumors of the lower genital tract. In: Fu YS, ed. *Pathology of the uterine cervix, vagina, and vulva*, 2nd ed., vol. 21 in *Major problems in pathology*. Philadelphia: Saunders, 2002:471–539.

117. **Nicklin JL, Hacker NF, Heintze SW, van Eijkeren M, Durham NJ.** An anatomical study of inguinal lymph node topography and clinical implications for the surgical management of vulvar cancer. *Int J Gynecol Cancer* 1995;5:128–133.

118. **Micheletti L, Levi AC, Bogliatto F, Preti M, Massobrio M.** Rationale and definition of the lateral extension of the inguinal lymphadenectomy for vulvar cancer derived from embryological and anatomical study. *J Surg Oncol* 2002;81:19–24.

119. **Dardarian TS, Gray HJ, Morgan MA, Rubin SC, Randall TC.** Saphenous vein sparing during inguinal lymphadenectomy to reduce morbidity in patients with vulvar carcinoma. *Gynecol Oncol* 2006;101:140–142.

120. **Zhang X, Sheng X, Niu J, Li H, Li D, Tang L, et al.** Sparing of saphenous vein during inguinal lymphadenectomy for vulvar malignancies. *Gynecol Oncol* 2007;105:722–726.

121. **Micheletti L, Borgno G, Barbero M, Preti M, Cavanna L, Nicolaci P, et al.** Deep femoral lymphadenectomy with preservation of the fascial lata. *J Reprod Med* 1990;35:1130–1133.

122. **Gaarenstroom KN, Kenter GG, Trimbos JB, Agous I, Amant F, Peters AAW, et al.** Postoperative complications after vulvectomy and inguinofemoral lymphadenectomy using separate groin incisions. *Int J Gynecol Cancer* 2003;13:522–527.

123. **Ryan M, Stainton C, Slaytor EK, Jaconelli C, Watts S, MacKenzie P.** Aetiology and prevalence of lower limb lymphoedema following treatment for gynaecological cancer. *Aust N Z J Obstet Gynecol* 2003;43:148–151.

124. **Origoni M, Sideri M, Garsia S, Carinelli SG, Ferrari AG.** Prognostic value of pathological patterns of lymph node positivity in squamous cell carcinoma of the vulva stage III and IVA FIGO. *Gynecol Oncol* 1992;45:313–316.

125. **Paladini D, Cross P, Lopes A, Monaghan JM.** Prognostic significance of lymph node variables in squamous cell carcinoma of the vulva. *Cancer* 1994;74:2491–2496.

126. **van der Velden J, van Lindert ACM, Lammes FB, ten Kate FJW, Sie-Go DMS, Oosting H, et al.** Extracapsular growth of lymph node metastases in squamous cell carcinoma of the vulva. *Cancer* 1995;75:2885–2890.

127. **Dvoretsky PM, Bonfiglio TA, Helmkamp BF.** The pathology of superficially invasive, thin vulvar squamous cell carcinoma. *Int J Gynecol Pathol* 1984;3:331–342.

128. **de Hulla JA, Pruim J, Qué TH.** Noninvasive detection of inguinofemoral lymph node metastases in squamous cell cancer of the vulva by tyrosine positron emission tomography. *Int J Gynecol Cancer* 1999;9:141–146.

129. **Land R, Herod J, Moskovic E, King M, Sohaib SA, Trott P, et al.** Routine computerized tomography scanning, groin ultrasound with or without fine needle aspiraton cytology in the surgical management of primary squamous cell carcinoma of the vulva. *Int J Gynecol Cancer* 2006;16:312–317.

130. **Mohammed DKA, Uberoi R, Lopes A de B, Monaghan JM.** Inguinal node status by ultrasound in vulvar cancer. *Gynecol Oncol* 2000;77:93–96.

131. **Cabanas RM.** An approach for the treatment of penile cancer. *Cancer* 1977;39:456–466.

132. **Morton DL, Wen DR, Wong JH, Economou JS, Cagk LA, Storm FR, et al.** Technical details of intraoperative lymphatic mapping for early stage melanoma. *Arch Surg* 1992;127:392–399.

133. **Raspagliesi F, Ditto A, Fontanelli R, Maccauro M, Carcangiu ML, Parazzini F, et al.** False-negative sentinel node in patients with vulvar cancer: a case study. *Int J Gynecol Cancer* 2003;13:361–363.

134. **Ansink AC, Sie-Go DM, van der Velden J.** Identification of sentinel lymph nodes in vulvar carcinoma patients with the aid of a patent blue dye injection. *Cancer* 1999;86:652–656.

135. **Louis-Sylvestre C, Evangelista E, Leonard F, Itti E, Meignan M, Paniel BJ.** Sentinel node localization should be interpreted with caution in midline vulvar cancer. *Gynecol Oncol* 2005;97:151–154.

136. **Moore RG, De Pasquale SE, Steinhoff MM, Gajewski W, Steller M, Noto R, et al.** Sentinel node identification and the ability to detect metastatic tumor to inguinal lymph nodes in squamous cell cancer of the vulva. *Gynecol Oncol* 2003;89:475–479.

137. **Moore RG, Granai CO, Gajewski W, Gordinier M, Steinhoff MM.** Pathologic evaluation of inguinal sentinel lymph nodes in vulvar cancer patients: a combination of immunohistochemical staining versus ultrastaging with hexatoxylin and eosin staining. *Gynecol Oncol* 2003;91:378–382.

138. **Molpus KL, Kelley MC, Johnson JE, Martin WH, Jones HW III.** Sentinel lymph node detection and microstaging in vulvar carcinoma. *J Reprod Med* 2001;46:863–869.

139. **de Hulla JA, Ansink AC, Tymstra T, van der Zee AGJ.** What doctors and patients think about false-negative sentinel lymph nodes in vulvar cancer. *J Psychosom Obstet Gynaecol* 2001;22:199–203.

140. **Gan S, Magarey C, Schwartz P, Papadatos G, Graham P, Vallentine J.** Women's choice between sentinel lymph node biopsy and axillary clearance. *ANZ J Surg* 2002;72:110–113.

141. **de Hulla JA, Oonk MH, Ansink AC.** Pitfalls in the sentinel node procedure in vulvar cancer. *Gynecol Oncol* 2004;94:10–15.

142. **Farrell R.** Personal communication.

143. **Montana GS, Thomas GM, Moore DH, Saxer A, Mangan CE, Lentz SS, et al.** Preoperative chemoradiation for carcinoma of the vulva with N_2/N_3 nodes. A Gynecologic Oncology Group Study. *Int J Radiat Oncol Biol Phys* 2000;48:1007–1013.

144. **Simonsen E, Johnsson JE, Trope C.** Radical vulvectomy with warm-knife and open-wound techniques in vulvar malignancies. *Gynecol Oncol* 1984;17:22–31.

145. **Trelford JD, Deer DA, Ordorica E, Franti CE, Trelford-Sauder M.** Ten-year prospective study in a management change of vulvar carcinoma. *Am J Obstet Gynecol* 1984;150:288–296.

146. **Low JJH, Hacker NF.** Vulvar reconstruction in gynecologic oncology. *Hungarian Journal of Gynecologic Oncology* 1999;3:105–112.

147. **Barnhill DR, Hoskins WJ, Metz P.** Use of the rhomboid flap after partial vulvectomy. *Obstet Gynecol* 1983;62:444–448.

148. **Ballon SC, Donaldson RC, Roberts JA.** Reconstruction of the vulva using a myocutaneous graft. *Gynecol Oncol* 1979;7:123–129.

149. **Chafe W, Fowler WC, Walton LA, Currie JL.** Radical vulvectomy with use of tensor fascia lata myocutaneous flap. *Am J Obstet Gynecol* 1983;145:207–213.

150. **Andersen BL, Hacker NF.** Psychosexual adjustment following pelvic exenteration. *Obstet Gynecol* 1983;61:457–461.

151. **Cavanagh D, Shepherd JH.** The place of pelvic exenteration in the primary management of advanced carcinoma of the vulva. *Gynecol Oncol* 1982;13:318–324.

152. **Grimshaw RN, Aswad SG, Monaghan JM.** The role of anovulvectomy in locally advanced carcinoma of the vulva. *Int J Gynecol Cancer* 1991;1:15–20.

153. **Boronow RC, Hickman BT, Reagan MT, Smith RA, Steadham RE.** Combined therapy as an alternative to exenteration for locally advanced vulvovaginal cancer: II. results, complications and dosimetric and surgical considerations. *Am J Clin Oncol* 1987;10:171–181.

154. **Thomas G, Dembo A, DePetrillo A, Pringle J, Ackerman I, Bryson P, et al.** Concurrent radiation and chemotherapy in vulvar carcinoma. *Gynecol Oncol* 1989;34:263–267.

155. **Jackson KS, Fankam EF, Das N, Nais R, Lopes AD, Godfrey KA.** Unilateral groin and pelvic irradiation for unilaterally node-positive women with vulval carcinoma. *Int J Gynecol Cancer* 2006;16:283–87.

156. **Parthasarathy A, Cheung MK, Osann K, Husain A, Teng NN, Berek JS, et al.** The benefit of adjuvant radiation therapy in simple node-positive squamous cell vulvar carcinoma. *Gynecol Oncol* 2006;103:1095–1099.

157. **Podratz KC, Symmonds RE, Taylor WF.** Carcinoma of the vulva: analysis of treatment failures. *Am J Obstet Gynecol* 1982;143:340–345.

158. **Malfetano J, Piver MS, Tsukada Y.** Stage III and IV squamous cell carcinoma of the vulva. *Gynecol Oncol* 1986;23:192–198.

159. **Faul CM, Mirmow D, Huang O, Gerszten K, Day R, Jones MW.** Adjuvant radiation for vulvar carcinoma: improved local control. *Int J Radiat Oncol Biol Phys* 1997;38:381–389.

160. **Stehman F, Bundy B, Thomas G, Varia M, Okagaki T, Roberts J, et al.** Groin dissection versus groin radiation in carcinoma of the vulva: a Gynecologic Oncology Group study. *Int J Radiat Oncol Biol Phys* 1992;24:389–396.

161. **Koh W-J, Chiu M, Stelzer KJ, Greer BE, Mastras D, Comsia N, et al.** Femoral vessel depth and the implications for groin node radiation. *Int J Radiat Oncol Biol Phys* 1993;27:969–974.

162. **van der Velden J, Ansink A.** Primary groin irradiation versus primary groin surgery for early vulvar cancer. *Cochrane Database of Systematic Reviews* 2001;4:Art.No.:CD002224.DOI:10.1002/14651858.CD002224.

163. **Lataifeh I, Nascimento MC, Nicklin JL, Perrin LC, Crandon AJ, Obermaier A.** Pattens of recurrence and disease-free survival in advanced squamous cell carcinoma of the vulva. *Gynecol Oncol* 2004;95:701–705.

164. **Hopkins MP, Reid GC, Morley GW.** The surgical management of recurrent squamous cell carcinoma of the vulva. *Obstet Gynecol* 1990;75:1001–1006.

165. **Weikel W, Schmidt M, Steiner E, Knapstein P-G, Koelbl H.** Surgical therapy of recurrent vulvar cancer. *Am J Obstet Gynecol* 2006;195:1293–1303.

166. **Hoffman M, Greenberg S, Greenberg H, Fiorica JV, Roberts WS, La Polla JP, et al.** Interstitial radiotherapy for the treatment of advanced or recurrent vulvar and distal vaginal malignancy. *Am J Obstet Gynecol* 1990;162:1278–1282.

167. **Marx GM, Friedlander ML, Hacker NF.** Cytotoxic drug treatment of vulval and vaginal cancer. *CME J Gynecol Oncol* 2001;6:67–72.

168. **Boutselis JG.** Radical vulvectomy for invasive squamous cell carcinoma of the vulva. *Obstet Gynecol* 1972;39:827–833.

169. **Japeze H, Garcia-Bunuel R, Woodruff JD.** Primary vulvar neoplasia: a review of the invasive carcinoma, 1935–1972l *Obstet Gynecol* 1977;49;404–410.

170. **Cavanagh D, Roberts WS, Bryson SCP, Marsden DE, Ingram JM, Anaderdon WR.** Changing trends in the surgical treatment of invasive carcinoma of the vulva. *Surg Gynecol Obstet* 1986;162;164–168.

171. **Beller U, Quinn MA, Benedet JL, Creasman WT, Ngan HYS, Maisonneuve P, et al.** Carcinoma of the vulva : In 26th Annual Report on the Results of Treatment in Gynecological Cancer. *Int J Gynecol Obstet* 2006;95:S7–S27.

172. **Kaern J, Iversen T, Trope C, Pettersen EO, Nesland JM.** Flow cytometric DNA measurements in squamous cell carcinoma of the vulva: an important prognostic method. *Int J Gynecol Cancer* 1992;2:169–174.

173. **Knopp S, Bjorge T, Nesland JM, Trope C, Scheistroen M, Holm R.** p16^{INK4a} and p27$^{Waf1/Cip1}$ expression correlates with clinical outcome in vulvar carcinomas. *Gynecol Oncol* 2004;95:37–45.

174. **Hyde SE, Ansink AC, Burger MPM, Schilthuis MS, van der Velden J.** The impact of performance status on survival in patients 80 years and older with vulvar cancer. *Gynecol Oncol* 2002;84:388–393.

175. **Blessing K, Kernohan NM, Miller ID, Al Nafussi AI.** Malignant melanoma of the vulva: clinicopathological features. *Int J Gynecol Cancer* 1991;1:81–88.

176. **Ragnarsson-Olding BK, Nilsson BR, Kanter-Lewensohn LR.** Malignant melanoma of the vulva in a nationwide, 25-year study of 219 Swedish females: predictors of survival. *Cancer* 1999;86:1285–1293.

177. **Chung AF, Woodruff JW, Lewis JL Jr.** Malignant melanoma of the vulva: a report of 44 cases. *Obstet Gynecol* 1975;45:638–644.

178. **Phillips GL, Twiggs LB, Okagaki T.** Vulvar melanoma: a microstaging study. *Gynecol Oncol* 1982;14:80–87.

179. **Podratz KC, Gaffey TA, Symmonds RE, Johansen KL, O'Brien PC.** Melanoma of the vulva: an update. *Gynecol Oncol* 1983;16:153–168.

180. **Clark WH, From L, Bernardino EA, Mihm MC.** The histogenesis and biologic behavior of primary human malignant melanomas of the skin. *Cancer Res* 1969;29:705–711.

181. **Breslow A.** Thickness, cross-sectional area and depth of invasion in the prognosis of cutaneous melanoma. *Ann Surg* 1970;172:902–908.

182. **Kim CJ, Reintgen DS, Balch CM for the AJCC Melanoma Staging Committee.** The new melanoma staging system. *Cancer Control* 2002;9:9–15.

183. **Aitkin DR, Clausen K, Klein JP, James AG.** The extent of primary melanoma excision: a re-evaluation. How wide is wide? *Ann Surg* 1983;198:634–641.

184. **Day CL, Mihm MC, Sober AJ, Fitzpatrick TB, Malt RA.** Narrower margins for clinical stage I malignant melanoma. *N Engl J Med* 1982;306:479–482.

185. **Dunton J, Berd D.** Vulvar melanoma, biologically different from other cutaneous melanomas. *Lancet* 1999;354:2013–2014.

186. **Rose PG, Piver MS, Tsukada Y, Lau T.** Conservative therapy for melanoma of the vulva. *Am J Obstet Gynecol* 1988;159:52–56.

187. **Davidson T, Kissin M, Wesbury G.** Vulvovaginal melanoma: should radical surgery be abandoned? *BJOG* 1987;94:473–479.

188. **Trimble EL, Lewis JL Jr, Williams LL, Curtin JP, Chapman D, Woodruff JM, et al.** Management of vulvar melanoma. *Gynecol Oncol* 1992;45:254–258.

189. **Verschraegen CF, Benjapibal M, Supakarapongkul W, Levy LB, Ross M, Atkinson EN, et al.** Vulvar melanomas at the M. D. Anderson Cancer Center: 25 years later. *Int J Gynecol Cancer* 2001;11:359–364.

190. **Phillips GL, Bundy BN, Okagaki T, Kucera PR, Stehman FB.** Malignant melanoma of the vulva treated by radical hemivulvectomy: a prospective study of the GOG. *Cancer* 1994;73:2626–2632.

191. Balch CM, Soong SJ, Bartolucci AA, Urist MM, Karakousis CP, Smith TJ, et al. Efficacy of an elective regional lymph node dissection of 1 to 4 mm thick melanomas for patients 60 years of age and younger. *Ann Surg* 1996;224:255–263.

192. de Hulla JA, Hollema H, Hoekstra HJ, Piers DA, Mourits MJE, Aalders JG, et al. Vulvar melanoma. Is there a role for sentinel lymph node biopsy? *Cancer* 2002;94:486–491.

193. Gershenwald JE, Colome MI, Lee JE, Mansfield PF, Tseng C, Lee J, et al. Patterns of recurrence following a negative sentinel lymph node biopsy in 243 patients with stage I and II melanomas. *J Clin Oncol* 1998;16:2253–2260.

194. Jaramillo BA, Ganjei P, Averette HE, Sevin B-U, Lovecchio JL. Malignant melanoma of the vulva. *Obstet Gynecol* 1985;66:398–401.

195. Beller U, Demopoulos RI, Beckman EM. Vulvovaginal melanoma: a clinicopathologic study. *J Reprod Med* 1986;31:315–321.

196. Kirkwood JM, Strawderman MH, Ernstoff MS, Smith TJ, Borden EC, Blum RH. Interferon alfa-2b adjuvant therapy of high-risk resected cutaneous melanoma: the Eastern Cooperative Oncology Group Trial EST 1684. *J Clin Oncol* 1996;14:7–17.

197. Kirkwood JM, Ibrahim JG, Sosman JA, Sondak VK, Agarwala SS, Ernstoff MS, et al. High-dose interferon alfa-2b significantly prolongs relapse-free and overall survival compared with the GM2-KLH/QS-21 vaccine in patients with resected stage IIB-III melanoma: results of the Intergroup Trial E1694/S9512/C509801. *J Clin Oncol* 2001;19:2370–2380.

198. Gray RJ, Pockaj BA, Kirkwood JM. An update on adjuvant interferon for melanoma. *Cancer Control* 2002;9:16–21.

199. Kim CJ, Dessureault S, Gabrilovich D, Reintgen DS, Slingluff CL. Immunotherapy for melanoma. *Cancer Control* 2002;9:22–30.

200. Scheistroen M, Trope C, Koern J, Pettersen EO, Abeler VM, Kristensen GB. Malignant melanoma of the vulva. *Cancer* 1995;75:72–80.

201. Copeland LJ, Sneige N, Gershenson DM, McGuffee VB, Abdul-Karim F, Rutledge FN. Bartholin gland carcinoma. *Obstet Gynecol* 1986;67:794–801.

202. Obermaier A, Koller S, Crandon AJ, Perrin L, Nicklin JL. Primary Bartholin gland carcinoma: a report of seven cases. *Aust N Z J Obstet Gynaecol* 2001;41:78–81.

203. Cardosi RJ, Speights A, Fiorica JV, Grendys EC, Hakam A, Hoffman MS. Bartholin's gland carcinoma: a 15-year experience. *Gynecol Oncol* 2001;82:247–251.

204. Lelle RJ, Davis KP, Roberts JA. Adenoid cystic carcinoma of the Bartholin's gland: the University of Michigan experience. *Int J Gynecol Cancer* 1994;4:145–149.

205. Yang S-YV, Lee J-W, Kim W-S, Jung K-L, Lee S-J, Lee J-H, et al. Adenoid cystic carcinoma of the Bartholin's gland: Report of two cases and review of the literature. *Gynecol Oncol* 2006;100:422–425.

206. De Pasquale SE, McGuinness TB, Mangan CE, Husson M, Woodland MB. Adenoid cystic carcinoma of Bartholin's gland: a review of the literature and report of a patient. *Gynecol Oncol* 1996;61:122–125.

207. Lopez-Varela E, Oliva E, McIntyre JF, Fuller AF Jr. Primary treatment of Bartholin's gland carcinoma with radiation and chemoradiation: a report on ten consecutive cases. *Int J Gynecol Cancer* 2007;17:661–667.

208. Rosenberg P, Simonsen E, Risberg B. Adenoid cystic carcinoma of Bartholin's gland: a report of 5 new cases treated with surgery and radiotherapy. *Gynecol Oncol* 1989;34:145–147.

209. Copeland LJ, Sneige N, Gershenson DM, Saul PB, Stringer CA, Seski JC. Adenoid cystic carcinoma of Bartholin gland. *Obstet Gynecol* 1986;67:115–120.

210. Underwood JW, Adcock LL, Okagaki T. Adenosquamous carcinoma of skin appendages (adenoid squamous cell carcinoma, pseudoglandular squamous cell carcinoma, adenoacanthoma of sweat gland of Lever) of the vulva: a clinical and ultrastructural study. *Cancer* 1978;42:1851–1857.

211. de Giorgi V, Salvini C, Massi D, Raspollini MR, Carli P. Vulvar basal cell carcinoma: retrospective study and review of literature. *Gynecol Oncol* 2005;97:192–194.

212. Dudzinski MR, Askin FB, Fowler WC. Giant basal cell carcinoma of the vulva. *Obstet Gynecol* 1984;63:575–579.

213. Benedet JL, Miller DM, Ehlen TG, Bertrand MA. Basal cell carcinoma of the vulva: clinical features and treatment results in 28 patients. *Obstet Gynecol* 1997;90:765–768.

214. Hoffman MS, Roberts WS, Ruffolo EH. Basal cell carcinoma of the vulva with inguinal lymph node metastases. *Gynecol Oncol* 1988;29:113–117.

215. Mulayim N, Silver DF, Ocal IT, Babalola E. Vulvar basal cell carcinoma: two unusual presentations and review of the literature. *Gynecol Oncol* 2002;85:532–537.

216. Partridge EE, Murad R, Shingleton HM, Austin JM, Hatch KD. Verrucous lesions of the female genitalia: II. verrucous carcinoma. *Am J Obstet Gynecol* 1980;137:419–424.

217. Gualco M, Bonin S, Foglia G, Fulcheri E, Odicino F, Prefumo F, et al. Morphologic and biologic studies on ten cases of verrucous carcinoma of the vulva supporting the theory of a discrete clinicopathologic entity. *Int J Gynecol Cancer* 2003;13:317–324.

218. Crowther ME, Lowe DG, Shepherd JH. Verrucous carcinoma of the female genital tract: a review. *Obstet Gynecol Surv* 1988;43: 263–280.

219. Gallousis S. Verrucous carcinoma: report of three vulvar cases and a review of the literature. *Obstet Gynecol* 1972;40:502–508.

220. Japaze H, Dinh TV, Woodruff JD. Verrucous carcinoma of the vulva: study of 24 cases. *Obstet Gynecol* 1982;60:462–466.

221. Haidopoulos D, Diakomanolis E, Rodolakis A, Voulgaris Z, Vlachos G, Michalas S. Coexistence of verrucous and squamous carcinoma of the vulva. *Aust NZJ Obstet Gynaecol* 2005;45: 60–63.

222. Demian SDE, Bushkin FL, Echevarria RA. Perineural invasion and anaplastic transformation of verrucous carcinoma. *Cancer* 1973; 32:395–399.

223. Ulutin HC, Zellars RC, Frassica D. Soft tissue sarcoma of the vulva: a clinical study. *Int J Gynecol Cancer* 2003;13:528–531.

224. Curtin JP, Saigo P, Slucher B, Venkatraman ES, Mychalczak B, Hoskins WJ. Soft tissue sarcoma of the vagina and vulva: a clinicopathologic study. *Obstet Gynecol* 1995;86:269–272.

225. Aartsen EJ, Albus-Lutter CE. Vulvar sarcomas: clinical implications. *Eur J Obstet Gynecol Reprod Biol* 1994;56:181–189.

226. Tavassoli FA, Norris HJ. Smooth muscle tumors of the vulva. *Obstet Gynecol* 1979;53:213–220.

227. Nielsen GP, Rosenberg AE, Koerner FC, Young RH, Scully RE. Smooth muscle tumors of the vulva. A clinicopathological study of 25 cases and review of the literature. *Am J Surg Pathol* 1996;20: 779–793.

228. Ulbright TM, Brokaw SA, Stehman FB, Roth LM. Epithelioid sarcoma of the vulva. *Cancer* 1983;52:1462–1465.

229. de Visscher SA, van Ginkel RJ, Wobbes T, Veth RP, Ten Heuvel SE, Suurmeijer AJ, et al. Epithelial sarcoma: still an only surgically curable disease. *Cancer* 2006;107:606–612.

230. Spillane AJ, Thomas JM, Fisher C. Epithelial sarcoma: clinicopathologic complexities of this rare soft tissue sarcoma. *Ann Surg Oncol* 2000;7:218–25.

231. Bell J, Averette H, Davis J, Toledano S. Genital rhabdomyosarcoma: current management and review of the literature. *Obstet Gynecol Sun* 1986;41:257–264.

232. Arndt CAS, Donaldson SS, Anderson JR, Andrassy RJ, Laurie F, Link MP, et al. What constitutes optimal therapy for patients with rhabdomyosarcoma of the female genital tract. *Cancer* 2001;91: 2454–2468.

233. Harris NL, Scully RE. Malignant lymphoma and granulocytic sarcoma of the uterus and vagina. *Cancer* 1984;53:2530–2545.

234. Khunamornpong S, Siriaunkgul S, Suprasert P, Chitapanarux I. Yolk sac tumor of the vulva: a case report with long-term disease-free survival. *Gynecol Oncol* 2005;97:238–242.

235. Bottles K, Lacy CG, Goldberg J, Lanner-Cusin K, Horn J, Miller TR. Merkel cell carcinoma of the vulva. *Obstet Gynecol* 1984;63:61S–65S.

236. Husseinzadeh N, Wesseler T, Newman N, Shbaro I, Ho P. Neuroendocrine (Merkel cell) carcinoma of the vulva. *Gynecol Oncol* 1988;29:105–112.

237. Bock JE, Andreasson B, Thorn A, Holck S. Dermatofibromasarcoma protuberans of the vulva. *Gynecol Oncol* 1985;20: 129–133.

238. Soergel TM, Doering DL, O'Connor D. Metastatic dermatofibrosarcoma protuberans of the vulva. *Gynecol Oncol* 1998;71: 320–324.

239. Dehner LP. Metastatic and secondary tumors of the vulva. *Obstet Gynecol* 1973;42:47–53.

14

Vaginal Cancer

Neville F. Hacker

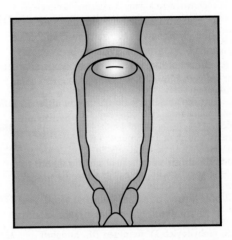

Primary carcinomas of the vagina represent 2% to 3% **of malignant neoplasms of the female genital tract. In the United States, it is estimated that there will be 2,160 new cases diagnosed in 2009, and 770 deaths from the disease** (1). More than 50% of patients are diagnosed in the seventh, eighth, and ninth decades, and squamous cell histology accounts for about 80% of cases (2).

Until the late 1930s, vaginal cancer was in general considered to be incurable. Most patients presented with disease that had spread beyond the vagina, and radiation therapy techniques were poorly developed. **With modern techniques for radiation therapy, cure rates of even advanced cases should now be comparable with those for cervical cancer** (3-5). According to the Annual Report, the overall 5-year survival rate has increased from 34.1% in 1959 to 1963 to 53.6% in 1999 to 2001 (2).

Fu (6) reported that **84% of carcinomas involving the vagina were secondary, usually from the cervix (32%); endometrium (18%); colon and rectum (9%); ovary (6%); or vulva (6%).** Of 164 squamous cell carcinomas, 44 (27%) were primary and 120 (73%) were secondary. Among the latter, 95 (79%) originated from the cervix; 17 (14%) from the vulva; and 8 (7%) from the cervix and the vulva (6). This apparent discrepancy is partly related to the International Federation of Gynecology and Obstetrics (FIGO) classification and staging of malignant tumors of the female pelvis. The staging requires that a tumor that has extended to the portio and reached the area of the external os should be regarded as a carcinoma of the cervix, whereas a tumor that involves the vulva and vagina should be classified as a carcinoma of the vulva. **Endometrial carcinomas and choriocarcinomas commonly metastasize to the vagina, whereas tumors from the bladder or rectum may invade the vagina directly.**

Primary Vaginal Tumors

The histologic types of primary vaginal tumors are shown in Table 14.1 (7-19). Squamous cell carcinomas are the most common, although adenocarcinomas, melanomas, and sarcomas are also seen. Sarcomas occasionally follow radiation therapy for cervical cancer.

Squamous Cell Carcinoma

Squamous cell carcinoma is the most common vaginal cancer. The mean age of the patients is approximately 67 years, although the disease occasionally is seen in the third and fourth decades of life (4,7,10,13). About 80% of patients are older than 50 years (2).

Table 14.1 Primary Vaginal Cancer: Reported Incidence of Histologic Types

Histologic Types	Number	Percentage
Squamous cell	1,054	82.6
Adenocarcinoma (including clear cell)	123	9.6
Melanoma	42	3.3
Sarcoma	40	3.1
Undifferentiated	8	0.6
Small cell	5	0.4
Lymphoma	4	0.3
Carcinoid	1	0.1
Total	**1,277**	**100.0**

Data compiled from **Perez et al.,** 1974 (7); **Pride and Buchler,** 1977 (8); **Ball and Berman,** 1982 (9); **Houghton and Iversen,** 1982 (10); **Benedet et al.,** 1983 (11); **Peters et al.,** 1985 (12); **Rubin et al.,** 1985 (13); **Sulak et al.,** 1988 (14); **Eddy et al.,** 1991 (15); **Ali et al.,** 1996 (16); **Tjalma et al.,** 2001 (17); and **Tewari et al.,** 2001 (18), **Hellman et al.,** 2006 (19).

Etiology

Women who have been treated for a prior anogenital cancer, particularly of the cervix, have a high relative risk of developing vaginal cancer, although the absolute risk is low (20).

In a population-based study of 156 women with *in situ* or invasive vaginal cancer, Daling et al. determined that they had many of the same risk factors as patients with cervical cancer, including a strong relationship with human papilloma virus (HPV) infection (20). The presence of antibodies to HPV 16 was strongly related to this risk. A study of 341cases from the Radiumhemmet reported that the disease seemed to be etiologically related to cervical cancer, and thus HPV infection, in young patients, but in older patients, there was no such association (21).

As many as 30% of patients with primary vaginal carcinoma have a history of *in situ* or invasive cervical cancer treated at least 5 years earlier (11–13). In a report from the University of South Carolina, a past history of invasive cervical cancer was present in 20% of the cases and of cervical intraepithelial neoplasia (CIN) in 7% (15). The median interval between the diagnosis of cervical cancer and the diagnosis of vaginal cancer was 14 years, with a range of 5 years, 8 months to 28 years. Sixteen percent of the patients had a history of prior pelvic irradiation.

There are three possible mechanisms for the occurrence of vaginal cancer after cervical neoplasia:

1. **Occult residual disease**
2. **New primary disease arising in an "at-risk" lower genital tract**
3. **Radiation carcinogenicity**

In the first instance, extension of intraepithelial neoplasia from the cervix to the upper vagina was not appreciated and an adequate vaginal cuff was not taken because vaginal colposcopy was not performed before surgical management of the cervical tumor. Surgical margins of the upper vaginal resection usually show *in situ* neoplasia, and these persistent foci eventually progress to invasive disease. In the second instance, vaginal colposcopy is negative, and the surgical margins of resection are free of disease.

There is controversy regarding the distinction between a new primary vaginal cancer and a recurrent cervical cancer. Many authorities use a 5-year cut-off because 95% of cervical cancers will recur within this period (22,23) but others prefer a 10-year interval (19).

Prior pelvic radiation therapy has been considered a possible cause of vaginal carcinoma (8). In the series of 314 patients with squamous cell carcinoma of the vagina reported from Sweden, previous pelvic radiation was reported by 44 patients (14%) on an average of 22 years earlier (range 5–55 years)(19). Judicious use of pelvic radiation may be particularly important

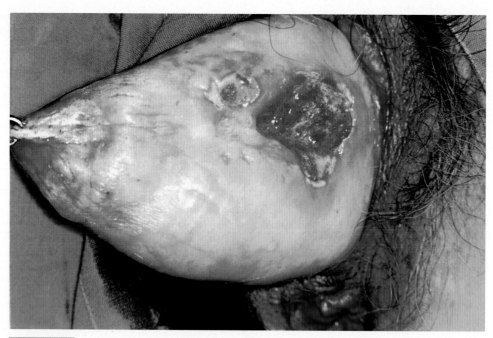

Figure 14.1   Squamous cell carcinoma of the vagina in a patient with a procidentia. The cancer was apparently related to long-term pessary use.

in young patients, who may live long enough to develop a second neoplasm in the irradiated vagina (24).

The true malignant potential of vaginal intraepithelial neoplasia is unclear because once diagnosed, the condition is usually treated. Benedet and Saunders (25) reviewed 136 cases of carcinoma *in situ* of the vagina seen over a 30-year period. Four cases (3%) progressed to invasive vaginal cancer in spite of various methods of treatment. Rome and England reported 9 cases (6.8%) of early invasive vaginal cancer detected during the initial management of 132 cases of vaginal intraepithelial neoplasia (VAIN) (26).

Chronic local irritation from long-term use of a pessary may also be of significance (6) (Fig. 14.1), although pessaries are used less commonly in modern gynecology.

Screening

For screening to be cost effective, the incidence of the disease must be sufficient to justify the cost of screening. In the United States, the age-adjusted incidence of vaginal cancer is 0.6 per 100,000 women, making routine screening of all patients inappropriate (27). However, **women with a history of cervical intraepithelial or invasive neoplasia are at increased risk and should be monitored carefully with Pap smears.**

As many as 59% of patients with vaginal cancer have had a prior hysterectomy (9). However, **when age and prior cervical disease are controlled for, there is no increased risk of vaginal cancer in women who have had a hysterectomy for benign disease** (28).

Symptoms and Signs

Most patients with vaginal cancer present with painless vaginal bleeding and discharge. The bleeding is usually postmenopausal but may be postcoital. In the large series reported from the Radiumhemmet, 14% of patients were asymptomatic, and the diagnosis was made either by routine examination (7%) or by abnormal cytology (7%) (19).

Because the bladder neck is close to the vagina, bladder pain and frequency of micturition occur earlier than with cervical cancer. Posterior tumors may produce tenesmus. Approximately 5% of patients present with pelvic pain because of extension of disease beyond the vagina.

Most lesions are situated in the upper one-third of the vagina, usually at the apex or on the posterior wall (19). Macroscopically, the lesions are usually exophytic (fungating, polypoid), but they may be endophytic. Surface ulceration usually occurs late in the course of the disease.

Diagnosis

The diagnosis of carcinoma of the vagina is often missed on first examination, particularly if the lesion is small and situated in the lower two-thirds of the vagina, where it may be covered by the blades of the speculum. Definitive diagnosis is usually made by biopsy of a gross lesion, which can often be performed in the office without anesthesia. Particularly in elderly patients or in those with some degree of vaginal stenosis, examination under anesthesia may be desirable to allow adequate biopsy and clinical staging. The latter may require cystoscopy or proctoscopy, depending on the location of the tumor.

In patients with an abnormal Pap smear and no gross abnormality, careful vaginal colposcopy and the liberal use of Lugol's iodine to stain the vagina are necessary. This is performed in the office initially, but may need to be repeated with the patient under regional or general anesthesia to allow excision of colposcopically abnormal lesions. **For definitive diagnosis of early vaginal carcinoma, it may be necessary to resect the entire vaginal vault and submit it for careful histologic evaluation because the lesion may be partially buried by closure of the vaginal vault at the time of hysterectomy.** This is usually done with a cold knife, but Fanning et al. have reported the successful use of the loop electrosurgical procedure for partial upper vaginectomy in 15 patients (29). Inadvertent cystotomy may occur occasionally, and this requires immediate repair.

Hoffman et al. (30) at the University of South Florida reported on 32 patients who underwent upper vaginectomy for VAIN 3. Occult invasive carcinoma was found in nine patients (28%). In five cases, the depth of invasion was less than 2 mm, but in four cases, invasion ranged from 3.5 mm to full-thickness involvement.

Staging

The FIGO staging (2009) for vaginal carcinoma is shown in Table 14.2. **Updated FIGO staging tables can be seen on pages 665 to 668.** The staging is clinical and is based on the findings at general physical and pelvic examination, cystoscopy, proctoscopy, chest x-ray, and possible skeletal radiographs if the latter are indicated because of bone pain.

Because it is difficult to determine accurately any spread into subvaginal tissues, particularly from anterior or posterior lesions, differences in observations are common. This is reflected in the wide range of stage distributions reported and the wide range of survivals within a given stage. The distribution by FIGO stage from 13 series is shown in Table 14.3. Fewer than one-third of patients present with disease confined to the vagina, although Hellman et al. reported that significantly more patients were diagnosed at an early stage in the last 20 years of their study, compared to the first 20 years (19).

Surgical staging for vaginal cancer has been used less commonly than for cervical cancer, but in selected premenopausal patients, a pretreatment laparotomy may allow better definition of the extent of disease, excision of any grossly enlarged lymph nodes, and placement of an ovary up into the paracolic gutter beyond the radiation field.

Table 14.2 Carcinoma of the Vagina: FIGO Nomenclature	
Stage I	The carcinoma is limited to the vaginal wall
Stage II	The carcinoma has involved the subvaginal tissue but has not extended to the pelvic wall
Stage III	The carcinoma has extended to the pelvic wall
Stage IV	The carcinoma has extended beyond the true pelvis or has involved the mucosa of the bladder or rectum; bullous edema as such does not permit a case to be allotted to stage IV
IVA	Tumor invades bladder and/or rectal mucosa and/or direct extension beyond the true pelvis
IVB	Spread to distant organs

FIGO Annual Report, *Int J Gynecol Obstet* 2006;95:S29, and *Int J Gynecol Obstet* 2009;105:3–4.

Table 14.3 Primary Vaginal Carcinoma: Distribution by Stage of Disease		
Stage	*Number*	*Percentage*
I	559	28.4
II	721	36.6
III	428	21.7
IV	262	13.3
Total	**1,970**	**100.0**

Data compiled from **Ball and Berman,** 1982 (9); **Houghton and Iversen,** 1982 (10); **Benedet *et al.,*** 1983 (11); **Peters *et al.,*** 1985 (12); **Rubin *et al.,*** 1985 (13); **Kucera *et al.,*** 1991 (31); **Eddy *et al.,*** 1991 (15); **Kirkbridge *et al.,*** 1995 (4); **Stock *et al.,*** 1995 (32); **Chyle *et al.,*** 1996 (3); **Ali *et al.,*** 1996 (16); **Perez *et al.,*** 1996 (33); **Tjalma *et al.,*** 2001 (17); and **Tewari *et al.,*** 2001 (18); **Hellman *et al.,*** 2006 (19).

Peters et al. (34) suggested criteria for microinvasive carcinoma of the vagina: focal invasion associated with VAIN 3, no lymph-vascular invasion, free margins on partial or total vaginec-tomy, and a maximum depth of invasion of less than 2.5 mm, measured from the overlying surface. However, Eddy et al. (35) reported six patients who met these criteria and were treated by either partial or total vaginectomy. In one of the six, a bladder recurrence developed at 35 months.

Patterns of Spread

Vaginal cancer spreads by the following routes:

1. **Direct extension** to the pelvic soft tissues, pelvic bones, and adjacent organs (bladder and rectum).
2. **Lymphatic dissemination** to the pelvic and later the paraaortic lymph nodes. Lesions in the lower one-third of the vagina metastasize directly to the inguinofemoral lymph nodes, with the pelvic nodes being involved secondarily.
3. **Hematogenous dissemination** to distant organs, including lungs, liver, and bone. Hematogenous dissemination is a late phenomenon in vaginal cancer, and the disease usually remains confined to the pelvis for most of its course.

There is little information available on the incidence of lymph node metastases in vaginal cancer because most patients are treated with radiation therapy. Rubin et al. (13) reported that 16 of 38 patients (42.1%) with all stages of disease had lymphangiographic abnormalities, but many of these abnormalities were not confirmed histologically. Al-Kurdi and Monaghan (36) performed lymph node dissections on 35 patients and reported positive pelvic nodes in 10 patients (28.6%). **Positive inguinal nodes were present in 6 of 19 patients (31.6%), with disease involving the lower vagina.** Stock et al. (32) reported positive pelvic nodes in 10 of 29 patients (34.5%) with all stages of disease who underwent bilateral pelvic lymphadenec-tomy as part of their therapy or staging. Positive paraaortic nodes were present in one of eight patients (12.5%) undergoing paraaortic dissection.

Van Dam et al. described sentinel node detection in three patients with primary vaginal cancer (37). Preoperatively, 60-mBq technetium-labeled nanocolloid was injected around the tumor, and sentinel nodes were detected using a laparoscopic or hand-held probe. Sentinel nodes could be found in two of the three patients. The first patient described had a 1-cm tumor in the distal anterior vagina. Lymphoscintigraphy revealed sentinel nodes in the groin and obturator fossa, but both were negative histologically. The second patient had squamous cell carcinoma at the vaginal vault, which followed an abdominal hysterectomy two years earlier for a stage Ia1 squamous cervical carcinoma. Regardless of whether this is considered a vaginal or a recurrent cervical cancer, lymphoscintigraphy demonstrated two sentinel nodes just below the common iliac bifurcation, and both were histologically positive.

Preoperative Evaluation

Apart from the standard staging investigations, a computed tomographic (CT) or magnetic resonance imaging (MRI) scan of the pelvis and abdomen is useful for evaluation of the status of the primary tumor, liver, pelvic and paraaortic lymph nodes, and ureters.

The group in St. Louis compared CT and F-18 fluorodeoxy glucose (FDG) positron emission tomography (PET) for the detection of the primary tumor and lymph node metastases in patients with carcinoma of the vagina (38). Of the 21 patients with an intact primary tumor, CT visualized the tumor in 9 patients (43%), whereas FDG-PET identified abnormal uptake in all 21 cases (100%). Similarly, CT demonstrated abnormally enlarged lymph nodes in 17% of cases, compared to abnormal uptake in 35% of patients with FDG-PET.

Treatment

Experience with the management of primary vaginal cancer is limited because of the rarity of the disease. Most gynecologic oncology centers in the United States see only two to five new cases per year, and even in some European centers, where referral of oncology cases tends to be more centralized, only approximately one new case per month can be expected (31). **Therapy must be individualized and varies depending on the stage of disease and the site of vaginal involvement, further limiting individual experience.**

Anatomic factors and psychological considerations place significant constraints on treatment planning. The proximity of the vagina to the rectum, bladder, and urethra limits the dose of radiation that can be delivered and restricts the surgical margins that can be attained unless an exenterative procedure is performed. **For most patients, maintenance of a functional vagina is an important factor in the planning of therapy.**

Surgery

Surgery has a limited role in the management of patients with vaginal cancer because of the radicality required to achieve clear surgical margins, but in selected cases, satisfactory results can be achieved (9,17,19,32,36,39,40,41). Surgery may be useful in the following circumstances:

1. **In patients with stage I disease involving the upper posterior vagina.** If the uterus is still *in situ*, these patients require radical hysterectomy, partial vaginectomy, and bilateral pelvic lymphadenectomy. If the patient has had a hysterectomy, radical upper vaginectomy and pelvic lymphadenectomy can be performed after development of the paravesicular and pararectal spaces and dissection of each ureter out to its point of entry into the bladder.

   A Chinese report described four patients who had laparoscopic radical hysterectomy, pelvic lymphadenectomy, and total vaginectomy for stage I vaginal carcinoma (39). Vaginal reconstruction was performed using the sigmoid colon. Mean operating time was 305 minutes (range 260–350 minutes), mean blood loss 325 mL (range 250–400 mL), and median number of resected lymph nodes 16 (range 13–20). The mean postoperative stay was 7 days (range 6–8) and all patients were clinically free of disease with a mean follow-up of 46 months (range 40–54 months).

   A surgical approach to conserve reproductive and sexual function was described from Italy (40). Three nulliparous women under 40 years of age with stage I squamous cell carcinoma confined to the upper third of the vagina underwent radical tumorectomy and pelvic lymphadenectomy. A fourth patient underwent partial hemivaginectomy plus ipsilateral paracolpectomy and pelvic lymphadenectomy. One patient with microscopic involvement of the paracolpium received adjuvant radiation after laparoscopic ovarian transposition. With a follow-up of 9 to 51 months, all patients were regularly menstruating, sexually active, and clinically free of disease.

   Although this approach has obvious appeal, the number of cases is very limited, and such an approach should probably be limited to small lesions, particularly if located in the upper vagina. The authors recommended more intensive follow-up, particularly aimed at early detection of any locoregional relapse and/or second tumor of the lower genital tract (40).

2. **In young patients who require radiation therapy.** Pretreatment laparotomy in such patients may allow ovarian transposition, surgical staging, and resection of any enlarged lymph nodes.

3. **In patients with stage IVA disease, particularly if a rectovaginal or vesicovaginal fistula is present.** Primary pelvic exenteration is a suitable treatment option for such patients, provided they are medically fit. Eddy et al. (15) reported a 5-year disease-free survival in three of six patients with stage IVA disease treated with preoperative radiation followed by anterior or total pelvic exenteration. In sexually active patients, vaginal reconstruction should be performed simultaneously.

4. **In patients with a central recurrence after radiation therapy.** Surgical resection, which usually necessitates pelvic exenteration, is the only option for this group of patients. Van Dam et al. reported a patient who recurred 6 months after chemoradiation for stage III carcinoma of the upper vagina (37). Sentinel nodes were detected in the obturator fossa which were histologically negative. The patient then underwent posterior pelvic exenteration.

Radiation Therapy

Radiation therapy is the treatment of choice for all patients except those listed previously, and comprises an integration of teletherapy and intracavitary/interstitial therapy (3,4,5,7,18,19,31,33). Selected stage I and II lesions can be treated adequately with brachytherapy alone (3,4,33,42). For larger lesions, treatment is usually started with approximately 5,000 cGy external irradiation to shrink the primary tumor and treat the pelvic lymph nodes. Intracavitary or interstitial treatment follows.

There is improved local control with total tumor doses of at least 7,000 cGy (3,43). If the uterus is intact and the lesion involves the upper vagina, an intrauterine tandem and ovoids can be used. If the uterus has been previously removed, a Bloedorn type of applicator or vaginal cylinder may be used. If the lesion is more deeply invasive (thicker than 0.5 cm), interstitial irradiation, alone or in conjunction with the intracavitary therapy, improves the dose distribution (18,33). Extended-field radiation has rarely been used for patients with vaginal cancer, but if positive paraaortic nodes are documented after either surgical staging, CT scanning and fine-needle aspiration cytologic evaluation, or PET scanning, this treatment should be given. **If the lower one-third of the vagina is involved, the groin nodes should be treated or dissected.**

There is limited reported experience with chemoradiation for vaginal cancer (4,44), although many centers now routinely use this combined therapy, as is being done for cervical carcinoma. In our center, *cisplatin* 35 mg/m^2 given on the first day of each week of external beam therapy is used. The small number of cases makes it virtually impossible to ever conduct a randomized, prospective study to compare standard radiation with chemoradiation for patients with vaginal cancer.

Complications of Therapy

Major complications of therapy are usually reported in 10% to 15% of patients treated for primary vaginal cancer, whether the treatment is by surgery or radiation. Workers at the M. D. Anderson Hospital reported serious complications in 39 of 311 patients (13%), but estimated an actuarial incidence of 19% at 20 years (3). **The close proximity of the rectum, bladder, and urethra predisposes these structures to injury, and radiation cystitis, radiation proctitis, rectovaginal or vesicovaginal fistulas, and rectal strictures or ulceration may occur.** Radiation necrosis of the vagina occasionally occurs, and radiation-induced fibrosis and subsequent vaginal stenosis are a constant concern.

Stryker reported vaginal morbidity in 9 of 15 patients (60%) undergoing external beam therapy plus intracavitary brachytherapy, and 3 of 10 patients (30%) undergoing external beam therapy plus interstitial brachytherapy. He suggested that when combining external beam therapy with brachytherapy, interstitial techniques were preferable (45).

Patients who are sexually active must be encouraged to continue regular intercourse, but those who are not sexually active or for whom intercourse is temporarily too painful should be encouraged to use topical estrogen and a vaginal dilator, at least every second night. There is inadequate documentation of the adequacy of vaginal function after radiation therapy for vaginal cancer.

Prognosis

The reported overall 5-year survival rate for vaginal cancer is approximately 52%, which is more than 15% poorer than that for carcinoma of the cervix or vulva, and reflects the difficulties involved in treating this disease and the late stage at presentation (Table 14.4). Even for patients with stage I disease, the 5-year survival rate in combined series is only approximately 74%. In the 26th volume of the *Annual Report on the Results of Treatment in Gynecological Cancer*, the 5-year survival for 224 patients with vaginal cancer was as follows: stage I, 77.6%; stage II, 52.2%; stage III, 42.5%; stage IVA, 20.5%; stage IVB, 12.9% (2).

Stage	No.	5-Year Survival	Percentage
I	509	378	74.3
II	622	333	53.5
III	377	128	34.0
IV	163	24	15.3
Total	**1,671**	**864**	**51.7**

Table 14.4 Primary Vaginal Carcinoma: 5-Year Survival Rates

Data compiled from **Pride et al.,** 1979 (46); **Houghton and Iversen,** 1982 (10); **Benedet et al.,** 1983 (11); **Rubin et al.,** 1985 (13); **Kucera et al.,** 1991 (31); **Eddy et al.,** 1991 (15); **Kirkbridge et al.,** 1995 (4); and **Tewari et al.,** 2001 (18); **Perez et al.,** (33); **Otton et al.,** 2004 (41); **Frank et al.,** 2005(5); **Hellman et al.,** 2006 (19); **Tran et al.,** 2007 (47).

Better results have been reported from individual centers. In a report of 193 cases of primary vaginal squamous cell carcinoma from the M. D. Anderson Hospital in Houston, Frank et al. reported 5-year disease-specific survival (DSS) rates of 85% for 50 patients with FIGO stage I disease, 78% for 97 patients with stage II, and 58% for 46 patients with stages III-IV(5). Five-year DSS rates were 82% and 60% for patients with tumors $\geq$4 cm and >4 cm respectively ($p = 0.0001$). Kirkbridge et al. (4) from the Princess Margaret Hospital in Toronto reported on 138 patients with invasive vaginal carcinoma. The 5-year cause-specific survival rates by stage were 77% for stages I/II and 56% for stages III/IV. In a multivariate analysis, only tumor size and stage of disease were significant variables.

Most recurrences are in the pelvis (48), so improved radiation therapy, which may include chemoradiation and/or increasing experience with interstitial techniques, may improve the results. Chyle et al. (2) reported that salvage after first relapse was uncommon, with a 5-year survival rate of only 12%.

Because of the rarity of the disease, patients with vaginal cancer should be referred centrally to a limited number of tertiary referral units so that increasing experience can be gained in their management.

Adenocarcinoma

Approximately 10% of primary vaginal carcinomas are adenocarcinomas, and they affect a younger population of women, regardless of whether exposure to *diethylstilbestrol (DES) in utero* has occurred (49). Adenocarcinomas may arise in areas of vaginal adenosis, particularly in patients exposed to *DES in utero,* but they probably also arise in Wolffian rest elements, periurethral glands, and foci of endometriosis. They have been reported to have a worse prognosis than squamous carcinomas (3,41) although this has not been confirmed by other groups (2,19).

Vaginal adenosis is the sequestration of müllerian glandular epithelium into the vaginal mucosa during embryogenesis. It is thought to arise as a consequence of disrupted development and has been reported in non–*DES*-exposed women from infancy to old age (50). Intestinal metaplasia occasionally occurs in tissues of müllerian origin, and primary vaginal adenocarcinoma of intestinal type has been described (51). **Secondary tumors from such sites as the colon, endometrium, or ovary should be considered when vaginal adenocarcinoma is diagnosed.**

Diethylstilbestrol Exposure In Utero

In 1970, Herbst and Scully (52) initially reported on seven women 15 to 22 years of age with clear cell adenocarcinoma of the vagina, seen over a 4-year period. Subsequently, Herbst et al. (53) reported an association with maternal *DES* ingestion during pregnancy in six of these seven cases. A Registry for Research on Hormonal Transplacental Carcinogenesis was established by Herbst and Scully in 1971 to investigate the clinical, pathologic, and epidemiologic aspects of clear cell adenocarcinoma of the vagina and cervix occurring in women born after 1940 (i.e., during the years when *DES* was used to maintain high-risk pregnancies). Such high-risk situations included diabetic and twin pregnancies in women with a history of spontaneous abortion. The use of *DES* for pregnant patients was discontinued in the United States in 1971.

More than 500 cases of clear cell carcinoma of the vagina or cervix have been reported to the registry, although **only approximately two-thirds of the completely investigated cases have a history of prenatal exposure to *DES*.** In all instances, the mother was treated in the first half of the pregnancy (54). An additional 10% of the mothers received some unknown medication, but in 25% of the cases, there was no indication of maternal hormone ingestion.

These cancers become most frequent after the age of 14 years, and the peak age at diagnosis is 19 years. The oldest reported *DES*-exposed patient with vaginal clear cell carcinoma was 52 years of age. **The estimated risk of clear cell adenocarcinoma in an exposed offspring is 1:1,000 or less. Approximately 70% of vaginal adenocarcinomas are stage I at diagnosis.**

Although *DES* exposure *in utero* rarely leads to vaginal adenocarcinoma, vaginal adenosis occurs in approximately 45% of such patients, and approximately 25% of exposed women have structural changes to the cervix and vagina. Such changes include a transverse vaginal septum, a cervical collar, a cockscomb (a raised ridge, usually on the anterior cervix), or cervical hypoplasia. The occurrence of these abnormalities is related to the dosage of medication given and the time of first exposure, the risk being insignificant if administration is begun after the 22nd week.

Two types of cells have been described in vaginal adenosis and cervical ectropion: the mucinous cell, which resembles the endocervical epithelium, and the tuboendometrial cell. Robboy et al. (55) reported foci of atypical tuboendometrial epithelium in 16 of 20 (80%) cases of clear cell adenocarcinoma of the cervix or vagina. The foci were almost immediately adjacent to the tumor, and they suggested that atypical vaginal adenosis and atypical cervical ectropion of the tuboendometrial type may be precursors of clear cell adenocarcinoma. Sandberg and Christian (56) reported the appearance of cervicovaginal clear cell adenocarcinoma in only one of a genetically identical (monozygotic) pair of twins, simultaneously exposed to *DES in utero*. Benign teratologic changes were present in both twins. This discordance suggests that factors other than embryonic exposure to *DES* may be operative in tumorigenesis.

Areas of vaginal adenosis and cervical ectropion are progressively covered with metaplastic squamous epithelium as the individual matures, and areas of adenosis may disappear completely and be replaced by normally glycogenated squamous epithelium. Structural abnormalities (e.g., cervical hoods) also tend to disappear progressively (57).

In addition to benign changes in the lower genital tract, a number of other abnormalities in the upper genital tract have been reported in *DES*-exposed female offspring. Kaufman et al. (58) reported abnormalities of the hysterosalpingogram in 185 of 267 (69%) exposed women. The most common abnormality was a T-shaped uterus, with or without a small cavity; less common abnormalities included constriction rings, uterine filling defects, synechiae, diverticulae, and uterus unicornis or bicornis. These abnormalities translate into an impaired reproductive experience for *DES*-exposed offspring, with an increased incidence of primary infertility, ectopic pregnancy, spontaneous abortion, and premature delivery (59).

It is recommended that a young woman exposed to *DES in utero* should be initially seen when she begins to menstruate, or at approximately 14 years of age. The most important aspects of the examination are careful inspection and palpation of the entire vagina and cervix, and cytologic sampling by direct scraping of the vagina and cervix. Colposcopy is not essential if clinical and cytologic evaluations are negative, but staining with half-strength Lugol's iodine delineates areas of adenosis.

Treatment

In general, *DES*-related tumors may be treated in a way similar to that for squamous carcinomas, except that in these young patients, every effort should be made to preserve vaginal and ovarian function. **For early-stage tumors, particularly those involving the upper vagina, the performance of radical hysterectomy, pelvic lymphadenectomy, vaginectomy, and replacement of the vagina with a split-thickness skin graft has been successful in a high percentage of cases.** A combination of wide local excision, retroperitoneal lymphadenectomy, and local irradiation can be effective therapy for stage I tumors (60). Local surgical excision alone for small primary tumors is associated with a higher incidence of local and regional recurrence. Approximately 16% of patients with stage I disease have positive pelvic nodes (61). If radiation alone is used, a pretreatment staging laparotomy to allow pelvic lymphadenectomy and ovarian transposition may facilitate an optimal functional outcome. Freezing of embryos with a view to a subsequent surrogate pregnancy may be considered if ovarian function is in jeopardy and the patient has a suitable partner.

Prognosis

The overall 5-year survival rate for registry patients with clear cell carcinoma of the vagina, regardless of the mode of therapy, is 78%. **The survival rate correlates well with stage of disease: 87% for patients with stage I disease, 76% for patients with stage II, and 30% for those with stage III** (61).

Small Cell Carcinoma

Primary small cell carcinoma of the vagina is extremely rare, but as many as 5% of such tumors arise in extrapulmonary sites. In the female genital tract, such tumors arise most commonly in the cervix, followed by the ovary, endometrium, vagina, and vulva (62). As with other primary sites, small cell carcinoma of the vagina has a proclivity for distant failure and a poor prognosis. Management should be with concurrent chemoradiation.

Verrucous Carcinoma

Verrucous carcinomas of the vagina are rare, but their clinical and pathologic features are similar to those of their vulvar counterparts (63). **They are large, warty tumors that are locally aggressive but have a minimal tendency to metastasize. Wide surgical excision of the tumor is the treatment of choice.** Crowther et al. (63), in a literature review, reported a successful outcome in four of five patients with small lesions treated by wide excision. Similarly, for larger lesions, exenteration or vaginectomy was successful in seven of seven patients, but there were three postoperative deaths. Regional lymphadenectomy is not required, provided there is no suspicious lymphadenopathy. **Radiation therapy has been implicated in the rapid transformation of such lesions to a more malignant tumor,** and Crowther et al. (63) reported recurrence in all four patients treated with primary radiation therapy.

Vaginal Melanoma

Malignant melanomas of the vagina are rare, with less than 250 reported cases to 2002 (64). The 26th Annual Report documents 13 cases (4%) among 324 cases of vaginal cancer (2). They presumably arise from melanocytes that are present in the vagina in 3% of normal women (65). The average age of the patients is 58 years, but vaginal melanomas have been reported from the third to the ninth decades of life (66). **Almost all cases occur in white women** (67).

Clinically, most patients present with vaginal bleeding, a vaginal mass, or vaginal discharge (66,67). **The lesions most commonly arise in the distal part of the vagina, particularly on the anterior wall** (67,68). They may be nonpigmented and are frequently ulcerated, making them easily confused with squamous carcinomas. Most are deeply invasive. Expressing the lesion in terms of Chung's level of invasion (as defined for vulvar melanomas [69]), Chung et al. (68) reported that 13 of 15 (87%) vaginal melanomas were at level IV. A more recent study from Houston reported that 20 of 26 cases (77%) were level IV lesions (70). Approximately 60% of Chung's cases exhibited spread of melanocytic cells into the adjacent epithelium, and in approximately 30% of the cases, the lateral spread was extensive (68).

Radical surgery has traditionally been the mainstay of treatment, and this has often involved anterior, posterior, or total pelvic exenteration, depending on the location of the lesion. Small upper vaginal lesions have been treated with radical hysterectomy, subtotal vaginectomy, and pelvic lymphadenectomy, whereas small distal vaginal lesions have been treated by partial vaginectomy, total or partial vulvectomy, and bilateral inguinofemoral lymphadenectomy.

More recently, conservative operations (e.g., wide local excision) have been used, followed frequently by pelvic radiotherapy (64,67,71,72,73), and there appears to be no significant benefit in terms of survival or disease-free interval for radical versus conservative surgery. The most important issue is to remove all gross disease whenever possible (73). Postoperative radiation therapy is effective for prevention of local recurrence, and **high-dose fractions (>400 cGy) may be preferable to conventional or low-dose fractions** (74). Chemotherapy (e.g., with *methyl-CCNU [semustine]* or *dacarbazine*) is disappointing, which is unfortunate because most patients die of distant metastases (70).

The overall prognosis for patients with vaginal melanoma is poor because most patients have deeply penetrating lesions at the time of diagnosis. Buchanan et al. (71) reviewed the literature and reported that only 18 of 197 patients (9.1%) survived for 5 years or longer. Six of the 18 patients were treated with radical operative procedures, 4 with radiation, 6 with wide local excision, and 1 with radiation plus wide excision. In one patient, the mode of therapy was unknown. Both reviews by Reid et al. (67) and Buchanan et al. (71) noted that **size of the lesion was the best prognostic indicator.** Among thirteen 5-year survivors who had their tumor size noted, 11 (84.6%) had lesions less than 3 cm in maximal diameter. Among ten 5-year survivors who had depth of invasion noted, only 2 (20%) had invasion of greater than 2 mm (71).

Adjuvant therapy with *interferon alfa-2b* has been shown to improve relapse-free and overall survival in patients with high-risk cutaneous melanomas (75), but there are as yet no data on this treatment for vaginal melanomas.

Once a recurrence is noted, prognosis is extremely poor, with a mean survival time of 8.5 months.

Vaginal Sarcomas

Leiomyosarcoma

Vaginal sarcomas, such as **fibrosarcomas** and **leiomyosarcomas,** are rare tumors. They are usually bulky lesions and occur most commonly in the upper vagina. Tavassoli and Norris (76) reported 60 smooth muscle tumors of the vagina, only 5 of which recurred. All recurrences were seen in tumors more than 3 cm in diameter with moderate to marked cytologic atypia and more than five mitoses per 10 high-power fields. A review of vaginal leiomyosarcomas in 2000 revealed fewer than 70 cases reported in the English literature (77). The average age at presentation was 47 years, and the overall 5-year survival was 43%.

Surgical excision is the mainstay of treatment. If the lesion is well differentiated and the surgical margins are not involved, as is likely with tumors of low malignant potential, the likelihood of cure is good. For frankly malignant lesions, lymphatic and hematogenous dissemination is common. Adjuvant pelvic radiation is indicated for such tumors (78).

Rhabdomyosarcoma

Rhabdomyosarcoma, a malignant tumor of the rhabdomyoblasts, is the most common soft tissue tumor in children. **Rhabdomyosarcoma of the female genital tract is one of the most curable forms of the disease, but accounts for less than 4% of all pediatric rhabdomyosarcomas** (79).

Sarcoma botryoides (embryonal rhabdomyosarcoma) is a highly malignant, grapelike tumor. The term *botryoides* comes from the Greek word *botrys,* which means "grapes," and, grossly, the tumor usually appears as a polypoid mass extruding from the vagina. Microscopically, the characteristic feature is the presence of cross-striated rhabdomyoblasts (strap cells). **More than 75% of vulvovaginal rhabdomyosarcomas are of the botryoid histological type** (80). **In the female genital tract, sarcoma botryoides is usually found in the vagina during infancy and early childhood, in the cervix during the reproductive years, and in the corpus uteri during the postmenopausal period.**

Approaches to management have varied over the years, but **radical surgery, including pelvic exenteration for primary management, has progressively been replaced by chemotherapy and more conservative surgery and radiation.** The most influential group in this regard has been the Intergroup Rhabdomyosarcoma Study Group (IRSG), which conducted four consecutive trials commencing in 1972 (79,81). The initial study (1972–1978) involved radical surgical resection followed by chemotherapy, with or without radiotherapy. In the second study (1978–1984), multiagent chemotherapy was given first to reduce tumor size, with the objective of allowing more conservative surgery and organ preservation. Radiotherapy was reserved for those patients with residual disease after surgery. In both the third (1984–1991) and fourth (1991–1997) studies, chemotherapy was intensified further, with the aim of reducing further the extent of surgery necessary. After induction chemotherapy, clinical and radiological response was closely monitored and local treatment given only if residual tumor persisted (79).

The IRSG grouping classification is shown in Table 14.5. Chemotherapy was given according to the tumor group. **Patients with group I, II, or III tumors received 12 months of treatment with either VAC** (*vincristine, actinomycin D,* and *cyclophosphamide*), **VAI** (*vincristine, actinomycin D,* and *ifosfamide*) **plus VAC, or VIE** (*vincristine, ifosfamide and etoposide*) **plus VAC.** Patients with group IV tumors were randomized to receive VM (*vincristine* and *melphelan*) or ID (*ifosfamide* and *doxyrubicin*) given as initial therapy, followed by VAC plus RT.

As with surgery, radiotherapy has been more limited in recent years with a view to decreasing morbidity and preserving reproductive capability. Since 1990, only residual disease has been included in the brachytherapy-treated volume at the Gustave Roussy Institute in Paris

Table 14.5 IRSG Grouping Classification

Group I	Localized disease, completely excised, no microscopic residual tumor
	A. Confined to site of origin, completely resected
	B. Infiltrating beyond site of origin, completely resected
Group II	Total gross resection
	A. Gross resection with evidence of microscopic local residual disease
	B. Regional disease with involved lymph nodes, completely resected with no macroscopic residual tumor
	C. Microscopic local and/or lymph node residual disease
Group III	Incomplete resection or biopsy with gross residual disease
Group IV	Distant metastases

IRSG: Intergroup Rhabdomyosarcoma Study Group.

(79). **Ovarian transposition should be undertaken surgically prior to radiation therapy.** Tumors larger than 40 mm after chemotherapy are not candidates for exclusive brachytherapy (79).

In a review of the records of 82 cases of vaginal rhabdomyosarcoma treated on IRSG protocols I–IV, **the estimated 5-year survival was over 85% for patients with locoregional tumors** (81).

Other Vaginal Sarcomas

A variety of other malignant mesodermal tumors have been described to arise in the vagina, including malignant fibrous histiocytoma (82); angiosarcoma (83); and hemangiopericytoma (84). Petur and Young suggested that the latter tumors probably represent extrauterine endometrial stromal sarcomas (85).

Endodermal Sinus Tumor (Yolk Sac Tumor)

These rare germ cell tumors are occasionally found in extragonadal sites such as the vagina. Leverger et al. (86) reported 11 such cases from the Institut Gustave-Roussy. The average age of the patients was 10 months, and the presenting symptom was vaginal bleeding. Diagnosis was made by examination and biopsy with the patient under anesthesia. All children had high serum alpha fetoprotein levels. From 1977 to 1983, six of eight children were cured, with an average follow-up of 3 years. Treatment consisted of primary chemotherapy to reduce the tumor volume, followed by either partial colpectomy, radiation therapy, or both.

Carcinoma of the Urethra

Primary carcinoma of the female urethra is a rare malignancy, accounting for less than 0.1% of all female genital malignancies (87). The disease has been reported from the third to the ninth decades of life, with a median age of approximately 65 years. The most common presenting symptoms are urethral bleeding, hematuria, dysuria, urinary obstruction, and a mass at the introitus (88). Uncommon presenting symptoms include urinary incontinence, perineal pain, and dyspareunia.

Most tumors involve the anterior or distal urethra and may be confused with a urethral carbuncle or mucosal prolapse. Histologically, these distal lesions are usually squamous cell carcinomas. Tumors involving the posterior or proximal urethra are usually adenocarcinomas or transitional cell carcinomas. The relative frequency of the various histologic variants is shown in Table 14.6. Urethral carcinomas occasionally arise in a urethral diverticulum (90).

There is no FIGO staging for the disease, and several staging classifications have been suggested (89,91,94,95). The TNM staging system is shown in Table 14.7. **Distal tumors spread to the lymph nodes of the groin, whereas proximal tumors spread to pelvic nodes, and treatment planning should take this into consideration.** Bladder neck involvement is a common cause of local recurrence, and examination under anesthesia, endoscopic evaluation, and biopsy of the bladder neck should be undertaken as part of the pretreatment workup.

The treatment of urethral cancer must be individualized (87) and multimodal (88,93,96). For small distal lesions, the distal half of the urethra can be excised without loss of urinary

Table 14.6 Histology of Urethral Carcinomas		
Type	*No.*	*Percentage*
Squamous cell	133	53.0
Adenocarcinoma	54	21.5
Transitional cell	48	19.1
Undifferentiated	8	3.2
Melanoma	5	2.0
Sarcoma	1	0.4
Non-Hodgkin's lymphoma	1	0.4
Unknown	1	0.4
Total	**251**	**100.0**

Data compiled from **Bracken *et al.,*** 1976 (89); **Benson *et al.,*** 1982 (90); **Weghaupt *et al.,*** 1984 (87); **Prempree *et al.,*** 1984 (91); **Grigsby,** 1998 (92); **Eng *et al.,*** 2003 (93) and **Thyarihally *et al.,*** 2005 (88).

continence. **Bilateral inguinofemoral lymphadenectomy should be performed for all but the most superficial lesions involving the distal half of the urethra.** Interstitial radiation may be satisfactory for more proximal early lesions.

The majority of patients present with advanced disease, and surgery alone is suboptimal. **Radiation therapy is considered to be the treatment of choice, although it may cause complications such as urinary stricture, fistula, or total incontinence.** Surgery may be used in conjunction with radiation for advanced lesions (91). Anterior exenteration and high-dose ^{192}iridium (^{192}Ir) intraoperative radiotherapy, followed several weeks later by external beam pelvic radiation, has been reported to give local control in four of six patients (67%), with a median follow-up of 21 months (range 12 to 47 months) (96). Four of the six patients were also treated with neoadjuvant or concomitant platinum-based chemotherapy. Klein et al. from Memorial Sloan-Kettering reported on five women who were treated with preoperative radiation followed by anterior exenteration combined with resection of the inferior pubic rami (97). Two died with distant metastases, and one died of surgical complications at 1 month. For medically unfit patients, external beam therapy followed by high dose-rate brachytherapy delivered with a remote afterloader, using a shielded vaginal applicator and modified urethral catheter, has been successfully used (98).

Experience with chemoradiation is limited to case reports, but the results appear to be favorable (99,100,101). Chemotherapeutic agents used have included *cisplatin, 5-fluorouracil,* and *mitomycin-C.* In view of the experience with other primary sites, this would seem to be an acceptable initial approach for locally advanced cases.

A Japanese case report described bladder-sparing urethrectomy with resection of the anterior vaginal wall and continent urinary diversion using the appendix (Mitrofanoff procedure) for a 2 cm × 2 cm distal urethral cancer invading the anterior vaginal wall. The patient was 77 years old and 4 years after surgery, she remained disease-free (102).

Prognosis

Bracken et al. (89) from the M. D. Anderson Hospital reported an overall 5-year survival rate of only 32% for 81 cases of carcinoma of the female urethra. When analyzed with respect to tumor size, 5-year survival rates were 60%, 46% and 13% for lesions <2, 2–4, and >4 cm respectively. Grigsby (92), from the Mallinckrodt Institute of Radiology in St. Louis, reported a 5-year survival rate of 42% for 44 cases. Stage distribution was as follows: T_1 in 8, T_2 in 5, T_3 in 22, and T_4 in 9. Treatment was with surgery in 7 cases, radiation therapy in 25 cases, and combined surgery and radiation therapy in 12. The severe complication rate was 29% for treatment with surgery, 24% for radiation therapy, and 8% for combined therapy. **The most important clinical factors affecting prognosis were tumor size and histologic type—none of 13 women with adenocarcinomas was alive at 5 years, and only 1 of 10 women with tumors greater than 4 cm diameter was a 5-year survivor. The main cause of treatment failure is local recurrence.**

Table 14.7 TNM Staging for Urethral Cancer

Stage		TNM	
Stage 0$_a$	T$_a$	N$_0$	M$_0$
Stage 0$_{is}$	T$_{is}$	N$_0$	M$_0$
Stage I	T$_1$	N$_0$	M$_0$
Stage II	T$_2$	N$_0$	M$_0$
Stage III	T$_1$	N$_1$	M$_0$
	T$_2$	N$_1$	M$_0$
	T$_3$	N$_0$	M$_0$
	T$_3$	N$_1$	M$_0$
Stage IV	T$_4$	N$_0$	M$_0$
	T$_4$	N$_1$	M$_0$
	Any T	N$_2$	M$_0$
	Any T	N$_3$	M$_0$
	Any T	Any N	M$_1$

TNM Classification

T:	Primary Tumor	M:	Distant Metastases
T$_a$	Noninvasive papillary, polypoid, or verrucous carcinoma		
T$_{is}$	Carcinoma *in situ*	M$_x$	Presence of distant metastasis cannot be assessed
T$_1$	Tumor invades subepithelial connective tissue	M$_0$	No distant metastasis
T$_2$	Tumor invades the periurethral muscle	M$_1$	Distant metastasis
T$_3$	Tumor invades the anterior vagina or bladder neck	**Histopathologic Type**	
T$_4$	Tumor invades other adjacent organs	Cell types can be divided into transitional, squamous, and glandular	

N:	Regional Lymph Nodes	G:	Histopathologic Grade
N$_x$	Regional lymph nodes cannot be assessed	G$_x$	Grade cannot be assessed
N$_0$	No regional lymph node metastasis	G$_1$	Well differentiated
N$_1$	Metastasis in a single lymph node, 2 cm or less in greatest dimension	G$_2$	Moderately differentiated
N$_2$	Metastasis in a single lymph node, more than 2 cm but not more than 5 cm in greatest dimension; or multiple lymph nodes, none more than 5 cm in greatest dimension	G$_{3-4}$	Poorly differentiated or undifferentiated
N$_3$	Metastasis in a lymph node more than 5 cm in greatest dimension		

Malignant Melanoma

This rare tumor accounts for 0.2% of all melanomas. Di Marco et al. reported the Mayo Clinic experience of 11 cases (mean age 68 years) treated from 1950 to 1999 (103). Most patients presented with hematuria or a urethral mass. Four patients were treated by radical surgery, including anterior exenteration in two patients. Two (50%) of the four patients undergoing radical surgery recurred at 4 and 34 months, respectively. The remaining seven patients underwent local excision with partial urethrectomy. This group experienced urethral recurrence in five of the seven patients (71%). No patient received any adjuvant therapy. The authors suggested that radical urethrectomy with bladder preservation and a continent catheterizable stoma may be a more appropriate option. The catheterizable stoma could be constructed using an appendicovesicostomy or an ileovesicostomy for urinary diversion.

References

1. **Jemal A, Siegel R, Ward E, Hao Y, Xu J, Murray T, et al.** Cancer statistics 2009. *CA Cancer J Clin* 2009; published online before print. doi:10.3322/caac.20006.
2. **Beller U, Benedet JL, Creasman WT, Ngan HYS, Quinn MA, Maisonneuve P, et al.** Carcinoma of the vagina: 26th Annual report on the results of treatment in gynecological cancer. *Int J Gynecol Obstet* 2006;95:S29–S42.
3. **Chyle V, Zagars GK, Wheeler JA, Wharton JT, Delclos L.** Definitive radiotherapy for carcinoma of the vagina: outcome and prognostic factors. *Int J Radiat Oncol Biol Phys* 1996;35:891–905.
4. **Kirkbridge P, Fyles A, Rawlings GA, Manchul L, Levin W, Murphy KJ, et al.** Carcinoma of the vagina: experience at the Princess Margaret Hospital (1974–1989). *Gynecol Oncol* 1995;56: 435–443.
5. **Frank SJ, Thingran A, Levenbach C, Eifel PJ.** Definitive radiation therapy for squamous cell carcinoma of the vagina. *Int J Radiat Oncol Biol Phys* 2005;62:138–147.
6. **Fu YS.** *Pathology of the uterine cervix, vagina, and vulva,* 2nd ed. Philadelphia: Saunders, 2002:531.
7. **Perez CA, Arneson AN, Dehner LP, Galakatos A.** Radiation therapy in carcinoma of the vagina. *Obstet Gynecol* 1974;44:862–872.
8. **Pride GL, Buehler DA.** Carcinoma of vagina 10 or more years following pelvic irradiation therapy. *Am J Obstet Gynecol* 1977; 127:513–518.
9. **Ball HG, Berman ML.** Management of primary vaginal carcinoma. *Gynecol Oncol* 1982;14:154–163.
10. **Houghton CRS, Iversen T.** Squamous cell carcinoma of the vagina: a clinical study of the location of the tumor. *Gynecol Oncol* 1982;13: 365–372.
11. **Benedet JL, Murphy KJ, Fairey RN, Boyes DA.** Primary invasive carcinoma of the vagina. *Obstet Gynecol* 1983;62:715–719.
12. **Peters WA III, Kumar NB, Morley GW.** Carcinoma of the vagina. *Cancer* 1985;55:892–897.
13. **Rubin SC, Young J, Mikuta JJ.** Squamous carcinoma of the vagina: treatment, complications, and long-term follow-up. *Gynecol Oncol* 1985;20:346–353.
14. **Sulak P, Barnhill D, Heller P, Weiser E, Hoskins W, Park R, et al.** Nonsquamous cancer of the vagina. *Gynecol Oncol* 1988;29: 309–320.
15. **Eddy GL, Marks RD, Miller MC III, Underwood PB Jr.** Primary invasive vaginal carcinoma. *Am J Obstet Gynecol* 1991;165: 292–298.
16. **Ali MM, Huang DT, Goplerud DR, Howells R, Lu JD.** Radiation alone for carcinoma of the vagina: variation in response related to the location of the primary tumor. *Cancer* 1996;77:1934–1939.
17. **Tjalma WAA, Monaghan JM, de Barros Lopes A, Naik R, Nordin AJ, Weyler JJ.** The role of surgery in invasive squamous carcinoma of the vagina. *Gynecol Oncol* 2001;81:360–365.
18. **Tewari KS, Cappuccini F, Puthawala AA, Kuo JV, Burger RA, Monk BJ, et al.** Primary invasive carcinoma of the vagina: treatment with interstitial brachytherapy. *Cancer* 2001;91:758–770.
19. **Hellman K, Lundell M, Silfversward C, Nilsson B, Hellstrom AC, Frankendal B.** Clinical and histopathological factors related to prognosis in primary squamous cell carcinoma of the vagina. *Int J Gynecol Cancer* 2006;16:1201–1211.
20. **Daling JR, Madeleine MM, Schwartz SM, Shera KA, Carter JJ, McKnight B, et al.** A population-based study of squamous cell vaginal cancer: HPV and cofactors. *Gynecol Oncol* 2002;84: 263–270.
21. **Hellman K, Silfversward C, Nilsson B, Hellstrom AC, Frankendal B, Pettersson F.** Primary carcinoma of the vagina: factors influencing the age at diagnosis: The Radiumhemmet Series 1956–96. *Int J Gynecol Cancer* 2004;14:491–501.
22. **Murad TM, Durant JR, Maddox WA, Dowling EA.** The pathologic behavior of primary vaginal carcinoma and its relationship to cervical cancer. *Cancer* 1975;35:787–794.
23. **Perez CA, Grigsby PW, Garipagaoglu M, Mutch DG, Lockett MA.** Factors affecting long-term outcome of irradiation in carcinoma of the vagina. *Int J Radiat Oncol Biol Phys* 1999;44:37–45.
24. **Choo YC, Anderson DG.** Neoplasms of the vagina following cervical carcinoma. *Gynecol Oncol* 1982;14:125–132.
25. **Benedet JL, Saunders BH.** Carcinoma *in situ* of the vagina. *Am J Obstet Gynecol* 1984;148:695–700.
26. **Rome RM, England PG.** Management of vaginal intraepithelial neoplasia: a series of 132 cases with long term follow-up. *Int J Gynecol Cancer* 2000;10:382–390.
27. **Cramer DW, Cutler SJ.** Incidence and histopathology of malignancies of the female genital organs in the United States. *Am J Obstet Gynecol* 1974;118:443–449.
28. **Herman JM, Homesley HD, Dignan MB.** Is hysterectomy a risk factor for vaginal cancer? *JAMA* 1986;256:601–606.
29. **Fanning J, Manahan KJ, McLean SA.** Loop electro-surgical excision procedure for partial upper vaginectomy. *Am J Obstet Gynecol* 1999;181:1382–1385.
30. **Hoffman MS, De Cesare SL, Roberts WS, Fiorica JV, Finan MA, Cavanagh D.** Upper vaginectomy for *in situ* and occult superficially invasive carcinoma of the vagina. *Am J Obstet Gynecol* 1992;166: 30–33.
31. **Kucera H, Vavra N.** Radiation management of primary carcinoma of the vagina: clinical and histopathological variables associated with survival. *Gynecol Oncol* 1991;40:112–116.
32. **Stock RG, Chen ASJ, Seski J.** A 30-year experience in the management of primary carcinoma of the vagina: analysis of prognostic factors and treatment modalities. *Gynecol Oncol* 1995;56: 45–52.
33. **Perez CA, Grigsby PW, Garipagaoglu M, Mutch PG, Lockett MA.** Factors affecting long-term outcome of irradiation in carcinoma of the vagina. *Int J Radiat Oncol Biol Phys* 1999;44:37–45.
34. **Peters WA III, Kumar NB, Morley GW.** Microinvasive carcinoma of the vagina: a distinct clinical entity? *Am J Obstet Gynecol* 1985; 153:505–507.
35. **Eddy GL, Singh KP, Gansler TS.** Superficially invasive carcinoma of the vagina following treatment for cervical cancer: a report of six cases. *Gynecol Oncol* 1990;36:376–379.
36. **Al-Kurdi M, Monaghan JM.** Thirty-two years experience in management of primary tumors of the vagina. *BJOG* 1981;88: 1145–1150.
37. **Van Dam P, Sonnemans H, van Dam P-J, Verkinderen L, Dirix LY.** Sentinel node detection in patients with vaginal carcinoma. *Gynecol Oncol* 2004;92:89–92.

38. **Lamoreaux WT, Grigsby PW, Dehdashti F, Zoberi I, Powell MA, Gibb RK, et al.** FDG-PET evaluation of vaginal carcinoma. *Int J Radiat Oncol Biol Phys* 2005;62:733–737.

39. **Ling B, Gao Z, Sun M, Sun F, Zhang A, Zhao W, et al.** Laparoscopic radical hysterectomy with vaginectomy and reconstruction of vagina in patients with stage I primary vaginal cancer. *Gynecol Oncol* 2008;109:92–96.

40. **Cutillo G, Gignini P, Pizzi G, Vizza E, Micheli A, Arcangeli G, et al.** Conservative treatment of reproductive and sexual women with squamous carcinoma of the vagina. *Gynecol Oncol* 2006;103: 234–237.

41. **Otton GR, Nicklin JL, Dickie GJ, Niedetzky P, Tripcony L, Perrin LC, et al.** Early-stage vaginal carcinoma—an analysis of 70 patients. *Int J Gynecol Cancer* 2004;14:304–310.

42. **Reddy S, Lee MS, Graham JE, Yordan EL, Phillips R, Saxena VS, et al.** Radiation therapy in primary carcinoma of the vagina. *Gynecol Oncol* 1987;26:19–24.

43. **Andersen ES.** Primary carcinoma of the vagina: a study of 29 cases. *Gynecol Oncol* 1989;33:317–320.

44. **Dalrymple JL, Russell AH, Lee SW, Scudder SA, Leiserowitz GS, Kinney WK, et al.** Chemoradiation for primary invasive squamous carcinoma of the vagina. *Int J Gynecol Cancer* 2004;14: 110–117.

45. **Stryker JA.** Radiotherapy for vaginal carcinoma: a 23-year review. *Brit J Radiol* 2000;73:1200–1205.

46. **Pride GL, Schultz AE, Chuprevich TW, Buehler DA.** Primary invasive squamous carcinoma of the vagina. *Obstet Gynecol* 1979;53:218–225.

47. **Tran PT, Su Z, Lee P, Lavori P, Husain A, Teng N, Kapp DS.** Prognostic factors for outcomes and complications for primary squamous cell carcinoma of the vagina treated with radiation. *Gynecol Oncol* 2007;105:641–649.

48. **Tabata T, Takeshima N, Nishida H, Hirai Y, Hasumi K.** Treatment failure in vaginal cancer. *Gynecol Oncol* 2002;84: 309–314.

49. **Ballon SC, Lagasse LD, Chang NH, Stehman FB.** Primary adenocarcinoma of the vagina. *Surg Gynecol Obstet* 1979;149:233–237.

50. **Robboy SJ, Hill EC, Sandberg EC, Czernobilsky B.** Vaginal adenosis in women born prior to the diethylstilbestrol (DES) era. *Human Pathol* 1986;17:488–492.

51. **Madhar HS, Smith JHF, Tidy J.** Primary vaginal adenocarcinoma of intestinal type arising from an adenoma: a case report and review of the literature. *Int J Gynecol Pathol* 2001;20:204–209.

52. **Herbst AL, Scully RE.** Adenocarcinoma of the vagina in adolescence. *Cancer* 1970;25:745–751.

53. **Herbst AL, Ulfelder H, Poskanzer DC.** Adenocarcinoma of the vagina: association of maternal stilbestrol therapy with tumor appearance in young women. *N Engl J Med* 1971;284:878–882.

54. **Herbst AL, Cole P, Norusis MJ, Welch WR, Scully RE.** Epidemiologic aspects and factors related to survival in 384 registry cases of clear cell adenocarcinoma of the vagina and cervix. *Am J Obstet Gynecol* 1979;135:876–886.

55. **Robboy SJ, Young RH, Welch WR, Truslow GY, Prat J, Herbst AL, et al.** Atypical vaginal adenosis and cervical ectropion. *Cancer* 1984;54:869–875.

56. **Sandberg EC, Christian JC.** Diethylstilbestrol-exposed monozygotic twins discordant for cervicovaginal clear cell adenocarcinoma. *Am J Obstet Gynecol* 1980;137:220–223.

57. **Antonioli DA, Burke L, Friedman EA.** Natural history of diethylstilbestrol associated genital tract lesions: cervical ectopy and cervicovaginal hood. *Am J Obstet Gynecol* 1980;137:847–853.

58. **Kaufman RH, Adam E, Binder GL, Gerthoffer E.** Upper genital tract changes and pregnancy outcome in offspring exposed in utero to diethylstilbestrol. *Am J Obstet Gynecol* 1980;137: 299–308.

59. **Herbst AL, Hubby MM, Aziz F, Mak II MM.** Reproductive and gynecologic surgical experience in diethylstilbestrol-exposed daughters. *Am J Obstet Gynecol* 1981;141:1019–1028.

60. **Senekjian EK, Frey KW, Anderson D, Herbst AL.** Local therapy in stage I clear cell adenocarcinoma of the vagina. *Cancer* 1987;60:1319–1324.

61. **Herbst AL, Robboy SJ, Scully RE, Poskanzer DC.** Clear-cell adenocarcinoma of the vagina and cervix in girls: analysis of 170 registry cases. *Am J Obstet Gynecol* 1974;119:713–724.

62. **Kaminski JM, Anderson PR, Han AC, Mitra RK, Rosenblum NG, Edelson MI.** Primary small cell carcinoma of the vagina. *Gynecol Oncol* 2003;88:451–455.

63. **Crowther ME, Lowe DG, Shepherd JH.** Verrucous carcinoma of the female genital tract: a review. *Obstet Gynecol Surv* 1988;43: 263–280.

64. **Piura B, Rabinovich A, Yanai-Inbar I.** Primary malignant melanoma of the vulva: a case report and literature review. *Eur J Gynecol Oncol* 2002;23:195–198.

65. **Nigogosyam G, De La Pava S, Pickren JW.** Melanoblasts in vaginal mucosa. *Cancer* 1964;17:912–917.

66. **Morrow CP, DiSaia PJ.** Malignant melanoma of the female genitalia: a clinical analysis. *Obstet Gynecol Surv* 1976;31:233–241.

67. **Reid GC, Schmidt RW, Roberts JA, Hopkins MP, Barrett RJ, Morley GW.** Primary melanoma of the vagina: a clinico-pathologic analysis. *Obstet Gynecol* 1989;74:190–199.

68. **Chung AF, Casey MJ, Flannery JT, Woodruff JM, Lewis JL Jr.** Malignant melanoma of the vagina: report of 19 cases. *Obstet Gynecol* 1980;55:720–727.

69. **Chung AF, Woodruff JW, Lewis JL Jr.** Malignant melanoma of the vulva: a report of 44 cases. *Obstet Gynecol* 1975;45:638–644.

70. **Gupta D, Malpica A, Deavers MT, Silva EG.** Vaginal melanoma: a clinicopathologic and immunohistochemical study of 26 cases. *Am J Surg Path* 2002;26:1450–1457.

71. **Buchanan DJ, Schlaerth J, Kurosaki T.** Primary vaginal melanoma: thirteen-year disease-free survival after wide local excision and recent literature review. *Am J Obstet Gynecol* 1998;178: 1177–1184.

72. **Tjalma WA, Monaghan JM, de Barros Lopes A, Naik R, Nordin A.** Primary vaginal melanomas and long-term survivors. *Eur J Gynaecol Oncol* 2001;22:20–22.

73. **Miner TJ, Delgado R, Zeisler J, Busam K, Alektiar K, Barakat R, et al.** Primary vaginal melanoma: a critical analysis of therapy. *Ann Surg Oncol* 2004;11:34–39.

74. **Harwood AR, Cumming BJ.** Radiotherapy for mucosal melanoma. *Int J Radiat Oncol Biol Phys* 1982;8:1121–1127.

75. **Gray RJ, Pockay BA, Kirkwood JM.** An update on adjuvant interferon for melanoma. *Cancer Control* 2002;9:16–21.

76. **Tavassoli FA, Norris HJ.** Smooth muscle tumors of the vagina. *Obstet Gynecol* 1979;53:689–695.

77. **Ciaravino G, Kapp DS, Vela AM, Fulton RS, Lum BL, Teng NNH, et al.** Primary leiomyosarcoma of the vagina: a case report and literature review. *Int J Gynecol Cancer* 2000;10:340–347.

78. **Curtin JP, Saigo P, Slucher B, Venkatraman ES, Mychalczak B, Hoskins WJ.** Soft tissue sarcoma of the vagina and vulva: a clinicopathologic study. *Obstet Gynecol* 1995;86:269–272.

79. **Magné N, Haie-Meder C.** Brachytherapy for genital tract rhabdomyosarcomas in girls: technical aspects, reports, and perspectives. *Lancet Oncol* 2007;8:725–729.

80. **Magné N, Oberlin O, Martelli H, Gerbaulet A, Chassagne D, Haie-Meder C.** Vulval and vaginal rhabdomyosarcoma in children: The Institute Gustave Roussy brachytherapy experience with particular attention on long-term outcomes. *Int J Gynecol Cancer* 2006;16(suppl 3):610 (Abst 0038).

81. **Arndt CAS, Donaldson SS, Anderson JR, Andrasy RJ, Laurie F, Link MP, et al.** What constitutes optimal therapy for patients with rhabdomyosarcoma of the female genital tract. *Cancer* 2001;91: 2454–2468.

82. **Webb MJ, Simmonds RE, Weiland LH.** Malignant fibrous histiocytoma of the vagina. *Am J Obstet Gynecol* 1974;119:190–192.

83. **McAdam JA, Stewart F, Reid R.** Vaginal epithelial angiosarcoma. *J Clin Pathol* 1998;51:928–930.

84. **Buscema J, Rosenshein NB, Taqi F, Woodruff JD.** Vaginal hemangiopericytoma: a histopathologic and ultrastructural evaluation. *Obstet Gynecol* 1985;21:376–384.

85. **Pertur NG, Young RH.** Mesenchymal tumors and tumor-like lesions of the female genital tract: a selective review with emphasis on recently described entities. *Int J Gynecol Pathol* 2001;20:105–127.

86. **Leverger G, Flamant F, Gerbaulet A, Lemerle J.** Tumors of the vitelline sac located in the vagina in children. *Arch Pediatr* 1983;40: 85–89.

87. **Weghaupt K, Gerstner GJ, Kucera H.** Radiation therapy for primary carcinoma of the female urethra: a survey over 25 years. *Gynecol Oncol* 1984;17:58–63.

88. **Thyavihally YB, Wuntkal R, Bakshi G, Uppin S, Tongoankar HB.** Primary carcinoma of the female urethra: single center experience of 18 cases. *Jpn J Clin Oncol* 2005;35:84–87.

89. **Bracken RB, Johnson DE, Miller LS, Ayala AG, Gomez JJ, Rudledge F.** Primary carcinoma of the female urethra. *J Urol* 1976;116:188–192.

90. **Benson RC, Tunca JC, Buchler DA, Uehling DT.** Primary carcinoma of the female urethra. *Gynecol Oncol* 1982;14:313–318.

91. **Prempree T, Amornmarn R, Patanaphan V.** Radiation therapy in primary carcinoma of the female urethra. *Cancer* 1984;54:729–733.

92. **Grigsby PW.** Carcinoma of the urethra in women. *Int J Radiat Oncol Biol Phys* 1998;41:535–541.

93. **Eng TY, Naguib M, Galang T, Fuller CD.** Retrospective study of the treatment of urethral cancer. *Am J Clin Oncol* 2003;26:558–562.

94. **Ampil FL.** Primary malignant neoplasms of the female urethra. *Obstet Gynecol* 1985;66:799–804.

95. **Grabstald H, Hilaris B, Henschke U, Whitmore WF Jr.** Cancer of the female urethra. *JAMA* 1966;197:835–842.

96. **Dalbagni G, Donat MS, Eschwege P, Herr HW, Zelefsky MJ.** Results of high dose rate brachytherapy, anterior pelvic exenteration and external beam radiotherapy for carcinoma of the female urethra. *J Urol* 2001;166:1759–1761.

97. **Klein FA, Whitmore WF, Herr HW, Morse MJ, Sogani PC.** Inferior pubic rami resection with en bloc radical excision for invasive proximal urethral carcinoma. *Cancer* 1983;51:1238–1242.

98. **Kuettel MR, Parda DS, Harter KW, Rodgers JE, Lynch JH.** Treatment of female urethral carcinoma in medically inoperable patients using external beam irradiation and high dose rate intracavitary brachytherapy. *J Urol* 1997;157:1669–1671.

99. **Shah AB, Kalra JK, Silber L, Molho L.** Squamous cell carcinoma of the female urethra: successful treatment with chemoradiotherapy. *Urology* 1985;25:284–286.

100. **Hara I, Hikosaka S, Eto H, Miyake H, Yamada Y, Soejima T, et al.** Successful treatment for squamous cell carcinoma of the female urethra with combined radio- and chemotherapy. *Int J Urol* 2004;11:678–682.

101. **Licht MR, Klein EA, Bukowski R, Montie JE, Saxton JP.** Combination radiation and chemotherapy for the treatment of squamous cell carcinoma of the male and female urethra. *J Urol* 1995;153:1918–1920.

102. **Kobayashi M, Nomura M, Yamada Y, Fujimoto N, Matsumoto T.** Bladder-sparing surgery and continent urinary diversion using the appendix (Mitrofanoff procedure) for urethral cancer. *Int J Urol* 2005;12:581–584.

103. **Di Marco DS, Di Marco CS, Zincke H, Webb MJ, Keeney GL, Bass S, et al.** Outcome of surgical treatment for primary malignant melanoma of the female urethra. *J Urol* 2004;171:765–767.

15 Gestational Trophoblastic Neoplasia

Ross S. Berkowitz
Donald P. Goldstein

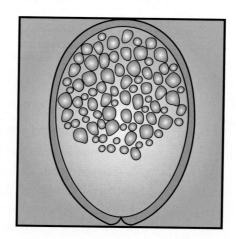

Gestational trophoblastic neoplasia (GTN) is among the rare human malignancies that can be cured even in the presence of widespread metastases (1–3). **GTN includes a spectrum of interrelated tumors—including hydatidiform mole, invasive mole, placental-site trophoblastic tumor, and choriocarcinoma—that have varying propensities for local invasion and metastasis.** Although persistent GTN most commonly ensues after a molar pregnancy, it may follow any gestational event, including therapeutic or spontaneous abortion and ectopic or term pregnancy. Dramatic advances have been made in the diagnosis, treatment, and follow-up of patients with GTN since the introduction of chemotherapy in 1956.

Hydatidiform Mole

Complete Versus Partial Hydatidiform Mole

Hydatidiform moles may be categorized as either complete or partial moles on the basis of gross morphology, histopathology, and karyotype (Table 15.1).

Complete Hydatidiform Mole

Pathology   Complete moles lack identifiable embryonic or fetal tissues, and the chorionic villi exhibit generalized hydatidiform swelling and diffuse trophoblastic hyperplasia.

Chromosomes   **Cytogenetic studies have demonstrated that complete hydatidiform moles usually have a 46XX karyotype, and the molar chromosomes are entirely of paternal origin** (4). Complete moles appear to arise from an ovum that has been fertilized by a haploid sperm, which then duplicates its own chromosomes, and the ovum nucleus may be either absent or inactivated (5). Although most complete moles have a 46XX chromosomal pattern, approximately 10% have a 46XY karyotype (6). Chromosomes in a 46XY complete mole also appear to be entirely of paternal origin, but in this circumstance, an apparently empty egg is fertilized by two sperm.

Table 15.1 Features of Complete and Partial Hydatidiform Moles

	Complete Mole	Partial Mole
Fetal or embryonic tissue	Absent	Present
Hydatidiform swelling of chorionic villi	Diffuse	Focal
Trophoblastic hyperplasia	Diffuse	Focal
Scalloping of chorionic villi	Absent	Present
Trophoblastic stromal inclusions	Absent	Present
Karyotype	46XX; 46XY	69XXY; 69XYY

Reproduced from **Berkowitz RS, Goldstein DP.** The management of molar pregnancy and gestational trophoblastic tumors. In: **Knapp RC, Berkowitz RS, eds.** *Gynecologic oncology.* New York: MacMillan, 1993:425, with permission.

Partial Hydatidiform Mole

Pathology   Partial hydatidiform moles are characterized by the following pathologic features (7):

1. Chorionic villi of varying size with focal hydatidiform swelling and cavitation
2. Marked villous scalloping
3. Focal trophoblastic hyperplasia with or without atypia
4. Prominent stromal trophoblastic inclusions
5. Identifiable embryonic or fetal tissues

Chromosomes   **Partial moles usually have a triploid karyotype (69 chromosomes), with the extra haploid set of chromosomes derived from the father** (8). When a fetus is present in conjunction with a partial mole, it usually exhibits the stigmata of triploidy, including growth retardation and multiple congenital malformations. In a careful review of our pathologic material, Genest et al. concluded that nontriploid partial moles probably do not exist (9).

Clinical Features

The presenting symptoms and signs of patients with complete and partial molar pregnancy are presented in Table 15.2 (10–12).

Complete Hydatidiform Mole

Vaginal Bleeding   **Vaginal bleeding** is the most common presenting symptom in patients with complete molar pregnancy and **occurs in 97% of cases.** Molar tissues may separate from the decidua and disrupt maternal vessels, and large volumes of retained blood may distend the

Table 15.2 Presenting Symptoms and Signs in Patients with Complete and Partial Molar Pregnancy

Sign	Complete Mole[a] N = 306 (%)	Partial Moles[b] N = 81 (%)
Vaginal bleeding	97	73
Excessive uterine size	51	4
Prominent ovarian theca lutein cysts	50	0
Toxemia	27	3
Hyperemesis	26	0
Hyperthyroidism	7	0
Trophoblastic emboli	2	0

Adapted from [a]**Berkowitz RS, Goldstein DP.** Pathogenesis of gestational trophoblastic neoplasms. *Pathobiology Annual* 1981;11:391, and [b]**Berkowitz RS, Goldstein DP, Bernstein MR.** Natural history of partial molar pregnancy. *Obstet Gynecol* 1985;66:677–681.

endometrial cavity. As intrauterine clots undergo oxidation and liquefaction, "prune juice"–like fluid may leak into the vagina. Because vaginal bleeding may be considerable and prolonged, half of these patients present with anemia (hemoglobin <10 g/100 mL).

Excessive Uterine Size   Excessive uterine enlargement relative to gestational age is one of the classic signs of a complete mole, although it is present in only **about half of the patients.** The endometrial cavity may be expanded by both chorionic tissue and retained blood. **Excessive uterine size is usually associated with markedly elevated levels of human chorionic gonadotropin (hCG)** because uterine enlargement results in part from exuberant trophoblastic growth.

Toxemia   Preeclampsia is **observed in approximately 27% of patients** with a complete hydatidiform mole. Although preeclampsia is often associated with hypertension, proteinuria and hyperreflexia, and eclamptic convulsions rarely occur. **Toxemia develops almost exclusively in patients with excessive uterine size and markedly elevated hCG levels.** The diagnosis of hydatidiform mole should be considered whenever preeclampsia develops early in pregnancy.

Hyperemesis Gravidarum   Hyperemesis requiring antiemetic and/or intravenous replacement therapy **occurs in one-fourth of the patients** with a complete mole, particularly those with excessive uterine size and markedly elevated hCG levels. Severe electrolyte disturbances may develop occasionally and require treatment with parenteral fluids.

Hyperthyroidism   Clinically evident hyperthyroidism is **observed in approximately 7% of patients** with a complete molar gestation. These patients may present with tachycardia, warm skin, and tremor, and the diagnosis can be confirmed by detection of elevated serum levels of free thyroxine (T_4) and triiodothyronine (T_3).

Laboratory evidence of hyperthyroidism is commonly detected in asymptomatic patients with hydatidiform moles. Galton et al. (13) reported 11 patients whose thyroid function test values were elevated before molar evacuation, and the thyroid function test values rapidly returned to normal in all patients after evacuation.

If hyperthyroidism is suspected, it is important to administer β-adrenergic blocking agents before the induction of anesthesia for molar evacuation because anesthesia or surgery may precipitate a thyroid storm. The latter may be manifested by hyperthermia, delirium, convulsions, atrial fibrillation, high-output heart failure, or cardiovascular collapse. Administration of β-adrenergic blocking agents prevents or rapidly reverses many of the metabolic and cardiovascular complications of a thyroid storm.

Some investigators have suggested that hCG is the thyroid stimulator in patients with a hydatidiform mole because positive correlations between serum hCG and total T_4 or T_3 concentrations have sometimes been observed. However, Amir et al. (14) measured thyroid function in 47 patients with a complete mole and reported no correlation between serum hCG levels and the serum free T_4 index or free T_3 index. Thus, **the identity of a thyrotropic factor in hydatidiform mole has not been clearly delineated.** Although some investigators have speculated about a separate chorionic thyrotropin, this substance has not yet been isolated.

Trophoblastic Embolization   **Respiratory distress develops in approximately 2% of patients** with a complete mole. **These patients may have chest pain, dyspnea, tachypnea, and tachycardia** and may experience severe respiratory distress after molar evacuation. Auscultation of the chest usually reveals diffuse rales, and the chest radiograph may demonstrate bilateral pulmonary infiltrates. The signs and symptoms of respiratory distress usually resolve within 72 hours with cardiopulmonary support. Respiratory insufficiency may result not only from trophoblastic embolization, but also from the cardiopulmonary complications of thyroid storm, toxemia, and massive fluid replacement.

Theca Lutein Ovarian Cysts   **Prominent theca lutein ovarian cysts (>6 cm in diameter) develop in approximately half the patients** with a complete mole. These cysts contain amber-colored or serosanguineous fluid and are usually bilateral and multilocular. Their formation may be related to increased serum levels of hCG and prolactin (15). **Ovarian enlargement occurs almost exclusively in patients with markedly elevated hCG values.** Because the uterus may also be excessively enlarged, theca lutein cysts may be difficult to palpate on physical examination; however, ultrasonography can accurately document their presence and size. After molar evacuation, theca lutein cysts normally regress spontaneously within 2 to 4 months.

Prominent theca lutein cysts frequently cause symptoms of marked pelvic pressure, and they may be decompressed by laparoscopic or transabdominal aspiration to relieve such symptoms. If acute pelvic pain develops, laparoscopy should be performed to assess possible cystic torsion or rupture, and laparoscopic manipulation may successfully manage incomplete ovarian torsion or cystic rupture (16).

Although in the 1960s, 1970s, and early 1980s, complete moles were usually diagnosed in the second trimester, in more recent years the diagnosis has commonly been made in the first trimester (17). Because of this, the diagnosis of complete mole is now often made before the classic clinical signs and symptoms develop. With earlier diagnosis, excessive uterine size, hyperemesis, anemia, and preeclampsia were observed at presentation in only 28%, 8%, 5%, and 1% of our patients, respectively. Between 1988 and 1993, none of our 74 patients with complete mole had respiratory distress or hyperthyroidism. However, patients continue to present with vaginal bleeding and markedly elevated hCG levels.

The histopathologic characteristics of complete mole are different in the first trimester (18). First trimester complete moles have less circumferential trophoblastic hyperplasia and smaller villi and their more subtle morphologic alterations may lead to misclassification as partial moles or nonmolar spontaneous abortions. **Immunohistochemistry for p57** (paternally imprinted, maternally expressed gene product) **is useful for confirming the diagnosis of a complete mole** (19). Nuclei of decidual cells (maternally derived tissue) and extra villous trophoblast of all types of gestations stain positively for p57. **Almost all complete moles have absent (or nearly absent) villous stromal and cytotrophoblastic nuclear activity for p57,** while all other types of gestations (including partial moles) show nuclear reactivity in more than 25 percent of cases. Fisher et al. (20) showed that maternal chromosomal 11 is retained in the rare case of complete mole exhibiting p57 staining. This helps to explain the rare occurrence of recurrent complete hydatidiform moles of biparental origin.

Partial Hydatidiform Mole

Patients with a partial hydatidiform mole usually do not have the clinical features characteristic of complete molar pregnancy. **In general, these patients present with the signs and symptoms of incomplete or missed abortion, and the diagnosis of partial mole may be made only after histologic review of the curettings** (21).

The main presenting symptom among 81 patients with a partial mole seen at the New England Trophoblastic Disease Center (NETDC) **was vaginal bleeding,** which occurred in 59 patients (72.8%). There was absence of a fetal heart beat in 12 patients (14.8%). Excessive uterine enlargement and preeclampsia were present in only three (3.7%) and two (2.5%) patients, respectively. **No patient presented with theca lutein ovarian cysts, hyperemesis, or hyperthyroidism.** The clinical diagnosis was incomplete or missed abortion in 74 patients (91.4%) and hydatidiform mole in only 5 patients (6.2%). Pre-evacuation hCG levels were measured in 30 patients and were greater than 100,000 mIU/mL in only 2 patients (10).

Natural History

Complete Hydatidiform Mole

Complete moles are well recognized to have a potential for local invasion and distant spread. **After molar evacuation, local uterine invasion occurs in 15% of patients and metastases in 4%** (11,12).

A review of 858 patients with complete hydatidiform mole revealed that **two-fifth of the patients had** the following signs of marked trophoblastic proliferation at the time of presentation:

1. **Human chorionic gonadotropin level greater than 100,000 mIU/mL**
2. **Excessive uterine enlargement**
3. **Theca lutein cysts larger than 6 cm in diameter**

Patients with any of these signs are at high risk for postmolar persistent tumor. The sequelae of 858 patients with low- and high-risk complete hydatidiform moles are shown in Table 15.3. After molar evacuation, local uterine invasion occurred in 31%, and metastases developed in 8.8% of the 352 high-risk patients. For the 506 low-risk patients, local invasion was found in only 3.4%, and metastases developed in 0.6%. **Older women are also at increased risk of postmolar GTN.** Tsukamoto et al. reported that 56% of women older than 50 years developed persistent GTN after molar evacuation (22).

Table 15.3 Sequelae of Low- and High-Risk Complete Hydatidiform Moles

	No. of Patients (%)	
Outcome	Low-Risk	High-Risk
Normal involution	486/506 (96.0)	212/352 (60.2)
Persistent GTN		
Nonmetastatic	17/506 (3.4)	109/352 (31.0)
Metastatic	3/506 (0.6)	31/352 (8.8)
Totals	**506/858 (59.0)**	**352/858 (41.0)**

GTN, gestational trophoblastic neoplasia.

All patients managed by evacuation without prophylactic chemotherapy.

Reproduced from **Goldstein DP, Berkowitz RS, Bernstein MR.** Management of molar pregnancy. *J Reprod Med* 1981;26:208, with permission.

Partial Hydatidiform Mole

Approximately 2% to 4% of patients with a partial mole have persistent postmolar tumor and require chemotherapy to achieve remission (23). Those patients in whom persistent disease develops have no distinguishing clinical or pathologic characteristics.

Diagnosis

Ultrasonography is a reliable and sensitive technique for the diagnosis of complete molar pregnancy. Because the chorionic villi exhibit diffuse hydatidiform swelling, complete moles produce a characteristic vesicular sonographic pattern, usually referred to as a **"snowstorm" pattern.** Ultrasonography continues to be useful in the detection of first trimester complete moles (24).

Ultrasonography may also contribute to the diagnosis of partial molar pregnancy by demonstrating focal cystic spaces in the placental tissues and an increase in the transverse diameter of the gestational sac (25).

Treatment

After molar pregnancy is diagnosed, the patient should be evaluated carefully for the presence of associated medical complications, including preeclampsia, hyperthyroidism, electrolyte imbalance, and anemia. After the patient has been stabilized, a decision must be made concerning the most appropriate method of evacuation.

Hysterectomy

If the patient desires surgical sterilization, a hysterectomy may be performed with the mole *in situ*. **The ovaries may be preserved at the time of surgery, even though theca lutein cysts are present.** Prominent ovarian cysts may be decompressed by aspiration. Although hysterectomy eliminates the risks associated with local invasion, it does not prevent distant spread.

Suction Curettage

Suction curettage is the preferred method of evacuation, regardless of uterine size, in patients who desire to preserve fertility. It involves the following steps:

1. **Oxytocin infusion**—This is begun in the operating room before the induction of anesthesia.
2. **Cervical dilatation**—As the cervix is being dilated, the surgeon frequently encounters increased uterine bleeding. Retained blood in the endometrial cavity may be expelled during cervical dilatation. However, active uterine bleeding should not deter the prompt completion of cervical dilatation.
3. **Suction curettage**—Within a few minutes of commencing suction curettage, the uterus may decrease dramatically in size, and the bleeding is usually well controlled. If the uterus is more than 14 weeks in size, one hand may be placed on top of the

Table 15.4 Prophylactic *Actinomycin D* (Act-D) After Evacuation for Molar Pregnancy		
	No. of Patients (%)	
Outcome	Act-D	No Act-D
Normal involution	237 (96.0)	698 (81.4)
Persistent GTN		
Nonmetastatic	10 (4.0)	126 (14.6)
Metastatic	0 (0)	34 (4.0)
Totals	247 (100)	858 (100)

GTN, gestational trophoblastic neoplasia.

Reproduced from **Goldstein DP, Berkowitz RS, Bernstein MR.** Management of molar pregnancy. *J Reprod Med* 1981;26:208, with permission.

fundus and the uterus massaged to stimulate uterine contraction and reduce the risk of perforation.

4. **Sharp curettage**—When suction evacuation is thought to be complete, sharp curettage is performed to remove any residual molar tissue.

The specimens obtained on suction and sharp curettage should be submitted separately for pathologic review.

Prophylactic Chemotherapy

The use of prophylactic chemotherapy at the time of evacuation of a complete mole is controversial (26). The debate concerns the wisdom of exposing all patients to potentially toxic treatment when only approximately 20% are at risk for development of persistent GTN.

In a study of 247 patients with complete molar pregnancy who received a single course of *actinomycin D (Act-D)* prophylactically at the time of evacuation, local uterine invasion subsequently developed in only 10 patients (4%), and in no case did metastases occur (Table 15.4). Furthermore, all 10 patients with local invasion achieved remission after only one additional course of chemotherapy. **Prophylactic chemotherapy, therefore, not only prevented metastases, it reduced the incidence and morbidity of local uterine invasion.** Kim et al. (27) and Limpongsanurak (28) performed prospective, randomized studies of prophylactic chemotherapy in patients with a complete mole and observed a significant decrease in persistent GTN in patients with high-risk mole who received prophylactic chemotherapy. Therefore, **prophylaxis may be particularly useful in the management of high-risk complete molar pregnancy, especially when hormonal follow-up is unavailable or unreliable.**

Follow-up

Human Chorionic Gonadotropin

Human chorionic gonadotropin is a predictable secretory product of the trophoblastic cell. Like the other glycoprotein hormones—luteinizing hormone (LH), follicle-stimulating hormone, and thyroid-stimulating hormone—hCG is composed of two polypeptide chains (α and β) attached to a carbohydrate moiety. **There is considerable cross-reactivity between hCG and LH because they share indistinguishable α chains.** Each of the β chains of these four glycoprotein hormones is biochemically unique and confers biologic and immunologic specificity. **The β-subunit radioimmunoassay is the most reliable assay available for the management of patients with GTN** and is particularly useful in quantitating low levels of hCG without substantial interference from physiologic levels of LH.

After molar evacuation or hysterectomy with the mole *in situ*, patients should be followed by weekly determinations of β-subunit hCG levels until these are normal for 3 consecutive weeks and then by monthly determinations until the levels are normal for at least 3 consecutive months. The normal postmolar β-hCG regression curve is presented in Figure 15.1. When a patient with molar pregnancy, either partial or complete, achieves a nondetectable hCG

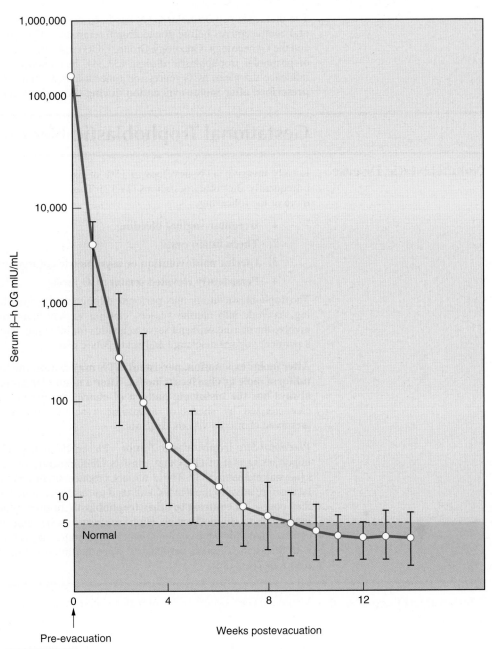

Figure 15.1 Normal regression curve of beta-subunit human chorionic gonadotropin (-hCG) after molar evacuation. (Reprinted from **Morrow CP, Kletzky OA, DiSaia PJ, Townsend DE, Mishell DR, Nakamura RM.** Clinical and laboratory correlates of molar pregnancy and trophoblastic disease. *Am J Obstet Gynecol* 1977;128:424–430, with permission.)

level, the risk of developing tumor relapse is very low (29–31). Based on these findings, **pregnancy is currently allowed after only three months of follow-up. This is particularly important for those older patients** who feel that their window of opportunity for successful pregnancy is closing.

Contraception

Patients are encouraged to use effective contraception during the entire interval of gonadotropin follow-up. Intrauterine devices should not be inserted until the patient achieves a normal hCG level because of the potential risk of uterine perforation, infection, and bleeding. If the patient does not desire surgical sterilization, the choice is to use either hormonal contraception or barrier methods.

The incidence of postmolar GTN has been reported to be increased among patients who use oral contraceptives before gonadotropin remission (32). However, data from both the NETDC and the Gynecologic Oncology Group (GOG) indicate that these agents do not increase the risk of postmolar trophoblastic disease (33,34). In addition, the contraceptive method does not influence the mean hCG regression time. It appears that **oral contraceptives may be safely prescribed after molar evacuation during the entire interval of hormonal follow-up.**

Gestational Trophoblastic Neoplasia

Nonmetastatic Disease

Locally invasive GTN develops in 15% of patients after evacuation of a complete mole and infrequently after other gestations (11,12). These patients usually present clinically with one or more of the following:

1. **Irregular vaginal bleeding**
2. **Theca lutein cysts**
3. **Uterine subinvolution or asymmetric enlargement**
4. **Persistently elevated serum hCG levels**

The trophoblastic tumor may perforate through the myometrium, causing intraperitoneal bleeding, or erode into uterine vessels, causing vaginal hemorrhage. Bulky, necrotic tumor may involve the uterine wall and serve as a nidus for infection. Patients with uterine sepsis may have a purulent vaginal discharge and acute pelvic pain.

After molar evacuation, persistent GTN may exhibit the histologic features of either hydatidiform mole or choriocarcinoma. After a nonmolar pregnancy, however, persistent GTN always has the histologic pattern of choriocarcinoma. Histologically, choriocarcinoma is characterized by sheets of anaplastic syncytiotrophoblast and cytotrophoblast with no preserved chorionic villous structure.

Placental-Site Trophoblastic Tumor   Placental-site trophoblastic tumor is an uncommon but important variant of GTN that consists predominantly of intermediate trophoblast and a few syncytial elements (35). These tumors produce small amounts of hCG and human placental lactogen relative to their mass, and tend to remain confined to the uterus, metastasizing late in their course. **In contrast to other trophoblastic tumors, placental-site tumors are relatively insensitive to chemotherapy.** High cure rates can be achieved with early diagnosis and surgical resection. Intensive combination chemotherapy may achieve complete remission in patients with metastatic disease, particularly when the interval from the antecedent pregnancy is less than four years (36).

Metastatic Disease and Choriocarcinoma

Metastatic GTN occurs in 4% of patients after evacuation of a complete mole and is infrequent after other pregnancies (11,12). Metastasis is usually associated with choriocarcinoma, although **the precise histology is usually not determined because diagnosis and treatment are based on rising hCG** levels. Approximately one-half of choriocarcinomas occur following a hydatidaform mole and one-half after other pregnancies, including normal ones. Choriocarcinoma has a tendency toward early vascular invasion with widespread dissemination. Because trophoblastic tumors are often perfused by a network of fragile vessels, they are frequently hemorrhagic. Symptoms of metastases may therefore result from spontaneous bleeding at metastatic foci. Sites of metastatic spread are shown in Table 15.5.

Pulmonary   At the time of presentation, 80% of the patients with metastatic GTN show lung involvement on chest radiographs. Patients with pulmonary metastases may have chest pain, cough, hemoptysis, dyspnea, or an asymptomatic lesion on a chest radiograph. Respiratory symptoms may be of acute onset, or they may be protracted over many months.

Gestational trophoblastic neoplasia produces four principal radiographic patterns in the lungs:

1. An alveolar or "snowstorm" pattern
2. Discrete, rounded densities
3. A pleural effusion
4. An embolic pattern caused by pulmonary arterial occlusion

Table 15.5 Relative Incidence of Common Metastatic Sites	
Lungs	80%
Vagina	30%
Pelvis	20%
Brain	10%
Liver	10%
Bowel, kidney, spleen	<5%
Other	<5%
Undetermined[a]	<5%

[a]Persistent human chorionic gonadotropin titer after hysterectomy.

Reproduced from **Berkowitz RS, Goldstein DP.** Pathogenesis of gestational trophoblastic neoplasms. *Pathobiol Annual* 1981;11:391, with permission.

Because respiratory symptoms and radiographic findings may be dramatic, the patient may be thought to have primary pulmonary disease. Some patients with extensive pulmonary involvement have minimal or no gynecologic symptoms and the diagnosis of GTN may be confirmed only after thoracotomy has been performed. This occurs particularly in patients with a nonmolar antecedent pregnancy.

Pulmonary hypertension may develop in patients with GTN secondary to pulmonary arterial occlusion by trophoblastic emboli. Although patients with pulmonary hypertension may be very symptomatic, the chest film may reveal only minimal changes.

Vaginal   Vaginal metastases are **present in 30% of patients with metastatic tumor**. These lesions are usually highly vascular and may appear reddened or violaceous. They can bleed vigorously if sampled for biopsy, so attempts at histologic confirmation of the diagnosis should be resisted. Metastases to the vagina may occur in the fornices or suburethrally and may produce irregular bleeding or a purulent discharge.

Hepatic   Liver metastases **occur in 10% of patients with disseminated trophoblastic tumor**. Hepatic involvement is encountered almost exclusively in patients with protracted delays in diagnosis and extensive tumor burdens. Epigastric or right upper quadrant pain may develop if metastases stretch Glisson's capsule. Hepatic lesions are hemorrhagic and friable and may rupture, causing exsanguinating intraperitoneal bleeding.

Central Nervous System   **Ten percent of metastatic trophoblastic disease involves the brain.** Virtually all patients with brain metastases have concurrent pulmonary and/or vaginal involvement. Because cerebral lesions may undergo spontaneous hemorrhage, patients may have acute focal neurologic deficits.

Staging

The current staging system for GTN (2000) combines both anatomic staging and a prognostic scoring system (Tables 15.6, 15.7). It is hoped that this staging system will encourage the objective comparison of data among various centers.

Table 15.6 Staging of Gestational Trophoblastic Neoplasia	
Stage I	Disease confined to uterine corpus
Stage II	GTN extends outside of uterus, but is limited to the genital structures (adnexa, vagina, broad ligament)
Stage III	GTN extends to the lungs, with or without known genital tract involvement
Stage IV	All other metastatic sites

FIGO, International Federation of Obstetrics and Gynecology. **FIGO Annual Report,** *Int J Gynecol Obstet* **2006;95:S29, and** *Int J Gynecol Obstet* **2009;105:3–4.**

Table 15.7 Scoring System Based on Prognostic Factors				
	Scores			
	0	1	2	4
Age (yr)	<40	≥40	—	
Antecedent pregnancy	Mole	Abortion	Term	
Interval months from index pregnancy	<4	4–<7	7–<13	≥13
Pretreatment serum hCG (IU/L)	$<10^3$	10^3–$<10^4$	10^4–$<10^5$	$>10^5$
Largest tumor size (including uterus)		3 cm–<5 cm	≥5 cm	
Site of metastases	Lung	Kidney/ Spleen	Gastrointestinal/ Liver	Brain
Number of metastases	—	1–4	5–8	>8
Previous failed chemotherapy	—	—	Single drug	2 or more drugs

Format for reporting to FIGO Annual Report: In order to stage and allot a risk factor score, a patient's diagnosis is allocated to a stage as represented by a Roman numeral I, II, III, and IV. This is then separated by a colon from the sum of all the actual risk factor scores expressed in Arabic numerals e.g., stage 11:4, stage IV:9. This stage and score will be allotted for each patient.

Stage I includes all patients with persistently elevated hCG levels and tumor confined to the uterine corpus.

Stage II comprises all patients with metastases to the vagina and/or pelvis.

Stage III includes all patients with pulmonary metastases with or without uterine, vaginal, or pelvic involvement. The diagnosis is based on a rising hCG level in the presence of pulmonary lesions on a chest film.

Stage IV patients have far advanced disease with involvement of the brain, liver, kidneys, or gastrointestinal tract. These patients are in the highest-risk category because they are most likely to be resistant to chemotherapy. In most cases, their disease follows a nonmolar pregnancy and has the histologic pattern of choriocarcinoma.

Prognostic Scoring System

In addition to anatomic staging, it is important to consider other variables to predict the likelihood of drug resistance and to assist in selection of appropriate chemotherapy. A prognostic scoring system, based on one developed by Bagshawe, reliably predicts the potential for resistance to chemotherapy (3).

When the prognostic score is 7 or more, the patient is categorized as high risk and requires intensive combination chemotherapy to achieve remission. Patients with stage I disease usually have a low-risk score, and those with stage IV disease have a high-risk score, so that the distinction between low and high risk applies mainly to patients with stage II or III disease.

Diagnostic Evaluation

Optimal management of persistent GTN requires a thorough assessment of the extent of the disease before the initiation of treatment. All patients with persistent GTN should undergo a careful pretreatment evaluation, including:

1. A complete **history and physical examination**
2. Measurement of the **serum hCG level**
3. **Hepatic, thyroid, and renal function tests**
4. Determination of baseline peripheral **white blood cell and platelet counts**

The metastatic workup should include:

1. A **chest radiograph** and/or chest computed tomographic (CT) scan
2. An **ultrasonogram or a CT scan of the abdomen and pelvis**
3. A **CT or** magnetic resonance imaging **(MRI) scan of the head**
4. **Selective angiography** of abdominal and pelvic organs, if indicated
5. **Whole body 18 FDG-PET scan to identify occult disease** (37)

Liver ultrasonography and/or CT scanning document most hepatic metastases in patients with abnormal liver function tests. CT or MRI of the head has facilitated the early diagnosis of asymptomatic cerebral lesions (38). In the absence of lung or vaginal metastasis, the risk of cerebral and hepatic spread is exceedingly low.

In patients with choriocarcinoma and/or metastatic disease, it has been traditional to measure hCG levels in the cerebrospinal fluid (CSF) to exclude cerebral involvement if the CT scan of the brain was negative (39,40). However, in this era of MRI and 18 FDG-PET scans, the need for csf hCG determination is limited.

Stool guaiac tests should also be routinely performed in patients with persistent GTN. If the guaiac test is positive or if the patient reports gastrointestinal symptoms, a complete radiographic evaluation of the gastrointestinal tract should be undertaken.

Pelvic ultrasonography appears to be useful in detecting extensive trophoblastic uterine involvement and may also aid in identifying sites of resistant uterine tumor (41). Because ultrasonography can accurately and noninvasively detect extensive uterine tumor, it may help to select patients who will benefit from hysterectomy. When the uterus contains large amounts of tumor, hysterectomy may substantially reduce the tumor burden and limit the requirement for chemotherapy, as well as eliminate the potential for hemorrhage or infection (42).

Management of Gestational Trophoblastic Neoplasia

Stage 1

The NETDC protocol for the management of stage I disease is presented in Table 15.8. The selection of treatment is based primarily on whether the patient wishes to retain fertility.

Hysterectomy Plus Chemotherapy

If the patient no longer wishes to preserve fertility, hysterectomy with adjuvant single-agent chemotherapy may be performed as primary treatment. Adjuvant chemotherapy is administered for three reasons:

1. To reduce the likelihood of disseminating viable tumor cells at surgery.
2. To maintain a cytotoxic level of chemotherapy in the bloodstream and tissues in case viable tumor cells are disseminated at surgery.
3. To treat any occult metastases that may already be present at the time of surgery. Occult pulmonary metastases may be detected by CT scan in about 40% of patients with presumed nonmetastatic disease (43).

Chemotherapy can be administered safely at the time of hysterectomy without increasing the risk of bleeding or sepsis. At the NETDC, 32 patients with stage I disease have been treated

Table 15.8 Protocol for Treatment of Stage I Gestational Trophoblastic Neoplasia	
Initial	*MTX-FA;* if resistant, switch to *Act-D* or hysterectomy with adjuvant chemotherapy
Resistant	Combination chemotherapy or hysterectomy with adjuvant chemotherapy; local uterine resection; pelvic intraarterial infusion
Follow-up hCG	Weekly until normal for 3 wks, then monthly until normal for 12 mos
Contraception	12 consecutive mos of normal hCG values

MTX, methotrexate; FA, folinic acid; Act-D, actinomycin D; hCG, human chorionic gonadotropin.

Modified from **Goldstein DP, Berkowitz RS, eds.** *Gestational trophoblastic neoplasms: clinical principles of diagnosis and management.* Philadelphia: WB Saunders, 1982:1–301, with permission.

with primary hysterectomy and a single course of adjuvant chemotherapy, and all have achieved complete remission with no additional therapy.

Hysterectomy is also performed in all patients with a placental-site trophoblastic tumor. Because placental-site tumors are relatively resistant to chemotherapy, hysterectomy for nonmetastatic disease is most prudent.

Chemotherapy Alone

Single-agent chemotherapy is the preferred treatment in patients with stage I disease who desire to retain fertility. Between July 1965 and June 2006, 502 patients were treated with primary single-agent chemotherapy at the NETDC. Of these patients, 419 **(83.4%) achieved complete remission with sequential *MTX/Act-D*.** The remaining 83 (16.6%) with *MTX/Act-D* resistant disease subsequently attained remission after combination chemotherapy or surgical intervention.

When patients are resistant to single-agent chemotherapy and wish to preserve fertility, combination chemotherapy should be administered. **If the patient is resistant to both single-agent and combination chemotherapy and wants to retain fertility, local uterine resection may be considered.** When local resection is planned, a preoperative ultrasonogram, MRI, arteriogram, or/and PET scan may help to define the site of the resistant tumor.

Follow-up

All patients with stage I lesions should be followed with:

1. **Weekly hCG levels until they are normal for 3 consecutive weeks**
2. **Monthly hCG levels until levels are normal for 12 consecutive months**
3. **Effective contraception** during the entire period of hormonal follow-up

Stages II and III

Low-risk patients are treated with primary single-agent chemotherapy, and high-risk patients are managed with primary intensive combination chemotherapy. A protocol for the management of patients with stage II and III disease is presented in Table 15.9.

All twenty-eight patients with stage II disease treated at the NETDC between July 1965 and June 2006 achieved remission. Single-agent chemotherapy induced complete remission in 16 (80%) of 20 patients with low-risk GTN. Four patients with resistant disease were cured with combination chemotherapy. In contrast, only two of eight patients with high-risk GTN achieved remission with single-agent treatment, the others requiring combination chemotherapy and local resection.

Table 15.9 Protocol for Treatment of Stages II and III Gestational Trophoblastic

	Neoplasia
Low-risk[a]	
Initial	*MTX-FA;* if resistant, switch to *Act-D*
Resistant to both single agents	Combination chemotherapy
High-risk[a]	
Initial	Combination chemotherapy
Resistant	Second-line combination chemotherapy
Follow-up hCG	Weekly until normal for 3 weeks, then monthly until normal for 12 months
Contraception	Until there have been 12 consecutive months of normal hCG levels

MTX, methotrexate; FA, folinic acid; Act-D, actinomycin D; hCG, human chorionic gonadotropin.

[a]Local resection optional.

Modified from **Goldstein DP, Berkowitz RS, eds.** *Gestational trophoblastic neoplasms: clinical principles of diagnosis and management.* Philadelphia: WB Saunders, 1982:1–301, with permission.

Vaginal Metastases

Vaginal metastases may bleed profusely because they are highly vascular and friable. Yingna et al. reported that 18 (35.3%) of 51 patients with vaginal metastases presented with vaginal hemorrhage (44). When bleeding is substantial, it may be controlled by packing of the hemorrhagic lesion or by wide local excision. Arteriographic embolization of the hypogastric arteries may also be used to control hemorrhage from vaginal metastases.

Pulmonary Metastases

Of 161 patients with stage III disease managed at the NETDC between July 1965 and June 2006, 160 (99.3%) attained complete remission. Gonadotropin remission was induced with single-agent chemotherapy in 90 of 110 (81.7%) patients with low-risk GTN. The remaining twenty patients with low-risk GTN resistant to single agent chemotherapy subsequently achieved remission with combination chemotherapy and/or local pulmonary resection. Fifty of the 51 (98%) stage III patients with high-risk scores treated with primary combination chemotherapy were cured.

Thoracotomy   Thoracotomy has a limited role in the management of stage III disease. However, **if a patient has a persistent viable pulmonary metastasis despite intensive chemotherapy, thoracotomy may be used to excise the resistant focus** (45). A thorough metastatic workup should be performed before surgery to exclude other sites of persistent disease. Fibrotic pulmonary nodules may persist indefinitely on radiographs of the chest, even after complete gonadotropin remission has been attained. In patients undergoing thoracotomy for resistant disease, postoperative chemotherapy should be administered to treat potential occult sites of micrometastases.

Hysterectomy

Hysterectomy may be required in patients with metastatic GTN to control uterine hemorrhage or sepsis. Furthermore, in patients with extensive uterine tumor, hysterectomy may substantially reduce the trophoblastic tumor burden and thereby limit the need for multiple courses of chemotherapy.

Follow-up

Follow-up monitoring for patients with stage II and III disease is the same as for patients with stage I disease.

Stage IV

A protocol for the management of stage IV disease is presented in Table 15.10. These patients are at greatest risk for development of rapidly progressive and unresponsive tumors despite intensive multimodal therapy. They should all be referred to centers with special expertise in the management of trophoblastic disease.

Table 15.10 Protocol for Treatment of Stage IV Gestational Trophoblastic Neoplasia	
Initial	Combination chemotherapy
Brain	Whole-head irradiation (3,000 cGy) Craniotomy to manage complications
Liver	Resection to manage complications
Resistant[a]	Second-line combination chemotherapy Hepatic arterial infusion
Follow-up hCG	Weekly until normal for 3 weeks, then monthly until normal for 24 months
Contraception	Until there have been 24 consecutive months of normal hCG levels

hCG, human chorionic gonadotropin.

[a]Local resection optional.

Modified from **Goldstein DP, Berkowitz RS, eds.** *Gestational trophoblastic neoplasms: clinical principles of diagnosis and management.* Philadelphia: WB Saunders, 1982:1–301, with permission.

All patients with stage IV disease should be treated with primary intensive combination chemotherapy and the selective use of radiation therapy and surgery. Before 1975, only 6 of 20 patients (30%) with stage IV disease treated at the NETDC attained complete remission. Since 1975, however, 17 of 21 patients (80.9%) with stage IV tumors have achieved gonadotropin remission. This improvement in survival has resulted from the use of primary combination chemotherapy in conjunction with radiation and surgical treatment.

Hepatic Metastases

The management of hepatic metastases is particularly challenging and problematic. If a patient is resistant to systemic chemotherapy, hepatic arterial infusion of chemotherapy may induce complete remission in selected cases. Hepatic resection may also be required to control acute bleeding or to excise a focus of resistant tumor.

Cerebral Metastases

If cerebral metastases are diagnosed, whole-brain irradiation (3,000 cGy in ten fractions) should be instituted promptly. Alternatively, localized external beam radiation may be given. Yordan and colleagues reported that deaths as a result of cerebral involvement occurred in 11 of 25 patients (44%) treated with chemotherapy alone, but in none of 18 patients treated with brain irradiation and chemotherapy (46). **The risk of spontaneous cerebral hemorrhage may be lessened by the concurrent use of combination chemotherapy and brain irradiation** because irradiation may be both hemostatic and tumoricidal.

Craniotomy   Craniotomy may be required to provide acute decompression or to control bleeding and should be performed to manage life-threatening complications in the hope that the patient ultimately will be cured with chemotherapy. **Infrequently, cerebral metastases that are resistant to chemotherapy may be amenable to local resection.** Fortunately, most patients with cerebral metastases who achieve sustained remission generally have no residual neurologic deficits (47).

Salvage Therapy for Drug Resistance

Despite the effectiveness of well-recognized regimens, there is a need to identify new agents that have the potential to treat resistant GTN. Although *ifosfamide* and *paclitaxel* have been used successfully, further studies are needed to define their potential role as either first or second-line therapy (48,49). Osborne et al. reported that a novel three-drug doublet regimen consisting of *paclitaxel, etoposide* and *cisplatin* (TE/TO) induced complete remission in two patients with relapsed high risk GTN (50). Wan et al. demonstrated the efficacy of *floxuridine (FUDR)-containing regimens* in drug resistant patients (51). Matsui et al. found that *5FU* in combination with *actinomycin D* could also be used effectively as salvage therapy (52).

There have been individual case reports of successful high-dose chemotherapy with autologous bone marrow or stem cell support in patients with otherwise refractory GTN (53,54).

Follow-up

Patients with stage IV disease should be followed with:

1. Weekly hCG levels until they are normal for 3 consecutive weeks
2. Monthly hCG levels until they are normal for 24 consecutive months
3. Effective contraception during the interval of hormonal follow-up

These patients require prolonged gonadotropin follow-up because they are at increased risk of late recurrence.

An algorithm for the management of GTN is presented in Fig. 15.2.

Many hCG assays have some cross-reactivity with luteinizing hormone. Following multiple courses of combination chemotherapy, ovarian steroidal function may be damaged, leading to rising luteinizing hormone levels. **Patients who receive combination chemotherapy should therefore be placed on oral contraceptives to suppress luteinizing hormone levels and prevent problems with cross-reactivity.**

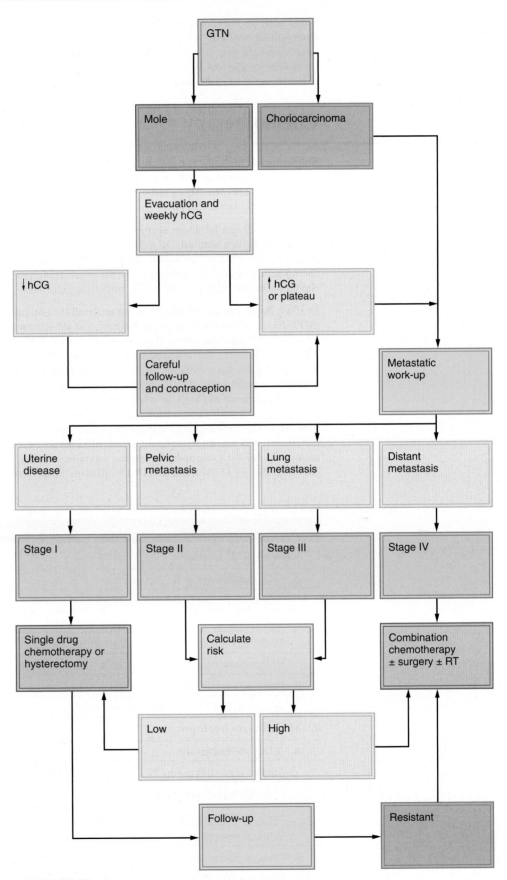

Figure 15.2 **Management of gestational trophoblastic neoplasia.** GTN, gestational trophoblastic neoplasia; hCG, human chorionic gonadotropin; RT, radiation therapy.

Some patients may have a false-positive elevation in serum hCG values due to circulating heterophilic antibody (55). Patients with phantom choriocarcinoma or phantom hCG often have no progressive rise in their hCG levels and no clear antecedent pregnancy. The possibility of false-positive hCG levels should be evaluated by sending both urine and serum samples to a reference hCG laboratory.

Chemotherapy

Single-Agent Chemotherapy

Single-agent chemotherapy with either *actinomycin D (Act-D)* or *methotrexate (MTX)* has achieved comparable and excellent remission rates in both nonmetastatic and low-risk metastatic GTN (56). There are several protocols available for the treatment of patients with *MTX* or *Act-D* (Table 15.11).

Actinomycin D can be given every other week in a 5-day regimen or in a pulse fashion, and *MTX* can be given similarly in a 5-day regimen or weekly in a pulse fashion. No study has compared all of these protocols with regard to success and morbidity. The selection of chemotherapy should be influenced by the associated systemic toxicity. An optimal regimen should maximize response rate while minimizing morbidity.

In 1964, Bagshawe and Wilde (57) first reported the administration of *MTX* with *folinic acid (MTX-FA)* in GTN to limit systemic toxicity, and subsequently it has been confirmed that *MTX-FA* is both effective and safe in the management of GTN (58) (Table 15.12). *Methotrexate* with *folinic acid* has been the preferred single-agent regimen in the treatment of GTN at the NETDC since 1974 (58). An evaluation of 185 patients treated in this manner revealed that complete remission was achieved in 162 patients (87.6%), and 132 of the 162 patients (81.5%) required only one course of *MTX-FA* to attain remission. **MTX-FA induced remission in 147 of 163 patients (90.2%) with stage I GTN and in 15 of 22 patients (68.2%) with low-risk stages II and III GTN**. Resistance to therapy was more common in patients with choriocarcinoma, metastases, and when pretreatment serum hCG levels exceeded 50,000 mIU/mL. After treatment with *MTX-FA*, thrombocytopenia, granulocytopenia, and hepatotoxicity developed in only 3 (1.6%), 11 (5.9%), and 26 (14.1%) patients, respectively. *MTX-FA* therefore achieved an

Table 15.11 Single-Drug Treatment
I. *Actinomycin D* treatment
A. 5-Day *actinomycin D*
Actinomycin D 12 µg/kg IV daily for 5 d
CBC, platelet count, aspartate aminotransferase daily
With response, retreat at the same dose
Without response, add 2 µg/kg to the initial dose or switch to *methotrexate* protocol
B. Pulse *actinomycin D*
Actinomycin D 1.25 mg/m^2 every 2 wk
II. *Methotrexate* treatment
A. 5-Day *methotrexate*
Methotrexate 0.4 mg/kg IV or IM daily for 5 d
CBC, platelet count daily
With response, retreat at the same dose
Without response, increase dose to 0.6 mg/kg or switch to *actinomycin D* protocol
B. Pulse *methotrexate*
Methotrexate 40 mg/m^2 IM weekly

CBC, complete blood count; IV, intravenous; IM, intramuscular.

Table 15.12 Protocol for Therapy with *Methotrexate* and Folinic Acid "Rescue"		
Day	**Time**	**Follow-up Tests and Therapy**
1	8 a.m.	CBC, platelet count, AST
	4 p.m.	*Methotrexate*, 1.0 mg/kg
2	4 p.m.	*Folinic acid*, 0.1 mg/kg
3	8 a.m.	CBC, platelet count, AST
	4 p.m.	*Methotrexate*, 1.0 mg/kg
4	4 p.m.	*Folinic acid*, 0.1 mg/kg
5	8 a.m.	CBC, platelet count, AST
	4 p.m.	*Methotrexate*, 1.0 mg/kg
6	4 p.m.	*Folinic acid*, 0.1 mg/kg
7	8 a.m.	CBC, platelet count, AST
	4 p.m.	*Methotrexate*, 1.0 mg/kg
8	4 p.m.	*Folinic acid*, 0.1 mg/kg

CBC, complete blood count; AST, aspartate aminotransferase.

Reproduced from **Berkowitz RS, Goldstein DP, Bernstein MR.** Ten years' experience with *methotrexate* and folinic acid as primary therapy for gestational trophoblastic disease. *Gynecol Oncol* 1986;23:111, with permission.

excellent therapeutic outcome with minimal toxicity and attained this goal with limited exposure to chemotherapy.

Administration of Single-Agent Treatment

The serum hCG level is measured weekly after each course of chemotherapy, and the hCG regression curve serves as the primary basis for determining the need for additional treatment.

After the first treatment:

1. Further chemotherapy is withheld as long as the hCG level is falling progressively.
2. Additional single-agent chemotherapy is not administered at any predetermined or fixed time interval.

A second course of chemotherapy is administered under the following conditions:

1. **If the hCG levels plateau** for more than 3 consecutive weeks or begin to rise again
2. **If the hCG level does not decline by 1 log within 18 days after completion of the first treatment**

If a second course of *MTX-FA* is required, the dosage of *MTX* is unaltered if the patient's response to the first treatment was adequate. **An adequate response is defined as a fall in the hCG level by 1 log after a course of chemotherapy.** If the response to the first treatment is inadequate, the dosage of *MTX* is increased from 1.0 to 1.5 mg/kg/day for each of the 4 treatment days. **If the response to two consecutive courses of *MTX-FA* is inadequate, the patient is considered to be resistant to *MTX*, and *Act-D* is promptly substituted in patients with nonmetastatic and low-risk metastatic GTN.** If the hCG values do not decline by 1 log after treatment with *Act-D*, the patient is also considered resistant to *Act-D* as a single agent. She must then be treated intensively with combination chemotherapy to achieve remission.

Combination Chemotherapy

MAC III

In the past, the preferred combination drug regimen at the NETDC was MAC III (triple therapy), which included *MTX-FA*, *Act-D*, and *cyclophosphamide (Cytoxan, CTX)* (59). However, triple therapy proved to be inadequate as an initial treatment in patients with metastases and a high-risk prognostic score. Data from the GOG, M. D. Anderson Hospital, and the NETDC indicated that triple therapy induced remission in only 21 (49%) of 43 patients with metastases and a high-risk score (score 7 or >) (60–62).

Table 15.13 EMA-CO Regimen for Patients With Gestational Trophoblastic Neoplasia
Regimen

Course 1 (EMA)

Day 1	VP-16 (etoposide), 100 mg/m², IV infusion in 200 mL of saline over 30 min
	Actinomycin D, 0.5 mg, IV push
	Methotrexate, 100 mg/m², IV push, followed by a 200 mg/m² IV infusion over 12 hr
Day 2	VP-16 (etoposide), 100 mg/m², IV infusion in 200 mL of saline over 30 min
	Actinomycin D, 0.5 mg, IV push
	Folinic acid, 15 mg, IM or orally every 12 hr for 4 doses beginning 24 hr after start of methotrexate

Course 2 (CO)

Day 8	Vincristine, 1.0 mg/m², IV push
	Cyclophosphamide, 600 mg/m², IV in saline

IV, intravenous; IM, intramuscular.

This regimen consists of two courses: (a) course 1 is given on days 1 and 2; (b) course 2 is given on day 8. Course 1 might require overnight hospital stay; course 2 does not. These courses can usually be given on days 1 and 2, 8, 15, and 16, 22, etc., and the intervals should not be extended without cause.

Reproduced from **Bagshawe KD.** Treatment of high-risk choriocarcinoma. *J Reprod Med* 1984;29:813, with permission.

EMA-CO

Etoposide was reported to induce complete remission in 56 (93%) of 60 patients with nonmetastatic and low-risk metastatic GTN (63). In 1984, Bagshawe (64) first described a new combination regimen that included *etoposide, MTX, Act-D, Cytoxan,* and *vincristine* (EMA-CO; Table 15.13), and reported an 83% remission in patients with metastases and a high-risk score. Bolis et al. confirmed that primary EMA-CO induced complete remission in 76% of the patients with metastatic GTN and a high-risk score (65). Bower et al. updated the data from Charing Cross Hospital and reported that EMA-CO induced complete remission in 130 of 151 patients (86.1%) with high-risk metastatic GTN (66). Furthermore, Newlands et al. reported remission using EMA-CO with intrathecal *MTX* in 30 of 35 patients (86%) with brain metastases (67).

The EMA-CO regimen is usually well tolerated, and treatment seldom has to be suspended because of toxicity, particularly with the judicious use of marrow stimulants. It is now the preferred primary treatment in patients with metastases and a high-risk prognostic score. If patients become resistant to EMA-CO, remission may still be achieved by substituting *etoposide* and *cisplatin* for *cyclophosphamide* and *vincristine* on day 8 (66). The optimal combination drug protocol will most likely include *etoposide, MTX,* and *Act-D* and perhaps other agents, administered in the most dose-intensive manner. *Vinblastine, bleomycin,* and *cisplatin* also effectively induced remission in four of seven patients who were resistant to triple therapy (68). Other regimens that have exhibited activity in patients with resistant GTN include the three-drug doublet regimen consisting of *paclitaxel, etoposide* and *cisplatin* (TE/TO) (50), *floxuridine (FUDR)*-containing regimens (51), and *5FU/Act-D* (52), as well as autologous marrow transplantation or stem cell rescue (53,54).

Duration of Therapy

Patients who require combination chemotherapy must be treated intensively to attain remission. Combination chemotherapy should be given as often as toxicity permits until the patient achieves three consecutive normal hCG levels. **After normal hCG levels are attained, at least two additional courses of chemotherapy are undertaken as consolidation therapy to reduce the risk of relapse.**

Secondary Tumors

Investigators have reported an increased risk of secondary tumors, including leukemia, colon cancer, melanoma, and breast cancer, in patients treated with chemotherapy for gestational trophoblastic tumors (69). **The increased risk of secondary tumors has been attributed to** the inclusion of *etoposide* in combination chemotherapy. The increased incidence of colon cancer, melanoma, and breast cancer was not apparent until more than 5, 10, and 25 years after therapy, respectively, and was limited to those patients who received a total dose of at least 2 gm/M2.

Subsequent Pregnancies

Pregnancies After Hydatidiform Mole

Patients with hydatidiform moles can anticipate normal reproduction in the future (70). From July 1, 1965 to December 31, 2007, patients who were treated at the NETDC for complete molar gestation had 1,337 subsequent pregnancies that resulted in 912 full-term live births (68.1%); 101 premature deliveries (7.6%); 11 ectopic pregnancies (0.9%); 7 stillbirths (0.5%); and 20 repeat molar pregnancies (1.5%). First- and second-trimester spontaneous abortions occurred in 245 pregnancies (18.3%). There were 41 therapeutic abortions (3.1%). Major and minor congenital malformations were detected in 40 of 1,020 infants (3.9%). Primary cesarean section was performed in 81 of 414 (19.6%) term or premature births from 1979 to 2007. **Therefore, patients with a complete molar pregnancy should be reassured that they are at no increased risk of prenatal or intrapartum obstetric complications in later pregnancies. Although data concerning subsequent pregnancies after a partial mole were available for only 294 pregnancies, the data were similarly reassuring.**

When a patient has had a hydatidiform mole, she is at increased risk of molar pregnancy in subsequent conceptions. **Approximately 1 in 100 patients has at least two molar gestations.** Some patients with repetitive molar pregnancies have a molar pregnancy with different male partners (71). Later molar pregnancies are characterized by worsening histologic type and increased risk of postmolar GTN. **After two episodes of molar pregnancy, patients may still achieve a normal full-term gestation in a later pregnancy.**

Therefore, for any subsequent pregnancy, the patient should have:

1. **A pelvic ultrasonogram during the first trimester** to confirm normal gestational development

2. **An hCG measurement 6 weeks post-partum** to exclude occult trophoblastic neoplasia

Pregnancies After Persistent Gestational Trophoblastic Neoplasia

Patients with GTN who are treated successfully with chemotherapy can expect normal reproduction in the future (70). Patients who were treated with chemotherapy at the NETDC from 1965 to 2007 reported 631 subsequent pregnancies that resulted in 422 term live births (66.9%); 42 premature deliveries (6.7%); 7 ectopic pregnancies (1.1%); 9 stillbirths (1.4%); and 9 repeat molar pregnancies (1.4%). First- and second-trimester spontaneous abortions occurred in 132 pregnancies (22.4%). There were 28 therapeutic abortions (4.4%). Major and minor congenital anomalies were detected in only 10 of 473 infants (2.1%). Primary cesarean section was performed in 81of 371 (21.8%) subsequent term and premature births from 1979 to 2007. **It is particularly reassuring that the frequency of congenital malformations was not increased,** although chemotherapeutic agents are known to have teratogenic and mutagenic potential.

References

1. **Berkowitz RS, Goldstein DP.** Chorionic tumors. *N Engl J Med* 1996;335:1740–1748.
2. **Goldstein DP, Berkowitz RS.** *Gestational trophoblastic neoplasms: clinical principles of diagnosis and management.* Philadelphia: WB Saunders, 1982:1–301.
3. **Bagshawe KD.** Risk and prognostic factors in trophoblastic neoplasia. *Cancer* 1976;38:1373–1385.
4. **Kajii T, Ohama K.** Androgenetic origin of hydatidiform mole. *Nature* 1977;268:633–634.
5. **Yamashita K, Wake N, Araki T, Ichinoe K, Makoto K.** Human lymphocyte antigen expression in hydatidiform mole: androgenesis following fertilization by a haploid sperm. *Am J Obstet Gynecol* 1979;135:597–600.
6. **Pattillo RA, Sasaki S, Katayama KP, Roesler M, Mattingly RF.** Genesis of 46,XY hydatidiform mole. *Am J Obstet Gynecol* 1981;141:104–105.
7. **Szulman AE, Surti U.** The syndromes of hydatidiform mole: I. cytogenetic and morphologic correlations. *Am J Obstet Gynecol* 1978;131:665–671.
8. **Lawler SD, Fisher RA, Dent J.** A prospective genetic study of complete and partial hydatidiform moles. *Am J Obstet Gynecol* 1991;164:1270–1277.
9. **Genest DR, Ruiz RE, Weremowicz S, Berkowitz RS, Goldstein DP, Dorfman DM.** Do nontriploid partial hydatidiform moles exist? *J Reprod Med* 2002;47:363–368.

10. **Berkowitz RS, Goldstein DP, Bernstein MR.** Natural history of partial molar pregnancy. *Obstet Gynecol* 1985;66:677–681.

11. **Berkowitz RS, Goldstein DP.** Presentation and management of molar pregnancy. In: **Hancock BW, Newlands ES, Berkowitz RS, eds.** *Gestational trophoblastic disease.* London: Chapman and Hall, 1997:127–142.

12. **Goldstein DP, Berkowitz RS.** Current management of complete and partial molar pregnancy. *J Reprod Med* 1994;39:139–146.

13. **Galton VA, Ingbar SH, Jimenez-Fonseca J, Hershman JM.** Alterations in thyroid hormone economy in patients with hydatidiform mole. *J Clin Invest* 1971;50:1345–1354.

14. **Amir SM, Osathanondh R, Berkowitz RS, Goldstein DP.** Human chorionic gonadotropin and thyroid function in patients with hydatidiform mole. *Am J Obstet Gynecol* 1984;150:723–728.

15. **Osathanondh R, Berkowitz RS, de Cholnoky C, Smith BS, Goldstein DP, Tyson JE.** Hormonal measurements in patients with theca lutein cysts and gestational trophoblastic disease. *J Reprod Med* 1986;31:179–183.

16. **Berkowitz RS, Goldstein DP, Bernstein MR.** Laparoscopy in the management of gestational trophoblastic neoplasms. *J Reprod Med* 1980;24:261–264.

17. **Soto-Wright V, Bernstein M, Goldstein D, Berkowitz RS.** The changing clinical presentation of complete molar pregnancy. *Obstet Gynecol* 1995;86:775–779.

18. **Mosher R, Goldstein DP, Berkowitz RS, Bernstein M, Genest DR.** Complete hydatidiform mole—comparison of clinicopathologic features, current and past. *J Reprod Med* 1998;43:21–27.

19. **Thaker HM, Berlin A, Tycko B, et al.** Immunochemistry for the imprinted gene product IPL/PHLDA2 for facilitating the differential diagnosis of complete hydatidiform mole. *J Reprod Med* 2004;49:630–636.

20. **Fisher R, Nucci MR, Thaker HM, et al.** Complete hydatidiform mole retaining a chromosome 11 of maternal origin: analysis of a case. *Mod Pathol* 2004;17:1155–1158.

21. **Szulman AE, Surti U.** The clinicopathologic profile of the partial hydatidiform mole. *Obstet Gynecol* 1982;59:597–602.

22. **Tsukamoto N, Iwasaka T, Kashimura Y, Uchino H, Kashimura M, Matsuyama T.** Gestational trophoblastic disease in women aged 50 or more. *Gynecol Oncol* 1985;20:53–61.

23. **Feltmate CM, Growdon WB, Wolfberg AJ, Goldstein DP, Genest DR, Chichilla ME, et al.** Clinical characteristics of persistent gestational trophoblastic neoplasia after partial hydatidiform molar pregnancy. *J Reprod Med* 2006;51:902–906.

24. **Benson CB, Genest DR, Bernstein MR, Soto-Wright V, Goldstein DP, Berkowitz RS.** Sonographic appearance of first trimester complete hydatidiform moles. *Ultrasound Obstet Gynecol* 2000;16:188–191.

25. **Fine C, Bundy AL, Berkowitz RS, Boswell SB, Beregin AF, Doubilet PM.** Sonographic diagnosis of partial hydatidiform mole. *Obstet Gynecol* 1989;73:414–418.

26. **Goldstein DP, Berkowitz RS.** Prophylactic chemotherapy of complete molar pregnancy. *Semin Oncol* 1995;22:157–160.

27. **Kim DS, Moon H, Kim KT, Moon YJ, Hwang YY.** Effects of prophylactic chemotherapy for persistent trophoblastic disease in patients with complete hydatidiform mole. *Obstet Gynecol* 1986;67:690–694.

28. **Limpongsanurak S.** Prophylactic *actinomycin D* for high-risk complete hydatidiform mole. *J Reprod Med* 2001;46:110–116.

29. **Feltmate CM, Batorfi J, Fulop V, Goldstein DP, Doszpod J, Berkowitz RS.** Human chorionic gonadotropin follow-up in patients with molar pregnancy: a time for reevaluation. *Obstet Gynecol* 2003;101:732–736.

30. **Wolfberg AJ, Feltmate C, Goldstein DP, Berkowitz RS, Lieberman E.** Low risk of relapse after achieving undetectable hCG levels in women with complete molar pregnancy. *Obstet Gynecol* 2004;104:551–554.

31. **Growdon WB, Wolfberg AJ, Feltmate CM, Goldstein DP, Genest DR, Chinchilla ME, et al.** Postevacuation hCG levels and risk of gestational trophoblastic neoplasia among women with partial molar pregnancies. *J Reprod Med* 2006;51:871–874.

32. **Stone M, Dent J, Kardana A, Bagshawe KD.** Relationship of oral contraception to development of trophoblastic tumor after evacuation of a hydatidiform mole. *BJOG* 1976;83:913–916.

33. **Berkowitz RS, Goldstein DP, Marean AR, Bernstein M.** Oral contraceptives and postmolar trophoblastic disease. *Obstet Gynecol* 1981;58:474–477.

34. **Curry SL, Schlaerth JB, Kohorn EI, Boyce JB, Gore H, Twiggs LB, et al.** Hormonal contraception and trophoblastic sequelae after hydatidiform mole (a Gynecologic Oncology Group study). *Am J Obstet Gynecol* 1989;160:805–811.

35. **Feltmate CM, Genest DR, Wise L, Bernstein MR, Goldstein DP, Berkowitz RS.** Placental site trophoblastic tumor: a 17-year experience at the New England Trophoblastic Disease Center. *Gynecol Oncol* 2001;82:415–419.

36. **Papadopoulos AJ, Foskett M, Seckl MJ, McNeish I, Paradinas FJ, Rees H, et al.** Twenty-five years' clinical experience with placental site trophoblastic tumors. *J Reprod Med* 2002;47:460–464.

37. **Dhillon T, Palmieri C, Sebirre NJ, et al.** Value of whole body 18 FDG_PET to identify the active site of gestational trophoblastric neoplasia. *J Reprod Med* 2006;51:879–883.

38. **Athanassiou A, Begent RH, Newlands ES, Parker D, Rustin GJ, Bagshawe KD.** Central nervous system metastases of choriocarcinoma: 23 years' experience at Charing Cross Hospital. *Cancer* 1983;52:1728–1735.

39. **Bagshawe KD, Harland S.** Immunodiagnosis and monitoring of gonadotropin-producing metastases in the central nervous system. *Cancer* 1976;38:112–118.

40. **Bakri YN, Al-Hawashim N, Berkowitz RS.** Cerebrospinal fluid/serum beta-subunit human chorionic gonadotropin ratio in patients with brain metastases of gestational trophoblastic tumor. *J Reprod Med* 2000;45:94–96.

41. **Berkowitz RS, Birnholz J, Goldstein DP, Bernstein MR.** Pelvic ultrasonography and the management of gestational trophoblastic disease. *Gynecol Oncol* 1983;15:403–412.

42. **Soper JT.** Surgical therapy for gestational trophoblastic disease. *J Reprod Med* 1994;39:168–174.

43. **Garner EIO, Garrett A, Goldstein DP, Berkowitz RS.** Significance of chest computed tomography findings in the evaluation and treatment of persistent gestational trophoblastic neoplasms. *J Reprod Med* 2004;49:422–427.

44. **Yingna S, Yang X, Xiuyu Y, Hongzhao S.** Clinical characteristics and treatment of gestational trophoblastic tumor with vaginal metastasis. *Gynecol Oncol* 2002;84:416–419.

45. **Fleming EI, Garrett LA, Growdon WB, Callahan M, Nevadunsky N, Ghosh S, et al.** The changing role of thoracotomy in gestational trophoblastic neoplasia at the New England Trophoblastic Disease Center. *J Reprod Med* 2008;53:493–498.

46. **Yordan EL Jr, Schlaerth J, Gaddis O, Morrow CP.** Radiation therapy in the management of gestational choriocarcinoma metastatic to the central nervous system. *Obstet Gynecol* 1987;69:627–630.

47. **Newlands ES, Holden L, Seckl MJ, McNeish I, Strickland S, Rustin GJS.** Management of brain metastases in patients with high-risk gestational trophoblastic tumors. *J Reprod Med* 2002;47:465–471.

48. **Jones WB, Schneider JT, Blessing JA, Lewis JL Jr.** Treatment of resistant gestational choriocarcinoma with Taxol; report of two cases. *Gynecol Oncol* 1996;61:126–129.

49. **Sutton GP, Soper JT. Blessing JA, et al.** Ifosfamide alone and in combination in the treatment of refractory malignant gestational trophoblastric disease. *Am J Obstet Gynecol* 1992;167:489–493.

50. **Osborne R, Covens AS, Mechandani DE, Gerulath AS.** Successful salvage of relapsed high-risk gestational trophoblastic neoplasia patients using a novel *paclitaxel*-containing doublet. *J Reprod Med* 2004;49:655–659.

51. **Wan X, Yang Y, Wu Y, et al.** Floxuridine-containing regimens in the treatment of gestational trophoblastic tumor. *J Reprod Med* 2004;49:453–457.

52. **Matsui H, Itsuka Y, Suzuka K, et al.** Salvage chemotherapy for high-risk gestational trophoblastic tumor. *J Reprod Med* 2004;49:438–441.

53. **Giacalone PL, Benos P, Donnadio DF, Laffargue F.** High-dose chemotherapy with autologous bone marrow transplanation for refractory metastatic gestational trophoblastic disease. *Gynecol Oncol* 1995;58:383–387.

54. **Van Besien K, Vershcragen C, Mehra R, et al.** Complete remission of refractory gestational trophoblastic disease with brain metastases treated with multicycle ifosfamide, *carboplatin* and *etoposide* (ICE) and stem cell rescue. *Gynecol Oncol* 1997;67:366–370.

55. **Cole LA, Butler S.** Detection of hCG in trophoblastic disease: the USA hCG Reference Service Experience. *J Reprod Med* 2002;47:433–444.

56. **Garrett AP, Garner EO, Goldstein DP, Berkowitz RS.** *Methotrexate* infusion and folinic acid as primary therapy for nonmetastatic and low-risk metastatic gestational trophoblastic tumors: 15 years of experience. *J Reprod Med* 2002;47:355–362.

57. **Bagshawe KD, Wilde C.** Infusion therapy for pelvic trophoblastic tumors. *J Obstet Gynaecol Br Commonw* 1964;71:565–570.

58. **Berkowitz RS, Goldstein DP, Bernstein MR.** Ten years' experience with *methotrexate* and folinic acid as primary therapy for gestational trophoblastic disease. *Gynecol Oncol* 1986;23:111–118.

59. **Berkowitz RS, Goldstein DP, Bernstein MR.** Modified triple chemotherapy in the management of high-risk metastatic gestational trophoblastic tumors. *Gynecol Oncol* 1984;19:173–181.

60. **Curry SL, Blessing JA, DiSaia PJ, Soper JT, Twiggs LB.** A prospective randomized comparison of *methotrexate,* dactinomycin and *chlorambucil* versus *methotrexate, dactinomycin, cyclophosphamide, doxorubicin, melphalan, hydroxyurea* and *vincristine* in "poor prognosis" metastatic gestational trophoblastic disease: a Gynecologic Group study. *Obstet Gynecol* 1989;73:357–362.

61. **Gordon AN, Gershenson DM, Copeland LJ, Stringer CA, Morris M, Wharton JT.** High-risk metastatic gestational trophoblastic disease: further stratification into two clinical entities. *Gynecol Oncol* 1989;34:54–56.

62. **DuBeshter B, Berkowitz RS, Goldstein DP, Cramer DW, Bernstein MR.** Metastatic gestational trophoblastic disease: experience at the New England Trophoblastic Disease Center, 1965 to 1985. *Obstet Gynecol* 1987;69:390–395.

63. **Wong LC, Choo YC, Ma HK.** Primary oral *etoposide* therapy in gestational trophoblastic disease: an update. *Cancer* 1986;58:14–17.

64. **Bagshawe KD.** Treatment of high-risk choriocarcinoma. *J Reprod Med* 1984;29:813–820.

65. **Bolis G, Bonazzi C, Landoni F, Mangili G, Vergadoro F, Zanaboni F, et al.** EMA/CO regimen in high-risk gestational trophoblastic tumor (GTT). *Gynecol Oncol* 1988;31:439–444.

66. **Bower M, Newlands ES, Holden L, Short D, Brock C, Rustin GJS, et al.** EMA/CO for high-risk gestational trophoblastic tumors: Results from a cohort of 272 patients. *J Clin Oncol* 1997;15: 2636–2643.

67. **Newlands ES, Bagshawe KD, Begent RH, Rustin GJ, Holden L.** Results with the EMA/CO (*etoposide, methotrexate, actinomycin D, cyclophosphamide, vincristine*) regimen in high risk gestational trophoblastic tumors, 1979 to 1989. *BJOG* 1991;98:550–557.

68. **DuBeshter B, Berkowitz RS, Goldstein DP, Bernstein MR.** *Vinblastine, cisplatin* and *bleomycin* as salvage therapy for refractory high-risk metastatic gestational trophoblastic disease. *J Reprod Med* 1989;34:189–192.

69. **Rustin GJ, Newlands ES, Lutz JM, Holden L, Bagshawe KD, Hiscox JG, et al.** Combination but not single-agent *methotrexate* chemotherapy for gestational trophoblastic tumors increases the incidence of second tumors. *J Clin Oncol* 1996;14:2769–2773.

70. **Garrett LA, Garner EIO, Feltmate CM, Goldstein DP, Berkowitz RS.** Subsequent pregnancy outcomes in patients with molar pregnancy and persistent gestational trophoblastic neoplasia. *J Reprod Med* 2008;53:481–486.

71. **Tuncer ZS, Bernstein MR, Wang J, Goldstein DP, Berkowitz RS.** Repetitive hydatidiform mole with different male partners. *Gynecol Oncol* 1999;75:224–226.

16 Breast Disease

Laura Kruper
Armando E. Giuliano

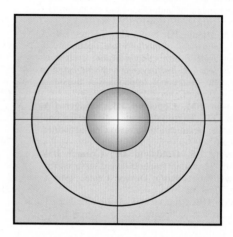

Essential tools for the practicing gynecologist are an understanding of benign and malignant breast diseases, the ability to detect and diagnose breast cancer, and an appreciation of the various treatment options for the breast cancer patient. In this chapter, benign conditions that can masquerade as malignancy, as well as the diagnosis and management of *in situ* and invasive breast cancers, are discussed.

Detection

Physical Examination

Breast malignancies are usually asymptomatic and are discovered only by physical examination or screening mammography. Any physical findings on a routine breast examination must be recorded in the medical record for future reference.

For the breast and nodal examination, the patient should be examined in both the upright and supine positions. Examination should begin with inspection of the breasts with the patient seated comfortably, arms relaxed at her sides. Differences in symmetry or contour of the breasts should be noted, as well as any skin changes such as edema or erythema. Skin dimpling or nipple retraction may become apparent by having the patient raise her arms above her head then press her hands on her hips (Fig. 16.1). Next, the cervical, supraclavicular and axillary areas should be palpated for enlarged nodes. With the patient still seated, each breast is examined by using the nondominant hand to support the breast while palpating with the dominant hand using the flat portion of the fingers rather than the tips. The upper outer quadrant of the breast up to the clavicle, the axillary tail of Spence, and the axilla are palpated for possible masses. The nipples should also be assessed for nipple discharge.

The patient is then asked to lie down and raise one arm over her head while keeping the other arm at her side. The breast examination commences on the side with the raised arm. Once again, the breast is systematically palpated from the clavicle to the costal margin. The manner in which the breast is examined is not as important as consistency and diligence; it is important to choose one method that allows for examination of the entire breast that can be repeated methodically. One technique that many clinicians use is to palpate the breast in enlarging concentric circles. Placement of a pillow or towel beneath the scapula to elevate the side examined is important for women with large, pendulous breasts, which tend to fall laterally, making palpation of the lateral breast challenging.

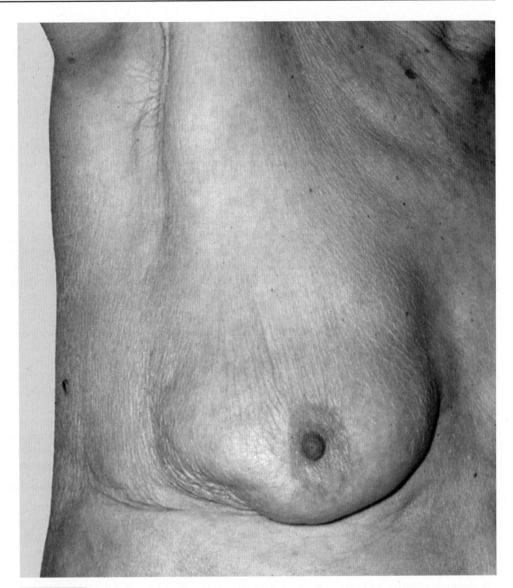

Figure 16.1   Retraction of the skin of the lower, outer quadrant seen only on raising the arm. A small carcinoma was palpable.

The major features in a breast examination to be identified are nodularity, tenderness, and dominant masses. Any abnormalities should be documented by identifying the area of concern as the position on the face of a clock and its distance from the nipple, e.g., a right breast lesion at 10 o'clock, 5 cm from the nipple is located in the upper outer quadrant. Many patients, particularly young, premenopausal women, have nodular breast parenchyma. Nodularity is frequently diffuse although it tends to be more prevalent in the upper outer quadrants where there is more breast tissue. Nodules are small, indistinct, and similar in size. Conversely, **breast cancers tend to present as nontender, firm masses with unclear margins, often feeling distinct from the surrounding nodularity. Malignant masses may also be fixed to the chest wall (underlying fascia) or to the skin.** However, not all breast cancers possess these characteristics so **any dominant mass in the breast requires further evaluation.**

Around the time of menses, many women have increased nodularity and engorgement of the breast, which occasionally obscures an underlying lesion. If a patient presents to the physician with concern about a mass that she has palpated and the physician cannot confirm the patient's finding due to engorgement of the breasts, the examination should be repeated after the patient's menstrual period. Further imaging such as mammography or ultrasonography is also a useful adjunct in cases where the patient has palpated a mass, yet the clinician is unable to confirm the patient's finding.

Breast Self-examination

Although there is no evidence to date that breast self-examination (BSE) leads to a decreased mortality rate by diagnosing breast cancers at an early stage, its utilization is still advocated by many organizations (1,2). It is viewed as a surveillance tool for women to heighten awareness of the normal composition of the breast, as well as to detect changes that may occur. BSE can be useful in detecting interval cancers between screenings. It is important to note that BSE should not be used in isolation; it supplements screening by clinical breast examination (CBE) and mammography.

It is advocated by the American Cancer Society (ACS) as well as the National Comprehensive Cancer Network (NCCN) that BSE begin early, at age 20 years. Starting BSE at an early age allows women to familiarize themselves with the composition of their breasts, increases awareness of breast cancer surveillance, and establishes a good habit for when they are older. **Women should report any changes to their physicians.** As part of the ACS guidelines for the Early Detection of Breast Cancer, **clinical breast examination should be performed every 3 years starting at age 20,** with the option of monthly BSE also starting at age 20. **Premenopausal women may find that monthly examinations are most informative during the week after their menses.** There are complex reasons why many women do not perform BSE, but reassurance and patient education may encourage women to overcome psychological barriers. In women who have been treated for breast cancer, BSE can also be used as a supplemental method to aid in detecting recurrence.

Like clinical breast examination, the breast self-examination should begin with visual inspection. A woman should inspect her breasts while standing or sitting before a mirror, looking for asymmetry, nipple retraction or skin dimpling. Skin dimpling is highlighted by elevation of the arms over the head or by pressing the hands against the hips and performing a "squeezing" motion (to contract the chest muscles). While standing or sitting, she should carefully palpate her breasts using the finger pads of the opposite hand with first light pressure then with increasing firmness. This may be performed while showering with soapy hands to increase the sensitivity of palpation. Finally, she should lie down and again palpate each quadrant of the breast extending into the axilla. A good resource for instructions on BSE can be found on the Susan G. Komen for the Cure Web site (**http://cms.komen.org/komen/index.htm**).

Breast Imaging

The two most common and important imaging techniques for the early detection of malignancy are **mammography** and **ultrasonography**. Recently **magnetic resonance imaging** (MRI) has been incorporated as a screening tool in subsets of women at higher risk of breast cancer, as well as a diagnostic tool in certain clinical situations.

Screening Mammography

Screening of asymptomatic women for breast cancer has been shown to reduce the death rate by 20% to 30%, most likely due to earlier detection. Half of the reduction seen in breast cancer deaths in the United States has been attributed to screening mammography (3).

Several randomized controlled trials (RCTs) support the use of mammography for breast cancer screening in women older than 50 years of age. Controversy regarding the benefit of screening women aged 40 to 49 years was primarily due to the lack of RCTs designed specifically to evaluate the efficacy of screening in that particular age group. However, **when data regarding screening in women aged 40 to 49 years were pooled together from the various RCTs and analyzed in a meta-analysis, there was a significant reduction of 18% in the breast cancer mortality rate for this group of women** (4). In addition, the Swedish Two-Country Trial demonstrated a 23% reduction in mortality rate for this group of women with screening mammography with 18 years of follow-up (5). Furthermore, a UK study has shown a survival benefit in younger women equivalent to that seen in women over 50 years (6).

Currently, the American Cancer Society as well as the National Cancer Institute recommends that annual screening begin at age 40 for women at normal risk (7). Additional screening recommendations exist for women at increased risk of breast cancer; these recommendations include more frequent clinical breast examination, initiation of screening at ages younger than 40, and using other modalities as adjuncts to mammography including ultrasound and MRI. **There is no established upper age limit for breast cancer screening.**

Mammography is the best method of detection for a nonpalpable breast cancer but occasionally misses some palpable and nonpalpable or ultrasonographically detected

malignancies. Mammography should not be used in isolation. Neither the technology of mammography nor its interpretation by radiologists is infallible. **The basis of any screening program or work-up of breast abnormalities is the physical examination.** Mammography and CBE complement one another; it is recommended that women undergo CBEs around the time of their regularly scheduled annual mammograms (8). Patients should be cautioned that breast compression can be uncomfortable and that steady compression of the breast is necessary to obtain good images.

In addition to mammography used as a screening tool, there are circumstances in which bilateral mammography is mandatory:

1. **In any patient with a dominant mass,** even if biopsy is planned, to assess the ipsilateral lesion and to exclude disease in the contralateral breast.

2. **In any patient with enlarged axillary or supraclavicular nodes,** in order to search for an occult primary breast carcinoma.

3. **Before any cosmetic breast operation** (augmentation, implant exchange, breast reduction) to rule out occult disease.

Mammographic Abnormalities

Mammography, either used as a screening tool or used in the diagnostic work-up of a breast mass, can detect microcalcifications, breast densities, and architectural distortions (Fig. 16.2). To standardize the reporting of mammographic findings, **the American College of Radiology developed the Breast-Imaging Reporting and Data System (BI-RADS) classification** (9). There are six categories (1–6) for classifying findings, with category 0 representing an incomplete assessment with the need for additional studies (Table 16.1). Additional imaging recommendations may include magnification, spot compression, and ultrasonography. A patient may have a screening mammogram that shows a questionable abnormality, while spot compression views may indicate the finding is completely normal; this would fall into category 1 "negative."

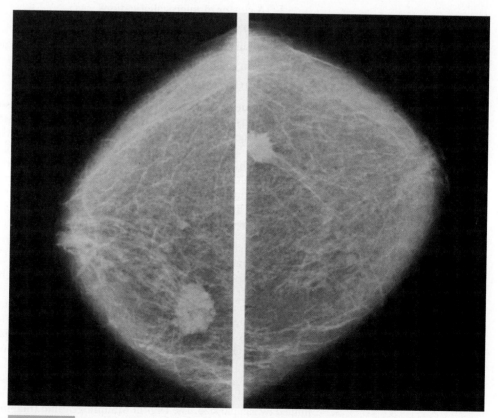

Figure 16.2 Bilateral film screen mammograms showing typical carcinoma in each breast, illustrating the importance of bilateral mammography in the workup of a clinically apparent mass.

Table 16.1 Mammographic Interpretations and the Breast Imaging Reporting and Data System Classification with Recommendations	
Category 0	Needs additional studies
Category 1	Negative; routine screening mammogram
Category 2	Benign finding; routine screening mammogram
Category 3	Probably a benign finding; repeat mammogram in 6 months
Category 4	Suspicious abnormality; biopsy
Category 5	Highly suggestive of malignancy; biopsy if palpable or needle localization biopsy if nonpalpable
Category 6	Known biopsy-proven malignancy

Mammographic Findings

Microcalcifications are the most frequent mammographic abnormalities necessitating biopsy. The evaluation of microcalcifications includes review of their size, number, location, distribution, and morphology. Microcalcifications that tend to be benign are smooth, round, solid, or lucent-centered spheres. Tubular or rod-shaped calcifications are often associated with ectatic ducts. If further analysis is required, magnification and spot compression views are the primary techniques used. Calcifications that are classified as benign do not require histologic confirmation. **Of concern, are calcifications that vary in size and shape.** The majority of calcifications in breast cancers form in the intraductal portion of the breast and are small and irregular with varying levels of maturation or density.

The most common signs of breast cancer seen on mammography are:

1. **A cluster of microcalcifications**
2. **A mass** seen as an area of increased radiodensity
3. **An area of architectural distortion** in the breast parenchyma
4. **Skin thickening or edema**
5. **Rarely, asymmetry alone**

These "common signs" can also be seen with benign lesions, leading to a false-positive mammography rate of 15% to 20% (10). For example, clusters of microcalcifications are also seen with benign processes such as hyperplasia, adenosis, fibroadenomas, and ductal papillomas. However, for accurate diagnosis, a stereotactic core or excisional biopsy may be required. **Mammography misses approximately 10% to 15% of cancers.** It has a low sensitivity for the detection of cancers in dense breasts, and infiltrating lobular cancers (11). False-negative mammograms occur particularly in young women with dense breast parenchyma and little fat (11). If there are suspicious findings on clinical examination, biopsy of the breast must be performed regardless of the mammographic findings; this will be discussed in more detail below (12).

Digital Mammography

Digital mammography (DM) was developed to address some of the limitations of film mammography (13). **Its advantages include speed and higher contrast resolution**, which in theory is better for detecting densities and masses in dense tissue. The image contrast can be manipulated to aid in the evaluation of dense breasts, which have low contrast. The advantage of film mammography (FM) is spatial resolution, which is better for detecting calcifications. Digital mammography also delivers a smaller dose of radiation than that of FM. However, given that the dose of radiation from FM is so low, the differences in radiation doses is of minor significance.

Results from previous trials have not demonstrated a significant difference in accuracy in breast cancer detection between digital and conventional mammography; however, these studies were limited by sample size. The **Digital Mammographic Imaging Screening Trial** (DMIST) **was designed to assess the performance of digital versus film mammography.** The study involved 49,500 female volunteers undergoing both conventional screening mammography and digital mammography. Subset analyses indicated that in women under age 50, as well as in women with dense breasts, digital mammography may be more accurate in detecting breast cancer (14). Because digital images can be stored electronically, many facilities plan to transition to DM in the future. At this time however, many centers still use conventional FM. Even though DM may be of benefit in certain subgroups of women, women should not forego annual screening mammograms if DM is not available to them.

Ultrasonography

Breast ultrasonography (US) is a popular imaging technique that is **primarily used as an adjunctive tool** and not as a screening modality. Currently, **there is an American College of Radiology Imaging Network Trial in progress to assess the screening capabilities of breast US,** but current clinical practices utilize US with accompanying mammography (15).

Although studies are examining the use of ultrasound for screening, currently there is no role for surveying the entire breast using ultrasound; the main use of ultrasound is to focus on an area of concern identified as abnormal by mammography or clinical examination. Ultrasonography can determine whether a lesion is present, or whether a clinical breast examination finding is within the spectrum of normal parenchyma, such as a prominent fat lobule. If a lesion does exist, US can be used to further characterize the finding.

There are clinical indications for the use of US as the primary imaging modality. These include evaluating palpable findings in young patients (teens and early 20s); **pregnant women; and women presenting with erythematous, tender breasts** (15). In the latter category, the diagnostic dilemma is between infection and inflammatory breast cancer; US allows for an initial evaluation of the breast when the breast is too tender for mammographic compression. Other uses for US are in the evaluation of axillary lymph nodes in breast cancer patients; post-operative examination of fluid collections (seroma, hematoma); and as an aid in interventional procedures such as in needle aspiration or biopsy and the preoperative localization of nonpalpable lesions.

Ultrasonography is 95% to 100% accurate in differentiating solid masses from cysts. **It can aid in the evaluation of a benign-appearing, nonpalpable density identified by mammography.** If such a lesion proves to be a simple cyst, no further workup is necessary if the patient is asymptomatic. There are certain criteria that must be met for a cyst to be classified as "simple," thus falling into the category of BI-RADS 2: benign finding. These criteria are: (i) anechoic; (ii) well-circumscribed round or oval mass with posterior enhancement; and (iii) thin bilateral edge shadows (16).

Magnetic Resonance Imaging

Magnetic resonance imaging (MRI) produces detailed cross-sectional images of tissues and structures utilizing magnetic fields. The use of screening and diagnostic MRI is gaining more recognition as an adjunct to mammography in specific clinical scenarios. However, as with mammography and other screening tools, MRI has associated false-negative rates depending on the specific clinical application. In studies evaluating MRI, **the specificity of MRI is significantly lower than that of mammography, resulting in an increased recall and biopsy rate,** due to the enhancement of benign lesions such as fat necrosis, fibroadenomas, and fibrocystic changes (17).

As the technology of MRI has become more sophisticated with dedicated breast MRI coils, contrast agents, and protocols (17), breast MRI is increasingly being used in the clinical setting. **MRI is a useful tool** in the setting of equivocal mammographic or ultrasonic findings, **particularly in patients with dense breasts, post-lumpectomy scarring, a strong suspicion of infiltrating lobular carcinoma, scattered calcifications suggestive of extensive ductal carcinoma *in situ* (DCIS) or extensive intraductal cancer, bloody nipple discharge, or silicone implants** (11).

In women who have an occult primary breast cancer presenting as axillary adenopathy, mammography is limited in its ability to identify the primary breast cancer. There is evidence that **MRI can identify occult breast lesions,** allowing for more accurate staging and the possibility of breast conserving surgery (18,19). Clinical studies have shown that **MRI can be beneficial in monitoring the response to neoadjuvant chemotherapy** (20) as well as determining the extent of disease in a breast cancer patient for staging purposes and for contralateral breast cancer screening (21). MRI is also used as an adjunct to mammography in high-risk women (22) (Table 16.2).

Table 16.2 Recommendations for Breast MRI Screening as Adjunct to Mammography

Recommend Annual MRI Screening (based on nonrandomized screening trials and observational studies)

- *BRCA* mutation

- Lifetime risk 20% to 25% or greater, as defined by risk assessment models largely dependent on family history

- First-degree relative of *BRCA* carrier, but untested

Recommend Annual MRI Screening (based on expert consensus opinion and evidence of lifetime risk of breast cancer)

- Li-Fraumeni syndrome and first-degree relatives

- Radiation to chest between age 10 and 30 years

- Cowden and Bannayan-Riley-Ruvalcaba syndromes and first-degree relatives

Saslow D, Boetes, Burke W, et al. American Cancer Society (ACS) Guidelines for breast screening with MRI as an adjunct to mammography. *CA: Cancer J Clin* 2007;57;75–89.

Benign Breast Conditions

Fibrocystic Disease

Fibrocystic disease is one of the most common breast problems seen in clinical practice. **The term "disease" is misleading and "change" or "condition" is a preferable,** more accurate description. **Fibrocystic change/condition (FCC) constitutes a spectrum of clinical signs, symptoms and histologic features.** In a woman with FCC symptoms, an important part of the evaluation is to exclude malignancy, because the diagnosis of FCC is otherwise of little clinical significance (23).

Clinical Presentation

Symptoms and Signs   **FCC is thought to be hormonally related** because it appears primarily in women between the ages of 30 and 50 years, subsides after menopause, and can fluctuate with menstrual cycles. Women may present with multiple, tender, palpable masses; usually the breasts are most tender and the masses largest just before the menses, with signs and symptoms abating after menstruation. **It is estimated that 60% of women have clinical findings compatible with the diagnosis of FCC** (23). FCC involves changes of both the stromal (fatty and fibrous tissue that give the breast support and shape) and glandular tissues (lobules and ducts).

Evaluation   Malignancy must be excluded in the evaluation of a woman with probable FCC. Often on physical examination, the breasts are diffusely nodular, with areas of increased density, mainly in the upper, outer quadrants, with no dominant masses. A mammogram should be performed, with possible ultrasound if there is concern about the presence of a mass on physical examination. **A repeat physical examination after the next menstrual cycle is often valuable** to document resolution of questionable areas. In the case of a dominant mass, a breast biopsy, preferably needle biopsy or aspiration cytology, is recommended to rule out malignancy. Large cysts may be aspirated if symptomatic.

Clear, watery, straw-colored, or greenish nipple discharge in patients with FCC should be tested for blood by means of a standard guaiac or Hemoccult test. If the discharge is from multiple ducts, bilateral and nonbloody, most likely the discharge is benign. Copious discharge may be a sign of malignancy.

Pathology   The histologic features of FCC are variable (23). Changes such as fibrosis, cyst formation, hyperplasia (overgrowth of the cells that line the ducts), adenosis (enlargement of breast lobules), and sclerosing adenosis can be seen microscopically. One or more of these histologic features can be found in 50% to 60% of asymptomatic women (23). **In the case of** epithelial hyperplasia, it is important to distinguish between usual and atypical hyperplasia. Atypical hyperplasia is associated with an increased risk of breast cancer in the future (see below).

Cancer and Fibrocystic Disease

The conclusion that there is an association between FCC and cancer was originally drawn because FCC and malignancy were commonly found together in the same breast (24). However, because 50% to 60% of women have FCC and one in every eight women has breast cancer in her lifetime, it is not surprising that these two entities frequently coexist.

Not all women with FCC are at an increased risk for cancer. Those with histologic features such as fibrosis, cysts, apocrine metaplasia, and mild hyperplasia are at no increased risk of developing breast cancer (25,26). Histologic features such as sclerosing adenosis and solid or papillary hyperplasia increase the risk slightly (1.5–2 times). **Women who have atypical hyperplasia, either lobular or ductal, have 5 times the average risk**.

Benign Tumors

Intraductal Papilloma

An intraductal papilloma is a benign lesion that can cause serous, serosanguinous, or bloody nipple discharge (27). It is the **most common etiology of bloody nipple discharge without an associated mass.** True polyps of epithelial-lined breast ducts, intraductal papillomas are often solitary and found in the subareolar location, arising in a major duct close to the nipple. Intraductal papillomas are most frequently observed in women aged 30 to 50 years, and typically are not palpable because they are rarely larger than 5 mm. Compression of the breast close to the nipple in the affected quadrant often produces discharge from the affected duct. Because malignancies may also present with bloody nipple discharge, mammography should be performed to rule out other abnormalities in the breast. **Biopsy is usually necessary to rule out malignancy.**

Fiber optic ductoscopy is an endoscopic technique that has been developed over the past 15 years for evaluating bloody nipple discharge; it allows direct visualization of the ductal system of the breast through a nipple orifice. For diagnosis of nipple discharge, fiber optic ductoscopy demonstrated 88% sensitivity, 77% specificity, 83% positive predictive value, and 82% negative predictive value (28). However, this technique is not widely used in clinical practice due to limited expertise, high cost, and poor reproducibility.

In addition to ductoscopy, ductal lavage is another screening procedure for women with nipple discharge. Ductal lavage involves irrigation of the duct with saline and cytologic evaluation of the irrigant. Cytologic analysis of ductal lavage alone has a positive predictive value of 72% and a negative predictive value of 50% but when combined with fiber optic ductoscopy, the positive predictive value increases to 86% and the negative predictive value increases to 87% (28). There are limitations to the utilization of this technique including patient discomfort, low cytologic yield, and limited accuracy

Treatment   **Local excision of the draining duct is the treatment of choice.** This can be performed using local anesthesia through a circumareolar incision by reflecting the nipple away from the breast tissue. A lacrimal probe can be used to assist in locating the offending duct. If it is not possible to identify the duct, total ductal excision of the subareolar duct can be performed through the same incision. **The subsequent risk of invasive breast cancer is increased with the presence of atypical hyperplasia in a papilloma,** with an increased risk similar to that of proliferative disease with atypia (29). **Papillomas may have malignant epithelium either *in situ* or invasive** (30).

Fibroadenoma

Fibroadenomas are the most common benign breast mass in women (23). They are noncancerous growths composed of epithelial and stromal elements. They rarely occur after menopause, but occasionally calcified fibroadenomas are found in postmenopausal women. It is believed that they are influenced by estrogenic stimulation (23).

Symptoms and Signs   Clinically, a young patient usually notices a mass while showering or dressing. **Most masses are 1 to 3 cm in diameter, but they can grow to an extremely large size**

(i.e., the giant fibroadenoma). On physical examination, they are firm, rubbery, smooth, and freely mobile. Fibroadenomas may be multiple. On mammography, they may appear as circumscribed oval or round masses. Occasionally, coarse calcifications can be seen within a fibroadenoma. On ultrasonography, they characteristically appear as circumscribed, homogeneous, hypoechoic oval masses with occasional lobulations and are wider rather than tall. On MRI, they typically appear as smooth masses with high signal intensity on T2-weighted images.

Although the risk of cancer in a fibroadenoma is extremely low, some clinicians choose to biopsy (with FNA, core needle, or excisional biopsy) any solid mass in patients older than 30 years for definitive diagnosis. A lesion that is benign on ultrasonography and mammography is benign more than 99% of the time. **Some clinicians will omit biopsies in younger women with lesions characteristic of fibroadenomas,** and will follow these patients with serial ultrasonography (23).

Complex fibroadenomas are fibroadenomas that contain cysts, sclerosing adenosis, papillary apocrine changes, or epithelial calcifications. In a clinical follow-up study by Dupont et al. (31), complex fibroadenomas were shown to be associated with a slightly increased risk of breast cancer. **Patients who have simple fibroadenomas without complex histologic features are at no increased risk for development of invasive cancer.**

Treatment Although complete excision under local anesthesia can treat the lesion and confirm the absence of malignancy, excision is not often necessary. A fibroadenoma diagnosed by clinical examination, imaging, and needle biopsy may be followed if the lesion remains stable. **If a fibroadenoma increases in size, it should be excised.** Also, excision is generally recommended for fibroadenomas that are greater than 2 cm or 3 cm to rule out phyllodes tumor. **Fibroadenomas may diminish in size or even totally resolve particularly in younger women, and therefore excision can be avoided** (32).

Benign Phyllodes Tumor

Phyllodes tumors are fibroepithelial breast tumors characterized by stromal overgrowth and hypercellularity combined with an epithelial component, grossly forming a leaflike structure. Clinically, phyllodes tumors tend to occur in women aged 35 to 55 years, and comprise less than 1% of breast tumors (33). These lesions usually appear as isolated masses that are difficult to distinguish from fibroadenomas (34). Size is not a diagnostic criterion, although phyllodes tumors tend to be larger than fibroadenomas, often with a history of rapid growth. Both appear as well circumscribed, oval or lobulated masses with round borders on mammography and ultrasonography. **There are no good clinical or radiographic criteria by which to distinguish a phyllodes tumor from a fibroadenoma** (33,34).

Pathology **Phyllodes tumors are classified as benign, borderline, or malignant** based on the histologic criteria first described in 1978 by Pietruszka and Barnes (35). These histologic criteria are based on features such as the number of mitoses, pushing or infiltrative tumor margins, degree of stromal overgrowth, and degree of stromal cellular atypia, which are all used in combination to distinguish between the benign and malignant spectrum (36). Even with histologic criteria, definitive distinction between fibroadenoma, benign phyllodes tumor, and malignant phyllodes tumor can be very difficult and the correlation of histologic grade to clinical behavior and outcome has been challenging. **Even "benign" phyllodes tumors tend to recur locally particularly if the tumor is simply enucleated. Malignant phyllodes tumors have a higher local recurrence rate but also can metastasize, usually to the lungs** (36,37); for this reason, these tumors were originally called cystosarcoma phyllodes. **Axillary lymph node metastases are extremely unusual** despite the large size of some phyllodes tumors that are classified as "malignant."

Treatment **Due to the high propensity for local recurrence, the treatment of phyllodes tumors should consist of a wide, local excision** (36–38). Large tumors not amenable to breast conservation and malignant tumors with particularly infiltrative margins may require total mastectomy without axillary node dissection; however, mastectomy should be avoided whenever possible. **These malignant tumors are rarely multicentric and rarely metastasize to lymph nodes.** Typically, a phyllodes tumor is discovered by histologic examination after a patient undergoes an excisional biopsy of a mass believed to be a fibroadenoma. When the pathologic diagnosis is phyllodes tumor, a complete reexcision of the area should be undertaken so that the prior biopsy site and any residual tumor are excised. **There is no role for adjuvant therapy, either radiation therapy or chemotherapy.**

Breast Cancer

Breast cancer is the most common cancer in women under the age of 60 and is second only to lung cancer as the leading cause of cancer deaths in women. It accounts for 26% of all new cancer cases in women. In 2009 in the United States, an estimated 192,370 new cases of invasive breast cancer and 62,280 cases of ductal carcinoma *in situ* (DCIS) will be diagnosed in women, with approximately 40,170 deaths (39). **The overall lifetime risk for development of breast cancer in women in the United States is one in eight or 12.5%** (39).

During the past 50 years, there has been a significant increase in the incidence of breast cancer in the United States. This correlates with the increased use of screening mammography (40). Breast cancer incidence rates increased after 1980, but decreased by 3.5% per year from 2001 to 2004 probably due to declining use of hormonal replacement therapy (HRT) by postmenopausal women, as well as delays in diagnosis due to a decrease in mammographic utilization (41).

The mortality rate has dropped slightly, thought to be due in part to mammographic screening and improvements in systemic therapy (3). Screening mammography has also resulted in a decrease in the size of breast cancer at diagnosis, with close to one-third of cancers being 1 cm or less in diameter (42). Not surprisingly, nodal involvement has decreased and the proportion of DCIS cases has increased. It is predicted that in the next decade, these trends will continue.

Predisposing Factors

One of the fundamental steps in determining a patient's risk for breast cancer is to obtain a detailed history. This allows the physician to plan preventive and diagnostic strategies, as well as to educate the patient about breast cancer. Intrinsic and extrinsic factors both contribute to increasing a woman's risk. Intrinsic characteristics include genetic and familial elements, age, endogenous hormonal exposures, and benign breast lesions with high-risk histologies. Extrinsic characteristics include environmental exposures, diet, and exogenous hormonal exposures.

Age

The risk of developing breast cancer increases steadily with age. Breast cancer is rare before the age of 25 years, accounting for less than 1% of all cases of breast cancer. After the age of 30 years, there is a sharp increase in the incidence, with a small plateau between the ages of 45 and 50 years, which points to the involvement of hormonal factors (43). From 1996 to 2000, the incidence of breast cancer in the U.S. for women aged 30 to 34 years was 25 per 100,000, 198 per 100,000 for women aged 45 to 49 years, and for women aged 70 to 74, the incidence was 476 per 100,000 (44).

Prior History of Breast Cancer

One of the strongest single risk factors for the development of a breast cancer is the previous diagnosis of a contralateral breast cancer. The risk of subsequent contralateral breast cancer in a patient with unilateral breast cancer has been reported to range from 0.5% to 1% per year (45–48). **Young age (45,46,48) and lobular histology (46–48) were found to be associated with a greater likelihood of contralateral breast cancer; adjuvant chemotherapy significantly decreased the rate** (47,48). In patients diagnosed with unilateral breast cancer, breast MRI has been shown to detect clinically and mammographically occult contralateral cancers in 3.1% of cases at the time of diagnosis (21).

Family History

A family history of breast cancer increases a patient's overall relative risk (49). However, the risk is not significantly increased for women with first-degree relatives (mother, sister) with post-menopausal breast cancers, whereas **women whose mothers or sisters had bilateral premenopausal breast cancer have a high likelihood of acquiring the disease.** If the patient's mother or sister had unilateral premenopausal breast cancer, the likelihood of the patient developing breast cancer is approximately 30%. If a woman has several first-degree relatives with breast cancer, the risk increases. The risk of breast cancer is substantially increased if there is a genetic component.

Inherited Syndromes of Breast Cancer

The majority of breast cancers occur sporadically without a recognizable genetic association, with only approximately 5% to 10% attributed to breast cancer susceptibility genes (50). Two breast cancer susceptibility genes, *BRCA1* mapped to chromosome 17q21, and *BRCA2* on chromosome 13q12-13, are high penetrance tumor suppressor genes inherited in an autosomal-dominant fashion (51,52). Mutations in these genes account for only about 15% of all familial breast cancers, suggesting that other breast cancer susceptibility genes may exist. (53).

The estimated lifetime risk of breast cancer for women who have *BRCA1* genetic mutations ranges from 36% to as high as 87%, with a pooled estimate of 65% (54–56). The cumulative risk of ovarian cancer in *BRCA1* carriers has been reported to be between 27% and 45% (56–58). Estimates for the risk of developing a contralateral breast cancer are 60% (58). An increased risk also exists for the development of additional cancers such as colon, pancreatic, uterine, and cervical cancers (57,58). Breast cancers that occur in women with *BRCA1* mutations are mostly estrogen-receptor (ER) negative (up to 90%) and of high nuclear grade. Lifetime estimated risk for *BRCA2* mutation carriers is 45% to 84% for breast cancer and 10% to 20% for ovarian cancer (49). *BRCA2* mutations are also associated with a 6% lifetime risk for male breast cancer.

The prevalence of *BRCA1* and *BRCA2* in the general population is unknown but is estimated to be less than 0.12% and 0.044%, respectively (53). In Ashkenazi Jewish women, the prevalence of these mutations is as high as 2% (59). In women diagnosed with breast cancer before the age of 32, the incidence of *BRCA1* or *BRCA2* mutations is approximately 12% and in Ashkenazi women diagnosed with breast cancer before age 40, the incidence is 20% (60,61). Both *BRCA1* and *BRCA2* are very large genes with numerous possible mutations. This accounts for the highly variable risks for the development of breast, ovarian, and other cancers (62).

There are other hereditary syndromes associated with breast cancer with mostly autosomal dominant transmission, such as Li-Fraumeni, Cowden's disease, Muir-Torre, a variant of hereditary nonpolyposis colon cancer (HNPCC), ataxia-telangiectasia (autosomal recessive), and Peutz-Jeghers syndromes. Each syndrome is associated with an abnormal gene responsible for producing a recognized phenotype. In clinical practice, these syndromes contribute to only a small fraction of hereditary breast cancers; however, it is important that clinicians recognize when patients should be considered candidates for genetic testing.

In 1996, the American Society of Clinical Oncology issued a statement regarding genetic testing for cancer susceptibility with an update released in 2003 (63,64). The guidelines are summarized in Table 16.3.

Table 16.3 American Society of Clinical Oncology: Genetic Testing for Cancer Susceptibility Guidelines*

ASCO recommends that genetic testing only be offered when:

- the patient has very early onset of cancer or a strong family history

- the test can be adequately interpreted

- medical management of the patient (or family member) will be influenced by the result

Patients must be given appropriate informed consent including information about the test performed and the implications of a negative and positive result.

There should be pre- and post-test counseling that includes a discussion about the options available to genetic carriers. Such options include surveillance and early detection with radiographic or physical examination, which have inherent limitations, and risk reduction strategies such as chemoprevention or prophylactic surgery, which have presumed but unproven efficacy.

Criteria defining patients at high risk of hereditary breast-ovarian cancer syndrome:

- Family with >2 breast cancers and one or more cases of ovarian cancer diagnosed at any age

- Family with >3 breast cancers diagnosed before age 50

- Sister pairs with 2 or more of the following cancers diagnosed before age 50:

  ○ 2 breast cancers, 2 ovarian cancers, one breast and one ovarian cancer

Adapted from a Statement of the American Society of Clinical Oncology: Genetic testing for cancer susceptibility. *J Clin Oncol* 1996;14:1730–1736; **American Society of Clinical Oncology policy statement update:** Genetic testing for cancer susceptibility. *J Clin Oncol* 2003;12:2397–2406.

The American Society of Breast Surgeons issued a statement in 2006 defining patients at high risk for breast cancer. Persons in this high-risk population are patients with early onset breast cancer (before age 50), two primary breast cancers, a family history of early onset breast cancer, a previously identified *BRCA1/BRCA2* mutation in the family, a personal or family history of ovarian cancer, or Ashkenazi Jewish heritage (http://www.breastsurgeons.org/brca.shtml). Patients included in this group are at a 10% or greater risk of harboring a *BRCA1* or *BRCA2* mutation, which is the traditional cutoff for testing.

Reproductive and Hormonal Factors

A number of studies have shown a relationship between early menarche, late menopause, and breast cancer. (65–67). It is thought that lifetime exposure to endogenous estrogen plays a promotional role in the development of breast cancer. Women with breast cancer begin menses at a younger median age, (67) and the **longer a woman's reproductive phase, the higher the risk for development of breast cancer** (65). There is no clear association between the risk of breast cancer and duration of menses or menstrual irregularity. Studies of the effect of lactation on the incidence of breast cancer have been inconclusive but childbearing definitely has an effect on breast cancer risk (66). **Women who have never been pregnant have an increased risk of breast cancer compared to women who are parous; additionally, late age at first birth also increases the risk of breast cancer** (66).

There have been conflicting reports concerning the effect of oral contraceptives on breast cancer incidence. **A large meta-analysis of 54 epidemiologic studies found convincing evidence that there was a small increased relative risk of breast cancer for women currently using oral contraceptives and for up to 10 years after stopping use** (68). Because breast cancer incidence rises steeply with age, the estimated excess number of cancers diagnosed increased with increasing age at last use. After 10 or more years from cessation of oral contraceptives, there was no excess risk. Additionally, breast cancers in women who had used oral contraceptives tended to be less advanced clinically and localized to the breast. No risk factors, such as reproductive history or family history of breast cancer, changed the results after current usage had been taken into account. Similarly, the duration of use, age at first use, and the dose and type of hormone had little additional effect on breast cancer risk.

The association between breast cancer and hormonal replacement therapy (HRT) in post-menopausal women has been investigated in two large randomized trials. In the Women's Health Initiative (WHI) study, investigators demonstrated that **women randomized to combination HRT, had a significantly increased incidence of breast cancer, stroke, and pulmonary embolus compared with those randomized to a placebo** (69). HRT significantly decreased the incidence of colorectal cancer and femoral neck fractures. The trial was stopped early after it became apparent that the risks outweighed the benefits. **The risk of breast cancer has been shown to be greater for combination versus estrogen-only HRT.** However, the WHI demonstrated that women receiving estrogen-only HRT after hysterectomy were at an increased risk for stroke (70). The Million Women Study in the United Kingdom recruited 1,084,110 women and also demonstrated that current use of HRT was associated with an increased risk of breast cancer (71).

Soon after the report of the Women's Health Initiative, the use of HRT in the United States decreased by 38% with approximately 20 million fewer prescriptions written in 2003 than 2002 (72). Analysis of data from the National Cancer Institute's Surveillance, Epidemiology, and End Results (SEER) registries indicate that the age-adjusted incidence rate of breast cancer in women fell by 6.7% in 2003. **This decrease in breast cancer incidence seems to be temporally related to the drop in HRT by post-menopausal women** (73).

In counseling women with complaints of post-menopausal symptoms, the decision to initiate combination HRT must be individualized. For some patients, the improved quality of life and protection against fractures outweigh the potential risks. The individual risk of breast cancer in a particular postmenopausal patient should be considered before initiating HRT. If HRT is to be prescribed, low dosage formulations should be used with the understanding that the risk for harm will likely increase with prolonged use, and the survival benefit will diminish over time. For women at high risk for fractures, bisphosphonates are a suitable alternative. **Any postmenopausal women on HRT should be aware of the increased risks of breast cancer and should be counseled to be particularly diligent regarding breast cancer awareness and screening.**

Diet, Obesity, and Exercise

Earlier studies linked marked differences in the incidence of breast cancer among women in different geographic areas to **high-fat diets** in particular, and to obesity in general (74). Current epidemiologic studies have linked obesity and increasing BMI to an increased risk in postmenopausal breast cancer, but have not been able to demonstrate the same increased risk in premenopausal breast cancer (75,76). Regarding diet and breast cancer, the majority of epidemiologic studies are case-control studies and cohort studies. Few randomized control trials have been conducted and are problematic because the randomized dietary plan has to be adhered to for a many years. **One large pooled analysis of seven cohort studies including 337,819 women found no evidence of a positive association between fat intake and risk of breast cancer when those in the highest quintile of total fat intake were compared with those in the lowest quintile** (77). In the same study, the type of fat intake and cholesterol also had no positive association with an increased risk. Similarly, a recent, large randomized controlled trial involving 40 U.S. clinical centers from the Women's Health Initiative followed 48,835 postmenopausal women for 8 years who were randomly assigned to a dietary modification group or control group (78). The dietary modifications included 5 servings of fruits and vegetables, 6 servings of grains and total fat to 20% of energy requirements daily. The results surprisingly showed that a low-fat diet did not prevent a statistically significant reduction in invasive breast cancer risk. However, results were confounded by relatively few women meeting the low-fat dietary target (only 14.4% at year 6). Future studies were encouraged because it may take years for the benefits of a low-fat diet to be manifested.

One large prospective study in the United States of 90,655 premenopausal women found no association between **fiber intake** and the risk of breast cancer, whereas a study in the United Kingdom of 35,792 women demonstrated a reduced risk of breast cancer for premenopausal women who consumed >30 gram of fiber day as compared to those who consumed <20 g/day (79,80). Studies of **dietary carotenoids, vitamins A, C, and E,** as measured by intake of fruits and vegetables, have also been conflicting. One large prospective cohort study involving 83,234 women in the Nurses' Health Study showed that premenopausal women who consumed more than five or more servings of fruits and vegetables had a modestly lower risk of breast cancer than those who had less than two servings per day (81). These findings are in contrast to a large prospective study of 285,526 women, which showed no significant association between **fruit or vegetable intake** and reduction in breast cancer risk (82). Similarly, a large pooled analysis of cohort studies involving 351,825 women showed no significant association between increased fruit and vegetable consumption and reduced breast cancer risk (83). It has been postulated that selected nutrients have an effect on DNA repair and metabolic detoxification by virtue of their antioxidant properties (84).

Exercise has been shown to reduce the risk of postmenopausal breast cancer in a large systematic review (85). A recent study of 64,777 women from the Nurses' Health Study Cohort II evaluated premenopausal exercise habits and showed that the most active women (running 3.25 hours or walking 13 hours per week) had a 23% reduction in the risk for premenopausal breast cancer (86). A large systematic review also supports the decreased risk of breast cancer with exercise: 62 studies were evaluated with the conclusion that increased **physical activity led to an overall risk reduction for breast cancer of 25%** with a dose-dependent effect noted in 28 of the studies (87). This reduction in risk was seen in both premenopausal and postmenopausal women.

Alcohol

Regular alcohol consumption has been linked to an increased risk of breast cancer. A large pooled analysis of seven prospective case-control studies from the United States (Nurses' Health Study, Iowa Women's Health Study, New York State Cohort); Canada (CNBSS); Sweden (Sweden Mammography Cohort); and the Netherlands (Netherlands Cohort Study) was conducted. With 322,647 women and up to 11 years of follow-up, this pooled study found a linear increase in the relative risk of breast cancer from 9% in women with a daily alcohol consumption of 10 g/day (approximately one drink per day) to 41% in women who consumed 60 g/day (approximately five drinks per day) compared with nondrinkers (88). **The type of alcoholic beverage was not shown to be of significance.**

Radiation Exposure

Prior radiation exposure, particularly to the thoracic area, has been shown to increase the risk of breast cancer. A study of Canadian women who received radiation from fluoroscopic examinations during the treatment of tuberculosis demonstrated that the risk of breast cancer associated with radiation was related to the age of exposure (89). The risk was highest for women who were exposed at ages 10–14. Similarly, Japanese women who survived the atomic bomb had an increased risk of breast cancer, and that risk was greatest for women who were exposed as children (90). Regarding the risk of breast cancer from radiation used for therapy, multiple studies demonstrate an increased risk for women who underwent treatment for Hodgkin's disease (HD) (91–94). **Survivors of Hodgkin's disease have an increased risk of breast cancer from radiation exposure that is primarily age-related, with the highest risk associated with treatment at ages 10 to 20 years.** In addition, the increased risk has been shown to have a late manifestation with a median time from treatment to breast cancer of 15 years.

Diagnosis

The majority of breast tumors are found in the upper, outer quadrant, where there is more breast tissue, although breast cancer may occur anywhere in the breast. Breast cancer is often discovered by the patient when she feels a painless mass. Less commonly, a physician discovers a mass during a routine breast examination. The findings on mammography may suggest that a palpable lesion is malignant. On the other hand, screening mammography may detect an abnormality without a palpable tumor. Rarely, the patient may present with an axillary mass and no obvious carcinoma in the breast.

A breast mass in a woman of any age must be approached as a possible carcinoma. Physical examination alone is inaccurate in evaluating palpable masses. At times, the only clue to an underlying malignancy may be a subtle finding of an area of thickening amid normal nodularity. Obvious clues to malignancy include nipple retraction, skin dimpling, involved nodes, or ulceration, but these are late signs and, fortunately, are not common at presentation.

After obtaining the history and physical examination, the "**triple test**" should be utilized to evaluate a palpable mass. Triple test refers to the combination of **physical examination, breast imaging** (usually mammogram +/− ultrasound), **and pathologic diagnosis** employing cytology by means of fine-needle aspiration (FNA), or histology by means of core-needle biopsy or excisional biopsy. The diagnostic accuracy is approximately 100% when all three are concordant (95,96). Indications for an excisional biopsy include cytologic or histologic atypia on needle biopsy, any discordance between any of the three modalities, or the patient's desire to eliminate a source for concern. Algorithms for the evaluation of breast masses in premenopausal and postmenopausal women are presented in Figs. 16.3 and 16.4. The American Cancer Society reports that 80% of breast biopsies are benign (http://www.cancer.org).

Fine-Needle Aspiration Cytologic Testing

Fine-needle aspiration is performed with a 20- or 22-gauge needle. The technique has a high diagnostic accuracy, with a **10% to 15% false-negative rate** and a rare but persistent false-positive rate often in association with epithelial proliferative lesions such as ductal or lobular hyperplasia (97,98).

Fine-needle aspiration can aid a clinician in discussing alternatives with a patient if a mass appears to be malignant on physical examination and/or breast imaging. A negative FNA cytologic diagnosis is usually discordant with other modalities and frequently must be followed with excisional biopsy. An FNA cytologic diagnosis of a fibroadenoma (without atypia) in a young woman can be used to safely follow the mass.

Biopsy

Core-Needle Biopsy   Core-needle biopsy (CNB) is a less invasive procedure than open biopsy to obtain tissue for accurate histopathologic diagnosis of palpable or nonpalpable mammographic or ultrasonographic lesions. It utilizes an 11- to 14-gauge needle to obtain specimens; abnormal architecture and invasion can be identified in these tissue samples which can provide more information than FNA and may be evaluated for specific tumor markers such as estrogen receptor (ER), progesterone receptor (PR), or HER-2/*neu*. **Indications for CNB are the same as for open biopsy** and may be performed handheld for palpable masses. Suspicious nonpalpable lesions seen on mammography or ultrasonography should be biopsied using an image-guided core biopsy technique (99,100).

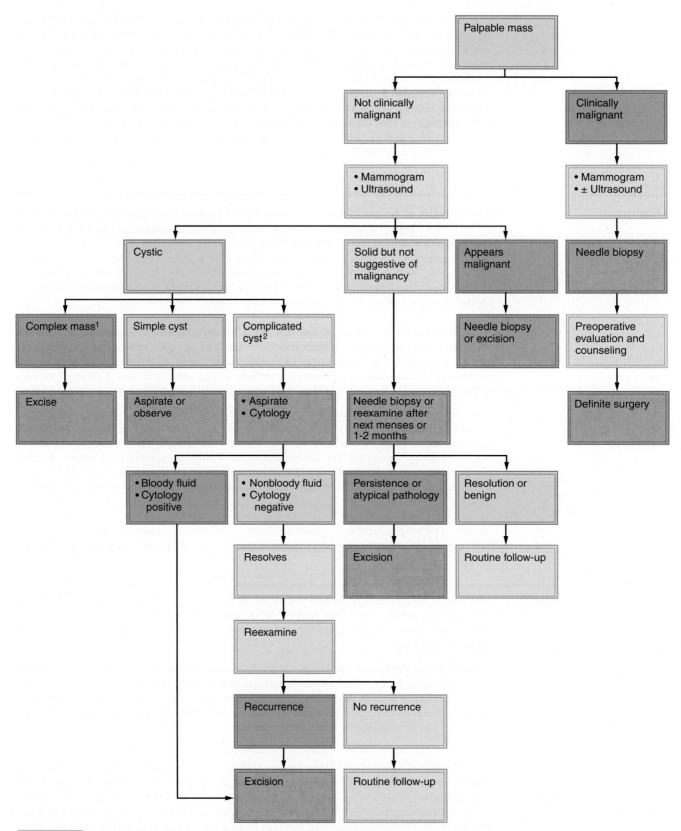

Figure 16.3   **Schematic evaluation of breast masses in premenopausal women.** 1 complex mass—a cystic mass with a solid component that may be malignant. 2 complicated cyst—usually multiple simple cysts or cysts with septations.

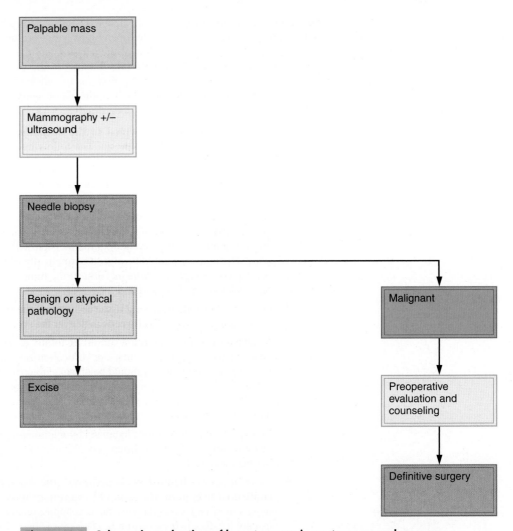

Figure 16.4   Schematic evaluation of breast masses in postmenopausal women.

A number of studies have shown sensitivity and specificity ranging from of 85% to 100% for image-guided CNB for diagnosing breast cancer. The sensitivity and negative predictive values of CNB are less for mammographic calcifications (.84 and .94, respectively) than for the diagnosis of masses (.96 and .99 respectively) (99,100). When CNB is used to sample microcalcifications, radiography must be performed of the specimen to ensure the calcifications are present in the tissue removed. A microclip is placed after CNB to indicate the biopsied area and a post-biopsy mammogram is obtained. CNB usually does not result in architectural distortion, which may alter the interpretation of future mammograms.

Certain technical issues may not allow CNB to be employed, such as very superficial or posterior lesions. **Mammographic lesions in a very small breast are usually not amenable to stereotactic core biopsy, and silicone implants can make CNB more challenging.** Depending on the location of the lesion in relation to the implant, open biopsy is sometimes recommended to avoid implant rupture. If a lesion is detectable on ultrasound, CNB using ultrasound guidance is simpler and less expensive than stereotactic CNB and does not require special equipment. Vacuum-assisted devices with CNB allow for multiple samples to be obtained without withdrawing and reinserting the needle.

Open Biopsy   A minority of patients require surgical biopsy if the lesion is not amenable to CNB, the sample is inadequate, or the pathologic results are equivocal. Likewise, follow-up open biopsy is indicated if benign diagnoses of a radial scar or atypical ductal hyperplasia are made after CNB because of the coexistence of malignancy in 20% to 30% of cases (99). As mentioned above, the biopsy results must correlate with the clinical and mammographic results. Any discordance requires an additional biopsy, either repeat CNB, or more commonly surgical biopsy.

Image-Guided Open-Biopsy   Nonpalpable lesions detected by a mammogram or ultrasound that are not amenable to CNB require open biopsy after pre-operative localization by imaging. This requires the collaborative effort of the surgeon and the radiologist and entails the placement of a needle or specialized wire into the area of the suspected abnormality in the breast parenchyma. To further assist in localization, many radiologists also inject a biologic dye. The surgeon then reviews the films and localizes the abnormality with respect to the tip of the wire or needle and plans his/her operation accordingly.

Open biopsy can usually be performed in the outpatient setting with the aid of intravenous (IV) sedation and local anesthesia. The following steps are undertaken:

1. **IV sedation** often aids in easing anxiety. **Local anesthesia** is used to infiltrate the skin and subcutaneous tissue surrounding the mass (if palpable) or wire-localized abnormality.

2. **An incision is made usually directly over the mass or localized area or at the site of the wire insertion.** The incision should be planned with future procedures in mind: if a mastectomy is required, the incision will be incorporated into the mastectomy. The incision should be placed cosmetically so that a partial mastectomy can be performed through the same incision. If the tumor is far from the areola, circumareolar incisions are best avoided.

3. Once the skin and underlying tissue are incised, **the mass can be gently grasped** with a stay suture or **with Allis forceps** to deliver the specimen into the operative field.

4. **Whenever possible, the mass should be totally excised.** An incisional biopsy may be obtained for large masses that are difficult to excise totally with local anesthesia. However, a frozen section should be obtained to confirm that malignant tissue has been obtained in the case of an incisional biopsy. It is important not to remove too much additional breast tissue from around a mass (or wire) because the main purpose of the procedure is to obtain a tissue diagnosis for clinical management and not result in deformity.

5. In the case of abnormalities localized by mammography, **a post-excisional mammogram of the surgical specimen** is performed to be certain that the lesion in question has been excised.

6. **After adequate hemostasis is achieved, the wound is irrigated, the specimen is confirmed to contain the lesion by mammography and the incision is closed.** The most superficial subcutaneous fat is reapproximated with fine, absorbable sutures, usually a 3-0 or 4-0 vicryl suture. The skin is best closed with an absorbable subcuticular suture, with either Steri-Strips or Dermabond to the incision to achieve the most cosmetically pleasing result.

Two-Step Approach   The two-step approach involves the initial biopsy, either by needle or open procedures, followed by subsequent definitive treatment. Women who are diagnosed with breast cancer on biopsy can discuss the various treatment options and seek out additional consultations, if desirable, before undergoing definitive treatment. For most patients, being engaged in the planning of therapy is an important psychological aspect in the healing process.

Pathology and Natural History

Breast cancer constitutes a heterogeneous group of histopathologic lesions (101). Regardless of the histologic type, most breast cancers arise in the terminal duct lobular unit. The most widely used classification of invasive breast cancers, that of the World Health Organization, recognizes invasive carcinoma as "ductal" and "lobular." This classification scheme is based on cytologic features and growth patterns of the invasive tumor cells, with the distinction between lobular and intraductal carcinoma based on the histologic appearance rather than the site of origin.

Breast cancer may be either **invasive** (infiltrating ductal carcinoma, infiltrating lobular carcinoma) which indicates invasion into the breast stroma with the potential for lymph node and distant metastases or *in situ* (ductal carcinoma *in situ* [DCIS] or lobular carcinoma *in situ* [LCIS]) which indicates the inability to spread to other sites.

The most common histologic diagnosis of invasive breast carcinoma is infiltrating ductal carcinoma. This histologic type accounts for 60% to 70% of the breast cancers in the United States (102). This diagnosis is actually a diagnosis by default because this tumor type is defined as a type of cancer that does not fall into any of the other categories of invasive mammary carcinoma (101) as recognized by defined histologic features (mucinous, tubular, medullary). Mammographically, it is often characterized by a stellate appearance with microcalcifications. The classic macroscopic appearance of infiltrating ductal carcinoma is a firm, often rock-hard mass that has gritty, chalky streaks within the substance of the tumor. This consistency is due to the fibrotic response of the surrounding stroma, not the neoplastic cells. Microscopically, the appearance is highly heterogeneous with regard to growth pattern, cytologic features, mitotic activity, and extent of *in situ* component.

The second most common histologic diagnosis of invasive breast carcinoma is infiltrating lobular carcinoma (ILC), which comprises 5% to 10% of breast cancers (102,103). It may present as a mammographic abnormality or palpable mass, as with invasive ductal carcinoma, but the extent of disease may be underestimated by the physical or radiographic findings (103). Invasive lobular carcinoma often presents as multicentric disease in the ipsilateral breast with **coexistent LCIS in approximately 5% to 15% of cases** (104,105). **The incidence of contralateral breast cancer in ILC patients is about 20%** (103). Macroscopically, some invasive lobular carcinomas may appear as firm, gray-white masses similar to invasive ductal cancers, or some may only have a rubbery consistency of the breast tissue. Microscopically, invasive lobular cancer is characterized by small, uniform neoplastic cells infiltrating the stroma in a single-file pattern (101) with little or no desmoplastic stromal reaction.

Other types of invasive breast carcinoma are far less common and are subtypes of infiltrating ductal carcinoma. **Medullary carcinoma accounts for approximately 2% to 5% of breast carcinomas** and may be a slow-growing, less aggressive malignancy than the usual infiltrating ductal carcinoma (101,102,106). These tumors are often well circumscribed grossly with a dense lymphocytic infiltrate microscopically. **Tubular carcinoma** is a well-differentiated breast cancer with limited metastatic potential and an excellent prognosis, occurring in about 1% of breast cancers (102,106,107). **Mucinous (colloid) carcinoma accounts for fewer than 5% of all breast cancers and is associated with a favorable prognosis** (102,106,107). Grossly, the tumors are well circumscribed and may have areas that appear mucinous or gelatinous. Microscopically, small clusters or sheets of tumor cells are dispersed in pools of extracellular mucin (101). **Papillary carcinoma** is used to describe a predominantly noninvasive ductal carcinoma; **invasive papillary carcinomas are rare, accounting for approximately 1% of breast cancers** (102,107). **An extremely rare form of breast cancer is adenoid cystic carcinoma,** which is similar histologically to the salivary gland tumor (108). They often present as a palpable mass with no clinico-radiological features. **These cancers metastasize late and tend to be well differentiated.**

Growth Patterns

The tumor growth rate of a breast cancer varies widely among patients and at different stages of the disease. Many mathematical models have been devised based on the natural history of breast cancer, assumptions of tumor growth rate, the probability of detecting a tumor of a given size, and the rate of clinical surfacing (109). Doubling time of breast cancer has been estimated to range from several weeks for rapidly growing tumors to months for slowly growing ones. **Based on seminal studies, the mean doubling time for mammary carcinomas has been estimated to be 5.4 months with a standard deviation of 4 months** (110). To give an example for clinical application, if it is assumed that the doubling time is 100 days, the doubling time is constant (which is not often the case), and the tumor originated from one cell, it would take 8 years to result in a 1-cm tumor (111) (Fig. 16.5). One primary concern is that during the time in which the tumor is growing before being clinically apparent, tumor cells may be circulating through the body.

On account of the long preclinical tumor growth phase and the early metastastic rate of some infiltrating carcinomas, **many clinicians view breast cancer as a systemic disease** at the time of diagnosis. **This pessimistic view is not justified.** A more realistic approach is to view breast cancer as a two-compartment disease: one consists of the primary breast tumor with its possible local and regional extension, and the other consists of the systemic metastases with their life-threatening consequences.

Biology of Breast Cancer

The biology of breast cancer is highly variable. **Some view breast cancer as a local disease** that progresses in a predictable manner to develop distant metastases over time, known as the **"Halstedian" theory,** named after the prominent surgeon who popularized the radical mastectomy. **With this view, aggressive local control is necessary for survival. Others view breast cancer as a "systemic" disease,** with distant metastases present before a patient is diagnosed.

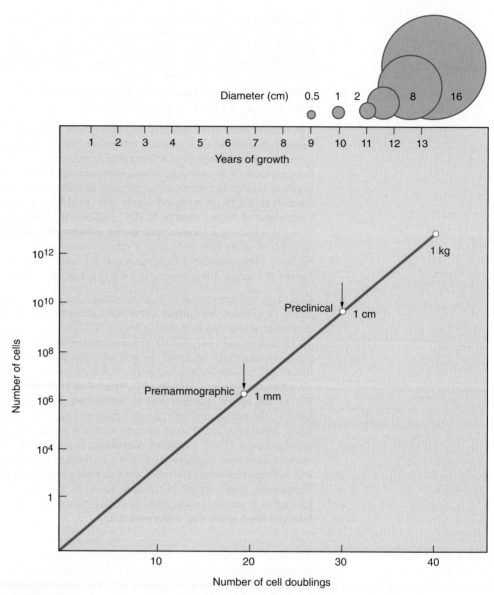

Figure 16.5 **Growth rate of breast cancer, indicating long preclinical phase.** (From **Gullino PM.** Natural history of breast cancer: progression from hyperplasia to neoplasia as predicted by angiogenesis. *Cancer* 1977;39:2699. Copyright 1977 American Cancer Society. Reprinted by permission of Wiley-Liss, Inc., a subsidiary of John Wiley & Sons, Inc.)

With the systemic view, it is thought that some tumors have the ability to metastasize and others do not; the emphasis is on systemic therapy with the belief that local recurrences are treated as they develop and have no bearing on the development of future distant disease or on survival. Another theory, known as the **"spectrum theory," is a synthesis of the two views: breast cancer is a heterogeneous disease** with some cancers that remain local throughout their course at one end of the spectrum while others are systemic from the outset at the other end (112). With this view, unless initial local control is sufficient, some tumors will gain the ability to disseminate to distant sites. However, it is acknowledged that if there is a high likelihood that a tumor has disseminated at the time of diagnosis, local control will have little overall impact.

Staging

After the diagnosis of breast cancer has been confirmed either by cytology or histology, the clinical stage of the disease should be determined. Clinical staging involves findings on physical examination, with incorporation of information gained from imaging. The **American Joint Committee on Cancer (AJCC) uses the TNM** (tumor–nodes–metastases) **system,** presented in Tables 16.4 and 16.5 (113). The advantage of this system is its use both

Table 16.4 TNM (Tumor–Nodes–Metastases) System for Staging of Breast Cancer

Primary Tumor (T)

TX	Primary tumor cannot be assessed
T_0	No evidence of primary tumor
T_{is}	Carcinoma *in situ* Tis (DCIS) Ductal carcinoma *in situ* Tis (LCIS) Lobular carcinoma *in situ* Tis (Paget) Paget's disease of the nipple with no tumor
T_1	Tumor 2 cm or less in greatest dimension
	T_{1mic} Microinvasion 0.1 cm or less in greatest dimension
	T_{1a} Tumor more than 0.1 cm but not more than 0.5 cm in greatest dimension
	T_{1b} Tumor more than 0.5 cm but not more than 1 cm in greatest dimension
	T_{1c} Tumor more than 1 cm but not more than 2 cm in greatest dimension
T_2	Tumor more than 2 cm but not more than 5 cm in greatest dimension
T_3	Tumor more than 5 cm in greatest dimension
T_4	Tumor of any size with direct extension to (a) chest wall or (b) skin, only as described below
	T_{4a} Extension to chest wall, not including pectoralis muscle
	T_{4b} Edema (including peau d'orange) or ulceration of the skin of the breast, or satellite skin nodules confined to the same breast
	T_{4c} Both (T_{4a} and T_{4b})
	T_{4d} Inflammatory carcinoma (see section on Inflammatory Carcinoma)

Regional Lymph Nodes (N)

NX	Regional lymph nodes cannot be assessed (e.g., previously removed)
N_0	No regional lymph node metastasis
N_1	Metastasis in movable ipsilateral axillary lymph node(s)
N_2	Metastasis in ipsilateral axillary lymph node(s) fixed or matted, or in clinically apparent[a] ipsilateral internal mammary nodes in the absence of clinically evident axillary lymph node metastasis
	N_{2a} Metastasis in ipsilateral axillary lymph nodes fixed to one another (matted) or to other structures
	N_{2b} Metastasis only in clinically apparent[a] ipsilateral internal mammary nodes and in the absence of clinically evident axillary lymph node metastasis
N_3	Metastasis in ipsilateral infraclavicular lymph node(s), or in clinically apparent[a] ipsilateral internal mammary lymph node(s) and in the presence of clinically evident axillary lymph node metastasis; or metastasis in ipsilateral supraclavicular lymph node(s) with or without axillary or internal mammary lymph node involvement
	N_{3a} Metastasis in ipsilateral infraclavicular lymph node(s) and axillary lymph node(s)
	N_{3b} Metastasis in ipsilateral internal mammary lymph node(s) and axillary lymph node(s)
	N_{3c} Metastasis in ipsilateral supraclavicular lymph node(s)

Pathologic Classification (pN)

pNX	Regional lymph nodes cannot be assessed (e.g., previously removed, or not removed for pathologic study)
PN_0	No regional lymph node metastasis histologically, no additional examination for isolated tumor cells
	$PN_{0(i-)}$ No regional lymph node metastasis histologically, negative IHC
	$PN_{0(i+)}$ No regional lymph node metastasis histologically, positive IHC, no IHC cluster greater than 0.2 mm
	$PN_{0(mol-)}$ No regional lymph node metastasis histologically, negative molecular findings (RT-PCR)
	$PN_{0(mol+)}$ No regional lymph node metastasis histologically, positive molecular findings (RT-PCR)
	PN^{1mi} Micrometastasis (>0.2 mm, none >2.0 mm)
pN_1	Metastasis in one to three axillary lymph nodes and/or in internal mammary nodes with microscopic disease detected by sentinel lymph node dissection but not clinically apparent
	PN_{1a} Metastasis in one to three axillary lymph nodes
	PN_{1b} Metastasis in internal mammary nodes with microscopic disease detected by sentinel lymph node dissection but not clinically apparent
	PN_{1c} Metastasis in one to three axillary lymph nodes and in internal mammary lymph nodes with microscopic disease detected by sentinel lymph node dissection but not clinically apparent

(Continued)

Table 16.4 TNM (Tumor–Nodes–Metastases) System for Staging of Breast Cancer (*Continued*)

Pathologic Classification (pN)

pN_2	Metastasis in four to nine axillary lymph nodes, or in clinically apparent internal mammary lymph nodes in the absence of axillary lymph node metastasis
PN_{2a}	Metastasis in four to nine axillary lymph nodes (at least one tumor deposit >2.0 mm)
PN_{2b}	Metastasis in clinically apparent internal mammary lymph nodes in the absence of axillary lymph node metastasis

pN_3	Metastasis in 10 or more axillary lymph nodes, or in infraclavicular lymph nodes, or in clinically apparent ipsilateral internal mammary lymph nodes in the presence of one or more positive axillary lymph nodes; or in more than three axillary lymph nodes with clinically negative microscopic metastasis in internal mammary lymph nodes; or in ipsilateral supraclavicular lymph nodes
pN_{3a}	Metastasis in 10 or more axillary lymph nodes (at least one tumor deposit >2.0 mm), or metastasis to the infraclavicular lymph nodes
pN_{3b}	Metastasis in clinically apparent ipsilateral internal mammary lymph nodes in the presence of one or more positive axillary lymph nodes; or in more than three axillary lymph nodes and in internal mammary lymph nodes with microscopic disease detected by sentinel lymph node dissection but not clinically apparent
pN_{3c}	Metastasis in ipsilateral supraclavicular lymph nodes

Distant Metastasis (M)

MX	Distant metastasis cannot be assessed
M_0	No distant metastasis
M_1	Distant metastasis

Note: Paget's disease associated with a tumor is classified according to the size of the tumor.
IHC, immunohistochemistry; RT-PCR, reverse transcription—polymerase chain reaction.
[a]"clinically apparent" is defined as detected by imaging studies (excluding lymphoscintigraphy) or by clinical examination.
Used with the permission of the American Joint Committee on Cancer (AJCC), Chicago, IL. The original source for this material is the *AJCC Cancer Staging Manual,* 6th ed. New York: Springer-Verlag, 2002 (113).

Table 16.5 TNM (Tumor–Nodes–Metastases) Stage Grouping of Breast Cancer

Stage 0	T_{is}	N_0	M_0
Stage I	T_1[a]	N_0	M_0
Stage IIA	T_0	N_1	M_0
	T_1[a]	N_1	M_0
	T_2	N_0	M_0
Stage IIB	T_2	N_1	M_0
	T_3	N_0	M_0
Stage IIIA	T_0	N_2	M_0
	T_1[a]	N_2	M_0
	T_2	N_2	M_0
	T_3	N_1	M_0
	T_3	N_2	M_0
Stage III B	T_4	N_0	M_0
	T_4	N_1	M_0
	T_4	N_2	M_0
Stage IIIC	Any T	N_3	M_0
Stage IV	Any T	Any N	M_1

[a]T_1 includes T_{1mic}.

Used with the permission of the American Joint Committee on Cancer (AJCC), Chicago, IL. The original source for this material is the *AJCC Cancer Staging Manual,* 6th ed. New York: Springer-Verlag, 2002 (113).

preoperatively for clinical staging as well as postoperatively for pathologic staging. In the most recent AJCC staging revision, new areas are incorporated regarding evaluation of the axilla and prognostic factors: the number of positive axillary nodes; the method used for detection (clinical examination or sentinel node biopsy); and the presence of micrometastatic disease.

Preoperative Evaluation

The initial stage of the disease dictates the extent of the preoperative workup (114). According to the National Comprehensive Cancer Network, for most patients with TNM stage I or II disease (small tumors, no palpable lymph nodes, and no symptoms of metastases), the preoperative evaluation should consist of: (http://www.nccn.org).

1. History and physical examination
2. Diagnostic bilateral mammography
3. Complete blood count
4. Screening blood chemistry tests (including liver function tests)
5. Pathology review
6. Optional breast MRI
7. Chest x-ray (usually required for general anesthesia)

A routine bone scan, abdominal CT scan (to evaluate the liver), and chest CT imaging are not necessary unless symptoms or abnormal blood chemistry suggest bone, liver, or pulmonary metastases. Chest CT imaging should be included for any patient presenting with clinical stage III or IV disease. Although the NCCN guidelines for clinical stage III workup recommends a bone scan or abdominal CT scan only if dictated by symptoms or laboratory values, most physicians will obtain these studies in patients with locally advanced breast cancer. **Patients with clinical stage IV disease should have both a bone scan and abdominal CT scan;** if metastases are evident on imaging or there is obvious bone marrow dysfunction, most physicians will recommend a bone marrow biopsy for confirmation of bony metastatic disease. **Routine bone marrow biopsy is viewed by some to be an important prognostic test for staging breast cancer patients that may supplant axillary dissection** (115).

Positron emission tomography (PET) uses a glucose analog tracer, fluorodeoxyglucose (FDG), which is taken up by cells in proportion to the rate of glucose metabolism (116); malignant cells have increased glucose uptake in comparison to normal tissue. As of November 2004, the Centers for Medicare and Medicaid Services approved coverage for FDG-PET scanning in breast cancer for the following indications: (i) staging patients with distant metastasis; (ii) restaging patients with locoregional recurrence; or (iii) monitoring response to therapy in women with either metastasis or locally advanced breast cancer when a change in treatment is planned. **Currently, FDG-PET should be used as an adjunct to standard imaging modalities.** At this time, **FDG-PET is not recommended for axillary staging in patients with an initial diagnosis of breast cancer** because research studies have produced mixed results and FDG-PET cannot detect small metastases (i.e., <1 cm) (116–119).

Treatment of Breast Cancer

Surgery

The traditional treatment of breast cancer was primarily surgical but has evolved over the years to a multidisciplinary approach, requiring the collaborative effort of surgeons, pathologists, radiologists, oncologists, and others.

The modern era of breast surgery began with Halsted and the development of the **radical mastectomy,** based on his understanding of breast cancer as a locally infiltrative process that spread primarily via the lymphatics (120). The radical mastectomy involved resection of the entire breast with overlying skin, the underlying pectoral muscles, and the axillary lymph nodes in continuity 121 (Fig. 16.6). However, this initial operation was designed to treat patients with palpable axillary lymph nodes and locally advanced disease. Although effective in local control of the tumor, this surgery failed to cure many patients, most likely because of their advanced stage at presentation.

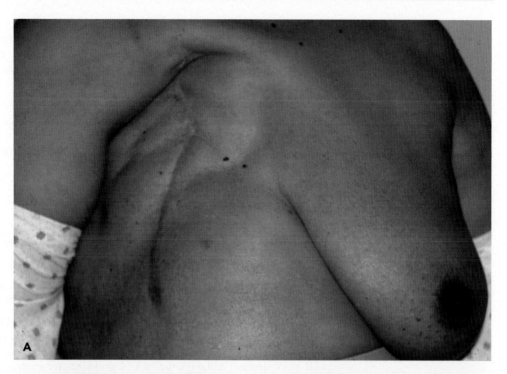

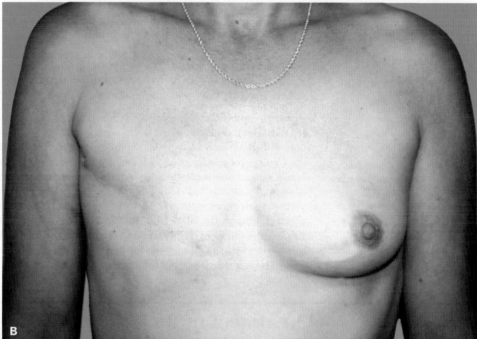

Figure 16.6 Defects after mastectomy (A) radical mastectomy (B) modified radical mastectomy.

During the 20th century, more extensive variations of the radical mastectomy were adopted in order to remove more regional tissue. Some of the variations included supraclavicular dissection (122) and supraclavicular, internal mammary, and mediastinal lymph node dissections, with resulting higher morbidity and mortality rates (123). The extended radical mastectomy, first described by Urban (124) added an *en bloc* internal mammary node dissection to the standard operation. This surgery did not improve survival rates but increased morbidity.

The **modified radical mastectomy (MRM) was gradually adopted as the operative treatment for invasive breast cancer when it was recognized that mortality after treatment was**

due to systemic dissemination of neoplastic cells before surgery rather than inadequate resection. In addition, MRM is functionally and cosmetically superior to more radical mastectomies. The MRM is similar to the radical mastectomy with complete removal of the breast and axillary nodes; however, there is less removal of the skin with no need for skin grafting, and the pectoralis muscles are preserved (Fig. 16.6B). The main advantage of the MRM is a better functional and cosmetic result.

Total or simple mastectomy is the removal of the entire breast, nipple, and areolar complex with preservation of the pectoralis muscles and axillary lymph nodes. Usually included in the specimen are the low-lying lymph nodes in the upper, outer portion of the breast and low axilla.

To refute the Halstedian concept that aggressive local control was necessary in the treatment of invasive breast cancer, the National Surgical Adjuvant Breast and Bowel Project (NSABP) B-04 study was a randomized trial comparing the Halsted mastectomy to less extensive surgery, with or without radiation therapy. In this trial, patients with clinically negative axillary nodes were randomly assigned to a radical mastectomy, total mastectomy with postoperative irradiation, or total mastectomy with delayed dissection if positive nodes developed. Patients with clinically positive axillary nodes were randomly assigned to radical mastectomy or total mastectomy with postoperative irradiation. After 25-year follow-up, there was no significant difference among the three groups of women with negative nodes or between the two groups of women with positive nodes with respect to disease-free survival, distant-disease free survival, or overall survival (125). Therefore, the **radical mastectomy was shown to have no advantage over total mastectomy in terms of local control or overall survival; in addition, the removal of lymph nodes was shown to have no effect on survival.**

Breast-Conserving Surgery

Breast-conserving surgery developed from the same desires as did the modified radical mastectomy: defining the extent of surgery required to treat invasive breast cancer without compromising outcome. One of the major goals of breast-conserving surgery is to preserve the cosmetic appearance of the breast. **Radiation therapy without surgical treatment was shown to result in high local failure rates** (126). Two pivotal prospective randomized trials compared standard surgery to a combination of less extensive surgery with or without radiation. In the **Milan study,** patients were randomly assigned to either (i) the standard Halsted radical mastectomy or (ii) quadrantectomy, axillary lymph node dissection (ALND), and postoperative radiation (127,128). **Patients with tumors less than or equal to 2 cm with clinically negative axillary nodes ($T_1N_0M_0$) were eligible for this trial;** the two groups (total of 701 women) were comparable (age, tumor size, menopausal status, nodal involvement) (128). **After 20 years of follow-up, there was no statistical significant difference between the two groups regarding contralateral breast cancer, second primary cancer, distant metastases, or overall survival (Table 16.6) (128); however there was a statistical difference of chest wall recurrences of 8.8% in the BCS group versus 2.3% in the radical mastectomy group.**

Table 16.6 Halsted Radical Mastectomy Versus Breast-Conserving Surgery: Results of 20-Year Follow-Up

	Halsted (%)	Quadrantectomy + RT (%)
No. of patients	349	352
Contralateral-breast carcinoma	9.7	8.2
Distant metastases	23.8	23.3
Other primary cancers	8.6	8.8
Overall survival	43.6	44.3

RT, radiation therapy.

From **Veronesi U, Cascinelli N, Mariani L, Greco M, Saccozzi R, Luini A, et al.** Twenty-year follow-up of a randomized study comparing breast-conserving surgery with radical mastectomy for early breast cancer. *N Engl J Med* 2002;347:1227–1232.

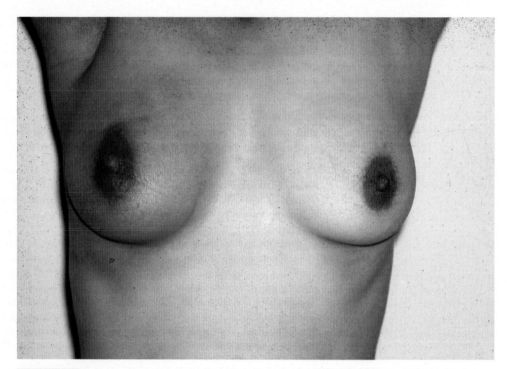

Figure 16.7 Appearance after lumpectomy, axillary dissection, and radiation therapy.

The NSABP conducted a similar trial, B-06 (129). Patients with tumors less than or equal to 4 cm either without palpable nodes or with palpable nonfixed axillary lymph nodes (i.e., stage I or II: T_1 or T_2, and N_0 or N_1) were eligible. Patients were assigned randomly to (i) the modified radical mastectomy (MRM); (ii) lumpectomy (segmental mastectomy) and ALND; or (iii) lumpectomy, ALND, and postoperative radiation therapy (Fig. 16.7). Tumor-free specimen margins were required to maintain eligibility. A total of 1,851 women were randomized among the three treatment arms, and the groups were comparable. **After 20-years of follow-up, the NSABP B-06 trial provides clear evidence that the combined lumpectomy, ALND, and postoperative radiation therapy is as effective as the modified radical mastectomy for the management of patients with early stage breast cancer** (130). Although there was no significant difference in overall survival among the three treatment arms, there were significant differences in local control. The in-breast recurrence rate for patients randomized to lumpectomy and radiation therapy was 14.3% versus 39.2% for patients randomized to lumpectomy alone. This trial also established the safety of breast-conserving surgery for early-stage breast cancer and showed the importance of postoperative radiation to reduce the risk of in-breast recurrences. The results of these trials led to a National Institute of Health (NIH) Consensus Conference in 1991 endorsing breast-conserving surgery as the preferred treatment for early-stage breast cancer (131).

Axillary Lymph Node Staging

Axillary nodal involvement remains the most significant prognostic factor for recurrence and survival for patients with early-stage breast cancer. Dissection of the axillary nodal basin provides excellent regional control if metastases are present, accurate prognostic information, and allows appropriate management decisions regarding additional therapy.

As part of breast-conserving surgery, the axillary dissection preferably is performed through a separate incision in the axilla. For accurate staging and the prevention of axillary recurrences in early-stage breast cancer, an NIH Consensus Development Conference concluded that removal of level I and II nodes should be routine (131). The three levels of nodes in the axilla are based on their relationship to the pectoralis minor muscle. Level I and II axillary dissection involves removal of all the fatty and lymph node-bearing tissue lateral and posterior to the medial border of the pectoralis minor muscle. It is very rare for so-called "skip metastases" to be present in the higher levels of the axilla without involvement of the lower levels (132). If palpable nodes are encountered medial to the pectoralis minor (level III) during surgery, a complete dissection involving all three levels should be performed, usually necessitating transection of the pectoralis minor muscle.

Although axillary nodal dissection is accurate for staging, there are known morbidities associated with the procedure such as paresthesias, wound complications, and lymphedema. The latter occurs in approximately 10% to 20% of patients. **Since the advent of mammography, breast cancer size and positive nodal involvement at diagnosis have been diminishing. Only 30% of breast cancer patients have involved axillary nodes detected by standard pathologic techniques** (42). This has led some authorities to question the value of routine ALND in patients with early stage breast cancer (42).

The technique of sentinel lymph node biopsy (SNB), a minimally invasive procedure, is based on the observation that specific areas drain via lymphatic channels to one or two primary nodes before involving other lymph nodes within a nodal basin. By injecting radioisotope and/or blue dye into the region of the tumor or under the areola and performing a limited axillary dissection, these primary or sentinel nodes can be identified either by visual inspection or by the use of a hand-held gamma counter. Only these sentinel nodes are removed and analyzed using routine hematoxylin and eosin (H&E) staining and/or immunohistochemistry (IHC) to identify small foci of metastases. When the H&E-stained slides are negative, most institutions perform IHC.

Studies have shown that if the sentinel node is free of tumor histopathologically, the rest of the axillary nodes are theoretically free of tumor, thereby avoiding the need for a complete ALND (133-135). In experienced hands the false-negative rate is low and can be nearly 0% with proper patient selection and adherence to technical detail (134). If the sentinel node is positive for metastases, then the standard treatment is to undergo complete axillary dissection of levels I and II.

In 2005, the American Society of Clinical Oncology (ASCO) published guideline recommendations for SNB in early-stage breast cancer (136). These guidelines were based on 69 studies in which SNB was compared to ALND. There was sufficient evidence to show that a negative sentinel lymph node (SLN) was predictive of negative axillary nodes for the panel to **recommend the use of SNB in early-stage breast cancer patients with clinically negative nodes, provided the procedure was performed by an experienced team.** The panel also recommended that suspicious palpable nodes found during dissection should be submitted as SLNs. Also advised was a completion ALND for any patient with SLN metastases including micrometastasis (>0.2 mm to <2.0 mm).

The panel also gave recommendations regarding the use of SNB in certain clinical circumstances. Regarding cases involving DCIS, the panel **recommended SNB for mastectomy patients with DCIS, in DCIS with microinvasion, or in cases with DCIS larger than 5 cm.** Although DCIS is noninvasive in nature, in 10% to 20% of patients diagnosed with DCIS by core biopsy, invasive disease will subsequently be found upon excision due to a sampling error (137). If invasion is discovered after a mastectomy, the opportunity to stage the axilla with SLND will be lost. Other special clinical circumstances in which SNB is recommended are (i) in elderly patients; (ii) obese patients; (iii) male patients;(iv) multicentric tumors; and (v) after prior excisional biopsy. **Scenarios in which SNB is not recommended include (i) patients with a clinically positive axilla (N_1); (ii) pregnant patients; (iii) prior axillary surgery; (iv) inflammatory breast cancer; (v) after preoperative systemic therapy; and (vi) in patients with tumors larger than 5 cm.**

There is increasing evidence supporting the use of SNB in some of these circumstances. There are limited reports of the safe use of radioisotopes in pregnant patients (138,139). However, a recent review concluded that SNB should not be offered to pregnant patients under 30 weeks' gestation (140).

Regarding the technical aspects of the procedure, the panel supports the Guidelines for Performance of Sentinel Lymphadenectomy for Breast Cancer developed by the American Society of Breast Surgeons (ASBS) (**http://www.breastsurgeons.org/officialstmts/sentinel.shtml**). The ASBS maintains that a SLN identification rate of 85% and a false-negative rate of 5% or less are necessary in order to abandon axillary dissection. The ASBS also recommends that surgeons perform a minimum of 20 SNB cases followed by completion ALND, or have proper mentoring, before relying on the procedure to avoid ALND. The ASCO panel points out that the lowest false-negative rates in general were obtained with the combined methods of isotope and blue dye, but do not believe that ASCO should present separate guidelines for the technical performance of the procedure.

Adjuvant Radiation Therapy

Adjuvant radiation after breast-conserving procedures is essential for the achievement of recurrence rates equivalent to those obtained with mastectomy. Radiation therapy, when combined with radical surgery, improves local control, but overall survival rates are not affected (129,130,141). In B-06, the in-breast recurrence rate for patients randomized to lumpectomy and radiation therapy was 14.3% versus 39.2% for patients randomized to lumpectomy alone.

Although overall survival rates were not different between patients who were treated with BCS and those treated with more extensive mastectomies, as shown in B-06 and the Milan Group study, some small randomized trials have shown small but clinically relevant differences in survival. Pooled analyses of multiple trials, or meta-analyses, can often provide enough statistical power to detect these small differences. **In 2005, the Early Breast Cancer Trialists' Collaborative Group (EBCTCG) presented the findings from 78 randomized clinical trials evaluating the extent of surgery and the use of radiation** (142). This large meta-analysis investigated the effect of local recurrence on breast cancer mortality by analyzing data on 42,000 women, divided into groups based on a 5-year local recurrence risk, whether the risk was <10% or exceeded 10%. **This study was able to show that improved local control with radiotherapy at 5 years resulted in significant improvement in breast cancer survival at 15 years: For every four local recurrences that could be avoided over 15 years,** one breast cancer death would be avoided. Local treatments to improve local control had the greatest effects in the patients who were at greatest risk for local recurrence.

Postoperative radiation therapy is recommended as part of BCS to reduce local recurrence rates; however, there are also indications for its use in post-mastectomy patients who are at higher risk for locoregional failure. Studies, some included in the EBCTCG overview analysis, have shown that the risk of locoregional failure is reduced and disease-specific survival is improved by post-mastectomy radiotherapy (PMRT) (111, 143–145). A literature review recommended post-mastectomy radiation for women with greater than 4 positive nodes and women with tumors greater than 5 cm in diameter (146). The review concluded that there was insufficient evidence at this time for post mastectomy radiation for patients with high-risk, node-negative disease, including premenopausal women with tumors greater than 2 cm in diameter, evidence of vascular invasion, invasion of the skin or pectoral fascia, or close/positive margins.

Clinical trials evaluating breast-conserving surgery and intraoperative radiation therapy (IORT) for localized breast cancer are ongoing (147). The rationale for IORT is based on the desire to minimize length of treatment and the finding that 85% of recurrent breast cancer is confined to the same quadrant of breast as the primary tumor. The use of IORT requires wide mobilization of the breast tissue and can prolong operative times. Whether the therapeutic effect of IORT is equivalent to traditional whole breast radiation therapy remains to be determined.

Accelerated Partial Breast Irradiation (APBI)   The observation that most recurrences after breast-conserving surgery occur in close proximity to the surgical site led to investigation into the delivery of radiation therapy only to the lumpectomy cavity and the immediately adjacent tissue over a shortened period of time, referred to as **accelerated partial-breast irradiation** (148,149). Results from studies using interstitial catheter brachytherapy to deliver APBI have shown good local tumor control rates, but the technique can be cumbersome and difficult to learn. **The MammoSite balloon catheter was developed as a single catheter delivery device** that allows a shorter period of radiation treatment, usually 5 days instead of 5 to 6 weeks, as an alternative to external beam radiation or seed brachytherapy. **The balloon catheter is placed in the lumpectomy cavity** and filled with saline/contrast. Before treatment is initiated, the position of the balloon is checked to ensure adequate conformity to the lumpectomy cavity. The radiation source is advanced into the catheter and radiation therapy is delivered twice a day for five days. The radiation source is removed between treatments. After completion of therapy, the balloon catheter is removed.

The ASBS recommendations for eligibility criteria are age greater than 45, invasive ductal carcinoma or DCIS, tumor size of 3 cm or less, negative microscopic surgical margins and negative nodal status (**http://www.breastsurgeons.org.apbi.shtml**). Additional factors to be considered for MammoSite use are adequate skin-spacing (usually 7 mm) and catheter conformity to surgical cavity. **Early results have been promising with 5-year local recurrence rates comparable**

to those achieved with conventional whole-breast radiation, with decreased toxicity and good to excellent cosmetic results in the majority of patients (150–151). Randomized studies currently in progress will determine the role of accelerated partial breast irradiation.

Adjuvant Systemic Therapy

Patients may have clinically undetectable systemic micrometastases during primary surgery that are responsible for later recurrences, as evidenced by the lower survival rates for women with metastatic nodal disease. The objective of systemic adjuvant therapy is to control microscopic disease, reduce the risk of recurrence and improve long-term survival.

The results of many well-designed, randomized trials support the use of adjuvant systemic therapy, with reductions demonstrated in recurrence rates and breast cancer mortality. These reductions are most evident when data from various trials are pooled together and analyzed, such as in The Early Breast Cancer Trialists' Collaborative Group (EBCTCG) overview (152).

Adjuvant Systemic Chemotherapy

In the 2005 EBCTCG overview, meta-analyses were initiated on 194 randomized trials of adjuvant chemotherapy or hormonal therapy that began in 1995. Many of the trials involved *anthracycline*-based combinations, *cyclophosphamide, methotrexate,* and *5-fluorouracil,* (CMF) *tamoxifen,* or ovarian suppression. None of the trials involved the newer agents such as *taxanes, raloxifene, trastuzumab,* or *aromatase* inhibitors.

There was a significant reduction in the annual breast cancer death rate for patients allocated to a 6-month regimen of *anthracycline*-based polychemotherapy (primarily *doxorubicin* or *epirubicin*), which was independent of the use of *tamoxifen,* nodal status, estrogen-receptor (ER) status, or other tumor characteristics. The benefits were greater in younger women, with reductions in annual breast cancer death rates of 38% for women diagnosed under the age of 50 and 20% for women aged 50-69 years. The *anthracycline* regimens were also more effective than the CMF regimens, with moderate, but highly significant reductions in the annual recurrence rate of 11% ($p = 0.001$) and annual breast cancer death rate of 16% ($p < 0.00001$). **Four cycles of *doxorubicin* and *cyclophosphamide* (AC) have been shown to have an equivalent disease-free survival and overall survival to six months of traditional CMF in two NSABP trials (B-15 and B-23)** (153,154).

Newer chemotherapeutic agents have emerged as effective adjuvant systemic therapies for breast cancer, most notably, members of the *taxane* family, **including *paclitaxel (Taxol)* and *docetaxel (Taxotere)*.** The *taxanes* have been shown to have good activity in patients with metastatic breast cancer and are not cross-resistant to *anthracyclines.* For these reasons, the NSABP B-28 trial and other similar large, randomized trials have been conducted to evaluate the efficacy of the *taxanes.* Results from NASBP B-28 demonstrated that the addition of *paclitaxel* after *AC* resulted in a significant improvement in disease-free survival, but not overall survival (155). By contrast, both disease-free and overall survival rates were improved in node-positive patients who were randomized to receive *AC* in combination with sequential *paclitaxel* compared with *AC* alone in a large, cooperative, randomized study (156). **Early results from studies suggest that the combination of *docetaxel* and *cyclophosphamide* (TC) is associated with a superior disease-free survival than *AC* for patients with stage I-III breast cancer** (157). **Dose-dense regimens,** in which chemotherapeutic agents are given every 2 weeks with granulocyte colony-stimulating factor support rather than every 3 weeks, **have also been shown to improve clinical outcomes significantly** (158). These studies demonstrate that *taxanes* are valuable components of adjuvant chemotherapy for patients with early-stage breast cancer.

Amplification of the HER-2/*neu* gene, a member of the tyrosine-kinase pathway family, or overexpression of the HER-2/*neu* protein occurs in approximately 15% to 25% of breast cancers and is associated with aggressive tumor behavior (159). *Trastuzumab* **(Herceptin)** is a humanized monoclonal antibody against the HER-2/*neu* growth factor receptor which has been shown to have clinical activity in women with metastatic HER-2/*neu* positive breast cancer (160). **The Herceptin Adjuvant (HERA) Trial is** a large international, intergroup study to investigate whether the administration of *trastuzumab* is effective as adjuvant therapy for HER-2/*neu* positive breast cancer after surgical treatment and completion of chemotherapy (161). Interim analysis at one year indicated a significant reduction in disease-free survival events by almost half (48%, $p < 0.0001$) with an absolute benefit in disease-free survival of 8.4% at two years. **At two-year analysis, a significant survival benefit was seen with a 34% reduction in the risk of death with *trastuzumab* therapy given for one year** (162).

The available data from the EBCTCG overview support chemotherapy as adjuvant treatment for early breast cancer (152). However, some women will only derive a small benefit from such a regimen at the cost of excessive morbidity. A number of prognostic factors are used to predict the risk of future recurrence or death from breast cancer, factors including patient age, tumor size, number of involved axillary nodes, and HER-2-*neu* status (discussed below). One validated computer-based model (**Adjuvant! Online; http://www.adjuvantonline.com**) is available to the clinician to estimate 10-year disease-free and overall survival incorporating the above-mentioned prognostic factors in addition to patient comorbidity and tumor grade; HER-2/*neu* status is not included. The estimates for recurrence and death vary based on various treatment options from no additional therapy to the most aggressive form of polychemotherapy.

Although chemotherapy has been shown to benefit women with node-negative, estrogen-receptor-positive disease in large clinical trials such as NSABP B-14 and B-20 trials (163,164), there are many patients who would not derive much additional benefit from adjuvant chemotherapy and would in fact be over treated.

Two gene-based approaches are also available to the clinician to aid in determining those most likely to benefit from additional chemotherapy. One such tool is a 21-gene assay using reverse transcription polymerase chain reaction on RNA isolated from paraffin-embedded breast cancer tissue (**OncotypeDx**) (165). **This tool is able to quantify the 10-year risk of recurrence in *tamoxifen*-treated patients with node-negative, estrogen-receptor positive disease.** Women are given a recurrence score and stratified according to risk levels: low, intermediate and high. Another microarray-based tool analyzes a 70-gene expression profile from frozen breast tissue to predict those early-stage breast cancer patients who are more likely to develop distant recurrence (**Mammaprint**) (166).

Adjuvant Hormone Therapy

In the EBCTCG overview, the effects of hormonal therapy for early breast cancer on recurrence and 15-year survival were investigated (152). **For women with estrogen-receptor (ER) positive disease, adjuvant *tamoxifen* given for 5 years reduced the annual breast cancer rate by 31% independent of patient age, use of chemotherapy, or other tumor characteristics.** *Tamoxifen* therapy for 5 years was significantly more effective than only 1 or 2 years of therapy. **Among women with ER-positive disease who were allocated to 5 years of *tamoxifen*, there was a 41% reduction in the annual recurrence rate.** Most of the effect on recurrence was seen during the first 5 years; however, most of the effect on breast cancer mortality was seen after this time period.

For years, *tamoxifen* was the gold standard of hormonal therapy for patients with breast cancer. *Aromatase* inhibitors (AI) were first studied in the metastatic setting for postmenopausal women with hormone-receptor positive disease (122,167). These agents act to markedly reduce the circulating estrogen levels in postmenopausal women. In 1996, a randomized double-blind multicenter trial was initiated to investigate the efficacy of the *AI, anastrozole* (**Arimidex**) in the adjuvant setting. **The trial known as Arimidex, Tamoxifen, Alone or in Combination (ATAC)** compared *tamoxifen* with Arimidex alone and in combination with *tamoxifen* as adjuvant endocrine therapy for postmenopausal patients with operable, invasive, early stage (stage I and II) breast cancer. **Results of the ATAC trial demonstrated *Arimidex* to be better tolerated and more effective in improving disease-free survival and time to recurrence than *tamoxifen* after median follow-up of 100 months** (168). There was a yearly increased fracture episode rate with *anastrozole* over *tamoxifen* (2.93% versus 1.90%, respectively), but this effect did not continue after therapy was completed. **None of the known associated risks of *tamoxifen*, thromboembolism, endometrial cancer, or vaginal bleeding, were seen with *anastrazole*.**

Other *aromatase* inhibitors, such as *letrozole* (Femara), and *exemestane* (Aromasin), are additional alternatives for postmenopausal patients with hormone-sensitive breast cancer. In 2004, ASCO published a status report on the use of *aromatase* inhibitors as adjuvant therapy (169). Based on the results of multiple large randomized trials, the ASCO practice guidelines recommend incorporating *aromatase* inhibitors into adjuvant regimens. AIs are also recommended as initial treatment for women intolerant of *tamoxifen*. Conversely, women intolerant of *AIs* should receive *tamoxifen*. Additionally, **women with hormone receptor-negative tumors should not receive adjuvant hormonal therapy.**

Endocrine therapy in combination with chemotherapy further increases the relative benefits. ***Anthracycline*-based chemotherapy reduces 15-year mortality rates for women with**

Table 16.7 Prognostic Factors in Node-Negative Breast Cancers	
Factor	Increased Risk of Recurrence
Size	Larger tumors
Histologic grade	High-grade tumors
DNA ploidy	Aneuploid tumors
Labeling index	High index (>3%)
S-phase fraction	High fraction (>5%)
Lymphatic/vascular invasion	Present
p53 tumor suppressor gene	High expression
HER-2/neu oncogene expression	High expression
Epidermal growth factor	High levels
Angiogenesis	High microvessel density

ER-positive disease (the most common form of breast cancer). The 2005 meta-analysis demonstrated that **5 years of** *tamoxifen* **after** *anthracycline*-**based chemotherapy further reduced the 15-year mortality rates;** for patients with ER-positive disease and age less than 50, the final mortality reduction was almost 60% and for patients aged 50–69, the reduction in mortality was almost cut in half (152). The authors suggested that the effects might even have been stronger had there been full compliance with the allocated treatments.

In practice, oncologists are using systemic adjuvant therapy for most patients with early-stage breast cancer >1 cm and patients with nodal disease. Factors that determine the patient's risk of recurrence are tumor size, ER and PR status, HER-2/*neu* status, nuclear grade, histologic type, and proliferative rate (170–172). Other biochemical and biologic factors such as ploidy, S-phase fraction, and cathepsin D levels appear to have some prognostic significance (Table 16.7), especially in node-negative patients **(170). The NCCN guidelines recommend considering OncotypeDx testing in cases of tumors 0.6 cm to 1.0 cm with unfavorable features and in certain cases of tumors >1 cm.** OncotypeDx testing is best used in patients who would receive questionable benefit from the addition of chemotherapy. In patients with large tumors or tumors with aggressive features, such as HER-2/*neu* over-expression, the decision to offer adjuvant chemotherapy is obvious without the need for further testing. Patients with nodal disease should be considered for adjuvant chemotherapy. Most patients with tumors larger than 0.5 cm (or larger than 1 cm in the cases of tubular or mucinous tumors) and positive ER status should be offered hormonal therapy. Table 16.7 summarizes these prognostic factors and their effect on recurrence (170–172).

To aid in the discussion with patients regarding the use of adjuvant therapy, risk reductions in breast cancer mortality should be translated into absolute benefits by calculating the number of deaths avoided per 100 women (173). For instance, if the 10-year risk of death from breast cancer is 10%, and if adjuvant chemotherapy reduces the mortality rate by 30%, the absolute increase in the number of patients alive will be three per one hundred treated. On the other hand, if the 10-year risk of death is 50%, the same proportional reduction in mortality would mean 15 extra lives saved.

The current recommendations for adjuvant chemotherapy and hormonal therapy in breast cancer can be summarized as follows (Table 16.8):

1. **Premenopausal women who have ER-negative tumors should be treated with adjuvant chemotherapy.**
2. **Premenopausal women with ER-positive tumors should be treated with hormonal therapy (*tamoxifen*) in addition to chemotherapy.**
3. **Postmenopausal patients who have negative lymph nodes and positive hormone receptor levels should be treated with adjuvant endocrine therapy (preferably *aromatase* inhibitors) or both chemotherapy and endocrine therapy. Those with positive lymph nodes should receive both endocrine therapy and chemotherapy.**

Table 16.8 Summary of Adjuvant Systemic Therapy for Women With Breast Cancer			
Patient Age	Estrogen-Receptor Status	Level of Risk	Adjuvant Systemic Therapy
<50 years	Negative	Any	Chemotherapy
	Positive	Low	Hormonal therapy or Chemotherapy or Chemotherapy and hormonal therapy
	Positive	Moderate or high	Chemotherapy and hormonal therapy or Investigational therapies
	Unknown	Any	Chemotherapy and hormonal therapy
≥50 years	Negative	Any	Chemotherapy
	Positive	Low	Tamoxifen or Chemotherapy and hormonal therapy
	Positive	Moderate or high	Chemotherapy and hormonal therapy or Investigational therapies
	Unknown	Any	Chemotherapy and hormonal therapy

aChemotherapy consists of *fluorouracil, doxorubicin,* and *cyclophosphamide* (FAC); *doxorubicin* and *cyclophosphamide (AC);* or *cyclophosphamide, methotrexate,* and *fluorouracil* (CMF). Hormonal therapy consists of *tamoxifen* or ovarian ablation (either surgical or chemical). From **Hortobagyi GN.** Drug therapy: treatment of breast cancer. *N Engl J Med* 1998;339:974–984. Copyright ©1998. Massachusetts Medical Society. All rights reserved.

4. **Postmenopausal women who have negative hormone receptor levels may be treated with adjuvant chemotherapy.**

5. **All women with invasive breast cancer and HER-2/*neu* over-expression should undergo chemotherapy treatment with trastuzumab.**

In spite of all of the evidence, the decision for adjuvant therapy resides with a well-educated and well-informed patient.

Metastatic Disease

Although the natural history of breast cancer can involve metastases to any organ, 85% of women with metastatic breast cancer have involvement of bone, lungs, or liver (174), with bone as the most common site. Bone metastases can give rise to pathologic fractures and/or hypercalcemia.

Treatment for metastatic disease may include surgery (if locally recurrent disease), chemotherapy, hormonal therapy, and radiation treatment if indicated. There are therapeutic regimens specific to each site of metastases. Work-up for metastatic disease is also tailored to specific complaints. If any one site is involved, metastases in other organs are highly likely which requires careful detailed work-up. The initial work-up for patients presenting with recurrent or stage IV disease should include liver function tests, chest imaging, bone scan, x-rays of symptomatic bones, biopsy documentation of first recurrence if possible, and possible CT scan/PET imaging and/or MRI. Whether a patient received prior chemotherapy or endocrine therapy also determines future treatment options. **For patients with systemic recurrence of breast cancer, cure is no longer possible and the goal of treatment is to prolong survival without jeopardizing quality of life.**

The treatment algorithm and various therapeutic options in metastatic breast disease are complex; to discuss them in any great detail is beyond the scope of this chapter, however, a few notable therapies will be addressed.

Bisphosphonates

According to the NCCN guidelines for recurrent or metastatic breast cancer, patients are initially stratified according to the presence or absence of bony metastases. The two subsets of patients are then further stratified by HER-2/*neu* and hormone receptor status. **Women with bone metastasis, especially with lytic lesions, should be offered a bisphosphonate with calcium and vitamin D**. The use of bisphosphonates in this setting has no impact on overall survival but is of value in that it provides supportive care (175).

Hormonal Therapies

Metastatic disease may respond to hormonal manipulation. The latter may involve ovarian ablative surgery, radiation, (not frequently used), chemical ablation, drugs that block synthesis of hormones, or drugs that block hormonal receptor sites (176). The usual course of metastatic disease is progression after initial response to hormonal therapy, indicating the drug is no longer effective. Sequential therapy using other drugs is instituted in a stepwise fashion with responses typically diminishing with each new line of therapy. Even patients with ER/PR negative disease who have metastasis limited to bone or soft tissue may be considered for a trial of endocrine therapy, but the response rate is extremely low. Women with bulky, progressive visceral metastases should receive initial cytotoxic chemotherapy, not hormonal therapy even if ER-positive.

In premenopausal patients, who progress on *tamoxifen*, the preferred second-line therapy is oophorectomy, radiation, or chemical ovarian ablation using a luteinizing hormone-releasing hormone (LHRH) agonist, such as *goserelin (Zoladex)*. The combination of *tamoxifen* and *goserelin* has been shown in a meta-analysis of four randomized trials to provide a significant survival and progression-free benefit, with a 30% reduction in the risk of an event with the combined therapy (177). Premenopausal women with ER-positive disease who have undergone ovarian ablation/suppression should be treated following postmenopausal guidelines.

Many postmenopausal women with hormone-receptor positive breast cancer benefit from sequential endocrine therapies. There are several *aromatase* inhibitors that are effective and well tolerated in metastatic disease, such as ***anastrozole (Arimidex), letrozole (Femara) or exemestane (Aromasin). Fulvestrant (Faslodex)*** is a new estrogen receptor antagonist that down-regulates the ER and has none of the estrogen agonist effects of *tamoxifen* (i.e., endometrial proliferation). It is indicated for postmenopausal patients with metastatic breast cancer previously treated with an antiestrogen, who progress on therapy. *Fulvestrant* appears to be at least as effective as *anastrozole* for the second-line treatment of patients with metastatic breast cancer (178).

Targeted Therapies

Patients who have **HER-2/*neu*** positive metastatic disease may benefit from treatment with ***trastuzumab*** as a single agent or ***lapatinib (Tykerb)*** in combination with ***capecitabine (Xeloda)***, an oral form of *5-FU* (179). ***Lapatinib***, also an oral agent, is a tyrosine kinase inhibitor of HER-2/*neu* and epidermal growth factor receptor. In a phase III open-label trial, **the combination of *lapatinib* plus *capecitabine* was superior to *capecitabine* alone in women with HER-2-positive metastatic breast cancer that had progressed after therapies including *trastuzumab*, *anthracycline* and a *taxane*** (179). Time to progression was increased by 50% in patients receiving combination therapy, with median time to progression of 8.4 months compared to 4.4 months with *capecitabine* alone.

Other Breast Diseases

Preinvasive (*In Situ*) Breast Carcinoma

Both lobular and ductal carcinomas may be confined by the basement membrane of the ducts or lobules. These preinvasive cancers by definition do not invade the surrounding tissue and, in theory, lack the ability to spread. The goal of treatment for pure *in situ* disease is preventing invasive disease from occurring or diagnosing developing invasive disease that is localized to the breast. If microinvasion or invasion is found on pathologic review, re-excision, or mastectomy, then the patient should be treated appropriately for invasive disease.

Lobular Carcinoma In Situ (LCIS)   LCIS is typically an incidental finding at biopsy for a mass, or mammographic abnormality unrelated to the LCIS. The true incidence of LCIS is unknown due to the lack of clinical and mammographic signs. Most cases occur in premenopausal women. **It is viewed as a marker of increased risk for breast cancer, not limited to the side involved with LCIS.** Most subsequent cancers that develop are invasive ductal carcinomas, with infiltrating lobular carcinomas representing the minority. The risk of developing invasive cancer is approximately 1% annually, a risk which indefinitely persists (136,137).

Biopsy-proven LCIS is usually managed after biopsy with surveillance by careful observation, clinical breast examination bi-annually, and yearly mammography and possibly breast MRI. **Patients should be informed that they have a higher risk for development of invasive breast cancer, and bilateral prophylactic mastectomy should be considered in certain cases such as in women with strong family histories of breast cancer or women with a *BRCA 1/2* mutation.**

Tamoxifen **is approved by the Food and Drug Administration (FDA) as a chemopreventive in women with LCIS.** In the NSABP P-1 Study, women at an increased risk for breast cancer were given *tamoxifen* as a chemopreventive agent for 5 years. Women with LCIS who took *tamoxifen* had over a 50% reduction in the occurrence of invasive cancer compared to women in the placebo group. Women who are found to have LCIS on biopsy should be counseled regarding chemoprevention (see below) (180).

Ductal Carcinoma In Situ   **Ductal carcinoma *in situ* typically occurs in postmenopausal women.** The incidence of ductal carcinoma *in situ* has increased by a factor of 10 in two decades since the implementation of mammography as a screening tool (181). The incidence has increased from approximately 5,000 cases annually in the 1980s to more than 50,000 cases annually currently (39). Mammographically, DCIS typically appears as a cluster of branched or Y-shaped microcalcifications, although it sometimes presents as a palpable mass. DCIS is characterized by a clonal proliferation of malignant epithelial cells that do not invade beyond the basement membrane.

Unlike patients with LCIS, **30% to 60% of patients with DCIS will develop invasive cancer in the same breast when treated with excisional biopsy alone** (182). Axillary metastases occur in fewer than 5% of patients. The occurrence of metastases indicates that an invasive component has been missed on biopsy. **Approximately 15% to 20% of patients with DCIS diagnosed with initial core-needle biopsy will be upstaged during excision due to the discovery of infiltrating ductal carcinoma** (137).

For years the standard treatment for DCIS was total mastectomy. Currently, most women in the United States with ductal carcinoma *in situ* are treated with breast-conserving surgery owing to the shift toward this approach for invasive cancer (181). However, there have been no randomized trials comparing mastectomy with breast-conserving surgery for DCIS.

The NSABP B-17 randomized trial compared lumpectomy with or without postoperative radiation for DCIS. After 8 years of follow-up, the overall recurrence rate for either DCIS or invasive carcinoma in the ipsilateral breast was reduced by more than half, from 26.8% to 12.1% in the patients who received radiation (183). The benefit of radiation was greatest for recurrent invasive carcinoma, with an 8-year reduction from 13.4% to 3.9%. The benefit of radiation was seen with all patient subgroups, including those with small nonpalpable tumors detected by mammography.

The NSABP-24 randomized clinical trial evaluated adjuvant *tamoxifen* therapy in addition to lumpectomy and radiation. The trial involved 1,800 women with DCIS who were randomly assigned to lumpectomy and radiation therapy, followed by 5 years of *tamoxifen* or placebo. **After 7 years of follow-up, the addition of tamoxifen significantly reduced the rate of all breast cancer events** (ipsilateral and contralateral, *in situ* and invasive) by 39%, from 16% in the placebo group to 10% in the *tamoxifen* group ($p = 0.0003$) (184).

Paget's Disease

Paget's disease of the breast, first described in 1874, is a rare manifestation of breast cancer with associated nipple changes similar to eczema, with itching and ulceration (185). Characteristic large cells with irregular nuclei, called **Paget's cells,** invade the nipple and surrounding areola. There is debate as to the origin of Paget's cells: either the cells originate from underlying carcinoma in the breast and then migrate into the major ducts of the nipple–areolar complex, or the cells originate in the epidermis. Initially there may be no visible changes with invasion of the nipple. Patients often notice a nipple discharge, a combination of serum and blood from the involved ducts. Paget's disease is often mistaken for a dermatitis, which can lead to a delay in diagnosis.

The underlying malignancy determines the overall prognosis for patients with Paget's disease. Paget's associated with DCIS alone has a very favorable prognosis, whereas those cases with infiltrating ductal carcinoma and involved lymph nodes do poorly.

Traditional treatment has been total mastectomy and lymph node dissection, although breast-conserving surgery is being performed at some institutions. Results of studies of breast-conserving surgery have generally been translated to the treatment of Paget's disease with underlying DCIS only. One small study treated patients with Paget's disease presenting without a palpable mass or radiographic abnormality with segmentectomy of the nipple–areolar complex followed by radiotherapy. The local control rate at 10 and 15 years was 87%, with a cause-specific survival of 97% (186). Another single institutional study showed breast-conserving surgery in Paget's cases to be equivalent to mastectomy regarding recurrence-specific, disease-specific, and overall survival with proper patient selection (187).

Inflammatory Carcinoma

Inflammatory breast carcinoma (IBC) is a rare but aggressive form of breast cancer, characterized by the rapid onset of inflammation of the breast with accompanying redness, warmth and edema. The differential diagnosis includes mastitis and cellulitis of the breast. The distinguishing pathologic finding associated with IBC is metastatic invasion of the dermal and subdermal lymphatics. However, **the diagnosis of IBC is primarily clinical** and absence of lymphatic invasion does not exclude the diagnosis. **Mammographically, the breast shows skin thickening with an infiltrative process.** Often there is no detectable palpable mass because the tumor, which is often very poorly differentiated, infiltrates through the breast with ill-defined margins. According to the AJCC staging guidelines, 6th edition, (113) (Tables 16.4 and 16.5), even if no mass is apparent, IBC by definition is classified a T4d lesion (the primary tumor size). Then, depending on the degree of nodal involvement and presence of distant metastasis, patients with IBC are staged as stage IIIb, IIIc, or IV.

The initial step in management is a skin biopsy with excision of a small portion of underlying tissue, followed by complete staging with diagnostic labs, bilateral mammograms (± ultrasound), bone scan, CT imaging, and optional breast MRI. **Primary surgical treatment in the face of inflammatory carcinoma is associated with high local failure rates and survival is not improved. The treatment of IBC involves a combined-modality approach using chemotherapy, radiation therapy, and at times surgery.** If a good response is achieved with induction chemotherapy, one of the combined-modality options includes a modified radical mastectomy with postoperative radiation therapy to the chest wall, internal mammary nodes, and supraclavicular nodes, followed by additional chemotherapy (188). If there is no response to induction chemotherapy, mastectomy is not recommended. Despite the improvements in IBC treatment, **the prognosis for patients with IBC remains poor.**

Future Fertility

Approximately 25% of breast cancer cases occur in premenopausal women (189). For premenopausal women diagnosed with breast cancer, counseling regarding future childbearing is important. Infertility can be a significant problem for those patients treated with adjuvant systemic chemotherapy and endocrine therapy. In premenopausal patients, the rates of amenorrhea may be as high as 40% to 70% (190). Even if amenorrhea resolves and patients resume menstrual cycles, **many cancer survivors have limited ovarian reserve** with significantly reduced ability to become pregnant (191).

It is important to discuss fertility preservation for patients, if desired by the patient. In the recommendations set forth by ASCO, the only option not considered experimental is to undergo a cycle of ovarian stimulation, oocyte retrieval, and creation of embryos for cryopreservation and subsequent *in vitro* fertilization before starting chemotherapy (192). Another option, not as successful as *in vitro* fertilization, but which is rapidly gaining popularity, is **cyropreservation of oocytes. For** breast cancer survivors, there can be concern about the risk of recurrence due to the high levels of circulating hormones during a subsequent pregnancy. Epidemiologic data have not found a detrimental effect of subsequent pregnancy after treatment of breast cancer, even if conception takes place six months after therapy (193).

Prognosis

The most reliable predictor of survival for patients with breast cancer is the stage of disease at the time of diagnosis. Based on recent data collected on women diagnosed with breast cancer from 1995 to 1998 from the American College of Surgeons National Cancer Data Base, **the 5-year survival rates for stage I disease is almost 100%.** For patients with stage IIA disease, prognosis is favorable with a 5-year survival rate of 92%, and 82% for those with stage IIB disease. As the level of nodal involvement increases and/or tumor size increases, the survival rates are lower. Patients with stage IIIA breast cancer have a 5-year survival rate of 67%, stage IIIB 54% and those with distant metastasis, stage IV, have a 20% 5-year survival rate.

As primary components of staging, **two significant prognostic indicators are the presence or absence of axillary nodal involvement and tumor size** (170,171). **Histologic subtype is also a prognostic factor;** certain subtypes of breast cancer have more favorable prognosis, such as tubular or mucinous (106,107). Nuclear grade, lymphovascular invasion, younger age at diagnosis, and proliferation indices such as mitotic index, S-phase fraction, Ki-67 have all been shown to be of prognostic significance in breast cancer (170,171,194–197).

The presence of estrogen and progesterone receptors (ER/PR-positive) may indicate less aggressive disease, although these factors are more predictive than prognostic. The main utility of these factors is in determining which patients should receive hormonal therapy. Her-2/*neu* oncogene amplification is associated with more aggressive disease, and its presence in an invasive breast cancer indicates that *trastuzumab* therapy would be of benefit.

Chemoprevention

In an NSABP trial of adjuvant *tamoxifen* for breast cancer, *tamoxifen* was found to decrease the incidence of contralateral breast cancers as a secondary end point (198). As a consequence, the NSABP conducted a randomized, controlled trial, the Breast Cancer Prevention Trial (BCPT), which investigated the efficacy of *tamoxifen* as a chemopreventive agent in women who were at high risk for breast cancer based on their risk profile. **With over 13,000 women enrolled, the group of women who received *tamoxifen* for 5 years experienced a 50% reduction in both noninvasive and invasive breast cancers compared with those women taking a placebo** (199). Offsetting these benefits were a 2- to 3-fold increase in the risk of endometrial cancer as well as increased risk of deep venous thrombosis, particularly in postmenopausal women.

Raloxifene, **a second-generation selective estrogen receptor modulator,** has been used for the prevention of osteoporosis in postmenopausal women. It exhibits antiestrogenic properties in the breast and possibly in the endometrium, as well as protective, estrogenic properties in the bone. Secondary endpoints from studies of *raloxifene* demonstrated its ability to reduce the risk of invasive breast cancer. This led to the development of the multicenter, randomized, double-blind trial named **Study of *Tamoxifen* and *Raloxifene* (STAR)** NSABP P-2 to directly compare the effectiveness of *raloxifene* with that of *tamoxifen* in postmenopausal women who are at increased risk for developing breast cancer (200,201). **Initial results show that *raloxifene* is as effective as *tamoxifen* in reducing the risk of invasive breast cancer and has a lower risk of thromboembolic events and cataracts (202).**

References

1. **Semiglazov VF, Moiseyenko VM, Bavli JL, Migmanova NS, Seleznyou NK, Popova RT, et al.** The role of breast self-examination in early breast cancer detection (results of the 5-years USSR/WHO randomized study in Leningrad). *Eur J Epidemiol* 1992;8:498–502.
2. **Thomas DB, Gao DL, Ray RM, Wang WW, Allison CJ, Chen FL, et al.** Randomized trial of breast self-examination in Shanghai: final results. *J Natl Cancer Inst* 2002;94:1445–1457.
3. **Berry DA, Cronin KA, Plevritis SK, Fryback DG, Clarke L, Zelen M, et al.** Effect of screening and adjuvant therapy on mortality from breast cancer. *N Engl J Med* 2005;353:1784–1792.
4. **Hendrick RE, Smith RA, Rutledge JH, Smart CR.** Benefit of screening mammography in women aged 40–49: a new meta-analysis of randomized controlled trials. *J Natl Cancer Inst Monogr* 1997;22:87–92.
5. **Larsson LG, Andersson I, Bjurstam N, Fagerberg G, Frisell J, Tabar L, et al.** Updated overview of the Swedish randomized trials on breast cancer screening with mammography: age group 40–49 at randomization. *J Natl Cancer Inst Monogr* 1997;22:57-61.
6. **UK trial of early detection of Breast Cancer Group.** 16-year mortality from breast cancer in the UK Trial of Early Detection of Breast Cancer. *Lancet* 1999;353:1909–1914.
7. **National Cancer Institute and American Cancer Society.** Joint statement on breast cancer screening for women in their 40s. The Cancer Information Service, 1997.
8. **Leitch AM, Dodd GI, Costanza M.** American Cancer Society guidelines for the early detection of breast cancer: update1997. *CA Cancer J Clin* 1997;47:150–153.
9. **American College of Radiology.** *Breast-imaging reporting and data system (BI-RADS) mammography*, 4th ed. Reston, Virginia: American College of Radiology, 2003.
10. **Christiansen CL, Wang F, Barton MB, Kreuter W, Elmore JG, Gelfand AE, et al.** Predicting the cumulative risk of false-positive mammograms. *J Natl Cancer Inst* 2000;92:1657–1666.

11. **Bleicher RJ, Morrow M.** MRI and breast cancer: role in detection, diagnosis and staging. *Oncol* 2007;21:1521–1530.

12. **Mann BD, Giuliano AE, Bassett LW, Barber MS, Hallauer W, Morton DL.** Delayed diagnosis of breast cancer as a result of normal mammograms. *Arch Surg* 1983;118:23–24.

13. **Shtern F.** Digital mammography and related technologies: a perspective from the National Cancer Institute. *Radiology* 1992;183:629–630.

14. **Pisano ED, Gatsonis C, Hendrick E, Yaffe M, Baum JK, Acharyya S, et al.** Diagnostic performance of digital versus film mammography for breast cancer screening. *N Engl J Med* 2005;353:1773–1783.

15. **Yang W, Dempsey PJ.** Diagnostic breast ultrasound: current status and future directions. *Radiol Clin N Am* 2007;46:845–861.

16. **Levy L, Suissa M, Chiche JF, Teman G, Martin B.** BIRADS ultrasonography. *Eur J Radiol* 2007;61:202–211.

17. **Orel SG, Schnall MD.** MR imaging of the breast for the detection, diagnosis, and staging of breast cancer. *Radiology* 2001;200:13–30.

18. **Esserman L, Wolverton D, Hylton N.** MR imaging and breast cancer. *Endocr Relat Cancer* 2002;9:141–153.

19. **Orel S.** Who should have breast magnetic resonance imaging evaluation? *J Clin Oncol* 2008;26:703–711.

20. **Segara D, Krop IE, Garber JE, Winer E, Harris L, Bellon JR, et al.** Does MRI predict pathologic tumor response in women with breast cancer undergoing preoperative chemotherapy? *J Surg Oncol* 2007;96:474–480.

21. **Lehman CD, Gatsonis C, Kuhl CK, Hendrick RE, Pisano ED, Hanna L, et al.** MRI Evaluation of the contralateral breast in women with recently diagnosed breast cancer. *N Engl J Med* 2007;356:1295–1303.

22. **American Cancer Society (ACS).** Guidelines for breast screening with MRI as an adjunct to mammography. *CA Cancer J Clin* 2007;57:75–89.

23. **Santen RJ, Mansel R.** Benign breast disorders. *N Engl J Med* 2005;353:275–285.

24. **Page DL, Dupont WD.** Anatomic markers of human premalignancy and risk of breast cancer. *Cancer* 1990;66:1326–1335.

25. **Morrow M, Jordan VC eds.** *Managing breast cancer risk.* Ontario: BC Decker, 2000.

26. **Hartman LC, Sellers TA, Frost MH, Lingle WL, Degnim AC, Gosh K, et al.** Benign breast disease and the risk of breast cancer. *N Engl J Med* 2005;353:329–337.

27. **Schnitt SJ, Connolly JL.** Pathology of benign breast disorders. In: *Diseases of the breast.* Harris JR, Lippman ME, Morrow M, Osborne CK, eds. Philadelphia: Lippincott Williams & Wilkins, 2004:77–99.

28. **Shen KW, Wu J, Lu JS, Han QX, Shen ZZ, Nguyen M, et al.** Fiberoptic ductoscopy for patients with nipple discharge. *Cancer* 2000;89:1512–1519.

29. **Page DL, Salhany KE, Jensen RA, Dupont WD.** Subsequent breast carcinoma risk after biopsy with atypia in a breast papilloma. *Cancer* 1996;78:258–266.

30. **Mulligan AM, O'Malley FP.** Papillary lesions of the breast. *Adv Anat Pathol* 2007;14:108–119.

31. **Dupont WD, Page DL, Parl FF, Vnencak-Jones CL, Plummer WD, Rados MS, et al.** Long-term risk of breast cancer in women with fibroadenoma. *N Engl J Med* 1994;331:10–15.

32. **Dixon JM, Dobie V, Lamb J, Walsh JS, Chetty U.** Assessment of the acceptability of conservative management of fibroadenoma of the breast. *Br J Surg* 1996;83:264–265.

33. **Jacklin RK, Ridgway PF, Ziprin P, Healy V, Hadjiminas D, Darzi A, et al.** Optimizing preoperative diagnosis in phyllodes tumour of the breast. *J Clin Pathol* 2006;59:454–459.

34. **Krishnamurthy S, Ashfaq R, Shin HJ, Sneige N.** Distinction of phyllodes tumor from fibroadenoma. *Cancer* 2000;90:342–449.

35. **Pietruszka M, Barnes L.** Cystosarcoma phyllodes: A clinicopathologic analysis of 42 cases. *Cancer* 1978;41:1974–1983.

36. **Zissis C, Apostolikas N, Konstantinidou A, Griniatsos J, Vassilopoulos PP.** The extent of surgery and prognosis of patients with phyllodes tumor of the breast. *Breast Cancer Res Treat* 1998;48:205–210.

37. **Chen WH, Cheng SP, Tzen CY, Yang TL, Jeng KS, Liu CL, et al.** Surgical treatment of phyllodes tumors of the breast: Retrospective review of 172 cases. *J Surg Oncol* 2005;91:185–194.

38. **Taira N, Takabatake D, Aogi K, Ohsumi S, Takashima S, Nishimura R, et al.** Phyllodes tumor of the breast: Stromal overgrowth and histological classification are useful prognosis-predictive factors for local recurrence in patients with a positive surgical margin. *Jpn J Clin Oncol* 2007;37:730–736.

39. **Jemal A, Siegel R, Ward E, Hao Y, Xu J, Murray T, et al.** Cancer statistics, 2009. *CA Cancer J Clin* 2009; published online. doi: 10.3322/caac.20006.

40. **Hoeksema MJ, Law C.** Cancer mortality rates fall: a turning point for the nation. *J Natl Cancer Inst* 1996;88:1706–1707.

41. **Jemal A, Ward E, Thun MJ.** Recent trends in breast cancer incidence rates by age and tumor characteristics among U.S. women. *Breast Cancer Res* 2007;9:R28.

42. **Cady B, Stone MD, Schuler JG, Thakur R, Wanner MA, Lavin PT.** The new era in breast cancer: invasion, size, and nodal involvement dramatically decreasing as a result of mammographic screening. *Arch Surg* 1996;131:301–308.

43. **Pike MC, Spicer DV, Dahmoush L, Press MF.** Estrogens, progestogens, normal breast cell proliferation, and breast cancer risk. *Epidemiol Rev* 1993;15:48–65.

44. **Ries L, Eisner M, Kosary C, Hankey B, Miller B, Clegg L, et al.** *SEER cancer statistics review 1975-2000.* Bethesda MD: National Cancer Institute, 2003.

45. **Healey EA, Cook EF, Orav EJ, Schnitt SJ, Connolly JL, Harris JR.** Contralateral breast cancer: Clinical characteristics and impact on prognosis. *J Clin Oncol* 1993;11:1545–1552.

46. **Mariani L, Coradini D, Biganzoli E, Boracchi P, Marubini E, Pilotti S, et al.** Prognostic factors for metachronous contralateral breast cancer: A comparison of the linear Cox regression model and its artificial neural network extension. *Breast Cancer Res* 1997;44:167–178.

47. **Bernstein JL, Thompson WD, Risch N, Holford TR.** Risk factors predicting the incidence of second primary breast cancer among women diagnosed with first primary breast cancer. *Am J Epidemiol* 1992;136:925–936.

48. **Broët P, de la Rochefordière A, Scholl SM, Fourquet A, Mosseri V, Durand JC, et al.** Contralateral breast cancer: Annual incidence and risk parameters. *J Clin Oncol* 1995;13:1578–1583.

49. **Tchou J, Morrow M.** Overview of clinical risk assessment. In: *Managing breast cancer risk.* Ontario: BC Decker, 2000:3–25.

50. **Claus EB, Schildkraut JM, Thompson WD, Risch NJ.** The genetic attributable risk of breast and ovarian cancer. *Cancer* 1996;77:2318–2324.

51. **Miki Y, Swensen J, Shattuck-Eidens D, Futreal PA, Harshman K, Tavtigian S, et al.** A strong candidate for the breast and ovarian susceptibility gene *BRCA1*. *Science* 1994;266:66–71.

52. **Wooster R, Bignell G, Lancaster J, Swift S, Seal S, Mangion J, et al.** Identification of the breast cancer susceptibility gene *BRCA2*. *Nature* 1995;378:789–792.

53. **Antoniou AC, Pharoah PD, McMullan G, Day NE, Stratton MR, Peto J, et al.** A comprehensive model for familial breast cancer incorporating *BRCA1*, *BRCA2*, and other genes. *Br J Cancer* 2002;86:76–83.

54. **Fodor FH, Weston A, Bleiweiss IJ, McCurdy LD, Walsh MM, Tartter PI, et al.** Frequency and carrier risk associated with common *BRCA1* and *BRCA2* mutations in Ashkenazi Jewish breast cancer patients. *Am J Hum Genet* 1998;63:45–51.

55. **Antoniou A, Pharoah PD, Narod S, Risch HA, Eyfjord JE, Hopper JL, et al.** Average risks of breast and ovarian cancer associated with *BRCA1* and *BRCA2* mutations detected in case series unselected for family history: a combined analysis of 22 studies. *Am J Hum Genet* 2003;72:1117–1130.

56. **Easton D, Bishop D, Ford D, Crockford G.** Genetic linkage analysis in familial breast and ovarian cancer: results from 214 families. *Am J Hum Genet* 1993;52:678–701.

57. **Brose MS, Rebbeck TR, Calzone KA, Stopfer JE, Nathanson KL, Weber BL.** Cancer risk estimates for *BRCA1* mutation carriers identified in a risk evaluation program. *J Natl Cancer Inst* 2002;94:1365–72.

58. **Ford D, Easton D, Bishop D, Narod S, Goldgar D.** Risks of cancer in *BRCA1*-mutation carriers. *Lancet* 1994;343:692–695.

59. **Struewing JP, Hartge P, Wacholder S, Baker SM, Berlin M, McAdams M, et al.** The risk of cancer associated with specific mutations of *BRCA1* and *BRCA2* among Ashkenazi Jews. *N Engl J Med* 1997;336:1401–1408.

60. Krainer M, Silva-Arrieta S, FitzGerald MG, Shimada A, Ishioka C, Kanamaru R, et al. Differential contributions of *BRCA1* and *BRCA2* to early-onset breast cancer. *N Engl J Med* 1997;336: 1416–1421.

61. Fitzgerald MG, Macdonald DJ, Krainer M, Hoover I, O'Neil E, Unsal H, et al. Germ-line mutations in Jewish and non-Jewish women with early-onset breast cancer. *N Engl J Med* 1996;334:143–149.

62. Shattuck-Eidens D, McClure M, Simard J, Labrie F, Narod S, Couch F, et al. A collaborative survey of 80 mutations in the *BRCA1* breast and ovarian cancer susceptibility gene. *JAMA* 1995;273: 535–541.

63. American Society of Clinical Oncology. Genetic testing for cancer susceptibility. *J Clin Oncol* 1996;14:1730–1736.

64. American Society of Clinical Oncology. Policy statement update: genetic testing for cancer susceptibility. *J Clin Oncol* 2003;12: 2397–2406.

65. Pike MC, Krailo MD, Henderson BD, Casagrande JT, Hoel DG. Hormonal risk factors, "breast tissue age" and the age incidence of breast cancer. *Nature* 1983;303:767–770.

66. Trapido EJ. Age at first birth, parity, and breast cancer risks. *Cancer* 1983;51:946–948.

67. Hsieh CC, Trichopoulos D, Katsouyanni K, Yuasa S. Age at menarche, age at menopause, height and obesity as risk factors for breast cancer: associations and interactions in an international case-control study. *Int J Cancer* 1990;46:796–800.

68. Collaborative Group on Hormonal Factors in Breast Cancer. Breast cancer and hormonal contraceptives: collaborative reanalysis of individual data on 53,297 women with breast cancer and 100,239 women without breast cancer from 54 epidemiological studies. *Lancet* 1996;347:1713–1727.

69. Writing Group for the Women's Health Initiative Investigators. Risks and benefits of estrogen plus progestin in healthy post-menopausal women: principal results from the Women's Health Initiative randomized controlled trial. *JAMA* 2002;288:321–333.

70. Women's Health Initiative Steering Committee. Effects of conjugated equine estrogen in postmenopausal women with hysterectomy: the Women's Health Initiative Randomized controlled trail. *JAMA* 2004;291:1701–1712.

71. Beral V; Million Women Study Collaborators. Breast cancer and hormone-replacement therapy in the Million Women Study. *Lancet* 2003;362:419–427.

72. Hersh AL, Stefanick ML, Stafford RS. National use of post-menopausal hormone therapy: annual trends and response to recent evidence. *JAMA* 2004;291:47–53.

73. Ravdin PM, Cronin KA, Howlader N, Berg CD, Chlebowski RT, Feuer EJ, et al. The decrease in breast-cancer incidence in 2003 in the United States. *N Engl J Med* 2007;356:1670–1674.

74. Van Veer P, Van Leer EM, Rietdijk A, Kok FJ, Schouten EG, Hermus RJ, et al. Combination of dietary factors in relation to breast cancer occurrence. *Int J Cancer* 1991;47:649–653.

75. Reeves GK, Pirie K, Beral V, Green J, Spencer E, Bull D. Cancer incidence and mortality in relation to body mass index in the Million Women Study: cohort study. *BMJ* 2007;335:1134.

76. Lahmann PH, Hoffmann K, Allen N, van Gils CH, Khaw KT, Tehard B, et al. Body size and breast cancer risk: Findings from the European Prospective Investigation into Cancer and Nutrition (EPIC). *Int J Cancer* 2004;111:762–771.

77. Hunter DJ, Spiegelman D, Adami H-O, Beeson L, van den Brandt PA, Folsom AR, et al. Cohort studies of fat intake and the risk of breast cancer: a pooled analysis. *N Engl J Med* 1996;334:356–361.

78. Prentice RL, Thomson CA, Caan B, Hubbell FA, Anderson GL, Beresford SA, et al. Low-fat dietary pattern and risk of invasive breast cancer. *JAMA* 2006;295:629–642.

79. Cho E, Spiegelman D, Hunter DJ, Chen WY, Colditz GA, Willett WC. Premenopausal dietary carbohydrate. Glycemic index, glycemic loan, and fiber in relation to risk of breast cancer. *Cancer Epidemiol Biomarkers Prev* 2003;12:1153–1158.

80. Cade JE, Burley VJ, Greenwood DC; UK Women's Cohort Study Steering Group. Dietary fibre and risk of breast cancer in the UK Women's Cohort Study Steering Group. *Int J Epidemiol* 2007;36:431–438.

81. Zhang S, Hunter DJ, Forman MR, Rosner BA, Speizer FE, Colditz GA, et al. Dietary caretoniods and vitamins A, C and E and risk of breast cancer. *J Natl Cancer Inst* 1999;91:547–556.

82. van Gils CH, Peeters PH, Bueno-de-Mesquita H, Boshuizen HC, Lahmann PH, Clavel-Chapelon F, et al. Consumption of vegetables and fruits and risk of breast cancer. *JAMA* 2005;293:183–193.

83. Smith-Warner SA, Spiegelman D, Yaun SS, Adami HO, Beeson WL, van den Brandt PA, et al. Intake of fruits and vegetables and risk of breast cancer: a pooled analysis of cohort studies. *JAMA* 2001;285:769–776.

84. Michels KB, Mohllajee AP, Roset-Bahmanyar E, Beehler GP, Moysich KB. Diet and breast cancer. *Cancer* 2007;109:2712–2749.

85. Monninkhof EM, Elias SG, Vlems FA, van der Tweel I, Schuit AJ, Voskuil DW, et al. Physical activity and breast cancer: A systematic review. *Epidemiology* 2007;18:137–57.

86. Maruti SS, Willett WC, Feskanich D, Rosner B, Colditz GA. A prospective study of age-specific physical activity and premenopausal breast cancer. *J Natl Cancer Inst* 2008;100:728–737.

87. Friedenreich CM, Cust AE. Physical activity and breast cancer risk: Impact of timing, type and dose of activity and population subgroup effects. *Brit J Sports Med* 2008;0:1–12.

88. Smith-Warner SA, Spiegelman D, Yaun S-S, van den Brandt PA, Folsom AR, Goldbohm RA, et al. Alcohol and breast cancer in women: a pooled analysis of cohort studies. *JAMA* 1998;279:535–540.

89. Miller AB, Howe GR, Sherman GJ, Lindsay JP, Yaffe MJ, Dinner PJ, et al. Mortality from breast cancer after irradiation during fluoroscopic examinations in patients being treated for tuberculosis. *N Engl J Med* 1989;321:1285–1289.

90. Land CE, Tokunaga M, Koyama K, Soda M, Preston DL, Nishimori I, et al. Incidence of female breast cancer among atomic bomb survivors, 1950-1985. *Radiat Res* 1994;138:209–223.

91. Hancock SL, Tucker MA, Hoppe RT. Breast cancer after treatment of Hodgkin's disease. *J Natl Cancer Inst* 1993;85:25–31.

92. Yahalom J, Petrek JA, Biddinger PW, Kessler S, Dershaw DD, McCormick B, et al. Breast cancer in patients irradiated for Hodgkin's disease: a clinical and pathologic analysis of 45 events in 37 patients. *J Clin Oncol* 1992;10:1674–1681.

93. Bhatia S, Robison LL, Oberlin O, Greenberg M, Bunin G, Fossati-Bellani F, et al. Breast cancer and other second malignant neoplasms after childhood Hodgkin's disease. *N Engl J Med* 1996;334:745–751.

94. Yahalom J. Breast cancer after Hodgkin disease: Hope for a safer cure. *JAMA* 2003;290:529–531.

95. Morris A, Pommier RF, Schmidt WA, Shih RL, Alexander PW, Vetto JT, et al. Accurate evaluation of palpable masses by the triple test score. *Arch Surg* 1998;133:930–934.

96. Kaufman Z, Shpitz B, Shapiro M, Rona R, Lew S, Dinbar A. Triple approach in the diagnosis of dominant breast masses: combined physical examination, mammography, and fine-needle aspiration. *J Surg Oncol* 1994;56:254–257.

97. Ariga R, Bloom K, Reddy VB, Kluskens L, Francescatti D, Dowlat K, et al. Fine-needle aspiration of clinically suspicious palpable breast masses with histopathologic correlation. *Am J Surg* 2002;184:410–413.

98. Ishikawa T, Hamaguchi Y, Tanabe M, Momiyama N, Chishima T, Nakatani Y, et al. False-positive and false-negative cases of fine-needle aspiration cytology for palpable breast lesions. *Breast Cancer* 2007;14:388–392.

99. Bassett L, Winchester DP, Caplan RB, Dershaw DD, Dowlatshahi K, Evans WP, et al. Stereotactic core-needle biopsy of the breast: a report of the Joint Task Force of the American College of Radiology, American College of Surgeons, and College of American Pathologists. *CA Cancer J Clin* 1997;47:171–190.

100. Fajardo LL, Pisano ED, Caudry DJ, Gatsonis CA, Berg WA, Connolly J, et al. Stereotatic and sonographic large-core biopsy of nonpalpable breast lesions: results of the Radiologic Diagnostic Oncology Group V study. *Acad Radiol* 2004;11:293–308.

101. World Health Organization. *Histological typing of breast tumors*, 2nd edition. *Am J Clin Pathol* 1982;78:806–816.

102. Northridge ME, Rhoadds GG, Wartenberg D, Koffman D. The importance of histologic type on breast cancer survival. *J Clin Epidemiol* 1997;50:283–290.

103. Arpino G, Bardou VJ, Clark GM, Elledge RM. Infiltrating carcinoma of the breast: tumor characteristics and clinical outcomes. *Breast Cancer Res* 2004;6:149–156.

104. Abner AL, Connolly JL, Recht A, Bornstein B, Nixon A, Hetelekidis S, Silver B, et al. The relation between the presence and

extent of lobular carcinoma *in situ* and the risk of local recurrence for patients with infiltrating lobular carcinoma of the breast treated with conservative surgery and radiation therapy. *Cancer* 2000;88: 1072–1077.

105. **Jolly S, Kestin LL, Goldstein NS, Vicini FA.** The impact of lobular carcinoma *in situ* in association with invasive breast cancer on the rate of local recurrence in patients with early-stage breast cancer treated with breast-conserving therapy. *Int J Radiat Oncol* 2006;66:365–371.

106. **Diab SG, Clark GM, Osborne CK, Libby A, Allred DC, Elledge RM.** Tumor characteristics and clinical outcome of tubular and mucinous breast carcinomas. *J Clin Oncol* 1999;17:1442–1448.

107. **Berg JW, Hutter RV.** Breast cancer. *Cancer* 1995;75:257–269.

108. **Soon SR, Yong WS, Ho GH, Wong CY, Ho BC, Tan PH.** Adenoid cystic breast carcinoma: A salivary gland-type tumour with excellent prognosis and implications for management. *Pathology* 2008;40: 413–415.

109. **Plevritis SK.** A mathematical algorithm that computes breast cancer sizes and doubling times detected by screening. *Math Biosci* 2001;171: 155–178.

110. **Kusama S, Spratt JS, Donegan WL, Watson FR, Cunningham C.** The gross rates of growth of human mammary carcinoma. *Cancer* 1972;30:594.

111. **Tubiana M, Pejovic JM, Renaud A, Contesso G, Chavaudra N, Gioanni J, et al.** Kinetic parameters and the course of the disease in breast cancer. *Cancer* 1981;47:937–943.

112. **Punglia RS, Morrow M, Winer EP, Harris JR.** Local therapy and survival in breast cancer. *N Engl J Med* 2007;356:2399–2405.

113. **Greene FL, Page DL, Fleming ID, Fritz A, Balch CM, Haller DG, Morrow M, eds.** *AJCC cancer staging manual,* 6th ed. New York: Springer-Verlag, 2002.

114. **National Comprehensive Cancer Network.** Breast cancer: in NCCN clinical practice guidelines in oncology. V.2.2008; http://www.nccn.org.

115. **Diel IJ, Kaufmann M, Costa SD, Holle R, von Minckwitz G, Solomayer EF, et al.** Micrometastatic breast cancer cells in bone marrow at primary surgery: prognostic value in comparison with nodal status. *J Natl Cancer Inst* 1996;88:1652–1664.

116. **Quon A, Gambhir SS.** FDG-PET and beyond: Molecular breast cancer imaging. *J Clin Oncol* 2005;23:1664–1673.

117. **Wahl RL, Siegel BA, Coleman RE, Gatsonis CG; PET Study Group.** Prospective multicenter study of axillary nodal staging by positron emission tomography in breast cancer: a report of the staging of breast cancer with the PET Study Group. *J Clin Oncol* 2004;22:277–285.

118. **Fehr MK, Hornung R, Varga Z, Burger D, Hess T, Haller U, et al.** Axillary staging using positron emission tomography in breast cancer patients qualifying for sentinel lymph node biopsy. *Breast J* 2004;10:89–93.

119. **Gil-Rendo A, Zornoza G, García-Velloso MJ, Regueira FM, Beorlegui C, Cervera M.** Fluorodeoxyglucose positron emission tomography with sentinel lymph node biopsy for evaluation of axillary involvement in breast cancer. *Br J Surg* 2006;93:707–712.

120. **Halsted WS.** The results of radical operation for cure of cancer of the breast. *Ann Surg* 1907;46:1–19.

121. **Meyer W.** Carcinoma of the breast: ten years experience with my method of radical operation. *JAMA* 1905;45:219–313.

122. **Dahl-Iversen E, Tobiassen T.** Radical mastectomy with parasternal and supraclavicular dissection for mammary carcinoma. *Ann Surg* 1969;170:889–891.

123. **Lewis FJ.** Extended or super radical mastectomy for cancer of the breast. *Minn Med* 1953;36:763–766.

124. **Urban JA.** Extended radical mastectomy for breast cancer. *Am J Surg* 1963;106:399.

125. **Fisher B, Jeong JH, Anderson S, Bryant J, Fisher ER, Wolmark N.** Twenty-five-year follow-up of a randomized trial comparing radical mastectomy, total mastectomy, and total mastectomy followed by irradiation. *N Engl J Med* 2002;347:567–575.

126. **Prosnitz LR, Goldenberg IS, Packard RA, Levene MB, Harris J, Hellman S, et al.** Radiation therapy as initial treatment for early stage cancer of the breast without mastectomy. *Cancer* 1977;39:917–923.

127. **Veronesi U, Saccozzi R, Del Veccio M, Banfi A, Clemente C, De Lena M, et al.** Comparing radical mastectomy with quadrantectomy, axillary dissection and radiotherapy in patients with small cancers of the breast. *N Engl J Med* 1981;305:6–11.

128. **Veronesi U, Cascinelli N, Mariani L, Greco M, Saccozzi R, Luini A, et al.** Twenty-year follow-up of a randomized study comparing breast-conserving surgery with radical mastectomy for early breast cancer. *N Engl J Med* 2002;347:1227–1232.

129. **Fisher B, Bauer M, Margolese R, Poisson R, Pilch Y, Redmond C, et al.** Five-year results of a randomized clinical trial comparing total mastectomy and segmental mastectomy with or without radiation in the treatment of cancer. *N Engl J Med* 1985;312:665–673.

130. **Fisher B, Anderson S, Bryant J, Margolese RG, Deutsch M, Fisher ER, et al.** Twenty-year follow-up of a randomized trial comparing total mastectomy, lumpectomy, and lumpectomy plus irradiation for the treatment of invasive breast cancer. *N Engl J Med* 2002;347:1233–1241.

131. **NIH Consensus Conference.** Treatment of early-stage breast cancer. *JAMA* 1991;265:391–395.

132. **Veronesi U, Rilke F, Luini A, Sacchini V, Galimberti V, Campa T, et al.** Distribution of axillary node metastases by level of invasion: an analysis of 539 cases. *Cancer* 1987;59:682–687.

133. **Giuliano AE, Kirgan DM, Guenther JM, Morton DL.** Lymphatic mapping and sentinel lymphadenectomy for breast cancer. *Ann Surg* 1994;220:391–401.

134. **Giuliano AE, Jones RC, Brennan M, Statman R.** Sentinel lymphadenectomy in breast cancer. *J Clin Oncol* 1997;15:2345–2350.

135. **Giuliano AE, Haigh PI, Brennan MB, Hansen NM, Kelley MC, Ye W, et al.** Prospective observational study of sentinel lymphadenectomy without further axillary dissection in patients with sentinel node-negative breast cancer. *J Clin Oncol* 2000;18:2553–2559.

136. **Lyman GH, Giuliano AE, Somerfield MR, Benson AB 3rd, Bodurka DC, Burstein HJ, et al.** ASCO guideline recommendations for sentinel lymph node biopsy in early-stage breast cancer. *J Clin Oncol* 2005;23:7703–7720.

137. **Yen TW, Hunt KK, Ross MI, Mirza NQ, Babiera GV, Meric-Bernstam F, et al.** Predictors of invasive breast cancer in patients with an initial diagnosis of ductal carcinoma *in situ*: A guide to selective use of sentinel lymph node biopsy in management of ductal carcinoma *in situ*. *J Am Coll Surg* 2005;200:516–526.

138. **Keleher A, Wendt R 3rd, Delpassand E, Stachowiak AM, Kuerer HM.** The safety of lymphatic mapping in pregnant cancer patients using Tc-99m sulfur colloid. *Breast J* 2004;10:492–495.

139. **Gentilini O, Cremonesi M, Trifirò G, Ferrari M, Baio SM, Caracciolo M, et al.** Safety of sentinel node biopsy in pregnant patients with breast cancer. *Ann Oncol* 2004;15:1348–51.

140. **Filippakis GM, Zografos G.** Contraindications of sentinel node biopsy: are there really any? *World J Surg Oncol* 2007;29:5–10.

141. **Arrigada R, Le MG, Rochard F, Contesso G.** Conservative treatment versus mastectomy in early breast cancer: patterns of failure with 15 years of follow-up data. Institut Gustave-Roussy Breast Cancer Group. *J Clin Oncol* 1996;14:1558–1564.

142. **Clarke M, Collins R, Darby S, Davies C, Elphinstone P, Evans E, et al.** Effects of radiotherapy and of differences in the extent of surgery for early breast cancer on local recurrence and 15-year survival: an overview of the randomized trials. *Lancet* 2005;366:2087–106.

143. **Overgaard M, Hansen PS, Overgaard J, Rose C, Andersson M, Bach F, et al.** Postoperative radiotherapy in high-risk premenopausal women with breast cancer who receive adjuvant chemotherapy. *N Engl J Med* 1997;337:949–955.

144. **Overgaard M, Jensen MB, Overgaard J, Hansen PS, Rose C, Andersson M, et al.** Postoperative radiotherapy in high-risk postmenopausal breast-cancer patients given adjuvant tamoxifen: Danish Breast Cancer Cooperative Group DBCG 82c randomized trial. *Lancet* 1999;353:1641–1648.

145. **Ragaz J, Olivotto IA, Spinelli JJ, Phillips N, Jackson SM, Wilson KS, et al.** Locoregional radiation therapy in patients with high-risk breast cancer receiving adjuvant chemotherapy: 20-year results of the British Columbia randomized trial. *J Natl Cancer Inst* 2005:116–126.

146. **Pierce LJ.** The use of radiotherapy after mastectomy: a review of the literature. *J Clin Oncol* 2005;23:1706–1717.

147. **Veronesi U, Gatti G, Luini A, Intra M, Orecchia R, Borgen P, et al.** Intraoperative radiation therapy for breast cancer: technical notes. *Breast J* 2003;9:106–112.

148. **Fowble B.** Ipsilateral breast tumor recurrence following breast-conserving surgery for early-stage invasive cancer. *Acta Oncol Suppl* 1999;13:9–17.

651

149. **Pawlik TM, Bucholz TA, Kuerer HM.** The biologic rationale for and emerging role of accelerated partial breast irradiation for breast cancer. *J Am Coll Surg* 2004;199:479–492.

150. **Benitez PR, Keisch ME, Vicini F, Stolier A, Scroggins T, Walker A, et al.** Five-year results: the initial clinical trial of Mammosite balloon brachytherapy for partial breast irradiation in early-stage breast cancer. *Am J Surg* 2007;194:456–462.

151. **Chao KK, Vicini FA, Wallace M, Mitchell C, Chen P, Ghilezan M, et al.** Analysis of treatment efficacy, cosmesis, and toxicity using the Mammosite breast brachytherapy catheter to deliver accelerated partial-breast irradiation: the William Beaumont Hospital experience. *Int J Rad Oncol* 2007;69:32–40.

152. **Early Breast Cancer Trialists' Collaborative Group.** Effects of chemotherapy and hormonal therapy for early breast cancer on recurrence and 15-year survival: an overview of the randomized trials. *Lancet* 2005;365:1687–1717.

153. **Fisher B, Brown AM, Dimitrov NV, Poisson R, Redmond C, Margolese RG, et al.** Two months of *doxorubicin-cyclophosphamide* with and without interval reinduction therapy compared with 6 months of *cyclophosphamide, methotrexate,* and fluorouracil in tamoxifen-nonresponsive tumors: results from the National Surgical Adjuvant Breast and Bowel Project B-15. *J Clin Oncol* 1990;8:1483–1496.

154. **Fisher B, Anderson S, Tan-Chiu E, Wolmark N, Wickerham DL, Fisher ER, et al.** Tamoxifen and chemotherapy for axillary node-negative, estrogen-receptor negative breast cancer: findings from National Surgical Adjuvant Breast and Bowel Project B-23. *J Clin Oncol* 2001;19:931–942.

155. **Mamounas EP, Bryant J, Lembersky B, Fehrenbacher L, Sedlacek SM, Fisher B, et al.** Paclitaxel after *doxorubicin* plus *cyclophosphamide* as adjuvant chemotherapy for node-positive breast cancer: results from NSABP B-28. *J Clin Oncol* 2005;23:3686–3696.

156. **Henderson IC, Berry DA, Demetri GD, Cirrincione CT, Goldstein LJ, Martino S, et al.** Improved outcomes from adding sequential *paclitaxel* but not from escalating *doxorubicin* dose in an adjuvant chemotherapy regimen for patients with node-positive primary breast cancer. *J Clin Oncol* 2003;976–983.

157. **Jones SE, Savin MA, Holmes FA, O'Shaughnessy JA, Blum JL, Vukelja S, et al.** Phase III trial comparing *doxorubicin* plus *cyclophosphamide* with *docetaxel* plus *cyclophosphamide* as adjuvant therapy for operable breast cancer. *J Clin Oncol* 2006;24:5381–5387.

158. **Citron ML, Berry DA, Cirrincione C, Hudis C, Winer EP, Gradishar WJ, et al.** Randomized trial of dose-dense versus conventionally scheduled and sequential versus concurrent combination chemotherapy as postoperative adjuvant treatment of node-positive primary breast cancer: first report of Intergroup trial C9741/Cancer and Leukemia Group B Trial 9741. *J Clin Oncol* 2003;21:1431–1439.

159. **Slamon DJ, Godolphin W, Jones LA, Holt JA, Wong SG, Keith DE, et al.** Studies of the HER-2/*neu* proto-oncogene in human breast and ovarian cancer. *Science* 1989;244:707–712.

160. **Slamon DJ, Leyland-Jones B, Shak S, Fuchs H, Paton V, Bajamonde A, et al.** Use of chemotherapy plus a monoclonal antibody against HER2 for metastatic breast cancer that overexpresses HER2. *N Engl J Med* 2001;344:783–792.

161. **Piccart-Gebhart MJ, Procter M, Leyland-Jones B, Goldhirsch A, Untch M, Smith I, et al.** Trastuzumab after adjuvant chemotherapy in HER-2 positive breast cancer. *N Engl J Med* 2005;353:1659–1672.

162. **Smith I, Procter M, Gelber RD, Guillaume S, Feyereislova A, Dowsett M, et al.** 2-year follow-up of trastuzumab after adjuvant chemotherapy in HER2-positive breast cancer: a randomized controlled trial. *Lancet* 2007;369:29–36.

163. **Fisher B, Dignam J, Bryant J, DeCillis A, Wickerham DL, Wolmark N, et al.** Five versus more than five years of tamoxifen therapy for breast cancer patients with negative lymph nodes and estrogen receptor-positive tumors. *J Natl Cancer Inst* 1996;88:1529–1542.

164. **Fisher B, Dignam J, Wolmark N, DeCillis A, Emir B, Wickerham DL, et al.** Tamoxifen and chemotherapy for lymph node-negative, estrogen receptor-positive breast cancer. *J Natl Cancer Inst* 1997;89:1673–1682.

165. **Paik S, Shak S, Tang G, Kim C, Baker J, Cronin M, et al.** A multigene assay to predict recurrence of tamoxifen-treated, node-negative breast cancer. *N Engl J Med* 2004;351:2817–2826.

166. **van de Vijver MJ, He YD, van't Veer LJ, Dai H, Hart AA, Voskuil DW, et al.** A gene-expression signature as a predictor of survival in breast cancer. *N Engl J Med* 2002;347:1999–2009.

167. **Buzdar AU, Jonat W, Howell A, Jones SE, Blomqvist CP, Vogel CL, et al.** Anastrozole versus megestrol acetate in the treatment of postmenopausal women with advanced breast carcinoma: results of a survival update based on a combined analysis of data from two mature phase III trials. Arimidex Study Group. *Cancer* 1998;83:1142–1152.

168. **Forbes JF, Cuzick J, Buzdar A, Howell A, Tobias JS, Baum M, et al.** Effect of anastrozole and tamoxifen as adjuvant treatment for early-stage breast cancer: 100-month analysis of the ATAC trial. *Lancet* 2008;9:45–53.

169. **Winer EP, Hudis C, Burstein HJ, Wolff AC, Pritchard KI, Ingle JN, et al.** American Society of Clinical Oncology Technology Assessment on the use of aromatase inhibitors as adjuvant therapy for postmenopausal women with hormone receptor-positive breast cancer: status report 2004. *J Clin Oncol* 2005;23:619–629.

170. **Cianfrocca M, Goldstein LJ.** Prognostic and predictive factors in early-stage breast cancer. *Oncologist* 2004;9:606–616.

171. **Fisher ER, Anderson S, Tan-Chiu E, Fisher B, Eaton L, Wolmark N.** Fifteen-year prognostic discriminants for invasive breast carcinoma: National Surgical Adjuvant Breast and Bowel Project Protocol-06. *Cancer* 2001;91:1679–1687.

172. **Fisher ER, Redmond C, Fisher B, Bass G.** Pathologic findings from the National Surgical Adjuvant Breast and Bowel Projects (NSABP): prognostic discriminants for eight-year survival for node-negative invasive breast cancer patients. *Cancer* 1990;65:2121–2128.

173. **Early Breast Cancer Trialists' Collaborative Group.** Systemic treatment of early breast cancer by hormonal, cytotoxic, or immune therapy: 133 randomised trials involving 31,000 recurrences and 24,000 deaths among 75,000 women (Part 2). *Lancet* 1992;339:71–85.

174. **Lee Y-T.** Breast carcinoma: pattern of metastasis at autopsy. *Surg Oncol* 1983;23:175–180.

175. **Hillner BE, Ingle JN, Chlebowski RT, Gralow J, Yee GC, Janjan NA, et al.** American Society of Clinical Oncology 2003 update on the role of bisphosphonates and bone health issues in women with breast cancer. *J Clin Oncol* 2003;21:4042–4057.

176. **Taylor CW, Green S, Dalton WS, Martino S, Rector D, Ingle JN, et al.** Multicenter randomized clinical trial of goserelin versus surgical ovariectomy in premenopausal patients with receptor-positive metastatic breast cancer: an Intergroup study. *J Clin Oncol* 1998;16:994–999.

177. **Klijn JG, Blamey RW, Boccardo F, Tominaga T, Duchateau L, Sylvester R, et al.** Combined tamoxifen and luteinizing hormone-releasing hormone (LHRH) agonist versus LHRH agonist alone in premenopausal advanced breast cancer: a meta-analysis of four randomized trials. *J Clin Oncol* 2001;19:343–353.

178. **Robertson JF, Osborne CK, Howell A, Jones SE, Mauriac L, Ellis M, et al.** Fulvestrant versus anastrozole for the treatment of advanced breast carcinoma in postmenopausal women. *Cancer* 2003;98:229–238.

179. **Geyer CE, Forster J, Lindquist D, Chan S, Romieu CG, Pienkowski T, et al.** Lapatinib plus capecitabine for HER2-positive advanced breast cancer. *N Engl J Med* 2006;355:2733–2743.

180. **Fisher B, Costantino JP, Wickerham DL, Redmond CK, Kavanah M, Cronin WM, et al.** Tamoxifen for prevention of breast cancer: Report of the National Surgical Adjuvant Breast and Bowel Project P-1 Study. *J Natl Cancer Inst* 1998;90:1371–1388.

181. **Burstein HJ, Polyak K, Wong JS, Lester SC, Kaelin CM.** Ductal carcinoma *in situ* of the breast. *N Engl J Med* 2004;350:1430–1441.

182. **Page DL, Dupont WD, Rogers LW, Landenberger M.** Intraductal carcinoma of the breast: follow-up after biopsy only. *Cancer* 1982;49:751–758.

183. **Fisher B, Dignam J, Wolmark N, Mamounas E, Costantino J, Poller W, et al.** Lumpectomy and radiation therapy for the treatment of intraductal breast cancer: findings from the NSABP B-17. *J Clin Oncol* 1998;16:441–452.

184. **Fisher B, Land S, Mamounas E, Dignam J, Fisher ER, Wolmark N.** Prevention of invasive breast cancer in women with ductal carcinoma *in situ*: an update of the national surgical adjuvant breast and bowel project experience. *Semin Oncol* 2001;28:400–418.

185. **Paget J.** Disease of the mammary areola preceding cancer of the mammary gland. *St. Bartholomew's Hospital Report* 1874;10:89.

186. **Marshall JK, Griffith KA, Haffty BG, Solin LJ, Vicini FA, McCormick B, et al.** Conservative management of Paget disease of the breast with radiotherapy. *Cancer* 2003;97:2142–2149.

187. **Kawase K, Dimaio DJ, Tucker SL, Buchholz TA, Ross MI, Feig BW, et al.** Paget's disease of the breast: there is a role for breast-conserving therapy. *Ann Surg Oncol* 2005;12:1–7.

188. **Colozza M, Gori S, Mosconi AM, Anastasi P, de Angelis V, Giansanti M, et al.** Induction chemotherapy with *cisplatin, doxorubicin*, and *cyclophosphamide* (CAP) in a combined modality approach for locally advanced and inflammatory breast cancer: long-term results. *Am J Clin Oncol* 1996;19:10–17.

189. **Schover LR.** Premature ovarian failure and its consequences: vasomotor symptoms, sexuality, and fertility. *J Clin Oncol* 2008;26:753–758.

190. **Bines J, Oleske DM, Cobleigh MA.** Ovarian function in premenopausal women treated with adjuvant chemotherapy for breast cancer. *J Clin Oncol* 1996;14:1718–1729.

191. **Lutchman Singh K, Muttukrishna S, Stein RC, McGarrigle HH, Patel A, Parikh B, et al.** Predictors of ovarian reserve in young women with breast cancer. *Br J Cancer* 2007;96:1806–1816.

192. **Lee SJ, Schover LR, Partridge AH, Patrizio P, Wallace WH, Hagerty K, et al.** American Society of Clinical Oncology recommendations on fertility preservation in cancer patients. *J Clin Oncol* 2006;24:2917–2931.

193. **Ives A, Saunders C, Bulsara M, Semmens J.** Pregnancy after breast cancer: population-based study. *BMJ* 2007;334:194.

194. **Brown RW, Allred CD, Clark GM, Osborne CK, Hilsenbeck SG.** Prognostic value of Ki-67 compared to S-phase fraction in axillary node-negative breast cancer. *Clin Cancer Res* 1996;2:585–592.

195. **Neville AM, Bettelheim R, Gelber RD, Säve-Söderbergh J, Davis BW, Reed R, et al.** Factors predicting treatment responsiveness and prognosis in node-negative breast cancer. The International (Ludwig) Breast Cancer Study Group. *J Clin Oncol* 1992;10: 696–705.

196. **Wegner CR, Clark GM.** S-phase fraction and breast cancer–a decade of experience. *Breast Cancer Res Treat* 1998;51:255–265.

197. **Nixon AJ, Neuberg D, Hayes DF, Gelman R, Connolly JL, Schnitt S, et al.** Relationship of patient age to pathologic features of the tumor and prognosis for patients with stage I or II breast cancer. *J Clin Oncol* 1994:12;888–894.

198. **Fisher B, Costantino J, Redmond C, Poisson R, Bowman D, Couture J, et al.** A randomized clinical trial evaluating tamoxifen in the treatment of patients with node-negative breast cancer who have estrogen-receptor-positive tumors. *N Engl J Med* 1989;320: 479–484.

199. **Fisher B, Constantino JP, Wickerham DL, Redmond CK, Kavanah M, Cronin WM, et al.** Tamoxifen for prevention of breast cancer: report of the National Surgical Adjuvant Breast and Bowel Project P-1 study. *J Natl Cancer Inst* 1998;90:1371–1388.

200. **Dunn BK, Ford LG.** From adjuvant therapy to breast cancer prevention: BCPT and STAR. *Breast J* 2001;7:144–157.

201. **Rhodes DJ, Hartmann LC, Perez EA.** Breast Cancer Prevention Trials. *Curr Oncol Rep* 2000;2:558–565.

202. **Vogel VG, Costantino JP, Wickerham DL, Cronin WM, Cecchini RS, Atkins JN, et al.** Effects of tamoxifen vs raloxifene on the risk of developing invasive breast cancer and other disease outcomes. *JAMA* 2006;295:2727–2741.

17 Cancer and Pregnancy

Amreen Husain
Maurice Druzin

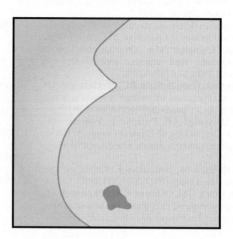

The diagnosis of cancer during pregnancy is a serious medical and psychological challenge to the woman, her family, and her caregivers. Pregnancy is normally a happy time with great expectations for the future, and the diagnosis of a life-threatening illness may lead to inappropriate responses by the patient, her family, and the medical team. When faced with a diagnosis of cancer in pregnancy, the single most important question that the obstetrician must ask of the oncologist is: "What would the optimal therapy be for this patient with this diagnosis if she were not pregnant?" The answer will almost always be appropriate for the pregnant patient.

Cancer in pregnancy presents many challenges and requires management by a team which should include a gynecologic oncologist, a maternal-fetal medicine specialist, a medical oncologist, a radiation oncologist, and a neonatal pediatrician. **The issues relate to the type of cancer with which the woman is diagnosed, the gestational age at which the diagnosis is made, the stage at which the cancer is diagnosed, the social and ethical attitudes of the woman with respect to pregnancy termination, and the ongoing management of the pregnancy.**

Cancer complicates approximately 1 in 1,000 pregnancies. The most commonly diagnosed cancers in pregnancy are cancer of the breast and cervix, melanoma, and Hodgkin's disease (1). The diagnostic and therapeutic management of cancer in pregnancy needs to take several matters into consideration, including the risk of diagnostic procedures to the unborn fetus, the risks of therapeutic interventions to the ongoing pregnancy, and the social implications of child bearing and motherhood for the woman. **Ideally, the cancer and the pregnancy must be managed without negatively affecting outcomes for the baby or the mother. This is not always possible, and appropriate counseling in these situations is essential.**

Diagnosis

Overall, the outcomes of cancer in pregnancy are not worse than in the nonpregnant state. While it has been speculated that cancer outcomes in pregnancy are worse than in nonpregnant patients, this impression has not been supported by multiple studies over the last four decades, and suboptimal treatment of the cancer in pregnancy may be responsible for this erroneous assumption (2).

The most critical issue in the diagnosis and treatment of cancer in pregnancy is to avoid unnecessary delay. Delay may cause more harm than well-planned diagnostic and therapeutic interventions, which for the most part pose minimal risk to the unborn fetus after the first trimester. Many signs and symptoms of cancer can be misinterpreted as being due to the pregnancy, leading frequently to delayed evaluation. If a physical symptom is found in a pregnant woman that may indicate a malignancy, the best principle to follow is to investigate it in the same manner as for a non-pregnant woman.

Diagnostic Testing

With few exceptions, most diagnostic modalities are safe in pregnancy. Ultrasound has a long safety record during pregnancy, and most radiologic procedures will cause insignificant amounts of fetal radiation exposure when used judiciously and with appropriate shielding. It is inappropriate to delay necessary diagnostic procedures based on theoretical and unproven risks to the fetus. Magnetic resonance imaging is ideal for scanning the pelvis and abdomen during pregnancy, as it delivers no radiation. Diagnostic imaging in pregnancy must be used judiciously—the axiom of "do not perform a test unless you are going to use the information for expediting the care of the patient" is most relevant under these circumstances.

Effects of Cancer Therapy on the Fetus

The majority of cytotoxic agents can cross the placenta and reach the fetus and thus the concern regarding effects of chemotherapy on the unborn child. **Chemotherapy during the first trimester has been shown to increase the risk of spontaneous abortions, major malformations, and fetal demise and thus should be avoided unless termination of pregnancy is planned. Second and third trimester exposure is associated primarily with intrauterine growth restriction and low birth weight as well as potentially preterm deliveries and neonatal myelosuppression** (3–5).

Of the different types of chemotherapeutic agents, the antimetabolites are more likely to be teratogenic than *alkylating agents* or anthracyclines. Long-term studies of infants born to mothers treated with chemotherapy for hematologic malignancies in pregnancy have reported normal physical, neurological, and psychological development as well as no increased risk of childhood malignancies (3–5).

The use of radiotherapy in pregnancy has been reported much less frequently but with appropriate treatment planning and shielding of the fetus, tumors not involving the pelvis or abdomen which require radiation therapy can be treated, with good overall outcomes (6).

Management of the Ongoing Pregnancy

Gestational age of the pregnancy is a critical component of the information required to offer optimal therapy (Fig. 17.1). For example, in a patient diagnosed with cancer in the first or early second trimester, termination should be discussed with the patient and her family as a therapeutic option if the treatment would otherwise disrupt the pregnancy. If the decision is made to continue the pregnancy, careful counseling concerning the risks, benefits, and alternatives to diagnostic and therapeutic intervention must be thoroughly discussed with the patient.

Surgical removal of tumors is often possible with minimal risk of disrupting the pregnancy. Surgery during the early second trimester is ideal, but surgery at any gestational age is reasonable if it will maximize the chance of cure and long-term survival (7). Delivery of the fetus is often advocated but rarely necessary. Each case is unique and therapy must be carefully individualized.

If surgery is performed after 24 weeks, which is considered the lower limit of viability, careful attention must be paid to adequate fluid replacement and prevention of hypotension. **Fetal monitoring is recommended,** with emergency cesarean section being reserved for imminent fetal compromise.

Antenatal corticosteroid therapy for induction of fetal lung maturity should be considered in all cases after 24 weeks of gestation (8,9). The beneficial effects of steroids on fetal lung, brain, and bowel development allow the obstetric and oncologic teams to plan interventions and to have flexibility to perform an early delivery if necessary.

Fetal surveillance should be instituted after 28 weeks. This should include serial obstetrical ultrasonography to evaluate fetal growth and placental function, and a combination of nonstress testing, biophysical profile testing, and umbilical artery Doppler measurements.

Consideration for Delivery After 32 Weeks' Gestation

The method of delivery should be determined by obstetrical indications. **The presence of a malignancy is not an indication for cesarean delivery** *per se.* In a modern neonatal intensive care unit, the neonatal survival rate at 28 weeks' gestation following antenatal corticosteroid administration is well above 90%. In addition, long-term neurologic outcome is near normal in

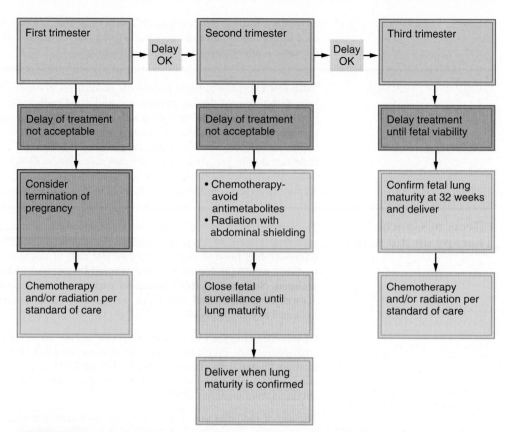

Figure 17.1 **Figure 17.1** Management of a non-gynecologic cancer during the three trimesters of pregnancy.

over 90% of survivors (10). These encouraging neonatal statistics afford the obstetric and oncologic teams the flexibility to institute optimal maternal therapy, while also allowing for a successful pregnancy outcome.

Specific Cancers in Pregnancy

Cervical Intraepithelial Neoplasia and Invasive Carcinoma of the Cervix	Pregnancy represents an opportunity to screen women for a variety of conditions and often this represents the only occasion when some women will have cytologic screening for cervical cancer. **The reported incidence of cervical cancer is 1.2 per 10,000 pregnancies** (1).
Management of an Abnormal Pap Test in Pregnancy	**Currently the recommendations for addressing abnormal Pap tests during pregnancy favor a conservative approach in the absence of frankly malignant cells.** The ASCCP guidelines (11) generally recommend that women with an abnormal pap smear concurrently have HPV testing performed. **An algorithm for the management of the abnormal Pap test in pregnancy is presented in Fig. 17.2.**
Positive High-Risk HPV	**In women with negative cervical cytology and a positive high-risk HPV test, a repeat of both tests is recommended at 12 months. For pregnant women, it is recommended that this be repeated at the 6-week postpartum visit** (11).
ASC-US	**In women with an ASC-US Pap smear but high-risk HPV negative test, the recommendation is also to repeat both at the 6-week postpartum visit** (11). The chance of finding an invasive lesion following a minimally abnormal Pap smear antepartum or postpartum is less than 1% in women with an ASC-US Pap smear and a positive high-risk HPV test. **The current guidelines recommend that for women older than 21 years of age, ASC-US and a positive HPV test may be managed by colposcopy at the time of diagnosis, or colposcopy may be deferred until the postpartum evaluation** (11).

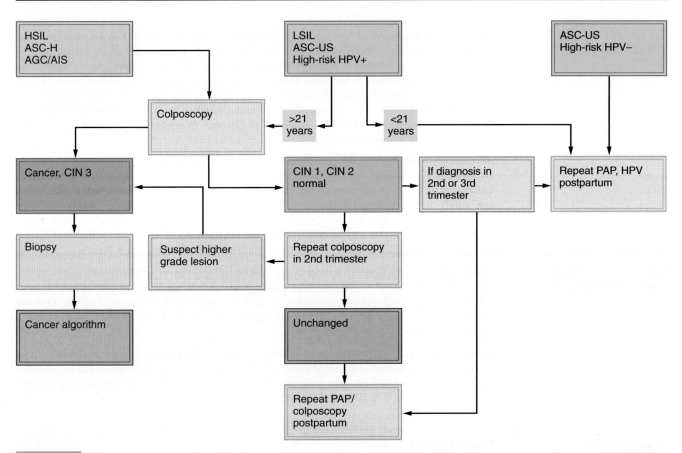

Figure 17.2   Management of abnormal Pap test in pregnancy as per ASCCP guidelines. (CIN = cervical intraepithelial lesion, HPV = human papilloma virus, LSIL = low-grade squamous intraepithelial lesion, HSIL = high-grade intraepithelial lesion, ASC-US = atypical squamous cells of undetermined significance. ASC-H = atypical squamous cells, cannot exclude high-grade, AGC = atypical glandular cells, AIS = adenocarcinoma *in situ*)

LSIL	Patients with LSIL on cervical cytology are extremely unlikely to have an invasive lesion and a study by Jain et al. found none of 287 patients had an invasive lesion on antepartum biopsy (12). Thus, **the current ASCCP guidelines state that colposcopy is preferred for the nonadolescent pregnant woman with LSIL, but deferring this procedure until at least 6 weeks postpartum is an option provided there is no cytologic or macroscopic evidence of a more invasive process** (11–14).
HSIL	**Patients with HSIL on a Pap smear should undergo colposcopy** (11). Because of the increased vascularity of the cervix during pregnancy, the colposcopic findings are exaggerated, and are more difficult to interpret. Therefore, those with an expertise in this area should perform colposcopy during pregnancy.
	Women with HSIL on a Pap smear should be referred antepartum for expert colposcopic evaluation and they should undergo colposcopically directed biopsies of any suspicious findings. There is a risk of excessive bleeding from the cervix, but most studies have reported no significant adverse outcomes from colposcopically directed biopsies during pregnancy (13,14). The general recommendation is to defer colposcopy until the second trimester, although the vascularity of the cervix is significantly increased after the first trimester. **In all cases, endocervical curettage should be avoided, although this is primarily because there have been no trials to evaluate the risk** (13,14).
Atypical Glandular Cells	Atypical glandular cells (AGC) on a Pap smear should be thoroughly evaluated at any time during pregnancy and the pregnant woman with atypical glandular cells or adenocarcinoma *in situ* on a Pap smear should undergo colposcopically directed biopsies and if indicated, cervical conization or loop electrosurgical excision procedure (LEEP) (14).

Treatment of CIN 2-3

The risk of progression of cervical intraepithelial neoplasia (CIN) 2-3 to microinvasive or frankly invasive carcinoma is minimal, and the rate of spontaneous postpartum regression of CIN 2-3 is relatively high, so the treatment of CIN during pregnancy should be observation unless there is a strong suspicion of microinvasive or invasive disease (15). If indicated, a LEEP procedure can be performed in pregnancy but significant bleeding may occur and the practitioner should be prepared to deal with this potential. **LEEP should primarily be reserved for patients in the early stages of pregnancy in whom the presence of invasive disease is strongly suspected** (15).

All patients with abnormal Pap smears or cervical dysplasia during pregnancy should be reevaluated 6 to 8 weeks postpartum with repeat Pap testing and colposcopic evaluation. Patients with cervical intraepithelial neoplasia in the absence of other contraindications can safely undergo vaginal delivery. Furthermore, an increased rate of regression after vaginal delivery (as opposed to cesarean section) for LSIL and HSIL has been reported, which may obviate the need for an excisional procedure postpartum (15,16).

Invasive Cervical Cancer in Pregnancy

Worldwide, invasive cervical cancer is the most common cancer of the female reproductive tract with approximately half a million annual cases and 250,000 deaths (17). Most of these cases are seen in developing countries in reproductive-age women, which explains the high rate of cervical cancer in pregnancy. Though relatively uncommon in the United States, this is a significant international health problem.

Cervical cancer is one of the most common cancers diagnosed during pregnancy. The diagnosis and treatment of cervical cancer during pregnancy should be managed by a multidisciplinary team, and treatment will depend on the stage and the gestational age at diagnosis, and the patient's desires and beliefs regarding continuation versus termination of the pregnancy (18).

Management

Stages IA1/IA2

Early stage cervical cancer can often be managed conservatively. If stage IA1 disease is diagnosed on the basis of a cone biopsy with negative margins, it is reasonable to follow the pregnancy until term and anticipate vaginal delivery.

In patients with stage IA2 disease identified before 20 to 24 weeks' gestation, pelvic lymphadenectomy should be performed. If the nodes are positive, standard therapy should be recommended. If the nodes are negative, a cone biopsy with clear margins should be sufficient treatment for the primary lesion. After 24 weeks, it is reasonable to await lung maturity, deliver the baby by caesarian section, and treat the cancer postpartum.

The complications associated with cervical conization in pregnancy are significant. Cervical conization has been associated with significant hemorrhage in 5% to 15% of patients and miscarriage rates as high as 25% (19,20). **Delaying treatment of an occult lesion probably has no impact on overall survival, as the likelihood of significant progression during a pregnancy is small** (21). Most earlier reports pertained to squamous cell carcinomas, and management of adenocarcinomas of the cervix remains somewhat controversial, but several recent reports have described conservative management of adenocarcinoma *in situ* and early invasive adenocarcinoma in pregnancy (22,23).

Stages IB/IIA

In patients with frankly invasive carcinomas, the gestational age at diagnosis impacts more significantly on the treatment recommendations, as well as the patient's desire to continue the pregnancy (24,25).

In the first and early second trimester, treatment options for patients with Stage IB or Stage IIA disease include radical hysterectomy with the fetus *in situ* versus standard chemoradiation therapy. The survival rates for patients having stage IB or IIA cervical carcinoma treated in early pregnancy are similar to nonpregnant patients (24,25).

If the patient selects to undergo conservative management, or if the diagnosis is not made until after 24 weeks, she should be followed until fetal lung maturity has been achieved, then delivered by classical cesarean section followed immediately by a radical hysterectomy and pelvic

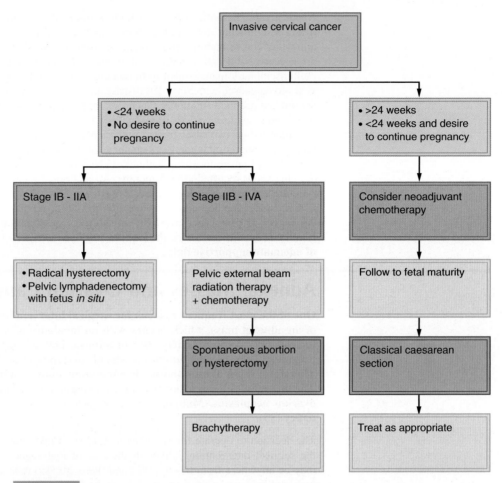

Figure 17.3 Management of cervical cancer in pregnancy.

lymphadenectomy (24–26). **Delivery by classical cesarean section is recommended and may have better outcomes as seen in the report by Sood et al. (26) who reported a 14% recurrence rate (1 in 7) among patients delivered by cesarean section versus a 56% recurrence (10 in 17) among those patients delivered vaginally. Others though have found no benefit to cesarean versus vaginal delivery (27). The later has a significantly higher risk of hemorrhage, infection, and potential for episiotomy site metastasis.**

Advanced Disease

Patients with stage IB2 to IVA disease, should be offered pelvic radiation including external beam with concurrent chemotherapy if diagnosed in the first 20 weeks of pregnancy (28). An algorithm for the treatment of advanced stage cervical cancer is presented in Fig. 17.3. Treatment should be given with the fetus *in situ*. After several treatments of external beam therapy, a spontaneous termination of pregnancy should occur. However, for patients in whom the psychological impact of this approach would be potentially devastating, it is reasonable to offer termination of pregnancy by hysterotomy or by *in utero* intracardiac injection (28) which will then result in spontaneous expulsion of the fetus or potentially require uterine evacuation. Radiation can be started prior to evacuation of the fetus particularly if it is needed to control bleeding from a bulky tumor.

Management of advanced cervical cancer diagnosed after 20 to 24 weeks will usually be conservative. A delay of treatment for 6 to 8 weeks will significantly improve fetal outcome, without impacting negatively on maternal outcome (29,30). Therefore, if there is no significant urgency because of heavy bleeding or ureteric obstruction, it is reasonable to observe until acceptable fetal maturity has been reached, then undertake classical cesarean section. Chemoradiation should be commenced as soon as possible post-cesarean section, usually within 2–3 weeks.

Neoadjuvant chemotherapy in patients with locally advanced cervical cancer who strongly desire a significant delay in treatment has been reported. This approach has the potential to allow the fetus to mature before instituting delivery and definitive radiotherapy, but the reports are anecdotal and data regarding safety and outcome are limited. Appropriate counseling and multidisciplinary management in these cases is essential. Maran et al. reported a case of a 26-year-old diagnosed with Stage IIB disease at 14 weeks' gestation who delivered a healthy infant at term and declined additional cancer treatment after being treated with *cisplatin* 50 mg/m2 on days 2 and 3 and *bleomycin* 30 mg on day 1 for three cycles every 3 weeks (29). Tewari et al. (30) reported on two cases treated with *cisplatin* and *vincristine* with successful regression of tumor allowing completion of pregnancy followed by radical hysterectomy. One patient with Stage IB2 (7 cm lesion) was without evidence of disease at 2 years but the other (stage IIA, 4.5 cm lesion) recurred after 5 months. An additional paper reported one patient treated with *cisplatin* and *vincristine* for four cycles between 23 to 33 weeks' gestation with good long-term outcome (31). The literature has three additional case reports (32–34). **This approach to cervical cancer in pregnancy must be considered experimental and used only in very exceptional circumstances where the woman has been extensively counseled regarding the lack of adequate supportive data.**

Adnexal Masses and Ovarian Cancer in Pregnancy

One of the most frequent reasons for surgical intervention in pregnancy is the diagnosis of an adnexal mass, which occurs with an incidence of between 0.2% and 2% of pregnancies (35). Approximately 90% of adnexal masses diagnosed in the first trimester of pregnancy are corpus luteum cysts of pregnancy, and will resolve spontaneously. Therefore, surgical intervention is not recommended until early in the second trimester. The majority of lesions that persist are benign, and include teratomas and other benign ovarian neoplasms. Malignant and borderline ovarian tumors are rare during pregnancy (35).

The decision to operate for an adnexal mass must take into account the risks and benefits of the surgical intervention. Although the risk of malignancy is very low, the risk of torsion may be anywhere from 6% to 20%, and there are also risks of obstructed labor or an abnormal fetal lie.

The overall risk of surgical intervention during pregnancy is thought to be low and in a review of about 12,000 cases of surgery during pregnancy, Cohen-Kerem and colleagues concluded that surgery does not increase the risk for miscarriage or congenital anomalies. Premature deliveries occurred in 3.5% of cases, mainly after abdominal surgery and peritonitis in the third trimester (36).

Laparoscopic surgery has also been reported during pregnancy and has been found to be safe. Although it does offer advantages, only limited data are available and it should only be performed by a very experienced gynecologist (37,38). The management of an adnexal mass in pregnancy should be a collaboration between a gynecologic surgeon and a maternal-fetal medicine specialist, giving careful consideration to the size and ultrasonic features of the mass, and the gestational age at diagnosis.

Leiserowitz et al. (39) reported a population-based study of 4,846,505 obstetrical patients using the California hospital discharge records from 1991 to 1999. There were 9,375 women (0.2%) who had a hospital diagnosis of an ovarian mass associated with pregnancy. The California Cancer Registry database identified 87 ovarian cancers (0.93% of adnexal masses) and 115 ovarian low malignant potential tumors (1.2% of adnexal masses) in the same cohort. Thirty-four of the 87 ovarian cancers (39%) were germ cell tumors. Malignant ovarian tumors had an adverse affect on maternal morbidity including increased need for cesarean section, hysterectomy, blood transfusion, and extended hospitalization. There did not appear to be any adverse affect on neonatal outcomes.

Schmeler et al. (40) reviewed the records of pregnant patients diagnosed with adnexal masses 5 cm or greater in diameter and compared patients who had surgical intervention with those having observation. At the Women's & Infant's Hospital of Rhode Island, Brown University Medical School, Providence, RI, between 1990 and 2003, adnexal masses 5 cm or larger were diagnosed in 63 of 127,000 pregnant women for a rate of 0.05%. Antepartum surgery was performed in 17 patients (29%), the majority for ultrasonic findings suggestive of malignancy.

In four patients, the surgery was performed because of an ovarian torsion. The remaining patients were observed and surgery was performed in the postpartum period or at the time of cesarean delivery when a cesarean was performed for obstetric indications. They found four patients (6.8%) with an ovarian cancer and one patient (1.7%) with a tumor of low malignant potential. The ultrasonic findings in all five patients prompted surgical intervention. Thus no case of malignancy was missed. They recommend observation with postpartum surgery provided the ultrasonic findings were not highly suspicious for malignancy.

Yen et al. (41) followed 174 pregnant patients presenting with adnexal tumors ≥4 cm diameter. Fourteen percent of patients experienced torsion, and these occurred primarily in adnexal masses between 6 and 8 cm. **Sixty percent of torsions occurred between 10 and 17 weeks of gestation and only 6% occurred after 20 weeks. The incidence of malignancy was 3.4% with the greatest risk being in tumors larger than 10 cm at initial diagnosis.** Tumor growth greater than 3.5 cm per week was also associated with a significantly higher risk of malignancy. The authors recommended surgical intervention for tumors between 6 and 8 cm if diagnosed before the 20th week of gestation and for any adnexal mass with sonographic findings suspicious for malignancy or undergoing significant growth rate during ongoing observation.

The incidence of ovarian malignancy is very low in pregnancy; however, the potential for missing a malignant tumor of the ovary certainly exists in these reproductive-age women, and **a suspicious ovarian mass should be removed surgically in the second trimester of pregnancy. Surgical outcomes in a well-controlled setting are excellent during pregnancy** (39).

The majority of cancers are early stage, and chemotherapy can usually be withheld until after delivery for stage I epithelial tumors (42,43). Germ cell tumors are uncommon, but if there is an indication for chemotherapy, then treatment should be undertaken as soon after expedited delivery, as possible or during the second or third trimester. Most of these cancers have a good prognosis for both the woman and the infant (42,43).

Breast Cancer in Pregnancy

Breast cancer is the most commonly diagnosed invasive malignancy during pregnancy and the postpartum period. The incidence has been reported to be 1 in 10,000 to 1 in 3,000 and it is thought that with the trend toward delayed child-bearing, the incidence of breast cancer diagnosed during pregnancy will increase further (44). Overall 3% of women diagnosed with breast cancer will be lactating or pregnant at the time of diagnosis (44). The diagnosis may be delayed due to physiologic changes which may obscure a breast mass, or lead to a mass being attributed to the pregnancy or lactation.

Frequently the stage of breast cancer diagnosis during pregnancy is higher than in nonpregnant patients, either due to delayed diagnosis or to a promotional effect of gestational hormones on breast tumors, causing an intrinsic biological aggressiveness. When controlled for stage, pregnancy *per se* does not confer a worse prognosis (45,46).

Any woman who presents with a breast abnormality should have it completely investigated, regardless of pregnancy or lactation. Diagnostic mammography can be performed with minimal risk to the fetus with the use of abdominal shielding, but mammography may be of limited value due to the denseness of breast tissue during pregnancy and lactation. Ultrasonography can be an accurate method of identifying cystic and solid lesions, and can be used to guide fine needle aspiration (47).

Once the initial diagnosis and metastatic workup has been accomplished, treatment should be instituted immediately. Pregnancy termination does not need to be routinely recommended, but some women may choose to terminate the pregnancy in order to expedite the treatment options (48).

The treatment strategies for pregnant women should be the same as for nonpregnant women with breast cancer. Initial surgical resection followed by postoperative adjuvant therapy is the standard of care and should be undertaken with minimal delay. If the diagnosis is made in the first trimester any chemotherapy should be delayed until the second or third trimester. If necessary, therapeutic radiation treatment may be instituted during pregnancy, with appropriate shielding to reduce fetal exposure. The level of ionizing radiation to the fetus that is absolutely safe is not known (48).

Any patient diagnosed with breast cancer during pregnancy should be managed by a multidisciplinary team, and the patient should be counseled regarding possible pregnancy outcomes related to the diagnostic and treatment methodologies employed (48).

Malignant Melanoma in Pregnancy

The incidence of cutaneous malignant melanoma has been increasing by 3% to 5% per year, with an increased incidence in women (49). **The skin changes that occur in pregnancy can make diagnosis more difficult but any suspicious lesion should be fully evaluated and treated appropriately.** The effects of pregnancy hormones on malignant melanoma remain controversial, though recent studies have shown no significant difference in survival between pregnant and nonpregnant women with melanoma, given similar prognostic factors, including tumor thickness (49). With early diagnosis and treatment excellent outcomes can be expected without any negative impact of the pregnancy on the disease.

O'Meara et al. from California reported the largest population based study of pregnant women with malignant melanoma (50). They recruited patients from 1991 to 1999, and compared women who had pregnancy associated melanoma with age matched controls. In their database, the incidence of pregnancy associated melanoma in California was 8.5 per 100,000 pregnant women. This was compared to the national SEER statistics from 1975 to 2000 which showed that the incidence of melanoma in women aged 20 to 45 years ranged from 6 to 21.2 per 100,000. **They reported no difference in stage, tumor thickness, lymph node involvement, or survival between the two groups.** The study was somewhat limited by the fact that the women who terminated their pregnancy prior to 20 weeks may not have been included, and there were very small numbers of women with advanced melanoma in the study group. The most important prognostic factor was tumor thickness, which is the same for nonpregnant women. A large Swedish study also found no differences in outcome for pregnant versus nonpregnant women with melanoma (51).

The potential for metastasis to the placenta in pregnant women with melanoma warrants careful histologic evaluation by pathologists. With placental involvement, fetal risk of melanoma metastasis is approximately 22%. Neonates delivered with concomitant placental involvement should be considered at high risk, must be followed with vigilance (52).

Lymphoma and Leukemia in Pregnancy

The median age of presentation of Hodgkin's disease is 30 years and given that this is the peak reproductive age, the diagnosis of Hodgkin's disease in pregnancy occurs in one in 6,000 pregnancies. Diagnosis by lymph node biopsy can be performed safely in the pregnant patient and any suspicious adenopathy should be assessed regardless of the gestational status.

Hodgkin's lymphoma and non-Hodgkin's lymphoma should be treated as in nonpregnant patients. Second and third trimester exposure to chemotherapeutic agents is not associated with fetal malformations, but there is an increase in the risk of fetal or neonatal death, intrauterine growth restriction (IUGR), preterm delivery, and low birth weight.

If the diagnosis of lymphoma is made during the first trimester, termination of pregnancy is recommended as there is a 10% to 20% incidence of congenital anomalies with first trimester exposure to chemotherapeutic agents. In cases of low grade or indolent lymphoma or if a patient desires to maintain the pregnancy, treatment should be instituted in the second trimester (53).

Women treated for lymphoma during pregnancy have the same recurrence rate and survival as their nonpregnant counterparts (53).

Leukemia in pregnancy is extremely rare but presents a very difficult challenge for both the patient and the treating physicians. **Treatment for leukemia should be started as soon as possible after the diagnosis has been made regardless of the gestational age.** In early pregnancy, termination is considered to be the best course of action, given the teratogencity of antineoplastic agents and the potential for maternal complications during periods of extreme pancytopenia and immunosuppression (54).

Summary

The diagnosis of a malignant neoplasm in pregnancy is devastating, but the oncologist and obstetrician must be able to appropriately determine the best treatment options, and counsel the patient regarding the potential outcome for the pregnancy, and the likely prognosis for these various treatment options (55). Termination of pregnancy is unlikely to improve the maternal outcome, except for patients with invasive cervical cancer diagnosed in the first or early second trimester. Oncologic treatment modalities including surgery, chemotherapy, and radiation therapy (except to the pelvis or abdomen) can safely be given after the first trimester.

References

1. **Pavlidis NA.** Coexistence of pregnancy and malignancy. *Oncologist* 2002;7:279–287.

2. **Pereg D, Koren K, Lishner M.** Cancer in pregnancy: gaps, challenges and solutions. *Cancer Treat Rev* 2008;34:302–312.

3. **Cardonick E, Iacobucci A.** Use of chemotherapy during human pregnancy. *Lancet Oncol* 2004;5:283–291.

4. **Avilés A, Díaz-Maqueo JC, Talavera A, Guzmán R, García EL.** Growth and development of children of mothers treated with chemotherapy during pregnancy: current status of 43 children. *Am J Hematol* 1991;36:243–248.

5. **Avilés A, Neri N.** Hematological malignancies and pregnancy: a final report of 84 children who received chemotherapy in utero. *Clin Lymphoma* 2001;2:173–177.

6. **Kal HB, Struikmans H.** Radiotherapy during pregnancy: fact and fiction. *Lancet Oncol* 2005;6:328–333.

7. **Mazze RI, Källén B.** Reproductive outcome after anesthesia and operation during pregnancy: a registry study of 5405 cases. *Am J Obstet Gynecol* 1989;161:1178–1185.

8. **Wright LL, Horbar JD, Gunkel H, Verter J, Younes N, Andrews E, et al.** Evidence from multicenter networks on the current use and effectiveness of antenatal corticosteroids in low birthweight infants. *Am J Obstet Gynecol* 1995;173:263–269.

9. **Wright LL, Verter J, Younes N, Stevenson DK, Fanaroff AA, Shankaran S, et al.** Antenatal corticosteroid administration and neonatal outcome in very low birthweight infants: the NICH Neonatal Research Network. *Am J Obstet Gynecol* 1995;173:269–274.

10. **Fanaroff AA, Stoll BJ, Wright LL, Carlo WA, Ehrenkranz Ran, Stark A, et al. for the NICHD Neonatal Research Network.** Trends in neonatal morbidity and mortality for very low birthweight infants. *Am J Obstet Gynecol* 2007;196:147.e1–8.

11. **Wright TC, Massad LS, Dunton CJ, Spitzer M, Wilkinson EJ, Solomon D.** 2006 consensus guidelines for the management of women with cervical intraepithelial neoplasia or adenocarcinoma *in situ. J Low Genit Tract Dis* 2007;11:223–239.

12. **Jain AG, Higgins AV, Boyle MJ.** Management of low-grade squamous intraepithelial lesions during pregnancy. *Am J Obstet Gynecol* 1997;177:298–302.

13. **Economos K, Perez Veridiano N, Delke I, Collado ML, Tancer ML.** Abnormal cervical cytology in pregnancy: a 17-year experience. *Obstet Gynecol* 1993;1:915–918.

14. **Hunter MI, Krishnansu T, Monk B.** Cervical neoplasia in pregnancy. Part 1: screening and management of preinvasive disease. *Am J Obstet Gynecol* 2008;199:3–9.

15. **Frega A, Scirpa P, Corosu R, Verrico M, Scarciglia ML, Primieri MR, et al.** Clinical management and follow-up of squamous intraepithelial cervical lesions during pregnancy and postpartum. *Anticancer Res* 2007;27:2743–2746.

16. **Siristatidis Ch, Vitoratos N, Michailidis E, Syciotis C, Panagiotopoulos N, Kassanos D, et al.** The role of the mode of delivery in the alteration of intrapartum pathological cervical cytologic findings during the postpartum period. *Eur J Gynaecol Oncol* 2002;23:358–360.

17. **Parkin DM, Bray F, Ferlay J, Pisani P.** Global cancer statistics, 2002. *CA Cancer J Clin* 2005;55:74–108.

18. **Hunter MI, Krishnansu T, Monk B.** Cervical neoplasia in pregnancy. Part 2: current treatment of invasive disease. *Am J Obstet Gynecol* 2008;199:10–18.

19. **Averette HE, Nasser N, Yankow SL, Little WA.** Cervical conization in pregnancy. Analysis of 180 operations. *Am J Obstet* Gynecol 1970;106:543–549.

20. **Hannigan EV, Whitehouse HH, Atkinson WD, Becker SN.** Cone biopsy during pregnancy. *Obstet Gynecol* 1982;60:450–455.

21. **Sood AK, Sorosky JI.** Invasive cervical cancer complicating pregnancy. *Obstet Gynecol Clin N Am* 1998;25:343.

22. **Yahata T, Numata M, Kashima K, Sekine M, Fujita K, Yamamoto T, et al.** Conservative treatment of stage IA1 adenocarcinoma of the cervix during pregnancy. *Gynecol Oncol* 2008;109:49–52.

23. **Lacour RA, Garner EI, Molpus KL, Ashfaq R, Schorge JO.** Management of cervical adenocarcinoma in situ during pregnancy. *Am J Obstet Gynecol* 2005;192:1449–1451.

24. **Amant F, van Calsteren K, Halaska MJ, Beijnen J, Lagae L, Hanssens M, et al.** Gynecologic cancers in pregnancy: guidelines of an international consensus meeting. *Int J Gynecol Cancer* 2009;19: S1–S12.

25. **Takushi M, Moromizato H, Sakumoto K, Kanazawa K.** Management of invasive carcinoma of the uterine cervix associated with pregnancy: outcome of intentional delay in treatment. *Gynecol Oncol* 2002;82:185–189.

26. **Sood AK, Sorosky JI, Mayr N, Andersen B, Buller RE, Niebyl J.** Cervical cancer diagnosed shortly after pregnancy: Prognostic variables and delivery routes. *Obstet Gynecol* 2000;95:832–838.

27. **van der Vange N, Weverling GJ, Ketting BW, Ankum WM, Samlal R, Lammes FB.** The prognosis of cervical cancer associated with pregnancy: a matched cohort study. *Obstet Gynecol* 1995;85: 1022–1026.

28. **Sood AK, Sorosky JI, Mayr N, Krogman S, Anderson B, Buller RE, et al.** Radiotherapeutic management of cervical carcinoma that complicates pregnancy. *Cancer* 1997;80:1073–1078.

29. **Marana HR, de Andrade JM, da Silva Mathes AC, Duarte G, da Cunha SP, et al.** Chemotherapy in the treatment of locally advanced cervical cancer and pregnancy. *Gynecol Oncol* 2001;80:272–274.

30. **Tewari K, Cappuccini F, Gambino A, Kohler MH, Pecorelli S, DiSaia PJ.** Neoadjuvant chemotherapy in the treatment of locally advanced cervical carcinoma in pregnancy: a report of two cases and review of issues specific to the management of cervical carcinoma in pregnancy including planned delay of therapy. *Cancer* 1998;82: 1529–1534.

31. **Bader AA, Petru E, Winter R.** Long-term follow-up after neoadjuvant chemotherapy for high-risk cervical cancer during pregnancy. *Gynecol Oncol* 2007;105:269–272.

32. **Giacalone PL, Laffargue F, Benos P, Rousseau O, Hedon B.** Cisplatinum neoadjuvant chemotherapy in a pregnant woman with invasive carcinoma of the uterine cervix. *Br J Obstet Gynaecol* 1996;103:932–934.

33. **Caluwaerts S, Van Calsteren K, Mertens L, Lagae L, Moerman P, Hanssens M, et al.** Neoadjuvant chemotherapy followed by radical hysterectomy for invasive cervical cancer diagnosed during pregnancy: report of a case and review of the literature. *Int J Gynecol Cancer* 2006;16:905–908.

34. **Karam A, Feldman N, Holschneider C.** Neoadjuvant cisplatin and radical cesarean hysterectomy for cervical cancer in pregnancy. *Nat Clin Pract Oncol* 2007;4:375–380.

35. **Sherard GB, Hodson CA, Williams HJ, Semer DA, Hadi HA, Tait DL.** Adnexal masses and pregnancy: a 12-year experience. *Am J Obstet Gynecol* 2003;84:179–182.

36. **Cohen-Kerem R, Railton C, Oren D, Lishner M, Koren G.** Pregnancy outcome following non-obstetric surgical intervention. *Am J Surg* 2005;190:467–473.

37. **Bunyavejchevin S, Phupong V.** Laparoscopic surgery for presumed benign ovarian tumor during pregnancy. *Cochrane Database Syst Rev* 2006;18:CD005459.

38. **Mathevet P, Nessah K, Dargent D, Mellier G.** Laparoscopic management of adnexal masses in pregnancy: a case series. *Eur J Obstet Gynecol Reprod Biol* 2003;108:217–222.

39. **Leiserowitz GS, Xing G, Cress R, Brahmbhatt B, Dalrymple JL, Smith LH.** Adnexal masses in pregnancy: how often are they malignant? *Gynecol Oncol* 2006;101:315–321.

40. **Schmeler KM, Mayo-Smith WW, Peipert JF, Weitzen S, Manuel MD, Gordinier ME.** Adnexal masses in pregnancy: surgery compared with observation. *Obstet Gynecol* 2005;105:1098–1103.

41. **Yen CF, Lin SL, Murk W, Wang CJ, Lee CL, Soong YK, et al.** Risk analysis of torsion and malignancy for adnexal masses during pregnancy. *Fertil Steril* 2009;91:1895–1902.

42. **Machado F, Vegas C, Leon J, Perez A, Sanchez R, Parrilla JJ, et al.** Ovarian cancer during pregnancy: analysis of 15 cases. *Gynecol Oncol* 2007;105:446–450.

43. **Boulay R, Podczaski E.** Ovarian cancer complicating pregnancy. *Obstet Gynecol Clin N Am* 1998;25:385–399.

44. **Hoover HC.** Breast cancer during pregnancy and lactation. *Surg Clin North Am* 1990;70:1151–1163.

45. **Middleton LP, Amin M, Gwyn K, Theriault R, Sahin A.** Breast carcinoma in pregnant women: assessment of clinicopathologic and immunohistochemical features. *Cancer* 2003;98:1055–1060.

46. **Mulvihill JJ, McKeen EA, Rosner F, Zarrabi MH.** Pregnancy outcome in cancer patients: experience in large cooperative groups. *Cancer* 1987;60:1143–1150.

47. **Yang WT, Dryden MJ, Gwyn K, Whitman GJ, Theriault R.** Imaging of breast cancer diagnosed and treated with chemotherapy during pregnancy. *Radiology* 2006;239:52–60.

48. **Loibl S, von Minckwitz G, Gwyn K, Ellis P, Blohmer JU, Schlegelberger B, et al.** Breast carcinoma during pregnancy: international recommendations from an expert meeting. *Cancer* 2006; 106:237–246.

49. **MacKie RM, Bufalino R, Morabito A, Sutherland C, Cascinelli N.** Lack of effect of pregnancy on outcome of melanoma. For The World Health Organisation Melanoma Programme. *Lancet* 1991;337: 653–655.

50. **O'Meara AT, Cress R, Xing G, Danielsen B, Smith LH.** Malignant melanoma in pregnancy. *Cancer* 2005;103:1217–1226.

51. **Lens MB, Rosdahl I, Ahlbom A, Farahmand BY, Synnerstad I, Boeryd B, et al.** Effect of pregnancy on survival in women with cutaneous malignant melanoma. *J Clin Oncol* 2004;22:4369–4375.

52. **Alexander A, Samlowski WE, Grossman D, Bruggers CS, Harris RM, Zone JJ, et al.** Metastatic melanoma in pregnancy: risk of transplacental metastases in the infant. *J Clin Oncol.* 2003;21: 2179–2186.

53. **Pereg D, Koren G, Lishner M.** The treatment of Hodgkin's and non-Hodgkin's lymphoma in pregnancy. *Haemotologica* 2002;92: 1230–1237.

54. **Shapira T, Pereg D, Lishner M.** How I treat acute and chronic leukemia in pregnancy. *Blood Rev* 2008;22:247–259.

55. **Amant F, Van Calsteren K, Vergote I, Ottevanger N.** Gynecologic oncology in pregnancy. *Crit Rev Oncol Hematol* 2008;67:187–195.

Updated - 2008 FIGO Staging Tables

Addendum: The following tables contain the updated 2008 FIGO staging for cancer of the uterine cervix, endometrium, and vulva, and new staging for uterine sarcomas. The FIGO staging for gestational trophoblastic neoplasia and for cancers of the ovary, fallopian tube, and vagina remains unchanged.

Table 9.1A Carcinoma of the Cervix Uteri (2008)	
Stage I	The carcinoma is strictly confined to the cervix (extension to the corpus would be disregarded)
IA	Invasive carcinoma which can be diagnosed only by microscopy, with deepest invasion ≤5 mm and largest extension ≤7 mm
IA1	Measured stromal invasion of ≤3.0 mm in depth and extension of ≤7.0 mm
IA2	Measured stromal invasion of >3.0 mm and not >5.0 mm with an extension of not >7.0 mm
IB	Clinically visible lesions limited to the cervix uteri or pre-clinical cancers greater than stage IA*
IB1	Clinically visible lesion ≤4.0 cm in greatest dimension
IB2	Clinically visible lesion >4.0 cm in greatest dimension
Stage II	Cervical carcinoma invades beyond the uterus, but not to the pelvic wall or to the lower third of the vagina
IIA	Without parametrial invasion
IIA1	Clinically visible lesion ≤4.0 cm in greatest dimension
IIA2	Clinically visible lesion >4 cm in greatest dimension
IIB	With obvious parametrial invasion
Stage III	The tumor extends to the pelvic wall and/or involves lower third of the vagina and/or causes hydronephrosis or non-functioning kidney**
IIIA	Tumor involves lower third of the vagina, with no extension to the pelvic wall
IIIB	Extension to the pelvic wall and/or hydronephrosis or non-functioning kidney
Stage IV	The carcinoma has extended beyond the true pelvis or has involved (biopsy proven) the mucosa of the bladder or rectum. A bullous edema, as such, does not permit a case to be allotted to Stage IV
IVA	Spread of the growth to adjacent organs
IVB	Spread to distant organs

FIGO Committee on Gynecologic Oncology. Revised FIGO staging for carcinoma of the vulva, cervix, and endometrium. *Int J Gynecol Obst* 2009;105:103–104.

*All macroscopically visible lesions—even with superficial invasion—are allotted to stage IB carcinomas. Invasion is limited to a measured stromal invasion with a maximal depth of 5.00 mm and a horizontal extension of not >7.00 mm. Depth of invasion should not be >5.00 mm taken from the base of the epithelium of the original tissue—squamous or glandular. The depth of invasion should always be reported in mm, even in those cases with "early (minimal) stromal invasion" (~1 mm). The involvement of vascular/lymphatic spaces should not change the stage allotment.

**On rectal examination, there is no cancer-free space between the tumor and the pelvic wall. All cases with hydronephrosis or non-functioning kidney are included, unless they are known to be due to another cause.

Table 10.6A Carcinoma of the Endometrium (2008)	
Stage I*	Tumor confined to the corpus uteri
IA*	No or less than half myometrial invasion
IB*	Invasion equal to or more than half of the myometrium
Stage II*	Tumor invades cervical stroma, but does not extend beyond the uterus**
Stage III*	Local and/or regional spread of the tumor
IIIA*	Tumor invades the serosa of the corpus uteri and/or adnexae[#]
IIIB*	Vaginal and/or parametrial involvement[#]
IIIC*	Metastases to pelvic and/or para-aortic lymph nodes[#]
IIIC1*	Positive pelvic nodes
IIIC2*	Positive para-aortic lymph nodes with or without positive pelvic lymph nodes
Stage IV*	Tumor invades bladder and/or bowel mucosa, and/or distant metastases
IVA*	Tumor invasion of bladder and/or bowel mucosa
IVB*	Distant metastases, including intra-abdominal metastases and/or inguinal lymph nodes

FIGO Committee on Gynecologic Oncology. Revised FIGO staging for carcinoma of the vulva, cervix, and endometrium. *Int J Gynecol Obst* 2009;105:103–104.

*Either G_1, G_2, or G_3.

**Endocervical glandular involvement only should be considered as Stage I and no longer as Stage II.

[#]Positive cytology has to be reported separately without changing the stage.

Table 10.26 Staging for Uterine Sarcomas (Leiomyosarcomas, Endometrial Stromal Sarcomas, Adenosarcomas, and Carcinosarcomas) (2008)

(1) Leiomyosarcomas

Stage	Definition
Stage I	Tumor limited to uterus
IA	<5 cm
IB	>5 cm
Stage II	Tumor extends to the pelvis
IIA	Adnexal involvement
IIB	Tumor extends to extrauterine pelvic tissue
Stage III	Tumor invades abdominal tissues (not just protruding into the abdomen).
IIIA	One site
IIIB	> one site
IIIC	Metastasis to pelvic and/or para-aortic lymph nodes
Stage IV	
IVA	Tumor invades bladder and/or rectum
IVB	Distant metastasis

(2) Endometrial stromal sarcomas (ESS) and adenosarcomas*

Stage	Definition
Stage I	Tumor limited to uterus
IA	Tumor limited to endometrium/endocervix with no myometrial invasion
IB	Less than or equal to half myometrial invasion
IC	More than half myometrial invasion
Stage II	Tumor extends to the pelvis
IIA	Adnexal involvement
IIB	Tumor extends to extrauterine pelvic tissue
Stage III	Tumor invades abdominal tissues (not just protruding into the abdomen).
IIIA	One site
IIIB	> one site
IIIC	Metastasis to pelvic and/or para-aortic lymph nodes
Stage IV	
IVA	Tumor invades bladder and/or rectum
IVB	Distant metastasis

(3) Carcinosarcomas

Carcinosarcomas should be staged as carcinomas of the endometrium.

FIGO Committee on Gynecologic Oncology. FIGO staging for uterine sarcomas. *Int J Gynecol Obst* 2009;104:179.

*Note: Simultaneous tumors of the uterine corpus and ovary/pelvis in association with ovarian/pelvic endometriosis should be classified as independent primary tumors.

Table 13.7A Carcinoma of the Vulva (2008)	
Stage I	Tumor confined to the vulva
IA	Lesions ≤2 cm in size, confined to the vulva or perineum and with stromal invasion ≤1.0 mm*, no nodal metastasis
IB	Lesions >2 cm in size or with stromal invasion >1.0 mm*, confined to the vulva or perineum, with negative nodes
Stage II	Tumor of any size with extension to adjacent perineal structures (1/3 lower urethra, 1/3 lower vagina, anus) with negative nodes
Stage III	Tumor of any size with or without extension to adjacent perineal structures (1/3 lower urethra, 1/3 lower vagina, anus) with positive inguino-femoral lymph nodes
IIIA	(i) With 1 lymph node metastasis (≥5 mm), or
	(ii) 1–2 lymph node metastasis(es) (<5 mm)
IIIB	(i) With 2 or more lymph node metastases (≥5 mm), or
	(ii) 3 or more lymph node metastases (<5 mm)
IIIC	With positive nodes with extracapsular spread
Stage IV	Tumor invades other regional (2/3 upper urethra, 2/3 upper vagina), or distant structures
IVA	Tumor invades any of the following:
	(i) upper urethral and/or vaginal mucosa, bladder mucosa, rectal mucosa, or fixed to pelvic bone, or
	(ii) fixed or ulcerated inguino-femoral lymph nodes
IVB	Any distant metastasis including pelvic lymph nodes

FIGO Committee on Gynecologic Oncology. Revised FIGO staging for carcinoma of the vulva, cervix, and endometrium. *Int J Gynecol Obst* 2009;105:103–104.

*The depth of invasion is defined as the measurement of the tumor from the epithelial-stromal junction of the adjacent most superficial dermal papilla to the deepest point of invasion.

MEDICAL AND SURGICAL TOPICS

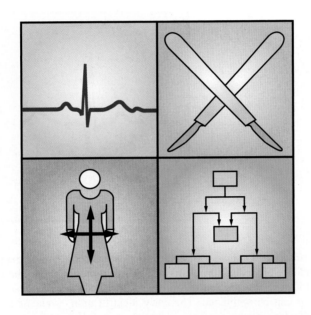

18 Preoperative Evaluation, Medical Management, and Critical Care

M. Iain Smith
Roger M. Lee
Spencer R. Adams
Samuel A. Skootsky

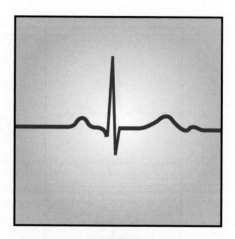

Because most patients with gynecological cancer are middle-aged to elderly, they have a high incidence of medical problems at the time of presentation. These need to be carefully assessed, and if necessary treated before the patient undergoes aggressive surgery, so that her medical status can be optimized. The early identification, evaluation, and management of emerging medical problems are also essential, especially in the perioperative period. This chapter discusses the most frequently encountered problems in patients with gynecologic cancers.

Preoperative Evaluation

The cornerstone of all perioperative medical management is the anticipation of specific problems. It is always better to have a management plan than to react to complications. Careful assessment of risk and monitoring of patients in the perioperative period minimizes morbidity and mortality.

Cardiovascular

Surgery can represent a major cardiovascular stress because of depression in myocardial contractility, changes in sympathetic tone induced by general anesthetic agents, and rapid changes in intravascular volume that occur due to blood loss and "third spacing" of fluids. The magnitude of cardiovascular stress depends on patient characteristics, the nature and site of the operation, the duration of the operation, and whether it is elective or emergent.

Cardiovascular Risk Factors

Multiple studies have been published over the last 30 years assessing clinical risks for cardiac events during surgery (1–5). A commonly used "simple index" called the **Revised Cardiac Risk Index** (Table 18.1) has been incorporated in the 2007 revision of the American College of Cardiology (ACC) and the American Heart Association (AHA) guidelines on perioperative cardiovascular evaluation and care for noncardiac surgery (5,6).

The recently revised ACC/AHA 2007 guidelines offer a simplified yet comprehensive approach to the assessment of cardiac risks for patients undergoing surgery (6). An algorithm based on this approach is shown in Fig. 18.1. This approach represents a consensus view derived from a review of the literature to date and is periodically updated on the ACC Web site

Table 18.1 Revised Cardiac Risk Index

1. Ischemic heart disease (history of myocardial infarction, history of positive cardiac stress test, use of nitroglycerin, current chest pain thought secondary to coronary ischemia, or ECG with abnormal Q waves).

2. Congestive heart failure (history of heart failure, pulmonary edema, paroxysmal nocturnal dyspnea, peripheral edema, bilateral rales, S_3, or x-ray with pulmonary vascular redistribution).

3. Cerebral vascular disease (history of transient ischemic attack [TIA] or stroke).

4. Diabetes mellitus treated preoperatively with insulin.

5. Chronic kidney disease with a preoperative creatinine greater than 2 mg per dL.

6. High-risk surgery (abdominal aortic aneurysm or other vascular surgery, thoracic, abdominal, or orthopedic surgery).

Adapted from **Lee TH, Marcantonio ER, Mangione CM, Thomas EJ, Polanczyk CA, Cook EF, et al.** Derivation and prospective validation of a simple index for prediction of cardiac risk of major noncardiac surgery. *Circulation* 1999;100:1043–1049.

(http://www.acc.org). **An important overriding theme of these guidelines is that cardiac stress testing and/or interventions (such as coronary stenting or coronary bypass graft surgery) are rarely necessary simply to lower the risk of surgery. In fact, such interventions are likely unnecessary unless they would have been performed even if the patient were not undergoing surgery.** Additionally, no test should be performed unless it likely to influence patient treatment.

If the patient has an active cardiac condition that indicates major clinical risk (Table 18.2), the surgery likely will be delayed or cancelled until the condition is stabilized unless the surgery is emergent (6,7). For stable patients, the algorithm can be used as follows: Obtain information from the patient and then use the **Revised Cardiac Risk Index** to determine how many of the clinical risk factors (from Table 18.1) that the patient has. **One point is assigned for each of the six possible clinical risk factors. Based on how many points are assigned, patients can be characterized as high risk (3 or more points), intermediate risk (1–2 points), or low risk (0 points).**

The first step is to determine the urgency of surgery. If emergent surgery is needed there is no time for any cardiac assessment beyond what history is available and the patient should proceed immediately to the operating room. For urgent or elective surgery, there is more time to assess a patient's cardiac risks. **If the patient has an active cardiac condition (Table 18.2), all but emergency surgeries should be delayed until the cardiac condition is properly evaluated and treated.**

Often patients need very little evaluation. In general, patients who are undergoing low-risk surgery (Table 18.3) do not need further evaluation. In addition, patients with good functional capacity (metabolic equivalents [METs] levels greater than or equal to 4) (Table 18.4) without symptoms and active conditions can proceed with typical gynecologic surgery without further evaluation (8) (Fig. 18.1).

Table 18.2 Major Active Cardiac Conditions

1. Unstable coronary syndromes (unstable or severe angina (Canadian class III or IV), acute (<7 days) or recent (7–30 days) myocardial infarction with evidence of important ischemic risk by clinical symptoms or noninvasive study)

2. Decompensated heart failure

3. Significant, uncontrolled arrhythmias (high-grade atrioventricular block, symptomatic ventricular arrhythmias in the presence of underlying heart disease)

4. Severe valvular heart disease (especially severe aortic stenosis)

Table 18.3 Cardiac Risk Stratification for Noncardiac Surgical Procedures
High (Reported cardiac risk often greater than 5%)
Emergent major operations, particularly in the elderly
Aortic and other major vascular surgery
Peripheral vascular surgery
Anticipated prolonged surgical procedures associated with large fluid shifts and/or blood loss
Intermediate (Reported cardiac risk generally less than 5%)
Carotid endarterectomy
Head and neck surgery
Intraperitoneal and intrathoracic surgery
Orthopedic surgery
Prostate surgery
Low (Reported cardiac risk generally less than 1%)
Endoscopic procedures
Superficial procedure
Cataract surgery
Breast surgery

If the patient has poor or unknown functional capacity, then the presence of clinical risk factors from the Revised Cardiac Risk Index help determine the need for further evaluation. For those patients undergoing intermediate risk surgeries (most gynecological surgeries), the presence of any clinical risk factor should prompt consideration of cardiology consultation and/or noninvasive stress testing if it will change management (9). Perioperative beta blockade will be discussed in more detail below, but given the results of recent studies, caution should be used when newly prescribing these drugs to patients with intermediate risk. *Dipyridamole-thallium* imaging or *dobutamine* stress echocardiography can be considered for noninvasive testing in these patients (10,11). If noninvasive testing shows only minor abnormalities, the patient can likely proceed with surgery with appropriate medical management including beta blockade. If moderate or severe abnormalities are found, subsequent care should include cardiology consultation. The cardiologist may recommend cancellation or delay of surgery, coronary revascularization followed by noncardiac surgery, or intensified care in such patients (6).

Myocardial Infarction

Even with the best preoperative assessment and preparation, postoperative myocardial infarction (MI) can still occur after surgery under general anesthesia. The risk factors for perioperative MI are related to the underlying risk of ischemic heart disease. Before the advent of more modern management of ischemic heart disease, the risk of a second MI after anesthesia and general surgery was considered too high during the first few months post myocardial infarction (12). Current cardiologic practice, including revascularization, angioplasty, or very aggressive medical therapy with lipid-lowering agents and use of β-blockers, makes this rule less useful. **It is now commonly believed that with proper treatment, patients can undergo surgery 6 weeks after myocardial infarction if necessary.**

Traditionally, it was felt that coronary artery bypass surgery lowered the risk in patients with coronary artery disease (CAD) (13,14). Recent evidence, however, suggests that **only certain patients with severe coronary artery disease benefit from coronary revascularization** (significant left main stenosis, 3-vessel CAD with a decreased left ventricular ejection fraction [<50%], 2-vessel CAD with proximal left anterior descending artery stenosis and either EF <50% or ischemia on stress-testing, or active acute coronary syndromes such as acute MI) (6). **If none of the factors listed above are present, aggressive medical therapy, including β-blockade, is likely as effective as revascularization at reducing surgical risk even in high-risk ischemic patients** (e.g. patients with significantly abnormal preoperative *dobutamine* stress echocardiograms) (15).

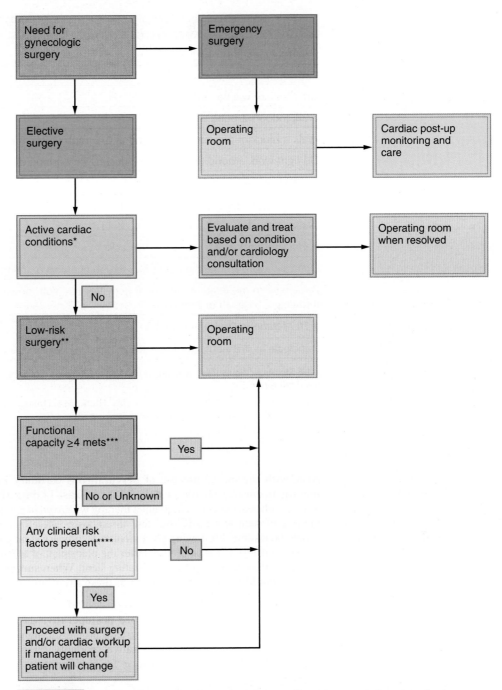

Figure 18.1   **Stepwise approach to preoperative cardiac assessment in gynecologic surgery.**
*Active cardiac conditions refers to Table 18.2; **Risk of surgery is shown in Table 18.3
***MET, metabolic equivalent (see Table 18.4) ****Clinical Risk Factors refers to Table 18.1.
From the following source: **Fliesher LA, Beckman JA, Brown KA, Calkins H, Chaikof E, et al.**
ACC/AHA 2007 guidelines on perioperative cardiovascular evaluation and care for noncardiac surgery: a report of the American College of Cardiology/American Heart Association Task Force on Practice Guidelines (Writing Committee to Revise the 2002 Guidelines on Perioperative Cardiovascular Evaluation for Noncardiac Surgery). *Circulation* 2007;116:e418–e499.

Table 18.4 Estimated Energy Requirements for Various Activities

1-4 Metabolic Equivalents (METs)

Can you take care of yourself?

Eat, dress, or use the toilet?

Walk indoors around the house?

Walk a block or two on level ground at 2–3 mph (3.2–4.8 km/hr)?

Do light work around the house like dusting or washing dishes?

5–10 Metabolic Equivalents (METs)

Climb a flight of stairs or walk up a hill?

Walk on level ground at 4 mph (6.4 km/hr)?

Run a short distance?

Do heavy work around the house like scrubbing floors or lifting or moving heavy furniture?

Participate in moderate recreational activities like golf, bowling, dancing, doubles tennis, or throwing a baseball or football?

>10 Metabolic Equivalents (METs)

Participate in strenuous sports like swimming, singles tennis, football, basketball, or skiing?

MET, Metabolic Equivalent, which can be used as a measure of energy requirements and may be used in treadmill reports.

Adapted from the Duke Activities Status Index. **Hlatky MA, Doineau RE, Higginbotham MB, Lee KL, Mark DB, Califf RM, et al.** *Am J Cardiol* 1989;64:651–654.

Also, with the increasing use of percutaneous coronary intervention (PCI), elective or nonurgent surgery should be delayed for at least 14 days after balloon angioplasty. When a stent is placed, dual oral antiplatelet therapy with *aspirin* and *clopridogrel* is needed to reduce the risk of stent restenosis and stent thrombosis. Therefore, *clopidigrel* and *aspirin* therapy should be instituted following placement of a coronary stent and elective or nonurgent surgery should be delayed at least 30 days after the placement of a bare-metal coronary stent, and 365 days after the placement of a drug-eluting stent. **When surgery is undertaken, perioperative** *aspirin* **should be continued in each of these situations** (6).

Postoperative MI can be painless. The risk of MI is throughout the first week, but the incidence is thought to peak on the third postoperative day. Additionally, diagnosis of a perioperative MI has both short- and long-term prognostic significance. Perioperative MI has been associated with significant perioperative mortality (30% to 50%) and reduced long-term survival (16,17). Hence, surveillance for perioperative MI is likely prudent in high-risk patients.

Electrocardiography (ECG), beginning in the immediate postoperative period and continuing at least through postoperative day 3, is the most well-established method of surveillance (18,19). Several studies suggest that serum troponin assays may be helpful for surveillance of perioperative MI as well, but their use is not yet well established (6,20,21). Because the risk of perioperative MI is increased in patients who are subjected to intraoperative hypotension, measures must be taken to maintain high-risk patients in a normotensive state during surgery. **If intraoperative hypotension occurs, the patient should be considered at high-risk of postoperative MI and monitored appropriately.**

Theoretically, β-blockers would be expected to facilitate the development of intraoperative hypotension because of the additive myocardial depressive effect of these medications with general anesthesia. However, **abrupt discontinuation of β-blocker medication can be associated with a dangerous rebound syndrome (i.e., acute hypertension and coronary ischemia), with the incidence of the syndrome peaking at 4 to 7 days after discontinuation of the drug** (22,23). Patients tolerate general anesthesia in the presence of continued β-blocker treatment. While several studies in the 1990s suggested that perioperative β-blocker use reduced postoperative nonfatal MI and mortality in many patients including those with intermediate risk, subsequent research has cast doubt on this claim (24,25,26). In fact, **the largest placebo-controlled trial of perioperative β-blocker use** to date was recently published and **showed an increase in mortality and stroke in those receiving β-blockers compared with placebo** (26).

Given the current controversy surrounding β-blockers, their use can only be strongly recommended in high-risk patients (at least 3 points on the Revised Cardiac Risk Index) undergoing vascular surgery (6). In addition, as stated previously, β-blockers should be continued in patients already taking them before surgery, because ischemia can be precipitated if a β-blocker is abruptly discontinued (22,23).

If β-blockers are prescribed, the recommended target heart rate for effective β-blockade is below 65, but not lower than 50 beats per minute. The appropriate duration of β-blockade is also currently being debated, but should certainly begin before surgery and continue throughout the hospitalization. If possible, there may be additional benefit if β-blockers can be started one month before surgery to titrate the heart rate, and be continued after hospitalization for at least 30 days if adequate postoperative medical follow up can be arranged (25,27).

Congestive Heart Failure

Heart failure is well known to be associated with a poorer outcome after noncardiac surgery (1,2,5). The cause of heart failure should be identified if possible as this may have implications concerning perioperative risk (6). Also, it may be reasonable to perform a noninvasive evaluation of left ventricular function (e.g., echocardiogram) in symptomatic patients, but the utility of this is still questionable (28). Patients with moderate or severe congestive heart failure should be treated before surgery with appropriate medications to optimize their cardiovascular status.

Perioperative use of a pulmonary artery (Swan-Ganz) catheter was previously advocated to allow cardiac function to be optimized and to aid in the intraoperative management of fluids and cardiac medications. Recent studies, however, have not shown clear benefit to these devices in managing high-risk surgical patients, and this procedure **is generally no longer recommended** (29).

Arrhythmias

Cardiac arrhythmias that are hemodynamically significant or symptomatic should be treated and stabilized prior to elective or nonurgent surgery. Atrial fibrillation is the most frequently seen arrhythmia and may require electrical or pharmacological cardioversion. Alternatively, a rate-control strategy can be attempted with β-blockers, calcium channel blockers, or *digoxin*. Ventricular arrhythmias, such as simple premature ventricular contractions, complex ventricular ectopy, or nonsustained tachycardia usually require no therapy unless they are associated with hemodynamic compromise or occur in the presence of left ventricle dysfunction or ongoing cardiac ischemia (30,31). However, **careful evaluation for underlying cardiopulmonary disease, drug toxicity, metabolic disturbances, and infection should be undertaken in patients who have any arrhythmia in the perioperative period.**

Conduction Disturbances

High-Grade Conduction Abnormalities

Patients who do not have permanent pacemakers and who have third-degree heart block at the time of presentation are at substantial risk of cardiopulmonary arrest during surgery. Typically, they are unable to mount an appropriate pulse response to the vasodilatation and decreased myocardial contractility induced by general anesthesia or to the volume depletion induced by surgical blood loss. Patients with high-grade conduction abnormalities including complete heart block may require temporary or permanent transvenous pacing.

Bifascicular Block

In patients with lower degrees of heart block, specifically bifascicular block (right heart block with left axis deviation), the risk of development of a higher degree of ventricular block during surgery is not significantly increased, provided there is no history of previous third-degree heart block or syncope. Such patients rarely require insertion of a temporary pacemaker (32). Patients with bifascicular block who have a history of third-degree heart block should be managed for complete heart block with preoperative cardiology evaluation and likely pacemaker insertion.

A new bifascicular block developing in the setting of acute MI carries a high risk of progression to complete heart block. Therefore, if this problem occurs after surgery, the patient should be considered at significant risk for the development of complete atrioventricular block. Such patients require a cardiology consultation and insertion of a temporary pacemaker.

Pacemakers

Patients with permanently implanted pacemakers should have a preoperative pacemaker evaluation to allow examination of all pacemaker functions. This precaution ensures that backup demand pacemaker failure will not be uncovered unexpectedly with the vagotonic stimuli associated with general anesthesia in abdominal surgery. Patients with implanted defibrillators typically have their devices turned off shortly before surgery and then turned back on shortly afterward.

Even newer pacemakers and defibrillators can sense the electromagnetic impulses created by electrocautery, especially when the electrocautery plate is close to the pacemaker unit. It is prudent to place the indifferent electrocautery electrode as far as possible from the chest and to use electrocautery sparingly. An added precaution consists of keeping a magnet available in the operating room to convert a pacemaker rapidly from the demand to a fixed pacing mode. Inappropriate discharges from the implanted defibrillator are avoided by having the device turned off during the time of surgery (33). Those with permanent pacemakers should also have their device assessed for proper function after surgery (6).

Endocarditis Prophylaxis

Recently revised guidelines for infective endocarditis (IE) do not recommend administration of antibiotics solely to prevent endocarditis for patients who undergo a genitourinary (GU) or gastrointestinal (GI) tract procedure. As a result of a lack of published data demonstrating a benefit from prophylaxis, current guidelines differ substantially from previous guidelines and far fewer patients should be recommended for IE prophylaxis than previously thought (34). Very few data exist on the risk or prevention of IE with a GI or GU tract procedure. Enterococci are part of the normal flora of the GI tract and are the primary bacteria from this area likely to cause IE. In patients with the highest risk cardiac conditions (prosthetic cardiac valve, previous IE, or congenital heart disease) who are to receive antibiotic therapy to prevent wound infection, it may be reasonable to include an antibiotic that is active against enterococci, such as penicillin, ampicillin, or vancomycin. However, no published studies demonstrate that such therapy will prevent enterococcal IE (34).

Hypertension

The significance of mild to moderate hypertension (stage 1 or 2 with systolic blood pressure below 180 mm Hg and diastolic blood pressure below 110 mm Hg) in patients undergoing surgery remains controversial. This controversy stems from the difficulty in sorting out the risk of hypertension *per se* from the risk of hypertension in the setting of hypertensive or atherosclerotic heart disease.

Numerous studies have shown that uncomplicated mild to moderate hypertension (stage 1 or 2), regardless of treatment status, is not an independent risk factor for perioperative complications (1,2,35,36). However, the presence of hypertension may be of consequence because it has been reported that patients with preoperative hypertension may demonstrate marked intraoperative blood pressure lability and postoperative hypertensive episodes (37). Certain medications used for the treatment of chronic hypertension including angiotensin-converting enzyme (ACE) inhibitors and angiotensin II receptor antagonists (ARBs) seem to make intraoperative hypertension more likely (38,39). It is also generally agreed that **severe hypertension** (stage 3 with systolic pressure greater than 180 mm Hg, diastolic greater than 110 mm Hg) **should be controlled with effective oral medications in the days to weeks before an elective operation.** Another option for severe hypertension is the use of rapidly acting intravenous agents, which usually can bring blood pressure under control in a few hours. **One randomized trial was unable to demonstrate a benefit to delaying surgery in a select patient group with severe hypertension** (40).

The causes of perioperative hypertension are presented in Table 18.5. Patients with both hypertensive and atherosclerotic heart disease may be at greater risk than those with uncomplicated

Table 18.5 Causes of Perioperative Hypertension

Cause	Recognition
Chronic hypertension	History, medication review
Laryngoscopy and intubation	Situation
Inadequate anesthesia	Situation
Inadequate ventilation	Arterial blood gas
Pain or anxiety	Patient examination and interview
Bladder distension	Bladder palpation
Emergence from anesthesia	Situation
Excessive fluid administration	Operating room records, patient examination
Postoperative fluid mobilization	Situation, patient examination
Acute cardiac events (e.g., congestive heart failure)	Patient examination, electrocardiogram, chest radiograph
Pheochromocytoma (rare—can be occult)	Unusual clinical responses
Malignant hyperthermia	Unusual clinical responses, fever

hypertension alone. As is the case for cardiac complications, the type of surgery is important in understanding the risk of hypertension. Hypotension due to any cause remains a concern in patients with coronary artery disease.

Hypertensive management begins with identification, followed by development of a plan for control. In general, most antihypertensive medications should be given on the morning of surgery. β-blockers and *clonidine* continue to be used in patients with hypertension in spite of many newer agents. It is especially important to continue β-blockers and *clonidine* to avoid withdrawal and potential heart rate or blood pressure rebound. Because of the possible problem of intraoperative hypotension, several authors have suggested holding ACE inhibitors and ARBs the morning of surgery (41,42). Most clinicians also hold diuretics to avoid volume depletion. Although diuretic use is associated with volume depletion and hypokalemia, the importance of correcting mild degrees of diuretic-induced hypokalemia in the absence of significant heart disease is controversial (43). Repletion should never be rapid and is safest by the oral route or by adjustment of medication.

In the postoperative period, many patients, especially the elderly, need less antihypertensive medication because of the salutary effects of bed rest and relative sodium restriction. If blood pressure is not elevated, it is wise to plan on reinstating drugs stepwise, beginning with the most active agent at approximately half the usual dose and finally adding the diuretic, if used, sometime later. An exception to this would be the use of β-blockers, which, because of their possible benefit in decreasing cardiac events and concern about rebound hypertensive effects and cardiac ischemia if they are stopped abruptly, should be continued in the postoperative setting. Likewise, *clonidine* should be continued in the perioperative period to avoid rebound hypertension. Patients whose only antihypertensive drugs are *thiazide* diuretics are best observed in the immediate postoperative period. **In general, patients who need additional antihypertensive therapy in the immediate preoperative period should not be treated with diuretics because of the risk of associated hypovolemia and hypokalemia.**

Pulmonary

It has been estimated that pulmonary complications are at least as common as cardiac complications after noncardiac surgery (44). Atelectasis, postoperative pneumonia, respiratory failure, and exacerbation of underlying pulmonary condition can all develop after abdominal and pelvic surgery. In fact, pulmonary complications are often associated with the longest hospital stays after abdominal surgery (45). Clinicians should attempt to identify patients at

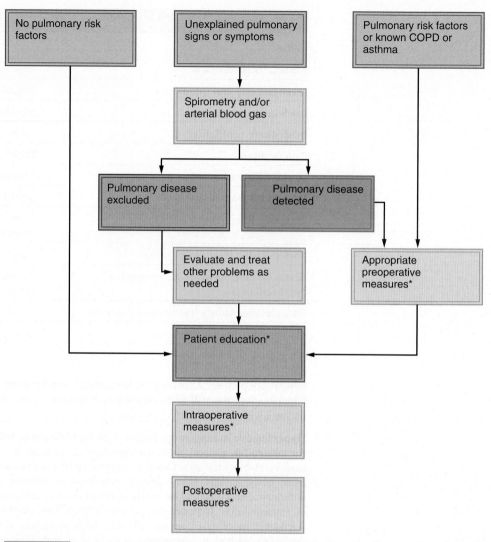

Figure 18.2   **Pulmonary evaluation and postoperative care.** *Refers to measures to reduce pulmonary complications (see Table 18.6). COPD, chronic obstructive pulmonary disease.

increased risk for pulmonary complications from surgical procedures, and reduce these risks whenever possible (Fig. 18.2).

Pulmonary Risk Factors

Pulmonary risk factors are typically grouped as "procedure related" or "patient related." For "procedure-related" risks, a large literature review recently confirmed the traditional teaching that **procedures closest to the diaphragm increase perioperative pulmonary risks** (46). This observation is presumably due to the higher likelihood of diaphragmatic dysfunction, or related postoperative pain and shallow inspiration. For this reason **upper abdominal surgeries create more postoperative risk than lower abdominal procedures.**

General anesthesia, emergency surgery, and prolonged surgeries (greater than 3 hours in duration) also increase the risk of postoperative pulmonary complications (46). There is some evidence that the use of shorter-acting neuromuscular blockers during an operation can reduce postoperative pulmonary complications (47). **Most clinicians believe that epidural anesthetics and analgesia, and the use of laparoscopic rather than open surgeries should reduce postoperative pulmonary risks.** Comparative data about these techniques and their association with pulmonary complications, though, is still limited (48,49).

A review of multiple studies over the last several years has confirmed several **patient-related risk factors** for postoperative pulmonary complications: **advanced age; ASA** (American

Society of Anesthesiologists) **class ≥2; heart failure; functional dependence; and chronic obstructive pulmonary disease (COPD). A serum albumin level <3.5 mg/dL** and overt malnutrition were also associated with increased risk. **Current smoking** also seems to increase postoperative pulmonary risks (50).

Although, COPD is a known risk factor for postoperative pulmonary complications, there has been considerable debate about the routine use of spirometry to screen for this condition before nonthoracic surgery. The American College of Physicians (ACP) recommends spirometry only if the history and physical examination suggest an undefined lung condition (51). **A history of prolonged cigarette smoking, dyspnea, chronic cough, sputum production, wheezing, or prolonged expiration and hyperinflation noted on examination would all be suggestive findings for COPD.** Patients with these findings would typically receive pulmonary function testing with spirometry (and possibly a blood gas), whether an operation was intended or not.

Although COPD increases the risk of postoperative complications, it does not typically make these risks prohibitive. Even patients with severe COPD can tolerate abdominal surgery when properly prepared (52). When patients with COPD are identified before elective operations, every effort should be made to optimize their lung function and minimize any other perioperative risks.

Interestingly, **studies have not identified asthmatic patients as having significant risks of serious postoperative complications when managed appropriately** (53). Isolated obesity has also not been associated with increased pulmonary risks. However, many of the attendant comorbidities with obesity, such as obstructive sleep apnea, are known to increase perioperative risk (54). Sleep apnea patients are often prescribed positive pressure airway masks to assist their breathing at home during the night. This equipment should be available in the postoperative period to assist with any apneic breathing episodes. **Obese patients** (as well as other patients with unusual upper airway anatomy) **may present difficulties for intubation,** and fiber optic instruments may be needed in the operating room. **Pulmonary hypertension,** whether associated with sleep apnea or not, **has also been associated with increased postoperative risks** in noncardiac surgery (55).

Pulmonary Risk Reduction

Physicians should attempt to reduce perioperative risks whenever possible (Table 18.6). Some identified risks (such as location of surgery, type of anesthesia, age, poor general health status, and fixed airways obstruction) cannot be improved. Smoking cessation, however, should be encouraged. **At least one study has shown that 6 weeks of smoking abstinence is needed to reduce smoking-related pulmonary risks** (56). Patients with airway obstruction (COPD and asthma) should be optimized to their baseline pulmonary status before surgery. This may involve bronchodilator use, inhaled steroids, or possibly antibiotics and/or oral steroids. As an example, **a one-week course of preoperative oral steroids in severe asthmatics has been shown to be safe in reducing the risks of postoperative bronchospasm** (57).

Both COPD and asthmatic patients should continue their home medications during their postoperative course. Modern ambulatory therapy for asthma emphasizes the use of inhaled steroids as well as inhaled beta agonists. Exacerbations during the postoperative period can be treated with additional doses of inhaled bronchodilators, and intravenous steroids if necessary.

COPD management typically involves both inhaled β-agonists and anticholinergics. Exacerbations can also be treated with additional doses of inhaled medications or steroids. **Noninvasive ventilation has been used successfully in postoperative patients with COPD exacerbations** (58).

There is good evidence that lung expansion maneuvers decrease postoperative pulmonary complications (59). Because low lung volumes produced by anesthesia, operative site pain, and bowel distension all contribute to respiratory dysfunction in the postoperative period, clinicians have prescribed deep-breathing exercises, intermittent positive pressure breathing (IPPB), and simple incentive spirometry for years to attempt lung expansion in the postoperative period. Continuous positive airway pressure has also been used with success to decrease postoperative pulmonary complications after abdominal surgeries (60). Adequate pain control is also important to improve deep breathing and lung expansion after abdominal surgery. **Recent reviews have also emphasized more judicious use of nasogastric tubes in the postoperative period to reduce postoperative pneumonia and atelectasis** (60). Recent guidelines

Table 18.6 Measures to Reduce Pulmonary Complications
Preoperative
Identification of patients at risk
Patient education to ensure optimal preoperative and postoperative compliance and performance
Cessation of smoking for at least 6 wks
Instruction in incentive spirometry
Bronchodilation (e.g., β-adrenergic agonist by inhaler)
Inhaled or possibly oral steroids for asthmatics
Antibiotics for bronchitis
Control of secretions
Intraoperative
Avoidance of prolonged anesthesia (>3 hr)
Possible use of regional anesthesia
Use of shorter acting neuromuscular blockers
Maintenance of bronchodilation
Possible use of laparoscopic procedures
Postoperative
Lung expansion maneuvers: incentive spirometry. Possible use of intermittent or continuous positive pressure breathing techniques
Early ambulation
Pain control, possible use of regional analgesia
Attention to the effects of analgesia on respiration

suggest that these tubes be used selectively for nausea and vomiting, inability to tolerate oral intake, or for symptomatic abdominal distension.

Diabetes Mellitus

Diabetes mellitus affects approximately 7.8% of the adult population in the United States. Type I diabetes is an autoimmune disease that attacks pancreatic beta cells. People with type I diabetes have a near-total lack of *insulin* due to pancreatic beta cell destruction and become ketoacidotic if *insulin* is withheld. Although common in juveniles, type I diabetes can occur in adults. **People with type II diabetes are not insulin deficient in an absolute sense** and thus are not generally prone to ketoacidosis. The problem in type II diabetes is usually one of relative *insulin* resistance. *Insulin* treatment is not limited to type I disease because **many patients with type II do require some *insulin* therapy.** Patients with type II diabetes are usually older and overweight. Both groups may experience the complications listed in Table 18.7. Many elderly patients have mild type II diabetes of recent onset related to obesity, are well controlled with diet or oral hypoglycemic drugs, and have few overt complications, but may have occult atherosclerotic vascular disease.

The management of diabetes begins with some understanding of the factors that influence perioperative glucose metabolism. *Insulin* is the principal glucose-lowering hormone; cortisol, glucagon, growth hormone, and catecholamines are the principal glucose-raising hormones. In the preoperative period, stress and the "dawn" phenomenon may elevate blood glucose. The dawn phenomenon is early-morning hyperglycemia resulting from nocturnal surges of growth hormone. **During surgery, cortisol, epinephrine, and growth hormone levels rise. In this period, there is hyperglycemia in diabetic and nondiabetic patients alike.** This is caused by glycogenolysis, inhibition of glucose uptake, and decreased insulin release. After surgery, in nondiabetic patients, the hyperglycemia is brought under control by increased endogenous

Table 18.7 Complications of Diabetes Mellitus

Complication	Importance
Cataracts	Decreased vision
Retinopathy	Decreased vision
Nephropathy	Nephrotic syndrome, hyperkalemia, metabolic acidosis, reduced glomerular filtration rate
Peripheral neuropathy	Decreased peripheral nociception, susceptibility to infection
Autonomic neuropathy	Orthostatic hypotension, gastropathy (delayed gastric emptying, diarrhea), uropathy (urinary retention, overflow incontinence, infection), cardiorespiratory arrest
Coronary artery disease	Silent ischemia, myocardial infarction
Vascular disease	Peripheral arterial insufficiency, coronary artery disease, stroke

insulin release over a period of 4 to 6 hours. Patients with diabetes may need additional exogenous *insulin*.

In addition to these hormonal factors, several other factors are important in modulating the blood glucose level in the perioperative period. **Inactivity, stress, and intravenous glucose infusions tend to raise blood glucose. Decreased caloric intake and semistarvation tend to lower blood glucose.** Because the net effect of these factors is sometimes difficult to anticipate, it is important frequently to monitor blood glucose levels.

Oral Hypoglycemics

There are many more oral agents being used to treat diabetes than in the past (Table 18.8). **Sulfonylureas such as *glyburide (Diabeta)* remain the most popular.** Most sulfonylureas are primarily excreted by the liver. These drugs are typically withheld 24 to 48 hours before surgery, depending on their half-life. They can be restarted when the patient starts eating. **The biguanide *metformin (Glucophage)* is being used more frequently.** However, *metformin* should not be used in the perioperative period and probably should be avoided altogether in systemically ill gynecologic oncology patients. There is a serious risk of lactic acidosis if renal function declines as a result of chemotherapy, dehydration, congestive heart failure, sepsis, radiologic contrast agents, or third spacing. It should not be used in patients with liver disease. *Acarbose (Precose)* is a complex oligosaccharide glucosidase inhibitor that delays the digestion of ingested carbohydrates. There is little use for this drug in the perioperative period. *Repaglinide (Prandin)* is a meglitinide that stimulates release of insulin from the pancreas. It is generally used to cover mealtime blood sugar and may have limited role in blood sugar management during the perioperative period when patients are not eating. Its safe use depends on stable renal and hepatic function. The thiazolidinedione *rosiglitazone (Avandia)* improves peripheral use of glucose by improving *insulin* sensitivity. This class of medication has a risk of fluid retention. It is generally not recommended for patients with NYHA class III or IV status. The use of thiazolidinediones around the perioperative period should be exercised with caution, especially in patients with cardiac disease and/or in those who have received more intravenous fluids during the perioperative period.

The newest oral diabetic medication is dipeptidyl peptidase-4 (DPP-4) enzyme inhibitor, *Sitagliptin (Januvia)*. DDP-4 breaks down incretin hormones. *Sitagliptin* therefore increases the level of incretin hormones (glucose-dependent insulinotropic polypeptide [GIP] and glucadon-like peptide-1 [GLP-1]) by inhibiting their breakdown. Incretins enhance glucose-dependent insulin secretion, glucose-dependent suppression of inappropriately high glucagon secretion, slowing of gastric emptying, reduction of food intake, and promotion of beta-cell activity. This medication is generally not useful during the perioperative period if patients are nil per os (NPO). Dose adjustment is needed for renal insufficiency patients.

Insulin

Insulin **is the mainstay of in-hospital management of diabetes because it is easily titrated during management.** In spite of newer therapies, *insulin* also remains an important tool in the

Table 18.8 Characteristics of Oral Hypoglycemics

Agent	Brand	Dose Range (mg)	Duration (hr)	Metabolism
Sulfonylureas				
Tolbutamide	Orinase	500–3,000	6–12	Liver
Chlorpropamide	Diabinese	100–500	60	Liver/renal
Acetohexamide	Dimelor	250–1,500	12–24	Liver
Tolazamide	Tolinase	100–1,000	10–18	Liver
Glyburide	DiaBeta	2.5–30	10–30	Liver
Glipizide	Glucotrol	5.0–4.0	18–30	Liver
Glimepiride	Amaryl	1.0–8.0	8–12	Liver/renal
Biguanide				
Metformin	Glucophage	850–2,300	18	Renal
Glucosidase inhibitors				
Acarbose	Precose	25–30	2	Gastrointestinal
Miglitol	Glyset	75–300	2	Renal
Meglitinides				
Repaglinide	Prandin	0.5–16	1	Liver/renal
Nateglinide	Starlix	180–720	4	Liver/renal
Thiazolidinediones				
Rosiglitazone	Avandia	4.0–8.0	3–4	Liver
Pioglitazone	Actos	15–45	16–24	Liver/renal
DDP-4 inhibitor				
Sitagliptin	Januvia	50–100	24	Renal

DDP-4—dipeptidyl peptidase-4.

ambulatory management of diabetes. There are various types of *insulin* available for treatment of diabetes (Table 18.9). The use of different *insulin* types depends on the goals of treatment. **Long-acting *insulins* like *glargine* and *detemir*** are used to cover basal blood sugar needs. **Short-acting *insulins* like ultrashort-acting *insulin* or regular *insulin*** are used to cover mealtime blood sugar or any elevated blood sugar not covered by the basal *insulin*.

Management

Hyperglycemia is known to impair neutrophil function, wound healing, and to increase the risk of wound infection (61–66). In addition, it also impairs cardiac ischemic preconditioning (a protective mechanism for ischemic insult), enhances neuronal damage following ischemia, decreases nitric oxide, increases platelet activation, increases inflammatory markers, and increases reactive oxygen species (67), all of which have significant impact on a patient's morbidity and mortality. Several observational studies have shown that hyperglycemic patients have a higher mortality, increased risk of infection, poorer functional recovery, and longer length of stay (68–75). **Tight glycemic control has been shown to improve mortality, decrease risk of infection, and decrease length of ICU stay** (76–80). In one study of critically ill surgical ICU patients (77), it was shown that **tight glycemic control with blood glucose at or around 110 mg/dL reduced blood stream infections, acute renal failure requiring dialysis, blood transfusion, length of mechanical ventilation and critical care, and in-hospital mortality.** Mortality at 12 months was reduced as well in the intensive *insulin* therapy patient (77). The American Diabetic Association and American College of Endocrinology

Table 18.9 Characteristics of Insulin

Type of Insulin	Brand	Onset of Action	Time of Peak Effect	Duration of Action
Ultra Short Acting				
Lispro	*Humulog*	5–15 minutes	30–90 minutes	4–6 hours
Aspart	*Novolog*	5–15 minutes	30–90 minutes	4–6 hours
Glulisine	Apidra	5–15 minutes	30–90 minutes	4–6 hours
Short Acting				
Regular	*Humulin R*	30–60 minutes	2–3 hours	8–10 hours
	Novolin R			
Intermediate Acting				
NPH	*Humulin*	2–4 hours	4–10 hours	12–18 hours
	Novolin			
Long Acting				
Glargine	*Lantus*	2–4 hours	No peak	20–24 hours
Detemir	*Levemir*	2–4 hours	No Peak	6–24 hours

NPH—neutral protamine Hagedorn.

recommend controlling preprandial blood sugar around 110 mg/dL in critical care patients, but differ in noncritical care patients, recommending 90 to 130 mg/dL and 110 mg/dL, respectively (Table 18.10). **In considering the merits of tight glucose control, the increased risk of hypoglycemia also needs to be considered.**

Details of the management of the diabetic patient who is taking an oral hypoglycemic agent are presented in Table 18.11. A patient with well-controlled diabetes who takes sulfonylureas is at risk of hypoglycemia if sulfonylureas are given while the caloric intake is reduced. Sulfonylureas should be held on the morning of surgery or longer if the medication has a long duration of action. **Dextrose infusion should be given to prevent any hypoglycemia.** However, glucose monitoring should be performed at regular intervals to ensure the blood sugar falls within acceptable range. **Any hyperglycemia can be treated with supplemental** *insulin.* When oral nutrition is reinstated, sulfonylureas can be resumed. Thiazolidinediones can be continued during the perioperative period, but should not be used if the patient has received excessive amount of fluids or developed NYHA Class III or IV heart failure. Glucosidase inhibitors, meglitinides, and DDP-4 inhibitor can be resumed only when the patient is on oral nutrition. *Metformin* is generally not used during the perioperative period for reasons mentioned above.

Table 18.10 Target Goals of Inpatient Blood Glucose Control

	American Diabetes Association	American College of Endocrinology
Critical Care Patients		
Preprandial	110 mg/dL	110 mg/dL
Postprandial	180 mg/dL	110 mg/dL
Noncritical Care Patients		
Preprandial	90–130 mg/dL	110 mg/dL
Postprandial	180 mg/dL	180 mg/dL

Table 18.11 Details of Perioperative Diabetes Management for Well-Controlled Patients Taking Oral Hypoglycemics

Preoperative

1. Plan for surgery early in the day

2. Hold oral hypoglycemic on day of surgery; long-acting drugs (e.g., *chlorpropamide*) should be held for 48 hours

3. Measure early a.m. glucose (use corrective dose insulin for glucose >140 mg/dL)

Intraoperative

4. Measure intraoperative glucose frequently (e.g., every 1 hour) and start insulin drip to keep blood glucose <140 mg/dL

Postoperative

5. Measure recovery room glucose (use corrective dose insulin for glucose >140 mg/dL)

6. Measure postoperative glucose every 6 hours (use corrective dose insulin to keep blood glucose <140 mg/dL)

7. Return to home regimen in a.m. if eating adequately

8. Alternatively, consider starting basal-bolus insulin regimen if concerns about resuming oral agents

Alternatively, patients can be started on basal-bolus *insulin* regimen perioperatively instead of resuming on oral hypoglycemic medications. Patients' oral nutritional intake is often unpredictable because of postoperative nausea and vomiting or NPO status for various studies. Total *insulin* need is between 0.3 and 0.6 U/kg/day depending on patients' insulin resistance status (81,82). Half of that *insulin* dose should be given as basal *insulin* with *glargine* or *detemir*. The other half should be divided into four doses given every 6 hours or before each meal and at bedtime using ultra short-acting or short-acting *insulin*. Any additional hyperglycemia should be covered with supplemental *insulin* with corrective scale. Basal *insulin* dosage can be increased daily by 10% to 20% if blood sugar is not controlled, or it can be decreased daily by 10% to 20% if patient has episodes of hypoglycemia.

Patients on *insulin* treatment should not be on sliding scale insulin, as that strategy produces fluctuating high and low blood sugars levels and the blood sugar may be still not adequately controlled (81,83–85). In a randomized control trial comparing sliding-scale *insulin* to a basal-bolus *insulin* regimen, the latter resulted in significantly improved glycemic control, without significant risk of hypoglycemia (81).

The management of the diabetic patient who routinely takes *insulin* at home is presented in Table 18.12. **Because caloric intake is reduced on the day of surgery, total daily *insulin* dose should be reduced. Usually, half the dose of basal *insulin* is given the night before or the morning of surgery to cover endogenous glucose production.** Patients should be started on a dextrose infusion to prevent hypoglycemia. Glucose monitoring should be performed to make sure the patient's blood sugar is within an acceptable range. Postoperatively, patients likely have increased stress hormone levels and are on a dextrose infusion; thus, hyperglycemia is often seen despite the patient being on nil orally. Frequent blood sugar monitoring is needed for management of these hyperglycemic episodes with corrective dose *insulin*. Once patients recover from the surgery and start to take oral nutrition, they can be resumed on their home *insulin* regimen. However, caution should be exercised with any changes in patients' nutritional status.

In critically ill patients or patients with uncontrolled diabetes, continuous *insulin* infusion is a better strategy for glycemic control (76–80). Continuous *insulin* infusion with glucose infusion maintains normal insulin sensitivity during the perioperative period and decreases blood cortisol, glucagons, fat oxidation, and free fatty acids when compared with controls (86). An *insulin* infusion can be started at 1 U per hour and the rate titrated by 0.5 U per hour increments

Table 18.12 Details of Perioperative Insulin Management for Well-Controlled Patients Taking Insulin

Preoperative

1. Plan for surgery early in the day
2. Measure early a.m. glucose (use corrective dose *insulin* to keep glucose <140 mg/dL)
3. Use one-half of long acting basal insulin
4. Start D5W at 50–100 mL/hr

Intraoperative

5. Measure intraoperative glucose frequently (e.g., every 2 hours) and make adjustments

Postoperative

6. Measure recovery room glucose (use corrective dose *insulin* to keep glucose <140 mg/dL)
7. Measure postoperative glucose every 6 hrs (use corrective dose *insulin* to keep glucose <140 mg/dL)
8. Use rapid short-acting insulin according to corrective dose scale as needed
9. Use one-half of long acting basal insulin when NPO
10. Continue above regimen until patient begins to eat (usually next morning)
11. Return to home regimen incrementally beginning in a.m. if eating

D5W, dextrose in 5% water. NPO, nil per os.

to keep blood glucose levels below 140 mg/dL. Five percent dextrose infusion with or without potassium at rate of 50 to 100 mL/hour should be given as well to avoid any hypoglycemia. **With recent data showing improved morbidity and mortality outcomes with tight blood sugar control, many hospitals have instituted *insulin* drip protocols.** Using those protocols tailored to the particular institution is preferable to empirically adjusting *insulin* drip *de novo*.

Thyroid Disorders

Hypothyroidism

Hypothyroidism is common and may go undetected in patients being prepared for surgery (87). Symptoms include cold intolerance, recent or progressive constipation, hoarseness, fatigability, and changes in cognition. Signs include associated goiter, skin dryness, and a delayed relaxation phase of peripheral reflexes (best demonstrated in the Achilles tendon). Studies have suggested that unrecognized mild to moderate hypothyroidism is clinically important, but fears of hyponatremia, prolonged respirator dependency, hypothermia, delayed recovery from anesthesia, or death are probably unwarranted (88,89). One retrospective study suggested that such patients have more intraoperative hypotension, postoperative ileus, and confusion and that infection is less often accompanied by fever (88).

For patients who are suspected before surgery of being hypothyroid, thyroid hormone levels should be measured. **Hypothyroid patients should be treated with replacement hormone and rendered euthyroid before surgery.** In urgent situations, patients who are not myxedematous should be given 1 or 2 days of oral replacement before surgery, with careful postoperative follow-up (90,91).

Hyperthyroidism

Hyperthyroidism can be a dramatic illness, with tachycardia, fever, and exophthalmos associated with goiter. Other common symptoms and signs include frequent weight loss, fatigue, diarrhea, heat intolerance, tremor, hyperreflexia, and muscle weakness. **Hyperthyroidism may be occult in older patients.** Unexplained tachycardia, weight loss, arrhythmias, or fever may be the only clinical indicators and always raise suspicions of unrecognized hyperthyroidism in surgical patients. With proper preparation (92), hyperthyroid patients undergoing thyroid surgery do well. However, there are scant data concerning the problems of the hyperthyroid patient undergoing nonthyroidal surgery, such as radical hysterectomy. Exacerbation of the illness into a "thyroid storm" is the usual concern. Because of this, **when any patient is suspected before surgery of being hyperthyroid, thyroid hormone levels should be measured. If the diagnosis is confirmed, elective surgery should be delayed until treatment has produced a euthyroid state.** (93) In the postoperative period, thyroid hormone levels should be measured when any patient has persistent unexplained tachycardia, fever, or tachyarrhythmias.

Corticosteroids

Patients taking corticosteroids or those who have taken them in the recent past should be evaluated for the need of supplemental corticosteroid coverage. In general, patients taking less than the equivalent of 5 mg *prednisone* **daily should not have adrenal suppression** (94–96). There is variability between patients in their response to suppression of the hypothalamic–pituitary–adrenal (HPA) axis by exogenous steroid. In a prospective cohort study, 75 patients were given short-term, high-dose glucocorticoid treatment of at least 25 mg *prednisone* daily for 5 to 30 days (97). Forty-five percent of the patients experienced HPA suppression. Of those patients, the majority recovered within 14 days. However, a couple of patients remained suppressed at 3 and 6 months.

In a retrospective study, 279 patients were taking *prednisone* or its equivalent steroid at doses of 5 to 30 mg per day for between 1 week and 15 years (98). Human corticotropin-releasing hormone (CRH) was used to assess HPA suppression. **There was a trend toward an inverse correlation between dosage and duration of therapy and the plasma cortisol response to CRH.** On the other hand, there were numerous patients taking high-dose steroids for more than 100 weeks who still had an intact HPA axis. Despite this variability, **suppression of the HPA axis should be anticipated in patients taking more than 25 mg of** *hydrocortisone,* **5 mg of** *prednisone,* **or 0.75 mg** *dexamethasone* **per day for more than 3 weeks** (99).

To further clarify whether patients on chronic steroids have suppressed HPA axis, a **cortrosyn (ACTH) stimulation test** can be performed. Baseline cortisol and ACTH levels should be obtained. Immediately 250 μg of ACTH is given intramuscularly or intravenously. A cortisol level is obtained 30 minutes after ACTH is given. If the stimulated cortisol level does not rise above 18 μg/mL, the patient is suspected of having a suppressed HPA axis and stress dose steroid should be given perioperatively (97,100–102).

Corticosteroid supplementation for patients suspected of adrenal suppression will depend on the type of surgery performed. Patients having minor surgeries like hernia repair or colonoscopy should be able to take their usual dose of oral steroid on the day of surgery without additional supplementation. Patients undergoing moderate surgical stress, such as hysterectomy, should take their usual steroid dose on the morning of the surgery and be supplemented with 50 mg intravenous *hydrocortisone* on call to surgery followed by 25 mg intravenously every 8 hours for three doses and resume usual oral steroids on the following morning. Patients undergoing major surgery, such as primary cytoreduction for advanced ovarian cancer, should take their usual steroid dose on the morning of surgery and be supplemented with 100 mg intravenous *hydrocortisone* on call to surgery, followed by 50 mg intravenous every 8 hours, tapering the dose by half each day over the next 24 to 48 hours. The patient can then resume oral steroids in the morning after tapered off intravenous stress dose hydrocortisone (103,104). For those patients who continue to not be able to take oral medications, equivalent dose of intravenous hydrocortisone should be given in the mornings.

Thromboembolic Disease Prevention

Almost all hospitalized patients are at risk for venous thromboembolism (VTE), and should receive some type of prophylaxis. Surgical patients, in particular, are at increased risk for deep venous thrombosis and associated pulmonary embolism related to immobility and the operative stimulation of the coagulation cascade. One older analysis of historical data suggested nearly a third of hospitalized surgical patients might develop VTE, and perhaps 1% may develop fatal pulmonary embolism if no prophylaxis was given (105).

Although young, ambulatory patients without additional risks who undergo short (<30 minutes) surgeries may not need specific interventions other than early mobilization, almost all other postoperative patients should receive some type of thromboprophylaxis. Gynecologic surgery patients known to be at particularly high risk include those with malignant disease; open abdominal (versus vaginal or laparoscopic) surgeries; elderly

Table 18.13 Factors Related to Increased Risk of Thromboembolic Disease

Inherited Disorders (e.g., deficiency of antithrombin III, Factor C or S, or the Factor V Leiden Mutation)

Acquired or inherited thrombophillia

Nephrotic syndrome

Paroxysmal nocturnal hemoglobinuria

Cancer

Stasis (e.g., congestive heart failure)

Age >40 years

Estrogen therapy

Sepsis

Bed rest

Trauma

Stroke and/or lower extremity paralysis

Myeloproliferative disorder

Inflammatory bowel disease

Obesity

Prior thromboembolism

Central venous catheter

Erythropoiesis stimulating agents

Pregnancy and postpartum period

patients; and those who have had previous venous thrombotic events. A more complete list of risk factors for venous thromboembolic disease in hospitalized patients is shown in Table 18.13.

Preventive therapy for venous thrombosis **includes mechanical compression devices** placed on the lower extremities, and various subcutaneous anticoagulation regimens with **unfractionated** *heparin*, **low molecular weight** *heparins*, **and newer agents such as** *fondaparinux.* Higher doses of the latter agents may have associated risks for postoperative bleeding. There have been conflicting reports on the relative protective benefits of each of these treatments. At least one randomized trial has shown that proper use of compression stockings may be as effective as subcutaneous *heparin* in major surgeries for gynecologic malignancies (106). Other trials have suggested that higher doses of subcutaneous unfractionated *heparin* (three times a day) or low molecular weight heparin may be more protective than lower doses of unfractionated heparin (107). Some surgeons have even advocated the use of pneumatic compression devices and subcutaneous anticoagulants in their highest risk patients, although there is no clear data these treatments are additive in effectiveness. Thromboprophylaxis in hospitalized patients is typically continued until hospital discharge. **A recent consensus statement summarizes general recommendations for prevention of venous thromboembolism in postoperative gynecology patients** (see Table 18.14).

Preoperative Testing

The question of how much preoperative laboratory testing is warranted has been the subject of considerable interest and debate (108,109). It is important for the surgeon to recognize that data

---

Table 18.14 Recommendations for Venous Thromboembolic Prophylaxis in Gynecologic Surgery: Eighth (2008) American College of Chest Physicians Guidelines for Antithrombotic Therapy for Prevention and Treatment of Thrombosis

1. For low-risk gynecologic surgery patients who are undergoing minor procedures and have no additional risk factors, we recommend against the use of specific thromboprophylaxis other than early and frequent ambulation (Grade 1A).

2. For gynecology patients undergoing entirely laparoscopic procedures, we recommend against routine thromboprophylaxis, other than early and frequent ambulation (Grade 1B).

3. For gynecology patients undergoing entirely laparoscopic procedures in whom additional VTE risk factors are present, we recommend the use of thromboprophylaxis with one or more of LMWH, LDUH, IPC, or GCS (Grade 1C).

4. For all patients undergoing major gynecologic surgery, we recommend that thromboprophylaxis be used routinely (Grade 1A).

5. For patients undergoing major gynecologic surgery for benign disease without additional risk factors, we recommend LMWH (Grade 1A), LDUH (Grade 1A), or IPC started just before surgery and used continuously while the patient is not ambulating (Grade 1B).

6. For patients undergoing extensive surgery for malignancy and for patients with additional VTE risk factors, we recommend routine thromboprophylaxis with LMWH (Grade 1A), or LDUH three times daily (Grade 1A), or IPC, started just before surgery and used continuously while the patient is not ambulating (Grade 1A). Alternative considerations include a combination of LMWH or LDUH plus mechanical thromboprophylaxis with GCS or IPC, or fondaparinux (all Grade 1C).

7. For patients undergoing major gynecologic procedures, we recommend that thromboprophylaxis continue until discharge from hospital (Grade 1A). For selected high-risk gynecology patients, including some of those who have undergone major cancer surgery or have previously had VTE, we suggest that continuing thromboprophylaxis after hospital discharge with LMWH for up to 28 days be considered (Grade 2C).

Abbreviations: GCS = graduated compression stockings; IPC = intermittent pneumatic compression; LDUH = low-dose unfractionated heparin; LMWH = low-molecular-weight heparin; VTE = venous thromboembolism.

Evidence Grades: IA = Strong Recommendation, High Quality Evidence; 1B = Strong Recommendation, Moderate Quality Evidence; 1C = Strong Recommendation, Low Quality Evidence; 2C = Weak Recommendation, Low Quality Evidence.

Sources: Geerts WH, et al. Prevention of venous thromboembolism. *Chest* 2008;133:381S–453S; **Guyatt EH, et al.** Grades of recommendation for antithrombotic agents. *Chest* 2008;133:123S–131S.

---

from many studies confirm that **unless clinical indicators are present, preoperative test results will usually be normal, falsely positive, or truly positive with no significant clinical outcome on perioperative complications** (110–115).

The National Institute for Clinical Excellence of the United Kingdom developed guidelines in 2003 in an attempt to give some directions for clinicians on preoperative testing for elective surgery. The guidelines incorporated as much evidence as possible, but unfortunately, the evidence base is often lacking so that recommendations are frequently based on experts' opinions and consensus (116). These guidelines categorize patients by age; surgical grade (minor, intermediate, major, major+); anesthetic grade as per American Society of Anesthesiologists (ASA); and co-morbidity (cardiac, respiratory, and renal) (Tables 18.15 and 18.16). Preoperative test recommendations cover chest x-ray; complete blood count; electrocardiogram (ECG); coagulation studies; chemistry; renal function; and glucose, urine analysis, blood gas, and lung function tests. The complete guideline is available online (116).

Patients who are younger (<40 years old), healthy, without co-morbidity, and undergoing minor surgery generally do not need any preoperative testing. However, gynecologic oncology patients are at least Surgical Grade 3—major surgery. Such patients often have clinical indicators that support additional testing, particularly when they are older (>60 years old), have higher ASA Class, multiple co-morbidities, or with cancer. A preoperative ECG should be obtained on all women over 60 years of age or younger when patients have cardiac disease. Complete blood count and chemistries are recommended. Glucose level is not recommended by the guidelines in many patients, but is usually warranted to exclude diabetes due to the increased morbidity and mortality associated with

Table 18.15 Surgical Grade	
	Example
Grade 1 (minor)	Excision of skin, drainage of breast abscess
Grade 2 (intermediate)	Primary repair of inguinal hernia, knee arthroscopy, tonsillectomy/adenoidectomy, varicose vein stripping
Grade 3 (major)	Total abdominal hysterectomy, thyroidectomy, lumbar surgery, endoscopic resection of prostate
Grade 4 (major+)	Joint replacement, lung resection, radical neck surgery, colonic resection
Neurosurgery	—
Cardiovascular surgery	—

Adapted from http://www.nice.org.uk/Guidance/CG3/Guidance/pdf/English.

Table 18.16 American Society of Anesthesiologists (ASA) Class	
ASA Class 1	Healthy patient without clinical co-morbidity or medical conditions
ASA Class 2	Patients with mild systemic disease
ASA Class 3	Patients with severe systemic disease
ASA Class 4	Patients with severe systemic disease that is constant threat to life

Adapted from http://www.nice.org.uk/Guidance/CG3/Guidance/pdf/English.

inpatient hyperglycemia. Chest x-ray is generally not recommended, but can be considered if the patient has respiratory symptoms or abnormal chest examination. Urine analysis is considered in all gynecologic patients. Interestingly, coagulation studies are not recommended in the majority of the patients, except for those patients with renal co-morbidity or cardiac co-morbidity in ASA Class 3 status. In addition, for those patients with metastatic liver cancer or who are significantly malnourished, coagulation studies prior to surgery are reasonable. Blood gas can be considered in patients with multiple co-morbidities. Pulmonary function tests are not recommended for gynecologic patients even if they have respiratory co-morbidity (Tables 18.17, 18.18, and 18.19).

The guidelines on preoperative tests are merely a general roadmap for the clinicians. Combining patients' medical conditions and symptoms with the guidelines will provide clinicians with a more focused approach to preoperative testing when evaluating patients for elective surgery.

Screening for Hemostatic Defects

A good history and physical examination are often most helpful in screening patients for hemostatic defects before operations. Some of the most important information involves the outcome of prior hemostatic stress and the family history. Minor surgical procedures should not have required transfusion, and a history of postoperative bleeding 2 or 3 days after surgery is also suspicious. Many patients have had tooth extractions. Bleeding should not last more than 24 hours and should not start again after stopping. **A familial history of bleeding or suspected bleeding should be investigated.** Patients should be questioned about nosebleeds, intestinal bleeding, and heavy menstrual bleeding. Large ecchymosis and mucosal bleeding on examination can be a cause for concern.

Like other laboratory tests, some have suggested that in otherwise healthy patients, screening for hemostatic defects may not be warranted (117). For cancer patients undergoing surgery for which bleeding is expected, some laboratory screening seems prudent. **A platelet count, INR (international normalized ratio), and PTT (partial thromboplastin time) are the most commonly ordered screening tests for this purpose.** A low platelet count can be caused by decreased production, sequestration into the spleen, or increased destruction. For platelet counts less than 100,000/cc, platelet transfusions may be necessary before the operation,

Table 18.17 Grade 3 Surgery (Major)				
	Age (years)			
	≥16 to <40	≥40 to <60	≥60 to <80	≥80
Test	**ASA Class 2 with cardiovascular disease**			
Chest x-ray	C	C	C	C
ECG	Y	Y	Y	Y
CBC	Y	Y	Y	Y
Coagulation	N	N	N	N
Renal function	Y	Y	Y	Y
Glucose	N	N	N	N
Urine analysis	C	C	C	C
Blood gas	C	C	C	C
PFT	N	N	N	N
	ASA Class 3 with cardiovascular disease			
Chest x-ray	C	C	C	C
ECG	Y	Y	Y	Y
CBC	Y	Y	Y	Y
Coagulation	C	C	C	C
Renal function	Y	Y	Y	Y
Glucose	N	N	N	N
Urine analysis	C	C	C	C
Blood gas	C	C	C	C
PFT	N	N	N	N

ASA—American Society of Anesthesiologists, C—Considered, Y—Yes, N—No ECG—electrocardiogram, CBC—complete blood count, PFT—pulmonary function test
Adapted from http://www.nice.org.uk/Guidance/CG3/Guidance/pdf/English.

depending on additional risks. Certain commonly prescribed drugs (such as *aspirin* and *nonsteroidal antiinflammatory drugs* [NSAIDs]) can inhibit platelet function and should be held for a week before the operation if possible. Renal dysfunction is another common cause of acquired platelet dysfunction.

Elevated INR and PTT values often reflect blood coagulation protein deficiencies (or inhibitors). Patients with elevated values may require plasma factor replacement before surgery to minimize their bleeding risks.

There are some patients with normal screening laboratory tests who nonetheless have suggestive histories and/or examinations for hemostatic defects. One possible culprit might be **Von Willebrand's disease—an inheritable coagulation defect in platelet function.** Identification and perioperative management of this and other more uncommon bleeding disorders may require further laboratory testing and the expertise of a hematologist.

Perioperative Antibiotics for Wound Infection Prophylaxis

It is reasonable to administer 1 g *cefotetan* intravenously or intramuscularly just before surgery and then every 6 hours for two additional doses in patients undergoing extensive gynecologic oncology surgery. One study demonstrated that **preoperative antibiotics must be given within 2 hours of surgery to be effective** (118). In addition, if bowel resection is anticipated, mechanical cleansing of the bowel on the day before surgery is prudent, with or without oral *neomycin* and *erythromycin* base.

Table 18.18 Grade 3 Surgery (Major)				
	Age (years)			
	≥16 to <40	≥40 to <60	≥60 to <80	≥80
Test	**ASA Class 2 with respiratory disease**			
Chest x-ray	C	C	C	C
ECG	C	C	C	Y
CBC	Y	Y	Y	Y
Coagulation	N	N	N	N
Renal function	C	C	Y	Y
Glucose	N	N	N	N
Urine analysis	C	C	C	C
Blood gas	C	C	C	C
PFT	N	C	C	C
	ASA Class 3 with respiratory disease			
Chest x-ray	C	C	C	C
ECG	C	C	Y	Y
CBC	Y	Y	Y	Y
Coagulation	C	C	C	C
Renal function	Y	Y	Y	Y
Glucose	C	C	C	C
Urine analysis	C	C	C	C
Blood gas	C	C	C	C
PFT	C	C	C	C

ASA—American Society of Anesthesiologists, C—Considered, Y—Yes, N—No ECG—electrocardiogram, CBC—complete blood count, PFT—pulmonary function test Adapted from http://www.nice.org.uk/Guidance/CG3/Guidance/pdf/English.

Postoperative Management

Cardiovascular

Hypertension

High blood pressure, both labile and persistent, is a common problem for acutely ill patients. Perioperative hypertensive episodes occur commonly in hypertensive patients and occasionally in normotensive patients because of pain, anxiety, stress, medications, and other factors (see Table 18.5). Perioperative hypertension is most common during laryngoscopy and induction (primarily because of sympathetic stimulation) and immediately after surgery, often in the recovery room.

Patients with preexisting hypertension usually require some continuation of their daily anti-hypertensive medication when they are brought into the hospital or are critically ill, but the dosages may need titration, and diuretic use for blood pressure control is infrequent. Many agents can be converted to an intravenous form or administered with minimal fluid down a gastric tube if the patient is not eating or drinking. The use of β-blockers as antihypertensives in the acute care setting may have additional benefits by decreasing the risks of atrial fibrillation and myocardial ischemia in vulnerable patients, and these agents are often selected as first line agents for this reason. Some studies have suggested that routine use of these agents might decrease cardiovascular

Table 18.19 Grade 3 Surgery (Major)

Test	≥16 to <40	≥40 to <60	≥60 to <80	≥80
ASA Class 2 with renal disease				
Chest x-ray	C	C	C	C
ECG	C	C	Y	Y
CBC	Y	Y	Y	Y
Coagulation	C	C	C	C
Renal function	Y	Y	Y	Y
Glucose	C	C	C	C
Urine analysis	C	C	C	C
Blood gas	C	C	C	C
PFT	N	N	N	N
ASA Class 3 with renal disease				
Chest x-ray	C	C	C	C
ECG	C	C	Y	Y
CBC	Y	Y	Y	Y
Coagulation	C	C	C	C
Renal function	Y	Y	Y	Y
Glucose	C	C	C	C
Urine analysis	C	C	C	C
Blood gas	C	C	C	C
PFT	N	N	N	N

ASA—American Society of Anesthesiologists, C—Considered, Y—Yes, N—No ECG—electrocardiogram, CBC—complete blood count, PFT—pulmonary function test
Adapted from http://www.nice.org.uk/ Guidance/CG3/Guidance/pdf/English.

mortality after noncardiac surgery in patients at risk (119). At the minimum, care should be taken that β-blockers are not discontinued suddenly as this can cause rebound hypertension and associated problems. Sublingual, short-acting calcium channel blockers (e.g., *nifedipine*), on the other hand, should be avoided because their use can lead to reflex tachycardia and myocardial ischemia.

Corticosteroid medications can sometimes cause hypertension in susceptible patients. Mild antihypertensives may be necessary until the steroid dose is lowered or discontinued.

Many hypertensive episodes resolve spontaneously. **Patients with pain and anxiety are best treated with appropriate analgesics and anxiolytics.** When evaluating the hypertensive postoperative patient, adequacy of ventilation and stable cardiac status should be verified by examination, arterial blood gases, and ECG. **Bladder distension** can cause elevated blood pressure and should be relieved. **Occasionally, a patient may require a continuous intravenous infusion to control severe hypertension. Intravenous drugs with short half-lives** are chosen to allow safe titration (the vasodilator *nitroprusside* or short acting β-blockers are two popular choices), and the patient is changed over to longer-acting agents as their condition stabilizes (120).

Myocardial Injury and Ischemia

Patients undergoing oncologic treatment may have underlying coronary artery disease. The variable stresses in the postoperative period, such as inflammation, increased hypercoagulable state and hypoxemia, can lead to myocardial injury or ischemia. One study of unselected patients over age 50 years undergoing noncardiac surgery showed the risk of postoperative cardiac events was nearly

1.5% (5). Most postoperative myocardial infarcts (MI) occur during the first three days after surgery, at a time when patients may be receiving narcotics that may mask the symptoms of ischemia.

Patients experiencing postoperative MI have an increased hospital mortality. These patients need to be managed promptly by a surgeon and a consulting cardiologist, and observed closely in a monitored bed for any complicating features such as arrhythmia, pulmonary edema, and shock. In addition to correcting anemia, hypoxia, and starting β-blockers in those that can tolerate them, **the treatment of such acute coronary syndromes involves the use of anticoagulants such as** *aspirin* **and** *heparin.* The use of these agents must be balanced against the risk of postoperative bleeding. Myocardial infarcts are typically divided into ST segment or non-ST segment elevation injury depending on the ECG appearance. Myocardial infarction patients with ST elevation or with hemodynamic instability have improved outcomes if they can receive rapid angiography and angioplasty, while those in a stable condition with non-ST segment elevations can often be managed medically (at least initially). Unless contraindicated, **all patients with postoperative myocardial infarction should be on** *aspirin,* β**-blockers, HMG co A reductase inhibitors, and ACE inhibitors by the time of discharge** (121).

Arrhythmia

Every physician working in an acute care hospital should be familiar with the use of a defibrillator and the algorithms developed by the American Heart Association for Advanced Life Support (122). Fluid shifts, electrolyte changes, and myocardial ischemia can put the patient receiving treatment for gynecologic malignancy at increased risk for heart rhythm abnormalities.

The tachyarrhythmias, both ventricular and supraventricular, can be quite dangerous and should be electrically cardioverted immediately if the blood pressure is low or the patient is unstable. In less urgent situations, a variety of antiarrhythmic medications are available for chemical conversion and stabilization of these tachyarrhythmias. Many of these medications are proarrhythmic as well, and a search for an underlying cause of the rhythm disturbance is indicated to reduce the propensity for recurrence. **Often, when the electrolyte imbalance or other precipitant is corrected the heart rhythm normalizes,** and these agents can be discontinued. **Persistent or unstable ventricular arrhythmias are often managed in the acute setting with intravenous** *amiodarone.* **Supraventricular tachycardias** may respond to vagal maneuvers or a rapid bolus of *adenosine.*

Atrial fibrillation is the most common postoperative tachyarrhythmia and deserves special mention. Once the blood pressure is stabilized in a patient with atrial fibrillation, attempts should be made to control the heart rate. **Popular drugs for rate control include** β**-blockers** (if left ventricular function is preserved), *diltiazem,* or *digoxin.* If the rhythm persists once other precipitants have been corrected (e.g., hypokalemia, hypoxemia, fluid overload), many clinicians would attempt chemical or electrical conversion if the atrial fibrillation has not been present more than 48 hours. Restoration of normal sinus rhythm often improves cardiac output (CO) and mitigates the risk of stroke from left atrial thrombus forming in the fibrillating chamber. Patients with atrial fibrillation lasting longer than a few days, and who have no contraindication, should be considered for anticoagulation, to decrease their risk of a stroke (123).

Bradyarrhythmias often arise from excessive vagal stimulation. Nausea, bladder distension, pain, and endotracheal tube manipulation can all stimulate excessive vagal tone. As with tachyarrhythmias, attention to blood pressure is paramount. **Those patients who develop hypotension should receive** *atropine* **and/or catecholamines. Patients not responding to these agents may need urgent transvenous pacemaker placement.** Transcutaneous pacing can also be attempted if available at the bedside.

Shock

Shock is defined as a clinical syndrome in which the patient shows signs of decreased perfusion of vital organs. Typical findings include alterations in mental status, cold and clammy skin, oliguria, and metabolic acidosis. In general, patients with shock have a substantial decrease in blood pressure, but no absolute value is used to define shock.

The therapeutic approach to these patients is facilitated by a functional classification of shock states. Each class of shock has its own pathophysiologic process and requires a different management strategy. Traditionally, four varieties of shock are described:

1. **Hypovolemic shock**—secondary to fluid losses and decreased cardiac filling pressures (e.g., postoperative bleeding or intravascular fluid redistribution).

2. **Distributive shock**—secondary to inappropriate "vasodilation" and venous pooling (e.g., sepsis syndrome, anaphylaxis, decreased vasomotor tone from spinal anesthesia, and adrenal insufficiency from steroid withdrawal).

3. **Cardiogenic shock**—secondary to decreased myocardial contractility and function (e.g., acute myocardial infarction or ischemia and/or congestive cardiac failure).

4. **Obstructive shock**—secondary to mechanical obstructions in the cardiovascular circuit (e.g., pulmonary embolism, cardiac tamponade).

Common causes of shock in the perioperative management of gynecologic malignancy include:

1. **Hemorrhage (hypovolemic).**

2. **Sepsis (distributive)**

3. **Postoperative MI (cardiogenic)**

4. **Pulmonary embolus (obstructive)**

A careful physical examination, review of laboratory and test results, as well as consideration of the clinical situation often suggests the etiology of a particular shock syndrome. Therapy should begin promptly, as information is being gathered. In the past, invasive hemodynamic monitoring with pulmonary artery catheters was often used to diagnose and manage these conditions. There use, however, has declined as recent studies have shown they do not clearly improve patient outcomes (124). **There has been increased interest in recent years in using central venous catheters and echocardiograms to gather this information noninvasively.** The pulmonary catheter may still be useful in certain clinical situations where the diagnosis and treatment for shock remains uncertain.

Regardless of whether measured directly with a pulmonary catheter, or deduced from less invasive data, each of the shock states has an expected hemodynamic profile. Therapy is therefore targeted to the underlying defect in cardiovascular performance:

1. **Hypovolemic shock** is treated with crystalloid or colloid infusion to increase cardiac filling and therefore cardiac output and perfusion to vital organs. There is no clear evidence that colloids have any benefits over crystalloids for this purpose (125). Hypovolemic shock is the most common form of shock in the surgical patient, and treatment of the hypotensive, oliguric patient typically begins with a "fluid trial."

2. **Distributive shock** often requires vasopressor management with catecholamines active at the alpha receptors on the vasculature. This helps restore adequate resistance to create a perfusing blood pressure. Equally important, however, is to commence treatment of the presumed cause of the vasodilation: prompt antibiotics and source control for cases of suspected sepsis, steroids if secondary adrenal insufficiency is a possibility, or withdrawal of the offending agent and antiinflammatory treatment if an allergic reaction is suspected. There are published guidelines for the treatment of septic shock (126).

3. **Cardiogenic shock** is characterized by inadequate cardiac output, such that inotropic management with catecholamine and dopaminergic compounds is often necessary to maintain adequate contractility. Vasodilator therapy can be helpful in cardiogenic shock because it unburdens the failing heart's afterload. This allows contractility to improve without excessive cardiac work, which might exacerbate myocardial ischemia.

4. **Obstructive shock** can be difficult to manage and might require a combination of measures to maintain adequate filling pressures and contractility. Like distributive shock, it is important to attempt reversal of the precipitant quickly (e.g., anticoagulation for pulmonary embolism, pericardiocentesis for tamponade) because the patient's ultimate outcome depends on this.

An algorithm for the management of shock syndromes is shown in Fig. 18.3, although critically ill patients may often develop mixed shock states.

Respiratory Failure

Respiratory failure can be defined as a failure of gas exchange, that is, failure of the respiratory system to accomplish the exchange of oxygen and carbon dioxide between ambient air and red blood cells in amounts required to meet the body's metabolic needs. **Respiratory syndromes characterized by difficulty in oxygenation of the blood** are grouped under the umbrella term, **hypoxic respiratory failure,** and **those with difficulty removing carbon dioxide** from the blood are described **as ventilatory failure.** It is often helpful for assessment and therapy to consider these as separate entities, although in reality they are closely connected. The arterial blood gas is used to determine the degree and type of gas exchange failure and should be performed as part of the initial evaluation. Patients with respiratory failure commonly have abnormal mental

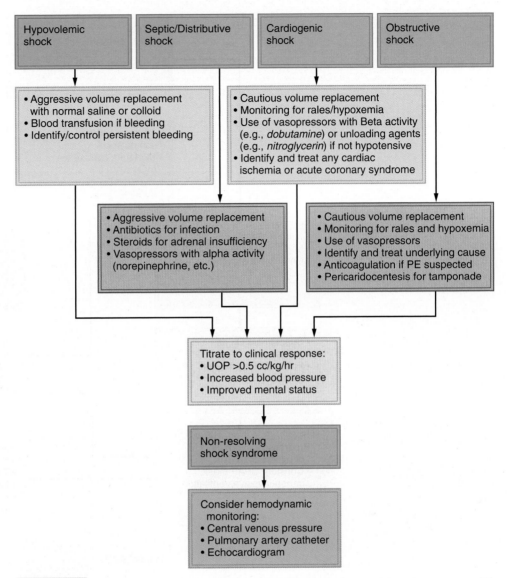

Figure 18.3 **Algorithm for the management of hypotension.** UOP, urine output; PE, pulmanory embolism.

status (agitation, somnolence, and disorientation), and physical findings may include tachycardia, hypertension, and occasionally cyanosis and sweating (Fig. 18.4).

Common causes of respiratory failure in the perioperative management of gynecologic cancer patients include:

1. **Nervous system depression secondary to sedative or analgesic medications**
2. **Bronchospasm**
3. **Pneumonia**
4. **Pulmonary edema**
5. **Lymphangitic spread of cancer**
6. **Respiratory muscle weakness**

Hypoxic Respiratory Failure

Hypoxic respiratory failure is usually caused by a mismatch between inhaled gas and blood circulation in the lung parenchyma. Blood circulating in areas of mismatch is relatively deoxygenated. The degree of hypoxic respiratory failure can be characterized by the alveolar–arterial oxygen gradient. This value is determined by measuring the arterial oxygen tension with a

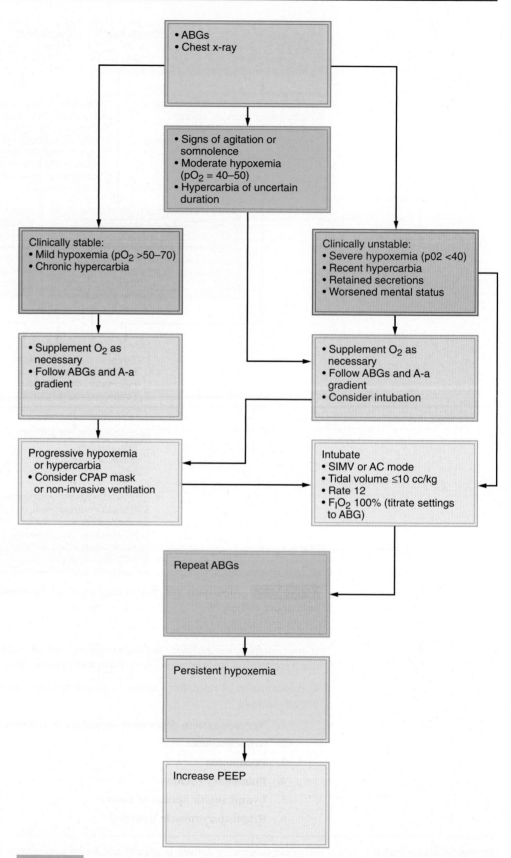

Figure 18.4   Management of respiratory failure. ABG, arterial blood gases; CPAP, continuous positive airway pressure; PEEP, positive end-expiratory pressure; SIMV, synchronized intermittent mandatory ventilation; AC, assist control; F_IO_2, fraction of inspired oxygen; A-a gradient, alveolar-arterial gradient.

blood gas, and then calculating the alveolar oxygen tension using known values for the fraction of inspired air that consists of oxygen (dependent on ambient barometric pressure and amount of oxygen supplementation) and the amount of carbon dioxide tension in the alveolus (calculated by measuring the arterial carbon dioxide tension on blood gas and adjusting for the expected exchange into the alveolus to maintain metabolic processes). This calculation is frequently performed at the bedside using the following alveolar gas equation:

$$\text{Alveolar } P_{O_2} = \text{Inspired } O_2 \text{ concentration} - \text{alveolar } CO_2 \text{ concentration}$$
$$\text{Alveolar } P_{O_2} = (F_{IO_2} \times [\text{barometric pressure} - \text{water vapor pressure*}])$$
$$- ([Pa_{CO_2} \text{ arterial}] \times 1.25)$$

*713 mm Hg at sea level

Without oxygen supplementation at sea level, the inspired oxygen concentration is approximately 150 mm Hg. Normal Pa_{CO_2} is 40 mm Hg in arterial blood. Therefore, the alveolar oxygen concentration in a healthy patient breathing ambient air by the preceding equation is approximately 100 mm Hg. This would then be compared with the measured arterial oxygen concentration on a blood gas sample to describe the **alveolar–arterial gradient (alveolar P_{O_2} – arterial P_{O_2}).** The alveolar–arterial difference in oxygen concentration increases with age, but typically does not exceed 20 mm Hg. **A gradient wider than 20 mm Hg is the hallmark of hypoxic respiratory failure.**

Treatment of hypoxic respiratory failure involves improving oxygenation of arterial blood as well as attempting correction of the underlying mismatch in lung function. **Interventions to improve oxygenation include supplemental oxygen by nasal cannula or mask, or by positive-pressure breathing for refractory hypoxemia.** Positive airway pressure serves in part to inflate partially or totally collapsed regions of the lung, often with a dramatic improvement in oxygenation. On a mechanical ventilator, different manipulations can be made to increase airway pressures. Most commonly, this is done by increasing positive end-expiratory pressure (PEEP). Additional measures to help reverse underlying ventilation-perfusion mismatch in hypoxic respiratory failure are as follows:

1. **Bronchodilators for bronchospasm**
2. **Diuretics for excess lung edema**
3. **Antibiotics for pneumonia**
4. **Chest physiotherapy for atelectasis**
5. **Anticoagulants for pulmonary embolism**

Ventilatory Failure

Ventilatory failure occurs in patients who fail to "excrete" adequate carbon dioxide from their lungs. These problems typically do not arise from mismatch at the alveolar–capillary level, but more likely from failure of the lungs to effectively pump gas out of the respiratory circuit. As P_{CO_2} builds up in the alveoli, the arterial P_{CO_2} begins to rise as well. **Hypercarbia on the blood gas measurement is the hallmark of ventilatory failure.** "Pump" dysfunction can occur anywhere from the medulla, to the diaphragm, to the thickened or destroyed airways of the patient with COPD. Typical scenarios for the oncologic patient include the oversedated patient with an inadequate respiratory rate, or the weakened patient unable to pump air adequately through diseased lungs.

Treatment of ventilatory failure consists of reversing any precipitants, and if these are not readily correctable, providing an adequate tidal volume and respiratory rate with a mechanical ventilator. This is typically administered through an endotracheal tube with a mechanical ventilator, although there is increasing interest in the use of noninvasive masks to administer continuous or phasic positive airway pressure in certain situations (58).

Chronic Respiratory Failure

Some patients with gynecologic malignancy may have adapted to chronic respiratory insufficiency. These patients with chronic lung disease may have abnormal alveolar–arterial oxygen gradients or carbon dioxide tensions as their baseline equilibrium. Chronic hypoxemia leads to elevated hemoglobin and improved oxygen delivery chemistry, and these patients are not in acute distress unless their P_{O_2} dips into the 50 mm Hg range. Chronic lung disease can lead to carbon dioxide retention, which is compensated by a metabolic alkalosis. Increasing oxygen supplementation beyond that necessary to maintain hemoglobin saturations at the patient's baseline can sometimes lead to worsening pump function in patients with chronic CO_2 retention. Likewise, improving ventilation by mechanical means to a "normal" Pco_2 on blood gas measurement may lead to dangerous alkalemia in a patient with chronic lung disease who was in acid–base balance at a higher Pco_2. The goal of oxygenation and ventilation in patients with chronic respiratory insufficiency should be to maintain their baseline status.

Adult Respiratory Distress Syndrome

One pattern of severe respiratory failure that deserves special mention is the adult respiratory distress syndrome (ARDS). **This is a pattern of lung injury that can be precipitated by direct damage (aspiration) or can occur as part of a septic syndrome and resulting lung inflammation. It is characterized by severe hypoxemia and decreased lung compliance thought to be secondary to diffuse capillary leakage into the lung parenchyma.** The chest radiograph has the appearance of pulmonary edema, although direct measurement with a pulmonary catheter typically shows low or normal left sided filling pressures. Management typically involves mechanical ventilation with lower tidal volumes to minimize lung distension and to avoid fluid overload (127,128). Despite aggressive support, the mortality rate from this syndrome remains high (129).

Mechanical Ventilation

Physicians working with critically ill patients need to understand the principles of mechanical ventilation. Postoperative patients sometimes remain on mechanical ventilation until they are stabilized. Even apparently stable oncologic patients on the wards are often at risk for hypoxic and ventilatory failure that can progress to the need for mechanical ventilation.

Mechanical ventilation is typically performed by placement of an endotracheal tube, although tight-fitting masks are sometimes used in patients who are awake enough to protect their airways (noninvasive positive-pressure ventilation) (58). There has been a proliferation in both the types and terminology for mechanical ventilation over the years, often leading to some confusion. Despite the many modalities, little is known about improved benefits of one ventilator setting versus another in terms of long-term patient outcome.

A basic understanding of ventilator management can be divided into two realms (much like the understanding of respiratory failure)—ventilation and oxygenation. **Management of ventilation requires adjusting when and how often the machine delivers a breath** (with every patient effort or on a timer), and how it delivers that breath (either as a preset volume or applying a preset pressure). These settings are chosen to help the clinician accomplish two goals: full or partial support of the patient's breathing efforts, and adequate ventilation without excessive airway pressures. **Management of oxygenation requires adjustment of the fraction of inspired oxygen delivered into the lungs and the end-expiratory airway pressure settings.** These values are also set to achieve adequate blood oxygen saturation without damaging the lungs.

When the machine is set to deliver a full mechanical breath with each patient effort, the patient is receiving fully supported ventilation. Typically, a backup respiratory rate is set, but the patient can breathe as often as she wants and receive a fully supported tidal breath each time. This is typically called **assist control (AC) ventilation.** When the machine is set to deliver only a certain number of breaths each minute, the patient needs to breathe without full machine support for any additional respirations above the set rate. This is considered partially supported ventilation and is most typically set as **synchronized intermittent mandatory ventilation (SIMV).**

The mechanical breath itself can be delivered as a preset volume with each breath, so-called volume control ventilation. This ensures an adequate tidal volume but risks increased airway pressures if the lungs become difficult to inflate because of increased airway resistance or lung stiffness. High airway pressures can cause barotrauma, such as pneumothorax, and it is recommended to keep peak airway pressures less than 35 cm H_2O if possible (130). **Instead of volume control, the mechanical breath can be administered as a preset pressure**; this is usually termed **pressure control** (or in a slightly different mode, **pressure support**). This avoids the risks of increased airway pressures but may provide smaller (or larger) tidal volumes with each breath if lung mechanics (or patient effort) changes. Some of the more sophisticated ventilators can adjust pressures with each breath to meet a targeted volume in a mode called **pressure regulated volume control.** Regardless of which mode is chosen, arterial blood gases are typically followed for patients on mechanical ventilation, and adjustments are made in the aforementioned settings to keep the patient's arterial carbon dioxide level near her baseline value.

When adjusting oxygenation settings on the ventilator, most critical care physicians attempt to lower the fraction of inspired oxygen (F_IO_2) to below 65%. Values above this for prolonged periods are believed to be damaging to lung parenchyma (131). The addition of PEEP often increases the functional reserve capacity of the diseased lung and allows F_IO_2 reductions. PEEP should be titrated to maximize oxygenation in respiratory failure, although some caution is needed because higher values can begin to precipitate barotrauma from increased peak pressures. In some forms of acute respiratory failure, such as ARDS, additional measures may be tried for refractory hypoxemia, including lengthening the inspiratory time on the ventilator cycle or changing patients to the prone position. Unfortunately, these interventions have not been shown in any prospective trials to improve long-term outcomes (128).

Once the cause of respiratory failure is improved or improving, and the patient is judged hemodynamically stable, attempts to remove the patient from mechanical ventilation should begin. This process has become known as weaning, although it does not need to be as slow as this appellation suggests. Although clinicians have looked at many screening methods for identifying patients who are ready to come off mechanical ventilation, none offers perfect sensitivity or specificity. Traditional weaning criteria such as negative inspiratory force less than 25 cm and minute ventilation less than 10 L/minute have shown poor predictive value. Many physicians think the bedside test with best predictive accuracy may be the **rapid shallow breathing index,** which divides respiratory rate (breaths per minute) by tidal volume (liters) measured with the patient removed briefly from ventilatory support. **A rapid shallow breathing index value less than 100 breaths/minute/L showed the best predictive value for successful extubation** in a recent review of multiple different predictors (132).

In the end, **the most useful test to determine a patient's readiness for extubation is probably a trial of spontaneous breathing with little or no support from the ventilator.** This is often performed with minimal pressure support (7 cm of H_2O per breath or less) or by having the patient breathe through the endotracheal tube without any ventilator support at all. Patients who can tolerate 30 minutes to 2 hours of such unsupported breathing should be considered for extubation if they can protect their airways, manage their secretions, and maintain oxygenation and ventilation (133). Early extubation can help avoid nosocomial pneumonia as well as other complications associated with the mechanical ventilator and a prolonged ICU stay.

Renal Insufficiency, Fluids, and Electrolytes

Acute Renal Failure

Acute renal failure (ARF) or acute renal injury remains a serious postoperative complication in surgical patients. Surgical patients are particularly predisposed to ARF due to the physiologic insult induced by the surgical procedure, preexisting comorbidity, and sepsis. **The overall incidence of ARF in surgical patients has been estimated at 1% to 2%, although it is higher in at-risk groups** (Table 18.20), and mortality rates remain high despite advances in dialysis and supportive care (134). The most consistent preoperative factor contributing to ARF is preexisting renal impairment (135). At present the best form of treatment is prevention.

While a number of definitions of acute renal failure exist in the literature, the first sign of new or worsening renal dysfunction is a rising serum creatinine concentration or a low urinary output. **Oliguria is defined as a urine output of less than 400 mL/day. Acute renal failure typically**

Table 18.20 Risk Factors for Developing Perioperative Acute Renal Failure
1. Preexisting renal impairment (chronic kidney disease)
2. Hypertension
3. Cardiac disease
4. Diabetes mellitus
5. Jaundice or liver disease
6. Advanced age

Table 18.21 Common Causes of Acute Renal Failure in Surgical Cancer Patients*
I. Prerenal
a. Hypotension
b. Hypovolemia (diarrhea, vomiting, anemia)
c. Heart failure
d. Sepsis
e. Drugs: angiotensin converting enzyme (ACE) inhibitors, nonsteroidal antiinflammatory drugs (NSAIDs)
II. Intrinsic (Renal)
a. Acute tubular necrosis
1. ischemia (shock, severe sepsis)
2. nephrotoxic agents (radiographic contrast, aminoglycosides, *cisplatin,* amphotericin)
3. pigment nephropathy—rhabdomyolysis (myoglobin)
b. Acute interstitial nephritis
1. allergic nephritis (drugs such as antibiotics)
2. cancer infiltration
c. Glomerulonephritis
1. amyloidosis
2. IgA nephropathy
3. membranous glomerulonephritis
d. Renal tubular obstruction—
1. urate crystals (tumor lysis syndrome)
2. light chains (multiple myeloma)
3. drugs—*acyclovir, methotrexate*
III. Postrenal
a. Bladder dysfunction—drugs, nerve injury
b. Uretral obstruction—cancer

*Adapted from **Carmichael P, Carmichael AR.** Acute renal failure in the surgical setting. *ANZ J Surg* 2003;73:144–153; and **Darmon M, Ciroldi M, Thiery G, Schlemmer B, Azoulay E.** Clinical review: specific aspects of acute renal failure in cancer patients. *Crit Care* 2006;10:211–217.

reflects an abrupt loss and sustained decline in the glomerular filtration rate, which manifests as an increasing serum creatinine to twice its baseline value (136). In the hospital setting, acute oliguria or renal failure is usually caused by hypovolemia, decreased cardiac output, postoperative kidney injury, or the use of nephrotoxic drugs (137). **Prerenal causes (see below) are responsible for the majority of cases (up to 90%) of ARF in surgical patients** (135). Patients are also at increased risk for acute kidney injury from etiologies arising from cancer treatment such as severe vomiting or diarrhea, nephrotoxic chemotherapy, or tumor lysis syndrome. The cancer itself may also cause ureteral obstruction (Table 18.21) (138).

The causes of acute renal failure are grouped into three categories: prerenal, intrinsic, and postrenal (Table 18.21). Initial evaluation attempts to group the patient into one of these classes. **Prerenal failure and intrinsic renal failure due to ischemia and nephrotoxins (acute tubular necrosis) are responsible for most cases** (135). The physical examination should exclude orthostatic blood pressure changes, evidence of liver disease, a palpable bladder, and an elevated postvoid residual urine volume as determined by bladder catheterization. Laboratory evaluation should include determinations of urinary and serum sodium and creatinine concentrations (to calculate the fractional excretion of sodium [$F_{ex}Na$]; see below), urine osmolality, and microscopic urinalysis. Unfortunately, the results of urinary electrolytes may be unreliable and should be interpreted with caution in patients with glycosuria, preexisting renal disease, and those receiving diuretics.

Postrenal causes of oliguria or acute renal failure arise from obstruction of the urinary tract. If this remains a suspicion even after a urethral catheter is placed, a renal ultrasound can be ordered, which may show characteristic dilation of the collection system (hydronephrosis) above the obstruction. Although quite specific, this finding may not be present in all cases of ureteral obstruction, and additional radiographic tests may be needed (139). Percutaneous or cystoscopic stenting is often performed for cases of acute ureteral obstruction.

Prerenal azotemia can often be diagnosed with urinary indices. It tends to be associated with high urine osmolality, low urinary sodium, and a high urine-to-plasma creatinine ratio. It was shown many years ago that **the best discriminator between prerenal and other causes of acute renal failure is the $F_{ex}Na$** (140). This can be easily calculated from serum and urine sodium and creatinine concentrations as follows:

$$F_{ex}Na = \frac{\text{Urine sodium} \times \text{plasma creatinine}}{\text{Plasma sodium} \times \text{urine creatinine}} \times 100$$

Prerenal azotemia is associated with a $F_{ex}Na$ of less than 1%, whereas obstructive uropathy (postrenal) and most forms of intrinsic renal failure (except pigment- or radiocontrast-induced acute tubular necrosis) are associated with $F_{ex}Na$ levels greater than 2%. Patients with a history or physical examination suggestive of volume depletion, or urinary indices consistent with prerenal azotemia, should be treated with aggressive fluid administration and frequent examination for evidence of volume overload. Characteristic urinary indices for prerenal and other causes of acute renal failure are listed in Table 18.22.

If prerenal and postrenal causes of renal dysfunction are excluded, the patient likely has intrinsic disease of the kidney. Most of these cases are caused by acute tubular necrosis (ATN), although a small percentage of patients may have interstitial nephritis or a form of glomerulonephritis (136). Urinalysis in conjunction with urine microscopy may suggest the etiology. **Red blood cell casts** in the sediment are diagnostic of **glomerulonephritis, "muddy" and cellular casts are suggestive of ATN,** and **eosinophils** in the urine (stained with Wright's stain) **are often indicative of interstitial nephritis** induced by drugs.

Acute tubular necrosis is usually caused by either ischemia or nephrotoxic agents. Many drugs are known nephrotoxins, including radiocontrast agents and many chemotherapeutic drugs. Clinicians should attempt to avoid nephrotoxicity by careful dosing and avoidance of hypovolemia. Administration of intravenous fluids (isotonic saline or sodium bicarbonate) shortly before administering radiocontrast dye, for instance, has been shown to decrease the risk of nephropathy from contrast agents. While still controversial, studies have suggested a

	Prerenal Azotemia	Acute Oliguric Renal Failure	Acute Nonoliguric Renal Failure	Acute Obstructive Uropathy	Acute Glomerulonephritis
Urine osmolality, mOsm/kg H$_2$O	518 ± 35	369 ± 20	343 ± 17	393 ± 39	385 ± 61
Urine sodium, mEq/L	18 ± 3	68 ± 5	50 ± 5	69 ± 10	22 ± 6
Urine/plasma urea nitrogen	18 ± 7	3 ± 0.5	7 ± 1	8 ± 4	11 ± 4
Urine/plasma creatinine	45 ± 6	17 ± 2	17 ± 2	16 ± 4	43 ± 7
Fractional excretion of filtered sodium	0.4 ± 0.1	7 ± 1.4	3 ± 0.5	6 ± 2	0.6 ± 0.2

Table 18.22 Urinary Diagnostic Indices[a]

[a]Values are expressed as mean ± standard error of the mean (SEM).

Adapted from **Miller TR, Anderson RJ, Linas SC, Henrich WL, Berns AS, Gabow PA, et al.** Urinary diagnostic indices in acute renal failure: a prospective study. *Ann Intern Med* 1978;89:47, with permission.

possible reduction in nephrotoxicity of contrast agents with the use of *N-acetylcysteine* (141,142).

One cause of intrinsic renal failure that should be considered in any oncologic patient being treated with chemotherapy is **tumor lysis syndrome. This condition is caused by the rapid destruction of large numbers of tumor cells (often just after the initiation of chemotherapy) and results in the sudden release of intracellular phosphate and other intracellular ions** (138). Metabolic abnormalities including hyperphosphatemia, hypocalcemia, hyperkalemia, hyperuricemia, and increased serum creatinine can be seen. **Acute renal failure develops due to uric acid crystal formation in the renal tubules.** The syndrome is most commonly seen in high-grade hematological malignancies such as lymphoma, but it can occur in solid malignancies that respond dramatically to chemotherapeutic agents. Prophylactic measures include hydration and drugs that reduce uric acid levels such as allopurinol and urate oxidases. Urgent hemodialysis is often indicated (143).

Management of patients with acute renal failure includes discontinuation of any nephrotoxic agents and appropriate adjustment of continuing medications to the patient's new creatinine clearance. Adequate fluid resuscitation to ensure euvolemia is critical. Careful attention to volume status, serum electrolytes, and acid–base status is also warranted. Nephrology consultation is recommended for all patients in whom the diagnosis is uncertain or the acute renal failure persists. Many clinicians use diuretics to maintain urine output (144). This strategy may make volume management easier, but is controversial as several studies suggest that diuretics are potentially detrimental and do not improve mortality or make it less likely that the patient will require renal replacement therapy with dialysis (145).

Sometimes the use of renal replacement therapy (hemodialysis) is needed, as there are no effective pharmacological agents for the treatment of established acute renal failure. Indications for hemodialysis include hyperkalemia; pulmonary edema and volume overload that cannot be corrected; acidemia; and uremic symptoms (encephalopathy, bleeding from platelet dysfunction, or pericarditis). The selection of modality of renal replacement therapy (intermittent versus continuous) and the optimal timing of initiation and dose of therapy remain unclear (146). Patients who are hemodynamically unstable might benefit from continuous renal replacement techniques (continuous venovenous hemodialysis or ultrafiltration) rather than intermittent therapy (147). An algorithm for managing oliguria and/or rising serum creatinine (ARF) is shown in Fig. 18.5.

Prevention of acute renal failure in the surgical setting is key. Several preventative measures are essential for high-risk patients (especially those with preexisting impairment). These include (i) optimizing volume status; (ii) keeping the mean arterial pressure >80 mmHg; (iii) reducing the risk of nosocomial infections by rapid removal of intravascular and bladder catheters; (iv) appropriate use of antibiotics; (v) aggressive treatment of any sepsis; and (vi) restricted use or avoidance of potentially nephrotoxic agents (134).

Acid–Base Disorders

Disorders of acid–base homeostasis are common in critical care medicine, and accurate interpretation of these disorders is important for successful management. For an exhaustive review of acid–base disorders, the reader is referred to several excellent summaries (148–150).

The human body requires tight regulation of acid–base balance despite ongoing metabolic processes that produce substantial acid loads. It does this with several buffering systems, all of which are in balance and correct any disturbances. The most important (and most easily measured) is the bicarbonate–carbonic acid equilibrium. **This buffering system is reflected in serum bicarbonate levels and carbon dioxide tension** (which is in equilibrium with serum carbonic acid). Changes in these measurements from baseline reflect changes in acid or base balance.

Changes in serum carbon dioxide tension (Pco_2) reflect either primary lung disorders (hyperventilation or hypoventilation) with resulting respiratory disturbances in acid–base balance, or attempts by the lungs to compensate for metabolic disturbances causing changes in bicarbonate concentration in the blood. Hyperventilation as a primary disturbance results in a low Pco_2 in the blood and resulting **respiratory alkalemia.** Hypoventilation as a primary disturbance raises Pco_2 in the blood and causes a **respiratory acidemia.** On the other hand, **when the primary acid–base disturbance is caused by a metabolic disturbance, the patient's ventilatory system attempts to keep the pH balanced by hyperventilation or**

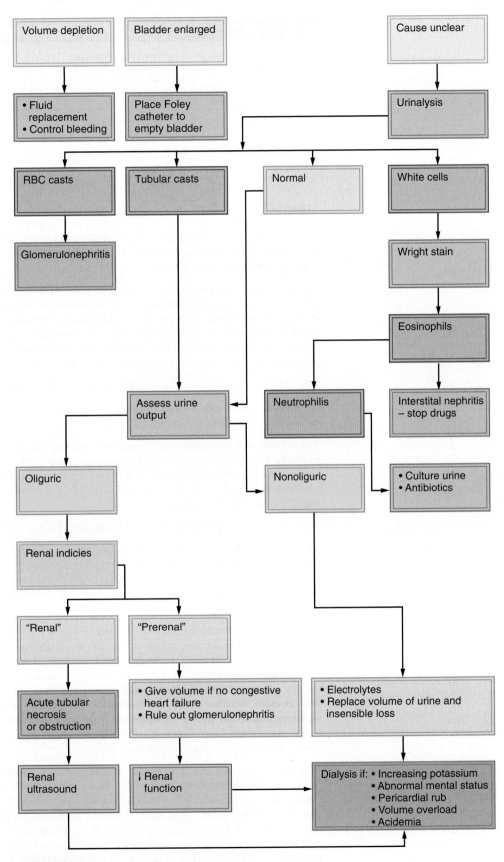

Figure 18.5 **Management of a rising serum creatinine.**

Table 18.23 Causes of Metabolic Acidosis		
Elevated Anion Gap	*Normal Anion Gap*	*Normal-Hyperkalemic Acidosis*
Renal failure	Renal tubular acidosis	Early renal failure
Ketoacidosis	Diarrhea	Hydronephrosis
Lactic acidosis	Posthypocapnic acidosis Carbonic anhydrase inhibitors Ureteral diversions	Addition of HCl Sulfur toxicity

hypoventilation, thereby creating compensatory changes in the Pco_2. By studying the serum pH and comparing changes in the serum Pco_2 to changes in the serum bicarbonate concentration, the clinician is often able to distinguish primary respiratory alkalemia and acidemia (as well as their duration) from secondary compensation (150,151). Bedside nomograms have been designed for this purpose as well.

Primary changes in the serum bicarbonate concentration often reflect metabolic processes initially less obvious than primary lung disturbances. **Metabolic acidosis is defined as a decrease in serum bicarbonate level and occurs as a primary disorder or as a compensation for a respiratory disturbance. Typically, the first step in evaluating a patient with a primary metabolic acidosis is to measure serum electrolytes and calculate the anion gap.** A formula for the anion gap using serum electrolyte concentrations is:

$$\text{Anion gap} = (Na^+) - (Cl^- + HCO_3^-)$$

A "normal" anion gap is 10 to 14 mEq/L. Selected causes of metabolic acidosis with elevated and normal anion gaps are presented in Table 18.23.

The second step in evaluating a metabolic acidosis is assessment of the adequacy of the patient's ventilatory response. The normal mechanism of compensation for decreased serum bicarbonate is hyperventilation, which lowers the Pco_2 and offsets the impact of the decreased bicarbonate on serum pH. The expected response to a primary metabolic acidosis can be estimated by the following equation (151):

$$\text{Expected Pco}_2 = 1.5 \text{ (measured HCO}_3^-) + 8 \text{ (range} \pm 2)$$

Patients who have metabolic acidosis and whose measured Pco_2 levels fall below those expected on the basis of this equation should be suspected of having a second disturbance (i.e., an additional respiratory alkalosis). In patients with a Pco_2 higher than this expected level, additional respiratory acidosis should be suspected as complicating their metabolic disturbance (151).

The treatment of metabolic acidosis depends on its severity. In most cases, identification and treatment of the underlying cause is the only direct therapy necessary. In patients who have profound disturbances and bicarbonate levels less than 10 or pH less than 7.2, especially if there is associated hypotension or if the underlying disease is expected to worsen, bicarbonate therapy can be considered. **Bicarbonate therapy is controversial and should be undertaken with caution, because there is a theoretical risk of causing a transient worsening of the cerebrospinal fluid pH or of inducing fluid overload and rebound metabolic alkalosis.** Some researchers have suggested the administration of exogenous bicarbonate may even worsen the outcome in lactic acidosis (152,153).

Metabolic alkalosis can also occur in hospitalized patients. Perhaps most commonly, metabolic alkalosis is associated with volume contraction. In such conditions, sodium reabsorption by the kidney is linked to bicarbonate resorption. Metabolic alkalosis does not resolve until the patient regains intravascular volume. To determine the primary precipitant of metabolic alkalosis and the appropriate treatment, the clinician can use urinary chloride measurements to divide patients into two groups (provided the patient has not received recent diuretic therapy): (i) **patients with very low urinary chlorides. These include those who have received nasogastric drainage, diuretic therapy, have been vomiting, or have lingering alkalosis after hypercapnic lung failure. These "chloride-responsive" patients are treated with normal saline solution;** (ii) patients with higher urinary chloride concentrations. These

Table 18.24 Differential Diagnosis to Metabolic Alkalosis in Gynecologic Oncology Patients
A. Sodium chloride responsive (urinary chloride <10 mmol/L)
1. Gastrointestinal disorders
Vomiting
Gastric drainage
Diarrhea
2. Diuretic therapy
3. Correction of chronic hypercapnia
B. Sodium chloride resistant (urinary chloride >15 mmol/L)
1. Profound potassium depletion
C. Unclassified
1. Alkali administration
2. Milk-alkali syndrome
3. Massive blood or plasma transfusion
4. Nonparathyroid hypercalcemia
5. Glucose ingestion after starvation
6. Large doses of *carbenicillin or penicillin*

Adapted from **Schrier RW, ed.** *Renal and electrolyte disorders,* 2nd ed. Boston: Little Brown, 1980:146.

patients do not respond to *sodium chloride* and must be managed by treatment of the underlying disease (149). Table 18.24 lists the causes of metabolic alkalosis.

Maintenance Fluids

Proper management of water and electrolyte therapy is an integral component in the care of surgical and oncologic patients, particularly those who are not taking oral hydration or nourishment. In the average adult who is taking fluids orally, the average daily loss of water is approximately 3 L (2 L as urine and 1 L as insensible losses from perspiration, respiration, and feces). The condition of critically ill patients may be complicated by additional ongoing losses, derangements in renal function, increased insensible losses, and disturbances in free water metabolism induced by the underlying disease. **Successful management of these patients requires frequent monitoring of volume status and serum electrolytes.** Predictable losses of fluids and electrolytes must be replaced, particularly those from nasogastric suctioning and the increased insensible losses associated with fever and diarrhea (154).

Several simple guidelines can be kept in mind when managing fluid replacement in the hospitalized patient. **In a patient with no preexisting renal disease and no disorder of water or electrolyte metabolism, a reasonable maintenance fluid regimen is 3 L daily of a half-normal saline solution with 20 mEq of potassium chloride in each liter. In the presence of significant renal impairment (glomerular filtration rate <25 mL/minute), potassium therapy should not be given routinely, replacement being based on serial determinations of serum potassium.** In patients suspected of having a defect in free water excretion (see below), it is prudent to decrease the free-water content of the initial maintenance fluids (typically by giving normal saline at half the rate). Gastric fluid is composed of hypotonic saline solution (one-fourth to one-half normal saline) with 5 to 10 mEq/L of potassium. Gastric fluid losses should be replaced with replacement fluids in addition to the maintenance prescription.

Hyponatremia and Hypernatremia

Hyponatremia is a common disorder in gynecologic oncology patients. Serum sodium concentration reflects total body water content. Total body sodium content is reflected in extracellular fluid volume. **Hyponatremia represents a relative water excess.** Disorders of sodium excess or deficit are expressed as either extracellular volume overload or depletion. Hyponatremia is common, affecting up to 15% of hospitalized patients. The most common causes of hyponatremia in hospitalized patients are hypovolemia and the syndrome of inappropriate diuretic hormone secretion (SIADH) (155). **Hyponatremic conditions are best grouped into three different categories:**

1. **Hyponatremia associated with extracellular volume depletion (hypovolemia).** Hypovolemic patients block free water excretion by increasing antidiuretic hormone secretion. All forms of intravascular volume depletion in patients with normal renal function predispose to this form of hyponatremia, especially when losses have been replaced with hypotonic fluids. Typically, the urinary sodium level is low (<20 mEq/L), and signs of volume depletion are present (156).

2. **Hyponatremia with normal volume status (euvolemia).** This is seen in patients with SIADH and patients with hypothyroidism. The cause of SIADH should be determined and can include certain malignancies, intrathoracic disorders, central nervous system disorders, and a variety of drugs including several chemotherapeutic agents. In SIADH, urinary sodium levels are typically greater than 30 to 35 mEq/L (156).

3. **Hyponatremia with increased total-body sodium and increased extracellular volume (hypervolemia).** The hallmark of these disorders is edema, and urinary sodium levels are often low reflecting the decreased effective arterial volume in these conditions. Patients with this category of hyponatremia usually have congestive heart failure, nephrotic syndrome, or cirrhotic liver disease (156).

The treatment of hyponatremia is tailored to its pathophysiology. Immediate treatment depends on the patient's symptoms, the rate at which the hyponatremia has developed, and the absolute serum sodium concentration. **Patients with diminished extracellular volume are treated with an infusion of normal saline. Patients with normal or increased extracellular volume can be managed initially with free water restriction** (157). Those with persisting or worsening hyponatremia and adequate extracellular volume can be managed acutely with *furosemide* to induce a hypotonic diuresis, and then with replacement of urine output with normal saline infusion. **Therapy with hypertonic saline is rarely necessary,** and reserved for patients with profound hyponatremia typically associated with seizures and/or markedly diminished mental status. An algorithm detailing an approach to the patient with hyponatremia is presented in Fig. 18.6.

Hypernatremia, less commonly encountered in hospitalized patients, represents relative total-body water deficit (158). Usually it is the result of inadequate water replacement in a patient unable to take fluids spontaneously. This might be exaggerated or precipitated by failure of the kidneys to adequately reabsorb water (concentrate urine), a condition termed *nephrogenic diabetes insipidus*. Hypercalcemia affects the kidney's ability to concentrate. Hyperglycemia can also worsen water losses by causing an osmotic diuresis. Treatment of hypernatremia is directed at providing adequate hypotonic fluids (often as "free water" or fluids with very minimal solute) and treating hypercalcemia and/or hyperglycemia. Rare patients may have disorders of antidiuretic hormone manufacture and secretion in the hypothalamus and posterior pituitary **(central diabetes insipidus)** and must receive exogenous hormone to maintain water balance.

Hypokalemia and Hyperkalemia

Disturbances in serum potassium concentration are common and important because of the pivotal role played by this ion in maintaining transmembrane potentials of the heart. Because 98% of total-body potassium is intracellular, small changes in serum potassium concentration may reflect very large excesses or deficits in total-body potassium content. For instance, a decrease in the plasma potassium concentration to 3 mEq/L can reflect a 100- to 200-mEq deficit in total-body potassium content; a decrease to 2 mEq/L can reflect a total-body deficit of 300 to 500 mEq of potassium.

Changes in hydrogen ion concentration can have an impact on the distribution of potassium between the intracellular and extracellular spaces. **In acidemic patients, there is a shift in potassium from intracellular to extracellular sites.** In a patient who is acidemic and hypokalemic, the plasma potassium concentration is not appropriately diminished, and the total-body potassium deficit will be underestimated.

Possible causes of hypokalemia include decreased dietary intake or insufficient replacement in maintenance fluids, often worsened by diarrhea, nasogastric suction, or diuretic therapy. Hypokalemia can present as weakness, ileus, and muscular cramps. Of most concern,

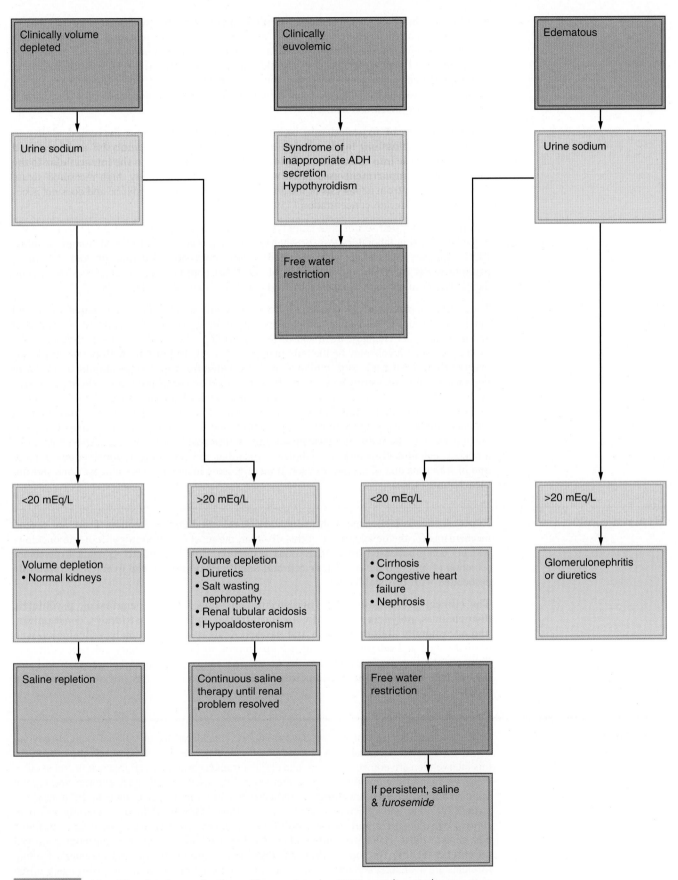

Figure 18.6   Algorithm for the evaluation of hyponatremia. ADH, antidiuretic hormone.

hypokalemia increases myocardial irritability and can precipitate dangerous arrhythmias (159). Treatment involves reversal of the underlying cause and repletion of the potassium deficit. Potassium is replaced relatively slowly in most circumstances to allow cell membranes to equilibrate. **In general, patients should not receive more than 10 mEq/hour intravenously.** Patients undergoing potassium therapy in the presence of renal failure have a diminished capacity to excrete potassium, and therefore added caution is needed to avoid the dangers of hyperkalemia (discussed below).

Common causes of hyperkalemia include renal insufficiency and decreased ability to excrete daily potassium load, cellular breakdown (including hemolysis) and increased potassium release into extracellular fluids, and redistribution from the intracellular to the extracellular compartment associated with acidemia. Occasionally, high measured serum potassium results from hemolysis of the drawn blood sample in the test tube and does not accurately reflect the serum concentration (159).

Patients with elevated serum potassium typically have no symptoms. The condition is usually noted on screening laboratory tests or when changes are noted on an ECG. **Although variable, ECG changes associated with elevated serum potassium include peaked T waves, prolonged PR interval, and widening of the QRS complex.** These changes often herald dangerous serum potassium levels that need correction to avert cardiac arrest.

The initial approach to hyperkalemia is to identify and remove the precipitating cause and rapidly assess any ECG changes. In patients with mild hyperkalemia (serum $K^+ < 6$ mEq/L) and minimal ECG changes, treatment of the underlying cause and careful monitoring of the serum potassium levels may be the only therapy necessary. **In patients with potassium levels greater than 6.5 mEq/L and evidence of QRS widening, rapid steps should be taken to decrease serum potassium levels with the use of oral or rectal potassium exchange resins such as sodium polystyrene sulfonate (*Kayexalate*) and a loop diuretic such as *furosemide*. If there is associated renal failure, urgent arrangements for dialysis are indicated.** In patients with prolonged QRS duration approaching sine-wave configuration, or in patients who are hypotensive, **the following treatments can "temporize"** until more definitive treatment is arranged: **calcium gluconate** to stabilize myocardial cell membranes, **intravenous glucose and *insulin*** (one unit of *insulin* for each gram of glucose in an ampule of glucose), and **sodium bicarbonate** (156).

Hypercalcemia

Hypercalcemia is associated with malignant disease and deserves mention. There are several mechanisms for the development of this disorder, the most common in gynecologic oncology patients being increased osteoclastic bone resorption. This is believed to result from tumor secretion of humoral factors. **Clear cell and small cell tumors of the ovary are commonly associated with this syndrome.**

The clinical presentation of hypercalcemia includes lethargy, confusion, psychiatric disturbances, polyuria (caused by a concentrating defect in the kidney), constipation, and occasionally abdominal pain and nausea. Acute management includes hydration with normal saline and administration of a loop diuretic to increase urinary calcium excretion. Subsequent treatment is targeted to the underlying cause (treatment of the tumor) and also may include the use of **intravenous bisphosphonates** to control the elevated calcium level (159).

Nutrition

Patients who cannot eat for several days should be considered for nutritional support (beyond the minimal calories available in glucose-based maintenance fluids). Although the criteria for this intervention are not well defined, and clinical trials have shown variable results, most clinicians would consider this intervention after several days without adequate calories and several more anticipated. **Enteral feeding is preferred** because it may protect patients from gastrointestinal bleeding and infectious complications (160). **Parenteral feeding usually requires central line placement and carries additional risks. One large trial in postsurgical patients has shown these risks are outweighed by benefits only when the patients required parenteral feeding for longer than 14 days** (161). Various enteral and parenteral feeding formulas are available, and adjustments in constituents are often needed to avoid many of the fluid and electrolyte problems described previously.

Blood Replacement

Anemia/Red Blood Cells

Anemia can be an additional stress on the cardiovascular system and may worsen myocardial ischemia or heart failure. Appropriate preoperative or perioperative transfusion may reduce cardiac morbidity in patients with significant coronary artery disease or heart failure (6). Some studies suggest that even mild preoperative anemia is associated with increased risk of postoperative cardiac events and mortality in elderly patients undergoing noncardiac surgery (162).

The evidence base for what threshold to use and which patients benefit from transfusion is poor (163). One study suggested that restricting red cell transfusion to patients with hemoglobin levels less than 7.0 g/dL (and who were not actively losing blood) did not worsen outcomes (164). **Other investigators have demonstrated harm in transfused patients including increased rates of infection, myocardial ischemia, and postoperative morbidity and mortality** (165). In addition, there are risks of transfusion reactions and transmission of communicable diseases. Due to these factors, **a conservative or "restrictive" approach with respect to transfusion may be at least as effective and possibly safer than a more liberal transfusion policy** (166). Patients with unstable angina and risks for cardiac ischemia or other evidence of inadequate perfusion of vital organs (see below) may require more liberal blood transfusion. Some studies suggest that **patients with acute coronary syndromes do better with hemoglobin levels kept closer to 10.0 g/dL** (167). Current guidelines on perioperative transfusion practices have been recently published (163).

Red blood cells can be transfused in the form of **whole blood** or **packed red blood cells.** Whole blood contains red cells as well as platelets and plasma. Packed red blood cells are red cell concentrates that are prepared by removal of most platelets and all but approximately 100 mL of plasma from a unit of whole blood. In addition, red cells can be washed to remove leukocytes and contaminating plasma proteins for transfusion to selected patients who have had febrile reactions to them.

With the possible exception of the patient with massive exsanguination, there is little advantage to transfusion of whole blood and, as a practical rule, packed red blood cells should be used when red cell therapy is indicated. The possible indications for transfusion of red blood cells include:

1. **A decreasing hematocrit** value in a patient who, because of bone marrow failure, is unlikely to begin producing red blood cells in the near future. Unfortunately, there is no information available in the literature to define exactly when a transfusion should be given. Furthermore, despite many trials, the data is insufficient to define a transfusion trigger in surgical patients with blood loss (166). Experts agree that red blood cells should probably be transfused if the hemoglobin is less than 6 g/dL and that red blood cells are usually unnecessary for most patients when the level is greater than 10 g/dL (163). However, for levels between these parameters, no solid evidence is available and the decision to transfuse should be individualized.

2. **Anemia in a patient with such symptoms as shortness of breath or chest pain or evidence of inadequate perfusion and oxygenation of major organs.** Monitoring such parameters as blood pressure, heart rate, oxygen saturation, urine output, and electrocardiography is recommended to assess whether vital organs have adequate perfusion (163). In general, patients have no symptoms and should have adequate perfusion if hemoglobin levels are above 10 g/dL.

Acute Hemolytic and Nonhemolytic Reactions

Acute hemolytic and nonhemolytic transfusion reactions are also possible. Nonhemolytic transfusion reactions are often characterized by fever, chills, or urticaria. Hemolytic transfusion reactions can be life threatening because of associated hypotension, disseminated intravascular coagulation (DIC), and renal failure. It is often manifested by fever, chest pain, back pain, hypotension, tachycardia, and red urine indicating hemoglobinuria (163). **When a patient undergoing a red cell transfusion has any signs or symptoms suggestive of a hemolytic transfusion reaction, the transfusion should be stopped immediately and the remaining aliquot of blood sent to the blood bank, along with a sample of the patient's blood for culture and repeat cross-matching.** A screening for DIC, a urinalysis for hemoglobin, and a blood sample for bilirubin also should be obtained. In patients with symptoms of a hemolytic transfusion reaction who, on analysis, show no evidence of hemolysis, a hypersensitivity reaction to transfused leukocytes or plasma proteins contaminating the red cells should be suspected. The incidence of hemolytic transfusion reactions can be minimized by careful attention to clerical information, ensuring that the patient is receiving blood cross-matched to her blood sample, and careful cross-matching in the blood bank.

Platelets

Platelet concentrates are prepared by removal of platelets from whole-blood fractions. Platelets can be stored for 5 days, and each 50-mL platelet "unit" from a whole blood fraction contains approximately 6×10^{10} platelets. Platelets may also be obtained by pheresis from a single donor, and each "unit" of single donor platelet pheresis is equivalent to 5 or 6 whole blood fraction units.

Platelet transfusions are indicated in patients with:

1. **Platelet counts less than 50,000/mL^3 who show evidence of bleeding** (163).

2. **In certain patients (see below) with platelet counts less than 10,000/mL^3 as prophylaxis against acute bleeding.**

Each whole blood fraction unit of platelets should be expected to raise the recipient's platelet count approximately 5,000 to 10,000/mL^3. In general, prophylactic platelet transfusions are indicated only in patients whose platelet count is expected to recover in the future because platelets express human leukocyte antigens and hence induce antibodies in the recipient. After prolonged platelet therapy, most patients become resistant to platelet transfusions, presumably because of immune destruction of all transfused platelets.

Plasma Fractions

Several plasma fractions are available for transfusion. The two most commonly used fractions are fresh frozen plasma and cryoprecipitate.

Fresh Frozen Plasma (FFP)   All the blood-clotting proteins present in the original unit of blood are contained in fresh frozen plasma, and it is an adequate source of all coagulation factors for the treatment of mild coagulation factor deficiencies. **FFP may be used to rapidly reverse *warfarin* toxicity if bleeding is present.** FFP should also be given in bleeding patients if the international normalized ratio (INR) or activated partial thromboplastin time (aPTT) is elevated (163). Plasma may also be used in reversing the coagulopathy associated with massive blood loss and red cell replacement by restoring the lost coagulation factors. **In patients undergoing transfusion of multiple units of red blood cells, the INR and aPTT should be monitored for evidence of coagulopathy and FFP given as needed to correct this.** It may require several "units" of fresh frozen plasma to restore clotting factors to adequate levels. The half-life of transfused clotting factors is measured in hours, and bleeding risks can recur when these factors are consumed.

Cryoprecipitate   Cryoprecipitate is produced by freezing of plasma, followed by thawing, and produces a precipitate **rich in factor VIII and fibrinogen.** This cryoprecipitate fraction contains approximately 250 mg of fibrinogen per unit and 80 clotting units of factor VIII. Cryoprecipitate units are smaller in volume than fresh frozen plasma and can be useful adjuncts in treating certain bleeding conditions such as DIC (see below). Cryoprecipitate should be given to bleeding patients when fibrinogen concentrations are less than 80 mg/dL (163).

Clotting Disorders

Massive Blood Transfusion

Pelvic surgeons may at times encounter unexpected and dramatic intraoperative bleeding. This may require large amounts of transfused blood, typically given as packed red blood cell (RBC) units. **"Massive transfusion" is typically defined as replacing the entire blood volume (5–6 L in a 70-kg patient) over a 24-hour period, or half the blood volume over a 3-hour period.** Such **"washout" coagulopathy has been shown in some studies to begin when greater than 10 units of packed red cells have been transfused** (168,169). Such rapid blood transfusion can result in a **dilutional coagulopathy,** as these transfused units do not contain adequate amounts of blood proteins or platelets. **This can be worsened by the hypothermia and acidosis** brought on by hypovolemic shock.

The INR, aPTT, fibrinogen concentration, and platelet counts should be followed closely in these cases. In general, INR and aPTT levels should be kept less than 1.5 times control values, fibrinogen maintained greater than 100 mg/dL, and platelet count supported to greater than 50,000.

Disseminated Intravascular Coagulation

Disseminated intravascular coagulation is a syndrome that complicates the course of a variety of disease states and is characterized by the pathologic activation of the coagulation cascade and the fibrinolytic system. It occurs most commonly in critically ill patients with sepsis and/or liver disease. **In gynecologic oncology patients, it might also be associated with certain mucin-producing adenocarcinomas** (170).

In its acute form, DIC appears rapidly and is manifested by bleeding from multiple sites, including venipunctures, surgical wounds, gingiva, gastrointestinal tract, and skin. More rarely, DIC can take a chronic course over a period of months, with thrombotic complications more common than bleeding complications. This form is more typical for the syndrome associated with adenocarcinomas.

Direct evidence of DIC requires demonstration of intravascular fibrin deposition. The laboratory diagnosis of DIC depends on indirect evidence of coagulation activity. **The most common laboratory abnormalities in this disorder are decreased platelet count; elevated INR and aPTT; elevated D-dimer (a breakdown product of fibrin); and decreased fibrinogen concentration** (170,171).

The primary treatment of DIC is aimed at controlling the underlying cause. **Typical treatment would include empiric antibiotic therapy when sepsis is suspected, treatment of other conditions adversely affecting coagulation, and replacement with appropriate clotting factors** in patients with active bleeding. **Some of the controversial options,** such as anticoagulation, factor replacement, *epsilon aminocaproic acid* with *heparin,* and antiplatelet drugs, might also be considered (170).

Adverse Effects of Blood Transfusions

Some adverse effects of transfusions include bacterial contamination, transfusion-related lung injury (TRALI), transmission of infectious diseases, and transfusion reactions. Bacterial contamination, most commonly from platelets, is the leading cause of death from blood transfusion and often presents with a fever within 6 hours of the transfusion. TRALI is noncardiogenic pulmonary edema from an immune response of the recipient to leukocyte antibodies in the transfused blood. Hypoxia, fever, and dyspnea typically appear a few hours after transfusion. No specific therapy is available and treatment is limited to stopping the transfusion and supportive measures (163).

Blood products have become much safer with the development of better screening techniques. Transmission of infectious diseases, including hepatitis and human immunodeficiency virus, is rare but still occurs. **While not zero, the risk of tranfusion-transmitted viral infections, Hepatitis B and C and human immunodeficiency virus (HIV), is very low. Currently, bacterial contamination and sepsis are the most common infectious complications of blood transfusions** (172). **Cytomegalovirus can still be a problem,** although seroconverters are typically asymptomatic. The use of pooled products, such as platelets and plasma, increases the risks because multiple donors are required. **Autologous blood donation may be considered for elective surgery in certain patients.**

Thromboembolism

Detection of Deep Venous Thrombosis

Clinical signs and symptoms of venous thromboembolism (VTE) are notoriously unreliable, and detection of thromboembolic disease once it occurs is a challenging problem in acute care medicine. Deep venous thrombosis (DVT) of the lower extremity classically presents as a swollen, painful leg, but this may be completely absent in some patients. Lower-extremity venous clot is now **typically screened with compression ultrasonography of the femoral, popliteal, and calf vein trifurcation.** This method is greater than 90% sensitive for proximal thrombosis, but much less sensitive for calf thrombosis. Clinicians should perform serial testing with this method or use **contrast venography (gold standard test)** if clinical suspicion remains high (173).

Detection of Pulmonary Embolus

Pulmonary embolism (PE) can be a life-threatening emergency. Autopsy studies suggest that pulmonary embolism may account for as many as 5% of unexpected deaths in hospitalized patients (174). Presenting symptoms and signs of pulmonary embolism can include pleuritic chest pain, shortness of breath, cough with or without hemoptysis, and, in the case of a very large embolus, acute clinical decompensation or syncope, and hypotension. Patients are often tachycardic and hypoxic, the ECG may show evidence of right heart strain, and the chest radiograph may show an infarct with effusion. Unfortunately, these same symptoms and signs may be present in other conditions, such as pneumonia and myocardial ischemia. Conversely, a pulmonary embolism can occur with only a few, or even none of these clinical features. **Because of this variable presentation, clinicians must be vigilant, particularly in their relatively immobile postoperative patients** (175).

Once they suspect it, most clinicians attempt to confirm pulmonary embolism with radiographic testing. **The reference standard for diagnosis of pulmonary embolism remains direct angiography, although this test is rarely performed today. The two most commonly performed tests for pulmonary embolism are the ventilation-perfusion (VQ) scan of the lung and the CT angiogram of the chest.** These tests are most valuable when combined with pretest suspicion. Unfortunately, in the case of VQ scanning, a large study in hospitalized patients as compared to conventional pulmonary angiogram showed that **VQ test results were often not conclusive.** An entirely negative test was helpful in excluding a pulmonary embolus (risk of pulmonary embolism <1%), and a classic positive test obviated further testing, but, unfortunately, the test results were more typically intermediate or low probability. Combining results of the ventilation–perfusion scan with pretest clinical probability did improve its accuracy if clinical suspicion correlated with the scan results (176). **One advantage of VQ scanning is the absence of the contrast nephropathy risk associated with CT angiography; VQ scanning is often preferred in patients with marginal renal function.**

CT angiography performed with multi-detector CT scanners and delayed venography of the thighs has been shown to be both sensitive and specific for VTE detection in recent trials. If the patient's renal function can tolerate angiography dye, this test has largely supplanted VQ scanning at many centers. The predictive value of this test (like the VQ scan) does decrease if the test result conflicts with pretest suspicion (177).

In the outpatient or emergency room setting, assays for increased blood levels of D-dimer (one of the byproducts of the coagulation cascade) **are sensitive tests for VTE,** and can be used to screen for DVT or PE. **Unfortunately, this test is relatively nonspecific in the hospitalized, postoperative, and cancer patients** who often have many other reasons for elevated d-dimer levels (178).

Treatment

Once documented, DVT or PE requires immediate treatment to decrease the risk of complications (pulmonary embolism or recurrent embolism). Patients who do not have an overriding contraindication to anticoagulation should be treated immediately with *heparin* **even before the diagnosis is confirmed.** Traditionally this has been treated with intravenous *unfractionated heparin* in a large initial bolus, followed by a continuous *heparin* infusion adjusted to achieve an aPTT approximately two to three times that of the control value. **More recently, several trials have shown that treatment with** *low-molecular-weight heparin* **is equal to, if not better than, treatment with standard** *unfractionated heparin* **for pulmonary embolism** (179). Postsurgical and intensive care unit patients, however, are more often treated with unfractionated heparin infusions that are more easily reversed because of shorter drug half-lives.

Thrombolytic therapy can be considered in cases of acute pulmonary embolism with hypotension. Many postoperative patients, however, are at high risk for bleeding from lytic therapy, and this treatment should be carefully considered.

If patients with pulmonary embolism have active bleeding, or a high risk of bleeding and cannot be anticoagulated, a filter can be inserted into the inferior vena cava (IVC) to prevent recurrent pulmonary emboli. A percutaneously placed filter into the IVC can also be used for those patients who develop recurrent pulmonary emboli despite adequate anticoagulation (179). Temporary IVC filters have been developed that can be removed several months after placement, and their role in the treatment of pulmonary embolism is likely to increase (180).

Once a patient with pulmonary embolism is stabilized, treatment with intravenous *heparin* is often transitioned to **oral vitamin K antagonists (such as** *Coumadin***)** for continued outpatient treatment. The *Coumadin* oral dosage is titrated to an INR of 2.0 to 3.0. **Alternatively** a patient may go home on subcutaneous injections **of low molecular weight** *heparin* **or** *fondaparinux.*

The optimal duration of anticoagulation for deep venous thrombosis and/or pulmonary embolism remains controversial, but in general, these **medications are continued for at least 3 to 6 months.** Recent studies have suggested the risk of recurrent thrombosis can persist indefinitely, particularly in patients with underlying malignancy (181). For select patients, clinicians now consider lengthy or even lifelong treatment with anticoagulation.

Infection

In general, infections in patients with gynecologic malignancies should be managed as in all hospitalized patients—that is, with antibiotics chosen initially on the basis of possible infecting organisms and changed if necessary when the results of culture and sensitivity testing are known (182). Clinicians should be particularly alert to possible central venous catheter infections because many oncologic patients require these devices for treatment. **Central venous catheter infection rates range up to 5%** depending on the type of catheter inserted (183,184).

Fever in the Neutropenic Patient

Febrile neutropenia is one of the most serious adverse events related to antineoplastic chemotherapy and causes significant morbidity and mortality. When the absolute granulocyte count falls below 1,000/mm³, the incidence of infection rises and infected patients frequently decompensate rapidly. Many clinicians use prophylactic antibiotics in an attempt to decrease the frequency and mortality of this condition. While the most recent guidelines advise against the use of prophylactic antibiotics (185), several more recent studies have provided evidence for the benefit of prophylactic *levofloxacin* (186,187). In patients with solid tumors receiving moderately myelosuppressive chemotherapy, prophylactic *levaquin* has been shown to reduce the incidence of febrile neutropenia and all-cause mortality in the first cycle of treatment (188). Controversy about issues such as cost, toxicity, and antibiotic resistance remain.

Patients with established neutropenia who become febrile can decompensate rapidly and should be treated immediately with empiric broad-spectrum intravenous antibiotics, regardless of whether focal signs of infection or a positive culture result is present. Frequently encountered pathogens in the neutropenic patient include *Staphylococcus aureus* and gram-negative enteric organisms such as *Escherichia coli, Klebsiella,* and *Pseudomonas.*

There are many combinations of empiric antibiotics that achieve the goal of covering likely pathogens in the febrile neutropenic patient (185,189,190). **For hospitalized, low-risk patients who have fever and neutropenia during cancer chemotherapy, empiric therapy with oral *ciprofloxacin* and *amoxicillin-clavulanate* appears to be safe and effective** (189). This approach is as effective as intravenous therapy and may therefore be the preferred approach (190). If intravenous antibiotics are considered necessary, a broad-spectrum semi-synthetic *penicillin,* sometimes combined with an aminoglycoside and *vancomycin,* may be used. **If febrile neutropenia persists despite several days of broad-spectrum antibiotics, guidelines suggest the empiric addition of antifungal agents** (185). Meticulous daily follow-up and adjustment of antibiotic coverage is critical and likely more important than the precise initial combination chosen.

Use of growth factor rescue for febrile neutropenia has been studied, and the use of *granulocyte colony-stimulating factor (G-CSF)* can shorten the duration of neutropenia. G-CSF is sometimes prescribed prophylactically during courses of chemotherapy, although this usage remains controversial in many treatment regimens (191,192).

Fungemia

Fungemia is a life-threatening postoperative complication of surgery and severe medical illness. **Typical patients at risk include those receiving multiple antibiotics and hyperalimentation.** Central venous access lines and Foley catheters can provide entry sites for fungal organisms. Additional important risk factors are cancer, chemotherapy, corticosteroids, and hyperglycemia (193,194). **The clinical presentation of disseminated disease is identical to that of gram-negative sepsis.** These patients may have signs of local fungal disease, such as oral thrush. The principal organisms found are *Candida* species. There are now several antifungal agents available to treat invasive disease (195). Patients with localized fungal infections should be aggressively treated with topical agents.

References

1. **Goldman L, Caldera DL, Nussbaum SR, Southwick FS, Krogstad D, Murray B, et al.** Multifactorial index of cardiac risk in noncardiac surgical procedures. *N Engl J Med* 1977;297:845–850.
2. **Detsky AS, Abrams HB, McLaughlin JR, Drucker DJ, Sasson Z, Johnston N, et al.** Predicting cardiac complications in patients undergoing non-cardiac surgery. *J Gen Intern Med* 1986;1:211–219.
3. **Hollenberg M, Mangano DT, Browner WS, London MJ, Tubau JF, Tateo IM.** Predictors of postoperative myocardial ischemia in patients undergoing noncardiac surgery: the Study of Perioperative Ischemia Research Group. *JAMA* 1992;268:205–209.
4. **Mangano DT, Browner WS, Hollenberg M, London MJ, Tubau JF, Tateo IM.** Association of perioperative myocardial ischemia

with cardiac morbidity and mortality in men undergoing noncardiac surgery: the Study of Perioperative Ischemia Research Group. *N Engl J Med* 1990;323:1781–1788.

5. **Lee TH, Marcantonio ER, Mangione CM, Thomas EJ, Polanczyk CA, Cook EF, et al.** Derivation and prospective validation of a simple index for prediction of cardiac risk of major noncardiac surgery. *Circulation* 1999;100:1043–1049.

6. **Fleisher LA, Beckman JA, Brown KA, Calkins H, Chaikof E, Fleischmann KE, et al.** ACC/AHA 2007 guidelines on perioperative cardiovascular evaluation and care for noncardiac surgery: a report of the American College of Cardiology/American Heart Association Task Force on Practice Guidelines (Writing Committee to Revise the 2002 Guidelines on Perioperative Cardiovascular Evaluation for Noncardiac Surgery). *Circulation* 2007;116: e418–e499.

7. **Mangano DT, Goldman L.** Preoperative assessment of patients with known or suspected coronary disease. *N Engl J Med* 1995;333:1750–1756.

8. **Romero L, de Virgilio C.** Preoperative cardiac risk assessment. *Arch Surg* 2001;136:1370–1376.

9. **American College of Physicians.** Guidelines for assessing and managing the perioperative risk from coronary artery disease associated with major noncardiac surgery. *Ann Intern Med* 1997;127: 309–312.

10. **Palda VA, Detsky AS.** Perioperative assessment and management of risk from coronary artery disease. *Ann Intern Med* 1997;127: 313–328.

11. **Kertai MD, Boersma E, Bax JJ, Heijenbrok-Kal MH, Hunink MG, L'talien GJ, et al.** A meta-analysis comparing the prognostic accuracy of six diagnostic tests for predicting perioperative cardiac risk in patients undergoing major vascular surgery. *Heart* 2003;89: 1327–1334.

12. **Steen PA, Tinker JH, Tarhan S.** Myocardial infarction after anesthesia and surgery. *JAMA* 1978;239:2566–2570.

13. **Mahar LJ, Steen PA, Tinker JH, Vleitstra RE, Smith HC, Pluth JR.** Preoperative myocardial infarction in patients with coronary artery disease with and without aorta-coronary bypass grafts. *J Thorac Cardiovasc Surg* 1978;76:533–537.

14. **McCollum CH, Garcia-Rinald R, Graham JM, DeBakay ME.** Myocardial revascularization prior to subsequent major surgery in patients with coronary artery disease. *Surgery* 1977;81:302–304.

15. **McFalls EO, Ward HB, Moritz TE, Goldman S, Krupski WC, Littooy F, et al.** Coronary-artery revascularization before elective major vascular surgery. *N Engl J Med* 2004;351:2795–2804.

16. **Mangano DT, Browner WS, Hollenberg M, London MJ, Tubau JF, Tateo IM.** Association of perioperative myocardial ischemia with cardiac morbidity and mortality in men undergoing noncardiac surgery. The Study of Perioperative Ischemia Research Group. *N Engl J Med* 1990;323:1781–1788.

17. **Mangano DT, Browner WS, Hooenberg M, Li J, Tateo IM.** Long-term cardiac prognosis following noncardiac surgery. The Study of Perioperative Ischemia Research Group. *JAMA* 1992;268:233–239.

18. **Devereaux PJ, Goldman L, Yusuf S, Gilbert K, Leslie K, Guyatt GH.** Surveillance and prevention of major perioperative ischemic cardiac events in patients undergoing noncardiac surgery: a review. *CMAJ* 2005;173:779–788.

19. **Charlson ME, MacKenzie CR, Ales K, Gold JP, Fairclough G Jr, Shires GT.** Surveillance for postoperative myocardial infarction after noncardiac operations. *Surg Gynecol Obstet* 1988;167:407–414.

20. **Lee TH, Thomas EJ, Ludwig LE, Sacks DB, Johnson PA, Donaldson MC, et al.** Troponin T as a marker for myocardial ischemia in patients undergoing major noncardiac surgery. *Am J Cardiol* 1996;77:1031–1036.

21. **Lopez-Jimenez F, Goldman L, Sacks DB, Thomas EJ, Johnson PA, Cook EF, Lee TH.** Prognostic value of cardiac troponin T after noncardiac surgery: 6 month follow-up data. *J Am Coll Cardiol* 1997;29: 1241–1245.

22. **Psaty BM, Koepsell TD, Wagner EH, LoGerfo JP, Inui TS.** The relative risk of incident coronary artery disease associated with recently stopping the use of beta-blockers. *JAMA* 1990;263: 1653–1657.

23. **Shammash JB, Trost JC, Gold JM, Berlin JA, Golden MA, Kimmel SE.** Perioperative beta-blocker withdrawal and mortality in vascular surgery patients. *Am Heart J* 2001;141:148–153.

24. **Mangano DT, Layug EL, Wallace A, Tateo I.** Effect of atenolol on mortality and cardiovascular morbidity after non-cardiac surgery. *N Engl J Med* 1996;335:1713–1720.

25. **Poldermans D, Boersma E, Bax JJ, Thompson IR, van de Ven LL, Blakensteijn JD, et al.** The effect of bisoprolol on perioperative mortality and myocardial infarction in high-risk patients undergoing vascular surgery: Dutch Echocardiographic Cardiac Risk Evaluation Applying Stress Echocardiograph Study Group. *N Engl J Med* 1999;341:1789–1794.

26. **POISE Study Group.** Effect of extended-release metoprolol succinate in patients undergoing non-cardiac surgery (POISE trial): a randomized controlled trial. *Lancet* 2008;371:1839–1847.

27. **Auerbach AD, Goldman L.** β-blockers and reduction of cardiac events in noncardiac surgery, scientific review. *JAMA* 2002;287: 1435–1444.

28. **Halm EA, Browner WS, Tubau JF, Tateo IM, Mangano DT.** Echocardiography for assessing cardiac risk in patients having noncardiac surgery. Study of Perioperative Ischemia Research Group (published correction appears in *Ann Intern Med* 1997;126:494). *Ann Int Med* 1996;125:433–441.

29. **Sandham JD, Hull RD, Brant RF, Know L, Pineo GF, Doig CJ, et al.** A randomized, controlled trial of the use of pulmonary-artery catheter in high-risk surgical patients. *N Engl J Med* 2003;348:5–14.

30. **O'Kelly B, Browner WS, Massie B, Tubau J, Ngo L, Mangano DT.** Ventricular arrhythmias in patients undergoing noncardiac surgery. The Study of Preoperative Ischemia Research Group. *JAMA* 1992;268:217–221.

31. **Mahla E, Rotman B, Rehak P, Fruhwald S, Pürstner P, Metzler H.** Perioperative ventricular dysrhythmias in patients with structural heart disease undergoing noncardiac surgery. *Anesth Analg* 1998;86:16–21.

32. **Pastore JO, Yurchak PM, Janis KM, Murphy JD, Zir LM.** The risk of advanced heart block in surgical patients with right bundle branch block and left axis deviation. *Circulation* 1978;57:677–680.

33. **American Society of Anesthesiologists Task Force on Perioperative Management of Patients with Cardiac Rhythm Management Devices.** Practice advisory for the perioperative management of patients with cardiac rhythm management devices: pacemakers and implantable cardioverter-defibrillators. *Anesthesiology* 2005; 103:186–198.

34. **Wilson W, Taubert KA, Gewitz M, Lockhart PB, Baddour LM, Levison M, et al.** Prevention of infective endocarditis: guidelines from the American Heart Association: a guideline from the American Heart Association Rheumatic Fever, Endocarditis, and Kawasaki Disease Committee, Council on Cardiovascular Disease in the Young, and the Council on Clinical Cardiology, Council on Cardiovascular Surgery and Anesthesia, and the Quality of Care and Outcomes Research Interdisciplinary Working Group. *Circulation* 2007;116:1736–1754.

35. **Bedford RF, Feinstein B.** Hospital admission blood pressure: a predictor for hypertension following endotracheal intubation. *Anesth Analg* 1980;59:367–370.

36. **Ashton CM, Petersen NJ, Wray NP, Kiefe CI, Dunn JK, Wu L, Thomas M.** The incidence of perioperative myocardial infarction in men undergoing noncardiac surgery. *Ann Intern Med* 1993;118: 504–510.

37. **Charlson ME, MacKenzie CR, Gold JP, Ales KL, Topkins M, Shires GT.** Preoperative characteristics predicting intraoperative hypotension and hypertension among hypertensives and diabetics undergoing noncardiac surgery. *Ann Surg* 1990;212:66–81.

38. **Brabant SM, Bertrand M, Eyraud D, Darmon PL, Coriat P.** The hemodynamic effects of anesthetic induction in vascular surgery patients chronically treated with angiotensin II receptor antagonists. *Anesth Analg* 1999;89:1388–1392.

39. **Colson P, Saussine M, Seguin JR, Cuchet D, Chaptal PA, Roquifeuil B.** Hemodynamic effects of anesthesia in patients chronically treated with angiotensin-converting enzyme inhibitors. *Anesth Analg* 1992;74:805–808.

40. **Weksler N, Klein M, Szendro G, Rozentsveig V, Schily M, Brill S, et al.** The dilemma of immediate preoperative hypertension: to treat and operate, or to postpone surgery? *J Clin Anesth* 2003;15:179–183.

41. **Comfere T, Sprung J, Kumar MM, Draper M, Wilson DP, Williams BA, et al.** Angiotensin system inhibitors in a general surgical population. *Anesth Analg* 2005;100:636–644.

42. Bertrand M, Godet G, Meersschaert K, Brun L, Salcedo E, Coriat P. Should the angiotensin II antagonists be discontinued before surgery? *Anesth Analg* 2001;92:26–30.

43. Vitez TS, Soper LE, Wong KC, Soper P. Chronic hypokalemia and intraoperative dysrhythmias. *Anesthesiology* 1986;63:130–133.

44. Fleischmann KE, Goldman L, Young B. Association between cardiac and noncardiac complications in patients undergoing noncardiac surgery: outcomes and effects o length of stay. *Am J Med* 2003; 115:515–520.

45. Lawrence VA, Hilsenbeck SG, Mulrow CD. Incidence and hospital stay for cardiac and pulmonary complications after abdominal surgery. *J Gen Intern Med* 1995;10:671–678.

46. Smetana GW, Lawrence VA, Cornell JE, for the American College of Physicians. Preoperative pulmonary risk stratification for noncardiothoracic surgery: systemic review for the American College of Physicians. *Ann Intern Med* 2006;144:581–595.

47. Berg H, Roed J, Viby-Morgenson J, Mortensen CR, Engbaek J, Skovgaard LT, Krintel JJ. Residual neuromuscular block is a risk factor for postoperative pulmonary complications: a prospective, randomized, and blinded study of postoperative pulmonary complications after atracurium, vecuronium and pancuronium. *Acta Anaesthesiol Scand* 1997;41:1095–1103.

48. Rodgers A, Walker N, Schug S. Reduction of postoperative mortality and morbidity with epidural or spinal anaesthesia: results from overview of randomized trials. *BMJ* 2000;321:1493.

49. Abraham NS, Young J, Solomon M. Meta-analysis of short-term outcomes after laporoscopic resection for colorectal cancer. *Br J Surg* 2004;91:1111–1124.

50. Qassem T. Risk assessment for and strategies to reduce perioperative pulmonary complications. *Ann Intern Med* 2006;145: 553.

51. American College of Physicians. Preoperative pulmonary function testing. *Ann Intern Med* 1990;112:793–794.

52. Wong DH, Weber EC, Schell MJ. Factors associated with postoperative pulmonary complications in patients with severe chronic obstructive disease. *Anesth Analg* 1995;80:276–284.

53. Warner DO, Warner MA, Barnes RD. Perioperative respiratory complications in patients with asthma. *Anesthesiology* 1996;85: 460–467.

54. Gross JB, Bachenberg KL, Nanumof JL. Practice guidelines for the perioperative management of patients with obstructive sleep apnea: a report of the American Society of Anesthesiologists Task force on Perioperative Management of Patients with Obstructive Sleep Apnea. *Anesthesiology* 2006;104:1081–1093.

55. Ramakrishna G, Sprung J, Ravi BS. Impact of pulmonary hypertension on the outcomes of noncardiac surgery: predictors of perioperative morbidity and mortality. *J Am Coll Cardiol* 2005;45: 1691–1699.

56. Muller AM, Villebro N, Pederson, T. Effect of preoperative smoking intervention o postoperative complications: a randomized clinical trial. *Lancet* 2002;359:114–117.

57. Kabalin CS, Yarnold PR, Grammar LC. Low complication rate of corticosteroid-treated asthmatic undergoing surgical procedures. *Arch Intern Med* 1995;155:1379–1384.

58. Leisching T, Kwok H, Hill N. Acute applications of noninvasive positive pressure ventilation. *Chest* 2003;124:699–713.

59. Thomas JA, McIntosh JM. Are incentive spirometry, intermittent positive pressure breathing, and deep breathing exercises effective in the prevention of post-operative pulmonary complications after upper abdominal surgery? A systematic overview and meta-analysis. *Phys Ther* 1994;74:3–10.

60. Nelson R, Tse B, Edwards S. Systematic review of prophylactic nasogastric decompression after abdominal operations. *Br J Surg* 2005;92:673–680.

61. Marhoffer W, Stein M, Maeser E, Federlin K. Impairment of polymorphonuclear leukocyte function and metabolic control of diabetes. *Diabetes Care* 1992;15:256–260.

62. Alexiewicz JM, Kumar D, Smogorzewski M, Klin M, Massry SG. Polymorphonuclear leukocytes in non-insulin-dependent diabetes mellitus: abnormalities in metabolism and function. *Ann Intern Med* 1995;123:919–924.

63. Rassias AJ, Marrin CA, Arruda J, Whalen PK, Beach M, Yeager MP. Insulin infusion improves neutrophil function in diabetic cardiac surgery patients. *Anesth Analg* 1999,88:1011–1016.

64. Pozzilli P, Leslie R. Infections and diabetes: mechanism and prospects for prevention. *Diabet Med* 1994;11:935–941.

65. Loots M, Lamme E, Mekkes J, Bos JD, Middlekoop E. Cultured fibroblasts from chronic diabetic wounds on the lower extremity (non-insulin-dependent diabetes mellitus) show disturbed proliferation. *Arch Dermatol Res* 1999;291:93–99.

66. Turina M, Fry DE, Polk HC. Acute hyperglycemia and the innate immune system: clinical, cellular, and molecular aspects. *Crit Care Med* 2005;33:1624–1633.

67. Clement S, Braithwaite SS, Magee MF, Ahmann A, Smith EP, Schaefer RG, Hirsch IB, for the American Diabetes Association Diabetes in Hospitals Writing Committee. Management of diabetes and hyperglycemia in hospitals. *Diabetes Care* 2004;27: 553–591.

68. Bolk J, van der Ploeg T, Cornel JH, Arnold AE, Sepers J, Umans VA. Impaired glucose metabolism predicts mortality after a myocardial infarction. *Int J Cardiol* 2001;79:207–214.

69. William LS, Rotich J, Qi R, Fineberg N, Espay A, Bruno A, et al. Effects of admission hyperglycemia on mortality and costs in acute ischemic stroke. *Neurology* 2002;59:67–71.

70. Pomposelli JJ, Baxter JK 3rd, Babineau TJ, Pomfret AE, Driscoll DF, Forse RA, Bistrian BR. Early postoperative glucose control predicts nosocomial infection rate in diabetic patients. *JPEN J Parenter Enteral Nutr* 1998;22:77–81.

71. Umpierrez GE, Isaacs SD, Barzargan N, You X, Thaler LM, Kitabchi AE. Hyperglycemia: an independent marker of in-hospital mortality in patients with undiagnosed diabetes. *J Clin Endocrinol Metab* 2002;87:978–982.

72. Suleiman M, Hammerman H, Boulos M, Kapeliovich MR, Suleiman A, Agmon Y, et al. Fasting glucose is an important independent risk factor for 30-day mortality in patient with acute myocardial infarction: a prospective study. *Circulation* 2005;111:754–760.

73. Krinsley JS. Association between hyperglycemia and increased hospital mortality in a hertogeneous population of critically ill patients. *Mayo Clin Proc* 2003;78:1471–1478.

74. Finney SJ, Zekveld C, Elia A, Evans TW. Glucose control and mortality in critically ill patients. *JAMA* 2003;290:2041–2047.

75. Vilar-Compte Diana, Alvarez de Iturbe I, Martín-Onraet A, Pérez-Amador M, Sánchez-Hernández C, Volkow P. Hyperglycemia as a risk factor for surgical site infections in patients undergoing mastectomy. *Am J Infect Control* 2008;36:192–198.

76. Furnary A, Zerr K, Grunkemeier G, Starr A. Continuous intravenous insulin infusion reduces the incidence of deep sternal wound infection in diabetic patients after cardiac surgical procedures. *Ann Thorac Surg* 1999;67:352–362.

77. van den Berghe G, Wouters P, Weekers F, Verwaest C, Bruyninckx F, Schetz M, et al. Intensive insulin therapy in critically ill patients. *N Engl J Med* 2001;345:1359–1367.

78. van den Berghe G, Wiler A, Hermans G, Meersseman W, Wouters PJ, Milants I, et al. Intensive insulin therapy in the medical ICU. *N Engl J Med* 2006;354:449–461.

79. Kirnsley JS. Effect of intensive glucose management protocol on the mortality of critically ill adult patients. *Mayo Clin Proc* 2004;79:992–1000.

80. Lazar HL, Chipkin SR, Fitzgerald CA, Bao Y, Cabral H, Apstein CS. Tight glycemic control in diabetic coronary artery bypass graft patients improves perioperative outcomes and decreases recurrent ischemic events. *Circulation* 2004;109:1497–1502.

81. Umpierrez GE, Smiley D, Zisman A, Prieto LM, Palacio A, Ceron M, et al. Randomized study of basal-bolus insulin therapy in the in-patient management of patients with type 2 diabetes (RABBIT 2 trial). *Diabetes Care* 2007;30:2181–2186.

82. Inzucchi S. Management of hyperglycemia in the hospital setting. *N Engl J Med* 2006;355:1903–1911.

83. Queale WS, Seidler AJ, Brancati FL. Glycemic control and sliding scale insulin use in medical in-patients with diabetes mellitus. *Arch Intern Med* 1997;157:545–552.

84. Baldwin D, Villanueuva G, McNutt R, Bhatnagar S. Eliminating inpatient sliding-scale insulin: a reeducation project with medical house staff. *Diabetes Care* 2005;28:1008–1011.

85. Golightly LK, Jones MA, Hamamura DH, Stolpman NM, McDermott MT. Management of diabetes mellitus in hospitalized patients: efficiency and effectiveness of sliding-scale insulin therapy. *Pharmacotherapy* 2006;26:1421–1432.

86. **Nygren J, Thorell A, Soop M, Efendic S, Brismar K, Karpe F, et al.** Perioperative insulin and glucose infusion maintains normal insulin sensitivity after surgery. *Am J Physiol Endocrinol Metab* 1998;275:E140–E148.

87. **Drucker DJ, Burrow GN.** Cardiovascular surgery in the hypothyroid patient. *Arch Intern Med* 1985;145:1585–1587.

88. **Ladenson PW, Levin AA, Ridgway ED, Daniels GH.** Complications of surgery in hypothyroid patients. *Am J Med* 1984; 77:261–266.

89. **Weinberg AD, Brennan MD, Gorman CA, Maish HM, O'Fallon WM.** Outcome of anesthesia and surgery in hypothyroid patients. *Arch Intern Med* 1983;143:893–897.

90. **Schiff RL, Welsh GA.** Perioperative evaluation and management of the patient with endocrine dysfunction. *Med Clin N Am* 2003;87: 175–192.

91. **Stathatos, N, Wartofsky L.** Perioperative management of patients with hypothyroidism. *Endocrinol Metab Clin N Am* 2003;32: 503–518.

92. **Lennquist S, Jörtsö E, Anderberg B, Smeds S.** Beta-blockers compared with antithyroidal drugs as preoperative treatment in hyperthyroidism: drug tolerance, complications, and postoperative thyroid function. *Surgery* 1985;98:1141–1147.

93. **Langley RW, Burch HB.** Perioperative management of the thyrotoxic patient. *Endocrinol Metab Clin N Am* 2003;32:519–534.

94. **Bromberg JS, Alfrey EJ, Barker CF, Chavin KD, Dafoe DC, Holland T, et al.** Adrenal suppression and steroid supplementation in renal transplant recipients. *Transplantation* 1991;51:385–390.

95. **LaRochelle GE, LaRochelle AG, Ratner RE, Borenstein DG.** Recovery of the hypothalamic-pituitaryadrenal (HPA) axis in patients with rheumatic diseases receiving low-dose prednisone. *Am J Med* 1993;95:258–264.

96. **Glowniak JV, Loriaux DL.** A double-blind study of perioperative steroid requirements in secondary adrenal insufficiency. *Surgery* 1997;121:123–129.

97. **Henzen C, Suter A, Lerch E, Urbinelli R, Schorno X, Briner V.** Suppression and recovery of adrenal response after short-term, high-dose glucocorticoid treatment. *Lancet* 2000;355:542–545.

98. **Schlaghecke R, Kornelly E, Santen R, Ridderskamp P.** The effect of long-term glucocorticoid therapy on pituitary-adrenal responses to exogenous corticotropin-releasing hormone. *N Engl J Med* 1992; 326:226–230.

99. **Cooper M, Stewart P.** Corticosteroid insufficiency in acutely ill patients. *N Engl J Med* 2003;348:727–734.

100. **Dickstein G, Shechner C, Nicholson WE, Rosner I, Shen-Orr Z, Adawi F, Lahav M.** Adrenocorticotropin stimulation test: effects of basal cortisol level, time of day, and suggested new sensitive low dose test. *J Clin Endocrinol Metab* 1991;72:77–78.

101. **Oelkers W.** Adrenal insufficiency. *N Engl J Med* 1996;335: 1206–1212.

102. **Dorin RI, Qualls CR, Crapo LM.** Diagnosis of adrenal insufficiency. *Ann Intern Med* 2003;139:194–204.

103. **Salem M, Tainsh RE, Bromberg J, Loriaux DL, Chernow B.** Perioperative glucocorticoid coverage: a reassessment 42 years after emergence of a problem. *Ann Surg* 1994;219:416–425.

104. **Coursin D, Wood K.** Corticosteroid supplementation for adrenal insufficiency. *JAMA* 2002;287:236–340.

105. **Clagett GP, Reisch JS.** Prevention of venous thromboembolism in general surgical patients: results of meta-analysis. *Ann Surg* 1988;208:227–240.

106. **Maxwell GL, Synan I, Dodge R, Carroll B, Clarke-Pearson DL.** Pneumatic compression versus low molecular weight heparin in gynecologic oncology surgery: a randomized trial. *Obstet Gynecol* 2001;98,989–995.

107. **Heilmann L, von Tempelhoff GF, Schneider D.** Prevention of thrombosis in gynecologic malignancy. *Clin Appl Thromb/Hemost* 1998;4,153–159.

108. **Smetana GW, Macpherson DS.** The case against routine preoperative laboratory testing. *Med Clin North Am* 2003;89:7–40.

109. **Pasternack LR.** Preoperative screening for ambulatory patients. *Anesthesiol Clin North Am* 2003;21:229–242.

110. **Munro J, Booth A, Nicholl J.** Routine preoperative testing: a systematic review of the evidence. *Health Technol Assess* 1997;1:i–iv;1–62.

111. **Ajimura FY, Maia AS, Hachiya A, Watanabe AS, Nunes Mdo P, Martins Mde A, Machado FS.** Preoperative laboratory evaluation of patients aged over 40 years undergoing elective non-cardiac surgery. *Sao Paulo Med J* 2005;123:50–53.

112. **Joo HS, Wong J, Naik VN, Svoldelli GL.** The value of screening preoperative chest x-rays: a systematic review. *Can J Anesth* 2005; 52:568–574.

113. **Reynolds TM.** National Institute for Health and Clinical Excellence guidelines on preoperative tests: the use of routine preoperative tests for elective surgery. *Ann Clin Biochem* 2006;43:13–16.

114. **Schein O, Katz J, Bass E.** The value of routine preoperative testing before cataract surgery. *N Engl J Med* 2000;342:168–175.

115. **Narr BJ, Warner ME, Schroeder DR, Warner MA.** Outcomes of patients with no laboratory assessment before anesthesia and a surgical procedure. *Mayo Clin Proc* 1997;72:505–509.

116. **CG3 Preoperative Tests.** Available at: http://www.nice.org.uk/ Guidance/CG3/Guidance/pdf/English. Accessed September 19, 2008.

117. **Suchman A, Mushin A.** How well does the activated partial thromboplastin time predict post operative hemorrhage? *JAMA* 1986;256: 750–753.

118. **Classen DC, Evans RS, Pestotnik RL, Burke JP.** The timing of prophylactic administration of antibiotics and the risk of surgical wound infection. *N Engl J Med* 1992;326:281–286.

119. **Lindenauer PK.** Perioperative beta-blocker therapy and mortality after major noncardiac surgery. *N Engl J Med* 2005;353:349–361.

120. **Chobanian AV.** The Seventh Report of the Joint National Committee on Prevention, Detection, Evaluation, and Treatment of High Blood Pressure: the JNC 7 report. *JAMA* 2003;289: 2560–2572.

121. **Adebola OA.** Management of perioperative myocardial infarction in noncardiac surgical patients. *Chest* 2006;130:584–596.

122. **Advanced life support: Part 4.** *Circulation* 2005;112 (22 suppl 22); III–25–III–54.

123. **Fuster V.** ACC/AHA/ESC guidelines for management of patients with atrial fibrillation: executive summary. *Circulation* 2001;104: 2118–2150.

124. **Shah MR, Hasselblad V, Stevenson LW, Binanay C, O'Connor CM, Sopko G, Califf RM.** Impact of the pulmonary artery catheter in critically ill patients: meta-analysis of randomized clinical trials. *JAMA* 2005;294:1664–1670.

125. **Finfer S, Bellomo R, Boyce N, French J, Myburgh J, Norton R.** A comparison of albumin and saline for fluid resuscitation in the intensive care unit. *N Engl J Med* 2004;350:2247–2256.

126. **Dellinger RP, Levy MM, Carlet JM, Bion J, Parker MM, Jaeschke R, et al.** Surviving Sepsis Campaign: international guidelines for management of severe sepsis and septic shock: 2008. *Crit Care Med* 2008;36:296–327.

127. **Calfee CS, Matthay MA.** Nonventilatory treatments for acute lung injury and ARDS. *Chest* 2007;131:913–920.

128. **Girard T, Bernard GR.** Mechanical ventilation in ARDS: A state of the art review. *Chest* 2007;131:921–929.

129. **Bersten AD, Edibam C, Hunt T, Moran J, for the Australian and New Zealand Intensive Care Society Clinical Trials Group.** Incidence and mortality of acute lung injury and the acute respiratory distress syndrome in three Australian States. *Am J Respir Crit Care Med* 2002;165:443–448.

130. **Slutsky AS.** Mechanical ventilation. American College of Chest Physicians' Consensus Conference. *Chest* 1993;104:1833–1859.

131. **Jenkinson SJ.** Oxygen toxicity. *New Horizons* 1993;1: 504–511.

132. **Tobin MJ, Jubran A.** Variable performance of weaning-predictor tests. Variable performance of weaning-predictor tests: role of Bayes' theorem and spectrum and test-referral bias. *Intensive Care Med* 2006;32:2002–2012.

133. **MacIntyre NR, Cook DL, Ely EW Jr, Epstein SK, Fink JB, Heffner JE, et al.** Evidence-based guidelines for weaning and discontinuing ventilatory support: a collective task force facilitated by the American College of Chest Physicians; the American Association for Respiratory Care; and the American College of Critical Care Medicine. *Chest* 1993;120:375s–395s.

134. **Carmichael P, Carmichael AR.** Acute renal failure in the surgical setting. *ANZ J Surg* 2003;73:144–153.

135. **Novis BK, Roizen MF, Aronson S, Thisted RA.** Association of preoperative risk factors with postoperative acute renal failure. *Anesth Analg* 1994;78:143–149.

136. **Thadhani R, Pascual M, Bonvnetre J.** Acute renal failure. *N Engl J Med* 1996;334:1448–1460.

137. **Hou SH, Bushinsky DA.** Hospital acquired renal insufficiency: a prospective study. *Am J Med* 1983;74:243–248.

138. **Darmon M, Ciroldi M, Thiery G, Schlemmer B, Azoulay E.** Clinical review: specific aspects of acute renal failure in cancer patients. *Crit Care* 2006;10:211–217.

139. **Millet PJ, Pelle-Francoz D.** Nondilated obstructive acute renal failure: diagnostic procedures and therapeutic management. *Radiology* 1986;160:659–662.

140. **Miller TR, Anderson RJ, Linas SL, Henrich WL, Berns AS, Gabow PA, Schrier RW.** Urinary diagnostic indices in acute renal failure: a prospective study. *Ann Intern Med* 1978;89:47–50.

141. **Barrett JB, Parfrey PS.** Preventing nephropathy induced by contrast medium. *N Engl J Med* 2006;354:379–386.

142. **Tepel M, van der Giet M, Schwarzfeld C.** Prevention of radiographic-contrast agent-induced reductions in renal function by acetylcysteine. *N Engl J Med* 2000;343:180–184.

143. **Tiu RV, Mountantonakis SE, Dunbar AJ, Schreiber MJ Jr.** Tumor lysis syndrome. *Semin Thromb Hemost* 2007;33:397–407.

144. **Klahir S, Miller S.** Acute oliguria. *N Engl J Med* 1998;338:671–675.

145. **Bagshaw SM, Delaney A, Haase M, Ghali WA, Belloma R.** Loop diuretics in the management of acute renal failure: a systematic review and meta-analysis. *Crit Care Resusc* 2007;9:60–68.

146. **Weisbord SD, Palevsky PM.** Acute renal failure in the intensive care unit. *Semin Respir Crit Care Med* 2006;27:262–273.

147. **Yagi N, Paginini E.** Acute dialysis and continuous renal replacement: the emergence of new technology involving the nephrologist in the intensive care setting. *Semin Nephrol* 1997;17:306–320.

148. **Adrogué HJ, Madias NE.** Management of life-threatening acid-base disorders. First of two parts. *N Engl J Med* 1998;338:26–34.

149. **Adrogué HJ, Madias NE.** Medical progress: management of life-threatening acid-base disorders. Second of two parts. *N Engl J Med* 1998;338:107–111.

150. **Ayers P, Warrington L.** Diagnosis and treatment of simple acid-base disorders. *Nutr Clin Pract* 2008;23:122–127.

151. **Narins RG, Emmett M.** Simple and mixed acid base disorders. *Medicine (Baltimore)* 1980;59:161–187.

152. **Cooper DJ, Walley KR, Wiggs BR, Russell JA.** Bicarbonate does not improve the hemodynamics in critically ill patients who have lactic acidosis. A prospective, controlled study. *Ann Intern Med* 1990;112:492–498.

153. **Stacpoole PW.** Lactic acidosis: the case against bicarbonate therapy. *Ann Intern Med* 1986;105:276–279.

154. **McLaughlin ML, Kassirer JP.** Rational treatment of acid-base disorders. *Drugs* 1990;39:841–855.

155. **Kumar S, Berl T.** Sodium. *Lancet* 1998;352:220–228.

156. **Adrogue HJ, Madias NE.** Hyponatremia. *N Engl J Med* 2000;342:1581–1589.

157. **Goh KP.** Management of hyponatremia. *Am Fam Physician* 2004;69:2387–2394.

158. **Adrogue HJ, Madias NE.** Hypernatremia. *N Engl J Med* 2000;342:1493–1499.

159. **Kapoor M, Chan GZ.** Fluid and electrolyte abnormalities. *Crit Care Clin* 2001;17:503–529.

160. **Souba WW.** Nutritional support. *N Engl J Med* 1997;336:41–48.

161. **Sanstrom R, Drott C, Hyltander A, Arfvidsson B, Scherstén T, Wickström I, Lundholm K.** The effect of postoperative intravenous feeding (TPN) on outcome following major surgery evaluated in a randomized study. *Ann Surg* 1993;217:185–195.

162. **Wu WC, Schifftner TL, Henderson WG, Eaton CB, Poses RM, Uttley G, et al.** Preoperative hematocrit levels and postoperative outcomes in older patients undergoing noncardiac surgery. *JAMA* 2007;297:2481–2488.

163. **Nuttall GA, Brost BC, Connis RT, Gessner JS, Harrison CR, Miller RD, et al. Practice guidelines for perioperative blood transfusion and adjuvant therapies:** An Updated Report by the American Society of Anesthesiologists Task Force on Perioperative Blood Transfusion and Adjuvant Therapies. *Anesthesiology* 2006;105:198–208.

164. **Hébert PC, Wells G, Blajchman MA, Marshall J, Martin C, Pagliarello G, et al.** A multicenter, randomized, controlled clinical trial of transfusion requirements in critical care. Transfusion Requirements in Critical Care Investigators, Canadian Critical Care Trials Group. *N Engl J Med* 1999;340:409–417.

165. **Murphy GJ, Barnaby CR, Rogers CA, Rizvi SI, Culliford L, Angelini GD.** Increased mortality, postoperative morbidity, and cost after red blood cell transfusion in patients having cardiac surgery. *Circulation* 2007;116:2544–2552.

166. **Carson JL, Hill S, Carless P, Hébert P, Henry D.** Transfusion triggers: a systematic review of the literature. *Transfus Med Rev* 2002;16:187–199.

167. **Wu WC, Rathores SS, Wang Y, Radford MJ, Krumholz HM.** Blood transfusion in elderly patients with acute myocardial infarction. *N Engl J Med* 2001;345:1230–1236.

168. **Hellstern P, Haubelt H.** Indications for plasma in massive transfusion. *Thromb Res* 2002;107:s19–s22.

169. **Stainsby, D, Maclennan S, Hamilton PJ.** Management of massive blood loss: a template guideline. *Br J Anaesth* 2000;85:487–491.

170. **Levi M.** Disseminated intravascular coagulation. *Crit Care Med* 2007;35:2191–2195.

171. **Levi M, ten Cate H, van der Poll, van Deventer SJ.** Pathogenesis of disseminated intravascular coagulation in sepsis. *JAMA* 1993;270:975–979.

172. **Sandler SG, Yu H, Rassai N.** Risks of blood transfusion and their prevention. *Clin Adv Hematol Oncol* 2003;1:307–313.

173. **Hirsch J.** How we diagnose and treat deep vein thrombosis. *Blood* 2002;99:3102–3110.

174. **Alikhan R.** Fatal pulmonary embolism in hospitalized patients; a necrosopy review. *J Clin Pathol* 2004;57:1254–1257.

175. **Tapson VF.** Acute pulmonary embolism. *N Engl J Med* 2008;358:1037–1052.

176. **The PIOPED Investigators.** Value of the ventilation/perfusion scan in acute pulmonary embolism. Results of the Prospective Investigation of Pulmonary Embolism Diagnosis (PIOPED). *JAMA* 1990;263:2753–2759.

177. **Stein PD, Fowler SE, Goodman LR, Gottschalk A, Hales CA, Hull RD, et al.** Multidetector computed tomography for acute pulmonary embolism. *N Engl J Med* 2006;354:2317–2327.

178. **Goodacre S, Sampson FC, Sutton AJ, Mason S, Morris F.** Variation in the diagnostic performance of D-Dimer for suspected deep vein thrombosis. *QJM* 2005;98:513–27.

179. **Kearon C, Kahn SR, Agnelli G, Goldhaber S, Raskob GE, Comerota AJ.** Antithrombotic therapy for venous thrombembolic disease. American College of Chest Physicians Evidence-Based practice guidelines (8th ed). *Chest* 2008;133:454S–545.

180. **Dentali F, Ageno W, Imberti D.** Retrievable vena caval filters: clinical experience. *Curr Opin Pulm Med* 2006;12:304–309.

181. **Baglin T, Luddington R, Brown K, Baglin C.** Incidence of recurrent venous thromboembolism in relation to clinical and thrombophilic risk factors: a prospective cohort study. *Lancet* 2003;362:523–526.

182. **O'Grady NP, Bade PS, Bartlett J, Bleck T, Garvey G, Jacobi J, et al. for the Task Force of the American College of Critical Care Medicine of the Society of Critical Care Medicine in collaboration with the Infectious Disease Society of America.** Practice parameters for evaluating new fever in critically ill adult patients. *Crit Care Med* 1998;26:392–408.

183. **McGee DC, Gould MD.** Preventing complications of central venous catheterization. *N Engl J Med* 2003;348:1123–1133.

184. **Raad I, Hanna H, Maki D.** Intravascular catheter-related infections: advances in diagnosis, prevention, and management. *Lancet Infect Dis* 2007;7:645–657.

185. **Hughes WT, Armstrong D, Bodry GP.** 2002 guidelines for the use of antimicrobial agents in neutropenic patients with cancer. *Clin Infect Dis* 2002;34:730–751.

186. **Bucaneve G, Micozzi A, Menichetti F, Martino P, Dionisi MS, Martinelli G, et al. for the Gruppo Italiano Malattie Ematologiche dell'Adulto (GIMEMA) Infection Program.** Levofloxacin to prevent bacterial infection in patients with cancer and neutropenia. *N Engl J Med* 2005;353:977–987.

187. **Cullen M, Steven N, Billingham L, Gaunt C, Hastings M, Simmonds P, et al. for the Simple Investigation in Neutropenic Individuals of the Frequency of Infection after Chemotherapy +/- Antibiotic in a Number of Tumours (SIGNIFICANT) Trial Group.** Antibiotic prophylaxis after chemotherapy for solid cell tumors and lymphomas. *N Eng J Med* 2005;353:988–998.

188. **Gafter-Gvili A, Fraser A, Paul M, Leibovici L.** Meta-analysis: antibiotic prophylaxis reduces mortality in neutropenic patients. *Ann Int Med* 2005;142:979–995.

189. **Freifeld A, Marchigiani D, Walsh T, Chanock S, Lewis L, Hiemenz J, et al.** A double-blind comparison of empirical oral and intravenous antibiotic therapy for low-risk febrile patients with neutropenia during cancer chemotherapy. *N Engl J Med* 1999;341:305–311.

190. **Kern WV, Cometta A, de Bock R, Langenaeken J, Paesmans M, Gaya H, for the International Antimicrobial Therapy Cooperative Group of the European Organization for the Research and Treatment of Cancer.** Oral versus intravenous empirical antimicrobial therapy for fever in patients with granulocytopenia who are receiving cancer chemotherapy. *N Engl J Med* 1999;341:312–318.

191. **Ozer H, Armitage JO, Bennett CL, Crawford J, Demetri GD, Pizzo PA, et al. for the American Society of Clinical Oncology.** 2000 update of recommendations for the use of hematopoietic colony-stimulating factors: evidence based, clinical practice guidelines. American Society of Clinical Oncology Growth Factors Expert Panel. *J Clin Oncol* 2002;18:3558–3585.

192. **Lyman G.** Guidelines of the National Comprehensive Cancer Network on the use of myeloid growth factors with cancer chemotherapy: a review of the evidence. *J Natl Compr Canc Netw* 2005;3:557–571.

193. **Wey SB, Mori M, Pfaller MA, Woolson RF, Wenzel RP.** Risk factors for hospital-acquired candidemia: a matched case-control study. *Arch Intern Med* 1989;149:2349–2353.

194. **Faser VJ, Jones M, Dunkel J, Storfer S, Medoff G, Dunagan WC.** Candidemia in a tertiary care hospital: epidemiology, risk factors, and predictors of mortality. *Clin Infect Dis* 1992;15:414–421.

195. **Pappas PG, Rex JH, Sobel JD, Filler SG, Dismukes WE, Walsh TJ, Edwards JE, for the Infectious Diseases Society of America.** Guidelines for treatment of candidiasis. *Clin Infect Dis* 2004;38:161–189.

19 Nutritional Therapy

Carlos Brun
Norman Rizk

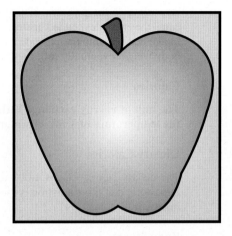

The impact of nutritional support on the outcome and quality of life of the gynecologic oncology patient has been widely recognized. To facilitate the appropriate institution of nutritional support, an understanding of the classification of malnutrition and its diagnosis is essential. Physicians should also be familiar with enteral and parenteral nutrition, their means of delivery, and their associated complications. There should also be appropriate monitoring of the response to therapy. A team approach by physician, nutritionist, and pharmacist is ideal for achieving these goals.

Malnutrition

About 40% to 55% of adult hospitalized patients in the United States are malnourished or at risk for malnutrition, and 12% are severely malnourished (1–3). Similar percentages of malnutrition have been documented in thousands of hospitalized patients throughout the world (4). A study of 67 consecutively hospitalized gynecologic oncology patients found a 54% prevalence of malnutrition (95% confidence interval, 41% to 66%) (3). In 2004, the same investigators evaluated gynecologic oncology patients in a prospective cohort trial (5). Subjective assessment utilized the Subjective Global Assessment (SGA), while objective assessment utilized the Prognostic Nutrition Index (PNI). They showed an incidence of malnutrition of 61% and 70% respectively.

It is important to screen patients to remain in accordance with the Joint Commission for Accreditation of Health Care Organizations (JCAHO) 1995 and the 2006 National Institute for Clinical Excellence recommendations (6). The time to identify a patient as needing nutritional support is not upon hospital admission, but at the time of diagnosis of cancer (7,8).

Risk Factors

Predisposing conditions frequently found in malnourished hospitalized patients include:

1. Heart failure
2. Chronic obstructive pulmonary disease
3. Infection
4. Gastrointestinal (GI) disorders
5. Psychiatric disorders
6. Renal insufficiency
7. Malignancy

It is typical for undernourished patients to have more than one predisposing condition (9).

Undernourished patients also commonly have vitamin and trace element deficiencies, particularly of vitamins A, D, E, B_{12}, and iron. Decreased stores of these vitamins can be detected in early malnutrition. Because vitamins are stored in small amounts, the provision of only dextrose and water intravenously leads to their rapid depletion, abnormal enzyme function, and clinical signs of vitamin deficiency.

Normal Body Metabolism

According to the first law of thermodynamics, the energy derived from ingested food must equal the energy expended or stored in the body at equilibrium. Although the quantity of energy intake and the amount expended and stored in any 24-hour period do not correspond exactly, body weight eventually reflects the balance between energy intake and energy expenditure.

Calories

The unit of energy exchange is the *calorie*, which is the amount of heat required to raise the temperature of 1 mL of water 1 degree C at 1 atmosphere of pressure.

Dietary Calories

The dietary calorie equals 1,000 calories. Thus, 1,500 dietary calories are equal to a 1,500-kilocalorie diet. This notation is used to describe body stores of energy and the quantity of food ingested.

Body Stores

Although diets are variable, all foods are broken down through digestion into monosaccharides, amino acids, fatty acids, and glycerol. These are then redistributed to body stores or metabolized for energy.

The body stores of energy are very different from the composition of the diet. The average diet has from 30% to 50% fat calories, 40% to 60% carbohydrate calories, and 15% to 20% protein calories. **Roughly 1,200 carbohydrate calories are stored as glycogen in muscle and liver, whereas 130,000 to 160,000 calories are contained in fat;** one pound of fat represents 3,500 stored calories. The body also contains approximately 54,000 calories as protein in muscle and organs, but only 30% to 50% of this is available to be burned for energy. **Greater than a 50% depletion of total body protein is incompatible with life** (9).

Metabolism During Starvation

During starvation, the body adapts to spare vital protein stores. Carbohydrate stores are depleted within 3 days of total starvation at rest, or more rapidly if the requirements are elevated by the metabolic effects of catabolic illnesses. Many organs use glucose in large amounts, obligating the breakdown of 75 g/day of muscle early in starvation (10). If the muscle were to continue to be broken down at this rate, starvation would lead to death in 45 to 60 days, but **adaptation from a fed to a fasting state over 2 to 3 days occurs** instead (Fig. 19.1). **In this adaptation, peripheral tissues and organs use ketone bodies, a breakdown product of fat, in place of glucose.** Because the fat stores contain an average of 160,000 calories, survival can be extended to 140 to 160 days. Some muscle breakdown continues, limiting survival, because the brain and the red blood cells require glucose, necessitating the breakdown of 20 g/day of muscle even after full adaptation.

Clinical Features

Regardless of the metabolic features of malnutrition, weight loss is usually the presenting sign. **Severe malnutrition can be defined as >10% weight loss over 2 to 3 months or a history of inadequate oral intake >7 days.** It is essential to know the patient's usual weight and ideal body weight (IBW).

Ideal Body Weight

For the purposes of assessment for malnutrition in gynecologic patients, a practical formula to use for determining the IBW is the following:

Hamwi equation for women: Ideal body weight = 100 lb for 5 ft + 5 lb/inch > 5 ft

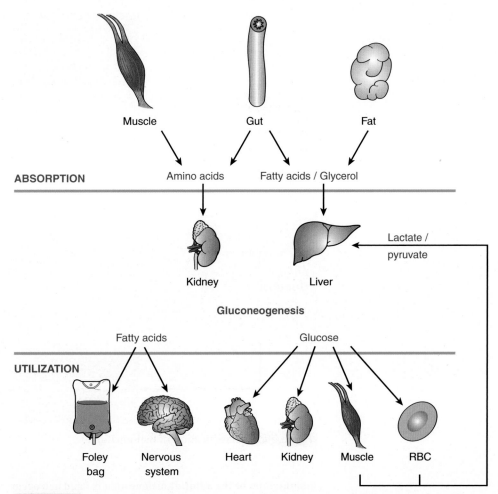

Figure 19.1   **The metabolic adaptation to starvation.** (From **Cahill GF, Owen OE.** Some observations on carbohydrate metabolism in man. In: **Dickens F, Randle PJ, Whelan WI, eds.** *Carbohydrate metabolism and its disorders.* New York: Academic Press, 1968:497, with permission.)

For example, a woman whose height is 5 feet, 4 inches would have an IBW of 120 pounds. This equation has never been validated, but was compared to the body mass index of 4.2 million people from life insurance tables in 1964. Overall it is equivalent to other predictive formulas of IBW (11). Some sources recommend that small frames subtract 10 pounds and large frames add 10 pounds, although no definition of frame measurement has been made.

For many common cancers, loss of as little as 6% of usual body weight can have significant prognostic effects on survival (12). Weight loss often mirrors declining performance status. Because some patients can be 70% of ideal body weight all their lives as a result of differences in frame size or habits such as chronic smoking, knowledge about usual body weight is important.

Weight Loss

Weight loss results from loss of body fat, body protein, or body water. Each liter of body water lost represents a weight loss of 2.2 pounds, but this weight loss can be corrected rapidly with rehydration. The degree to which losses of body protein or fat dominate the clinical picture is a reflection of the body's ability to adapt to a fat fuel economy in the face of inadequate nutrition (13). **There are three basic types of malnutrition: kwashiorkor, marasmus, and a combination of the two, cachexia** (Fig. 19.2).

Kwashiorkor   **This form of malnutrition is variously termed protein caloric malnutrition, hypoalbuminemic malnutrition, protein energy malnutrition, or kwashiorkor-like**

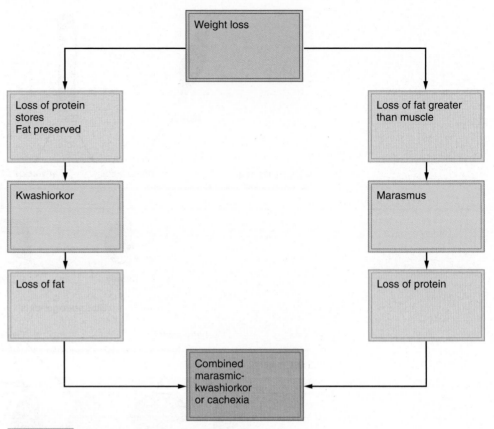

Figure 19.2 Classification of malnutrition.

malnutrition of the adult. If malnutrition is rapid and occurs in the face of disease factors that affect nutrition, a rapid depletion of protein stores can occur out of proportion to the loss of body weight. Kwashiorkor originally referred to a tropical pediatric disease and meant "separation from the breast" in Swahili.

In hospitalized patients, the major signs of protein depletion are:

1. **Decrease in serum albumin** to less than 3.5 mg/dL
2. **Decrease in absolute lymphocyte count** to less than 1,500/mm^3
3. **Decrease in serum transferrin** to less than 150 mg/dL
4. **Loss of reactivity to common skin test antigens**

It is possible for this form of malnutrition to occur in the absence of weight loss if the hypoalbuminemia leads to ascites or edema.

Marasmus   **The other major form of malnutrition in adults is called marasmus, starvation, or chronic inanition.** Primary malnutrition due to anorexia or dietary inadequacy is the most common form. **It is characterized by a depletion of fat stores and the obvious appearance of malnutrition with visible loss of muscle and fat in the arms and legs.** Although weight loss is often significant in these thin patients, protein stores can be remarkably preserved. It is not uncommon for the starved patient to have normal serum albumin and transferrin levels, a normal lymphocyte count, and normal skin test responses.

Cachexia   **When the two major forms of malnutrition occur together in patients with advanced malnutrition, the condition is called cachexia.** Cachexia is a life-threatening condition and has also been termed **combined marasmic-kwashiorkor or mixed-form malnutrition of the adult.**

Cancer-induced cachexia is related to proinflammatory cytokines such as IL-1, IL-2, IFNγ, and TNFα. Cytokines serve to decrease protein synthesis and increase proteolysis. Increased proteolysis releases amino acids to be utilized by the liver for energy production and as precursors in formation of C reactive protein and serum amyloid peptide. Cytokines also stimulate release of cortisol and catecholamines. Cachectic behavior further decreases patient's activity (14). **In this advanced condition, there is depletion of body fat stores and body protein stores, which produce visible emaciation** with loss of body muscle and fat, as well as decreased serum proteins.

The exact contribution of malnutrition to mortality in hospitalized gynecologic oncology patients is difficult to quantify. The additive effects of malnutrition include impaired immunity, poor wound healing, and cardiorespiratory dysfunction, which all impact negatively on patient survival (15).

Diagnosis

To diagnose malnutrition, **all patients should be at least minimally screened (8) or preferably assessed, for malnutrition upon diagnosis of cancer.** Low levels of circulating serum proteins can reflect impaired function of the liver and other organs, even in the absence of marked depletion of visceral and muscle protein (16). This usually occurs in the setting of excessive metabolic demands caused by specific illnesses that impair the body's ability to conserve protein. Similarly, protein and fat stores can be depleted markedly, while circulating proteins remain in the normal range. This in turn reflects a gradual adaptation to starvation in adults with anorexia and primary malnutrition.

A nutritionist can provide the nutritional assessment, which should include a history, physical examination, and laboratory evaluation. The assessment should include current medical problems/treatments; social support and functional status; anthropomorphic measurements; calculation of IBW; body mass index (BMI); and visceral protein measurement. **The nutritional assessment can identify the current degree of malnutrition, determine the nutritional support required, and set the goals of therapy.** Assaying immune function also contributes to an understanding of the nutritional status.

Anthropometry, in which body stores are estimated by direct measurements, **and biochemical markers** that assess circulating proteins, **must be used in concert to determine the specific type of malnutrition** in any given patient (Table 19.1).

Anthropometric techniques include the measurement of body weight and height in adults. The patient's normal weight can be obtained from the history. The Hamwi formula described above is used to calculate the percentage of IBW. **The BMI is calculated by dividing weight in kg by height in meters squared (kg/m^2).** Normal BMI is 18.5 to 25, overweight is 25 to 29.9, with obesity being >30, and underweight being <18.5.

Fat stores can be measured by assessing skin-fold thickness. The most commonly used skin fold in practice is the triceps. For this measurement, the patient sits with the right arm hanging freely at the side. For bedridden patients, the right arm is flexed at the shoulder while the forearm crosses the chest. The midpoint between the acromion and the olecranon posteriorly over the triceps muscle is marked. The skin and subcutaneous tissue at the midpoint are then pinched and pressure-regulated calipers are applied for 3 seconds before a reading is taken (17). The calipers are designed to deliver a pressure of 10 g/mm^2 regardless of the fold thickness and can be used to compare the same patient's progress over time as well as to assess the severity of malnutrition.

Table 19.1 Physical/Biochemical Markers of Malnutrition			
	Marasmus	*Kwashiorkor*	*Cachexia*
Albumin	Normal	↓	↓
Transferrin	Normal	↓	↓
White blood cell count	Normal	↓	↓
Skin tests	Normal	Negative	Negative
Body weight	↓	Normal	↓
Body fat	↓	Normal	↓

There are a number of other means of body fat assessment such as bioelectrical impedance analysis, and submersion measurements, but each institution should be capable of providing at least one type of assessment.

Protein Store Assessment

Midarm circumference and midarm muscle circumference can help estimate lean body mass/protein stores. Midarm muscle circumference = pi × triceps skin-fold thickness. It is an attempt to estimate lean body mass. Protein stores can also be assayed by a number of circulating proteins, most of which are secreted by the liver (18,19). Their synthesis and secretion are inhibited rapidly in the presence of protein malnutrition, and they decrease to a variable extent in the circulation according to their metabolic half-lives. **The most widely used markers are albumin and transferrin.** Each has advantages and disadvantages (18).

Albumin   Albumin has a half-life of 21 days, so that significant decreases may not occur for up to 1 month after the onset of starvation. **Albumin may also be decreased by rapid loss of serum proteins** (e.g., excessive losses from the gastrointestinal [GI] tract) **by dilution by volume resuscitation, or by fluid shifts into ascites.** Restoration of the serum albumin to normal levels by nutritional means is slow and often lags behind clear improvement in nutritional status by other criteria.

Transferrin   Transferrin is synthesized in the liver and other sites, where it can act as a growth-promoting peptide. **In the liver, synthesis is modulated by the iron stores in the hepatocytes, as well as by the overall protein status.** The half-life of the protein is 9 days, and the body pool is only 5 g. The synthetic rate is the major factor determining serum levels, and serum transferrin increases within 9 days of nutritional repletion. The problems with the interpretation of transferrin levels are that degradation rates increase during illness, and iron deficiency falsely elevates the serum levels.

For these reasons transferrin and albumin must be interpreted within the context of anthropometric determinations of body weight and triceps skin-fold thickness.

Retinol- and Thyroxine-Binding Proteins   Retinol-binding protein and thyroxine-binding prealbumin also are synthesized in the liver, with half-lives of 10 hours and 2 to 3 days, respectively. Their levels drop acutely with metabolic stress, and retinol-binding protein is also filtered and broken down by the kidney. These factors complicate the interpretation of serum levels for the diagnosis of malnutrition, but **they can be used in a research setting to assess more quickly the response to nutritional support.**

Inflammation causes a ≥25% decrease in all of the aforementioned serum transport proteins (20). The serum half-lives of these circulating proteins are listed in Table 19.2.

Immune Function

The total lymphocyte count and delayed cutaneous hypersensitivity responses to skin test antigens are nonspecific markers of impaired immune function in malnourished patients (21) (Fig. 19.3). In areas of endemic starvation, malnourished patients are at increased risk of opportunistic infections in the hospital and ambulatory settings because of the following:

1. Depressed levels of complement components, including C3.
2. Reduced amounts of secretory immunoglobulin A in external body secretions.
3. Abnormal T-cell function.
4. Impairment of nonspecific defenses, including decreased epithelial integrity, decreased mucus production, and decreased ciliary motility.

Table 19.2 Serum Half-Life of Circulating Proteins Decreased in Malnutrition	
Protein	*Half-life*
Albumin	3–4 wk
Transferrin	1 wk
Thyroxine-binding prealbumin	2 days
Retinol-binding protein	10 hr

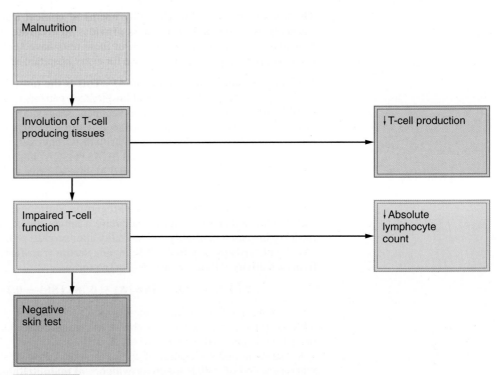

Figure 19.3   **Immunologic alterations associated with malnutrition.**

Most patients with protein and caloric malnutrition have multiple deficiencies, and **almost any single nutritional deficiency, if severe enough, can affect immune function** (22). Correction of malnutrition improves immune function; this is especially true in the gynecologic oncology patient, whose immune function can be impaired by therapy as well as by the tumor itself.

Absolute Lymphocyte Count (ALC)   The ALC is calculated by multiplying the percentage of lymphocytes by the total white blood cell count. The ALC and skin tests are the most widely used immune markers of nutritional status. The normal lymphocyte count is greater than 2,000/mm^3 in patients who are not receiving chemotherapy. **The ALC is not considered valid unless the white blood cell count is normal.**

Most circulating lymphocytes are T cells, and involution of the tissues producing T cells occurs early in the course of malnutrition. **The delayed hypersensitivity skin test response reflects three processes:**

1. **Processing of the antigen by macrophages resulting in the generation of both effector and memory T cells.**

2. **Recognition of antigen rechallenge** resulting in blast transformation, cellular proliferation, and generation of lymphokine-producing effector cells.

3. **Production of a local wheal and flare** secondary to the actions of lymphokines and chemotactic factors at the skin site.

Antigens that are frequently tested include purified protein derivative, streptokinases-treptodornase, mumps, *Candida, Trichophyton,* **and coccidioidin.** The prevalence of nonreactivity to skin test antigens is approximately 50% in patients whose serum albumin level is less than 3.0 g/dL, but it can be as high as 30% in patients whose serum albumin level exceeds 3.0 g/dL. Other problems with interpretation of skin tests include:

1. **Only about 60% of healthy patients respond to most of the antigens,** so that failure to respond to one or two antigens may not be predictive.

2. **Primary illnesses, including sarcoidosis and lymphoma,** as well as immunosuppressive drugs, **produce anergy.**

The delayed hypersensitivity (DH) and absolute lymphocyte count (ALC) are useful in uncomplicated nutritional deficiencies, but are not typically considered useful in this patient population.

The assessment of malnutrition by means of clinical examination in combination with routinely available laboratory tests provides an accurate estimation in more than 70% of patients (23). Difficulties with each of these tests have kept the nutritional assessment from becoming part of the routine database for every hospitalized patient.

Subjective Global Assessment (SGA)   This is the most commonly utilized tool by nutritionists in both surgical and medical hospitalized patients to assess the risk for malnutrition. It is subjective in that it does not rely on calipers or laboratory values, but rather on the patient's history of weight change, dietary change, gastrointestinal symptoms, functional status, and primary disease, coupled with the nutritionist's physical examination and global rating. A variant of this, the Patient Generated SGA (PGSGA) has been developed for assessment of the oncology patient and is considered highly sensitive (>90%) and specific for detection of malnutrition (24,25).

Prognostic Nutritional Index   The Prognostic Nutritional Index (PNI) combines anthropometric and laboratory tests to calculate a single index number. It is a linear predictive model of increased morbidity and mortality after surgical procedures, and uses serum albumin (A) in g/dL; triceps skin fold (TSF) in mm; serum transferrin (TFN) in mg/dL; and delayed hypersensitivity (DH) response (0–2). The formula is:

$$\text{PNI \%} = 158 - 16.6 \text{ (A)} - 0.78 \text{ (TSF)} - 0.2 \text{ (TFN)} - 5.8 \text{ (DH)}$$

For example, a well-nourished patient with A = 4.8, TSF = 14, TFN = 250, and DH = 2 has a PNI of 158.0 – 152.2, or a 5.8% chance of complications. On the other hand, a malnourished patient with abnormal indexes (A = 2.8, TSF = 9, TFN = 180, and DH = 1) has a PNI of 158 – 95.3, or a 62.7% chance of complications. A PNI of <40 is taken as well nourished, whereas a PNI of >40 is taken as evidence of malnutrition. In one study of 76 gynecologic oncology patients, serum albumin could be substituted for PNI to detect malnutrition (3). The Prognostic Nutritional Index describes surgical risk reliably based on nutritional status.

Impact of Disease on Malnutrition

Many systemic illnesses, including cancer, predispose patients to malnutrition (Fig. 19.4). Although abnormalities of metabolism, digestion, absorption, and utilization of nutrients all contribute to malnutrition in such patients, decreased nutrient intake is still an almost universal finding in malnourished patients, with the exception of those with uncomplicated hyperthyroidism. Many changes that occur in cancer patients are similar to those seen in inflammatory diseases. In particular, tumor necrosis factor (TNF), interleukins 1 and 6 (IL-1 and IL-6), and interferon-γ are etiologic agents of anorexia and cachexia (23).

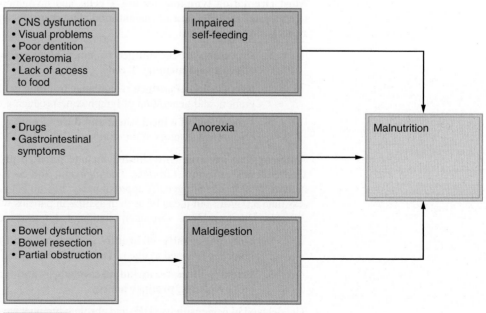

Figure 19.4   Impact of disease factors on nutrition.

Anorexia

Decreased appetite, or **anorexia, is the major factor contributing to decreased intake in many disease processes.** During tumor growth, anorexia and reduced food intake markedly contribute to the development of malnutrition. **Serotonin plays a key role in the control of appetite,** and there is evidence that administration of neutral amino acids can counteract anorexia mediated by the increased tryptophan concentrations observed in cancer patients with anorexia (16).

Although anorexia can be a feature of cancer, it can also be a side effect of many drugs, including antineoplastic drugs. A number of other commonly used drugs (e.g., anticholinergics, antihistamines, *methyldopa*, sympathomimetics, *clonidine*, and tricyclic antidepressants) may cause a dry mouth, which decreases sensation and food palatability. **Another common type of anorexia is a learned aversion to food when it is known to cause adverse physical symptoms. GI diseases,** including reflux esophagitis, gastritis, and peptic ulcer, frequently cause dyspepsia. Irritable bowel syndrome, food allergies, lactose intolerance, diverticulae, and biliary disease **can cause diarrhea or flatulence that may contribute to anorexia.**

All of these GI problems cause patients to avoid foods altogether or to ingest an unbalanced diet. Improvements in the pharmacotherapy of nausea have lessened the anorexia associated with chemotherapy. **The pharmacologic classes for possible cancer cachexia treatment include appetite stimulants, metabolic inhibitors, anabolic agents, and anticytokine agents.** *Megestrol acetate*, a progestational appetite stimulant, is an FDA-approved treatment for anorexia. This progestational steroid increases appetite through both central nervous system and peripheral mechanisms, analogous to the increased appetite that women note during the luteal phase of the menstrual cycle. **Body weight gains are from fat alone** and may not improve survival. *Megestrol* dosing begins at 160 mg/d and may advance to 480–800 mg/d. There may be a trend toward an increased risk of thromboembolism or adrenal insufficiency. **ASPEN guidelines recommend consideration of *megestrol* as a first-line agent. If this fails, a corticosteroid trial for several weeks may be warranted** (27).

Intestinal Dysfunction

Mechanical malfunction of the bowel is a particularly common problem among patients who have undergone abdominal radiation or extensive abdominal surgery. Postoperative or postirradiation adhesions can lead to partial or complete bowel obstruction. **In patients with a disseminated intraabdominal malignancy such as ovarian cancer, an adynamic ileus or intestinal pseudoobstruction can result in a nonfunctional GI tract.** Impaired capacity for self-feeding can also markedly decrease food intake. Imaging or exploratory laparotomy may be indicated to define the nature, severity, and location of intestinal dysfunction.

Metabolic Disturbances

Cancer specifically affects nutrient metabolism. Patients with metastatic and localized cancer have increased rates of hepatic glucose production, insulin resistance, whole-body glucose metabolism, lipolysis, and whole-body protein breakdown (28). Improved nutrition often fails to correct such abnormalities, once severe malnutrition is present, despite continuous parenteral or enteral alimentation with adequate nutrients (28–30). Specific metabolic disturbances and their consequences are presented in Table 19.3.

Nutritional Support

Nutritional support is an adjunct to primary therapy for the gynecologic oncology patient. The aim is to prevent deterioration of nutritional status during planned primary therapy, such as radiation, surgery, and chemotherapy. **Early initiation of nutritional support before any**

Table 19.3 Metabolic Consequences of Cancer	
Host Metabolic Abnormality	*Consequence*
Increased glucose production	Rapid weight loss, muscle breakdown
Increased lipid mobilization	Hypertriglyceridemia, rapid wasting
Insulin resistance	Hyperglycemia, hypertriglyceridemia
Hypoglycemia secondary to tumor humoral factors	Syncope, fatigue
Diarrheal syndromes due to tumor humoral factors	Electrolyte disturbances

deterioration of nutritional status is desirable. This goal necessitates early evaluation, the proper choice of nutritional therapeutic modalities, and an accurate assessment of requirements.

Once protein deficiency occurs, it is difficult to reverse, inasmuch as less than 5% of the protein is replaced per day, regardless of the amount of substrate provided. Vitamins and minerals are replaced more easily, but there is no substitute for adequate planning to meet caloric and protein requirements essential for nutritional maintenance of vital functions. The first intervention is dietary counseling.

Caloric Requirements

The protein and caloric requirements can be estimated at 0.8 g/kg/day and 20 to 35 kcal/kg/day for healthy adults,[12] respectively. If malnutrition exists or if the patient's metabolism is elevated by infection or other metabolic stresses, then 1.5 to 2.5 g/kg/day of protein and 35 to 45 kcal/kg/day should be supplied. More exact formulas are available for pediatric patients and patients at the extremes of height and weight.

Need for Support

There are two key aspects of the patient's nutritional status that affect decisions about nutritional support:

1. The degree of prior malnutrition at the time of assessment.
2. The degree of hypermetabolism or metabolic abnormality expected to interfere with nutritional rehabilitation.

If the degree of prior malnutrition is minimal and the patient has only mild hypermetabolism after elective surgery, a temporary form of nutritional support can be used. On the other hand, if the patient requires additional calories to restore preexisting severe malnutrition, forced intake of calories by an enteral or parenteral route must be used. The following guidelines can be used:

1. **If a patient is to be without nutrition for a period of 7 days, some form of nutritional support should be used.**
2. **If nutritional support is to be continued enterally for more than 4 weeks, a permanent intestinal access should be considered.** If more than 2 weeks of parenteral nutritional support is required, long-term central access should be placed. Arrangements should be made for home enteral or parenteral nutrition (31).

Method of Support

The choice between parenteral and enteral therapy should be made on the basis of the availability and functional status of the GI tract (Fig. 19.5). **If the GI tract is functioning normally, the expense and complications of parenteral nutrition are not warranted.** Swallowing evaluation and nutritional assessment are useful in determining whether the enteral route is the best alternative. Intake may also be improved by the pharmacologic therapies described previously. **If the GI tract is functional, but oral intake remains inadequate, a feeding device should be placed to assist intake.** Patients complaining of depression or pain should have these symptoms addressed concurrently.

Enteral Feeding

In view of the difficulties inherent in the use of parenteral nutritional support, every effort should be made to use the enteral route whenever possible. Enteral access may be obtained at the bedside by placement of a nasal feeding tube, by a gastroenterology consultant endoscopically, by an interventional radiologist under fluoroscopic or ultrasonic guidance, or by a surgeon in the operating room, depending upon the anticipated complexity of placement. **If a long-term nasal feeding tube is required, it should be changed to alternating nostrils every 4 to 6 weeks** (32). If enteral access is required beyond 4 weeks, consideration should be given to a gastrostomy or jejunostomy.

The gastrostomy port can be used at night for enteral support therapy by continuous infusion of isotonic enteral supplements at a rate no greater than 100 kcal/hour. The next day, the patient can cover the port with a dressing and go through her usual daily activities. This approach is often more acceptable to patients than a nasogastric tube, which is visible and irritating.

In some patients, the gastrostomy port has the added advantage that the stomach can be used as a reservoir for bolus feeding, which is more convenient. In cases of abnormal gastric motility, esophageal reflux, or possible aspiration of gastric contents, continuous slow infusion of

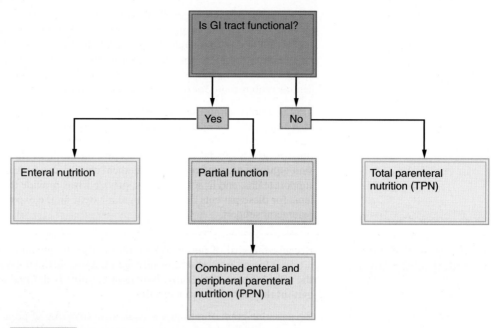

Figure 19.5   **Parenteral versus enteral nutrition.**

supplement should be used, or a tube passed beyond the pylorus into the jejunum. **The gastrostomy tube may also be used as a venting port if nausea and vomiting should develop.**

If the GI tract is atrophied from prior malnutrition, a period of rehabilitation with special formula diets can be used to renourish the patient gradually, so that routine formula diets can be used (33). The epithelium of the GI tract is directly nourished by the infused nutrients in the formula diet bathing these cells, and ultimately a complete formula diet can be used.

If the patient is already severely malnourished and hypermetabolic, with a nonfunctional GI tract, careful consideration should be given to initiation of concurrent parenteral nutrition to provide calories and protein during the period of nutritional rehabilitation of the GI tract. Tapering of parenteral nutrition may begin once tube feeds are between 33% and 50% of the goal for enteral feeds, and may be discontinued when tube feeds are between 50% and 75% of the goal (34).

The transition from tube feeding to oral feeding may require swallowing evaluation, holding tube feeding prior to meals, giving a bolus down the tube after each oral meal or giving nighttime feeds. When oral intake is approximately 50% for 2 days, tube feeding may be tapered by time and volume.

Parenteral Feeding

Total parenteral nutrition (TPN) is the provision of all required calories in an intravenous solution of dextrose, amino acids, and emulsified lipids via a centrally located catheter. **Parenteral nutrition, although appearing more definitive, should not be used in the malnourished patient with a functional GI tract.** In some patients receiving chemotherapy or radiation therapy, mucosal inflammation, nausea, and vomiting impair normal intake. In such patients, TPN may be needed as an adjunct to restore functional status and allow continuation of therapy. Patients with mid- to distal GI fistulae often require avoidance of enteral feeding.

Moderate to severely malnourished patients should receive more than 7 days of parenteral nutrition before surgery for the therapy to be of benefit. Additionally, life expectancy should be evaluated for those with advanced cancer. As per ASPEN guidelines, **only those with a life expectancy of greater than 3 months should be considered for specialized nutritional support** (35).

Peripheral parenteral nutrition (PPN) is composed of similar elements to TPN, but combined in lesser concentrations so that infusion of the less hyperosmolar (<900 to 1,000 mOsm/L) solution may be tolerated by peripheral veins. If PPN is needed for not more than

5 days, parenteral support probably is not warranted. Alternatively, if PPN is needed for 14 days or more, TPN should be given (35). Criteria for PPN administration include good peripheral access and ability to tolerate 2.5 to 3 L of fluid daily. Over time, PPNs 10% glucose solution may cause a chemical phlebitis, limiting the use of any single peripheral vein to a period of about 10 days. In patients receiving chemotherapy, peripheral veins are often sclerosed, and a central venous route for nutrition and medications must be used.

TPN is usually administered through a central venous catheter surgically placed in the subclavian vein, although other sites can be used, as described in Chapter 20. A large central vein is required for the ≥20% glucose solution plus added amino acids required for TPN. **The patient must be given special training in aseptic handling of the catheter site and use of the infusion equipment required.** Many medical centers also have special home parenteral nutritional support teams, and in some regions, private firms provide this service. Potential medical problems for these patients depend to a great extent on the experience of the team providing home parenteral support.

Evaluation of Response to Nutritional Support

Because the goal of nutritional support is the attainment of an anabolic state or reduction of nitrogen losses, **assessment of nitrogen balance is the most useful clinical tool to determine the effectiveness of therapy. Nitrogen balance is defined as the difference between nitrogen intake and nitrogen excretion.**

Because one gram of nitrogen is equivalent to 6.25 g of protein, **nitrogen intake** can be determined by dividing protein intake, as determined from dietary records, by 6.25. **Nitrogen excretion** is defined as the urinary nitrogen excreted per 24 hours, plus a fixed estimate of 4.0 g per 24 hours for unmeasured nitrogen losses from cellular sloughing into the feces (1 g); losses from the skin (0.2 g); and nonurea nitrogen losses in the urine (2 g) (36). Because nitrogen balance is most usefully applied in a serial fashion in the same patient, the particular constants used to estimate unmeasured excretion are important only for comparison of published results.

At any given level of nitrogen intake, nitrogen balance improves with increased administration of nonprotein calories. The maximum benefit is achieved when the ratio of nonprotein calories to grams of nitrogen is 150:1 (37).

To assess adequacy of protein intake, patients with stable renal function, consistent protein intake and the ability to collect a 24-hour urine sample, may benefit from a **urine urea nitrogen study (UUN), where UUN = (protein (grams)/6.25) minus UUN (excretion in grams) plus 4.** The goal is +2 to +4 or the least negative balance attainable. If the UUN is negative, increasing the protein delivered, assisting its absorption, and increasing the total calories given should be considered.

Proteins also vary in their biologic value, according to their mixture of essential and nonessential amino acids. Albumin has the ideal mixture of amino acids for optimal use of protein and is assigned a biologic value of 100. Casein is close to albumin in its biologic quality, whereas meat proteins, such as those found in steak or tuna, have a biologic value of 80. Corns and beans, each with biologic values of 40 or less, can be combined in a protein mixture with a biologic value of 80, because the amino acid mixtures of the two proteins are complementary. **The protein requirement for normal people is 0.55 g/kg for protein with a high biologic value, such as milk or albumin, but 0.8 g/kg for the mixture of proteins found in the average American diet** (38).

Effect of Nutritional Support on Prognosis

Although it is easy to demonstrate the impact of renutrition in simple starvation, it is much more difficult to demonstrate the beneficial effect of nutritional support in a patient with a chronic illness such as cancer (39). Often the course of the underlying illness masks the beneficial effects of nutritional therapy.

In patients with mild disease or elective surgery, malnutrition is relatively well tolerated from a clinical standpoint. In such cases, nutritional rehabilitation usually occurs without any special effort as the underlying medical or surgical condition runs its course. In patients with severe disease, nutrition is often relegated to the secondary list of problems, because the progress of the primary illness dictates therapeutic decisions. In both of these instances, however, nutritional therapy may play a beneficial role in either preventing or retarding malnutrition in individual patients (40). On the other hand, **an extensive meta-analysis of 53 published studies of parenteral and enteral nutrition showed that survival was improved in 6 studies,** unchanged in 43, and worse in 2 (41). **Nonetheless, the judicious application of nutritional support for gynecologic oncology patients may lead to an improvement in the quality of life and prognosis.**

Nutrition usually is an adjunct to primary medical and surgical therapy. Prior to beginning a nutritional support regimen, the patient's current clinical status and expected outcome must be discussed with the patient and her loved ones, especially in cases of end-stage disease. Broaching end-of-life topics should be done openly and early. According to the American Medical Association's Web site, **the decision to use any medical therapy "should be based on the best interests of the patient (what outcome would most likely promote the patient's well-being)".** Given the social and emotional value of nutrition, ultimately the autonomy of the patient should be guided by sound advice on what benefits, potential complications, and responsibilities come with specialized nutritional support. If there is any doubt as to whether nutrition should be provided, consultation with an ethicist may be of value.

Complications

Complications can occur after either enteral or parenteral nutrition. Complications can be mechanical, infectious, or metabolic (42).

Enteral Feeding

Tubes placed via the nares may cause nasal mucosal damage, septal necrosis, sinusitis, otitis, vocal cord dysfunction, and ulceration. Use of a smaller size (i.e., 5–12F) tube helps minimize complications. **Overall complication rates approach 10% and include epistaxsis, aspiration, and respiratory distress** (43). Cardiopulmonary complications for the transnasal route were 4%, while the transoral tubes had a 15% rate in nonintubated patients in one study. Additionally in less than 5% of patients, nasotracheal tube placement occurred. In these patients the malpositioning was unsuspected in 80%, and caused a pneumothorax in half of the patients. **Dislodgement of nasoenteral tubes has been documented in 16% to 41% of placements.** A nasal bridle may be useful (e.g., AMT, Brecksville, OH) to help prevent this occurrence. **Tubal occlusion occurs in up to 20% of cases.** Flushing regularly and using center specific protocols for declogging (e.g., *viokase* and *sodium bicarbonate*) may decrease the risk of occlusion. **Finally, up to 20% of patients with enteric tubes will experience dysphagia.**

The alternative approach of enterostomies may be associated with hemorrhage, perforation and bowel leakage, and bowel obstruction with necrosis. Aspiration risk may increase due to sedation and ileus associated with the placement procedure itself. **Pneumoperitoneum occurs in up to 50% of tube placements** and may delay diagnosis of a perforation, if present. The ostomy site should be observed for leakage or buried bumper syndrome. Inadvertent ostomy removal may occur and must be urgently addressed.

Since **enteral feeding increases the risk of aspiration,** identifying patients with gastroesophageal reflux, gastric dysmotility, or progressive obstruction and intolerance can help minimize the risk. Other ways to decrease aspiration risk include head of bed elevation, evaluation of swallowing, assessment of tolerance to tube feeding, and frequent monitoring of the airway. The ASPEN guidelines for gastric residual volumes are to check every 4 to 5 hours until at goal, and to hold feeds if residual volumes are greater than 200 mL. Unfortunately, nausea and/or vomiting develop in 12% to 20% of patients receiving enteral nutrition (35).

Diarrhea is the most common complication associated with tube feeding (44) and should be assessed and treated in the following ways:

1. **Infectious diarrhea should first be excluded,** including *C. difficile* pseudomembranous colitis secondary to antibiotics.

2. **The rate of infusion can be decreased.** If the GI tract dysfunction is due to atrophy of the epithelial cells, a gradual increase in infusion rate is often tolerated, starting with an initial rate of 25 mL/hour and increasing by twofold increments every 48 hours.

3. **The type of enteral formula can be changed to an isosmolar formula.** Many of the high-calorie or high-nitrogen supplements are hyperosmolar. Changing to an isotonic formula often decreases intestinal hypermotility. It is important to review medication lists to rule out any medications with a laxative effect. Stool anion gap may be sent to rule in osmotic rather than secretory diarrhea. Fecal fat should be checked if fat malabsorption is suspected. The patient's medical history should be reviewed for lactose and gluten intolerance.

4. **A number of specific medications can be used to decrease intestinal motility.** The presence of an obstruction or infectious diarrhea should be determined first, since these are contraindications to hypomotility agents.

5. The level of enteral support can be decreased and temporarily combined with peripheral parenteral alimentation until intestinal motility problems respond to the maneuvers discussed previously.

While evaluation of diarrhea is ongoing, attention should be kept on the clinical status of the patient as **dehydration may rapidly occur.** Dehydration with hypernatremia can be a problem in the elderly, in whom inadequate fluid intake can occur during the administration of a hypertonic enteral formula. When high-carbohydrate enteral formulas are used, glucosuria can occur even in patients without a prior history of diabetes.

Parenteral Feeding

The complications of parenteral nutrition are often more serious than those associated with enteral nutrition (45). **Pneumothorax and subclavian venous thrombosis are the most common catheter-related complications for temporary and permanent central venous catheters (CVC).** Pneumothorax should occur in only 1% to 2% of CVC insertions, but this rate is higher when transthoracic puncture is used rather than open surgical placement, or when less experienced personnel insert the catheter (46). A chest radiograph to confirm proper catheter placement and to exclude a pneumothorax is essential. A pneumothorax often resolves spontaneously, but a chest tube or pigtail catheter may be required in some cases. **Peripherally inserted central catheters (PICC) are another option for TPN. The lumen for TPN should be dedicated for TPN** only to minimize the risk of infection. Femoral CVCs should be avoided due to an increased risk of infection and thrombosis.

Permanent catheters, such as Hickman or Port catheters provide ready access for parenteral nutrition, blood products, and chemotherapy, but can also be malpositioned, cause thrombosis, or become infected. Thrombosis of the catheter in the central veins has been reported in 5% to 10% of patients receiving parenteral nutrition, especially with the hypercoagulable states of sepsis or cancer (47). In most patients, the catheter should be flushed with *heparin* solution (300 U/mL) to prevent this complication, predisposing the patient to the risk of *heparin*-induced thrombocytopenia (HIT). When venous thrombosis occurs, the catheter must be removed. Peripheral parenteral nutrition may be used, while a course of full intensity anticoagulation is given to treat the thrombosis and a new site for a central venous catheter is selected. A minimum of a three-month course of full-dose anticoagulation should be prescribed, and that access site should be avoided in the future.

In patients committed to lifelong parenteral nutrition, the CVC site choice must be made carefully because only nine external sites are available for central venous catheter placement: internal jugular veins, subclavian veins, femoral veins, and in some centers, the inferior vena cava.

Infections occur in 2% to 5% of central catheters placed for parenteral nutrition. Mortality of catheter related blood stream infections is 12% to 25% (48). When the patient is febrile and a peripheral source of infection is not found within 96 hours, the catheter should be removed and cultured for evidence of catheter-related infection. **Infections most commonly occur from skin contaminants, such as gram-positive organisms, but can include fungi and unusual bacteria, especially if acquired during hospitalization. Fevers in patients requiring TPN should always prompt investigation of potential blood stream infection.**

Infected catheters can also be a source of life-threatening septic phlebitis. Blood-borne infections from sources other than the catheter can be treated with intravenous antibiotics without removal of the catheter, but the patient should be observed carefully because the catheter may become seeded with bacteria. The subcutaneous tunnel of a permanent catheter may be a source of infection as well.

In patients treated with broad-spectrum antibiotics, systemic candidiasis can occur. The retina should be examined by an ophthalmologist for the presence of cotton-wool exudates that are pathognomonic of systemic candidiasis, and blood cultures should be sent for special fungal isolation procedures if candidiasis is suspected. *Caspofungin* (70 mg IV first day, then 50 mg IV daily) is a reasonable first-line agent in patients with suspected candidemia. In addition to holding TPN, the CVC should be removed and consideration given to evaluation for endocarditis (49).

A variety of metabolic complications can occur during parenteral nutrition. **The most common is overfeeding, which results in excess CO_2 production and occasionally hypercapnia** in patients with pulmonary disease (50). Blood sugars must be checked regularly as hyperglycemia or even hyperosmolar nonketotic coma can occur as a result of transient insulin resistance, relative insulin deficiency, or more rarely, chromium deficiency. Sliding scale subcutaneous insulin, an insulin drip, or insulin added to the parenteral solutions are appropriate measures (51). **Hypoglycemia sometimes occurs with abrupt cessation of TPN** as well. To avoid this, TPN should be tapered to half the standing infusion rate for one hour, before discontinuing it completely. Alternatively a D10W infusion can be substituted for the TPN at the same rate for one hour. Basic metabolic panels should be monitored for **metabolic acidosis, a less common problem** since acetate buffers have been used in parenteral solutions. **Abnormalities of phosphate, potassium, calcium, and magnesium can occur** because of excessive or inadequate administration, particularly in the presence of underlying disorders, such as renal failure or GI fistulae, which themselves predispose to electrolyte abnormalities (52,53).

Deficiencies of trace minerals such as zinc, copper, and chromium used to occur but are now rare, because these are now added routinely to parenteral solutions (54). Because multivitamin solutions are the same source for vitamin K, **the prothrombin time and partial prothrombin time should be monitored weekly.**

The most serious metabolic complication of TPN is refeeding syndrome, an acute state of electrolyte imbalance due to initiation of nutritional support. It is most likely to occur when TPN is commenced in the severely malnourished patient. Concern for this syndrome requires daily serum electrolytes initially, and often electrolyte supplementation (55).

Renal abnormalities are sometimes troubling. Azotemia may worsen in patients with renal failure or when there is excessive administration of amino acids relative to nonprotein calories, and this may treated by reduction of the amino acid load. However amino acid requirements may be higher in patients on hemodialysis. Daily weights and a strict fluid balance chart are mandatory for volume monitoring.

Hepatobiliary complications occur as well. Steatosis is associated with dextrose overfeeding, and a mild transaminitis may occur that typically resolves in 2 weeks. The latter can also reflect sepsis. **Cholestasis** manifests as a nonjaundiced patient (with bilirubin <2), with a mild increase in alkaline phosphatase, GGT, and direct bilirubin. Finally, **gallbladder stasis occurs in almost all TPN patients,** but consideration should be given to the possible development of cholangitis or cholecystitis.

Essential fatty acid (EFA) deficiency now rarely occurs because of the use of intravenous lipid emulsions (57). In animal studies, EFA deficiency occurs after 12 days without lipid supplementation. In humans this complication can be avoided by providing 1 to 3 days per week of lipid infusion. **EFA deficiency clinically manifests as scaly skin, alopecia, hepatomegaly, or thrombocytopenia.** To avoid hypertriglyceridemia due to lipid administration or dextrose overfeeding, **weekly triglyceride levels should be checked.** Rarely patients with egg allergy will react to the lipid infusion.

In most cases, the metabolic complications associated with parenteral nutrition respond to careful fluid and electrolyte management with daily monitoring of input and output. Complications can be avoided with effective communication between the physician, nutritionist, pharmacist, and patient.

Nutritional Support in Multiple Organ Failure Syndrome

Multiple organ failure syndrome (MOSF) can develop in critically ill patients secondary to a decline in cellular oxygen consumption, inflammatory cytokines, or sepsis (58). Cascading events, including at different times hypoperfusion/hypoxia, immunodysfunction, endocrine dysfunction, acute starvation, and metabolic derangements, may lead to early organ failure within 5 to 7 days after the initial insult, but can occur as late as 21 days.

The nutritional therapy provided for such patients has been called metabolic support to differentiate it from the nutritional support given to more stable patients with chronic anorexia and starvation. In nutritional support, the goals are simply to provide adequate calories and nutrients to restore nutritional deficiencies and to maintain protein synthesis, positive nitrogen balance, and lean body mass (59). **Metabolic support of the critically ill patient at risk of multiple organ failure syndrome is directed at partial caloric replacement, sustenance of** important cellular and organ metabolism, and the avoidance of overfeeding. Metabolic costs of overfeeding include lipogenesis, gluconeogenesis, thermogenesis, electrolyte imbalance, metabolic alkalosis, and hypervolemia. Excessive infusion rates and choice of the wrong mixture of macronutrients can be harmful in the critically ill patient (60).

A breakdown in the physical and immunologic barriers of the GI tract can promote multiple organ failure syndrome. The GI tract is particularly susceptible to ischemic and reperfusion injury. Glutamine, a preferred fuel for the gut epithelium, may promote healing of the GI tract epithelium after an injury (61). In animal studies, an enteral formula containing glutamine has been shown to maintain muscle glutamine metabolism without stimulating tumor growth, while also improving GI mucosal integrity and nitrogen balance (62). Currently there are no recommendations for glutamine outside of burn or trauma patients (63). The critical therapeutic difference between multiple organ failure syndrome and chronic malnutrition is the need to avoid overfeeding by providing a hypocaloric protein-sparing nutritional regimen in the former.

Provision of Nutritional Support

There are many methods of estimating basal energy requirements. The following are guidelines:

1. **Obese patients maintain their body weight when given between 15 to 25 kcal/kg of actual body weight (ABW) per day.**

2. **Normal weight patients maintain their weight when given 35 kcal/kg of ABW per day.**

3. In patients with malnutrition, there is a cost of anabolism that involves the calories necessary for new protein synthesis. **For patients with very severe illnesses and in whom malnutrition may be combined with sepsis or trauma to elevate energy requirements, ≤45 kcal/kg/day may be required.**

There are many other formulas for estimating energy requirements that take the patient's height into consideration. Taller patients have a higher resting energy expenditure at the same weight than shorter patients, because they have larger livers and other vital organs. In older people, metabolic rates tend to fall, in part because of a decrease in lean body mass. Although these equations are useful for clinical nutritional research, they are generally unnecessary for clinical management. A more practical set of guidelines is given in the following sections.

Estimation of Total Caloric Requirement

Severity of Illness	Daily Caloric Requirement
Mild	**35 kcal/kg**
Moderate	**40 kcal/kg**
Severe	**45 kcal/kg**

Estimation of Protein Requirement

The protein requirement can be estimated at approximately 1.0 g/kg of actual body weight per day for normal individuals or 1.0 g/kg of ideal body weight per day for obese patients. Stressed normal weight patients require 1.5 to 2.5 g/kg of actual body weight/day while stressed obese patients require 1.5 to 2 g/kg of ideal body weight/day (34).

Estimation of Nonprotein Calories

One simple method of estimating nonprotein calories is to subtract the protein calories from the total number of calories required daily. **1 gram of protein = 4 calories.** The nonprotein caloric requirement may be estimated by initially estimating the amount of nitrogen administered according to the following formula: **1 g nitrogen = 6.25 g protein.** By either the parenteral or the enteral route, **150 nonprotein calories must be provided for each gram of nitrogen administered.** Therefore, estimation of nonprotein calories can be achieved as follows:

$$\text{Nonprotein calories} = \frac{\text{Protein requirement} \times 150}{6.25}$$

Determination of Carbohydrate Requirement

It is usual to give approximately half the total calories as carbohydrates. Most nutritional solutions are premixed, and the precise formulas available vary in different hospitals. **Custom TPN solutions are possible and may be useful to decrease hyperglycemia.** It is best to discuss custom solutions with a nutritionist and a pharmacist, as solution stability must be maintained, which limits the proportions of protein, fat, and carbohydrate that can be mixed.

Determination of Fat Requirement	**The absolute fat requirement for essential fatty acids (i.e., linoleic acid and linolenic acid) is only 4% of the total calories.** The amount of fat usually administered either enterally or parenterally exceeds this amount. The balance of the calories necessary to fulfill the total caloric requirement after the protein and carbohydrate calories have been calculated is often given as fat. In all cases, the number of calories given as fat should be far less than 60% of the total calories, which is the maximal fat allowance.

Sample Calculations

Sample calculations for both enteral and parenteral formulations are presented.

Enteral

A 50-year-old woman who weighs 45 kg has a usual body weight of 70 kg and is severely ill with sepsis and postsurgical stress. Her GI tract is functional, and enteral formulation must be prescribed. The following steps allow calculation of the specific requirements:

1. The total daily caloric requirement is estimated by multiplying the caloric requirement based on severity (in this case, 45 kcal/kg/day) by the patient's weight (i.e., 45 kg). Therefore, the caloric requirement is 45 kcal/kg × 45 kg = 2,025 kcal.

2. The minimum protein requirement is determined by multiplying the ideal body weight by 1.0 g/kg (e.g., in this case 70 kg), and 1.0 g/kg = 70 g. Because protein = 4 kcal/g, the protein caloric need is 280 kcal.

3. The estimation of nonprotein calories is determined by multiplying the protein requirement (70 g) by 150, and this figure is divided by 6.25. Therefore, the minimum nonprotein calories required = [70 g × 150] / 6.25 = 1,680 kcal.

4. The determination of specific carbohydrate and fat needs is empiric; that is, if approximately one-half the total caloric need is given in carbohydrates (in this case, 1,010 kcal), the remainder of the calories may be given as fat. Therefore, fat calories = 2,025 − (1,010 + 280) = 735 kcal.

5. An enteral formula that approximates these caloric requirements should be used. A standard formula containing 1.0 kcal/mL, 15% protein, 34% fat, and 51% carbohydrate would provide approximately 150 kcal of protein, 340 kcal of fat, and 510 kcal of carbohydrate for every liter of formula given to the patient. Therefore, this patient's caloric requirements would be met by giving her approximately 2 L of formula per day.

Parenteral

A 45-kg, 70-year-old woman has lost 15 kg as a result of postirradiation changes to the bowel. In view of her poor GI function, parenteral alimentation is appropriate. The estimation of her nutritional requirements is as follows:

1. The total daily caloric requirement is estimated by multiplying the caloric requirement based on severity by the patient's weight (i.e., 45 kcal/kg × 45 kg = 2,025 kcal).

2. The minimum protein requirement is determined by multiplying the usual body weight (60 kg) by 1.0 g/kg = 60 g. At 4 kcal/g, the protein caloric need is 240 kcal.

3. The nonprotein caloric requirement thus equals approximately 1,785 kcal, which should include approximately 775 kcal fat and 1,010 kcal carbohydrate.

4. A standard TPN formula containing 20% dextrose and 3.5% protein (e.g., *Travasol*) would provide 680 kcal of dextrose per liter and 35 g (140 kcal) of protein per liter. Therefore, 1.7 L of this formula would approximate the carbohydrate and protein needs of the patient. The parenteral solution is administered at a rate of 75 mL/hour.

5. A single unit of 10% intravenous fat emulsion provides 550 kcal/unit. Therefore, the usual amount of fat given would be provided by 1.4 units (or 700 mL). Because fat emulsions are available in single units, it is preferable to give this patient 2 units of fat emulsion per day or one unit of 20% lipid.

In this example, the intravenous fat emulsion provides needed additional calories, allowing for the more complete utilization of the administered protein. An additional reason to provide fat emulsions parenterally is the need to provide essential fatty acids at a minimum level of 4% of total calories. For example, 4% × 2,000 kcal = 80 kcal/day. One 550 kcal unit of intravenous fat emulsion per week can meet this requirement. **In the absence of any fat administration,**

				Table 19.4 Typical Parenteral Nutrition Solutions				
Solution	Na+ (mEq/L)	K+ (mEq/L)	Mg²⁺ (mEq/L)	Acetate (mEq/L)	Cl⁻ (mEq/L)	Protein (g/L)	Calories/L (D 20)ᵃ
FreAmine III 3%	35	24.5	5	44	40	29	800
Aminosyn 4.25%	70	66	10	142	98	85	850
Travasol 4.25%	70	60	10	135	70	89	850
Travasol 3.5%	25	15	5	54	25	37	820

ᵃIf admixed with a solution of 20% dextrose.

essential fatty acid deficiency develops in 4 to 6 weeks in most people, once endogenous stores of essential fatty acids are depleted. Because the cost of lipid emulsions has decreased considerably, fat is being used as a parenteral caloric source in amounts exceeding those needed to meet the minimal essential fatty acid requirements, as outlined in the previous example.

Standard mixtures of electrolytes per liter of solution are provided by most pharmacies, and they are designed together with acetate buffers to deliver a nonacid solution with a pH of between 5.3 and 6.8. In unusual fluid and electrolyte situations, the composition of the solution can be custom designed, but this significantly increases the cost of parenteral nutrition and increases the possibility of the solution becoming insoluble or "cracking." The use of standard fluid and electrolyte solutions with supplements as necessary is preferable. Typical parenteral nutritional solutions are shown in Table 19.4.

Osmolarity and caloric content of the parenteral solution are related to the glucose and protein concentrations. For lipid preparations, the osmolarity and caloric content are also related to the percentage of lipid in the solution (Table 19.5).

Recommended vitamins that should be provided on a daily basis in parenteral solutions are listed in Table 19.6. These substances are available in preformulated ampules, and 1 ampule per day added directly to the parenteral solution meets all the requirements in most patients. In patients who are especially stressed (e.g., septic wounds), 500 mg of vitamin C should be given. Patients receiving common medications such as *phenytoin (Dilantin)* may require additional specific vitamin supplements (e.g., vitamin D). The amount of vitamin K provided in daily parenteral nutrition should be routinely reviewed by a pharmacist.

Major mineral requirements are listed in Table 19.7. The daily requirement has a wide range that depends largely on the extent of GI and renal losses. In patients with an abnormally high excretion, the losses must be replaced aggressively.

Supplementation with zinc, copper, chromium, and selenium is essential in parenteral nutrition (Table 19.8). Deficiency states of these trace elements have been described in

Table 19.5 Osmolarity and Caloric Content of Glucose and Lipids in Parenteral Nutritional Solutions		
Glucose Concentration (wt/vol)	Osmolarity (mOsm/L)	Calories (kcal/dL)
5%	250	17
10%	500	34
20%	1,000	68
50%	2,500	170
70%	3,500	237
Lipid Concentration (wt/vol)		
10%	280	110
20%	340	200

Table 19.6 Guidelines for Daily Adult Parenteral Vitamin Supplementation

Vitamin	Daily Intravenous Dose
A	3,300 IU
D	200 IU
E	10 IU
B$_1$ (thiamin)	3.0 mg
B$_2$ (riboflavin)	3.6 mg
B$_3$ (pantothenic acid)	15.0 mg
B$_5$ (niacin)	40.0 mg
B$_6$ (pyridoxine)	4.0 mg
B$_7$ (biotin)	60.0 mg
B$_9$ (folic acid)	400.0 mg
B$_{12}$ (cobalam in)	5.0 mg
C (ascorbic acid)	100.0 mg
K	5.0 mg/wk[a]

[a]Parenteral vitamin K supplementation is not included in the official recommendation because some patients are receiving anticoagulants.

From **American Medical Association/Nutrition Advisory Group Guidelines,** *JPEN J Parenter Enteral Nutr* 1979;3:258, with permission.

patients who have been receiving parenteral nutrition without supplementation. These patients respond to the specific replacement of deficient trace elements. **Patients who require home TPN should have trace element levels measured prior to discharge.**

Iron supplementation is not recommended in the acutely ill patient. Iron levels should be documented. **Manganese has not been clearly established as an essential component of TPN solutions,** but it has been included in some recommended regimens. **Iodine is not normally supplemented** because the transdermal absorption of iodine-containing solutions that are used to clean catheter sites permits intake of the required amount of iodine. Iodine deficiency is associated with high TSH. **Chromium levels may be useful in the diabetic patient** as chromium is an insulin receptor cofactor and deficiency may cause hypo- or hyperglycemia.

In the presence of excessive GI losses (e.g., small bowel fistula), additional zinc should be given for replacement. It is recommended that 12.2 mg of additional zinc per liter of small bowel loss should be given.

Table 19.7 Range of Daily Requirements of Major Minerals and Electrolytes in Parenteral Solutions

Electrolyte	Daily Requirement Range
Sodium	50–250 mEq
Potassium	30–200 mEq
Chloride	50–250 mEq
Magnesium	10–30 mEq
Calcium	10–20 mEq
Phosphorus	10–40 mmol

Modified from **Alpers DH, Clouse RE, Stenson WF.** *Manual of nutritional therapeutics.* Boston: Little, Brown 1983:238.

Table 19.8 Suggested Daily Adult Intravenous Requirements of Essential Trace Elements and Associated Deficiency Syndromes

Trace Element	Requirement	Deficiency Syndrome
Iron	10–18 mg/day	Anemia
Copper[a]	30 µg/kg/day	Rare hemolysis
Zinc[a]	15 mg/day	Blepharitis, conjunctivitis, growth retardation, dermatitis, diarrhea
Selenium[a]	50–200 µg/day	Cardiomyopathy
Chromium[a]	20 µg/day	Glucose intolerance, hypercholesterolemia, hyperaminoacidemia
Manganese	3–5 mg/day	Dermatitis, hypocholesterolemia, hair color change, decreased hair and nail growth
Iodine	100 µg/day	Hypothyroidism
Fluoride	1.5–4.0 mg/day	Anemia, growth retardation
Molybdenum[b]	200–500 µg/day	Muscle cramps

[a]Required in total parenteral nutrition solutions.

[b]Not absolutely required but included in most formulations.

Adapted from **AMA Department of Foods and Nutrition.** Guidelines for essential trace element preparations for parenteral use: a statement by an expert panel. *JAMA* 1979;241:2051–2054, with permission.

In patients who are being given enteral supplementation, 2 L of formula per day includes all the recommended dietary allowance for vitamins, minerals, and trace elements.

Further information regarding nutritional support may be obtained from the American Society for Parenteral and Enteral Nutrition (ASPEN) at http://www.nutritioncare.org.

References

1. **Gallagher-Allred CR, Voss AC, Finn SC, McCamish MA.** Malnutrition and clinical outcomes: the case for medical nutrition therapy. *J Am Diet Assoc* 1996;96:361–366.
2. **Naber TH, Schermer T, de Bree A, Nusteling K, Eggink L, Krumiel JW, et al.** Prevalence of malnutrition in nonsurgical hospitalized patients and its association with disease complications. *Am J Clin Nutr* 1997;66:1232–1239.
3. **Santoso JT, Canada T, Latson B, Aaaadi K, Lucci JA III, Coleman RL.** Prognostic nutritional index in relation to hospital stay in women with gynecologic cancer. *Obstet. Gynecol* 2000;95: 844–846.
4. **Baccaro F, Moreno JB, Borlenghi C, Aquino L, Armesto G, Plaza G, et al.** Subjective global assessment in the clinical setting. *JPEN J Parenter Enteral Nutr* 2007;31:406–409.
5. **Santoso JT, Cannada T, O'Farrel B, Alladi K, Coleman RL.** Subjective versus objective nutritional assessment study in women with gynecological cancer: a prospective cohort trial. *Int J Gynecol Cancer* 2004;14:220–223.
6. **Kudsk KA, Reddy SK, Sacks GS, Lai HC.** Joint Commission for Accreditation of Health Care Organizations guidelines: too late to intervene for nutritionally at-risk surgical patients. *JPEN J Parenter Enteral Nutr* 2003;27:288–290.
7. **Marín Caro MM, Laviano A, Pichard C.** Impact of nutrition on quality of life during cancer. *Curr Opin Clin Nutr Metab Care* 2007; 10:480–487.
8. **Huhmann MB, August DA.** Review of American Society for Parenteral and Enteral Nutrition (A.S.P.E.N.) clinical guidelines for nutrition support in cancer patients: nutrition screening and assessment. *Nutr Clin Pract* 2008;23:182–188.
9. **McWhirter J, Pennington C.** Incidence and recognition of malnutrition in hospital. *BMJ* 1994;9:945–948.
10. **Moore FD, Brennan ME.** Surgical inquiry: body composition, protein metabolism and neuroendocrinology. In: **Ballinger WF, Collins JA, Drucker WR, et al., eds.** *Manual of Surgical Nutrition.* Philadelphia: WB Saunders, 1975:169–222.
11. **Shah B, Sucher K, Hollenbeck CB.** Comparison of ideal body weight equations and published height-weight tables with body mass index tables for healthy adults in the United States. *Nutr Clin Pract* 2006;21:312–319.
12. **Chlebowski RT, Palomares MR, Lillington L, Grosvenor M.** Recent implications of weight loss in lung cancer management. *Nutrition* 1996;12:S43–S47.
13. **Tisdale MJ.** Cancer cachexia: metabolic alterations and clinical manifestations. *Nutrition* 1997;17:477–498.
14. **Morley JE, Thomas DR, Wilson MM.** Cachexia: pathophysiology and clinical relevance. *Am J Clin Nutr* 2006;83:735–743.
15. **Alexander JW, Ogle CK, Nelson JL.** Diets and infection: composition and consequences. *World J Surg* 1998;22:209–212.
16. **Gough DB, Heys SD, Eremin O.** Cancer cachexia: pathophysiological mechanisms. *Eur J Surg Oncol* 1996;22:192–196.
17. **Jensen TG, Dudrick SJ, Johnston DA.** A comparison of triceps skinfold and upper arm circumference measurements taken in standard and supine positions. *JPEN J Parenter Enteral Nutr* 1981;5:519–521.
18. **Ottery FD.** Definition of standardized nutritional assessment and interventional pathways in oncology. *Nutrition* 1996;12:S15–S19.
19. **Tchekmedyian NS, Zahyna D, Halpert C, Heber D.** Assessment and maintenance of nutrition in older cancer patients. *Oncology* 1992;6:105–111.

20. **Gabay C, Kushner I.** Acute-phase proteins and other systemic responses to inflammation. *N Engl J Med* 1999;340:448–454.

21. **Chen MK, Souba WW, Copeland EM.** Nutritional support of the surgical oncology patient. *Hematol Oncol Clin North Am* 1991;5:125–145.

22. **Buzby GP, Mullen JL, Matthews DC, Hobbs CL, Rosato EF.** Prognostic Nutritional Index in gastrointestinal surgery. *Am J Surg* 1980;139:160–167.

23. **McNamara JM, Alexander R, Norton JA.** Cytokines and their role in the pathophysiology of cancer cachexia. *JPEN J Parenter Enteral Nutr* 1992;16:S50–S55.

24. **Barbosa-Silva MC, Barros AJ.** Indications and limitations of the use of subjective global assessment in clinical practice: an update. *Curr Opin Clin Nutr Metab Care* 2006;9:263–269.

25. **Kubrak C, Jensen L.** Critical evaluation of nutrition screening tools recommended for oncology patients. *Cancer Nurs* 2007;30:E1–6.

26. **Cangiano C, Laviano A, Muscaritoli M, Meguid MM, Cascino A, Fanelli FR.** Cancer anorexia: new pathogenic and therapeutic insights. *Nutrition* 1996;12:S48–S51.

27. **Inui A.** Cancer anorexia-cachexia syndrome: current issues in research and management. *CA Cancer J Clin* 2002;52:72–91.

28. **Heber D, Byerley LO, Chi J, Grosvenor M, Bergman RN, Coleman M, et al.** Pathophysiology of malnutrition in the adult cancer patient. *Cancer* 1986;58:1867–1873.

29. **Giannotti L, Braga M, Vignali A.** Effect of route of delivery and formulation of postoperative nutrition in patients undergoing major operations for malignant neoplasms. *Arch Surg* 1997;132:1222–1229.

30. **Laughlin EH, Dorosin NN, Phillips YY.** Total parenteral nutrition: a guide to therapy in the adult. *J Fam Pract* 1977;5:947–957.

31. Guidelines for the use of parenteral and enteral nutrition in adult and pediatric patients. *JPEN J Parenter Enteral Nutr* 2002;26(suppl 1):1SA–138SA.

32. **Stroud M, Duncan H, Nightingale J.** Guidelines for enteral feeding in adult hospital patients. *Gut* 2003;52(suppl 7):vii1–vii12.

33. **Sirbu ER, Margen S, Calloway DH.** Effect of reduced protein intake on nitrogen loss from the human integument. *Am J Clin Nutr* 1967;20:1158–1165.

34. **Russel M.** *A.S.P.E.N. nutrition support practice manual*, 2nd ed.; 2005.

35. **Gottschlich MM, ed.** *The American Society for Parenteral and Enteral Nutrition's nutrition support core curriculum: a case-based approach—the adult patient.* Silver Spring, MD:ASPEN,2007.

36. **Calloway D, Spector H.** Nitrogen balance as related to caloric and protein intake in active young men. *Am J Clin Nutr* 1954;2:405–411.

37. Dietary Reference Intakes for Energy, Carbohydrate, Fat, Fatty Acids, Cholesterol, Protein, and Amino Acids (2002). Available at: http://www.nap.edu.

38. **Pillar B, Perry S.** Evaluating total parenteral nutrition: final report and statement of the Technology Assessment and Practice Guidelines Forum. *Nutrition* 1990;6:314–318.

39. **Klein S, Simes J, Blackburn GL.** Total parenteral nutrition and cancer clinical trials. *Cancer* 1986;58:1378–1386.

40. **Klein S, Koretz RL.** Nutrition support in patients with cancer: what do the data really show? *Nutr Clin Pract* 1994;9:91–100.

41. **Bethel RA, Jansen RD, Heymsfield SB, Nixon DW, Rudman D.** Nasogastric hyperalimentation through a polyethylene catheter: an alternative to central venous hyperalimentation. *Am J Clin Nutr* 1979;32:1112–1120.

42. **Voitk AJ, Echave V, Brown RA, Gund FN.** Use of elemental diet during the adaptive stage of short gut syndrome. *Gastroenterology* 1973;65:419–426.

43. **Iyer KR CT.** Complications of enteral access. *Gastrointest Endosc Clin N Am* 2007;17:717–729.

44. **Heymsfield SB, Bethel RA, Ansley JD, Nixon DW, Rudman D.** Enteral hyperalimentation: an alternative to central venous hyperalimentation. *Ann Intern Med* 1979;90:63–71.

45. **Feliciano DV, Mattox KL, Graham JM, Beall AC Jr, Jordan GL Jr.** Major complications of percutaneous subclavian vein catheters. *Am J Surg* 1979;138;869–874.

46. **Ryan JA Jr, Abel RM, Abbot WM, Hopkins CC, Chesney TM, Colley R, et al.** Catheter complications in total parenteral nutrition: a prospective study of 200 consecutive patients. *N Engl J Med* 1974;290:757–761.

47. **Covelli HD, Black JW, Olsen MS, Beekman JF.** Respiratory failure precipitated by high carbohydrate loads. *Ann Intern Med* 1981;95:579–581.

48. **O'Grady NP, Alexander M, Dellinger EP, Gerberding JL, Heard SO, Maki DG, et al.** Guidelines for the prevention of intravascular catheter-related infections. *Infect Control Hosp Epidemiol* 2002;23:759–769.

49. **Pappas PG, Rex JH, Sobel JD, Filler SG, Dismukes WE, Walsh TJ, et al., for the Infectious Diseases Society of America.** Guidelines for treatment of candidiasis. *Clin Infect Dis* 2004;38:161–189.

50. **Ryan JA.** Complications of total parenteral nutrition. In: **Fischer JE, ed.** *Total parenteral nutrition.* Boston: Little Brown, 1976:55.

51. **Ruberg RL, Allen TR, Goodman MJ, Long JM, Dudrick SJ.** Hypophosphatemia with hypophosphaturia in hyperalimentation. *Surg Forum* 1971;22:87–88.

52. **Fleming CR, McGill DB, Hoffman HN, Nelson RA.** Total parenteral nutrition. *Mayo Clin Proc* 1976;51:187–199.

53. **Fleming CR, Hodges RE, Hurley LS.** A prospective study of serum copper and zinc levels in patients receiving total parenteral nutrition. *Am J Clin Nutr* 1976;29:70–77.

54. **Chen WJ, Oashi E, Kasai M.** Amino acid metabolism in parenteral nutrition: with special reference to the calorie: nitrogen ratio and the blood urea nitrogen level. *Metabolism* 1974;23:1117–1123.

55. **Marinella MA.** Refeeding syndrome in cancer patients. *Int J Clin Pract* 2008;62:460–465.

56. **Goodgame JT, Lowry SF, Brennan MF.** Essential fatty acid deficiency in total parenteral nutrition: time course of development and suggestions for therapy. *Surgery* 1978;84:271–277.

57. **Blackburn GL, Wan JM, Teo TC, Georgieff M, Bistrian BR.** Metabolic support in organ failure. In: **Behari DJ, Cerra FB, eds.** *New horizons: multiple organ failure.* Fullerton, CA: Society of Critical Care Medicine, 1989:337–370.

58. **Cerra FB.** Hypermetabolism, organ failure, and metabolic support. *Surgery* 1987;101:1–14.

59. **Windmueller HG.** Glutamine utilization by the small intestine. *Adv Enzymol Relat Areas Mol Biol* 1982;53:201–237.

60. **Fox AD, Kripke SA, DePaula JA.** Glutamine supplemented diets prolong survival and decrease mortality in experimental enterocolitis. *JPEN J Parenter Enteral Nutr* 1988;12(suppl 1):8S.

61. **Klimberg VS, Souba WW, Salloum RM, Plumley DA, Cohen FS, Dolson DJ, et al.** Glutamine-enriched diets support muscle glutamine metabolism without stimulating tumor growth. *J Surg Res* 1990;48:319–323.

62. **Nuutinen LS, Kauppila, A, Ryhanen P, Niinimaki A, Kivinen S, Saarela M.** Intensified nutrition as an adjunct to cytotoxic chemotherapy in gynecological cancer patients. *Clin Oncol* 1982;8:107–112.

63. **Jones NE, Heyland DK.** Pharmaconutrition: a new emerging paradigm. *Curr Opin Gastroenterol* 2008;24:215–222.

20 Surgical Techniques

Jonathan S. Berek
Margrit Juretzka

In order to surgically manage gynecological malignancies, it is frequently necessary to perform surgical procedures beyond the genital tract. These include selected operations on the intestinal and urologic tracts and plastic reconstructive operations, including the creation of a neovagina. In addition, central venous access is frequently required for hyperalimentation or chemotherapy.

Responsibilities for these procedures vary from one center to another. In some centers, most or all of the operations are performed by the gynecologic oncologist, while in other centers, the emphasis is on the development of a multidisciplinary team with involvement of colorectal surgeons, urologists, plastic surgeons, and anesthesiologists. The surgical techniques for these nongynecologic procedures are presented in this chapter.

Central Lines

Central venous-access catheters are often necessary in the critically ill gynecologic oncology patient for either central venous pressure monitoring or centrally administered hyperalimentation or chemotherapy (1–4). The most frequently used veins are the subclavian and the jugular. **The brachial veins are used for peripherally inserted central catheters (PICC lines) (5).**

Subclavian Venous Catheter

Infraclavicular Technique   Although there are many different techniques for the insertion of a central venous catheter into the subclavian vein, the **infraclavicular technique** remains the one most commonly employed and the simplest. The subclavian vein lies immediately deep to the clavicle within the costoclavicular triangle, where the vein is more commonly approached from the right side (Fig. 20.1A). The **costoclavicular-scalene triangle** is bounded by the medial end of the clavicle anteriorly, the upper surface of the first rib posteriorly, and the anterior scalene muscle laterally (1). The anterior scalene muscle separates the subclavian vein anteriorly from the subclavian artery posteriorly. Just deep to the subclavian artery are the nerves of the brachial plexus. The subclavian vein is covered by the medial 5 cm of the clavicle. Just deep to the medial head of the clavicle, the right internal jugular vein joins the right subclavian vein to form the innominate vein, which then descends into the chest, where it joins the left innominate vein to form the superior vena cava in the retrosternal space.

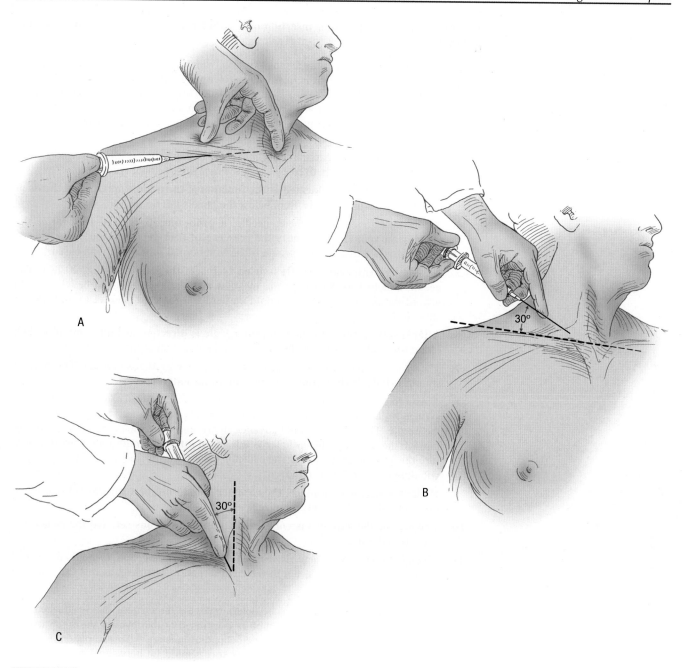

Figure 20.1   Central venous catheter insertion sites. The right subclavian and right internal jugular vein insertion sites are illustrated. The insertion sites for the subclavian venous catheter: **(A)** via the infraclavicular technique; **(B)** via the supraclavicular technique; **(C)** the site of insertion for the internal jugular vein. The needle is directed toward the suprasternal notch.

There are several other vital structures in the scalene triangle. The phrenic nerve courses anterior to the anterior scalene muscle and therefore lies immediately deep to the subclavian vein. If the deep wall of the vein is penetrated, the phrenic nerve can be injured. If the subclavian artery is penetrated, the brachial plexus, lying just deep to the vessel, can be injured. The right lymphatic duct and the thoracic duct on the left enter their respective subclavian veins near the junction with the internal jugular veins and therefore may be injured by a misplaced needle. The most common injury is to the pleura, the apex of which is just beneath the subclavian vein at the junction of the internal jugular vein.

741

The technique for infraclavicular insertion of a catheter into the right subclavian vein is as follows:

1. The patient is placed in the supine position, with the foot of the bed elevated about 1 foot so that **the patient is in the Trendelenburg position.** If possible, a bed that can be tilted into this position should be used. This position creates venous distention and increases the intraluminal pressure within the subclavian vein. The patient's head should be tilted away from the site of insertion so that the landmarks can be identified easily.

2. After careful skin preparation with *povidone–iodine* solution, **the skin and subjacent tissues are anesthetized** by means of *lidocaine* without *epinephrine.*

3. **The site of insertion is located at the junction of the middle and medial thirds of the clavicle,** approximately 1 cm below the bone's inferior margin.

4. Before insertion of the catheter needle, **a probe needle is used to localize the subclavian vein** and to identify the presence of dark venous blood. An 18-gauge needle attached to a 10-mL syringe filled with normal saline solution is used.

5. **A 14-gauge Intracath needle is used to insert the catheter** (Fig. 20.1A). The needle attached to the syringe is inserted into the skin with the bevel directed toward the heart. The needle should be held and directed parallel to the anterior chest wall.

6. **After insertion through the skin, the needle is directed medially and advanced along the undersurface of the clavicle** in the direction of the suprasternal notch.

7. The syringe is pulled gently to apply suction as the needle is inserted. **The patient should exhale during insertion to avoid an air embolus.**

8. After a free flow of blood has been obtained, the needle is held carefully in place, the syringe is detached, and the central venous catheter is advanced inside the lumen of the needle. The catheter should advance freely, and there should be blood returning through the catheter. **The catheter is advanced into the innominate vein and then into the superior vena cava.** The catheter should be aspirated, and if blood is easily withdrawn, the needle is removed.

9. **While the needle is in place, the catheter should not be withdrawn** because the tip can be sheared off and embolize.

10. **The end of the catheter is connected to an intravenous set,** and the catheter is sutured to the skin.

11. **The position of the catheter is verified by a chest radiograph.** It should be located in the superior vena cava, not in the right atrium or ventricle, as this can result in trauma to the heart.

If central venous pressure readings are to be determined, the intravenous line is attached to a manometer, and the base of the water column is positioned at the level of the right atrium, which is about 5 cm posterior to the fourth costochondral junction when the patient is in the supine position. **The normal central venous pressure should be between 5 and 12 cm of water.**

The complication rate for central venous catheter insertion through the subclavian route is about 1% to 2% (1–4). Most serious complications are related to puncture of the pleura and lung or perforation and laceration of vessels, resulting in a pneumothorax or hemothorax. **Catheter-related infection is seen in about 0.5% of patients, and the catheter should be removed if this source of infection is suspected.**

Supraclavicular Insertion   An alternative route of insertion into the subclavian vein is the supraclavicular route (Fig. 20.1B). Some prefer this to the infraclavicular route, but the morbidity of insertion is comparable with the two methods, and the preference is related to the technique that is most comfortable for the operator.

The technique for insertion is identical to that of the infraclavicular route, except that the needle is inserted above the clavicle, approximately 5 cm lateral to the midsternal notch. The angle of insertion is about 30 degrees from a line drawn between the two shoulders and directed caudally. The needle is aimed at the suprasternal notch.

Jugular Venous Catheterization

Another alternative for central venous access is the use of the jugular veins, either the internal or external vein. **Jugular venous catheterization is frequently the method of choice when the catheter is inserted intraoperatively and the catheter is to be used primarily for acute monitoring.** The advantage is that there is relatively easy access while the patient is anesthetized and draped for surgery, whereas the disadvantage is that it is more difficult to anchor the catheter because the neck is more mobile than the anterior chest wall. The location for the insertion site is illustrated in Fig. 20.1C.

The technique for insertion is as follows:

1. **The patient is placed in the Trendelenburg position.** With the patient's head turned away from the side of insertion, the needle is inserted just above the medial head of the clavicle between the medial and middle heads of the sternocleidomastoid muscle, where a small pocket is readily apparent and helps to localize the site for insertion.

2. **The angle of insertion is about 20 to 30 degrees from the sagittal median of the patient, and the direction is toward the heart.**

3. **As with subclavian catheterization, the use of a probe needle will help to localize the appropriate vessel.**

4. **The technique of catheter placement is the same as described above for the subclavian catheter.** However, the length of catheter that must be inserted is less, as the distance to the proper location in the superior vena cava is less.

5. **The position of the line inserted intraoperatively is checked with a chest radiograph** obtained in the recovery room if the catheter is to be left in place.

While individual studies have reported varying results, a meta-analysis of ultrasonic guidance for central venous cannulation reported a lower technical failure rate, reduction in the complication rate and faster access when using two dimensional ultrasonic guidance (5). The benefit was more significant for internal jugular versus subclavian venous catheterization.

External jugular catheters may also be used in patients who are under general anesthesia. Some patients have relatively prominent external jugular veins, and they are very easily catheterized. **The external jugular is not durable,** however, **and this route is not useful for central hyperalimentation.** The complication rate for jugular venous catheterization is essentially the same as that for the subclavian route.

Semipermanent Lines

The placement of semipermanent lines is useful in patients who require prolonged access to the central venous system, such as those with a chronic intestinal obstruction or fistula who are to receive hyperalimentation after discharge from the hospital (2).

Broviac, Hickman, and Quinton Catheters

The most common types of lines are catheters made of flexible, synthetic rubber (e.g., Broviac, Hickman, or Quinton catheters). The catheters are available in several sizes, although the adult type is used for most patients; the length is adapted by cutting the catheters as necessary. The catheters are available with either a single or double lumen. **The single-lumen catheters usually are sufficient for parenteral nutrition, whereas the double-lumen ones may be necessary for patients requiring frequent bolus medication, such as intravenous pain or antibiotic medications** (2,3).

The most common site for insertion of a semipermanent catheter is the right subclavian vein. The method of insertion is initially identical to the technique employed for the insertion of a temporary catheter, but an insertion cannula, called a Cook introducer, can simplify and facilitate insertion of the catheter (Fig. 20.2). It is preferable to insert the catheter under fluoroscopic guidance.

The technique is as follows:

1. After the patient has been properly positioned and the anterior chest and clavicular areas prepared, **the subclavian vein is identified in the manner described above.**

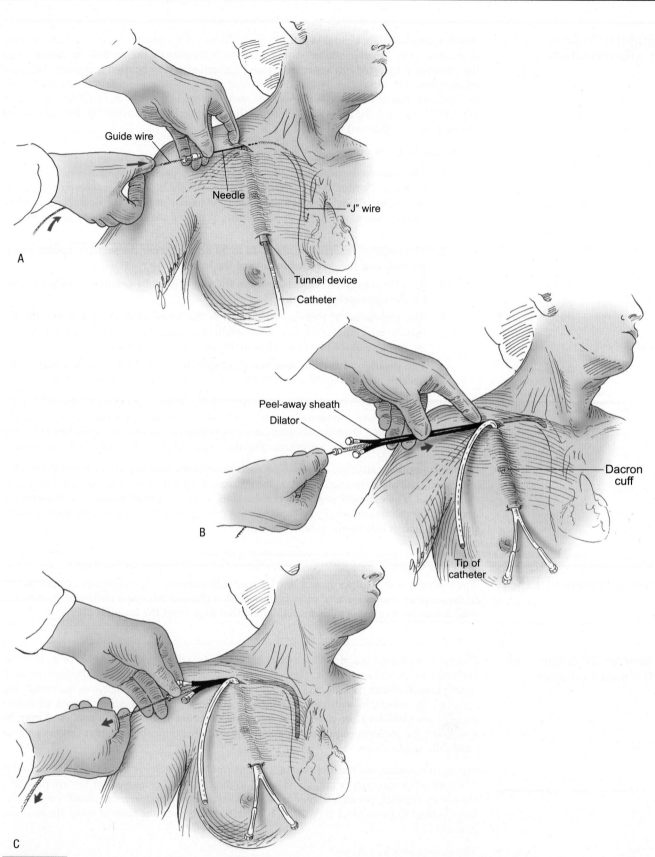

Figure 20.2 **Semipermanent catheter insertion.** The technique for insertion of the semipermanent (e.g., Hickman) catheter. **A:** A needle is inserted into the right subclavian vein, a guide wire is inserted through the needle, and the needle is withdrawn. **B:** The Cook introducer then is inserted over the guide wire. **C:** After the introducer with its outer sheath is in place in the right subclavian vein, the wire is withdrawn. *(Continued)*

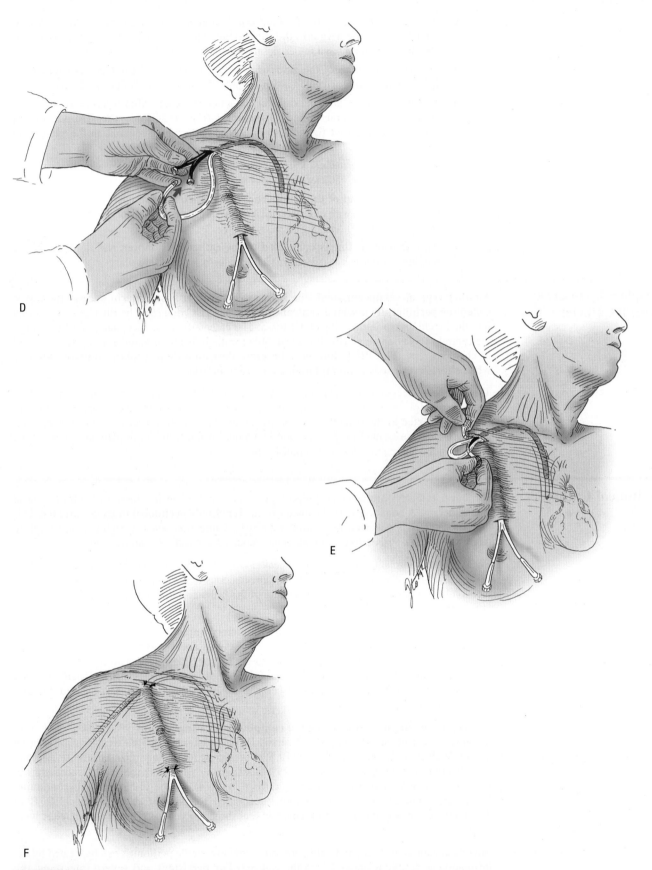

Figure 20.2   **D:** The central catheter of the Cook introducer is withdrawn, and the free end of the semipermanent catheter is inserted through the outer sheath. **E:** The outer sheath of the Cook introducer is peeled away. **F:** The semipermanent catheter is tunneled in the subcutaneous tissue under the skin of the right side of the chest, and the free end is exteriorized.

2. A premade kit is available for the Cook introducer. **An 18-gauge needle is used to introduce a guide wire into the subclavian vein, and the guide wire is passed into the superior vena cava** under fluoroscopy (Fig. 20.2A).

3. The proper position of the guide wire is documented, and **the Cook introducer is fed over the guide wire** and advanced into the subclavian vein (Fig. 20.2B).

4. The introducer has an inner catheter and an outer sheath. After insertion of the entire apparatus, the central cannula is removed (Fig. 20.2C) and **the semipermanent catheter is threaded through the outer sheath,** which remains in the subclavian vein (Fig. 20.2D).

5. After the semipermanent catheter has been inserted, **the outer sheath is peeled away,** leaving the catheter in place (Fig. 20.2E).

6. **The proximal end of the semipermanent catheter is tunneled under the skin** of the anterior chest wall **and exteriorized through a stab incision in the skin** as illustrated (Fig. 20.2F).

7. **An intravenous line is connected to the catheter's adapter,** and fluid is run into the line to establish its patency. The catheter is sutured into place.

Peripherally Inserted Central Catheter Lines

Another type of semipermanent line is inserted through a peripheral access site and is called the peripherally inserted central catheter or PICC line (6). The PICC line is inserted into the brachial vein in the antecubital fossa. The catheter is passed cephalad until it reaches the central subclavian vein. This line is suitable for the infusion of parenteral nutrition as well as chemotherapy. **The PICC line may be more desirable than a totally implantable line when short-term use is contemplated, e.g., 3 to 4 months.**

This approach is less durable than the centrally inserted catheters and somewhat more cumbersome because of the location of the insertion site. However, **its main advantage is that it can be easily inserted at the bedside.** Furthermore, it can be placed by a certified nurse or an intravenous technician trained in the insertion technique. Alternately, an implantable port can be inserted in the antecubital fossa by a physician.

Peritoneal Catheters

Peritoneal catheters are used in gynecologic oncology for the instillation of intraperitoneal chemotherapy. A commonly used catheter is the **Tenckhoff peritoneal dialysis catheter.** This dialysis catheter is designed to minimize the risk of infection, even though it is left in place many months (7). Alternatively, a Hickman venous access catheter can be used.

The catheter is implanted into the peritoneal cavity lateral to the midline laparotomy incision (Fig. 20.3). The catheter is tunneled in the subcutaneous tissue and brought out through a stab incision lateral to the fascial incision. The tip of the catheter in the peritoneal cavity is directed toward the pelvic cul-de-sac.

An alternative approach is the use of a completely implantable port which is attached directly to a fenestrated peritoneal catheter or venous access catheter. The port is inserted into the subcutaneous tissue and positioned in the left or right lower quadrant of the anterior abdomen, or over the lower anterior rib cage for ready access (Fig. 20.4). Both laparotomy and laparoscopy can be utilized for port placement. Postprocedure, the port is entered percutaneously with a 21-gauge needle.

The reported rate of catheter-related complications ranges from 3% to 34% (8–13). In the most recent phase III study of IP versus IV chemotherapy for the treatment of ovarian cancer, Walker et al. reported that 40 (19.5%) of 205 patients randomized to the IP arm had complications including infection ($n = 21$); blockage ($n = 10$); leakage ($n = 3$); access problems ($n = 5$); and vaginal leakage of fluid ($n = 1$) (8,14). Of the 119 patients discontinuing IP therapy, catheter-related complications accounted for 34% of cases (40 of 119). Both Tenckhoff or implantable ports with attached fenestrated or venous (Hickman) catheters were used.

Minor infections can be treated with antibiotics, and low-grade peritonitis can be treated by the instillation of antibiotics directly via the catheter. **For persistent and severe infections, the peritoneal catheter may require removal. In other studies, the most common problem associated with the catheters was blockage** (10,11), as there is no effective way to prevent

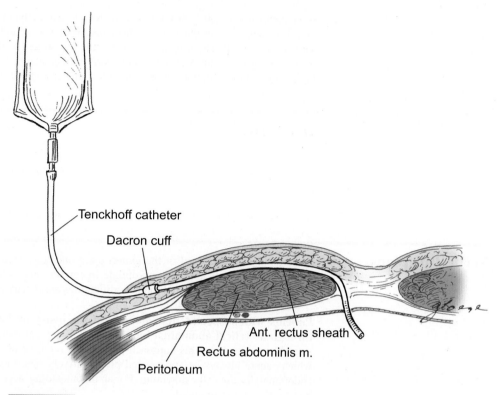

Figure 20.3 **Tenckhoff peritoneal catheter.** The placement of the Tenckhoff catheter into the peritoneal cavity is illustrated.

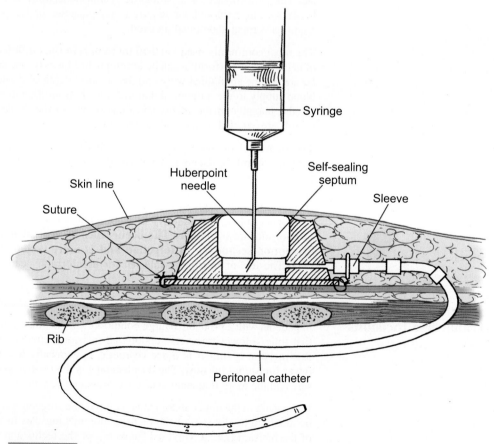

Figure 20.4 **Port-a-Cath peritoneal catheter.** The totally implantable peritoneal access catheter is tunneled through the subcutaneous tissues into the peritoneal cavity.

some deposition of fibrin around the catheter. Occasionally, this produces a "ball valve" effect; i.e., fluid will flow in but will not flow out. While some authors report higher fibrin sheath formation and adhesions in association with fenestrated catheters and dacron cuffs (15), a recent retrospective study of fenestrated peritoneal catheters reported that only 9 of 342 patients (3%) required discontinuation secondary to catheter complications (9).

Incisions

Particularly important in the operative plan for any patient is the determination of the type of incision to be made. The surgeon should have a general philosophy and *modus operandi* when planning the surgical procedure. There are certain incisions that are more appropriate in patients who are undergoing surgery for cancer rather than for benign conditions. In addition, special guidelines for the closure of incisions should be followed.

Vertical Incisions

Abdominal incisions used in the gynecologic oncology patient are most commonly vertical. Transverse incisions are also appropriate in certain circumstances. The indications and techniques for these incisions and their modifications are discussed.

Patients with suspected malignancies of the ovary or fallopian tube are best explored through a vertical abdominal incision. With a vertical incision, the patient's disease can be staged properly. Also, this approach permits the removal of any upper abdominal metastases, which cannot always be appreciated preoperatively. The most likely site of resectable upper abdominal disease is the omentum. For an omentectomy, access to the region of the splenic and hepatic flexures is required.

A vertical incision is also necessary in patients being explored for intestinal obstruction or fistulae. The performance of a paraaortic lymphadenectomy is facilitated by a vertical incision. Patients being explored for recurrent malignancies or for possible pelvic exenteration also require a vertical abdominal incision.

The most commonly used vertical incision is in the midline. This incision has the advantage of being easy to perform; it can be accomplished quickly, because the midline is the least vascular area of the abdominal wall, and the smallest depth of tissue must be divided. The principal blood supply to the anterior abdominal wall is from the inferior epigastric vessels, which are located laterally in the rectus sheath posterior to the rectus abdominis muscles, and these vessels are avoided by the mid-line incision.

The principal problem associated with the midline incision is that it has the highest rate of wound dehiscence when compared with all other incisions. The wound disruption rate is about 0.1% to 0.65% (16–21), although this rate may be higher in patients with cancer, particularly those with ascites and malnutrition, or those needing postoperative radiation. Dehiscence rates as high as 2% to 3% have been reported in obese, diabetic patients with cancer (18). The majority of wound dehiscences are associated with wound infection or poor closure technique. **The occurrence of ventral hernia is associated with wound disruption secondary to infection and is more common in patients with malignancy** (21). The use of prosthetic meshes for herniorraphy can significantly reduce the rate of recurrence of hernia.

Transverse Incisions

In patients with a probable benign condition who are undergoing abdominal exploration for the first time, a lower transverse abdominal incision is frequently employed. **The advantage of this incision is that it is more cosmetic, is generally less painful, and is associated with fewer incisional hernias.** The disadvantage is the relative problem of upper abdominal exposure and the more frequent occurrence of wound hematomas.

If exposure to the upper abdomen is required, the surgeon has several choices. The incision can be modified by division of the rectus abdominis muscles in a transverse direction at the level of the incision (i.e., **a Maylard incision**), or the rectus abdominis muscles may be detached from the symphysis pubis (i.e., **the Cherney incision**). After division or mobilization of the rectus muscles, the inferior epigastric vessels are ligated bilaterally and, if necessary, the incision is further extended laterally by incising (with the diathermy) the "strap" muscles of the anterior abdominal wall. The conversion of the incision to a Maylard or a Cherney incision always provides considerably more exposure in the pelvis and low paraaortic area.

If better access to the upper abdomen is required, the incision can be modified further by extending the incision cephalad to form a **"J,"** a reverse **"J,"** or **a "hockey stick" incision.** In general, any of these techniques is preferable to the making of a second incision, i.e., a midline incision coincident with the transverse incision, a so-called **"T"** incision. The principal difficulty with the latter approach is the weakness of the incision at the point of intersection of the two incisions.

In patients undergoing radical hysterectomy and pelvic lymphadenectomy for early-stage cervical cancer, a lower abdominal transverse incision is acceptable.

Incisional Closure

Of primary importance is the technique of incisional closure (16–21). The closure can be accomplished by closing the peritoneum, fascia, subcutaneous tissue, and skin individually, or a bulk closure can be performed that incorporates the peritoneum and the fascia together. **This bulk closure or internal retention suture, the "Smead-Jones" closure, is the strongest closure technique** (16). Mass closure with a continuous, single strand of polyglyconate monofilament absorbable suture (*Maxon*) or polydioxanone (*PDS*) has been shown to be an effective, safe alternative to the use of interrupted sutures, even in vertical midline incisions (22–27).

Internal Retention Suture

The Smead-Jones, or internal retention, technique uses interrupted sutures that are placed as illustrated in Fig. 20.5. The sutures are placed in a far-far, near-near distribution, which is a modified figure-of-eight. The first suture is placed through the anterior fascia, rectus muscle, posterior fascia, and peritoneum and the second through the anterior fascial layer only. The key

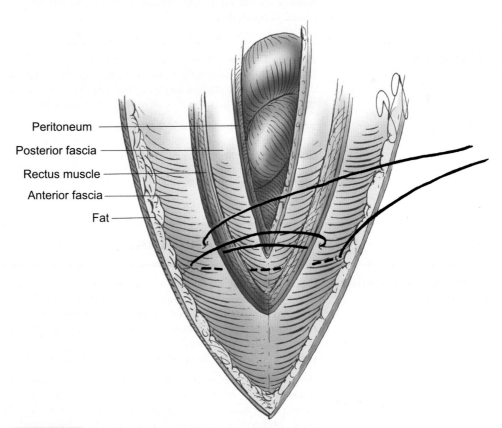

Peritoneum
Posterior fascia
Rectus muscle
Anterior fascia
Fat

Figure 20.5   Internal retention abdominal closure. The "Smead-Jones" far-far, near-near closure.

is to place the sutures at least 1.5 to 2.0 cm from the fascial edge and not more than 1 cm apart (16). **The disruption rate for midline incisions closed with this technique should be less than 0.2%.**

Suture Material

The choice of suture should be dictated by the circumstances (13–18). If there is evidence of significant infection, as with an abscess or an intestinal injury, a monofilament, nonabsorbable suture is most appropriate. The most frequently used substances are nylon sutures, such as *Prolene.*

For vertical incisions, an absorbable, long-lasting synthetic suture offers the best combination of strength, durability, and ease of use. Most suitable is either monofilament polyglyconate suture (*Maxon*) or monofilament polydioxanone (*PDS*) (24). Braided, polyglycolic acid (*PGA*) suture, such as *Vicryl* or *Dexon,* is suitable for transverse incisions. A grade 0 or 1 suture is necessary to provide a suitably strong closure. The tissue reactivity to these synthetic materials is less than that of chromic catgut. Nonabsorbable polyfilament materials, such as cotton and silk, are not used for incisional closure because of the higher potential for "stitch abscess" formation (27).

External Retention Suture

Retention sutures that are external can be used to prevent evisceration in patients who are at high risk of this potentially catastrophic occurrence. **The routine use of internal retention sutures has reduced the need for the external retention sutures.** However, in patients who are morbidly obese, patients who have a major wound infection, and patients whose incisions have eviscerated in the past, the addition of external retention sutures may be indicated. These sutures are placed in a manner similar to internal retention sutures, i.e., far-far, near-near, with the far sutures also placed through the skin so that the retention sutures are knotted externally. **The preferable suture material for this closure is nylon.** The external retention sutures are inserted through a rubber "bolster" that helps to protect the skin from injury from the suture. Sutures are placed at approximately 2 to 3 cm intervals, and interrupted fascial sutures are placed between them.

Skin Closure

Primary Closure   Skin closure of vertical incisions in cancer patients generally should be interrupted, generally with metal skin clips. Subcuticular closures are not appropriate in most circumstances for vertical incisions, but they are quite cosmetic and acceptable for small transverse incisions where the risk of wound infection is low.

Secondary Closure   A delayed or secondary skin closure is useful in patients whose incisions are infected, that is, after the drainage of an intraabdominal abscess or repair of an intestinal fistula. This is achieved by placement of interrupted mattress sutures in the skin, which are not tied, so that the skin remains unapproximated. Thus the skin can be closed later, usually after 3 to 4 days, when the infection is under control.

Intestinal Operations

Preoperative Intestinal Preparation

If bowel resection is planned or contemplated, a mechanical and antibiotic "bowel preparation" may be undertaken preoperatively. **If the intestine is prepared properly, the segment is well vascularized, and there is no sepsis, prior irradiation, or evidence of tumor at the site of anastomosis, colonic reanastomosis can be accomplished without leakage in 98% of the cases** (25). More proximal resection of the small intestine can be performed without a bowel preparation, because this portion of the intestine does not contain bacteria.

An effective protocol for bowel preparation is presented in Table 20.1. Recently, the FDA issued a Safety Alert discussing the risk of acute phosphate nephropathy, a rare type of renal failure associated with oral sodium phosphate bowel cleansing which may lead to permanent renal impairment. Increased risk has been associated with multiple factors including advanced age, kidney disease, and use of medications affecting renal perfusion and function. In response, over-the-counter oral sodium phosphate preparations such as *Fleet® Phospho-*

Table 20.1 Intestinal Preparation	
Preoperative Day 2	Clear liquid diet
Preoperative Day 1	Clear liquid diet
	Mechanical Prep
	Magnesium Citrate (one bottle of laxative 4 pm.)
	Fleet enemas until no solid stool in p.m. (Optional)
Day of Surgery	Fleet enemas until clear (Optional)

soda have been recalled. Bowel preparation regimens should be individualized for patients after assessment of risk factors. Alternative bowel preparation regimens include magnesium citrate and *Golytely*.

There is controversy regarding the use of bowel preparations in general as well as the optimal "bowel prep," as it is uncertain whether, in addition to the mechanical preparation, the antibiotic preparation is necessary (28). Several meta-analyses of patients undergoing elective colorectal procedures have found either no difference or increased rates of anastomotic leakage and wound infection when prophylactic mechanical bowel preparation is used (29–31). However, bowel resections for gynecologic malignancies are performed in a different patient population, often in the presence of ascites, extensive carcinomatosis, and multiple sites of bowel involvement. Lacking studies in the gynecologic oncology population, the use of mechanical bowel preparation and antibiotics are predominantly determined by surgeon preference. Before laparotomy for small intestinal obstruction caused by ovarian cancer, it is useful to insert a nasogastric (NG) tube for 24 to 48 hours preoperatively to avoid the possibility of vomiting and aspiration (32).

Minor Intestinal Operations

The most common intestinal operations are lysis of adhesions, repair of an enterotomy, and creation of an intestinal stoma.

Repair of Enterotomy

Intestinal enterotomy is a common inadvertent occurrence in abdominal surgery, and it can occur in the most experienced hands. Factors that predispose to serosal and mucosal injury include extensive adhesions, intraabdominal carcinomatosis, radiation therapy, chemotherapy, prior abdominal surgery, and peritonitis.

An enterotomy usually does not cause any problems, provided it is identified and repaired. **Any defect should be repaired when it occurs or marked with a long stitch so that it will not be overlooked later.** At the completion of any intraabdominal exploration necessitating significant lysis of adhesions, the surgeon must "run the bowel," carefully inspecting it to exclude either a serosal injury or an enterotomy.

Serosal defects through which the intestinal mucosa can be seen must be repaired. Less complete defects must be repaired in all patients who have had radiation treatment to the abdomen. When in doubt, the defect should be repaired to minimize the risk of intestinal breakdown, peritonitis, abscess, and fistula.

When there is an enterotomy, the repair should be made with interrupted 3-0 or 4-0 sutures on a gastrointestinal needle, placed at 2- to 3-mm intervals along the defect. The suture materials most commonly employed for this purpose are silk or PGA (*Vicryl* or *Dexon*). **The direction of closure should be perpendicular to the lumen of the bowel to minimize the potential for lumenal stricture** (Fig. 20.6).

With small defects (i.e., <5–6 mm), the closure can be accomplished with a single layer of sutures passed through both the serosa and the mucosa. However, it is preferable to close more extensive defects in two layers: an inner full-thickness layer covered with an outer

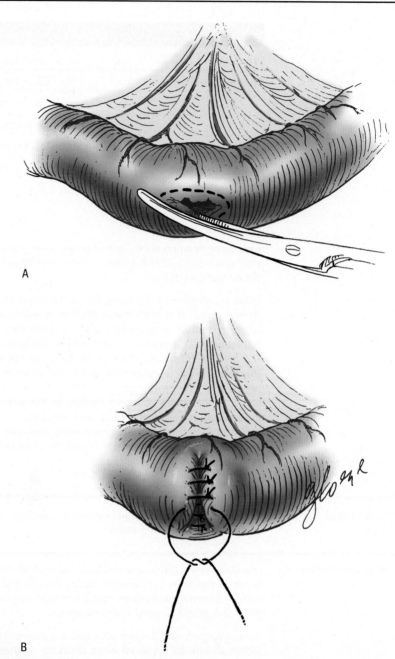

Figure 20.6 **Closure of an intestinal enterotomy. A:** The edges of the enterotomy are trimmed. **B:** The enterotomy is closed perpendicular to the lumen in two layers.

seromuscular layer. Care should be taken to approximate the tissues carefully without cutting through the fragile serosa.

Gastrostomy

A gastrostomy may be necessary in patients with chronic intestinal obstruction, usually from terminal ovarian cancer. It is particularly useful in those who require prolonged intestinal intubation and in whom the underlying intestinal blockage cannot be relieved adequately. This procedure may permit the removal of an uncomfortable nasogastric tube that is irritating to the nasopharynx. The two most common procedures are the Witzel and the Stamm gastrostomies (32).

Stamm Gastrostomy   The simplest technique is the Stamm gastrostomy, in which a small incision is made in the inferior anterior gastric wall. A Foley catheter with a 30-mL balloon is brought into the peritoneal cavity through a separate stab incision in the left upper outer quadrant of the abdomen. Two or three successive pursestring sutures, with 2-0 absorbable suture material, are used to invert the stomach around the tube. Interrupted 2-0 silk or PGA sutures are placed in the serosa, and the same material is used to suture the serosa to the peritoneum, approximating the gastric wall to the anterior abdominal wall in an effort to prevent leakage.

Witzel Gastrostomy   The Witzel technique is similar, but the catheter is tunneled within the gastric wall for several centimeters with Lembert sutures of 2-0 silk or PGA. This technique results in a serosal tunnel that may further reduce the risk of leakage. **The most important step in preventing gastrostomy leakage is approximation of the gastric serosa to the anterior abdominal wall.**

Percutaneous Gastrostomy   Another technique for gastrostomy in patients not otherwise undergoing laparotomy is the percutaneous placement of a catheter into the stomach. This method involves the initial passage of a gastroscope. The site for catheter insertion is illuminated by a fiberoptic light source through the gastroscope, and the catheter is introduced into the stomach percutaneously.

Cecostomy

The performance of a cecostomy may be useful in the occasional patient who has an obstruction of the colon and a grossly dilated cecum and in whom a simple palliative measure to relieve the obstruction is indicated. A more definitive procedure for relief of the obstruction may be appropriate when the patient's condition is more stable.

The cecostomy is performed by placement of a Foley catheter into the dilated portion of the cecum. The tube is sutured into place by the technique employed for a Stamm gastrostomy. The tube is exteriorized through a stab incision in the right lower quadrant of the abdomen and attached to gravity drainage.

Colostomy

Colostomies may be temporary or permanent. **A temporary colostomy may be indicated for "protection" of a colonic reanastomosis** in patients who have had prior radiation therapy or to palliate severe radiation proctitis and bleeding. It is indicated also in patients who have a large bowel fistula (e.g., rectovaginal fistula) to allow the inflammation to subside before definitive repair. **A permanent colostomy is indicated in patients who have an irreparable fistula or a colonic obstruction from a pelvic tumor that cannot be resected. A permanent colostomy is also indicated in patients undergoing total pelvic exenteration,** unless the distal rectum can be preserved and the colon reanastomosed, and in those who require anoproctectomy because of advanced vulvar cancer.

The site of the colostomy should be selected so that the stomal appliance and bag can be applied to the skin of the anterior abdominal wall without difficulty. The best site is approximately midway between the umbilicus and the anterior iliac crest. The most distal site possible should be employed in the large intestine. After selection of the stomal site, a circular skin incision is made to accommodate two fingers. The subcutaneous tissue is removed, and the fascia of the rectus sheath is incised similarly (Fig. 20.7). The end of the colon is brought through the stoma and sutured to fascia with interrupted 2-0 silk or PGA suture, and the stoma is everted to the skin to form a "rosebud" with the use of interrupted 2-0 or 3-0 absorbable braided suture.

Temporary

For patients who require temporary diversion, a transverse or sigmoid colostomy is usually created. The most distal portion of the colon should be used to allow the most formed stool possible. **A loop colostomy is usually created:** A loop of the colon is brought out through an appropriately placed separate incision in the abdominal wall. The loop is maintained by suturing it to the fascia beneath it. It can be reinforced with a rod of glass or plastic passed through a hole in the mesentery. The stoma can be opened immediately by means of an incision along the taenia coli in the longitudinal direction. Alternatively, the loop may be "matured" 1 to 2 days later to minimize the risk of sepsis if the bowel is unprepared.

The colon can be brought out as an end colostomy, which requires transection of the colon. This can be readily accomplished by means of a gastrointestinal anastomosis (GIA) stapler, which closes and transects the colon simultaneously. The distal end is sutured to the fascia, and

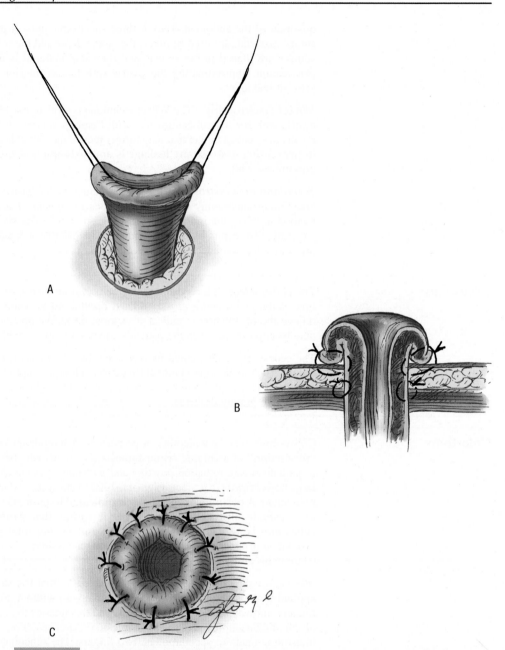

Figure 20.7 **The formation of a colostomy. A:** The end of the colon is brought through the abdominal wall. **B:** It is sutured to the fascia and skin. **C:** The "rosebud" stoma is formed.

the proximal end is brought out as the colostomy. If the distal colon must also be diverted (because of distal obstruction), a double-barrel colostomy can be created.

Permanent

A permanent colostomy is an end or terminal colostomy, performed as far distally as possible to allow the maximum amount of fluid reabsorption. The distal loop of the transected colon may be oversewn to create a **Hartman's pouch** if there is no distal obstruction. In patients in whom there is complete distal obstruction, a **mucous fistula** should be created.

| Enterostomy | If the colon is surgically inaccessible because of extensive carcinomatosis or radiation-induced adhesions, it may become necessary to palliate the bowel obstruction by the creation of a small intestinal stoma. Because the small-bowel contents are loose and irritating compared with colonic contents, **an ileostomy or a jejunostomy should be undertaken only when absolutely necessary.** |

Major Intestinal Operations

Intestinal Resection and Reanastomosis

After a segment of bowel, along with its wedge-shaped section of mesentery, has been resected, a reanastomosis may be performed (32–37). The most commonly used technique for reanastomosis is the **end-to-end anastomosis,** which is performed as either an open two-layered closure or a closed one-layered anastomosis. An **end-to-side anastomosis** may be used to create a J-pouch, i.e., a segment of bowel created to improve low colonic continence (38–49). A **side-to-side anastomosis** may be useful to increase the size of the lumen at the site of anastomosis. Increasingly, the use of surgical stapling devices has permitted more rapid performance of the reanastomosis, which is particularly useful when more than one resection is being carried out or when the duration of the procedure is of major concern.

Hand-Sewn Anastomosis

End-to-End Enteroenterostomy

When the reanastomosis is to be hand sewn, the proximal and distal ends are clamped with Bainbridge clamps (Fig. 20.8A), and the posterior interrupted, seromuscular **Lembert stitches** are placed with 3-0 silk or PGA sutures (*Vicryl* or *Dexon*) (Fig. 20.8B). The clamps are removed, the devitalized ends are trimmed, and an inner continuous full-thickness layer of 3-0 silk or PGA suture is placed to complete the posterior portion of the anastomosis. After the corner is reached, the needle is brought through the wall to the outside, and the continuous layer is completed anteriorly with a **Connell stitch** (outside-in, inside-out) to complete the inner layer (Fig. 20.8C). The anterior seromuscular layer is then placed with interrupted 3-0 silk or PGA sutures (Fig. 20.8D). The defect in the intestinal mesentery is repaired.

A single-layered closed technique is occasionally used for colonic reanastomosis in obstructed, unprepared bowel in an effort to minimize peritoneal contamination. In these circumstances, however, the use of the surgical staplers is now recommended (36).

Side-to-Side Enteroenterostomy

The side-to-side anastomosis is particularly useful in patients who are undergoing intestinal bypass rather than resection to palliate bowel obstruction, e.g., in patients with unresectable or recurrent tumor. The loops of intestine are aligned side to side, and linen-shod clamps are applied to prevent spillage of intestinal contents. A posterior row of 3-0 silk or PGA sutures is placed with interrupted Lembert sutures, and the lumina are created. An inner layer of continuous, full-thickness 3-0 PGA sutures is placed and continued anteriorly to complete the layer with a Connell stitch. The anastomosis is completed by placement of an anterior seromuscular layer with the use of interrupted 3-0 silk or PGA sutures.

Intestinal Staplers

The principal advantage of the gastrointestinal staplers is the speed with which they can be employed. There is no increase in the complication rate with the use of staplers as compared with hand-sewn anastomoses (32–37). The staplers are especially useful in facilitating reanastomosis after low resection of the rectosigmoid colon, because a hand-sewn anastomosis is technically difficult when performed deep in the pelvis. A disadvantage of the staplers is their increased cost, and staplers are difficult to use when the intestinal tissues are very edematous.

Types of Stapling Devices

The staplers are available in either reusable metal devices or in single-use disposable devices (Fig. 20.9A–C).

Thoracoabdominal Stapler   The thoracoabdominal (TA) stapler comes in several sizes, the TA-30, TA-55, TA-60, and TA-90, corresponding to the length, in millimeters, of the row of staples. Individual staples are either 3.5 or 4.8 mm long. The TA closes the lumen in an everting fashion. A TA device is available with a flexible, rotating end, called a Roticulator-55 that can be adjusted for placement into narrow areas (e.g., the deep pelvis).

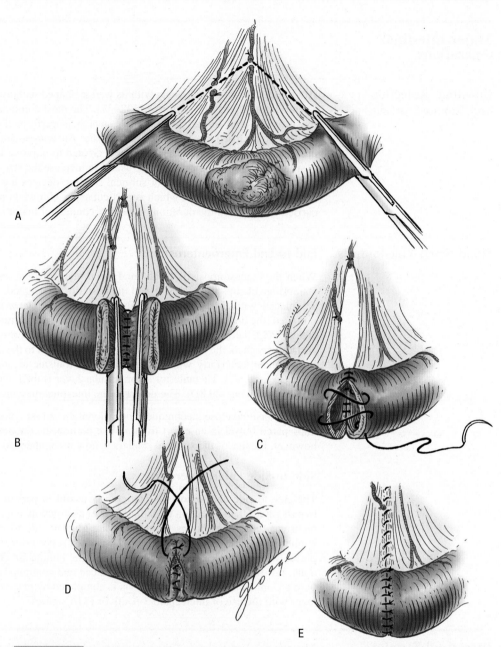

Figure 20.8 **Hand-sewn end-to-end enteroenterostomy. A:** The tumor and bowel are resected along with the mesentery. **B:** The posterior seromuscular layer is sutured. **C:** The Connell stitch is placed. **D:** The anterior seromuscular layer is placed. **E:** The completed anastomosis.

Gastrointestinal Anastomosis Stapler   The gastrointestinal anastomosis (GIA) device places two double rows of staples and then cuts the tissue between the two rows.

End-to-End Anastomosis Stapler   The end-to-end anastomosis (EEA) stapler is used primarily to approximate two ends of the colon, especially to facilitate the reanastomosis of the lower colon after pelvic exenteration or resection of pelvic disease in patients with ovarian cancer. The stapler places a double row of staples, approximates the two ends of the intestine, and cuts the devitalized tissue inside the staple line. It is available in diameters of 21, 25, 28, 31, and 35 mm, and a metal sizing device is used to measure the diameter of the intestinal lumen (37).

Intraluminal Stapler   The intraluminal stapler (ILS) is a disposable EEA stapler that has a detachable anvil. This removable feature can facilitate the placement of the anvil into a portion of one intestine that is difficult to mobilize. The anvil can be reattached to the rod of the ILS device after it has been placed in the anastomosis.

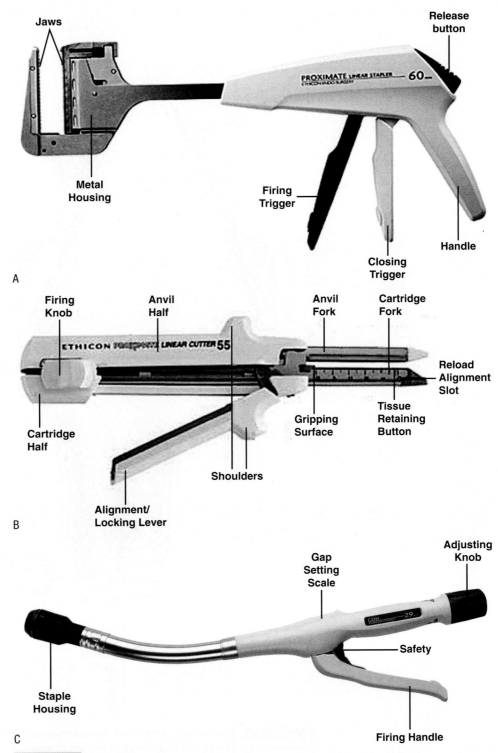

Figure 20.9 **Stapling devices for intestinal anastomosis.** The single-use staplers: (**A**) thoracoabdominal (TA); (**B**) gastrointestinal anastomosis (GIA); (**C**) end-to-end anastomosis (EEA).

Stapling Technique

Functional End-to-End Enteroenterostomy Anastomosis

This operation is illustrated in Fig. 20.10. The GIA stapler is used to staple and divide each end of the bowel segment to be resected. The antimesenteric borders of the bowel loops are approximated, and the corners are resected. A fork of the GIA device is inserted into each bowel lumen, and after alignment, the stapler is fired. The defect where the stapler was introduced then is closed with a TA stapler.

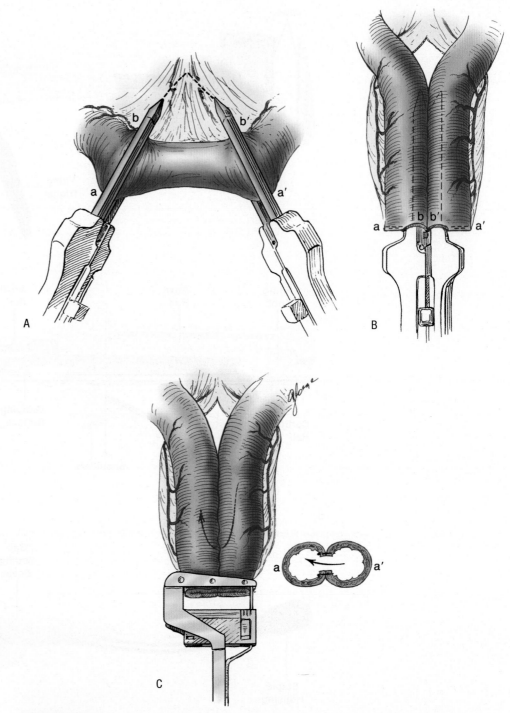

Figure 20.10 **Functional end-to-end anastomosis using the stapling technique. A:** The gastrointestinal anastomosis (GIA) stapler is used to resect the intestine. **B:** The segments of the transected intestine are placed side to side, and each antimesenteric corner is incised to create two holes into which the two forks of a second GIA stapler are placed. The GIA stapler is fired to create the new intestinal lumen. **C:** The thoracoabdominal (TA) stapler is placed over the end and "fired" to close the remaining defect. Note the cross section at a-a'.

Side-to-Side Enteroenterostomy Anastomosis

When a bypass enteroenterostomy is performed, the two loops of bowel to be anastomosed side to side are aligned, an enterotomy is created in each loop, and a fork of the GIA stapler is slid into each lumen, fired, and removed. This creates the lumen between the two bowel segments, and the enterotomy that is left when the instrument is withdrawn is then approximated with a TA stapler.

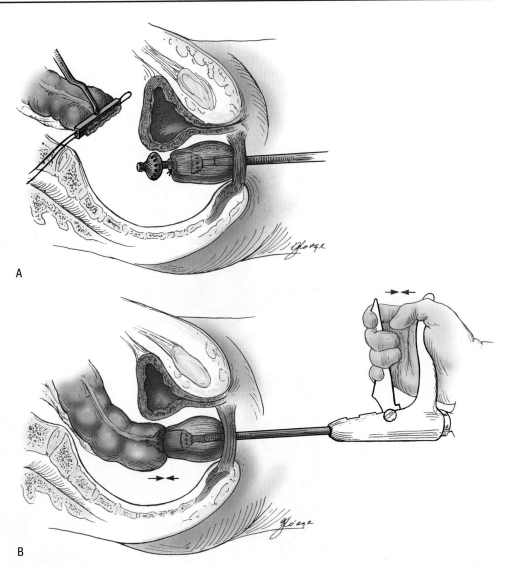

A

B

Figure 20.11   **Low colonic end-to-end anastomosis using the end-to-end anastomosis (EEA) stapler. A:** After resection of the rectosigmoid colon, the distal end of the descending colon is mobilized and a pursestring suture is placed by hand or with a special instrument (illustrated). A pursestring suture is also placed around the rectal stump. The open end of the EEA stapler is inserted through the anus, and the rectal pursestring is tied around the instrument. The end of the descending colon is placed over the end of the EEA, and the second pursestring is tied. **B:** The EEA device is closed and "fired."

Low Colonic End-to-End Anastomosis

A low colonic resection is performed by isolating and removing the portion of the rectosigmoid colon involved with disease. The EEA stapler is inserted through the anus and advanced to the site of the anastomosis. The instrument is opened to allow the anvil to accommodate the proximal colon, which is mobilized and tied over the distal end of the EEA. The distal colon is likewise tied over the EEA with a pursestring suture (Fig. 20.11). The EEA is then closed, approximating the two ends of the colon, and the instrument is fired and removed. A reinforcing layer of interrupted 3-0 silk or *Vicryl* Lembert sutures is placed anteriorly. The anastomosis is palpated to confirm that it is intact. Also, the pelvis can be filled with saline solution, and air can be insufflated through the rectum to search for bubbles, which would indicate a defect in the anastomosis (32).

Low Colonic End-to-Side Anastomosis: J-Pouch

An alternative end-to-side (functional end-to-end) low colonic anastomosis can be performed with the use of one of the newer disposable stapling devices, which has a removable distal one-piece anvil: the intraluminal stapler. In this manner, a J-pouch can be created, which has the potential to improve the continence of patients (Fig. 20.12A–D). **Studies comparing the colonic J-pouch with the direct end-to-end anastomosis have suggested that there is a lower**

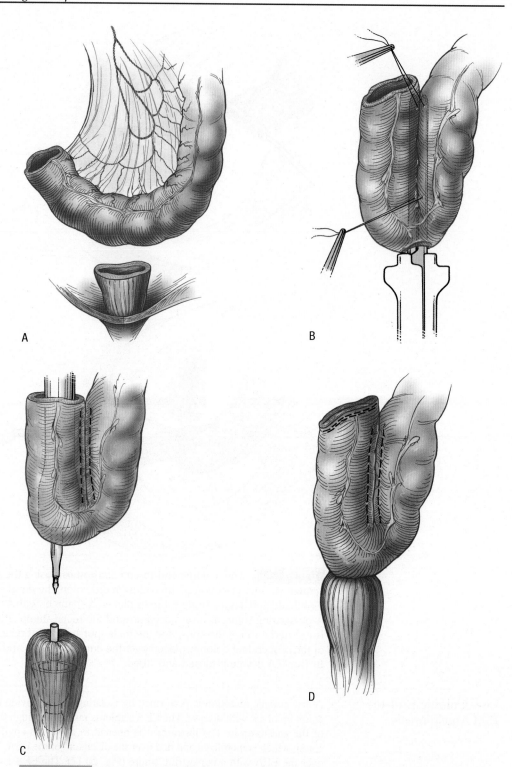

Figure 20.12   **Low colonic end-to-side anastomosis (EEA) to create a J-pouch. A:** The end-to-side anastomosis allows the mesocolon to be preserved and to cover the sacral hollow. **B:** The terminal end of the colon has the J-pouch created by stapling a loop side-to-side using a gastrointestinal anastomosis (GIA) stapler. **C:** The EEA device is then used to anastomose the rectal stump end-to-side with the pouch. **D:** The end of the pouch is stapled closed with a GIA or thoracoabdominal (TA) stapler.

leak rate, better continence rate, fewer stools per day, and better control of urgency and flatus (34,48). The problem with this approach is that some patients have more difficulty emptying the pouch, a problem that can be minimized by limiting the size of the pouch to about 5 centimeters in length (40).

The J-pouch is created by first folding the distal colon onto itself and stapling side to side with a GIA stapler (Fig. 20.12A). The pouch is then anastomosed to the rectal stump using an end-to-side technique with an EEA stapler (Fig. 20.12B) and by detaching the anvil, which is inserted in the proximal colon segment. The center rod of the open EEA instrument without the anvil is inserted through an opening in the bowel or through the anus (Fig. 20.12C). Then the rod is inserted through or near the staple line. In the other segment of bowel, a pursestring suture is placed, and the free anvil is inserted within the lumen of the bowel within the pursestring suture. The anvil is then screwed onto the rod, the device is closed, and the anastomosis is created (Fig. 20.12D).

Low Colonic Side-to-Side Anastomosis	An alternative side-to-side technique (functional end-to-end) anastomosis of the rectosigmoid colon can be used when the portion of removed bowel is proximal enough to permit this operation (i.e., 10 to 15 cm of preserved rectum). The GIA instrument is used to perform the colorectal anastomosis. After the segment of colon to be resected is mobilized, the proximal colon to be reanastomosed is closed with either the GIA or the TA-55 instrument. A stab wound is made in the antimesenteric border of the colon about 5 cm proximal to the staple line closure. A corresponding stab wound is made in the left anterolateral wall of the rectum at the proximal point of the planned site of anastomosis. The proximal colon is placed into the retrorectal space, side to side along the rectum; the GIA device is placed into the proximal and distal segments; and the instrument is closed and fired. The remaining single defect is closed with either a hand-sewn, double layer of 3-0 sutures or the rotating TA-55 device (Roticulator-55).
Low Colonic Coloplasty	A newer form of colorectal anastomosis is the coloplasty (see Chapter 22), which may have advantages over the colonic J-pouch for patients undergoing pelvic exenteration. The principal advantage is that this technique may be easier to perform in a narrow pelvis, such as in those patients undergoing a pelvic exenteration and simultaneous creation of a neovagina. In a randomized study of the three techniques, patients undergoing the coloplasty and colonic J-pouch had significantly more favorable compliance, reservoir volume, and fewer bowel movements per day than those having a straight anastomosis (49). The technique of coloplasty (Fig. 20.13) is illustrated. The lower part of the proximal colon is incised longitudinally and then reapproximated in the transverse direction (Fig. 20.13A). In this manner, a small, simple reservoir is created. The EEA stapler is used and then closed to create the anastomosis just as with the other techniques outlined above (Fig. 20.13B).
Postoperative Care	Historically, after resection of the small bowel, a nasogastric tube was usually placed for about 24 to 48 hours to reduce the volume of intestinal secretions that must pass through the site of anastomosis. However, numerous studies including a recent meta-analysis of 33 studies with 5,240 patients undergoing open abdominal procedures (including 14 studies of gastroduodenal or colorectal procedures) have demonstrated that prophylactic nasogastric decompression is associated with a slower return to bowel function and increased pulmonary complications, with no difference in anastomotic leaks (50,51). While prophylactic nasogastric decompression is often not indicated, it remains integral to the management of small bowel obstruction. Postoperative use is individualized based on preoperative diagnosis and intra-operative assessment. In patients who have received pelvic or abdominal irradiation, the upper intestinal tract may remain intubated until bowel function has returned, as signified by the passage of flatus or stool. Oral feeding can begin as patients develop an appetite, and **early feeding has been shown to be safe following both small and large bowel resection** (52–54). In patients who have undergone colonic resection and reanastomosis, enemas and cathartics should be avoided (49). Intravenous fluids must be continued while the patient is receiving nil by mouth. In patients whose recovery is likely to be prolonged beyond 7 days, such as those who have previously received whole-abdominal irradiation, consideration should be given to the use of parenteral nutrition, as discussed in Chapter 19. In such patients, a gastrostomy tube may be useful to avoid prolonged nasogastric intubation.

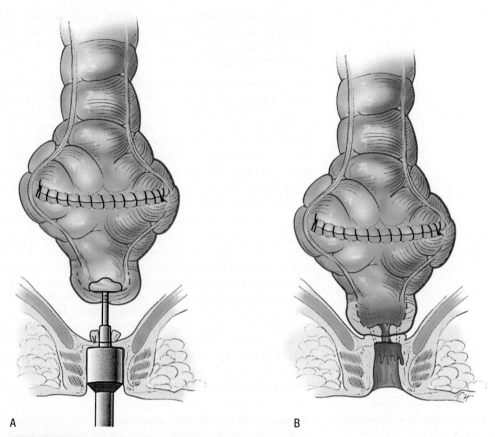

A   B

Figure 20.13   Low colonic coloplasty. A: The distal colon is incised in the longitudinal direction and resutured in the transverse direction to create a widening of the portion of the colon to be anastomosed to the rectum. **B:** The rectum is anastomosed to the distal colon using the end-to-end anastomosis (EEA) stapler.

Urinary Tract Operations

The preoperative evaluation of the urinary tract is important in patients with gynecologic malignancies because of the frequent involvement of the urinary organs, especially the bladder and the distal ureters (55–58). Renal function and ureteric patency must be assessed preoperatively.

Cystoscopy

Cystoscopy should be performed as part of the staging for cervical and vaginal cancers unless the disease has been diagnosed early (55). Cystoscopy is also indicated in patients with a lower urinary tract fistula or unexplained hematuria. Cystoscopic examination may demonstrate external compression of the bladder by a tumor, bullous edema produced by the blockage of lymphatic vessels from adjacent tumor growth, or mucosal involvement with tumor. When a mucosal lesion is seen, a biopsy can confirm the diagnosis.

Technique   Cystoscopy is performed with the patient in the dorsal lithotomy position. After preparation and draping of the area, the cystoscopic obturator and sheath are inserted into the urethra and carefully advanced into the bladder, after which the obturator is removed. The cystoscope is inserted into the sheath. About 250 to 400 mL of normal saline solution is instilled into the bladder to permit a thorough inspection of the entire mucosa.

Cystostomy

A suprapubic cystostomy catheter is useful in patients who require prolonged bladder drainage. This catheter may be useful in patients undergoing radical hysterectomy for cervical cancer or extensive resection of pelvic tumor because of the temporary disruption of bladder innervation that occurs with these dissections. The suprapubic catheter can be easier for the patient to manage than a transurethral Foley catheter, and the rate of bladder infection is lower (55). The other convenient aspect of this catheter is that it can facilitate trials of voiding. The patient can clamp the catheter for a specified interval, void, and then unclamp to check for residual urine. When the residual urine is less than 75 to 100 mL, the catheter can be removed. However, many patients are also managed successfully after radical hysterectomy with a period of continuous trnsurethral catheterization followed by intermittent self-catheterization (59,60).

Technique   The catheter used is an 18F Silastic Foley catheter with a 5- to 10-mL balloon. This catheter is well tolerated by patients, produces minimal local tissue irritation, and is of sufficient caliber that blockage of the catheter lumen is not a major problem.

The placement of a suprapubic catheter involves the following steps:

1. The catheter is inserted through a stab incision in the skin, subcutaneous tissue, and fascia, and a small hole is made in the dome of the bladder.

2. The tip of the catheter is inserted into the bladder, and a seromuscular pursestring suture is placed around the defect with 3-0 PGA sutures.

3. A second reinforcing layer consisting of either 2-0 absorbable braided PGA suture is placed in the bladder.

4. With the Foley balloon distended, the catheter is pulled up so that the bladder is applied snugly to the anterior abdominal wall.

5. The catheter can be attached to a urinary drainage bag, and it can also be attached to a smaller "leg bag," which is more portable and therefore easier for the patient to manage after discharge from the hospital.

Ureteral Obstruction

Ureteral obstruction is the most common urinary complication in patients with gynecologic malignancies. This problem is seen particularly in patients with cervical or vaginal cancer, either at the time of diagnosis or with recurrent disease. It may result from direct tumor extension into the bladder or distal ureters or from compression by lymph node metastases. In patients with intraabdominal carcinomatosis, most often from ovarian cancer, extensive pelvic tumor may cause significant progressive ureteral obstruction. **The most frequent site of lower urinary tract obstruction in gynecologic patients is the ureterovesical junction** (56).

Postoperative obstruction is usually incomplete and results from edema, possible infection, and partial devascularization of the distal ureter. However, the obstruction may be complete, and when it is, it most often results from inadvertent suture ligature of the distal ureter when the surgeon is attempting to ligate the blood vessels of the cardinal ligament (55). Chronic obstruction can result from stenosis after pelvic irradiation, particularly if pelvic surgery is also performed.

In patients who have a partial ureteral obstruction, the passage of a retrograde stent at the time of cystoscopy might bypass the site of blockage. The retrograde stent used is a 7F to 9F flexible, double "J" retrograde ureteral stent; it is inserted with the aid of a stent-placement apparatus that has an elevator attachment to the cystoscope. Great care must be taken, as **this procedure has the risk of ureteral perforation.** When the stent does not pass readily, the performance of a **percutaneous nephrostomy** is preferable.

In patients in whom complete ureteral obstruction is suspected (i.e., because of a rising serum creatinine level or the development of an acute unilateral hyelonephrosis), **a computed tomography urogram should be performed if the serum creatinine value is less than 2.0 mg/dL;** an ultrasonogram should be obtained if the level is higher. In patients with complete ureteral obstruction, the problem must be corrected immediately, either by temporary urinary diversion by means of a percutaneous nephrostomy or by reexploration and repair of the ureter. **Repair may be by either reanastomosis or reimplantation.**

Mild degrees of hydroureter are managed by bladder drainage alone in most patients, as these problems are usually temporary and resolve gradually as the edema subsides. Infection should be treated with appropriate antibiotics.

In patients undergoing radical hysterectomy and bilateral pelvic lymphadenectomy, postoperative ureteral damage from devascularization can be decreased by minimizing the collection of fluid in the retroperitoneal space by leaving the pelvic peritoneum open.

Retrograde Pyelography

If an excretory urogram cannot be performed (e.g., because of dye sensitivity) or if the study is inconclusive, retrograde pyelography may be necessary. This procedure is potentially morbid and should be performed only if the information to be gained is critical to the decision regarding diversion of the affected kidney (55–57). Contrast injected beyond a high-grade obstruction can produce pyelonephritis and sepsis and may require urgent drainage through a percutaneous nephrostomy. The attempted passage of a retrograde ureteral catheter or stent may be useful for diagnosis, and it will stent the ureter if the obstruction has not resulted from a misplaced suture ligature.

Percutaneous Nephrostomy

In patients with an obstructed ureter that cannot be decompressed by means of a retrograde ureteral stent, a percutaneous nephrostomy tube can be placed under fluoroscopic guidance (56). This procedure is relatively easy to perform, and the tube can be changed or replaced as necessary. In addition, an antegrade ureteral catheter or stent can occasionally be passed through a nephrostomy to allow removal of the percutaneous stent in patients in whom a retrograde catheter cannot be passed.

Ureteral Reanastomosis (Ureteroureterostomy)

When the ureter has been transected or damaged beyond repair, it will have to be revised and reanastomosed or reimplanted into the urinary bladder. If the ureteral injury is above the level of the pelvic brim, a simple reanastomosis is the procedure of choice. The two ends of the ureters are trimmed at a 45-degree angle. A double "J" ureteral stent is passed into the distal ureter with one "memory" end inserted into the bladder. The proximal end of the ureter is placed over the stent and sutured to its distal counterpart (58). Interrupted 4-0 absorbable PGA sutures are placed at close intervals in a circumferential fashion (Fig. 20.14). After several weeks, the absence of leakage can be established by means of intravenous pyelography, and the stent can be removed through a cystoscope.

Ureteroneocystostomy

The reimplantation of the distal ureter into the bladder is known as the **Leadbetter procedure, or ureteroneocystostomy** (44). This operation is preferred for the ureter that has been disrupted distal to the pelvic brim, as long as the bladder can be sufficiently mobilized on the side of reimplantation. Integral to successful ureteral reimplantation is the creation of a submucosal tunnel (Fig. 20.15). The tunnel minimizes the risk of vesicoureteral reflux and chronic, recurrent pyelonephritis (44).

The technique is as follows:

1. **The distal ureter is prepared by careful resection of any devitalized tissue** while the maximum length is preserved.
2. **The bladder base is mobilized, and the dome of the bladder is affixed laterally to the psoas muscle by means of a lateral cystopexy, a "psoas hitch"** (61). This permits stabilization of the bladder as well as extension of the bladder toward the end

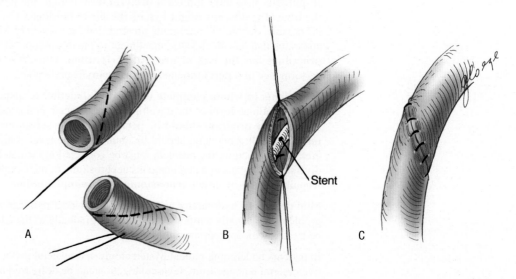

Figure 20.14   Ureteroureterostomy. A: The two ends of the ureters are cut diagonally. **B:** A ureteral stent is inserted into the proximal and distal ureter, and interrupted full-thickness sutures are placed. **C:** The completed anastomosis.

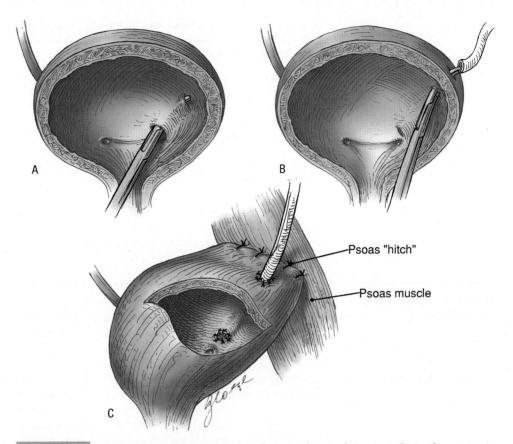

Psoas "hitch"

Psoas muscle

Figure 20.15   **Ureteroneocystostomy. A:** A submucosal tunnel is created. **B:** The ureter is brought into the bladder. **C:** The ureter is passed through the tunnel and sutured to the bladder serosa and mucosa. The serosa of the bladder is sutured to the psoas muscle to stabilize the anastomosis.

of the resected ureter, and it is especially important if the ureter is somewhat foreshortened.

3. **A cystotomy is made, and a tunnel is initiated by injection of the submucosal plane with saline solution to raise the mucosa.** The mucosa is incised, and a tonsil forceps is inserted submucosally for a length of 1 to 1.5 cm to the site where the serosa is to be incised. An incision in the serosa is made over the pointed tip of the clamp to create an opening to the tunnel that passes through the muscularis and mucosa of the bladder wall.

4. **The ureter is gently pulled through the submucosal tunnel, and mucosa-to-mucosa stitches are placed with interrupted 4-0 PGA suture material.** A ureteric stent, preferably a soft plastic double "J," is passed up the ureter into the renal calyx, and the other end is placed in the bladder lumen. The site of entrance of the ureter is sutured to the bladder serosa with 4-0 PGA.

5. **A suprapubic cystostomy is performed, and the cystotomy is closed with two layers of interrupted 2-0 absorbable suture.** The retroperitoneum is drained with a Jackson-Pratt drain. The ureteral stent is left in place 10 to 14 days and then removed through a cystoscope.

In cases where there is inadequate length of viable ureter, additional techniques can be utilized. The **Boari flap** utilizes a segment of bladder to bridge the defect to the remaining ureter (62). A U-shaped flap is created, turned superiorly and tabularized to create the additional length required. It should not be performed in patients with a history of prior radiation because of the increased risk of flap ischemia and failure. **Ileal interposition** can also be used to replace a portion of the ureter (63,64). First the required length of ileum is isolated and the ureter is anastomosed to the proximal end of the ileal segment in an end-to-side fashion with 4-0 delayed absorbable sutures. The ileum is then anastomosed in a tension-free fashion to the dome of the mobilized bladder.

In patients with a contracted, fibrotic bladder or when a portion of bladder requires resection for disease, the ileum can also be used for an **augmentation ileocystoplasty**. In this procedure, the isolated ileum is detubularized by opening it along its antimesenteric border and folding it into a "U" shape. The medial sides are sewn together using a running delayed absorbable suture, creating an ileal segment which can be anastomosed to the bladder (63).

Transureteroureterostomy

Another procedure that can be useful in the carefully selected patient is the transureter-oureterostomy (TUU) (65). When the distal ureter must be resected on one side, and the proximal ureter is too short to permit ureteroneocystostomy, it is possible to anastomose the distal end of the resected ureter into the contralateral side (66). The distal end of the partially resected ureter is tunneled under the mesentery of the sigmoid colon and approximated, end to side, to the recipient ureter. A ureteral stent is used to protect the anastomosis and is left in place for at least 7 to 10 days.

Permanent Urinary Diversion

Permanent urinary diversion must be performed after cystectomy or in patients who have an irreparable fistula of the lower urinary tract. Lower urinary tract fistulae can result from progressive tumor growth or from radical pelvic surgery and/or pelvic irradiation. The most common fistula is ureterovaginal.

Urinary Conduit

The most frequently employed techniques for urinary diversion are the creation of an **ileal conduit** (the **"Bricker procedure"**) (67), the creation of a **transverse colon conduit** (68), and the creation of a **"continent" urinary conduit** (e.g., the Koch, Miami, Indiana, Mainz, and Rome, pouch) (69–84). The ileal conduit has been the most widely used means of permanent urinary diversion, and it is suitable for most patients. A segment of transverse colon can be used if the ileum has been extensively injured (e.g., by radiation therapy). The transverse colon is usually away from the irradiated field, and thus its vascularity is not compromised.

The continent urinary conduit may be helpful for gynecologic oncology patients who require exenterative surgery. The first such conduit was the **continent ileal conduit (or "Koch pouch")**. It requires a longer portion of the ileum (up to 100 cm), a longer operative time (4 to 6 hours), and greater technical skills for the creation of the continence mechanism. It is now rarely performed (69).

The **continent colon conduit** utilizes the intestine from the terminal ileum to the mid-portion of the transverse colon and has been popularized in Indiana, Miami, and Mainz. These pouches are technically somewhat easier to perform than the Koch pouch. The type of continent conduit created is generally determined by the training and preference of the surgeon (70–78,82,83).

Technique   **The technique for the creation of an ileal conduit** involves the isolation of a segment of ileum at a site where the intestine appears healthy and nonirradiated. This is typically about 30 to 40 cm proximal to the ileocecal junction. The conduit requires a segment of ileum measuring approximately 20 cm and its associated mesentery (67). After isolation of the segment, the ileum is reanastomosed (Fig. 20.16). The ureters are implanted into the closed proximal end of the ileal segment, and double "J" ureteric stents are placed into both ureters. A no. 8 pediatric feeding tube made of soft flexible plastic can also be employed for the ureteric stent, as it is relatively atraumatic. The "butt" end of the conduit is sutured to the area of the sacral promontory.

The distal end of the conduit is brought through the anterior abdominal wall of the right lower quadrant, approximately midway between the umbilicus and the anterior superior iliac crest. The ureteral stents should be left in place for about 10 days.

When a **transverse-colon conduit** is selected, the technique is essentially the same. Care must be taken in both techniques to ensure that the vascularity of the intestinal mesentery is not interrupted. The mesentery of the reanastomosed bowel must be reapproximated to prevent herniation of intestinal loops through the defect.

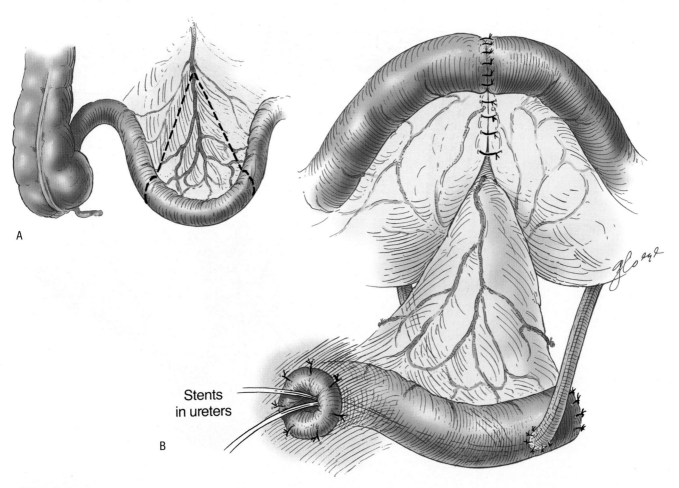

Figure 20.16 **Ileal urinary conduit. A:** A segment of nonirradiated ileum is used for the conduit. **B:** The ileum is reanastomosed, and the ureters are sewn into the "butt" end of the conduit. Note that ureters are stented individually.

The technique for creation of a continent Miami or Indiana pouch (70–76) involves resection of the intestine from the last 10 to 15 cm of ileum to the midportion of the transverse colon. The colon is opened along the antimesenteric border through the teniae coli (Fig. 20.17A). The ileum is used to create the continence mechanism (Fig. 20.17B). The ileal-cecal valve serves as the principal portion of the mechanism; the terminal ileum is narrowed, and several pursestring sutures are placed near the valve to reinforce the continence portion of the conduit (Fig. 20.17C). The ascending colon is sutured or stapled to the transverse colon to create a pouch. An ileotransverse anastomosis is performed to reconstitute the intestine (Fig. 20.17D).

Other modifications of the ileocolonic continent reservoir have been described. The **Rome pouch** utilizes multiple transverse teniamyotomies of the cecum instead of detubularization to create a low pressure reservoir (82,83). Bochner et al. describe the use of a **modified ureteroileocecal reservoir,** which **utilizes the appendix to create the cutaneous stoma** (85).

Skin Ureterostomy

In rare instances, a terminally ill patient undergoing exploratory surgery will have a bladder fistula. In such circumstances, one ureter can be ligated, and a skin ureterostomy can be created with the other ureter. The ureter is mobilized from its attachments and brought laterally through the retroperitoneal space to the lateral and anterior abdominal wall. The ureter is tunneled through the fascia and brought out through a stab incision in the skin, where it is affixed to create a small stoma (55).

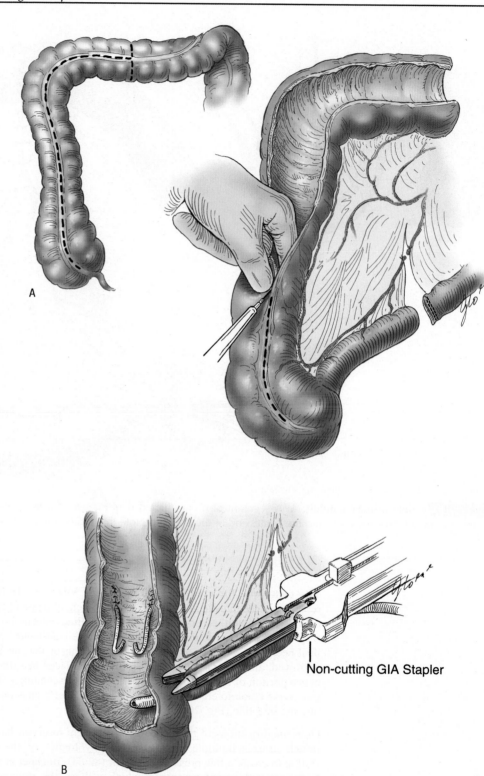

Figure 20.17   Colon continent urinary conduit: the "Miami" pouch. A: The segment of distal ileum and ascending and transverse colon is isolated, and the segment is opened on its antimesenteric border along the teniae coli. **B:** The ureters are reimplanted into the mesenteric side of the ascending colon, a continence mechanism is created with pursestring sutures near the ileal-cecal junction, and a noncutting double staple line is performed with a gastrointestinal anastomosis (GIA) stapler. *(Continued)*

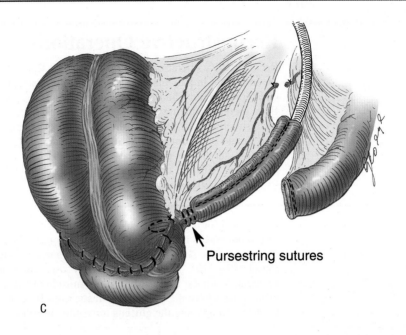

Pursestring sutures

C

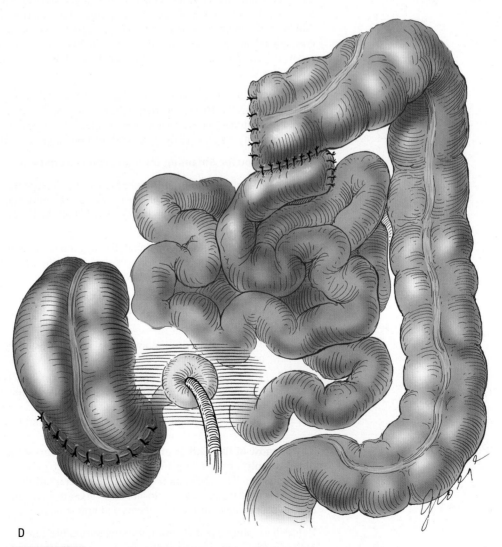

D

Figure 20.17   C: The conduit is closed with running sutures, and the ileal stoma is created.
D: The intestines are reconstituted with an ileal-transverse colon anastomosis.

Reconstructive Operations

Reconstructive operations, particularly pelvic floor reconstruction and creation of a neovagina, are important in patients who are undergoing extensive extirpative procedures, such as pelvic exenteration (see Chapter 22). Vaginal reconstruction helps to provide support to the pelvic floor, thereby reducing the prospect of perineal herniation. By helping to fill the pelvis, vaginal reconstruction also decreases the incidence of enteroperineal fistulae. Pelvic floor reconstruction should be performed in all patients undergoing a pelvic exenteration, and vaginal reconstruction should be performed simultaneously in most patients. The surgeon must be well acquainted with the types of graft that can be employed in the performance of these reconstructive operations and the techniques necessary to accomplish them (86).

Grafts

Grafts used for reconstructive operations in the pelvis are either **skin grafts,** which can be **full or partial (split) thickness** (86–90), or **myocutaneous grafts,** which are composed of the full thickness of the skin, its contiguous subcutaneous tissues, and a portion of a closely associated muscle (91–110). The most frequently used myocutaneous pedicle grafts contain muscle segments from the **rectus abdominis muscle** of the anterior abdominal wall, **gracilis muscle** of the inner thigh, the **bulbocavernosus muscle** of the vulva, the **tensor fascia lata muscle** of the lateral thigh, and the **gluteus maximus muscle.**

Skin Grafts

Skin grafts must be harvested under sterile conditions (61). The donor site most frequently used to obtain a split-thickness skin graft is either the anterior and medial thigh or the buttock. Although the thigh may be more readily accessible to the surgeon, the buttock donor site has cosmetic advantages; however, this latter site may be more uncomfortable in the postoperative recovery period. The selection of the donor site should be made preoperatively after discussion with the patient.

A dermatome is used to harvest the skin graft. Several different types of dermatome are available, including the Brown air-powered, electrically driven dermatome and the Padgett hand-driven dermatome. The surgeon should select the instrument with which he or she has the greatest facility, as an equally good graft can be harvested with either one.

The technique for obtaining the skin graft is as follows:

1. The graft width and thickness can be determined by adjusting the settings of the dermatome. A split-thickness graft can be obtained by setting the thickness between 14 and 16 one-thousandths of an inch. Full-thickness grafts are 20 to 24 one-thousandths of an inch.

2. When using the dermatome, the surgeon must apply firm, steady pressure in order to harvest a graft of uniform thickness. To minimize friction, mineral oil is applied to the skin over which the dermatome is to be passed.

3. The skin to be taken is stretched and flattened by the surgical assistant with the use of a tongue depressor. A second assistant picks up the leading edge of the graft as it is being harvested.

4. The harvested graft is kept moist in saline solution while the recipient site is being prepared.

5. The graft may be "pie crusted" by making small incisions in the surface. This technique maximizes the dimension of the graft while permitting the escape of fluid that might otherwise accumulate between the graft and the recipient site. However, extensive pie crusting may result in contracture when the graft is used to create a neovagina.

Pedicle Grafts

The purpose of the pedicle graft is to provide a substantial amount of tissue along with its blood supply either to repair an anatomic defect or to create a new structure, such as a neovagina (86–92). The pedicle graft can be either a full-thickness skin and subcutaneous tissue graft, as is used frequently for closure of a vulvar defect, e.g., a "Z-plasty" (a "rhomboid flap"), or a myocutaneous graft, e.g., a rectus abdominis or gracilis.

Before harvesting a pedicle graft, the surgeon should carefully outline the incisions on the skin with a marker pen. During the mobilization of the myocutaneous pedicle, the surgeon must carefully isolate and preserve the neurovascular bundle that supplies the muscle.

Vaginal Reconstruction

Vaginal reconstruction in the gynecologic oncology patient is performed either to revise or replace a vagina that has stenosed as a result of prior vaginal surgery and/or radiation or to create a neovagina when the vagina has been removed (87).

Split-Thickness Graft

When the vagina is fibrotic after irradiation, the scarred vaginal tissue first must be resected before placement of the split-thickness skin graft (87–90). The skin graft is placed over a vaginal stent that is then inserted into the space created by resection of the old, scarred vagina (Fig. 20.18A). The **Heyer-Schulte stent** is the vaginal stent preferred for this purpose, because it is inflatable, can be easily removed and replaced by the patient, and has its own drainage tube (Fig. 20.18B).

Split-thickness skin grafts can also be used in patients undergoing exenteration, but this approach is less satisfactory than the use of myocutaneous pedicle grafts, as discussed below. When an anterior exenteration is performed, or when a portion of the rectosigmoid colon is

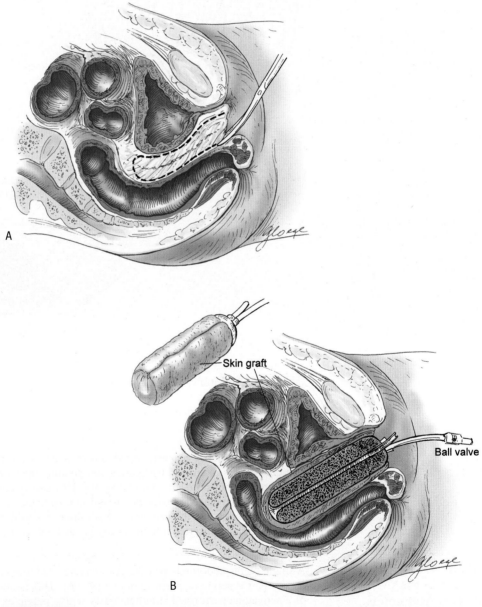

Figure 20.18   Creation of neovagina after radiation. A: The vaginal scar is resected in preparation for vaginal reconstruction with split-thickness skin grafts. **B:** A Heyer-Schulte vaginal stent has the skin graft placed around it, and this is inserted into the pelvic space to create a neovagina.

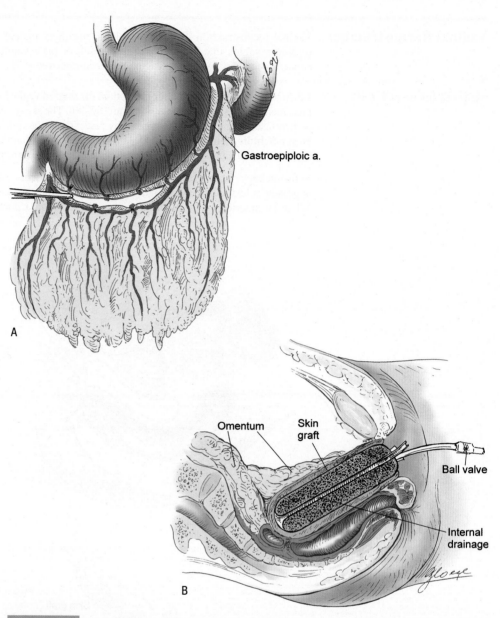

Gastroepiploic a.

Omentum   Skin graft   Ball valve   Internal drainage

Figure 20.19 **Mobilization of the omentum. A:** This is accomplished by ligating and dividing the right gastroepiploic artery and the short gastric arteries along the greater curvature of the stomach. **B:** The omentum is used to create a "pocket" for the placement of a split-thickness skin graft.

resected but primarily reanastomosed, a neovagina can be created with the use of skin grafts. The omentum is mobilized by ligating and dividing the short gastric vessels along the greater curvature of the stomach, preserving the left gastroepiploic pedicle (Fig. 20.19A). The omentum is then placed into the pelvis and sutured to the rectosigmoid posteriorly and laterally to create a pocket for the neovagina. Split-thickness skin graft(s) are harvested, sewn over a vaginal stent, and inserted into the newly created pelvic space (Fig. 20.19B).

Tranverse (TRAM) and Vertical (VRAM) Rectus Abdominis Myocutaneous Pedicle Grafts

A single rectus abdominis pedicle graft can be used to create a neovagina (91–97,111–115), or to repair a pelvic or perineal defect (95,96). This is our preferred technique for creation of a neovagina performed simultaneously with a pelvic exenteration (Fig. 20.20). The technique is relatively straightforward and has the advantage of a single pedicle harvested from the same site of the abdominal incision used to perform the exploratory surgery. This approach avoids the use of separate incisions on the inner aspects of the thigh as needed for the gracilis myocutaneous pedicle graft. The disadvantage is that the amount of tissue mobilized from the anterior abdominal is limited, and thus, the ability to adjust the size of the neovagina is somewhat limited. If too large a pedicle is created, there will be too much tension for the abdominal closure, and this can also create distortion of the anterior abdominal wall skin.

The pedicle location is shown in Fig. 20.20A. The oval-shaped pedicle should measure approximately 6 to 8 by 10 centimeters. The skin of the pedicle is incised, and the cephalad portion of

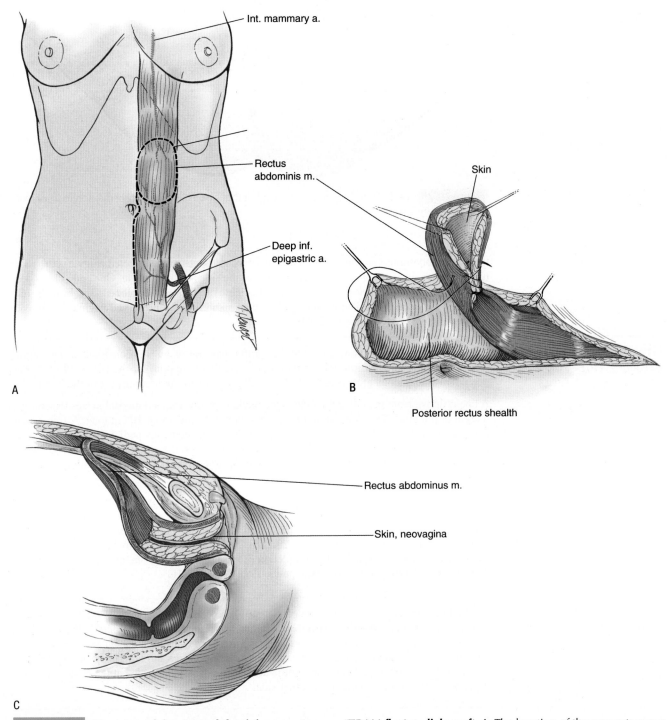

Int. mammary a.

Rectus abdominis m.

Deep inf. epigastric a.

A

Skin

Posterior rectus shealth

B

Rectus abdominus m.

Skin, neovagina

C

Figure 20.20   **The transpelvic rectus abdominis myocutaneous (TRAM flap) pedicle graft. A:** The location of the myocutaneous pedicle flap of the rectus abdominis muscle. **B:** The pedicle is harvested, and the tubular neovagina is created by suturing the full-thickness of the muscle, subcutaneous tissue, and skin of the anterior abdominal wall. **C:** The pedicle graft is brought down into the pelvis, and the leading edge is sutured to the preserved vaginal introitus. *(Continued)*

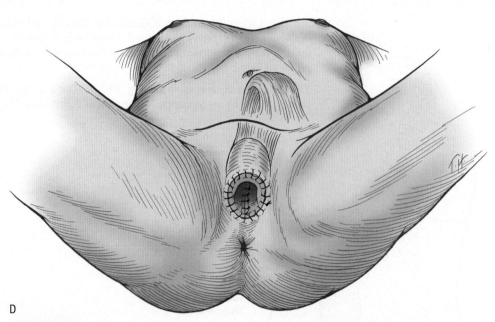

D

Figure 20.20   **D:** The final result is a neovagina that also helps to protect the pelvic floor from intestinal adhesions.

the rectus abdominis muscle and attached myofascial tissues are transected (Fig. 20.20B). The tubular neovagina is created by suturing together the sides of the pedicle. One end is left open, and this becomes the distal neovagina. The pedicle is harvested, mobilized, and brought into the pelvis (Fig. 20.20C). The pedicle graft is then sutured to the preserved vaginal introitus to complete the procedure (Fig. 20.20D).

Gracilis Myocutaneous Pedicle Grafts

Bilateral gracilis myocutaneous pedicle grafts can be used to construct a neovagina (86,87,102,103). In addition, the grafts provide excellent support for the pelvic viscera. The gracilis myocutaneous graft is harvested (Fig. 20.21A) from the inner aspect of the thigh.

A line is drawn from the pubic tubercle to the medial epicondyle, and this delineates the anterior margin of the graft. The graft should be about 5 cm wide and about 10 cm long. A skin bridge is preserved between the vulva and the pedicle. The myocutaneous pedicle graft is mobilized by transecting the gracilis muscle distally in continuity with the skin and subcutaneous tissue (Fig. 20.21B). **The vascular pedicle is proximal, and it must be carefully identified and preserved.**

The pedicle is "harvested," brought under the skin bridge of the vulva, and exteriorized through the introitus (Fig. 20.21C). The two grafts are sutured together to create a hollow neovagina (Fig. 20.21D, E). The entire neovagina is placed into the pelvis by posterior and upward rotation and sutured to the introitus (Fig. 20.21F). The apex is sutured to the symphysis pubis and/or the anterior sacrum. At the completion of the procedure, an omental pedicle is brought down over the graft to reconstruct the pelvic floor (Fig. 20.21G).

Bulbocavernosus Pedicle Grafts

The bulbocavernosus myocutaneous pedicle graft has been used for repair of radiation-induced rectovaginal fistulae (**Martius procedure**), but the procedure has been adopted for the creation of a neovagina (103,104,116). The procedure is performed by making an incision over the labium majus, isolating the bulbocavernosus muscle superiorly and anteriorly, and mobilizing it on a posterior vulvar pedicle. The graft is tunneled under a skin bridge at the posterior introitus and sutured to the pedicle of the other side.

Colonic Segment

Some authors have preferred to use a segment of colon to create a neovagina (86,105). This technique has had mixed success in the past, but an approach using a portion of the ascending colon may be an improvement over earlier procedures.

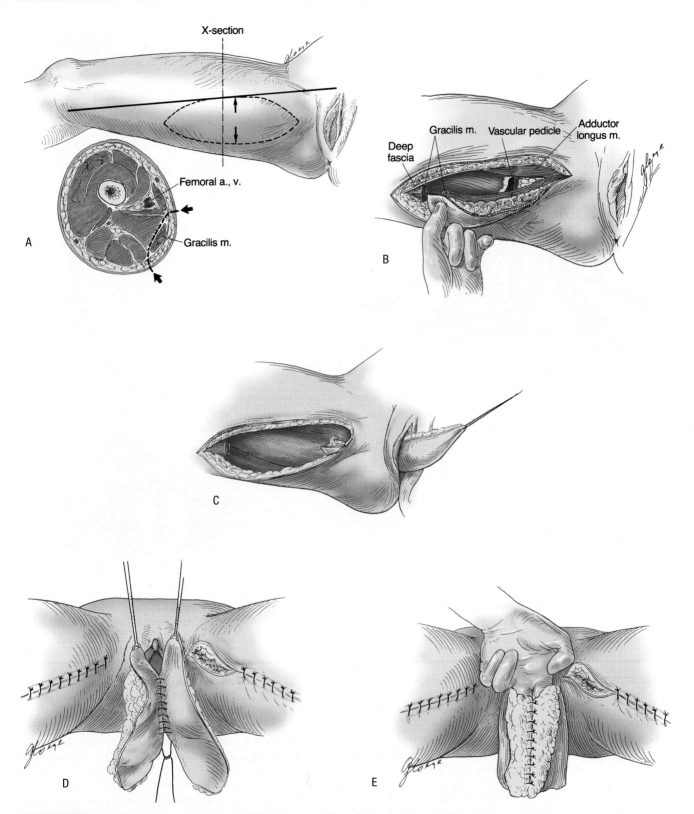

Figure 20.21   The gracilis myocutaneous pedicle graft. A: The pedicle graft is outlined on the inner thigh overlying the gracilis muscle. **B:** The myocutaneous pedicle graft is mobilized. **C:** The pedicle is brought under the skin bridge of the vulva. **D,E:** The two grafts are sutured together. *(Continued)*

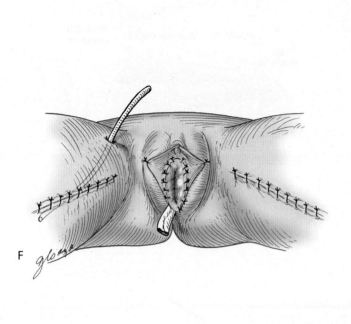

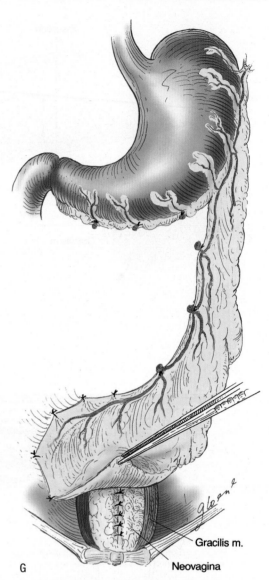

Gracilis m.

Neovagina

G

Figure 20.21   **F:** The neovagina is placed into the pelvis and sutured to the introitus. **G:** An omental pedicle is used to cover the graft. (Reproduced from **Berek JS, Hacker NF, Lagasse LD.** Vaginal reconstruction performed simultaneously with pelvic exenteration. *Obstet Gynecol* 1984;63:318, with permission from the American College of Obstetricians and Gynecologists.)

Vulvar and Perineal Reconstruction	Whenever feasible, the vulva should be closed primarily after radical vulvectomy (106–110,117). With radical local excision or a separate incision approach for the groin dissection, primary closure of the vulvar skin can be accomplished in almost all patients.
Rhomboid Pedicle Graft	If there is any tension on the skin edges, the skin can be mobilized by means of a Z-plasty using the adjacent skin and subcutaneous tissue. This is called a **rhomboid flap** (106). The technique (Fig. 20.22) involves the repositioning of a rhomboid flap of full-thickness skin and subcutaneous tissue. Use of these pedicle grafts will usually allow for the primary closure of vulvar defects after radical vulvar surgery, but if necessary, a split-thickness skin graft can be used. Myocutaneous pedicle grafts, such as a unilateral gracilis graft, can also be used to cover a large vulvar defect.
Tensor Fascia Lata Pedicle Graft	The tensor fascia lata pedicle graft, harvested from the lateral aspect of the thigh, can be useful in covering large defects of the lower abdomen, groin, and anterior vulva (107). The flap is particularly useful in patients who require extensive resection of large groin recurrences or large, fixed groin nodes.

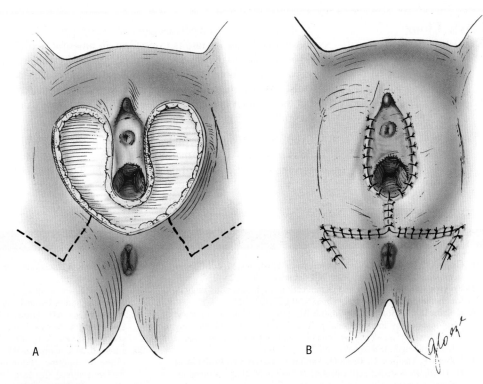

Figure 20.22 **A:** **The "rhomboid flap"** is used to close a posterior vulvar defect. **B:** The pedicle grafts are bilateral "Z-plasties" that are sutured together in the midline.

The graft is obtained by harvesting a myocutaneous pedicle from its proximal origin at the anterosuperior aspect of the iliac bone to its distal insertion on the lateral condyle of the tibia. The length of the proposed flaps is determined by measuring the distance from the muscle's vascular supply, located 6 to 8 cm distal to the anterior superior iliac spine, to the most inferior or distal point of the recipient site (e.g., the posterior vulva). The blood supply is from the lateral circumflex femoral artery located deep to the fascia lata between the rectus femoris and the vastus lateralis. The posterior border of the graft is defined as a line from the greater trochanter of the hip down to the knee, and the distal border is located about 5 cm proximal to the knee. The width of the flap is determined by the width of the defect to be covered, but typically it is 6 to 8 cm with a length of up to 40 cm.

The pedicle graft is harvested after the defect has been created in order to permit a more accurate measurement of the flap. The flap is first incised distally, and care is taken to avoid injury to the proximal blood supply. Once the flaps are elevated, they are rotated into place and sutured from their most distal point to the proximal. The donor site is closed primarily.

Gluteus Maximus Pedicle Grafts	The gluteus maximus muscles, or a portion thereof, can be used to reconstruct the pelvic floor and the perineum (109,110). This approach might be particularly useful for very large defects, such as for those patients who have undergone a total infralevator pelvic exenteration (see Chapter 22).
Vulvovaginoplasty	Although the preferred methods for vulvar and vaginal reconstruction are outlined above, there is occasionally a need to perform a vulvovaginoplasty, the so-called **William's procedure.** This procedure (117) involves the incision of a horseshoe-shaped flap on the vulva to create a marsupialized pouch that can be used as a neovagina. This operation has the advantage of being relatively simple to perform, and it does not require pelvic dissection. It has the disadvantage of being less anatomically suitable for vaginal intercourse, but its direction can improve with regular use. **It may be helpful in a patient who has undergone a pelvic exenteration without vaginal reconstruction.**

Pelvic Floor Reconstruction

At the completion of a pelvic exenteration, the pelvic floor must be reconstructed. Probably the most effective procedure is to perform an **omental pedicle graft** (provided there is sufficient omentum) and to use myocutaneous pedicle grafts whenever possible to reconstruct the vagina. In patients in whom this is not possible, alternatives include the use of **a variety of graft materials, either natural or synthetic** (118). A natural material that has been used is dura mater, but this is often unavailable (119,120). All areas that can be directly peritonealized should be carefully covered with peritoneal pedicle grafts.

Synthetic grafts using **Marlex** have been associated with a high incidence (>20%) of infectious morbidity and are therefore much less desirable. However, if a pedicle graft is not feasible, the synthetic material Gore-Tex may be the best alternative (121,122).

References

1. **Gajewski JL, Raad I.** Vascular access. In: **Haskell CM, ed.** *Cancer treatment,* 5th ed. Philadelphia: WB Saunders, 2001:225–235.
2. **Freytes CO.** Indications and complications of intravenous devices for chemotherapy. *Curr Opin Oncol* 2000;12:303–307.
3. **Kuizon D, Gordon SM, Dolmatch BL.** Single-lumen subcutaneous ports inserted by interventional radiologists in patients undergoing chemotherapy: incidence of infection and outcome of attempted catheter salvage. *Arch Intern Med* 2001;12:406–410.
4. **Volkow P, Vasquez C, Tellez O, Aguilar C, Barrera L, Rodriquez E, et al.** Polyurethane II catheter as long-indwelling intravenous catheter in patients with cancer. *Am J Infect Control* 2003;31:392–396.
5. **Hind D, Calvert N, McWilliams R, Davidson A, Paisley S, Beverley C, et al.** Ultrasonic locating devices for central venous cannulation: meta-analysis. *BMJ* 2003;327:361.
6. **Strahilevitz J, Lossos IS, Verstandig A, Sasson T, Kori Y, Gillis S.** Vascular access via peripherally inserted central venous catheters (PICCs): experience in 40 patients with acute myeloid leukemia at a single institute. *Leuk Lymphoma* 2001;40:365–371.
7. **Sakuragi N, Nakajima A, Nomura E, Noro N, Yamada H, Yamamoto R, et al.** Complications relating to intraperitoneal administration of cisplatin or carboplatin for ovarian carcinoma. *Gynecol Oncol* 2000;79:420–423.
8. **Walker JL, Armstrong DK, Huang HQ, Fowler J, Webster K, Burger RA, et al.** Intraperitoneal catheter outcomes in a phase III trial of intravenous versus intraperitoneal chemotherapy in optimal stage III ovarian and primary peritoneal cancer: a Gynecologic Oncology Group Study. *Gynecol Oncol* 2006;100:27–32.
9. **Black D, Levine DA, Nicoll L, Chou JF, Iasonos A, Brown CL, et al.** Low risk of complications associated with the fenestrated peritoneal catheter used for intraperitoneal chemotherapy in ovarian cancer. *Gynecol Oncol* 2008;109:39–42.
10. **Davidson SA, Rubin SC, Markman M, Jones WB, Hakes TB, Reichman B, et al.** Intraperitoneal chemotherapy: analysis of complications with an implanted subcutaneous port and catheter system. *Gynecol Oncol* 1991;41:101–106.
11. **Makhija S, Leitao M, Sabbatini P, Bellin N, Almadrones L, Leon L, et al.** Complications associated with intraperitoneal chemotherapy catheters. *Gynecol Oncol* 2001;81:77–81.
12. **Piccart MJ, Speyer JL, Markman M, ten Bokkel Huinink WW, Alberts D, Jenkins J, et al.** Intraperitoneal chemotherapy: technical experience at five institutions. *Semin Oncol* 1985;12:90–96.
13. **Fujiwara K, Sakuragi N, Suzuki S, Yoshida N, Maehata K, Nishiya M, et al.** First-line intraperitoneal carboplatin-based chemotherapy for 165 patients with epithelial ovarian carcinoma: results of long-term follow-up. *Gynecol Oncol* 2003;90:637–643.
14. **Armstrong DK, Bundy B, Wenzel L, Huang HQ, Baergen R, Lele S, et al.** Intraperitoneal cisplatin and paclitaxel in ovarian cancer. *N Engl J Med* 2006;354:34–43.
15. **Markman M, Walker JL.** Intraperitoneal chemotherapy of ovarian cancer: a review, with a focus on practical aspects of treatment. *J Clin Oncol* 2006;24:988–994.
16. **Gallup DG, Nolan TE, Smith RP.** Primary mass closure of midline incisions with a continuous polyglyconate monofilament absorbable suture. *Obstet Gynecol* 1990;76:872–875.
17. **Millikan KW.** Incisional hernia repair. *Surg Clin North Am* 2003;83: 1223–1234.
18. **Brolin RE.** Prospective, randomized evaluation of midline fascial closure in gastric bariatric operations. *Am J Surg* 1996;172:328–331.
19. **Niggebrugge AH, Hansen BE, Trimbos JB, van de Velde CJ, Zwaveling A.** Mechanical factors influencing the incidence of burst abdomen. *Eur J Surg* 1995;161:655–661.
20. **Carlson MA, Condon RE.** Polyglyconate (Maxon) versus nylon suture in midline abdominal incisional closure: a prospective randomized trial. *Am Surg* 1995;61:980–983.
21. **Gislason H, Grobech JE, Soreide O.** Burst abdomen and incisional hernia after major gastrointestinal operations-comparison of three closure techniques. *Eur J Surg* 1995;161:349–354.
22. **Hilgert RE, Dorner A, Wittkugel O.** Comparison of polydioxanone (PDS) and polypropylene (Prolene) for Shouldice repair of primary inguinal hernias: a prospective randomised trial. *Eur J Surg* 1999;165: 333–338.
23. **Outlaw KK, Vela AR, O'Leary JP.** Breaking strength and diameter of absorbable sutures after in vivo exposure in the rat. *Am Surg* 1998; 64:348–354.
24. **Osther PJ, Gjode P, Mortensen BB, Mortensen PB, Bartholin J, Gottrup E.** Randomized comparison of polyglycolic acid and polyglyconate sutures for abdominal fascial closure after laparotomy in patients with suspected impaired wound healing. *Br J Surg* 1995;82:1080–1082.
25. **Pfyger HL, Hakansson TU, Jensen LP.** Single layer colonic anastomosis with a continuous absorbable monofilament polyglyconate suture. *Eur J Surg* 1995;161:911–913.
26. **Trimbos JB, Niggebrugge A, Trimbos R, Van Rijssel EJ.** Knotting abilities of a new absorbable monofilament suture: poliglecaprone 25 (Monocryl). *Eur J Surg* 1995;161:319–322.
27. **Yaltirik M, Dedeoglu K, Bilgic B, Koray M, Ersev H, Issever H, et al.** Comparison of four different suture materials in soft tissues of rats. *Oral Dis* 2003;9:284–286.
28. **Yabata E, Okabe S, Endo M.** A prospective, randomized clinical trial of preoperative bowel preparation for elective colorectal surgery-comparison among oral, systemic, and intraoperative luminal antibacterial preparations. *J Med Dent Sci* 1997;44:75–80.
29. **Pineda CE, Shelton AA, Hernandez-Boussard T, Morton JM, Welton ML.** Mechanical bowel preparation in intestinal surgery: a meta-analysis and review of the literature. *J Gastrointest Surg* 2008;12:2037–2044.
30. **Wille-Jørgensen P, Guenaga KF, Matos D, Castro AA.** Pre-operative mechanical bowel cleansing or not? an updated meta-analysis. *Colorectal Dis* 2005;7:304–310.
31. **Guenaga KF, Matos D, Castro AA, Atallah AN, Wille-Jørgensen P.** Mechanical bowel preparation for elective colorectal surgery. *Cochrane Database Syst Rev*(1):2005;CD001544.
32. **Hacker NF, Berek JS, Lagasse LD.** Gastrointestinal operations in gynecologic oncology. In: **Knapp RC, Berkowitz RS, eds.** *Gynecologic oncology,* 2nd ed. New York: McGraw-Hill, 1993: 361–375.
33. **Shephard JH, Crawford RA.** Reconstructive procedures in benign and malignant gynecologic surgery. *Curr Opin Obstet Gynecol* 1994;6:206–209.

34. **Wheeless CR.** Recent advances in surgical reconstruction of the gynecologic cancer patient. *Curr Opin Obstet Gynecol* 1992;4:91–101.

35. **Wheeless CR.** Low colorectal anastomosis and reconstruction after gynecologic cancer. *Cancer* 1993;71:1664–1666.

36. **Hatch KD.** Low rectal anastomosis following pelvic exenteration. *CME J Gynecol Oncol* 1998;69:28–31.

37. **Hatch KD, Gelder MS, Soong SJ, Baker VV, Shingleton HM.** Pelvic exenteration with low rectal anastomosis: survival, complications, and prognostic factors. *Gynecol Oncol* 1990;38:462–467.

38. **Seow-Choen F, Goh HS.** Prospective randomized trial comparing J-colonic pouch-anal anastomosis and straight coloanal reconstruction. *Br J Surg* 1995;82:608–610.

39. **Hallbook O, Pahlman L, Krog M, Wexner SD, Sjodahl R.** Randomized comparison of straight and colonic J pouch anastomosis after low anterior resection. *Ann Surg* 1996;224:58–65.

40. **Hida J, Yasutomi M, Fujimoto K, Okuno K, Ieda S, Machidera N, et al.** Functional outcome after low anterior resection with low anastomosis for rectal cancer using the colonic J-pouch: prospective randomized study for determination of optimum pouch size. *Dis Colon Rectum* 1996;39:986–991.

41. **Furst A, Suttner S, Agha A, Beham A, Jauch KW.** Colonic J-pouch vs. coloplasty following resection of distal rectal cancer: early results of a prospective randomized pilot study. *Dis Colon Rectum* 2003;46:1161–1166.

42. **Machado M, Nygren J, Goldman S, Ljungqvist O.** Similar outcome after colonic pouch and side-to-side anastomosis in low anterior resection for rectal cancer: a prospective randomized trial. *Ann Surg* 2003;238:214–220.

43. **Mathur P, Hallan RI.** The colonic J-pouch in colo-anal anastomosis. *Colorectal Dis* 2002;4:304–312.

44. **Amin AI, Hallbook O, Lee AJ, Sexton R, Moran BJ, Heald RI.** A 5-cm colonic J pouch colo-anal reconstruction following anterior resection for low rectal cancer results in acceptable evacuation and continence in the long term. *Colorectal Dis* 2003;5:33–37.

45. **Dehni N, Parc R, Church JM.** Colonic J-pouch-anal anastomosis for rectal cancer. *Dis Colon Rectum* 2003;46:667–675.

46. **Moran BJ, Heald RJ.** Risk factors for and management of anastomotic leakage in rectal surgery. *Colorectal Dis* 2001;3:135–137.

47. **Schmidt O, Merkel S, Hohenberger W.** Anastomotic leakage after low rectal stapler anastomosis: significance of intraoperative anastomotic testing. *Eur J Surg Oncol* 2003;29:239–243.

48. **Berek JS, Hacker NF, Lagasse LD.** Rectosigmoid colectomy and reanastomosis to facilitate resection of primary and recurrent gynecologic cancer. *Obstet Gynecol* 1984;64:715–720.

49. **Mantyh CR, Hull TL, Fazio VW.** Coloplasty in low colorectal anastomosis. *Dis Colon Rectum* 2001;44:37–42.

50. **Nelson R, Edwards S, Tse B.** Prophylactic nasogastric decompression after abdominal surgery. *Cochrane Database Syst Rev*(3): 2007;CD004929.

51. **Yang Z, Zheng Q, Wang Z.** Meta-analysis of the need for nasogastric or nasojejunal decompression after gastrectomy for gastric cancer. *Br J Surg* 2008;95:809–816.

52. **Lewis SJ, Egger M, Sylvester PA, Thomas S.** Early enteral feeding versus "nil by mouth" after gastrointestinal surgery: systematic review and meta-analysis of controlled trials. *BMJ* 2001;323: 773–776.

53. **Petrilli NJ, Cheng C, Driscoll D, Rodriquez-Bigas MA.** Early postoperative oral feeding after colectomy: an analysis of factors that may predict failure. *Ann Surg Oncol* 2001;8:796–800.

54. **Bohm B, Haase O, Hofmann H, Heine G, Junghans T, Muller JM.** Tolerance of early oral feeding after operations of the lower gastrointestinal tract. *Chirurg* 2000;71:955–962.

55. **Kearney GP.** Urinary tract involvement in gynecologic oncology. In: **Knapp RC, Berkowitz RS, eds.** *Gynecologic oncology,* 2nd ed. New York: Macmillan, 1992:447–469.

56. **Kim SC, Kuo RL, Lingeman JE.** Percutaneous nephrolithotomy: an update. *Curr Opin Urol* 2003;13:235–241.

57. **Sherman ND, Stock JA, Hanna MK.** Bladder dysfunction after bilateral ectopic ureterocele repair. *J Urol* 2003;170:1975–1977.

58. **Thompson JD.** Operative injuries of the ureter: prevention, recognition, and management. In: **Rock JA, Thompson JD eds.** *Telinde's operative gynecology,* 8th ed. Philadelphia: Lippincott-Raven, 1997: 1135–1173.

59. **Naik R, Maughan K, Nordin A, Lopes A, Godfrey KA, Hatem MH.** A prospective randomised controlled trial of intermittent self-catheterisation vs. supra-pubic catheterisation for post-operative bladder care following radical hysterectomy. *Gynecol Oncol* 2005;99:437–442.

60. **Chamberlain DH, Hopkins MP, Roberts JA, McGuire EJ, Morley GW, Wang CC.** The effects of early removal of indwelling urinary catheter after radical hysterectomy. *Gynecol Oncol* 1991;43:98–102.

61. **Ahn M, Loughlin KR.** Psoas hitch ureteral reimplantation in adults—analysis of a modified technique and timing of repair. *Urology* 2001;58:184–187.

62. **Kishev SV.** Indications for combined psoas-bladder hitch procedure with Boari vesical flap. *Urology* 1975;6:447–452.

63. **Elkas JC, Berek JS, Leuchter R, Lagasse LD, Karlan BY.** Lower urinary tract reconstruction with ileum in the treatment of gynecologic malignancies. *Gynecol Oncol* 2005;97:685–692.

64. **Bonfig R, Gerharz EW, Riedmiller H.** Ileal ureteric replacement in complex reconstruction of the urinary tract. *BJU Int* 2004;93: 575–580.

65. **Joung JY, Jeong IG, Seo HK, Kim TS, Han KS, Chung J, et al.** The efficacy of transureteroureterostomy for ureteral reconstruction during surgery for a non-urologic pelvic malignancy. *J Surg Oncol* 2008;98:49–53.

66. **Sugerbaker PH, Gutman M, Verghese M.** Transureteroureterostomy: an adjunct to the management of advanced primary and recurrent malignancy. *Int J Colorectal Dis* 2003;18: 40–44.

67. **Bricker EM.** Bladder substitution after pelvic evisceration. *Surg Clin North Am* 1950;30:1511–1521.

68. **Schmidt JD, Buchsbaum HJ, Jacoby EC.** Transverse colon conduit for supravesical urinary tract diversion. *Urology* 1976;8: 542–546.

69. **Hart S, Skinner EC, Meyerowitz BE, Boyd S, Lieskovsky G, Skinner DG.** Quality of life after radical cystectomy for bladder cancer in patients with an ileal conduit, cutaneous or urethral Kock pouch. *J Urol* 1999;162:77–81.

70. **Rowland RG, Mitchell ME, Bihrle R, Kahnoski RJ, Piser JE.** Indiana continent urinary reservoir. *J Urol* 1987;137:1136–1139.

71. **Penalver MA, Bejany DE, Averette HE, Donato DM, Sevin BU, Suarez G.** Continent urinary diversion in gynecologic oncology. *Gynecol Oncol* 1989;34:274–288.

72. **Dottino PR, Segna RA, Jennings TS, Beddoe AM, Cohen CJ.** The stapled continent ileocecal urinary reservoir in the surgical management of gynecologic malignancy. *Gynecol Oncol* 1994;55: 185–189.

73. **Penalver M, Donato D, Sevin BU, Bloch WE, Alvarez WJ, Averette H.** Complications of the ileocolonic continent urinary reservoir (Miami pouch). *Gynecol Oncol* 1994;52:360–364.

74. **Penalver MA, Angioli R, Mirhashemi R, Malik R.** Management of early and late complications of ileocolonic continent urinary reservoir (Miami pouch). *Gynecol Oncol* 1998;69:185–191.

75. **Mannel RS, Manetta A, Buller RE, Braly PS, Walker JL, Archer JS.** Use of ileocecal continent urinary reservoir in patients with previous pelvic irradiation. *Gynecol Oncol* 1995;59: 376–378.

76. **Ramirez PT, Modesitt SC, Morris M, Edwards CL, Bevers MW, Wharton JT, et al.** Functional outcomes and complications of continent urinary diversions in patients with gynecologic malignancies. *Gynecol Oncol* 2002;85:285–291.

77. **El-Lamie IK.** Preliminary experience with Mainz type II pouch in gynecologic oncology patients. *Eur J Gynaecol Oncol* 2001;22: 77–88.

78. **Leissner J, Black P, Fisch M, Hockel M, Hohenfeller R.** Colon pouch (Mainz pouch III) for continent urinary diversion after pelvic exenteration. *Urology* 2000;56:798–802.

79. **Hartenbach EM, Saltzman AK, Carter JR, Fowler JM, Hunter DW, Carlson JW, et al.** Nonsurgical management strategies for the functional complications of ileocolonic continent urinary reservoirs. *Gynecol Oncol* 1995;59:358–363.

80. **Lentz SS, Homesley HD.** Radiation-induced vesicosacral fistula: treatment with continent urinary diversion. *Gynecol Oncol* 1995;58: 278–280.

81. **Kashif KM, Holmes SA.** The use of small intestine in bladder reconstruction. *Int Urogynecol J Pelvic Floor Dysfunct* 1998;9: 275–280.

82. **Salom EM, Mendez LE, Schey D, Lambrou N, Kassira N, Gómez-Marn O, et al.** Continent ileocolonic urinary reservoir

(Miami pouch): the University of Miami experience over 15 years. *Am J Obstet Gynecol* 2004;190:994–1003.

83. **Panici PB, Angioli R, Plotti F, Muzii L, Zullo MA, Manci N, et al.** Continent ileocolonic urinary diversion (Rome pouch) for gynecologic malignancies: technique and feasibility. *Gynecol Oncol* 2007;107:194–199.

84. **Angioli R, Zullo MA, Plotti F, Bellati F, Basile S, Damiani P, et al.** Urologic function and urodynamic evaluation of urinary diversion (Rome pouch) over time in gynecologic cancers patients. *Gynecol Oncol* 2007;107:200–204.

85. **Bochner BH, McCreath WA, Aubey JJ, Levine DA, Barakat RR, Abu-Rustum N, et al.** Use of an ureteroileocecal appendicostomy urinary reservoir in patients with recurrent pelvic malignancies treated with radiation. *Gynecol Oncol* 2004;94:140–146.

86. **Berek JS, Hacker NF, Lagasse LD.** Reconstructive pelvic surgery. In: Knapp RC, Berkowitz RS, eds. *Gynecologic oncology,* 2nd ed. New York: McGraw-Hill, 1993:420–431.

87. **Berek JS, Hacker NF, Lagasse LD.** Vaginal reconstruction performed simultaneously with pelvic exenteration. *Obstet Gynecol* 1984;63:318–323.

88. **Berek JS, Hacker NF, Lagasse LD, Smith ML.** Delayed vaginal reconstruction in the fibrotic pelvis following radiation or previous reconstruction. *Obstet Gynecol* 1983;61:743–748.

89. **Hyde SE, Hacker NE.** Vaginal reconstruction in the fibrotic pelvis. *Aust N Z J Obstet Gynaecol* 1999;39:448–453.

90. **Seccia A, Salgarello M, Sturla M, Loreti A, Latorre S, Farallo E.** Neovaginal reconstruction with the modified McIndoe technique: a review of 32 cases. *Ann Plast Surg* 2002;49:379–384.

91. **Jain AK, deFranzo AJ, Marks MW, Loggie BW, Lentz S.** Reconstruction of pelvic exenterative wounds with transpelvic rectus abdominis flaps: a case series. *Ann Plast Surg* 1997;38:115–122.

92. **Carlson JW, Carter JR, Saltzman AK, Carson LF, Fowler JM, Twiggs LB.** Gynecologic reconstruction with a rectus abdominis myocutaneous flap: an update. *Gynecol Oncol* 1996;61:364–368.

93. **Carlson JW, Soisson AP, Fowler JM, Carter JR, Twiggs LB, Carson LF.** Rectus abdominis myocutaneous flap for primary vaginal reconstruction. *Gynecol Oncol* 1993;51:323–329.

94. **Mirhashemi R, Averette HE, Lambrou N, Penalver MA, Mendez L, Ghurani G, et al.** Vaginal reconstruction at the time of pelvic exenteration: a surgical and psychosexual analysis of techniques. *Gynecol Oncol* 2003;90:690–691.

95. **De Haas WG, Miller MJ, Temple WJ, Kroll SS, Schusterman MA, Reece GP, et al.** Perineal wound closure with the rectus abdominis musculocutaneous flap after tumor ablation. *Ann Surg Oncol* 1995;2:400–406.

96. **McAllister E, Wells K, Chaet M, Norman J, Cruse W.** Perineal reconstruction after surgical extirpation of pelvic malignancies using the transpelvic transverse rectus abdominal myocutaneous flap. *Ann Surg Oncol* 1994;1:164–168.

97. **Niazi ZB, Kutty M, Petro JA, Kogan S, Chuang L.** Vaginal reconstruction with a rectus abdominis musculoperitoneal flap. *Ann Plast Surg* 2001;46:563–568.

98. **Rietjens M, Maggioni A, Bocciolone L, Sideri M, Youssef O, Petit JY.** Vaginal reconstruction after extended radical pelvic surgery for cancer: comparison of two techniques. *Plast Reconstr Surg* 2002;109:1592–1595.

99. **Jurado M, Bazan A, Elejabeita J, Paloma V, Martinez-Monge R, Alcazar JL.** Primary vaginal and pelvic floor reconstruction at the time of pelvic exenteration: a study of morbidity. *Gynecol Oncol* 2000;77:293–297.

100. **Horch RE, Gitsch G, Schultze–Seemann W.** Bilateral pedicled myocutaneous vertical rectus abdominis muscle flaps to close vesicovaginal and pouch-vaginal fistulas with simultaneous vaginal and perineal reconstruction in irradiated pelvic wounds. *Urology* 2002;60:502–507.

101. **Copeland LJ, Hancock KC, Gershenson DM, Stringer CA, Atkinson EN, Edwards CL.** Gracilis myocutaneous vaginal reconstruction concurrent with total pelvic exenteration. *Am J Obstet Gynecol* 1989;160:1095–1101.

102. **Lacey CG, Stern JL, Feigenbaum S, Hill EC, Braga CA.** Vaginal reconstruction after exenteration with use of gracilis myocutaneous flaps: the University of California San Francisco experience. *Am J Obstet Gynecol* 1988;158:1278–1284.

103. **Hatch KD.** Construction of a neovagina after exenteration using the vulvobulbocavernosus myocutaneous graft. *Obstet Gynecol* 1984;63:110–114.

104. **Wierrani F, Grunberger W.** Vaginoplasty using deepithelialized vulvar transposition flaps: the Grunberger method. *J Am Coll Surg* 2003;196:159–162.

105. **Parsons JK, Gearhart SL, Gearhart JP.** Vaginal reconstruction utilizing sigmoid colon: complications and long-term results. *J Pediatr Surg* 2002;37:629–633.

106. **Barnhill DR, Hoskins WJ, Metz P.** Use of the rhomboid flap after partial vulvectomy. *Obstet Gynecol* 1983;62:444–447.

107. **Chafe W, Fowler WC, Walton LA, Currie JL.** Radical vulvectomy with use of tensor fascia lata myocutaneous flap. *Am J Obstet Gynecol* 1983;145:207–213.

108. **Arkoulakis NS, Angel CL, DuBester B, Serletti JM.** Reconstruction of an extensive vulvectomy defect using the gluteus maximus fasciocutaneous V-Y advancement flap. *Ann Plast Surg* 2002;49:50–54.

109. **Loree TR, Hempling RE, Eltabbakh GH, Recio FO, Piver MS.** The inferior gluteal flap in the difficult vulvar and perineal reconstruction. *Gynecol Oncol* 1997;66:429–434.

110. **Germann G, Cedidi C, Petracic A, Kallinowski F, Herrfarth C.** The partial gluteus maximus musculocutaneous turnover flap: an alternative concept for simultaneous reconstruction of combined defects of the posterior perineum/sacrum and the posterior vaginal wall. *Br J Plast Surg* 1998;51:620–623.

111. **Sood AK, Cooper BC, Sorosky JI, Ramirez PT, Levenback C.** Novel modification of the vertical rectus abdominis myocutaneous flap for neovagina creation. *Obstet Gynecol* 2005;105:514–518.

112. **O'Connell C, Mirhashemi R, Kassira N, Lambrou N, McDonald WS.** Formation of functional neovagina with vertical rectus abdominis musculocutaneous (VRAM) flap after total pelvic exenteration. *Ann Plast Surg* 2005;55:470–473.

113. **Soper JT, Havrilesky LJ, Secord AA, Berchuck A, Clarke-Pearson DL.** Rectus abdominis myocutaneous flaps for neovaginal reconstruction after radical pelvic surgery. *Int J Gynecol Cancer* 2005;15:542–548.

114. **Soper JT, Secord AA, Havrilesky LJ, Berchuck A, Clarke-Pearson DL.** Rectus abdominis myocutaneous and myoperitoneal flaps for neovaginal reconstruction after radical pelvic surgery: comparison of flap-related morbidity. *Gynecol Oncol* 2005;97:596–601.

115. **Soper JT, Secord AA, Havrilesky LJ, Berchuck A, Clarke-Pearson DL.** Comparison of gracilis and rectus abdominis myocutaneous flap neovaginal reconstruction performed during radical pelvic surgery: flap-specific morbidity. *Int J Gynecol Cancer* 2007;17:298–303.

116. **Green AE, Escobar PF, Neubaurer N, Michener CM, Vongruenigen VE.** The Martius flap neovagina revisited. *Int J Gynecol Cancer* 2005;15:964–966.

117. **Hoffman MS, Fiorca JV, Roberts WS, Hewitt S, Shepard JH, Owens S, et al.** Williams' vulvovaginoplasty after supralevator total pelvic exenteration. *South Med J* 1991;84:43–45.

118. **Elaffandi AH, Khalil HH, Aboul Kassem HA, El Sherbiny M, El Gemeie EH.** Vaginal reconstruction with a greater omentum-pedicled graft combined with a vicryl mesh after anterior pelvic exenteration. Surgical approach with long-term follow-up. *Int J Gynecol Cancer* 2007;17:536–542.

119. **Donato D, Jarrell MA, Averette HE, Malinin TI, Sevin BU, Girtanner RE.** Reconstructive techniques in gynecologic oncology: the use of human dura mater allografts. *Eur J Gynaecol Oncol* 1988;9:135–139.

120. **Jarrell MA, Malinin TI, Averette HE, Girtanner RE, Harrison CR, Penalver MA.** Human dura mater allografts in repair of pelvic floor and abdominal wall defects. *Obstet Gynecol* 1987;70:280–285.

121. **Birch C, Fynes MM.** The role of synthetic and biological prostheses in reconstructive pelvic floor surgery. *Curr Opin Obstet Gynecol* 2002;14:527–535.

122. **Kohli N, Miklos JR.** Use of synthetic mesh and donor grafts in gynecologic surgery. *Curr Womens Health Rep* 2001;1:53–60.

21

Laparoscopy and Robotics

Margrit Juretzka
Kenneth D. Hatch

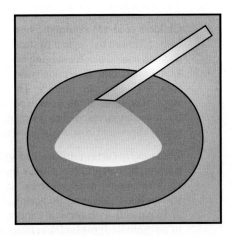

Laparoscopy has been widely accepted for numerous operative procedures. Laparoscopy performed with the assistance of video monitors has become the preferred technique because the surgeon can view the operation in real time.

Laparoscopic procedures such as **cholecystectomy** were adapted by surgeons and accepted by the public because of an associated short hospital stay, quick recovery time, and rapid return to full activity. However, **this procedure was incorporated into surgical practice before prospective trials could be established to evaluate its feasibility, morbidity, and cost-effectiveness compared with the standard laparotomy.** The same criticisms may be made in gynecology for such procedures as laparoscopically assisted vaginal hysterectomy, removal of adnexal masses, and management of endometriosis, which are widely performed by virtually thousands of gynecologists.

In gynecologic oncology, there has been a unique opportunity to study the use of operative laparoscopy in a prospective fashion because of the limited number of specialists performing the procedures, and the need to perform pelvic and/or paraaortic lymphadenectomy to stage several gynecologic malignancies. As surgeons adopt minimally invasive technologies, innovations in instrumentation from bipolar coagulation devices to large-scale robotic-assist devices continue to facilitate the use of laparoscopic approaches for increasingly complex surgical procedures.

Laparoscopic Pelvic and Paraaortic Lymphadenectomy

The performance of a pelvic and paraaortic lymphadenectomy, either a partial lymphadenectomy (lymph node sampling) or complete lymphadenectomy, is the key procedure for the staging of gynecologic malignancies.

In 1989, Dargent and Salvat (1) in France used the laparoscope to perform limited pelvic lymphadenectomy in women with cervical cancer. This was not widely accepted because of its limited access to the pelvic lymph nodes and the inability to evaluate the lymph nodes in the common iliac and paraaortic chains. In 1991, Childers and Surwit (2) described pelvic and paraaortic lymphadenectomy performed in conjunction with a laparoscopically assisted vaginal hysterectomy and bilateral salpingo-oophorectomy in two women with endometrial cancer. In 1992, Nezhat et al. (3) published a case of laparoscopic radical hysterectomy and pelvic and paraaortic lymphadenectomy, although the dissection went only 2 cm above the aortic bifurcation, an inadequate evaluation. **These early publications were limited case reports that gave no information on morbidity, mortality, or complications.**

Querleu et al. (4) performed transperitoneal laparoscopic pelvic lymphadenectomy on 39 patients with cervical cancer. Five patients had metastatic lymph nodes and were treated with radiation therapy. Thirty-two patients underwent abdominal radical hysterectomy and evaluation of the completeness of the laparoscopic lymphadenectomy. The sensitivity for node positivity by laparoscopy was 100%. However, the number of additional lymph nodes found at laparotomy was not stated.

Childers et al. (5) reported 59 patients with endometrial cancer who were staged laparoscopically, followed by vaginal hysterectomy and bilateral salpingo-oophorectomy. Of the 31 patients deemed candidates for staging based on criteria including high-grade or deep myometrial invasion, lymph node dissection was completed in 29 patients (obesity precluded it in two patients), for a feasibility rate of 93%. Three major and three minor complications were reported. The surgical complications were experienced early in the series and led to alternative techniques as the series progressed. The average hospital stay was 2.9 days, but the operative time, lymph node counts, and cost analysis were lacking.

These early series emphasized pelvic lymphadenectomy, but it remained necessary to do paraaortic lymphadenectomy for laparoscopy to be fully accepted as a technique to stage all gynecologic malignancies. In 1992, Childers et al. (6) reported their initial experience with pelvic and paraaortic lymphadenectomy extending from the duodenum to the bifurcation in 18 patients with cervical cancer. **They subsequently summarized the Arizona experience in paraaortic lymphadenectomy through 1993 with a report of 61 women with cervical, endometrial, or ovarian cancer (7). In three patients (5%), obesity prevented the completion of the surgery, and in one patient (0.8%), adhesions were responsible for failure.** Lymph node counts were available in 23 patients: For the right-sided dissection, there was an **average lymph node count of three.** The **operating time** for the six patients who underwent a bilateral paraaortic lymphadenectomy **ranged from 25 to 70 minutes, depending on whether or not a unilateral or bilateral procedure was performed (these times included only the time to complete the lymphadenectomy).** The hospital stay for the 33 patients undergoing laparoscopic lymphadenectomy was 1.3 days. There was **one vena caval injury** that required transfusion and laparotomy, a complication rate comparable with that of open surgery.

In 1995, Spirtos et al. (8) reported 40 patients who underwent bilateral partial paraaortic lymphadenectomy (sampling). Five laparotomies were performed: two to remove unsuspected metastases, two for control of hemorrhage, and one because of equipment failure. In two patients, the left-sided dissection was judged to be inadequate, which was an overall failure rate of 12.5%. An average of eight paraaortic lymph nodes were removed: four from the right side and four from the left side. Most of the patients also underwent a pelvic lymphadenectomy and hysterectomy. The mean operative time was 3 hours, 13 minutes, and the average hospital stay was 2.9 days.

In the early series (4–6,9), laparotomy was used to confirm the accuracy of the lymphadenectomy, and in each report, all positive lymph nodes were identified.

Possover et al. (10) reported 84 patients who underwent laparoscopic pelvic and paraaortic lymphadenectomy for cervical cancer. The surgeon classified the lymph nodes as positive or negative by visualization. The sensitivity and specificity of visualization was 92.3%. When frozen-section analysis was combined with laparoscopic assessment, 100% of the positive lymph nodes were identified. In 13 of the 84 patients (15.5%), the treatment plan was altered during surgery based on these findings.

Possover et al. (11) analyzed videotapes of 112 paraaortic lymphadenectomies and detailed the ventral tributaries of the infrarenal vena cava (Fig. 21.1). **They divided the vena cava into three levels based on the distribution of venous tributaries.** This is a significant contribution to anatomic knowledge and is an important guide for beginning laparoscopic surgeons.

A perforator of the inferior vena cava at the level of the bifurcation of the aorta is shown in Fig. 21.1A. A diagram of the most common sites where perforators are encountered during a paraaortic lymphadenectomy is shown in Fig. 21.1B.

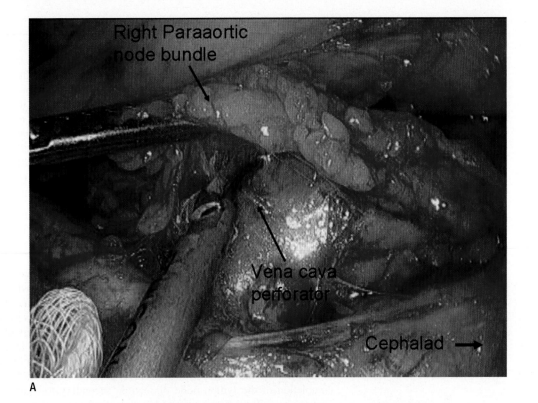

A

B

Figure 21.1 **Perforators of the vena cava. A: A vena cava perforator at the level of the bifurcation of the aorta. B. Diagram of the most common sites where perforators are encountered during the performance of a paraaortic lymphadenectomy.** The figure shows the anatomic distribution of 237 venous tributaries in 112 patients undergoing laparoscopic lymphadenectomy according to different levels of the inferior vena cava. (From **Possover M, Plaul K, Krause N, Schneider A.** Left-sided laparoscopic para-aortic lymphadenectomy: anatomy of the ventral tributaries of the infrarenal vena cava. *Am J Obstet Gynecol* 1998;179:1295–1297, with permission.)

Multiple recent studies continue to report the adequacy and safety of laparoscopic pelvic and paraaortic node dissections in gynecologic cancer (12–19). In one of the largest series to date, Koehler et al. reported on 650 patients undergoing laparoscopic transperitoneal pelvic ($n = 499$) or paraaortic ($n = 468$) (combined pelvic and paraarotic $n = 362$) lymphadenectomies (19). The mean number of pelvic lymph nodes removed from 1994 to 2003 remained fairly constant (16.9–21.9). However, the mean number of paraaortic lymph nodes increased from 5.5 in 1994 to 18.5 in 2003, reflecting improvements in technique and extensive training. Intraoperative complications (bowel or vessel injury) occurred in 2.9% of patients while 5.8% had postoperative complications for an overall complication rate of 8.7%. The authors reported that no major intraoperative complications were encountered during the last five years of the study.

Querleu et al. subsequently reported on their experience with transperitoneal and extraperitoneal lymph node dissections in 1,000 gynecologic cancer patients (18). This study included 777 pelvic (757 transperitoneal, 20 extraperitoneal) and 415 aortic lymphadenectomies (155 transperitoneal, 260 extraperitoneal) in patients with early cervical carcinoma ($n = 456$); advanced cervical carcinoma ($n = 219$); vaginal carcinoma ($n = 4$); endometrial carcinoma ($n = 182$); and ovarian carcinoma ($n = 139$). The mean number of pelvic lymph nodes removed was 18 via a transperitoneal approach and the mean number of paraaortic lymph nodes removed was 17 via a transperitoneal approach versus 21 via an extraperitoneal approach. **The authors reported an increase in the number of lymph nodes removed with increasing experience,** yielding an average of 24 pelvic and 22 aortic lymph nodes in 2003. Intraoperative complications occurred in 2% of patients including injury to vascular structures (1.1%); bowel (0.3%); ureter (0.3%); and nerves (0.3%). Five patients underwent conversion to laparotomy for completion of the lymph node dissection, secondary to fixed nodes or extensive adhesions. Conversion to laparotomy occurred in an additional two patients secondary to bowel or ureteric injury. Five patients required a second surgical intervention due to postoperative complications, most commonly bowel obstruction ($n = 4$).

These studies have demonstrated the ability of laparoscopic surgeons to perform pelvic and paraaortic lymphadenectomy. The American Medical Association Physicians Current Procedure Terminology (CPT 2007) lists a total of four laparoscopic lymph node dissection procedures, including total pelvic lymphadenectomy and paraaortic lymph node sampling. Laparoscopic surgery has been used by many oncologic surgeons, and has been applied to nearly every disease site in gynecologic oncology.

Indications for Laparoscopic Surgery

Endometrial Cancer

Most women with endometrial cancer present with disease confined to the uterus. The treatment consists of total hysterectomy, bilateral salpingo-oophorectomy, and surgical staging, which includes peritoneal washings, inspection of the abdomen, and retroperitoneal lymph node sampling. **Surgical staging with operative laparoscopy followed by vaginal hysterectomy or laparoscopic total hysterectomy has been proposed as an alternative to laparotomy** (2,12–15,20,21).

Childers et al. (5,6) reported two patients in 1992 who underwent laparoscopic staging of the retroperitoneal nodes followed by vaginal hysterectomy and bilateral salpingo-oophorectomy, and they presented the first large series in 1993 (7). Laparoscopic staging was performed successfully in 93% of the patients, with obesity noted as a limiting factor. Two patients had complications related to the hysterectomy: One had a transected ureter caused by the endoscopic stapler, and one had a cystotomy.

Spirtos et al. (20) reported 13 patients who underwent laparoscopic staging and hysterectomy and compared them with 17 patients who underwent laparotomy. The laparotomy group required significantly longer hospitalization, (6.3 vs. 2.4 days, $p < 0.001$), incurred higher overall hospital costs ($19,158 vs. $13,988, $p < 0.05$), and took longer to return to normal activity (5.3 weeks vs. 2.4 weeks, $p < 0.0001$). The patients having laparotomy were significantly more obese and had a higher body mass index (BMI) (30.2 vs. 24.2).

The effect of surgical experience has been demonstrated by Melendez et al. (21). In the first 100 patients with endometrial cancer, the operative time for staging decreased from a mean of 196 minutes for the first 25 patients to 128 minutes for the last 25 patients. Hospital stay decreased from 3.2 days to 1.8 days. The decrease in operative time and hospital stay, coupled

Table 21.1 Recurrence Rates for Laparoscopic Surgery versus Laparotomy For Endometrial Cancer

	Laparoscopy			Laparotomy		
	n	Months Follow-up	% Recurrence	*n*	Months Follow-up	% Recurrence
Gemignani *et al.* 1999 (15)	59	18	6%	235	30	7%
Eltabbakh 2002 (27)	100	27	7%	86	48	10%
Malur *et al.* 2001 (28)	37	16	3%	33	16	3%
Holub *et al.* 2002 (23)	177	33	6%	44	45	7%
Hatch 2003 (29)	111	33	7%	55	33	14%
Obermair *et al.* 2004 (30)	226	29[a]	4%	284	29	14%
Zapico *et al.* 2005 (31)	38	36	5%	37	53	5%
Kim *et al.* 2005 (32)	74	31	1%	168	37	1%
Frigerio *et al.* 2006 (33)	55	27	0%	55	33	5%
Kalogiannidis *et al.* 2007 (34)	69	51	9%	100	52	16%

[a]median follow-up for total study population

with the diminished use of expensive, disposable instruments, has led to a significant cost savings for laparoscopy. More important are the social benefits to the individual patient.

Subsequent publications have continued to show a decrease in operative time, hospital stay, and total cost for laparoscopic treatment of endometrial cancer (15,22,23).

Women with endometrial cancer are often obese with BMI greater than 35 (24). This has been thought to be a limiting factor in using laparoscopy to stage and treat endometrial cancer. As surgical skills have grown, **laparoscopy has been used successfully in these women.** Holub et al. (25) have completed staging and hysterectomies successfully in 94.4% of 33 patients with BMIs of 30 to 40. Eltabbakh et al. (26) have completed staging in 88% of 42 women with BMIs of 28 to 60. In both studies, the benefits of shorter hospital stay with faster recovery were verified. However, many retrospective studies comparing laparoscopy and laparotomy have reported a significantly lower BMI in patients undergoing laparoscopic management, reflecting a selection bias favoring open procedures in obese patients. Results of further prospective studies are awaited to assess the impact of BMI and obesity in laparoscopic versus open surgical approaches.

Long-term survival has been reported in several papers (Table 21.1; 15,23,27–34). In these series, more than 900 patients have been studied for a median of 16 to 53 months. Inclusion criteria were heterogeneous, with some authors reporting only on outcomes of patients with stage I and II disease. The recurrence rate following laparoscopic management ranged from 0% to 9%. When compared with historical controls undergoing laparotomy in these papers and adjusting for factors such as stage, grade, age, and weight, there was no difference in survival. **While these studies yield promising data, comparison of operative morbidity and short- and long-term outcomes between laparotomy and laparoscopy requires an adequately powered, randomized clinical study.**

To answer these questions, The Gynecologic Oncology Group (GOG) (35) conducted the LAP 2 trial, a large, prospective, randomized trial designed to determine equivalency in early-stage endometrial cancer outcomes in laparoscopically assisted vaginal hysterectomy and bilateral salpingo-oophorectomy with surgical staging, when compared with traditional open surgery. This study enrolled 2,616 patients, completing accrual in 2005. There were 1,696 patients randomized to laparoscopy and 920 to laparotomy in a two-to-one randomization ratio. Preliminary data were presented at the Annual Meeting of the Society of Gynecologic Oncologists in 2006. **Length of stay was shorter in the laparoscopic arm (median 3 days, range 0–95) versus laparotomy arm (median 4 days, range 1–49). Operative time was increased with laparoscopic procedures (3.3 hours versus 2.2 hours) and approximately 23% of patients randomized to laparoscopy required laparotomy to complete staging.**

Results of this important study will help answer many questions regarding feasibility, appropriate patient selection, and short- and long-term oncologic outcomes of laparoscopy in the management of endometrial cancer.

The concept of sentinel node removal has been studied in endometrial cancer in several small studies. Techniques utilized for the detection of sentinel lymph nodes include injection of blue dye, injection of a radiocolloid, or both. To date, studies in endometrial cancer have focused on injection of the tracer into the uterine corpus (subserosal or myometrial); the cervix; the endometrium using hysteroscopy; or combined sites (36). The sentinel lymph node detection rates using injection of the subserosal myometrium alone ranged from 0–92% (37–42). Altgassen reported the highest detection rate (92%) utilizing eight injection sites in contrast to the 1 to 3 sites reported by several other authors. Similarly, Li et al. (39) reported a 75% detection rate using three subserosal myometrial sites and two subserosal isthmic sites. Reported detection rates using cervical injection alone ranged from 80% to 100% (43–46). Holub et al. reported a detection rate using cervical and subserosal myometrial injections of 84% (47). Hysteroscopic injection of the endometrium has yielded detection rates of 50% to 100 % (48–51). While the possibility of laparoscopic assessment of sentinel lymph nodes and targeted sampling is interesting, sentinel lymph node detection in endometrial cancer remains investigational.

Cervical Cancer

The use of laparoscopy in the treatment of cervical cancer was initially limited by the fact that there was no apparent advantage to laparoscopic lymphadenectomy because the standard operation for the primary cervical tumor was radical abdominal hysterectomy.

Dargent (52) first suggested that laparoscopic pelvic lymphadenectomy could be followed by a Schauta radical vaginal hysterectomy and has published long-term results, reporting a 95.5% 3-year survival rate in 51 patients with negative pelvic lymph nodes. Querleu (53) reported eight patients and demonstrated an average blood loss of less than 300 mL, an average hospital stay of 4.2 days, and decreased pain from the elimination of an abdominal incision.

Hatch et al. (54) reported 37 patients treated by laparoscopic pelvic and paraaortic lymphadenectomy followed by radical vaginal hysterectomy. The mean operative time was 225 minutes, the mean blood loss was 525 mL, and the average hospital stay was 3 days. Blood transfusion was required in 11% of the patients, compared with the range of 35% to 95% reported in the literature for radical abdominal hysterectomy. Complications occurred early in the series and included two cystostomies repaired at surgery without an increase in hospital stay. In two patients (5.4%), ureterovaginal fistulae developed that were treated by ureteral stents. These were removed 6 weeks later without further operative intervention.

Schneider and colleagues (55) reported 33 patients in whom bipolar techniques were used for lymphadenectomy and to transect the cardinal ligaments and uterine vessels. Hysterectomy was completed by the Schauta-Stoeckel technique. There were five (15%) intraoperative injuries managed successfully without subsequent sequelae. Four patients required transfusion. Numerous retrospective studies comparing laparoscopically assisted radical hysterectomy versus radical abdominal hysterectomy have reported increased operative time but decreased blood loss, decreased transfusion rates, and hospital length of stay in patients undergoing the minimally invasive procedures (56–60).

Studies have shown that the complication rates go down as the operator's experience increases (61,62). Long-term survival has been reported by Hertel et al. (14) for 200 patients, with a mean follow-up of 40 months. The projected 5-year survival was 83%. For the 100 patients who were stage I, lymphovascular space–negative and lymph node–negative, the survival was 98%.

Laparoscopic Radical Hysterectomy

Although most initial reports in the literature detailed some form of laparoscopically assisted radical vaginal hysterectomy, there are increasing reports of laparoscopic radical hysterectomy. Spirtos et al. (13) reported laparoscopic radical hysterectomy (type III) with aortic and pelvic lymphadenectomy in 78 patients. The average operative time was 205 minutes, length of hospitalization was 3.2 days, and blood loss was 225 mL; one transfusion was necessary. There were acceptable intraoperative and postoperative complications. With a minimum of 3 years follow-up, the disease-free survival was 95%. Since then, numerous authors have reported similar findings (41,63–67). In one of the largest series, Puntambekar (65) reported on 248 patients with early stage cervical cancer, noting a median operative time of 292 minutes, median number of resected pelvic lymph nodes of 18, median blood loss of 165 mL, and a median length of stay of 3 days. Other studies generally have reported longer operating times ranging from 196 to 344 minutes (41,60,67,68).

The issue of blood loss and transfusion has become very important to patients and surgeons since the identification of the human immunodeficiency virus and other blood-borne pathogens. **Every report on laparoscopic lymphadenectomy and radical hysterectomy has noted a significant decrease in blood loss and transfusion rates.** Other societal advantages are the decreased hospital stay and rapid return to normal function, even with radical surgery.

Laparoscopic Nerve-Sparing Radical Hysterectomy

Preservation of the superior hypogastric nerve plexus, the hypogastric nerve and the inferior hypogastric plexus are important for function of the bladder and rectum. The superior hypogastric plexus is composed of sympathetic nerves that allow the bladder to store urine. If this is damaged, the bladder will have a small volume and high pressure under parasympathetic control. The inferior hypogastric plexus is composed of parasympathetic nerves that initiate urination. If the inferior hypogastric plexus is damaged, the patient will have lack of sensation and be unable to initiate urination. The hypogastric nerve connects the two plexes. If it is severed, the patient will have a mixed pattern, consisting of an initial small volume, high-pressure phase followed by a hypotonic high-residual state. This may lead to the need for chronic self-catheterization.

Damage to the superior hypogastric plexus can occur at the time of paraaortic node dissection or presacral node dissection. Injury to the hypogastric nerve may occur when clamping the cardinal or uterosacral ligaments. Injury to the inferior hypogastric plexus may occur with lateral dissection of the cardinal ligaments, dissection of the posterior vesicouterine ligament, or with removal of paravaginal tissue.

Recent description of the anatomy of these nerves and the surrounding blood vessels has established the role of nerve-sparing techniques in performing radical hysterectomy (69). The laparoscope is an excellent technique to identify and preserve the nerves, because it magnifies small vessels and nerves so that the surgeon can more easily identify them.

The technique performed at the University of Arizona is described below (Figs. 21.2–21.8).

1. **The patient is placed in the lithotomy position with Trendelenburg tilt to the table. A nasogastric tube is placed** to reduce the distention of the stomach. The four trocars are placed in the lower abdomen in a diamond shape.

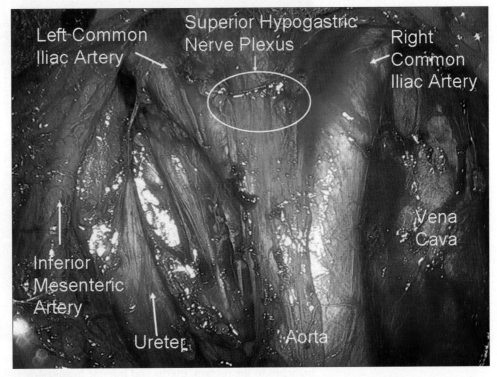

Figure 21.2 The superior hypogastric nerve plexus is preserved during the paraaortic node dissection.

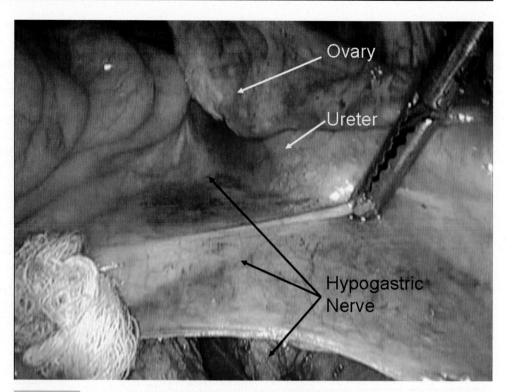

Figure 21.3   Traction on the peritoneum overlying the bifurcation of the aorta helps identify the course of the hypogastric nerve 2 to 3 centimeters medial to the ureter at the pelvic brim.

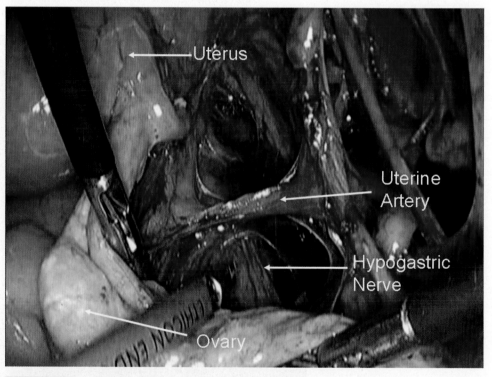

Figure 21.4   The hypogastric nerve continues into the pelvis along the ureter with branches to the rectum, uterus and inferior hypogastric plexus.

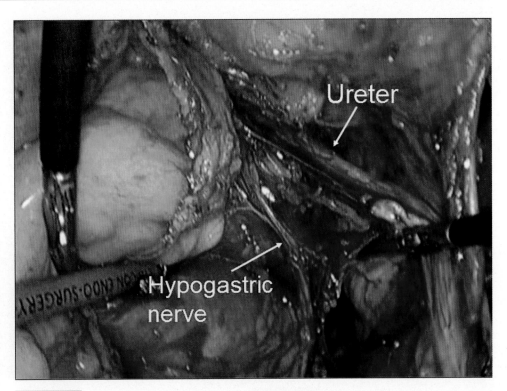

Figure 21.5   The hypogastric nerve is 1 to 2 centimeters dorsal to the uterine artery and can be preserved if mass ligature of the cardinal ligament is avoided.

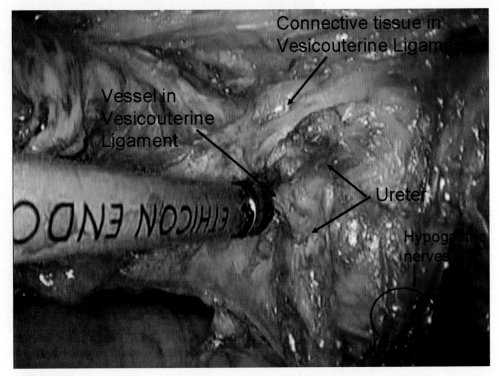

Figure 21.6   The vessels and connective tissue medial to the ureter is dissected so that the ureter can be retracted laterally out of the cardinal ligament tunnel.

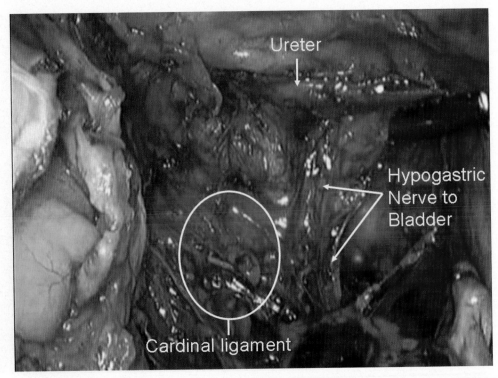

Figure 21.7   **The ureter is now retracted laterally with the hypogastric nerve.** The cardinal ligament can now be divided.

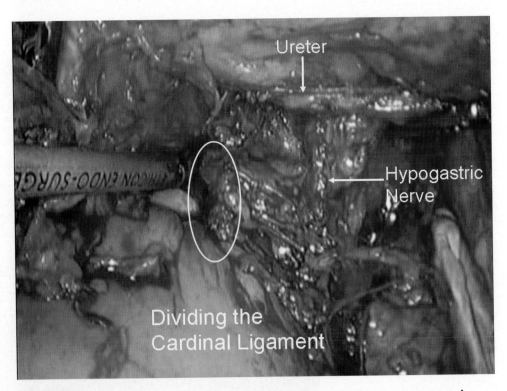

Figure 21.8   The anterior vesicouterine vessels and connective tissue are transected.

2. **The paraaortic node dissection is performed first when the tumor is 2 cm or greater in size.** This allows for exposure of the superior hypogastric plexus (Fig 21.2).

3. **The hypogastric nerve is located by opening the peritoneum between the ureter and the sigmoid colon mesentery** (Fig 21.3). The hypogastric nerve is dissected down into the pelvis and its location dorsal to the uterine artery is shown (Fig 21.4).

4. **The uterine artery is divided and the hypogastric nerve is dissected lateral and dorsal to the ureter** (Fig 21.5).

5. **The anterior vesicouterine ligament with its vessels and connective tissue is divided and the ureter dissected laterally** (Fig 21.6). The branch of the nerve following the ureter into the base of the bladder is preserved in the posterior vesicouterine ligament (Fig 21.7).

6. **The cardinal ligament can be divided medial to the nerve and ligament** (Fig 21.8).

The operation can be completed by the vaginal route or with further dissection through the laparoscope. The vaginal route allows more precise removal of the vaginal margin.

The urethral catheter is left in place for 48 hours. The patient is then allowed to void and a post-void residual is obtained. If she had good sensation of bladder fullness and a residual urine amount less than 60 cc, the catheter is left out. If she is unable to void, has no sensation of filling, or if the residual urine is over 60 cc, the catheter is left in place for 7 days. The nerve sparing operation has been performed in a total of 33 patients. Twenty-one of these patients had a laparoscopic node dissection and radical vaginal trachelectomy. Twelve had a laparoscopic node dissection and radical hysterectomy completed by laparoscopy or by vaginal assistance. Eight of the patients were unable to void with residual of less than 60 cc at 7 days. All of the patients were able to void at 21 days.

Laparoscopic staging of cervical cancer before treatment planning has been proposed (15,70,71). Vidaurreta et al. (69) staged 91 patients, stages IIB, IIIA, IIIB, and IVA. Computed tomography (CT) was performed in 49 patients, with 38 read as normal and 11 as positive. Histologic evaluation revealed metastases in 18 of the 38 (47.4%) patients with negative scans, and no metastases were found in 5 of the 11 (45.5%) with positive scans. Hertel et al. (71) compared laparoscopic surgical staging with magnetic resonance imaging (MRI) and CT scan in 101 patients, 91 of whom had a CT scan, 67 of whom had an MRI scan, and 49 of whom had both. False-positive or false-negative results were found in 22% of patients. Ten patients had false-positive paraaortic nodal metastases.

Sentinel Nodes	The initial studies of sentinel node detection showed sensitivity, negative predictive value, and accuracy of 100% (72–74). Subsequent studies have used both blue dye and Technetium 99m detection methods with varying success (74–86) (Table 21.2).
Radical Vaginal Trachelectomy with Laparoscopic Lymphadenectomy	Radical hysterectomy, with or without adjuvant therapy for patients with early cervical cancer, is associated with high cure rates. However, in young patients desiring fertility, alternative surgical options have been increasingly explored.

In 1994, Dargent et al. (87) first presented a series of 28 patients who underwent laparoscopic pelvic lymphadenectomy followed by radical vaginal trachelectomy. After a median follow-up of 36 months, there was only one recurrence in the paraaortic nodes of a 27-year-old patient with stage IB adenocarcinoma. The pelvic lymph nodes had been negative, and the margins were free. Among the eight patients who attempted pregnancy, three had cesarean section at 36 weeks gestation, and three had a spontaneous abortion.

The second report on radical vaginal trachelectomy was published in 1998 by Roy and Plante (88). Thirty patients underwent laparoscopic pelvic lymphadenectomy and radical vaginal trachelectomy; only six women had attempted pregnancy at the time of reporting, and four had healthy infants delivered by cesarean section.

Since these initial reports, several authors have now reported their experience with radical trachelectomy (Table 21.3; 89–98). **The indications commonly used are:**

1. **Desire for future childbearing**
2. **Stage IA1 disease with extensive lymph-vascular space invasion**
3. **Stage IA2 disease**

Table 21.2 Sentinel Node Detection for Patients with Cervical Cancer (Series with ≥30 Patients)

Reference	Number of Patients	Percent with Sentinel Nodes	Sensitivity	Negative Predictive Value	Detection Method
Malur et al. 2001 (74)[1]	50	78	83	97	BD, RC, or both
Malur et al. 2001 (74)[1]	20[a]	90	100	100	BD+RC
Levenback et al. 2002 (75)	39	100	87.5	97	BD + RC
Plante 2003 (76)	70	87		100	BD
Plante 2003 (76)	29[a]	93	93	100	BD + RC
Dargent, Enria 2003 (77)	70	NR[b]	100	NR	BD
Silva et al. 2005 (78)	56	93	82	92	RC
Rob et al. 2005 (79)	100	80	100	99	BD
Rob et al. 2005 (79)	83	96	100	100	BD+RC
Di Stefano et al. 2005 (80)	50	90	90	97	Blue dye
Angioli et al. 2005 (81)	37	70	100	100	RC
Lin et al. 2005 (82)	30	100	100	100	RC
Schwendinger et al. 2006 (83)	47	83	90	97	BD
Wydra et al. 2006 (84)	100	100	100	100	BD + RC
Hauspy et al. 2007 (85)	39	98	100	100	RC +/−BD
Yuan et al. 2007 (86)	81	94[c]		95	BD

NS, not stated.

BD = Blue Dye RC = Radiolabeled Colloid

[1]Total reported included BD alone (n = 9), RC alone (n = 21) and combined (n = 20). For combined technique, sensitivity = 100, NPV = 100.
[a]Subgroup using combined BD + RC technique
[b]90% rate of sentinel nodes found in 14 of 139 attempted dissections in 70 patients.
[c]Reported for subgroup of 49 patients with 4 mL of methylene blue. Subgroup of 28 patients with 2 to 3 mL injection = 66% detection.

4. **Stage IB1 ≤2 cm diameter with no involvement of the upper endocervix on MRI or intraoperative frozen section**

5. **Histology: squamous, adenocarcinoma, or adenosquamous**

6. **No metastases to regional lymph nodes**

Risk factors for recurrence include lesion size greater than 2 cm, depth of invasion greater than 1 cm, and lymph-vascular space invasion (76). However, some authors suggest that conservative fertility-sparing surgery may be appropriate for select patients with larger lesions that are clearly exophytic (99).

A recent systematic review of 504 women undergoing radical trachelectomy described the gestational outcomes of 200 pregnancies resulting in 133 third-trimester deliveries. The first trimester abortion rate was 19%, which is similar to the general population. **The second trimester spontaneous abortion rate was 9.5% (19 of 200) when defined as <24 weeks. Overall, 84 of 200 pregnancies (42%) resulted in term deliveries of viable infants, but 25% (49 of 200) of total pregnancies or 37% of third-term deliveries were preterm. Moreover, 13 of 133 (9.8%) patients delivered between 24 and 28 weeks and 14 (10.5%) delivered between 24 and 34 weeks (100).** These pregnancies should be managed by maternal fetal medicine specialists.

Ovarian Cancer

Laparoscopy has been used for several decades to manage adnexal masses and as a second-look procedure to avoid laparotomy in patients with persistent disease after primary chemotherapy. More recently, it has been reported to be useful for staging apparently early cancer of the ovary.

Table 21.3 Radical Trachelectomy for Fertility Preservation in Patients with Early-Stage Cervical Cancer: Oncologic Outcomes

Authors	Cases	Size		Histology		Intraop Complications n (%)	Aborted Procedure n/total[a] (%)	Follow-up (median, range)	Recurrences n (%)	Deaths n (%)
		<2 cm n (%)	>2 cm n (%)	Squamous n (%)	Adeno n (%)					
Dargent et al. 2001, 2002 (89, 90); Marchiole 2007 (91)	118	91 (81)[a]	21 (19)	90 (76)	25 (21)	3 (2.5)	17/135 (13)	95 (31–234)	7 (6)	4 (4)
Plante et al. 2004 (92)	72	64 (89)	8 (11)	42 (58)	30 (42)	5 (6)	10/82 (12)	60 (6–156)	2 (3)	1 (1)
Shepherd et al. 2006 (93)	123[c]	NR	NR	83 (66)	33 (27)	6 (5)	NR	45	5 (4)	4 (3)
Steed and Covens 2003 (94)	93	85 (91)	8 (9)	42 (48)	44 (52)		0/93 (0)	30 (1–103)	7 (7)	4 (4.2)
Burnett et al. 2003 (95)	19	19 (100)	0 (0)	10 (53)	9 (47)	0 (0)	2/21 (10)	31 (22–44)	0 (0)	0 (0)
Schlaerth et al. 2003 (96)	10	8 (80)	2 (20)	4 (40)	6 (60)	2 (17)	0 (0)	47 (28–84)	0 (0)	0 (0)
Sonoda et al. 2008 (97)	43[c]	43 (100)	0 (0)	24 (55)	19 (44)	0 (0)	2/43	21 (3–60)[d]	1 (3)	0 (0)
Chen et al. 2008 (98)	16	9 (56)	7 (44)	14 (88)	2 (13)	0 (0)	0 (0)	28 (8–50)	0 (0)	0 (0)

[a]Aborted cases/total number of cases attempted
[b]Excluding 6 patients with stage IIa disease (size not given)
[c]Total number of cases selected for radical trachelectomy
[d]Follow-up data for 36 patients without aborted procedure (2) or postop treatment (5)

The ability to perform retroperitoneal evaluation has seen it advocated again for second-look procedures.

Evaluation of the Suspicious Adnexal Mass

Laparotomy is accepted as the standard of care for management of the suspicious adnexal mass. However, it is possible to mismanage adnexal masses regardless of whether laparotomy or laparoscopy is used.

The incidence with which an unexpected malignancy is encountered when managing an adnexal mass is reported to be between 0.4% and 2.9% (101–103). Childers et al. (104) and Canis et al. (105) used laparoscopy for management of suspicious adnexal masses and reported malignancy rates of 14% and 15%, respectively. More than 80% of the masses were managed by laparoscopy. All of the malignancies were properly diagnosed and treated, including 13 staged by laparoscopy. A frozen section should be obtained so that surgical staging and appropriate treatment are not delayed.

Staging requires an infracolic omentectomy, peritoneal washings, multiple biopsies from the peritoneal surfaces and hemidiaphragms, and pelvic and paraaortic lymph node biopsies. Laparoscopic omentectomy has been described using a stapling technique (106) but has been simplified further with the advent of laparoscopic bipolar vessel sealing devices which incorporate both bipolar cautery and cutting functions.

Several investigators have reported their experiences with staging of early ovarian, fallopian tube, or primary peritoneal cancers. In 1994, Querleu and LeBlanc (107) described the first adequate laparoscopic surgical staging for ovarian carcinoma in eight patients undergoing pelvic and paraaortic lymph node sampling up to the level of the renal veins. An average of nine nodes (range 6–17) were removed, with an average operative time of 111 minutes, postoperative stay of 2.8 days, and blood loss of less than 300 mL. None of the lymph nodes were positive.

In 1995, Childers et al. (108) reported 14 patients undergoing staging for presumed early ovarian cancer. Metastatic disease was discovered in eight patients (57%) and the appropriate treatment instituted. Subsequent series by Pomel (n = 10) (109); Tozzi (n = 24) (110); Chi (n = 20) (111); Spirtos (n = 73) (112); and Leblanc (n = 44; 36 epithelial, 8 germ cell or granulosa cell) (113) have confirmed similar feasibility.

Results of these small series are encouraging and support the development of studies with larger sample sizes and long-term follow-up. However, the low incidence of early stage disease underscores the difficulty of clinical trial development in this patient group. **At this time, laparoscopy for the staging of ovarian cancer remains investigational. It may be considered for patients with apparent early stage disease at presentation, for staging of unstaged patients, or for patients who are candidates for fertility-sparing oophorectomy and staging alone.**

The two major concerns over the use of laparoscopy for adnexal masses are (i) delay in diagnosis and thus treatment; and (ii) rupture of the adnexal mass that is subsequently found to be malignant, which converts the stage from a possible IA to IC. Studies on laparotomy show that if the tumor is removed and proper treatment instituted, rupture does not affect the outcome (114–116), but it is prudent to avoid rupture to minimize any theoretical increase in the risk. If the tumor is ruptured, and the treatment is delayed, the prognosis is worsened (117). Thus, **the use of laparoscopy should be limited to suspicious masses that are small enough to be removed intact or utilizing endoscopic bags to allow for cyst aspiration without the leakage of cyst contents into the peritoneal cavity.**

Second-Look Laparoscopy   Laparoscopy was initially used before planned second-look laparotomy to identify residual disease and thus avoid the laparotomy. This strategy resulted in a reduction in the need for laparotomy in 50% of patients (118).

Improvements in laparoscopic equipment encouraged some investigators to perform the entire second-look procedure by laparoscopy. Childers et al. (108) reported 44 reassessment laparoscopies in 40 women. Twenty-four of the procedures were positive, including five that were only microscopically positive. Five patients (11%) had inadequate laparoscopies because of adhesions, and recurrent disease developed in all of them. Eight of the 20 patients (40%) who were negative later developed recurrent disease. All of these data were similar to those obtained with second-look laparotomy.

Abu-Rustum et al. (119) reported 31 women having second-look laparoscopy, and compared them with 70 patients who had laparotomy and 8 who had both. The rates of positivity were 54.8%, 61.4%, and 62.5%, respectively. The recurrence rates after a negative second look were 14.8% for laparoscopy versus 14.3% for laparotomy. Clough et al. (120) reported 20 patients who had laparoscopy followed by laparotomy at the same surgery, with a positive predictive value for laparoscopy of 86% (12 of 14 patients).

The effects of the CO_2 pneumoperitoneum and laparoscopy on the long-term survival of women undergoing second-look operations have been reported by Abu-Rustum and associates (121). Over an 11-year period, 289 patients had positive second-look operations. There were 131 laparoscopies using CO_2, 139 laparotomies, and 19 laparoscopies converted to laparotomy. The groups were controlled for age, stage, histology, grade, and size of disease found at second look. The median survival for patients who had laparoscopy was 41.1 months and for laparotomy 38.9 months ($p = 0.742$). Thus, **the overall survival was independent of the surgical approach.**

Second-look assessment has generally declined in practice, because approximately 50% of patients with negative second-look surgeries eventually recur (122). However, minimally invasive techniques continue to play a role in the management of patients with advanced ovarian cancer, including the placement of ports for intraperitoneal chemotherapy, if not performed at the initial surgery.

Complications

Complication rates of laparoscopy for malignant disease are higher than for benign disease (123). The rate depends on the type of case and the experience of the surgeon. Laparoscopic second looks have the highest rate of injury to bowel because of the adhesions from previous surgery. Vascular injuries from trocars or the dissection of lymph nodes can occur in any procedure.

Postoperative wound infection, ileus, and fever occur, but at lower rates than after laparotomy. Herniation of omentum or bowel into the trocar sites is a complication unique to laparoscopy. Boike et al. (124) reported 19 cases from 11 institutions. No patient had a hernia through a port smaller than 10 cm, and therefore it is recommended that all port sites greater than 10 mm be closed. Kadar et al. (125) reported a 0.17% rate of herniation among 3,560 laparoscopic operations.

Abdominal wall port-site implantations have been reported with nearly every tumor type, particularly ovarian cancer. However, in a review of 1,335 transperitoneal laparoscopies in 1,288 women with malignant disease, Abu-Rustum et al. reported that laparoscopy-related subcutaneous tumor implantation is rare, occurring in only 13 (0.97%) cases (126).

Technique

Preoperative Preparation

Patient preparation begins with a clear liquid diet the day before the surgical procedure. Evacuation of the bowel may be accomplished with a laxative or an oral gastrointestinal lavage solution. It is important for the bowel to be collapsed during the laparoscopic lymphadenectomy so that proper exposure can be obtained. This is particularly important if the patient is somewhat obese and paraaortic lymphadenectomy is planned.

Operative Approach

The recommended technique of laparoscopy is as follows:

1. **The patient is positioned in a dorsal lithotomy position with legs in stirrups that support the legs and decrease the tension on the femoral and peroneal nerves** (Fig. 21.9). It is helpful to have adjustable stirrups that allow for conversion from the low lithotomy to a leg-flexed position for vaginal surgery. The arms are tucked at the side, an endotracheal tube is positioned, and a Foley catheter is placed in the bladder.

2. **The first trocar is inserted into the umbilicus if the patient does not have a midline incision.** If there is a midline incision, then a left upper quadrant insufflation and 5-mm trocar are used. The left upper quadrant approach for patients with previous midline incisions allows the laparoscope to be placed away from possible adhesions that can then be dissected from the umbilicus before placing the 10-mm trocar.

3. **Additional trocars are placed in the right and left lower quadrants and in the suprapubic site.** Typically, a 10-mm trocar is placed in the suprapubic site so that the laparoscope can be placed in that port to help with packing the bowel or in dissecting adhesions from around the umbilical port (Fig. 21.9, Fig. 21.10).

4. **The bowel should be carefully packed into the upper abdomen so that adequate exposure of the paraaortic area and pelvis can be obtained.** Sponges or minilaparotomy packs can be placed around loops of bowel to aid in exposure and to blot

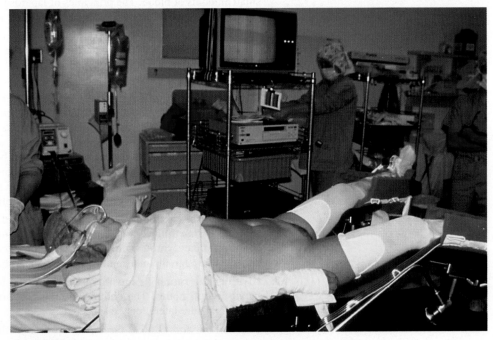

Figure 21.9   Patient position for laparoscopically assisted radical hysterectomy.

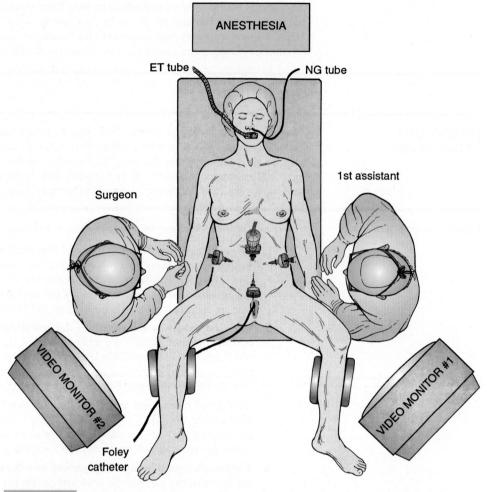

Figure 21.10   The position of the surgeons and placement of the trocars in the abdomen.

small amounts of blood. The principles of laparoscopic surgery are the same as those of laparotomy. There must be adequate exposure, identification of the anatomy, and removal of the appropriate tissue.

5. **The lymphadenectomy is best performed by the surgeon on the side opposite the side of dissection** (i.e., the surgeon on the patient's right side dissects the left pelvic lymph nodes). The peritoneal incisions are left open, and drains are not placed.

6. **The paraaortic lymphadenectomy is usually performed first.** Both the right- and left-sided aortic lymph nodes are sampled. The peritoneum is incised between the sigmoid mesentery and the mesentery of the cecum. The lymph node chain is isolated, and dissection is carried out. Monopolar surgery, bipolar surgery, harmonic scalpel, and the argon beam coagulator have all been used successfully. The landmarks are usually the reflection of the duodenum and inferior mesenteric vessel superiorly and the psoas muscles laterally. The ureter must be identified and placed on traction by the assistant to keep it out of the operative field (Fig. 21.11).

7. **The proximal common iliac lymph nodes are dissected through the retroperitoneal incision made from the paraaortic lymph nodes down to the middle common iliac lymph nodes.** The remaining common iliac lymph nodes are dissected through the incision for the pelvic lymphadenectomy.

8. **Dividing the round ligaments and finding the lateral pelvic space exposes the pelvic lymph nodes.** The obliterated umbilical artery is retracted medially, which opens the entire lateral pelvic space.

9. **The disease and clinical circumstances, as outlined previously, determine the extent of the pelvic lymphadenectomy.** To perform a **pelvic lymph node sampling,** the lymph nodes are removed medial to the external iliac and anterior to the obturator nerve. For a **complete lymphadenectomy,** the lymph nodes are also removed

from between the iliac vessels and the psoas muscle, and from the obturator fossa (Fig 21.12).

10. **All port sites 10 mm or larger should have the fascia and peritoneal layers closed to prevent herniation of bowel.** Several instruments are available to pass the suture through the skin incision lateral to the port and back up on the opposite side. The skin is closed, and a local anesthetic is injected around the port site to decrease postoperative pain.

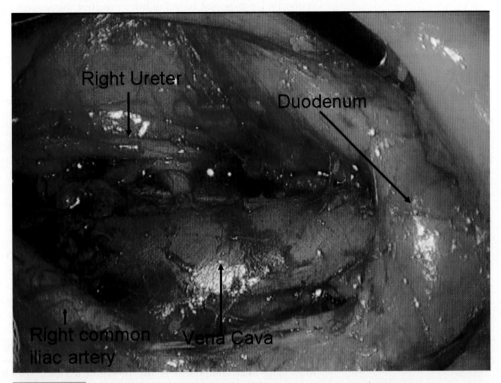

Figure 21.11   Completed right common iliac and paraaortic node dissection.

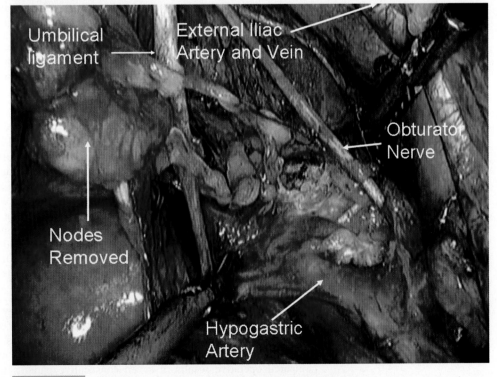

Figure 21.12   Partially completed right pelvic lymphadenectomy.

Detailed step-by-step images and details of the dissection can be found in the accompanying DVD. Video of the surgical procedure is available in *LWW Laparoscopy for Gynecology and Oncology* by Dr. Kenneth Hatch.

Postoperative Management

Patients are given liquids the day of surgery, and the diet is advanced rapidly. Early ambulation is encouraged. The patient's progress is usually rapid. Adynamic ileus is unusual after laparoscopic surgery, but any abdominal distention, worsening of pain, or vomiting must be taken seriously. Unsuspected bowel injuries manifest themselves by abdominal distention, pain, and free air in the peritoneal cavity. The CO_2 should be absorbed within hours, so any free air in the abdomen is highly suspicious.

Robotic-Assisted Laparoscopy

Traditional laparoscopy can be technically difficult in comparison with open procedures due to factors such as lack of depth perception, ergonomic difficulties with often counter-intuitive directional movements, tremor amplification, and relatively rigid instrumentation which lacks the flexibility of movement possible in open surgery. Even simple procedures such as suturing are associated with a much steeper learning curve, and can take longer to perform, hindering widespread adoption of minimally invasive techniques. More recently, **robotic-assisted surgical devices have been developed to address these issues.** It is hoped they will make minimally invasive techniques easier to learn, and will expand the scope of procedures that may be performed laparoscopically.

The DaVinci surgical system (Intuitive Surgical, Sunnyvale CA) **is currently the only commercially available robotic surgical system that is FDA approved** for gynecologic and other surgical procedures. It incorporates several components including a surgeon console, patient side cart, 3-D vision system, and proprietary EndoWrist instruments. **The surgeon console** is a remote unit that allows the seated surgeon to manipulate the robotic instruments while viewing a 3-D operative field. The next component is the **patient-side cart,** which provides three or four robotic arms, which in turn control the endoscope and two or three instrument arms. A major feature of the DaVinci system is the **EndoWrist instrumentation,** which provides seven degrees of motion, mimicking the full range of motion of a surgeon's hand and wrist. The final component is **the in-vision system, which allows for three-dimensional imaging.** The Vision System incorporates a high-resolution three-dimensional endoscope, which provides 3-D vision when the surgeon utilizes the stereoscopic viewer. An additional vision tower provides operative field visualization for the rest of the surgical team, although images are two dimensional.

Experience in gynecologic procedures is still limited, but increasing. Reynolds and Advincula reported their initial experience of 16 patients undergoing robotic-assisted laparoscopic-assisted vaginal hysterectomy (127). Oncologic indications included endometrial and ovarian carcinoma and cervical dysplasia. This series reported an operative time ranging from 270 to 600 minutes with a mean estimated blood loss (EBL) of 300 cc.

Several series have focused on the experience with hysterectomy for benign disease. Beste et al. reported on 11 patients undergoing robotic assisted total laparoscopic hysterectomy (128). Estimated blood loss ranged from 25 to 350 mL, with operative times ranging from 49 to 227 minutes. One patient required conversion to laparotomy because of bleeding at the level of the uterine arteries. Fiorentino et al. reported on 20 patients with a median EBL of 81 mL, median uterine weight of 98 gm, and median operative time of 200 minutes. Two patients were converted to laparotomy because of poor visualization, but 18 procedures were successful (129). Reporting their experience of 16 consecutive patients undergoing either complete laparoscopic hysterectomy or supracervical hysterectomy, Reynolds and Advincula similarly noted feasibility, with no conversions to laparotomy, a mean blood loss of 72.5 mL, and a mean operative time of 242 minutes (170 to 432 minutes). Thirteen of 16 patients required lysis of pelvic adhesions from prior pelvic surgeries (127).

More recently, the use of robotic radical hysterectomy in cervical cancer has been described. Kim reported on 10 patients with stage IA1–IB1 cervical cancer. The mean operative time was 207 minutes, mean docking time 26 minutes, mean EBL 355 mL, and mean pelvic lymph node count of 27.6. No conversions were required (130). Sert and Abeler compared operative results of seven consecutive patients undergoing robotic laparoscopic radical hysterectomy with eight previous laparoscopic procedures (131). Estimated blood loss (71 vs. 160 mL) and hospital stay (4 vs. 8 days) were decreased in the robotic vs. laparoscopic groups, while operative time (241 vs. 300 minutes) and lymph node count (13 vs. 15) were not significantly different.

In 2008, Magrina et al. described the prospective Mayo Clinic experience of 27 patients undergoing robotic radical hysterectomy (132). Patients were matched for age, BMI, type of malignancy, stage of disease, and type of radical hysterectomy. Patients who underwent robotic or laparoscopic surgery had decreased blood loss (133.1, 208.4 mL) and hospital stay (1.7, 2.4 days) when compared with laparotomy (443.6 mL, 3.6 days). However, operative time was shorter for open laparotomy (166.8 minutes) and robotic procedures (189.6 minutes) when compared with laparoscopy (220.4 minutes).

Challenges in robotic surgery include the lack of tactile sensation as well as the high cost of the system. However, while initial series are limited, these experiences suggest that robotics offer the same patient benefits afforded by traditional laparoscopy, while providing improved surgical dexterity and visualization. As with traditional laparoscopy, further prospective studies are required to determine appropriate indications, feasibility, and oncologic outcomes.

Summary

The skills to manage gynecologic malignancies by laparoscopic techniques are acquired through a commitment on the surgeon's part to learn the technique. It requires up-to-date equipment and a team familiar with the procedures. Hands-on experience in an animal laboratory and proctored learning in the operating suite are highly recommended. In the hands of experienced laparoscopic surgeons and with properly selected patients, laparoscopic surgery appears to result in shorter hospital stays, earlier return of function, and outcomes comparable with laparotomy. The results of prospective, randomized trials are awaited. Innovative technologies such as robotic-assisted surgical units may further expand the scope and use of minimally invasive techniques in the field of gynecologic oncology.

References

1. **Dargent D, Salvat J**. *Envahissenent ganglionnaire pelvien: place de la pelviscopie retroperitoneale.* Paris: Medsi, McGraw-Hill, 1989.
2. **Childers J, Surwit E.** A combined laparoscopic vaginal approach in the management of stage I endometrial cancer. *Gynecol Oncol* 1991;45:46–51.
3. **Nezhat C, Burrell M, Nezhat F.** Laparoscopic radical hysterectomy with para aortic and pelvic node dissection. *Am J Obstet Gynecol* 1992;166:864–865.
4. **Querleu D, LeBlanc E, Castelain B.** Laparoscopic pelvic lymphadenectomy in the staging of early carcinoma of the cervix. *Am J Obstet Gynecol* 1991;164:579–581.
5. **Childers J, Brzechffa P, Hatch K, Surwit E.** Laparoscopically assisted surgical staging (LASS) of endometrial cancer. *Gynecol Oncol* 1992;51:33–38.
6. **Childers J, Hatch K, Surwit E.** The role of laparoscopic lymphadenectomy in the management of cervical carcinoma. *Gynecol Oncol* 1992;47:38–43.
7. **Childers J, Hatch K, Tran A-H, Surwit E.** Laparoscopic paraaortic lymphadenectomy in gynecologic malignancies. *Obstet Gynecol* 1993;82:741–747.
8. **Spirtos NM, Schlaerth JB, Spirtos TW, Schlaerth AC, Indman PD, Kimball RE.** Laparoscopic bilateral pelvic and paraaortic lymph node sampling: an evolving technique. *Am J Obstet Gynecol* 1995;173:105–111.
9. **Fowler J, Carter J, Carlson JW, Maslonkowski R, Byers LJ, Carson LF, et al.** Lymph node yield from laparoscopic lymphadenectomy in cervical cancer: a comparative study. *Gynecol Oncol* 1993;51:187–192.
10. **Possover M, Krause N, Kuhne-Heid R, Schneider A.** Value of laparoscopic evaluation of paraaortic and pelvic lymph nodes for treatment of cervical cancer. *Am J Obstet Gynecol* 1998;178:806–810.
11. **Possover M, Plaul K, Krause N, Schneider A.** Left-sided laparoscopic para-aortic lymphadenectomy: anatomy of the ventral tributaries of the infrarenal vena cava. *Am J Obstet Gynecol* 1998;179:1295–1297.
12. **Kohler C, Tozzi R, Kelmm P, Schneider A.** Laparoscopic paraaortic left-sided transperitoneal infrarenal lymphadenectomy in patients with gynecologic malignancies: technique and results. *Gynecol Oncol* 2003;91:139–148.
13. **Spirtos NM, Eisenkop SM, Schlaerth JB, Ballon SC.** Laparoscopic radical hysterectomy (type III) with aortic and pelvic lymphadenectomy in patients with stage I cervical cancer: surgical morbidity and inter-mediate follow-up. *Am J Obstet Gynecol* 2002;187:340–348.
14. **Hertel H, Kohler C, Michels W, Possover M, Tozzi R, Schneider A.** Laparoscopic-assisted radical vaginal hysterectomy (LARVH): prospective evaluation of 200 patients with cervical cancer. *Gynecol Oncol* 2003;90:505–511.
15. **Gemignani ML, Curtin JP, Zelmanovich J, Patel DA, Venkatraman E, Barakat RR.** Laparoscopic-assisted vaginal hysterectomy for endometrial cancer: clinical outcomes and hospital charges. *Gynecol Oncol* 1999;73:5–11.
16. **Scribner, DR Jr, Walker JL, Johnson GA, McMeekin SD, Gold MA, Mannel RS.** Laparoscopic pelvic and paraaortic lymph node dissection: analysis of the first 100 cases. *Gynecol Oncol* 2001;82:498–503.
17. **Abu-Rustum NR, Chi DS, Sonoda Y, DiClemente MJ, Bekker G, Gemignani M, et al.** Transperitoneal laparoscopic pelvic and para-aortic lymph node dissection using the argon-beam coagulator and monopolar instruments: an 8-year study and description of technique. *Gynecol Oncol* 2003;89:504–513.
18. **Querleu D, Leblanc E, Cartron G, Narducci F, Ferron G, Martel P.** Audit of preoperative and early complications of laparoscopic

lymph node dissection in 1000 gynecologic cancer patients. *Am J Obstet Gynecol* 2006;195:1287–1292.

19. **Köhler C, Klemm P, Schau A, Possover M, Krause N, Tozzi R, et al.** Introduction of transperitoneal lymphadenectomy in a gynecologic oncology center: analysis of 650 laparoscopic pelvic and/or paraaortic transperitoneal lymphadenectomies. *Gynecol Oncol* 2004; 95:52–61.

20. **Spirtos N, Schlaerth J, Gross GM, Spirtos TW, Schlaerth AC, Ballon SC.** Cost and quality of life analyses of surgery for early endometrial cancer: laparotomy versus laparoscopy. *Am J Obstet Gynecol* 1996;174:1795–1799.

21. **Melendez TD, Childers JM, Nour M, Harrigill K, Surwit EA.** Laparoscopic staging of endometrial cancer: the learning experience. *J Soc Laparoendosc Surg* 1997;1:45–49.

22. **Scribner DR Jr, Mannel RS, Walker JL, Johnson GA.** Cost analysis of laparoscopy versus laparotomy for early endometrial cancer. *Gynecol Oncol* 1999;75:460–463.

23. **Holub Z, Jabor A, Bartos P, Eim J, Urbanek S, Pivovarnikova R.** Laparoscopic surgery for endome-trial cancer: long-term results of a multicentric study. *Eur J Gynaecol Oncol* 2002;23:305–310.

24. **Khosia I, Lowe C.** Indices of obesity derived from body weight and height. *Br J Prev Med Soc* 1967;21:122–124.

25. **Holub Z, Bartos P, Jabor A, Eim J, Fischlova D, Kliment L.** Laproscopic surgery in obese women with endometrial cancer. *J Am Assoc Gynecol Laparosc* 2000;7:83–88.

26. **Eltabbakh GH, Shamonki MI, Moody JM, Garafano LL.** Hysterectomy for obese women with endometrial cancer: laparoscopy or laparotomy? *Gynecol Oncol* 2000;78:329–335.

27. **Eltabbakh GH.** Analysis of survival after laparoscopy in women with endometrial carcinoma. *Cancer* 2002;95:1894–1901.

28. **Malur S, Possover M, Michels W, Schneider A.** Laparoscopic-assisted vaginal versus abdominal surgery in patients with endome-trial cancer—a prospective randomized trial. *Gynecol Oncol* 2001; 80:239–244.

29. **Hatch KD.** Clinical outcomes and long-term survival after laparoscopic staging and hysterectomy for endometrial cancer. *Proc Soc Gynecol Oncol* 2003;35(abst).

30. **Obermair A, Manolitsas TP, Leung Y, Hammond IG, McCartney AJ.** Total laparoscopic hysterectomy for endometrial cancer: patterns of recurrence and survival. *Gynecol Oncol* 2004; 92:789–793.

31. **Zapico A, Fuentes P, Grassa A, Arnanz F, Otazua J, Cortés-Prieto J.** Laparoscopic-assisted vaginal hysterectomy versus abdominal hysterectomy in stages I and II endometrial cancer. Operating data, follow up and survival. *Gynecol Oncol* 2005;98:222–227.

32. **Kim DY, Kim MK, Kim JH, Suh DS, Kim YM, Kim YT.** Laparoscopic-assisted vaginal hysterectomy versus abdominal hysterectomy in patients with stage I and II endometrial cancer. *Int J Gynecol Cancer* 2005;15:932–937.

33. **Frigerio L, Gallo A, Ghezzi F, Trezzi G, Lussana M, Franchi M.** Laparoscopic-assisted vaginal hysterectomy versus abdominal hysterectomy in endometrial cancer. *Int J Gynaecol Obstet* 2006; 93:209–213.

34. **Kalogiannidis I, Lambrechts S, Amant F, Neven P, Van Gorp T, Vergote I.** Laparoscopy-assisted vaginal hysterectomy compared with abdominal hysterectomy in clinical stage I endometrial cancer: safety, recurrence, and long-term outcome. *Am J Obstet Gynecol* 2007;196:248.e1–8.

35. **Walker J, Mannel R, Piedmonte M, Schlaerth J, Spirtos N, Spiegel G.** Phase III trial of laparoscopy versus laparotomy for surgical resection and comprehensive surgical staging of uterine cancer: a Gynecologic Oncology Group study funded by the National Cancer Institute. *Gynecol Oncol* 2006;101:S11, 22(abst).

36. **Khoury-Collado F, Abu-Rustum NR.** Lymphatic mapping in endometrial cancer: a literature review of current techniques and results. *Int J Gynecol Cancer* 2008 Jan 23. [Epub ahead of print]

37. **Burke TW, Levenback C, Tornos C, Morris M, Wharton JT, Gershenson DM.** Intraabdominal lymphatic mapping to direct selective pelvic and paraaortic lymphadenectomy in women with high-risk endometrial cancer: results of a pilot study. *Gynecol Oncol* 1996;62:169–173.

38. **Echt ML, Finan MA, Hoffman MS, Kline RC, Roberts WS, Fiorica JV.** Detection of sentinel lymph nodes with lymphazurin in

cervical, uterine, and vulvar malignancies. *South Med J* 1999;92: 204–208.

39. **Li B, Li XG, Wu LY, Zhang WH, Li SM, Min C, et al.** A pilot study of sentinel lymph nodes identification in patients with endometrial cancer. *Bull Cancer* 2007;94:E1–4.

40. **Frumovitz M, Bodurka DC, Broaddus RR, Coleman RL, Sood AK, Gershenson DM, et al.** Lymphatic mapping and sentinel node biopsy in women with high-risk endometrial cancer. *Gynecol Oncol* 2007;104:100–103.

41. **Frumovitz M, dos Reis R, Sun CC, Milam MR, Bevers MW, Brown J, et al.** Comparison of total laparoscopic and abdominal radical hysterectomy for patients with early-stage cervical cancer. *Obstet Gynecol* 2007;110:96–102.

42. **Altgassen C, Pagenstecher J, Hornung D, Diedrich K, Horneman A.** A new approach to label sentinel nodes in endometrial cancer. *Gynecol Oncol* 2007;105:457–461.

43. **Gargiulo T, Giusti M, Bottero A, Leo L, Brokaj L, Armellino F, et al.** Sentinel lymph node (SLN) laparoscopic assessment in early stage endometrial cancer. *Minerva Ginecol* 2003;55:259–262.

44. **Pelosi E, Arena V, Baudino B, Bellò M, Giusti M, Gargiulo T, et al.** Pre-operative lymphatic mapping and intra-operative sentinel lymph node detection in early stage endometrial cancer. *Nucl Med Commun* 2003;24:971–975.

45. **Barranger E, Cortez A, Grahek D, Callard P, Uzan S, Darai E.** Laparoscopic sentinel node procedure using a combination of patent blue and radiocolloid in women with endometrial cancer. *Ann Surg Oncol* 2004;11:344–349.

46. **Lelievre L, Camatte S, Le Frere-belda MA, Kerrou K, Froissart M, Taurelle R, et al.** Sentinel lymph node biopsy in cervix and corpus uteri cancers. *Int J Gynecol Cancer* 2004;14:271–278.

47. **Holub Z, Jabor A, Lukac J, Kliment L.** Laparoscopic detection of sentinel lymph nodes using blue dye in women with cervical and endometrial cancer. *Med Sci Monit* 2004;10:CR587–591.

48. **Niikura H, Okamura C, Utsonomiya H, Yoshinaga K, Akahira J, Ito K, et al.** Sentinel lymph node detection in patients with endometrial cancer. *Gynecol Oncol* 2004;92:669–674.

49. **Fersis N, Gruber I, Relakis K, Friedrich M, Becker S, Wallwiener D, et al.** Sentinel node identification and intraoperative lymphatic mapping. First results of a pilot study in patients with endometrial cancer. *Eur J Gynaecol Oncol* 2004;25:339–342.

50. **Raspagliesi F, Ditto A, Kusamura S, Fontanelli R, Vecchione F, Maccauro M, et al.** Hysteroscopic injection of tracers in sentinel node detection of endometrial cancer: a feasibility study. *Am J Obstet Gynecol* 2004;191:435–439.

51. **Maccauro M, Lucignani G, Aliberti G, Villano C, Castellani MR, Solima E, et al.** Sentinel lymph node detection following the hysteroscopic peritumoural injection of 99mTc-labelled albumin nanocolloid in endometrial cancer. *Eur J Nucl Med Mol Imaging* 2005;32:569–574.

52. **Dargent D.** A new future for Schauta's operation through a presurgical retroperitoneal pelviscopy. *Eur J Gynaecol Oncol* 1987;8: 292–296.

53. **Querleu D.** Laparoscopically assisted radical vaginal hysterectomy. *Gynecol Oncol* 1993;51:248–254.

54. **Hatch KD, Hallum AV III, Nour M.** New surgical approaches to treatment of cervical cancer. *J Natl Cancer Inst Monogr* 1996;21: 71–75.

55. **Schneider A, Possover M, Kamprath S, Endisch U, Krause N, Noschel H.** Laparoscopy-assisted radical vaginal hysterectomy modified according to Schauta-Stoeckel. *Obstet Gynecol* 1996;88: 1057–1060.

56. **Morgan DJ, Hunter DC, McCracken G, McClelland HR, Price JH, Dobbs SP.** Is laparoscopically assisted radical vaginal hysterectomy for cervical carcinoma safe? A case control study with follow up. *BJOG* 2007;114:537–542.

57. **Jackson KS, Das N, Naik R, Lopes AD, Godfrey KA, Hatem MH, et al.** Laparoscopically assisted radical vaginal hysterectomy vs. radical abdominal hysterectomy for cervical cancer: a match controlled study. *Gynecol Oncol* 2004;95:655–661.

58. **Steed H, Rosen B, Murphy J, Laframboise S, De Petrillo D, Covens A.** A comparison of laparascopic-assisted radical vaginal hysterectomy and radical abdominal hysterectomy in the treatment of cervical cancer. *Gynecol Oncol* 2004;93:588–593.

59. Sharma R, Bailey J, Anderson R, Murdoch J. Laparoscopically assisted radical vaginal hysterectomy (Coelio-Schauta): a comparison with open Wertheim/Meigs hysterectomy. *Int J Gynecol Cancer* 2006;16:1927–1932.

60. Malur S, Possover M, Schneider A. Laparoscopically assisted radical vaginal versus radical abdominal hysterectomy type II in patients with cervical cancer. *Surg Endosc* 2001;15:289–292.

61. Renaud MC, Plante M, Roy M. Combined laparoscopic and vaginal radical surgery in cervical cancer. *Gynecol Oncol* 2000;79: 59–63.

62. Querleu D, Narducci F, Poulard V, Lacaze S, Occelli B, LeBlanc E, et al. Modified radical vaginal hysterectomy with or without laparoscopic nerve-sparing dissection: a comparative study. *Gynecol Oncol* 2002;85:154–158.

63. Nezhat C, Nezhat F, Burrell MO, Benigno B, Welander CE. Laparoscopic radical hysterectomy with paraaortic and pelvic node dissection. *Am J Obstet Gynecol* 1994;170:699.

64. Canis M, Mage G, Wattiez A, Puly J, Chaptron C, Bruiat M. Vaginally assisted laparoscopic radical hysterectomy. *J Gynecol Surg* 1992;8:103–104.

65. Puntambekar SP, Palep RJ, Puntambekar SS, Wagh GN, Patil AM, Rayate NV, Agarwal GA. Laparoscopic total radical hysterectomy by the Pune technique: our experience of 248 cases. *J Minim Invasive Gynecol* 2007;14:682–689.

66. Gil-Moreno A, Puig O, Pérez-Benavente MA, Díaz B, Vergés R, De la Torre J, et al. Total laparoscopic radical hysterectomy (type II-III) with pelvic lymphadenectomy in early invasive cervical cancer. *J Minim Invasive Gynecol* 2005;12:113–120.

67. Malzoni M, Tinelli R, Cosentino F, Perone C, Vicario V. Feasibility, morbidity, and safety of total laparoscopic radical hysterectomy with lymphadenectomy: our experience. *J Minim Invasive Gynecol* 2007;14:584–590.

68. Pomel C, Atallah D, Le Bouedec G, Rouzier R, Morice P, Castaigne D, et al. Laparoscopic radical hysterectomy for invasive cervical cancer: 8-year experience of a pilot study. *Gynecol Oncol* 2003;91:534–539.

69. Fujii S, Takakura K, Matsumara N, Higuchi T, Yura S, Mandai M, et al. Anatomic identification and functional outcomes of the nerve sparing okabayashi radical hysterectomy. *Gynecol Oncol* 2007;107:4–13.

70. Vidaurreta J, Bermudez A, di Paola G, Sardi J. Laparoscopic staging in locally advanced cervical carcinoma: a new possible philosophy? *Gynecol Oncol* 1999;75:366–371.

71. Hertel H, Kohler C, Elhawary T, Michels W, Possover M, Schneider A. Laparoscopic staging compared with imaging techniques in the staging of advanced cervical cancer. *Gynecol Oncol* 2002;87:46–51.

72. Dargent D, Martin X, Mathevet P. Laparoscopic assessment of the sentinel lymph nodes in early stage cervical cancer. *Gynecol Oncol* 2000;79:411–415.

73. Lantzsch T, Wolters M, Grimm J, Mende T, Buchmann J, Sliutz G, et al. Sentinel node procedure in Ib cervical cancer: a preliminary series. *Br J Cancer* 2001;85:791–794.

74. Malur S, Krause N, Kohler C, Schneider A. Sentinel lymph node detection in patients with cervical cancer. *Gynecol Oncol* 2001;80: 254–257.

75. Levenback C, Coleman RL, Burke TW, Lin WM, Erdman W, Deavers M, et al. Lymphatic mapping and sentinel node identification in patients with cervix cancer undergoing radical hysterectomy and pelvic lymphadenectomy. *J Clin Oncol* 2002;20:688–693.

76. Plante M. Fertility preservation in the management of cervical cancer. *CME J Gynecol Oncol* 2003;8:128–138.

77. Dargent D, Enria R. Laparoscopic assessment of the sentinel lymph nodes in early cervical cancer. Technique—preliminary results and future developments. *Crit Rev Oncol Hematol* 2003;48:305–310.

78. Silva LB, Silva-Filho AL, Traiman P, Triginelli SA, de Lima CF, Siquiera CF, et al. Sentinel node detection in cervical cancer with (99m)Tc-phytate. *Gynecol Oncol* 2005;97:588–595.

79. Rob L, Strnad P, Robova H, Charvat M, Pluta M, Schlegerova D, et al. Study of lymphatic mapping and sentinel node identification in early stage cervical cancer. *Gynecol Oncol* 2005;98:281–288.

80. Di Stefano AB, Acquaviva G, Garozzo G, Barbic M, Cvjeticanin B, Meglic L, et al. Lymph node mapping and sentinel node detec-tion in patients with cervical carcinoma: a 2-year experience. *Gynecol Oncol* 2005;99:671–679.

81. Angioli R, Palaia I, Cipriani C, Muzii L, Calcagno M, Gullotta G, et al. Role of sentinel lymph node biopsy procedure in cervical cancer: a critical point of view. *Gynecol Oncol* 2005;96:504–509.

82. Lin YS, Tzeng CC, Huang KF, Kang CY, Chia CC, Hsieh JF. Sentinel node detection with radiocolloid lymphatic mapping in early invasive cervical cancer. *Int J Gynecol Cancer* 2005;15:273–277.

83. Schwendinger V, Müller-Holzner E, Zeimet AG, Marth C. Sentinel node detection with the blue dye technique in early cervical cancer. *Eur J Gynaecol Oncol* 2006;27:359–362.

84. Wydra D, Sawicki S, Wojtylak S, Bandurski T, Emerich J. Sentinel node identification in cervical cancer patients undergoing transperitoneal radical hysterectomy: a study of 100 cases. *Int J Gynecol Cancer* 2006;16:649–654.

85. Hauspy J, Beiner M, Harley I, Ehrlich L, Rasty G, Covens A. Sentinel lymph nodes in early stage cervical cancer. *Gynecol Oncol* 2007;105:285–290.

86. Yuan SH, Xiong Y, Wei M, Yan XJ, Zhang HZ, Zeng YX, et al. Sentinel lymph node detection using methylene blue in patients with early stage cervical cancer. *Gynecol Oncol* 2007;106:147–152.

87. Dargent D, Brun J, Roy M, Remy I. Pregnancies following radical trachelectomy for invasive cervical cancer. *Gynecol Oncol* 1994;52: 105(abst).

88. Roy M, Plante M. Pregnancies after radical vaginal trachelectomy for early stage cervical cancer. *Am J Obstet Gynecol* 1998;179:1491–1496.

89. Dargent D. Radical trachelectomy: an operation that preserves the fertility of young women with invasive cervical cancer. *Bull Acad Natl Med* 2001;185:1295–1304.

90. Dargent D, Franzosi F, Ansquer Y, Martin X, Marthevet P, Adeline P. Extended trachelectomy relapse: plea for patient involve-ment in the medical decision. *Bull Cancer* 2002;89:1027–1030.

91. Marchiole P, Benchaib M, Buenerd A, Lazlo E, Dargent D, Mathevet P. Oncological safety of laparoscopic-assisted vaginal radical trachelectomy (LARVT or Dargent's operation): a compara-tive study with laparoscopic-assisted vaginal radical hysterectomy (LARVH). *Gynecol Oncol* 2007;106:132–141.

92. Plante M, Renaud MC, François H, Roy M. Vaginal radical trach-electomy: an oncologically safe fertility-preserving surgery. An updated series of 72 cases and review of the literature. *Gynecol Oncol* 2004;94:614–623.

93. Shepherd JH, Spencer C, Herod J, Ind TE. Radical vaginal trach-electomy as a fertility-sparing procedure in women with early-stage cervical cancer-cumulative pregnancy rate in a series of 123 women. *BJOG* 2006;113:719–724.

94. Steed H, Covens A, Radical vaginal trachelectomy and laparoscpic pelvic lymphadenectomy for preservation of fertility. *Postgrad Obstet Gynecol* 2003;23:1–7.

95. Burnett AF, Roman LD, O'Meara AT, Morrow CP. Radical vaginal trachelectomy and pelvic lymphadenectomy for preservation of fertil-ity in early cervical carcinoma. *Gynecol Oncol* 2003;88:419–423.

96. Schlaerth JB, Spirtos NM, Schlaerth AC. Radical trachelectomy and pelvic lymphadenectomy with uterine preservation in the treat-ment of cervical cancer. *Am J Obstet Gynecol* 2003;188:29–34.

97. Sonoda Y, Chi DS, Carter J, Barakat RR, Abu-Rustum NR. Initial experience with Dargent's operation: the radical vaginal trach-electomy. *Gynecol Oncol* 2008;108:214–219.

98. Chen Y, Xu H, Zhang Q, Li Y, Wang D, Liang Z. A fertility-preserving option in early cervical carcinoma: laparoscopy-assisted vaginal radical trachelectomy and pelvic lymphadenectomy. *Eur J Obstet Gynecol Reprod Biol* 2008;136:90–93.

99. Plante M, Roy R. Fertility-preserving options for cervical cancer. *Oncology (Williston Park)* 2006;20:479–488; discussion 491–493.

100. Jolley JA, Battista L, Wing DA. Management of pregnancy after radical trachelectomy: case reports and systematic review of the literature. *Am J Perinatol* 2007;24:531–539.

101. Nezhat F, Nezhat C, Welander CE, Benigno B. Four ovarian cancers diagnosed during laparoscopic management of 1011 women with adnexal masses. *Am J Obstet Gynecol* 1992;167:790–796.

102. Canis M, Mage G, Pouly JL, Wattiez A, Manhes H, Bruhat MA. Laparoscopic diagnosis of adnexal cystic masses: a 12-year experience with long-term follow-up. *Obstet Gynecol* 1994;83: 707–712.

103. **Lehner R, Wenzl R, Heinzl H, Husslein R, Sevelda P.** Influence of delayed staging laparotomy after laparoscopic removal of ovarian masses later found malignant. *Obstet Gynecol* 1998;92:967–971.

104. **Childers JM, Nasseri A, Surwit EA.** Laparoscopic management of suspicious adnexal masses. *Am J Obstet Gynecol* 1996;175: 1451–1459.

105. **Canis M, Pouly JL, Wattiez A, Mage G, Manhes H, Bruhat MA.** Laparoscopic management of adnexal masses suspicious at ultrasound. *Obstet Gynecol* 1997;89:679–683.

106. **Boike GM, Graham JE Jr.** Laparoscopic omentectomy in staging and treating gynecologic cancers. *J Am Assoc Gynecol Laparosc* 1995;2–4(suppl):S4.

107. **Querleu D, LeBlanc E.** Laparoscopic infrarenal paraaortic lymph node dissection for restaging of carcinoma of the ovary or fallopian tube. *Cancer* 1994;73:1467–1471.

108. **Childers J, Lang J, Surwit E, Hatch K.** Laparoscopic surgical staging of ovarian cancer. *Gynecol Oncol* 1995;59:25–33.

109. **Pomel C, Provencher D, Dauplat J, Gauthier P, Le Bouedec G, Drouin P, et al.** Laparoscopic staging of early ovarian cancer. *Gynecol Oncol* 1995;58:301–306.

110. **Tozzi R, Köhler C, Ferrara A, Schneider A.** Laparoscopic treatment of early ovarian cancer: surgical and survival outcomes. *Gynecol Oncol* 2004;93:199–203.

111. **Chi DS, Abu-Rustum NR, Sonoda Y, Ivy J, Rhee E, Moore K, et al.** The safety and efficacy of laparoscopic surgical staging of apparent stage I ovarian and fallopian tube cancers. *Am J Obstet Gynecol* 2005;192:1614–1619.

112. **Spirtos NM, Eisekop SM, Boike G, Schlaerth JB, Cappellari JO.** Laparoscopic staging in patients with incompletely staged cancers of the uterus, ovary, fallopian tube, and primary peritoneum: a Gynecologic Oncology Group (GOG) study. *Am J Obstet Gynecol* 2005;193:1645–1649.

113. **Leblanc E, Sonoda Y, Narducci F, Ferron G, Querleu D.** Laparoscopic staging of early ovarian carcinoma. *Curr Opin Obstet Gynecol* 2006;18:407–412.

114. **Dembo AJ, Davy M, Stenwig AE, Berle EJ, Bush RS, Kjorstad K.** Prognostic factors in patients with stage I epithelial ovarian cancer. *Obstet Gynecol* 1990;75:263–273.

115. **Sevelda P, Vavra N, Schemper M, Salzer H.** Prognostic factors for survival in stage I epithelial ovarian carcinoma. *Cancer* 1990;65: 2349–2352.

116. **Vergote IB, Kaern J, Abeler VM, Pettersen EO, De Vos LN, Trope CG.** Analysis of prognostic factors in stage I epithelial ovarian carcinoma: importance of degree of differentiation and deoxyribonucleic acid ploidy in predicting relapse. *Am J Obstet Gynecol* 1993;160:40–52.

117. **Maiman M, Seltzer V, Boyce J.** Laparoscopic excision of ovarian neoplasms subsequently found to be malignant. *Obstet Gynecol* 1991;77:563–565.

118. **Ozols RF, Fisher RI, Anderson T, Makuch R, Young RC.** Peritoneoscopy in the management of ovarian cancer. *Am J Obstet Gynecol* 1981;140:611–619.

119. **Abu-Rustum NR, Barakat RR, Siegel PL, Venkatraman E, Curtin JP, Hoskins WJ.** Second-look operation for epithelial ovarian cancer: laparoscopy or laparotomy? *Obstet Gynecol* 1996; 88:549–553.

120. **Clough KB, Ladonne JM, Nos C, Renolleau C, Validire P, Durand JC.** Second look for ovarian cancer: laparoscopy or laparotomy? A prospective comparative study. *Gynecol Oncol* 1999;72: 411–417.

121. **Abu-Rustum NR, Sonoda Y, Chi DS, Teoman H, Dizon DS, Venkatrama E, et al.** The effects of CO2 pneumoperitoneum on the survival of women with persistent metastatic ovarian cancer. *Gynecol Oncol* 2003;90:431–434.

122. **Rubin SC, Randall TC, Armstrong KA, Chi DS, Hoskins WJ.** Ten-year follow-up of ovarian cancer patients after second-look laparotomy with negative findings. *Obstet Gynecol* 1999;93: 21–24.

123. **Abu-Rustum N, Barakat R, Curtin J.** Laparoscopic complications in gynecologic surgery for benign or malignant disease. *Gynecol Oncol* 1998;68:107(abst).

124. **Boike GM, Miller CE, Spirtos NM, Mercer LJ, Fowler JM, Summitt R, et al.** Incisional bowel herniations after operative laparoscopy: a series of nineteen cases and review of the literature. *Am J Obstet Gynecol* 1995;172:1726–1733.

125. **Kadar N, Reich H, Liu CY, Manko GF, Gimpelson R.** Incisional hernias after major laparoscopic gynecologic procedures. *Am J Obstet Gynecol* 1993;168:1493–1495.

126. **Abu-Rustum NR, Rhee EH, Chi DS, Sonoda Y, Gemignani M, Barakat RR.** Subcutaneous tumor implantation after laparoscopic procedures in women with malignant disease. *Obstet Gynecol* 2004; 103:480–487.

127. **Reynolds RK, Advincula AP.** Robot-assisted laparoscopic hysterectomy: technique and initial experience. *Am J Surg* 2006;191: 555–560.

128. **Beste TM, Nelson KH, Daucher JA.** Total laparoscopic hysterectomy utilizing a robotic surgical system. *JSLS* 2005;9:13–15.

129. **Fiorentino RP, Zepeda MA, Goldstein BH, John CR, Rettenmaier MA.** Pilot study assessing robotic laparoscopic hysterectomy and patient outcomes. *J Minim Invasive Gynecol* 2006; 13:60–63.

130. **Kim YT, Kim SW, Hyung WJ, Lee SJ, Nam EJ, Lee WJ.** Robotic radical hysterectomy with pelvic lymphadenectomy for cervical carcinoma: a pilot study. *Gynecol Oncol* 2008;108:312–316.

131. **Sert B, Abeler V.** Robotic radical hysterectomy in early-stage cervical carcinoma patients, comparing results with total laparoscopic radical hysterectomy cases. The future is now? *Int J Med Robot* 2007;3:224–228.

132. **Magrina JF, Kho RM, Weaver AL, Montero RP, Magtibay PM.** Robotic radical hysterectomy: comparison with laparoscopy and laparotomy. *Gynecol Oncol* 2008;109:86–91.

22

Pelvic Exenteration

Kenneth D. Hatch
Jonathan S. Berek

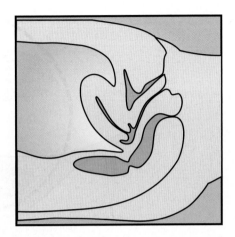

The first series of pelvic exenterations for gynecologic cancer was published in 1946 by Alexander Brunschwig (1). This initial report was of 22 patients, 5 of whom died of the operation itself. His original procedure included sewing both ureters into the colon, which was then brought out as a colostomy. Since these beginnings, there have been major improvements in the selection of patients, operative technique, blood product use, antibiotic availability, and intensive medical management.

The operation gained wider acceptance when Bricker (2) **published his technique of isolating a loop of ileum, closing one end, anastomosing the two ureters to this end,** and **bringing the other out as a stoma.** This eliminated the hyperchloremic acidosis and markedly diminished the recurrent pyelonephritis and renal failure that were experienced with the wet colostomy. The popularity of the Bricker ileal loop was aided by the development of watertight stomal appliances.

Failure of the small bowel anastomosis to heal because of radiation fibrosis in some patients led to the use of a segment of nonirradiated transverse colon for the conduit (3). Further reductions in bowel complications occurred with the use of surgical staplers, which also decreased the operative time, blood loss, and subsequent medical complications (4). Further refinements in the urinary diversion led to the continent urinary reservoir, which is described in Chapter 20.

As a higher percentage of patients became long-term survivors, the desire to improve quality of life led to reconstructive techniques for the vagina and the colon. Today, the patient undergoing pelvic exenteration may have a colonic J-pouch rectal anastomosis, vaginal reconstruction, and continent urinary diversion, allowing her to enjoy a near-normal quality of life without major alterations in her physical appearance.

The terminology of pelvic exenteration has changed as the operations have been tailored to remove the tumor and only those organs that are involved. The total exenteration performed by Brunschwig included the bladder, uterus, vagina, anus, rectum, and sigmoid colon (1). It usually included a large perineal phase (Fig. 22.1). This would lead to a permanent colostomy and urinary stoma. Rutledge et al. (5) and Symmonds et al. (6) reported decreased morbidity and acceptable survival when performing **anterior exenteration,** which removed the uterus, bladder, and various amounts of the vagina (Fig. 22.2). Total pelvic exenteration with rectosigmoid anastomosis (supralevator) became possible with the development of circular staplers. The rectum is excised to within 2 to 3 cm of the anal canal, and the levator support of the anal canal and perineal body is preserved (Fig. 22.3). The **posterior exenteration** removes the uterus, vagina, and portions of the rectosigmoid and anus. It is rarely performed today. Vaginal reconstructive techniques are discussed in Chapter 20.

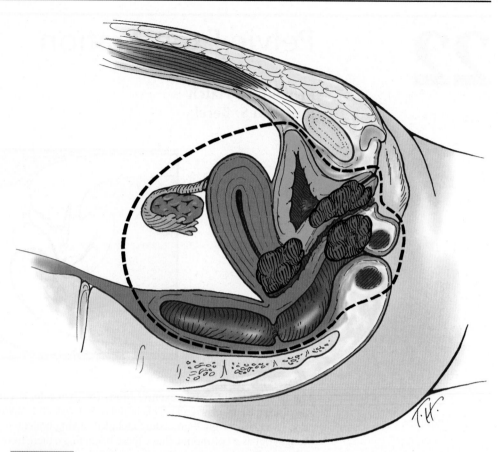

Figure 22.1   **Total pelvic exenteration with perineal phase.** This operation includes removal of the bladder, uterus, vagina, anus, rectum, and sigmoid colon, as well as performance of a perineal phase.

Indications

The most common indication for pelvic exenteration is recurrent or persistent cancer of the cervix after radiation therapy. Some of the early series reported exenterations as primary therapy for stage IVA cervical cancer and cancer of the vulva with urethral, vaginal, or rectal invasion. With modern radiation therapy, the use of exenteration as primary therapy is uncommon.

Exenteration has also been used for endometrial cancer, vaginal carcinoma, rhabdomyosarcoma, and other, miscellaneous rare tumors whenever ultraradical central resection of the cancer is feasible and there is no evidence of systemic or lymphatic spread.

Patients with endometrial cancer have a high likelihood of spread beyond the pelvis and are in general poor candidates for exenterative surgery. The survival rate for highly selected patients with endometrial cancer undergoing exenteration is less than 20% at 5 years (7). To debulk ovarian cancer optimally, a modified posterior exenteration is often performed, which includes *en bloc* resection of the pelvic peritoneum, uterus, tubes, ovaries, and a segment of rectosigmoid. It usually preserves most of the rectum and allows for a low rectal anastomosis. Because there is ovarian cancer left behind, the procedure violates the principle that exenterative surgery is meant to be curative. **In the treatment of ovarian cancer, modified exenteration is performed as part of a cytoreductive procedure and is followed by chemotherapy.**

Patient Selection

The medical evaluation begins with histologic confirmation that cancer is present. The patient should have no other potentially fatal disease, and her general medical condition must be adequate for a prolonged operative procedure (up to 8 hours) with considerable fluid shifts and blood loss.

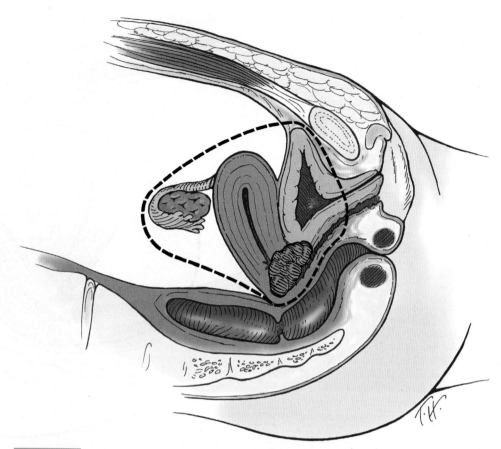

Figure 22.2   **Anterior pelvic exenteration.** This operation includes removal of the bladder, uterus, and varying amounts of the vagina, depending on the extent of disease.

The search for metastatic disease is imperative. The physical examination should include careful palpation of the peripheral lymph nodes and fine-needle aspiration (FNA) cytologic analysis if any suspicious nodes are found. Particular attention should be paid to the groin and supraclavicular nodes. A random biopsy of nonsuspicious supraclavicular lymph nodes has been advocated but is not routinely practiced (8). A computed tomographic (CT) scan of the lungs detects disease missed on routine chest radiography. An abdominal and pelvic CT scan is mandatory to detect liver metastasis and enlarged paraaortic nodes. CT-directed FNA cytologic analysis of any abnormalities should be undertaken. **CT scanning should not be relied on for determining resectability on the basis of apparent absence of fatty planes lateral to the tumor.**

Magnetic resonance imaging (MRI) has been evaluated for preoperative assessment of candidates for pelvic exenteration (9). Twenty-three patients were evaluated before pelvic exenteration for presence and location of the recurrent tumor; tumor extension to the bladder, rectum, or pelvic sidewall; and presence and location of lymphadenopathy. **In four patients (17.4%), the MRI was falsely positive for pelvic sidewall infiltration, and in one patient (4.3%), it was falsely negative.**

Lai and colleagues in Taipei evaluated the **PET scan for the restaging of cervical carcinoma at the time of first recurrence** (10). Forty patients had a PET scan, together with computed tomography and/or magnetic resonance imaging. Twenty-two patients (55%) had their treatment modified due to the PET findings. **PET was significantly superior to CT/MRI (sensitivity = 92% vs. 60%; $p < 0.0001$) in identifying metastatic lesions.** In addition, when compared with an earlier cohort of patients who did not undergo restaging with PET, there was a significantly better 2-year overall survival (72% vs. 36%; $p = 0.02$).

Husain et al. (11) used FDG PET to determine metastatic disease prior to pelvic exenteration or radical resection in 27 patients with recurrent cervical or vaginal cancers. They found that FDG PET had a high sensitivity (100%), and a specificity of 73% in detecting sites of extra-pelvic

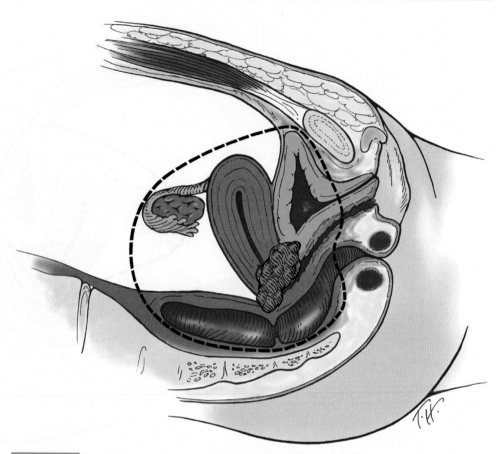

Figure 22.3 **Supralevator total pelvic exenteration.** This operation removes the uterus, vagina, and portions of the rectosigmoid colon with colonic reanastamosis.

metastasis. Chung (12) performed PET CT scans in 52 patients suspected of having recurrence of a cervical cancer. Twenty-eight of 32 patients (87.5%) with positive scans were proven to have recurrent disease. Seventeen of 20 patients (85%) with negative PET CT scans had no evidence of disease. The sensitivity was 90.2% and specificity 81.0%.

The high sensitivity of the PET CT scan may allow the clinician to perform needle-guided biopsies or minimally invasive procedures to confirm the metastatic disease and avoid an aborted exenteration attempt. On the other hand, the 70% to 80% specificity requires that patients undergo exploration if the minimally invasive techniques do not document metastatic disease. Thus, **the PET scan is an important addition to the preoperative investigation of a candidate for pelvic exenteration.**

Extension of the tumor to the pelvic sidewall is a contraindication to exenteration; however, this may be difficult for even the most experienced examiner to determine because of radiation fibrosis. If any question of resectability arises, the patient should be given the benefit of exploratory laparotomy and parametrial biopsies.

Laparoscopy has been described as useful in the assessment of lymph nodes as well as the resectability of disease in the pelvis. In the hands of highly skilled laparoscopic surgeons, this may be an option (13).

The clinical triad of unilateral leg edema, sciatic pain, and ureteral obstruction is nearly always indicative of unresectable cancer on the posterolateral pelvic sidewall.

Despite careful preoperative evaluation, there is approximately a 30% risk that patients will undergo exploratory laparotomy and be judged unsuitable candidates for exenteration. Miller et al. (14) reported that 111 of 394 patients (28.2%) undergoing exploration at the University of Texas M. D. Anderson Cancer Center had findings that led to abortion of the exenterative procedure. Reasons for aborting the procedure were peritoneal disease in

49 patients (44%); nodal metastasis in 45 (40%); parametrial fixation in 15 (13%); and hepatic or bowel involvement in 5 (4.5%).

Preoperative Patient Preparation

The patient must be counseled extensively concerning the seriousness of the operation. She should be prepared to spend several days in the intensive care unit and have a prolonged hospitalization of up to several weeks. She must understand that her sexual functioning will be permanently altered and that she may have one or two stomas. In addition, there is no guarantee of cure. The most difficult subject to broach is the possibility that she may have unresectable disease and that the procedure will need to be aborted.

At least a mechanical bowel preparation is given (see Chapter 20, Table 20.1). Intravenous fluids are started at the time of the bowel preparation to avoid dehydration. The patient should have the stoma sites marked by the ostomy team, and management of the ostomies should be discussed. **If the patient is severely malnourished, total parenteral nutrition (TPN) should be started in advance of surgery.** Because these patients may not have significant oral caloric intake for a week or longer, postoperative TPN is commonly given.

Operative Technique

The patient is placed in the low lithotomy position using stirrups that support the hips, knees, and thighs that can be repositioned during the surgery. This position allows the operators to perform the abdominal and perineal phases of the operation simultaneously. **Intermittent pneumatic compression devices are applied to the calves** as prophylaxis against deep venous thrombosis. **Combined epidural and general anesthesia** allow the epidural to be maintained after surgery for better pain control while keeping the patient alert and able to maintain better respiratory function.

The abdominal incision is made in the midline and should be adequate for exploration of the upper abdomen as well as for performing the pelvic surgery. The liver and omentum should be palpated carefully. The rest of the abdomen is explored, and the paraaortic nodes are palpated. Both the right and left paraaortic nodes are sent for frozen-section analysis. If these are negative, pelvic spaces are opened by dividing the round ligament at the pelvic sidewall. The prevesical, paravesical, pararectal, and presacral spaces are all developed and the ligaments are evaluated for resectability. Enlarged or suspicious pelvic lymph nodes should be removed and sent for frozen-section evaluation. **More than one positive pelvic node, positive paraaortic nodes, peritoneal breakthrough of tumor, or tumor implants in the abdomen or pelvis should lead to abandonment of the operation.**

The procedure begins by ligating the internal iliac artery just after it crosses the internal iliac vein. This sacrifices the uterine artery, vesical artery, and obliterated umbilical artery. The remainder of the hypogastric artery is left intact. It carries the internal pudendal and inferior hemorrhoidal arteries that are important in maintaining the blood supply to the anal canal and lower rectum, where a potential low rectal anastomosis will be performed. The obturator artery should also be preserved because it is the major blood supply to the gracilis muscle, and a gracilis neovagina may be planned. The cardinal ligaments are divided at the sidewall and the broad attachments of the rectum to the sacrum are divided. The vaginal attachments to the tendinous arch are divided. The vaginal arteries and vein are located at the lateral margin of this pedicle. The specimen is completely mobilized, and the penetration of the rectum and vagina through the pubococcygeal muscle can be identified. Various sites for ligation of pubococcygeal muscle for total exenteration versus anterior exenteration are identified (Fig. 22.4).

Anterior Exenteration

Anterior exenteration may be planned for lesions confined to the cervix and the anterior upper vagina. The uterus, cervix, bladder, urethra, and anterior vagina are removed, and the posterior vagina and rectum are preserved. Intraoperative bimanual palpation helps select the appropriate patient. The peritoneal reflection of the cul-de-sac can be incised and the rectum dropped away with a finger in the rectum and a finger in the vagina to ensure that the tumor is adequately resected. One surgeon conducts the perineal phase and the other surgeon conducts the abdominal phase.

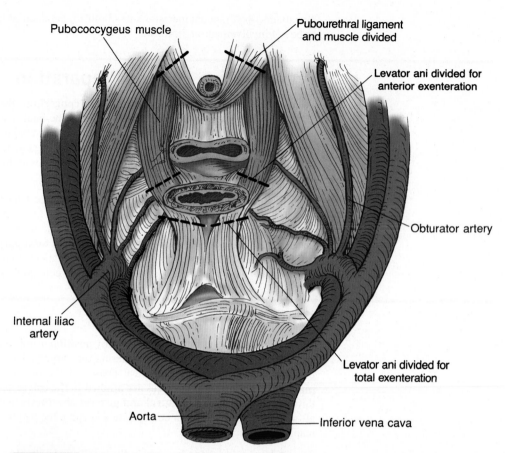

Pubococcygeus muscle

Pubourethral ligament
and muscle divided

Levator ani divided for
anterior exenteration

Obturator artery

Internal iliac
artery

Levator ani divided for
total exenteration

Aorta

Inferior vena cava

Figure 22.4   Cross-sectional diagram of pelvis showing lines of excision through the pubo-coccygeus muscle for anterior and total exenterations.

The perineal incision includes the urethral meatus and the anterior vagina. A long curved clamp is placed beneath the pubis and directed caudad and anterior to the urethra. Another clamp is placed lateral to the pubourethral ligaments and directed out under the symphysis pubis, first at 2 o'clock and then at 10 o'clock. This isolates the right and left pubourethral ligaments, which can be clamped, divided, and ligated. The posterior vaginal incision is made under direct vision from below, insuring a surgical margin of at least 4 cm. The specimen is then ready to be removed. Hemostasis is provided by suture ligatures, and a pelvic pack is placed while the urinary diversion is performed. **The omentum is mobilized and brought down the left paracolic gutter into the pelvis.** It is used to cover the denuded area of the rectum and may provide a receptacle for neovaginal construction by a split-thickness skin graft. The omentum is sewn to the posterior vaginal mucosa over the rectum and to the pelvic side-walls. The skin is harvested and placed around a sterile mold. It is then placed into the cylinder formed by the omentum. If there is not enough omentum, the bulbocavernosus flaps may be used (15).

Supralevator Total Exenteration

Supralevator total exenteration with low rectal anastomosis for patients whose disease extends off the cervix on to the posterior vagina should have the segment of rectum removed *en bloc* with the specimen. This usually entails resection of the rectum to within 6 cm of the anal verge (Fig. 22.3). To remove the specimen, it is best to divide the sigmoid with the stapler to allow for easier exposure to the presacral space. The space is developed in the median avascular plane down to where the rectum exits between the levator muscles. The superior rectal and middle rectal arteries are sacrificed. The incision in the vaginal mucosa is 1 to 2 cm inside the hymenal ring. The supralevator attachments of the bladder, urethra, and vagina are divided, leaving the specimen attached only by the rectum. The hand is placed to encircle the rectum, and traction is placed cephalad. The thoracoabdominal stapling device is then placed across the lower rectum with a 4-cm margin. **Preservation of some of the lower rectum is**

desirable for the patient to have better continence and stool storage functions. The specimen is then removed from the field. Hemostasis is provided, and a pack is placed while the urinary diversion is performed. The left colon is mobilized, sacrificing the sigmoidal arteries and leaving the inferior mesenteric vessels. **The sigmoid is then used for a colonic J-pouch,** and a low anastomosis is performed using the stapling device. The omentum should be mobilized and brought down to reinforce the stapled anastomosis and to cover the denuded area in the pelvis.

Because there is more of the vagina removed in this operation than in the anterior exenteration, the omentum may not be satisfactory for a split-thickness skin-grafted neovagina. **The patient is more likely to require a myocutaneous graft from the gracilis muscles in the medial thigh or the rectus abdominis muscle.** Because of the smaller opening in the vaginal introitus, the rectus abdominis myocutaneous graft is preferred.

Total Exenteration with Perineal Phase

If the tumor has extended down the lower vagina and involves the levator muscles, it is necessary to remove them for a chance of cure. The specimen is mobilized from above in a way similar to that described in the preceding operations (Fig. 22.5). The perineal incision is made around the anus and as far lateral as necessary to gain clearance from the tumor. The anococcygeal and pubococcygeal muscles are divided as necessary for margins. This leaves a large pelvic and perineal defect, which is best filled with bilateral gracilis myocutaneous flaps. Alternatively, the rectus abdominis muscle can be used. The omentum is harvested and used as a pedicle flap to provide additional blood supply and a barrier to bowel adhesions. A permanent colostomy is placed, and urinary diversion is undertaken.

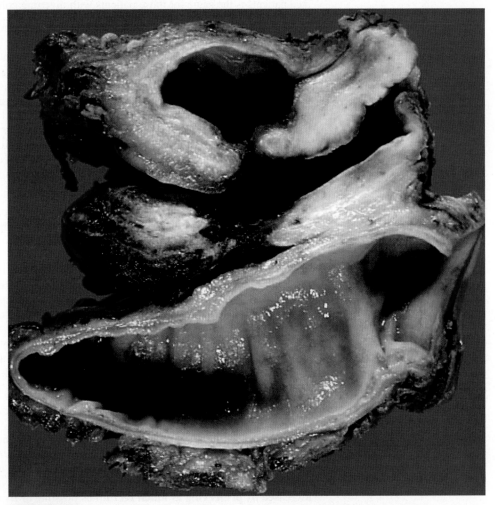

Figure 22.5 **A surgically removed specimen from a total pelvic exenteration.** Note the bladder above with a fistulous tract to the vagina, and the rectum below.

Posterior Exenteration

Posterior exenterations are now rarely performed except occasionally for cancer of the vulva involving the rectum after radiation therapy. When cervical cancer recurs after radiation therapy, even if it is confined to the posterior vagina and rectum, the distal ureters, bladder, and urethra should be removed to avoid the morbidity and mortality of urinary tract fistulae, stenosis, and denervation.

Low Rectal Anastomosis During Pelvic Exenteration

The introduction of the end-to-end circular stapling device has greatly facilitated and popularized the performance of low rectal resection and reanastomosis for a variety of general surgical and gynecologic malignancies. **The automatic circular stapling device has many advantages over the traditional hand-sewn anastomosis. It allows use of a shorter anal or rectal stump, causes less tissue inflammation, creates a higher collagen content, and facilitates faster healing** (16). These are most likely due to a better blood supply at the stapled anastomosis compared with a sutured anastomosis (17,18).

The anastomotic leak rate for low rectal anastomosis is reported to be less than 8% (19,20) in patients without previous radiation. **The most important variables in the anastomotic leak rate are the distance from the anus to the anastomosis, the vascularity of the cut ends, the tension on the anastomotic line, and the elimination of the pelvic cavity** (21,22). Graffner et al. (22) showed in a randomized series that the anastomotic leak rate in previously unirradiated patients is the same for those patients with diverting colostomies as for those without.

There are a few reports in the gynecologic literature concerning the low rectal anastomosis in women with previous pelvic radiation therapy. Berek et al. (23) reported 11 patients with no anastomotic leaks, and 7 of these patients had their bowel continuity reestablished with the end-to-end stapling device. Harris and Wheeless (24) reported 17 patients with a 12.4% anastomotic leak rate and a 12.4% stricture rate. Both groups advised using a diverting colostomy in the previously radiated patient. Hatch et al. (21) reported using a diverting colostomy in 12 of 31 previously irradiated patients. Six patients (50%) later had non–cancer-related rectovaginal fistulae requiring permanent colostomy. Of the 19 patients without protective colostomies, 6 (31.6%) had non–cancer-related rectovaginal fistulae. In the series of Hatch et al. (21), **the most important factor in fistula prevention was the use of an omental wrap to bring a new blood supply to the irradiated pelvis.** For patients who did not have a diverting colostomy, total parenteral nutrition was used for 14 to 21 days.

Mirhashemi et al. (20) conducted a risk factor analysis of 77 patients at the University of Miami who had low rectal anastomosis after exenterative surgery. The indications for the surgery were recurrent cervical cancer (33); ovarian cancer (27); recurrent vaginal cancer (7); recurrent endometrial cancer (4); colon cancer (3); and endometriosis (3). **Previous radiation was the major factor in anastomotic leak rate, with 35% of the irradiated patients and 7.5% of the nonirradiated patients having a leak or a fistula. Protective colostomy did not make a difference.** Of the 40 patients who had total pelvic exenteration with low rectal anastomosis, 36 had received pelvic radiation therapy. A protective colostomy was used in 12 of these patients, and 6 developed fistulae. Of the 24 who did not have protective colostomies, 6 developed an anastomotic leak or fistulae. Only 1 of the 37 patients who had posterior exenteration and low rectal anastomosis had previous radiation therapy, and this patient had an anastomotic leak. Of the remaining 36 patients, 3 had an anastomotic leak. Protective colostomies were not used on any of these patients (20).

Removal of the rectum alters the physiology of stool storage and defecation. The rectum is the reservoir for the collection of feces and transmits impulses to the sensory nerves to initiate the urge to defecate. Inhibitory reflexes from the rectum to the anus are necessary while the rectum is filling to ensure continence. After resection of most of the rectum, reservoir capacity, sensation, and recto-anal reflex are significantly altered (25). **The most important factor in restoring normal bowel function is restoration of the reservoir capacity. Capacity can be increased by preserving as much rectum as possible or by a colonic J-pouch.** The length of rectum necessary for return to acceptable function is 6 cm or more (26,27). When the anastomosis is above 12 cm, there is little alteration of function (28).

Table 22.1 Randomized Comparison of Colonic J-Pouch versus Coloanal Anastamosis in 100 Patients

Factor	Coloanal (n = 52)	J-Pouch (n = 45)	p Value
Anastomotic leak	8 (15%)	1 (2%)	0.03
Stool frequency	3.5	2	0.001
Incontinence score	5	2	0.001
Use of *Loperamide*	19	1	0.001
Medication to induce stooling	10	21	0.07

From **Hallbook O, Pahlman L, Krog M, Wexner SD, Sjodahl R.** Randomized comparison of straight and colonic J pouch anastomosis after low anterior resection. *Ann Surg* 1996;224:58–65, with permission (34).

The colonic J-pouch has been popularized by colorectal surgeons to treat rectal cancer with low rectal resection. It has replaced coloanal anastomosis because of its superior results. **Studies comparing colonic J-pouch with coloanal anastomosis have shown (i) a decreased anastomotic leak rate; (ii) a better continence rate; (iii) fewer stools per day; (iv) better control of urgency; and (v) better control of flatus** (29–32). Prospective, randomized trials have confirmed the observational studies (33,34) (Table 22.1).

The most significant drawback to the colonic J-pouch is the inability of some patients to empty the pouch. This is most likely because of the length of the staple line used to construct the pouch. Hida et al. (35) prospectively randomized patients to a 5-cm versus a 10-cm pouch and found the 5-cm pouch to be superior for evacuation without compromising the other parameters (Table 22.2). Most authors report using a diverting colostomy when creating the colonic J-pouch, which has led to a decrease in the anastomotic leak rate.

Harris et al. have reported the long-term function of J-pouch anal anastomosis in 119 consecutive randomized patients with colorectal cancer from the Cleveland Clinic. Patients who had J-pouch versus coloanal anastomosis had significantly better continence scores at 5 to 9 years after surgery and fewer nocturnal bowel movements (36).

A new procedure called a coloplasty has been developed at the Cleveland Clinic to improve on the poor bowel function after either a coloanal anastomosis or a colonic J-pouch anastomosis (37) (see Chapter 20). In a randomized study of the three techniques, the coloplasty and colonic J-pouch patients had significantly more favorable compliance, reservoir volume, and fewer bowel movements per day than the straight anastomotic group. The advantage of the coloplasty was that it could be used in a narrow pelvis. This may apply to the female

Table 22.2 Randomized Study of 5-cm J-Pouch versus 10-cm J-Pouch

	5 cm (n = 20)	10 cm (n = 20)	p Value
Sphincter function			
Resting pressure	97.8	90.6	NS
Squeeze pressure	214	194	NS
Reservoir function			
Threshold volume	40	70	<0.001
Maximum volume	98	129	0.003
Evacuation (mL within 5 min)	430	279	<0.001

NS, not significant.

From **Hida J, Yasutomi M, Fujimoto K, Okuno K, Ieda S, Machidera N, et al.** Functional outcome after low anterior resection with low anastomosis for rectal cancer using the colonic J-pouch: prospective randomized study for determination of optimum pouch size. *Dis Colon Rectum* 1996;39:986–991, with permission (35).

patient who is having vaginal reconstruction with myocutaneous graphs, where space for anastomosis is diminished (37).

There are some important anatomic considerations for patients undergoing pelvic exenteration with a continent urinary diversion. The continent urinary diversion uses the right colic artery up to its anastomosis with the middle colic artery. A colonic J-pouch uses the sigmoidal and left colic vessels. Adequate mobilization of the descending and left colon requires mobilization of the splenic flexure and rotation of the left colon into the pelvis. If a diverting loop colostomy is performed, it may interrupt the vascular supply from the marginal artery of Drummond. Care must be taken to preserve this vascular supply so that the colonic J-pouch and the resultant colorectal anastomosis have an adequate blood supply.

Husain et al. reported the experience at Memorial Sloan-Kettering in 13 patients who had total pelvic exenteration and low rectal anastomosis with a continent urinary diversion. Of these, seven leaked early and two had fistulae later, for a 30% success rate. They recommend against low rectal anastomosis when a continent diversion is used (38). Because of the vascular problems associated with a loop colostomy, the surgeon should consider a loop ileostomy for diversion of the fecal stream while the bowel anastomoses heal.

The overall survival rate for patients with pelvic exenteration and low rectal anastomosis at the University of Alabama at Birmingham was 68%. This was superior to that of patients with anterior exenteration (53%) (39), although the difference was not statistically significant. For both groups of patients, survival significantly improved if there was no spread of disease beyond the cervix and/or vagina. **Patients with disease confined to the cervix and/or vagina who underwent a total pelvic exenteration and a low rectal resection had a corrected survival rate of 94%, versus 70% for patients who underwent an anterior exenteration.** Although this difference is not statistically significant, it suggests that the more extensive procedure may improve survival by virtue of its larger tissue margin around apparently confined tumor. **The survival rate for patients with disease in the bladder, rectum, or parametria was 38%.**

Urinary Diversion

Techniques for urinary diversion are demonstrated in Chapter 20. The selection of the proper urinary diversion technique depends on a number of factors. The majority of women undergoing pelvic exenteration have had high doses of pelvic radiation therapy, which leads to fibrosis and lack of vascularity in the distal ileum. This increases the risk of anastomotic breakdown and both bowel and urinary fistulae.

Most centers currently prefer the transverse colon when a urinary conduit is chosen as the urinary diversion method in a patient who has had full dose radiotherapy. This leads to fewer bowel and ureterocolonic anastomotic leaks (40). The colon absorbs water, sodium, and chlorides. This may lead to hypochloremic acidosis with hyponatremia and hyperkalemia if there is urinary retention due to stomal stricture, or when a long segment of colon is used. **When a 10 to 15 cm length of colon is used and the stoma remains open, the complications of electrolyte imbalance are rarely encountered.**

Continent urinary diversion is preferred for those patients with motor skills and motivation to maintain the emptying and irrigation that it requires. It gives the advantage of avoiding the external appliance and helps restore the patient's self-image. **A greater degree of renal function is necessary for the continent reservoirs** versus the conduits. **The glomerular filtration rate (GFT) should be 40 mL/min. or greater.** The serum creatinine should be <2 mg/dL and there should be no urinary proteinuria. Because the cecum and ascending colon will absorb electrolytes, it is important that the patient empty the reservoir three times daily and irrigate once daily. The patient may experience diarrhea because the bowel has been shortened and the distal ileum has been taken out of the gastrointestinal stream. This leads to decreased bile acid absorption and steatorrhea. This can be treated with *cholestyramine* and with motility agents such as *Lomotil* and *Imodium*.

In the patients who have significant fibrosis in the pelvis after radiation therapy, the ureters should be cut above the pelvic brim so the ureterointestinal anastomosis has a lower fistula and stricture rate. The left ureter will need to be brought across the midline above the inferior mesenteric artery (IMA) to provide the appropriate length and to decrease the risk of stricture caused by the kinking at the level of the IMA. The continent reservoirs and the transverse colon conduit are ideal for patients with short ureters because the anastomosis is in the mid- to upper abdomen.

Postoperative Care

Patients are best managed in an intensive care unit with an arterial line and central venous catheter. Central catheter monitoring facilitates administration of blood products, colloids, and crystalloids, particularly in those patients whose urine output is not a reliable predictor of fluid status. Patients have a large abdominal and pelvic peritoneal defect that exudes serum, and they may have significant third-space fluid shifts. Inadequate fluid replacement may lead to intravascular compromise and decreased perfusion of the kidneys. The hematocrit should be kept stable above 30%, and the prothrombin and partial thromboplastin times should be kept normal with fresh frozen plasma. The central catheter can also be used for TPN.

A first-generation cephalosporin is given immediately before surgery for infectious prophylaxis. It is continued after surgery until the patient has remained afebrile for 48 hours. If febrile episodes persist or become severe, antibiotics are changed based on culture results. If no cultures are available, antibiotic therapy is extended to cover anaerobic and gram-negative organisms. If there is fecal spill during surgery, antibiotic coverage is usually extended to anaerobic and gram-negative organisms.

Complications

Although the mortality rate is less than 5%, as many as 50% of patients may have a major complication (41–43). The most significant intraoperative complication is hemorrhage, with blood loss of 1,500 to 4,000 mL being typical (44,45). Postoperative hemorrhage is often handled by percutaneous embolization because reexploration carries a high morbidity. The length of surgery (4 to 8 hours), large volume of blood loss, and inability to monitor urinary output because of the urinary diversion make the accurate replacement of fluids very difficult. The central catheter is invaluable in monitoring the replacement of blood, colloids, and crystalloids, which may reach 1,500 mL/hour during intraoperative management.

Nonsurgical complications, such as myocardial infarction, pulmonary embolism, heart failure, stroke, and multiorgan failure, account for a 2% to 3% mortality rate and are slightly more common in the elderly patient.

Gastrointestinal Complications

A small bowel anastomotic leak or fistula is a serious complication, with a mortality rate of 20% to 50%. **The incidence of small bowel fistulae ranged from 10% to 32% (41–46) in patients who had an ileo-ileal anastomosis in previously irradiated bowel.** Small bowel fistulae have been virtually eliminated by the use of transverse colon conduits and attention to pelvic floor reconstruction. Today, the continent urinary diversion commonly practiced uses an ileocolonic anastomosis with a low small bowel fistula rate.

The incidence of small bowel obstruction is 4% to 9%. Initially conservative management with nasogastric decompression and TPN should be attempted because reoperation has been associated with an 8% to 10% risk of mortality. The obstructions are most common in the distal ileum at the site of the ileal anastomosis. Avoiding the ileal anastomosis and using pelvic floor reconstruction has decreased the morbidity of small bowel obstruction.

Urinary Tract Complications

The standard urinary diversion for several decades was the urinary conduit using a segment of terminal ileum. The high complication rate of the ileo-ileal anastomosis led to development of the transverse colon conduit (47). There have been no bowel anastomotic leaks reported with this technique, and ureterocolonic anastomotic leaks also are rare.

The continent urinary diversion using the Miami pouch (see Chapter 20) also has a low rate of intestinal fistula formation and urinary leaks. If urinary leaks or fistulae do occur, conservative management with percutaneous drainage is recommended. The mortality rate from surgical reexploration for urinary complications may reach 50%.

The most common long-term complication is pyelonephritis, requiring rehospitalization in 14% of patients. The incidence of ureteral stricture has been decreased by the use of ureteral stents and is approximately 8% (48).

Results

The 5-year survival rate has improved significantly over time (Table 22.3) (5, 6, 41, 42, 46, 49–52). Patients who have had anterior exenterations have a better survival rate (30% to 60%) than those with total exenteration (20% to 46%), no doubt reflecting the smaller dimensions of the recurrent disease. **The clinical factors that have been reported to affect survival most significantly are length of time from initial radiation therapy to exenteration** (50), **size of the central mass** (51,53), **and preoperative pelvic sidewall fixation determined by clinical examination** (52).

The important pathologic factors are positive nodes, positive margins, and spread of tumor to adjacent organs. The occurrence of metastatic cancer in the pelvic lymph nodes after radiation therapy is a poor prognostic finding at the time of exenteration (Table 22.4). Stanhope and Symmonds (55) achieved the highest 5-year survival rate at 23%. In their analysis, they eliminated confounding high-risk factors, such as positive margins and metastasis to other peritoneal surfaces.

Table 22.3 Operative Mortality and 5-Year Survival Rates for Pelvic Exenteration

Author, Year	N	Operative Mortality (%)	5-Year Survival (%)
Brunschwig, 1965 (49)	535	16.0	20
Symmonds et al., 1975 (6)	198	8.1	33
Rutledge et al., 1977 (5)	296	13.5	42
Shingleton et al., 1989 (50)	143	6.3	50
Lawhead et al., 1989 (46)	65	9.2	23
Soper et al., 1989 (41)	69	7.2	40
Morley et al., 1989 (42)	100	2.0	61
Stanhope et al., 1990 (51)	133	6.7	41
Berek et al., 2003 (52)	75	4.0	54
Fleisch et al., 2007 (53)	203	1.8	21

Table 22.4 Survival of Patients With Positive Nodes at Time of Exenteration for Postirradiation Recurrence

Author, Year	Negative Nodes		Positive Nodes	
	N	5-Year Survival (%)	N	5-Year Survival (%)
Barber and Jones, 1971 (54)	299	21.7	97[a]	5.1
Symmonds et al., 1975 (6)	68	42	30	15
Rutledge et al., 1977 (5)[b]		—	30	6.6
Stanhope and Symmonds, 1985 (55)	—		26	23
Rutledge and McGuffee, 1987 (56)	—		41	26.3
Hatch et al., 1988 (39)	54	52	7	14
Morley et al., 1989 (42)	87	70	13	0
Berek et al., 2003 (52)	59	61	8	0
Fleisch et al., 2007 (53)	NS	35.3	NS	15.2

[a]Thirty-nine patients with gross disease unresected and 10 with metastasis to ovaries.
[b]Includes positive inguinal nodes.
NS, Not stated.

Rutledge et al. (5) in 1977 reported a 6.6% 5-year survival rate in 30 patients with positive nodes. This publication included patients who had positive pelvic and inguinal nodes and those who died of operative complications. Ten years later, Rutledge and McGuffee (56) reported a 26.3% survival rate in 41 patients with positive nodes. They noted an increase in the incidence of positive nodes in the later cases and suggested that the patients were more highly selected to eliminate other risk factors, and fewer died of operative complications. There was also a decrease in the number of posterior exenterations performed. These patients had vulvar, urethral, and rectal cancers and had been managed more aggressively despite significant risk factors for higher recurrence rates. The 5-year survival rate was 21.9% for recurrent cervical cancer after radiation therapy, after eliminating death from other causes. Given this rate of survival, **patients with positive pelvic nodes and no other poor prognostic factors can be considered candidates for exenteration.**

Morley et al. (42) reported a 73% 5-year survival rate for 57 patients with squamous cell cancer of the cervix versus 22% for 9 patients with cervical adenocarcinoma. Crozier et al. (57) reported a median survival of 38 months for 35 patients with adenocarcinoma and 25 months for 70 control patients with squamous cell carcinoma. They concluded that patients with cervical adenocarcinomas who meet the criteria for pelvic exenteration have results similar to those of patients with squamous carcinomas.

Chronologic age is not a contraindication to exenteration. Matthews et al. (45) compared 63 patients aged 65 years or older with 363 patients younger than 65 years who underwent pelvic exenteration. The operative mortality rates were 11% and 8.5%, and the 5-year survival rates were 46% and 45%, respectively.

Quality of Life

The quality of life after pelvic exenteration is significantly improved by organ reconstruction. Hawigorst-Knapstein et al. (58) reported 28 patients who were periodically assessed in a prospective study by examination, interview, and questionnaires in the postoperative period. The women were divided into groups of two, one, or no ostomies. A separate comparison was made of women with or without vaginal reconstruction. At all points of evaluation, the patients' quality of life was most affected by worries about progression of the tumor. One year after surgery, the patients with two ostomies reported a significantly lower quality of life and poorer body image than patients with no ostomy.

Those women with vaginal reconstruction reported fewer problems in all categories related to quality of life and significantly fewer sexual problems.

Ratliff et al. (59) prospectively evaluated 95 patients who underwent pelvic exenteration and gracilis myocutaneous vaginal reconstruction. Forty patients completed the study, and 21 (52.5%) reported that they had not resumed sexual activity after surgery. Of the 19 patients who resumed sexual activity, 84% did so within 1 year of surgery. The most common problems were in adjusting to the self-consciousness of the urostomy or colostomy. Vaginal dryness and vaginal discharge were also significant problems. These findings indicate the need for adequate counseling after the exenterative surgery.

Conclusions

While some European centers have advocated pelvic exenteration for patients with advanced primary cervical cancer (60), most centers restrict the operation to patients with a central recurrence following chemoradiation. The only exception would be patients with stage IVA disease and a recto- or vesico-vaginal fistula.

Pelvic exenteration provides the only hope for cure in women with recurrent pelvic malignancies after radiation therapy. Most procedures are done for recurrent cervical cancer. Operative morbidity and mortality can be decreased by careful patient selection, attention to intraoperative technique, excellent postoperative care, and early management of complications. The 5-year survival rate is acceptable given the lack of satisfactory alternative treatments. With modern reconstructive and rehabilitative techniques, the patient can maintain a near-normal lifestyle, but sexual functioning will always be significantly impaired.

References

1. **Brunschwig A.** Complete excision of pelvic viscera for advanced carcinoma. *Cancer* 1948;1:177–183.

2. **Bricker EM.** Bladder substitution after pelvic evisceration. *Surg Clin North Am* 1950;30:1511–1521.

3. **Orr JW Jr, Shingleton HM, Hatch KD, Taylor PT, Austin JM Jr, Partridge EE, et al.** Urinary diversion in patients undergoing pelvic exenteration. *Am J Obstet Gynecol* 1982;142:883–889.

4. **Orr JW Jr, Shingleton HM, Hatch KD, Taylor PT, Partridge EE, Soong SJ.** Gastrointestinal complications associated with pelvic exenteration. *Am J Obstet Gynecol* 1983;145:325–332.

5. **Rutledge FN, Smith JP, Wharton JT, O'Quinn AG.** Pelvic exenteration: analysis of 296 patients. *Am J Obstet Gynecol* 1977;129:881–892.

6. **Symmonds RE, Pratt JH, Webb MJ.** Exenterative operations: experience with 198 patients. *Am J Obstet Gynecol* 1975;121:907–918.

7. **Morris M, Alvarez RD, Kinney WK, Wilson TO.** Treatment of recurrent adenocarcinoma of the endometrium with pelvic exenteration. *Gynecol Oncol* 1996;60:288–291.

8. **Manetta A, Podczaski ES, Larson JE, Ge Geest K, Mortel R.** Scalene lymph node biopsy in the preoperative evaluation of patients with recurrent cervical cancer. *Gynecol Oncol* 1989;33:332–334.

9. **Popovich MJ, Hricak H, Sugimura K, Stern JL.** The role of MR imaging in determining surgical eligibility for pelvic exenteration. *Am J Roentgenol* 1993;160:525–531.

10. **Lai C-H, Huang K-G, See L-C, Yen T-C, Tsai C-S, Chang T-C, et al.** Restaging of recurrent cervical carcinoma with dual phase [18F] fluoro-2 deoxy-D-glucose positron emission tomography. *Cancer* 2004;100:544–552.

11. **Husain A, Akhurst T, Larson S, Alektiar K, Barakat R, Chi D.** A prospective study of the accuracy of ^{18}Fluorodeoxyglucose positron emission tomography (^{18}FDG PET) in identifying sites of metastasis prior to pelvic exenteration. *Gynecol Oncol* 2007;106:177–180.

12. **Chung H, Jo H, Kang W, Kim J, Park N-H, Song Y-S, et al.** Clinical impact of integrated PET/CT on the management of suspected cervical cancer recurrence. *Gynecol Oncol* 2006;104: 529–534.

13. **Plante M, Roy M.** Operative laparoscopy prior to a pelvic exenteration in patients with recurrent cervical cancer. *Gynecol Oncol* 1998;69:94–99.

14. **Miller B, Morris M, Rutledge F, Mitchell MF, Atkinson EN, Burke TW, et al.** Aborted exenterative procedures in recurrent cervical cancer. *Gynecol Oncol* 1993;50:94–99.

15. **Hatch KD.** Construction of a neovagina after exenteration using the vulvobulbocavernosus myocutaneous graft. *Obstet Gynecol* 1984;63:110–114.

16. **Ballantyne GH.** The experimental basis of intestinal suturing. *Dis Colon Rectum* 1984;27:61–71.

17. **Wheeless CR Jr, Smith JJ.** A comparison of the flow of iodine 125 through three different intestinal anastomoses: standard, Gambee and stapler. *Obstet Gynecol* 1983;62:513–518.

18. **McGinn FP, Gartell PC, Clifford PC, Brunton FJ.** Staples or sutures for low colorectal anastomoses: a prospective randomized trial. *Br J Surg* 1985;72:603–605.

19. **Hatch KD, Gelder MS, Soong SJ, Baker VV, Shingleton HM.** Pelvic exenteration with low rectal anastomosis: survival, complications and prognostic factors. *Gynecol Oncol* 1990;38:462–467.

20. **Mirhashemi R, Averette HE, Estape R, Angioli R, Mahran R, Mendez L, et al.** Low colorectal anastomosis after radical pelvic surgery: a risk factor analysis. *Am J Obstet Gynecol* 2000;183:1375–1380.

21. **Hatch KD, Shingleton HM, Potter ME, Baker VV.** Low rectal resection and anastomosis at the time of pelvic exenteration. *Gynecol Oncol* 1988;31:262–267.

22. **Graffner H, Fredlund P, Olsson SA, Oscarson J, Peterson BG.** Protective colostomy in low anterior resection of the rectum using the EEA stapling instrument: a randomized study. *Dis Colon Rectum* 1983;26:87–90.

23. **Berek JS, Hacker NF, Lagasse LD.** Rectosigmoid colectomy and reanastomosis to facilitate resection of primary and recurrent gynecologic cancer. *Obstet Gynecol* 1984;64:715–720.

24. **Harris WJ, Wheeless CR Jr.** Use of the end-to-end anastomosis stapling device in low colorectal anastomosis associated with radical gynecologic surgery. *Gynecol Oncol* 1986;23:350–357.

25. **Nakahara S, Itoh H, Mibu R, Ikeda S, Oohata Y, Kitano K, et al.** Clinical and manometric evaluation of anorectal function following low anterior resection with low anastomotic line using an EEA stapler for rectal cancer. *Dis Colon Rectum* 1988;31:762–766.

26. **Pedersen IK, Christiansen J, Hint K, Jensen P, Olsen J, Mortensen PE.** Anorectal function after low anterior resection for carcinoma. *Ann Surg* 1986;204:133–135.

27. **Karanjia ND, Schache DJ, Heald RJ.** Function of the distal rectum after low anterior resection for carcinoma. *Br J Surg* 1992;79:114–116.

28. **Lewis WG, Holdsworth PJ, Stephenson BM, Finan PJ, Johnston D.** Role of the rectum in the physiological and clinical results of coloanal and colorectal anastomosis after anterior resection for rectal carcinoma. *Br J Surg* 1992;79:1082–1086.

29. **Parc R, Tiret E, Frileux P, Moszkowski E, Loygue J.** Resection and colo-anal anastomosis with colonic reservoir for rectal carcinoma. *Br J Surg* 1986;73:139–141.

30. **Mortensen NJ, Ramirez JM, Takeuchi N, Humphreys MM.** Colonic J-pouch anal anastomosis after rectal excision for carcinoma: functional outcome. *Br J Surg* 1995;82:611–613.

31. **Joo JS, Latulippe JF, Alabaz O, Weiss EG, Nogueras JJ, Wexner SD.** Long-term functional evaluation of straight coloanal anastomosis and colonic J-pouch: is the functional superiority of colonic J-pouch sustained? *Dis Colon Rectum* 1998;41:740–746.

32. **Dehni N, Tiret E, Singland JD, Cunningham C, Schlegel RD, Guiguet M, et al.** Long-term functional outcome after low anterior resection: comparison of low colorectal anastomosis and colonic J-pouch anal anastomosis. *Dis Colon Rectum* 1998;41:817–822.

33. **Seow-Choen F, Goh HS.** Prospective randomized trial comparing J colonic pouch-anal anastomosis and straight coloanal reconstruction. *Br J Surg* 1995;82:608–610.

34. **Hallböök O, Påhlman L, Krog M, Wexner SD, Sjödahl R.** Randomized comparison of straight and colonic J pouch anastomosis after low anterior resection. *Ann Surg* 1996;224:58–65.

35. **Hida J, Yasutomi M, Fujimoto K, Okuno K, Ieda S, Machidera N, et al.** Functional outcome after low anterior resection with low anastomosis for rectal cancer using the colonic J-pouch: prospective randomized study for determination of optimum pouch size. *Dis Colon Rectum* 1996;39:986–991.

36. **Harris GJC, Lavery IC, Fazio VW.** Function of a colonic J pouch continues to improve with time. *Br J Surg* 2001;88:1623–1627.

37. **Mantyh CR, Hull TL, Fazio VW.** Coloplasty in low colorectal anastomosis. *Dis Colon Rectum* 2001;44:37–42.

38. **Husain A, Curtin J, Brown C, Chi D, Hoskins W, Poynor E, et al.** Continent urinary diversion and low-rectal anastomosis in patients undergoing exenterative procedures for recurrent gynecologic malignancies. *Gynecol Oncol* 2000;78:208–211.

39. **Hatch KD, Shingleton HM, Soong SJ, Baker VV, Gelder MS.** Anterior pelvic exenteration. *Gynecol Oncol* 1988;31:205–216.

40. **Chiva LM, Lapuente F, González-Cortijo L, González-Martín A, Rojo A, García JF, et al.** Surgical treatment of recurrent cervical cancer: State of the art and new achievements. *Gynecol Oncol* 2008;110:S60–66.

41. **Soper JT, Berchuck A, Creasman WT, Clarke-Pearson DL.** Pelvic exenteration: factors associated with major surgical morbidity. *Gynecol Oncol* 1989;35:93–98.

42. **Morley GW, Hopkins MP, Lindenauer SM, Roberts JA.** Pelvic exenteration, University of Michigan: 100 patients at 5 years. *Obstet Gynecol* 1989;74:934–943.

43. **Miller B, Morris M, Gershenson DM, Levenback CL, Burke TW.** Intestinal fistulae formation following pelvic exenteration: a review of the University of Texas M. D. Anderson Cancer Center experience, 1957–1990. *Gynecol Oncol* 1995;56:207–210.

44. **Magrina JF, Stanhope CR, Weaver AL.** Pelvic exenterations: supralevator, infralevator, and with vulvectomy. *Gynecol Oncol* 1997;64:130–135.

45. **Matthews CM, Morris M, Burke TW, Gershenson DM, Wharton JT, Rutledge FN.** Pelvic exenteration in the elderly patient. *Obstet Gynecol* 1992;79:773–777.

46. **Lawhead RA Jr, Clark DG, Smith DH, Pierce VK, Lewis JL Jr.** Pelvic exenteration for recurrent or persistent gynecologic malignancies: a 10-year review of the Memorial Sloan-Kettering Cancer Center experience (1972–1981). *Gynecol Oncol* 1989;33:279–282.

47. **Segreti EM, Morris M, Levenback C, Lucas KR, Gershenson DM, Burke TW.** Transverse colon urinary diversion in gynecologic oncology. *Gynecol Oncol* 1996;63:66–70.

48. **Beddoe AM, Boyce JG, Remy JC, Fruchter RG, Nelson JH.** Stented versus nonstented transverse colon conduits: a comparative report. *Gynecol Oncol* 1987;27:305–313.

49. **Brunschwig A.** What are the indications and results of pelvic exenteration? *JAMA* 1965;194:274.

50. **Shingleton HM, Soong SJ, Gelder MS, Hatch KD, Baker VV, Austin JM Jr.** Clinical and histopathologic factors predicting recurrence and survival after pelvic exenteration for cancer of the cervix. *Obstet Gynecol* 1989;73:1027–1034.

51. **Stanhope CR, Webb MJ, Podratz KC.** Pelvic exenteration for recurrent cervical cancer. *Clin Obstet Gynecol* 1990;33:897–909.

52. **Berek JS, Howe C, Lagasse LD, Hacker NF.** Pelvic exenteration for recurrent gynecologic malignancy: survival and morbidity analysis of the 45-year experience at UCLA. *Gynecol Oncol* 2005;99: 153–159.

53. **Fleisch MC, Panthe P, Beckman MW, Schnuerch HG, Ackermann R, Grimm MO, et al.** Predictors of long-term survival after interdisciplinary salvage surgery for advanced or recurrent gynecological cancers. *J Surg Oncol* 2007;95:476–84.

54. **Barber HR, Jones W.** Lymphadenectomy in pelvic exenteration for recurrent cervix cancer. *JAMA* 1971;215:1945–1949.

55. **Stanhope CR, Symmonds RE.** Palliative exenteration—what, when, and why? *Am J Obstet Gynecol* 1985;152:12–16.

56. **Rutledge FN, McGuffee VB.** Pelvic exenteration: prognostic significance of regional lymph node metastasis. *Gynecol Oncol* 1987;26: 374–380.

57. **Crozier M, Morris M, Levenback C, Lucas KR, Atkinson EN, Wharton JT.** Pelvic exenteration for adenocarcinoma of the uterine cervix. *Gynecol Oncol* 1995;58:74–78.

58. **Hawighorst-Knapstein S, Schonefussrs G, Hoffmann SO, Knapstein PG.** Pelvic exenteration: effects of surgery on quality of life and body image. A prospective longitudinal study. *Gynecol Oncol* 1997;66:495–500.

59. **Ratliff CR, Gershenson DM, Morris M, Burke TW, Levenback C, Schover LR, et al.** Sexual adjustment of patients undergoing gracilis myocutaneous flap vaginal reconstruction in conjunction with pelvic exenteration. *Cancer* 1996;78:2229–2235.

60. **Hockel M, Dornhofer N.** Pelvic exenteration for gynaecological tumours: achievements and unanswered questions. *Lancet Oncol* 2006;7:837–847.

QUALITY OF
LIFE

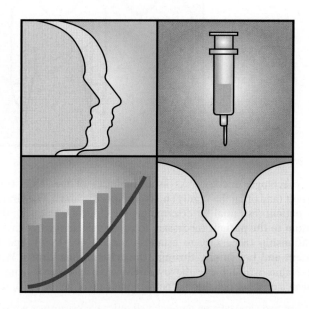

23 Communication Skills

Robert Buckman
Walter F. Baile

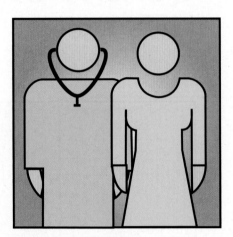

In gynecologic oncology, as in all branches of medicine, **the clinical encounter with the patient** (and often the family) **has four specific aims. The first is to gather information from the patient** (essential for determining the clinical diagnosis); **the second is to transmit information to the patient** (necessary to communicate the treatment plan); **the third is to build a relationship** (necessary to establish rapport and trust); and **the fourth is to support the patient and her family through the crisis of her illness.** When accomplished successfully, these aims will achieve the overarching goals of producing objective improvement in the patient's medical condition ("helping the patient get better"), if that is possible.

The last two aims take on particular significance because as a result of the increased survival rates of many cancers, the relationship with the oncologist and the clinical team now can extend over many years and encompass a progression of disease crises. The median survivals for women with advanced-stage ovarian cancer has increased substantially over the past 20 years, and it is not uncommon today for patients to experience remission and recurrence four or five times during the course of their cancer (1). However, **each disease recurrence can be a crisis in which the patient receives bad news again and must endure the rigors of a new round of treatment, uncertainty about the outcome, and the threat of death.** In these instances, the application of supportive communication skills in the context of a long-standing relationship with the patient can reduce anxiety, facilitate patient coping, and assist in providing the patient with hope (2–4,5).

Regardless of whether medical improvement is possible, accomplishment of these goals can produce amelioration of the patient's subjective symptoms ("helping the patient feel better"). Communication skills are essential for both. This chapter sets out a basic and practical approach to acquiring and improving effective communication skills.

Why Communication Skills Matter

Good communication skills facilitate the clinician's ability to take an accurate clinical history and therefore to make a correct diagnosis and formulate an appropriate plan of management. Hence, communication skills are a central component of every clinician's management skills. In addition, however, good communication skills change the patient's attitude to the entire medical intervention.

Effective communication changes the way a patient feels about the clinical outcome. Communication skills may affect what the patient perceives has happened to her, as well as her assessment (and feelings) about her management, her treatment, and her health care team (6). **Communication and interpersonal skills matter greatly to patients** and are an important determinant of satisfaction with care (7). In fact, the literature suggests that patients are both likely to choose and to change physicians based on how they perceive their physician communicates and interacts with them (8).

An important and related issue is one of medicolegal implications. Communication skills have been shown to be a determinant of more objective outcome measures, such as litigation. **Approximately three-fourths of complaints against medical practitioners are caused not by matters of medical management but by failures or obstacles in communication.** Levinson and Chaumeton (9) further showed that communication skills were a major factor in distinguishing those clinicians who were sued from those who were not.

Patients are very sensitive to communication messages from their oncologists. Using samples of dialogue from interactions between surgeons and their patients, Ambady et al. (10) were reliably able to predict those surgeons more likely to be sued. **Those whose voice communicated lack of empathy and concern toward the patient were more than twice as likely to have had a malpractice claim filed against them.** Furthermore, many insurance companies in North America now reduce their malpractice premiums for physicians who have attended specific programs in communication skills.

Communication skills are essential for ensuring informed consent, enlisting the family in the care of the patient, reducing the uncertainty associated with a new or recurrent illness, and increasing accrual to clinical trials (11,12).

Communication Skills as Learnable Techniques

Why Communication Skills Are So Difficult to Learn

Most oncologists have had little preparation in communicating with patients (11,13,14). Almost none have had any formal course work, and a fair number have learned by observing other clinicians (certainly no guarantee that anything useful will be learned!). Moreover, many clinical encounters, such as breaking bad news and making the transition to palliative care, are highly emotionally charged. The clinician is challenged not only to address the patient's feelings, but also his or her own, which can be characterized by the sense of helplessness and frustration in the face of incurable disease, or self-doubt about having done everything possible for the patient (12,15). **Sometimes these feelings may cause the doctor to offer false hope to the patient, avoid discussing issues important to the patient such as disease prognosis (16,17), or offer treatment when there is little or no chance of success** (18).

Acquiring Communication Skills

Since the late 1970s, clinicians have become increasingly aware of the need for improved communication skills, but it has been difficult to define and test techniques that can be acquired by practitioners. **In the late 1970s and early 1980s, it was widely believed that communication skills were intuitive—almost inherited—talents** ("You've either got the gift or you haven't"). This was coupled with the belief that somehow the physician would be able to feel or sense what the patient was thinking and to divine what the patient wanted, and would then be able to respond intuitively in an appropriate way. This belief alienated a large proportion of health care professionals who found the whole topic (as taught at that time) excessively "touchy-feely," intangible and amorphous, with no guidelines that could lead even a highly motivated practitioner to improve his or her skills.

Since the mid-1980s, researchers and educators have shown that communication skills can be taught and learned (and retained over years of practice), and that they are acquired skills, like any other clinical technique, and not inherited or granted as gifts from on high (19–23).

The main part of this chapter describes two practical protocols that can be used by any health care professional to improve her or his communication skills. They are **(i) a basic protocol, the CLASS protocol, that underlies all medical interviews; and (ii) a variation of that approach, the SPIKES protocol, for breaking bad news.**

Illustrations of Practical Techniques

The CLASS and SPIKES protocols are summarized briefly using simple and practical guidelines or rules. Both protocols have been published in greater detail elsewhere as a textbook (24), a booklet (25), and in illustrated form using videotaped scenarios of interactions between standardized patients (26). Review of this video material can enhance the understanding of these communication techniques.

CLASS: A Protocol for Effective Communication

There are probably an infinite number of ways of summarizing and simplifying medical interviews, but few (if any) are practical and easy to remember. The five-step basic protocol for medical communication set out in the following sections, which has the acronym *CLASS*, has the virtue of being easy to remember and to use in practice. Furthermore, it offers a relatively straightforward, technique-directed method for dealing with emotions. This is important, because one study showed that most oncologists (more than 85%) believe that dealing with emotions is the most difficult part of any clinical interview (27).

Trust and rapport are especially important to patients at times of illness crisis, and communication skills such as exemplified in the CLASS protocol underpin the establishment of confidence and a working relationship with the patient and her family.

In brief, the CLASS protocol identifies five essential components of the medical interview. They are **Context (the physical context or setting) and Connection (or building rapport), Listening skills, Acknowledgment of the patient's emotions, Strategy for clinical management, and Summary** (Table 23.1).

C—Context (or Setting) and Connection (or Building Rapport)

The context of the interview means the physical context or setting, and connection means the steps that are necessary to begin building rapport or a relationship with the patient. Both of these steps are important because they encourage trust on the part of the patient and family, an essential ingredient of any collaborative endeavor. They are especially important in the first encounter, during which often the most lasting impressions are formed. The essential components are listed in Table 23.2. **The first component is to arrange the space optimally. The second is to get your own body language right. It is important to pay attention to eye contact, to whether touch is helpful, and to making introductions.**

A few seconds spent establishing these features of the initial setup of the interview may save many minutes of frustration and misunderstanding later (for both the professional and the patient). These rules are not complex, but they are easy to forget in the heat of the moment.

Spatial Arrangements

The Setting

Try to ensure privacy. In a hospital setting, if a side room is not available, draw the curtains around the bed. In an office setting, shut the door. Get any physical objects out of the way—e.g., move any bedside tables, trays, or other impediments out of the line between you and the patient. Ask for the television or radio to be turned off for a few minutes. If you

Table 23.1 The CLASS Protocol
C—Physical **context** or setting and **connection**
L—**Listening** skills
A—**Acknowledge** emotions and explore them
S—Management **strategy**
S—**Summary** and closure

Table 23.2 The Elements of Physical Context	
Arrangement	Sitting down, placement of patient, appropriate distance.
Body language	Drop shoulders, sit comfortably and attentively.
Eye contact	Maintain eye contact except during anger or crying ("not when hot").
Touch (optional)	Touch patient's forearm if you and the patient are comfortable with touch.
Introductions	Tell the patient who you are and what you do. Introduce others.

are in an office or room, move your chair so that you are adjacent to the patient, not across the desk. There is evidence that conversations across a corner occur three times more frequently than conversations across the full width of a table (28).

Clear any clutter and papers away from the area of desk nearest to the patient. If you have the patient's chart open, make sure you look up from it and do not talk to the patient while reading the chart. If you find any of these actions awkward, state what you are doing *("It may be easier for us to talk if I move the table/if you turn the television off for a moment")*.

Then—the most important rule of all—sit down. This is an almost inviolable guideline. It is virtually impossible to assure a patient that she or he has your undivided attention and that you intend to listen seriously if you remain standing up. Only if it is absolutely impossible to sit should you try and hold a medical interview while standing. Anecdotal impressions suggest that when the doctor sits down, the patient perceives the period of time spent at the bedside as longer than if the doctor remains standing. Thus, not only does the act of sitting down indicate to the patient that he or she has control and that you are there to listen, but it saves time and increases efficiency. Before starting the interview itself, take care to get the patient organized if necessary. **If you have just finished examining the patient, allow or help her to dress to restore the sense of personal modesty.**

Distance

It is important to be seated at a comfortable distance from the patient. **This distance (sometimes called the "body buffer zone") seems to vary from culture to culture, but a distance of 2 to 3 feet between you usually serves the purpose for intimate and personal conversation** (28). This is another reason why the doctor who remains standing at the end of the bed ("six feet away and three feet up," known colloquially as "the British position") seems remote and aloof.

The height at which you sit can also be important; normally, your eyes should be approximately level with the patient's. If the patient is already upset or angry, a useful technique is to sit so that you are below the patient, with your eyes at a lower level. This often decreases the anger. It is best to try to look relaxed, particularly if that is not the way you feel.

Positioning

Make sure that whenever possible, you are seated closest to the patient and that any friends or relatives are on the other side of the patient. Sometimes relatives try to dominate the interview, and it may be important for you to send a clear signal that the patient has primacy.

Have Tissues Nearby

In almost all oncology settings, it is important to have a box of tissues nearby. If the patient or relative begins to cry, offer them tissues. This not only give overt permission to cry, but allows the person to feel less vulnerable when crying.

Your Body Language	**Try to look relaxed and unhurried.** To achieve an air of relaxation, sit down comfortably with both your feet flat on the floor. Let your shoulders relax and drop. Undo your coat or jacket if you are wearing one, and rest your hands on your knees. (In psychotherapy, this is often called "the neutral position.") Pay attention to your nonverbal behavior because it may communicate that you are listening or concerned. For example, if you are listening with your arms folded in front of you, the patient may feel that you have already made up your mind about things and are not open to further discussion.
Eye Contact	**Maintain eye contact for most of the time while the patient is talking.** If the interview becomes intense or emotionally charged—particularly if the patient is crying or is very angry—it is helpful to the patient for you to look away (to break eye contact) at that point.
Touching the Patient	**Touch may also be helpful during the interview** if (i) a nonthreatening area is touched, such as the hand or forearm; (ii) you are comfortable with touch; and (iii) the patient appreciates touch and does not withdraw.

Most clinicians have not been taught specific details of clinical touch at any time in their training (29). They are, therefore, likely to be ill at ease with touching as an interview technique until they have had some practice. Nevertheless, there is considerable evidence (although the data are somewhat "soft") that touching the patient (particularly above the patient's waist to avoid misinterpretation) is of benefit during a medical interview (30). **It seems likely that touching is a significant action at times of distress and should be encouraged, with the proviso that the professional should be sensitive to the patient's reaction.** If the patient is comforted by the contact, continue; if the patient is uncomfortable, stop. Touch can be misinterpreted (e.g., as lasciviousness, aggression, or dominance), so be aware that touching is an interviewing skill that requires extra self-regulation.

Starting Off

Introductions

Ensure that the patient knows who you are and what you do. Many practitioners, including the author, make a point of shaking the patient's hand at the outset, although this is a matter of personal preference. Often the handshake tells you something about the family dynamics as well as about the patient. Frequently the patient's spouse also extends his hand. It is worthwhile making sure that you shake the patient's hand before that of the spouse (even if the spouse is nearer) to demonstrate that the patient comes first, and the spouse (although an important member of the team) comes second. The "white coat syndrome" is a well-known phenomenon that describes how the medical setting induces anxiety in many patients (often even leading to blood pressure increases!), so that a friendly greeting may go a long way at putting the patient at ease. Also **remember to introduce others in the room** (e.g., medical students, nurse) that the patient may not know.

L—Listening Skills

As dialogue begins, the professional should show that she or he is in "listening mode." For a general review of interviewing skills, see Lipkin et al. (31). The four main points to attend to are covered in the following sections. **They are the use of open questions, facilitation techniques, the use of clarification, and the handling of time and interruptions** (Table 23.3).

Open-Ended Questions

Open questions are simply questions that can be answered in any way or manner of response. In other words, the question does not direct the respondent or require her to make a choice from a specific range of answers. In taking the medical history, of course, most of the questions are, appropriately, closed questions (*"Do you have swelling of the ankles?" "Have you had any bleeding after your menopause?"*). In therapeutic dialogue, when the clinician is trying to be part of the patient's support system, open questions are an essential way of finding out what the patient is experiencing as a way of tailoring support to the patient. Hence, open questions (*"What did you think the diagnosis was?" "How did you feel when you were told that . . ." "How did that make you feel?"*) are a mandatory part of the "nonhistory" therapeutic dialogue.

Facilitation Techniques

Silence

The first and most important technique in facilitating dialogue between the patient and clinician is silence (32). **If the patient is speaking, do not talk over her.** Wait for the patient to stop speaking before you start your next sentence. This, the simplest rule of all, is the one most often ignored, and it is most likely to give the patient the impression that the doctor is not listening.

Table 23.3 Fundamental Listening Skills

Switch on your listening skills and techniques to show that you are an effective listener.

1. **Open Questions**
   Questions that can be answered in any way (e.g., *"How are you?" "How did that make you feel?"*)

2. **Facilitating**
   Pausing or silence when patient speaks. Try not to interrupt. Nodding, smiling, saying *"mm hmm," "tell me more about that,"* and the like repetition (i.e., repeating one key word from patient's last sentence in your first sentence)

3. **Clarifying**
   Making overt any ambiguous or awkward topic

4. **Handling Time and Interruptions**
   With pagers and phones: acknowledge the patient who is with you as you answer Tell patient about any time constraints and clarify when discussion will resume

Silences also have other significance: they can be—and often are—revealing about the patient's state of mind. Often, a patient falls silent when she has feelings that are too intense to express in words. A silence, therefore, means that the patient is thinking or feeling something important, not that she has stopped thinking. If the clinician can tolerate a pause or silence, the patient may well express the thought in words a moment later.

If you have to break the silence, the ideal way to do so is to say *"What were you thinking about just then?"* or *"What is it that's making you pause?"* or something to that effect.

Other Simple Facilitation Techniques

Having encouraged the patient to speak, it is necessary to prove that you are hearing what is being said. The following techniques enhance your ability to demonstrate this.

In addition to silence, you can use any or all of the following simple facilitation techniques: nodding, pauses, smiling, saying *"Yes" "Mmm hmm,"* *"Tell me more,"* or anything similar.

Repetition and Reiteration

Repetition is probably the second most important technique of all interviewing skills (after sitting down).

To show that you are really hearing what the patient is saying, use one or two key words from the patient's last sentence in your own first one (*"I just feel so lousy most of the time." "Tell me what you mean by feeling lousy."*). Reiteration means repeating what the patient has told you, but in your words, not hers (*"Since I started those new tablets, I've been feeling sleepy." "So you're getting some drowsiness from the new tablets."*). Both repetition and reiteration confirm to the patient that she has been heard.

Reflection

Reflection is the act of restating the patient's statement in terms of what it means to the clinician. It takes the act of listening one step further and shows that you have heard and have interpreted what the patient said (*"If I understand you correctly, you're telling me that you lose control of your waking and sleeping when you're on these tablets."*).

Clarifying

Patients often have concerns about treatment or other issues related to their care. When not asked about them directly, they may hint or express them in nuances, protests, or questions that are not clear. Listed below are some examples of how important information may be indirectly communicated.

Statement: *"I don't know how my family can take any more of this."*

Patient means: *"I really feel guilty."*

Statement: *"I just couldn't stand another round of chemo."*

Patient means: *"I felt so awful when my hair fell out."*

Statement: *"Doctor, how long do you think I have to live?"*

Patient means: *"I wonder if I'll see my grandson graduate."*

Statement: *"What will the end be like?"*

Patient means: *"How much will I suffer?"*

As the patient talks, it is very tempting for the clinician to go along with what the patient is saying, even when the exact meaning or implication is unclear. This may lead very quickly to serious obstacles in the dialogue.

It is important to be honest when we do not understand what the patient means. Many different phrases can be used (*"I'm sorry—I'm not quite sure what you meant when you said . . ."* *"When you say . . . do you mean that . . . ?"*). Clarification gives the patient an opportunity to expand on the previous statement or to amplify some aspect of the statement, now that the clinician has shown interest in the topic. The key to addressing questions is to use clarifying statements that get at the issue underlying the concern.

Table 23.4 Acknowledgment of Emotions: The Empathic Response
Acknowledging the emotional content of the interview is the central skill of being perceived as sensitive and supportive.
The central technique is the empathic response.
1. Identify the emotion
2. Identify the cause or source of the emotion
3. Respond in a way that shows you have made the connection between (i) and (ii) (e.g., *"that must have felt awful," "this information has obviously come as quite a shock"*)
The empathic response is a technique or skill—not a feeling. It is not necessary for you to (i) experience the same feelings as the patient, or (ii) agree with the patient's view or assessment.

Handling Time and Interruptions

As clinicians, we seem to have a notorious reputation for being impolite in our handling of interruptions—by phone, pager, or other people. Too often, we appear abruptly to ignore the patient we are with and go immediately to the phone or respond immediately to the pager or to our colleague. Even though we may not realize it, this appears as a snub or an insult to the patient we are with.

If you cannot hold all calls or turn off your pager (and most cannot), at least indicate to the patient that you are sorry about the interruption and will return shortly (*"Sorry, this is another doctor that I must speak to very briefly—I'll be back in a moment." "This is something quite urgent about another patient—I won't be more than a few minutes."*). The same is true of time constraints (*"I'm afraid I have to go to the O.R. now, but this is an important conversation. We need to continue this tomorrow morning on the ward round . . ."*).

A—Acknowledgment (and Exploration) of Emotions

The Empathic Response

The empathic response is an extremely useful technique in an emotionally charged interview, yet is frequently misunderstood by students and trainees (Table 23.4).

The empathic response has nothing to do with your own personal feelings. If the patient feels sad, you are not required that moment to feel sad yourself. It is simply a technique of acknowledgment, showing the patient that you have observed the emotion she is experiencing. It consists of three mental steps:

1. **Identifying the emotion that the patient is experiencing.**
2. **Identifying the origin and root cause of that emotion.**
3. **Responding in a way that tells the patient that you have made the connection between steps 1 and 2.**

Often, the most effective empathic responses follow the format of *"You seem to be . . ."* or *"It must be . . ."* (e.g., *"It must be very distressing for you to know that all that therapy didn't give you a long remission"* or even *"This must be awful for you"*). **The objective of the empathic response is to demonstrate that you have identified and acknowledged the emotion that the patient is experiencing, and by doing so, you are giving it legitimacy as an item on the patient's agenda.** In fact, if the patient is experiencing a strong emotion (e.g., rage or crying), you must acknowledge the existence of that emotion or all further attempts at communication will fail. If strong emotions are not acknowledged in some way, you will be perceived as insensitive, and this will render the rest of the interaction useless.

S—Management Strategy

There are several useful techniques to ensure that you construct a management plan with which the patient concurs and will follow (Table 23.5). The following are useful guidelines:

1. **Determine what you judge to be the optimal medical strategy.** In your mind (or out loud), define the ideal management plan.

Table 23.5 Management Strategy

A reasonable management plan that the patient understands and will follow is better than an ideal plan that the patient will ignore.

1. **Think what is best medically, then . . .**

2. **Assess the patient's expectations of her condition, treatment, and outcome** (summarize this in your mind, or clarify and summarize aloud, if needed).

3. **Propose a strategy.**

4. **Assess the patient's response** (e.g., what stage of action is the patient in: precontemplation, contemplation, implementation, or reinforcement phase?).

5. **Agree on a plan** (as far as possible).

Table 23.6 Summary and Closure

Ending of the interview has three main components.

1. **A précis or summary of the main topics** you have discussed

2. **Identification of any important issues that need further discussion** (Even if you do not have time to discuss them in this interview, they can be on the agenda for the next.)

3. **A clear contract for the next contact**

2. **Assess (in your own mind or by asking the patient) what are her own expectations of her condition, treatment, and outcome.** Be aware if there is a marked "mismatch" between the patient's view of the situation and the medical facts, because you are going to have to work harder to make the plan appear logical and acceptable.

   Bearing in mind your conclusions from steps 1 and 2, propose your strategy. As you explain it to the patient;

3. **Assess the patient's response.** For example, make note of the patient's progress in forming an action plan (the stages are often defined as the precontemplation, contemplation, implementation, and reinforcement phases). Acknowledge the patient's emotions as they occur, and continue in a contractual fashion to arrive at a plan that the patient has "bought into" and that she will follow. Check the patient's understanding by asking her to repeat back to you what you have told her (don't just ask if she understood; most of the time she will say yes, even if she hasn't).

S—Summary

The summary is the closure of the interview. In gynecologic oncology, the relationship with the patient is likely to be a continuing one and a major component of the patient's treatment. The closure of the interview is an important time to emphasize that point.

It is relatively straightforward to cover three areas in the summary (Table 23.6). They are (i) a **précis** or reiteration of the main points covered in the dialogue; (ii) an **invitation** for the patient to ask questions; and (iii) **a clear arrangement for the next interaction** ("a clear contract for the contact"). This part of the interview is not necessarily long, but does require considerable focus and concentration.

SPIKES: A Variation of CLASS for Breaking Bad News

Among the various types of medical interviews, breaking bad news is a special case, and one of exceptional importance for both parties in the clinician–patient relationship (24,33,34).

Bad news can best be defined as "any news that seriously adversely affects the patient's view of her future" (35). In other words, the "badness" of bad news is the gap between the

Table 23.7 The SPIKES Protocol for Breaking Bad News[a]
S—**Setting** = **Context, connection** and listening skills
P—**Patient's perception** of condition and seriousness
I—**Invitation** from patient to give information
K—**Knowledge**—giving medical facts
E—**Explore emotions** and empathize as patient responds
S—**Strategy and summary**

[a]A variant of the basic CLASS approach.

patient's expectations of the future and the medical reality. This is crucially important because what is good news for one patient (e.g., "I'm really glad they could operate on this tumor,") may be very bad for another (e.g., "I don't think I can take another operation"). In gynecologic oncology, bad news is common at many stages in a patient's history: (i) initial diagnosis; (ii) recurrence or disease progression; (iii) clinical deterioration; (iv) development of new complications; and (v) change from therapeutic to palliative intent. It is necessary to have a protocol that will function in all of these circumstances.

The SPIKES protocol has been designed specifically for these purposes and allows assessment of the patient's expectations before sharing the information (Table 23.7).

S—Setting (= Context + Listening Skills)

In the SPIKES protocol, for the sake of convenience, we have combined two phases of the CLASS protocol—the **context** (see Table 23.2) and **listening skills** (see Table 23.3)—into "setting."

P—The Patient's Perception of the Situation

The cardinal rule of breaking bad news is to find out what the patient already knows or suspects before going on to share the information. To condense this into a slogan, one might say "Before you tell, ask."

The exact words used to find out how much the patient already understands are a personal choice (Table 23.8). (*"Before I go on to tell you about the results, why don't you tell me what you've been thinking?" "When you first developed that swelling of the abdomen, what did you think was going on?" "Had you been thinking this was something serious?"* or *"What did the referring medical team tell you about your medical condition?"*).

As the patient replies, pay particular attention to her **vocabulary** and **comprehension** of the subject. When starting to give information, it is very helpful if one can start at the same level of knowledge as the patient (36).

I—Getting a Clear Invitation to Share News

Next, try to get a clear invitation to share the information (Table 23.9). **Most patients want full disclosure.** There has been a steady increase in the desire for honest information from Oken's (37) study in 1961, when 95% of surgeons did not disclose to their patients a cancer diagnosis. Twenty years later, a study by Novack et al. (38) showed a dramatic reversal of this proportion. Regarding the proportion of patients who state they want to be informed, Jones's (391) study in 1981 showed that 50% of (British) patients wanted to know. Since then, there have been many studies that all put the proportion of patients who want full disclosure at above 90% (40–42).

Table 23.8 Patient's Perception of Condition
Ask the patient to say what she knows or suspects about the current medical problem (e.g., "What did you think when . . . ?" or "Did you think it might be serious . . . ?").
As the patient replies
Listen to the level of comprehension and vocabulary.
Note any mismatch between the actual medical information and the patient's perception of it (including denial).

Table 23.9 Invitation from Patient to Give Information
Find out from the patient if she wants to know the details of the medical condition or treatment (e.g., *"Are you the sort of person who . . . ?"*).
Accept patient's right not to know (but offer to answer questions as patient wishes later).

Disguising the information or lying to the patient is highly likely to be unsatisfactory. The phrase one uses to obtain a clear invitation is again a matter of personal choice and judgment (*"Are you the sort of person who'd like to know exactly what's going on?" "Would you like me to go on and tell you exactly what the situation is and what we recommend?"* or *"How would you like me to handle this information? Would you like to know exactly what's going on?"*) Once this is determined you can set goals for the interview, e.g., "So now I'm going to explain what the MRI showed."

It is important to respect cultural norms that may delineate how bad news is discussed. For example, in some Middle Eastern countries, the word "dying" is not used, and in others, bad information is felt to cause the progression of the patient's illness (e.g., in some Native American tribes, giving bad news is felt to make the situation worse) (43).

K—Knowledge (Explaining the Medical Facts)

Having obtained a clear invitation to share information, begin by giving the medical facts and simultaneously be aware of (and sensitive to) the patient's reaction to the information—in other words, giving the information and responding to the patient's emotions should proceed simultaneously.

The most important guidelines for giving the medical facts are shown in Table 23.10.

- **Begin at the level of comprehension and use the vocabulary that the patient indicated** (this is called **aligning**).
- **Use plain, intelligible English** (avoid the technical jargon of the medical profession—"medspeak"). Give information in small amounts.
- **Check that the patient understands the information before going further** (use phrases such as *"Do you follow what I'm saying?" "Is this clear so far?" "Am I making sense so far?"*).
- **Use a narrative approach to make sense of what has occurred:** Explain the sequence of events and how the situation seemed as events unfolded (*"When you became short of breath, we didn't know whether it was just a chest infection or something more serious. So that's when we did the chest x-ray . . ."*).
- **Respond to all emotions expressed by the patient as they arise** (see below).

E—Emotions (Exploration and Empathic Response)

The acknowledgment of emotions is more important in an interview about bad news than it is in most other interviews (see the "A—Acknowledgment" section in the CLASS protocol, previously; Table 23.4).

The doctor can effectively use an empathic response on his or her own feelings if they are becoming intense (*"I'm finding this very upsetting, too."*).

The value of all empathic responses lies in the fact that one is making an observation that is almost unemotional in itself about an issue that is heavily charged with emotion (whether the patient's or the doctor's). The fact that this is experienced by the patient as

Table 23.10 Knowledge: Giving Medical Facts
Bring the patient toward a comprehension of the medical situation, filling in any gaps.
Use language intelligible to the patient, and start at the level at which he or she finished.
Give information in small pieces.
Check the reception: Confirm that the patient understands what you are saying after each significant piece of information.
Respond to the patient's reactions as they occur.

supportive is why an empathic response cools the temperature of a fraught moment and facilitates the exploration of the situation without causing escalation.

S—Strategy and Summary

Close the interview with a management strategy and closure, as described in the "S—Strategy" and "S—Summary" sections for the CLASS protocol (see Table 23.5).

Dealing with Hope and False Hopes

Many clinicians and patients often say *"But you can't take away hope."* Frequently this is used by clinicians as an excuse for not telling the patient the truth. Usually, the real rationale behind this is to protect the clinician from discomfort, not the patient.

Clinicians are more likely to create major problems for themselves if they promise cure when that is not possible or hold out unrealistic hopes. Supporting the patient and reinforcing realistic hopes is part of the foundation of a genuinely therapeutic relationship. Setting realistic goals for treatment early on allows the patient to "hope for the best while preparing for the worst" (44,45).

The important thing is not whether to tell the truth (there is a moral, ethical, and legal obligation to do so if that is what the patient wants), but how to tell the truth. Insensitive and ineffective truth-telling may be just as damaging and counterproductive as insensitive lying. In practice, the preceding protocols allow the truth to be told at a pace determined by the patient and in a way that allows recruitment and reinforcement of the patient's coping strategies.

Communication in Palliative Care

In palliative care, communication skills are even more important than in acute care—and may sometimes be the only therapeutic modality available to the clinician (46). In palliative care, communication may have at least three distinct functions: (i) in taking the history; (ii) in breaking bad news; and (iii) as therapeutic dialogue (i.e., support of the patient).

Even when the prognosis is acknowledged to be grave, there may be stages in which some hoped-for improvement or stabilization is not achieved. In these circumstances, the SPIKES protocol can be helpful, even when the clinician and the patient already have a long-standing relationship.

At other times, simply listening to the patient and acknowledging the various emotions and reactions she is experiencing is in itself a therapeutic intervention. This is particularly true in discussions about dying. When a patient realizes and acknowledges that she is dying, there is no "answer" the clinician can give. Instead, listening to the questions, issues, and emotions is a valuable service.

Talking to Family Members

Family members are an important component of the psychological context surrounding the patient. Often they may assist the clinician in confirming the medical facts and supporting the patient as she responds to the information. **Sometimes, however, individual family members may be at a different phase of acceptance or understanding of the medical information than the patient. This is called discordance, and it can be a serious and additional problem for the clinician.** The important guideline is to seek and maintain clarity in talking to the relative. The clinician must stress that he or she is looking after the patient (not the relative), and empathic responses can be used to acknowledge and explore the emotions underlying the relative's state.

This is particularly true in a potential conflict, such as when a relative tells a clinician, "My mother is not to be told the diagnosis." This is a common and awkward situation, and it requires care and effort to emphasize the primacy of the patient's right to knowledge (if that is what she wants), while at the same time underlining the relative's importance and value as part of the patient's support system.

Another exceptionally difficult situation for the clinician is telling a relative that the patient has died. The central principle is to use a narrative approach to the events, but to be prepared at any instant to respond to the relative if he or she asks whether the patient has died.

Communication with Other Health Care Professionals

Medical professionals are only human. Sometimes under great stress, they may become short-tempered, rude, aggressive, or impatient. This is almost unavoidable. With good communication skills, the resulting damage can be minimized.

The two principles that are most useful are (i) clarication and (ii) acknowledgment of the situation (using empathic responses). **Whenever one responds to an emotion by acknowledging it with a relatively unemotional empathic response, the dispute will deescalate.** It is also worth remembering the old adage that "an ounce of prevention is worth a pound of cure." Giving information early (a "preemptive information strike") prefaced as a "for your information" discussion may prevent major disputes or discontent later *("Why didn't you tell me . . . ?").*

Motivation and Manners

Like any clinical intervention, effective communication requires motivation to be successful. If one is motivated to be a good clinical communicator, it is achievable. Some of it depends on having a basic strategy for the task, and the protocols presented here should be helpful. The rest is largely a matter of having an awareness of the effect of what one says and does on the patient and her family. There is a great deal of courtesy and common sense mixed in with the specific strategies. It is important to be mindful of the fact that if chosen poorly, words can be scalpels, but if chosen carefully, they can be perceived by the patient and family as a source of comfort and support.

Communication tasks are of enormous importance in the relationship between doctor and patient. As has been said, "Do this part of your job badly and they will never forgive you; do it well and they will never forget you."

References

1. **Armstrong DK.** Relapsed ovarian cancer: challenges and management strategies for a chronic disease. *Oncologist* 2002;7(suppl 5):20–28.
2. **Sardell AN, Trierweiler SJ.** Disclosing the cancer diagnosis: procedures that influence patient hopefulness. *Cancer* 1993;72: 3355–3365.
3. **Zachariae R, Pedersen CG, Jensen AB, Ehrnrooth E, Rossen PB, von der Maase H.** Association of perceived physician communication style with patient satisfaction, distress, cancer-related self-efficacy, and perceived control over the disease. *Br J Cancer* 2003;88: 658–665.
4. **Kerr J, Engel J, Schlesinger-Raab A, Sauer H, Holzel D.** Doctor-patient communication: results of a four-year prospective study in rectal cancer patients. *Dis Colon Rectum* 2003;46:1038–1046.
5. **Dimoska A, Butow PN, Dent E, Arnold B, Brown RF, Tattersall MH.** An examination of the initial cancer consultation of medical and radiation oncologists using the Cancode interaction analysis system. *Brit J Cancer* 2008;98:1508–1514.
6. **Kaplan SH, Greenfield S, Ware JE.** Impact of the doctor-patient relationship on the outcomes of chronic disease. In: **Stewart M, Roter D, eds.** *Communicating with medical patients.* Newbury Park, CA: Sage Publications, 1989:228–245.
7. **Bredart A, Bouleuc C, Dolbeault S.** Doctor-patient communication and satisfaction with care in oncology. *Curr Opin Oncol* 2005;17: 351–354.
8. **Gandhi IG, Parle JV, Greenfield SM, Gould S.** A qualitative investigation into why patients change their GPs. *Fam Pract* 1997;14: 49–57.
9. **Levinson W, Chaumeton N.** Communication between surgeons and patients in routine office visits. *Surgery* 1999;125:127–134.
10. **Ambady N, Laplante D, Nguyen T, Rosenthal R, Chaumeton N, Levinson W.** Surgeons' tone of voice: a clue to malpractice history. *Surgery* 2002;132:5–9.
11. **Albrecht TL, Ruckdeschel JC, Riddle DL, Blanchard CG, Penner LA, Coovert MD, et al.** Communication and consumer decision making about cancer clinical trials. *Patient Educ Couns* 2003;50:39–42.
12. **Stewart MA.** Effective physician-patient communication and health outcomes: a review. *CMAJ* 1995;152:1423–1433.
13. **Hoffman M, Ferri J, Sison C, Roter D, Schapira L, Baile W.** Teaching communication skills: an AACE survey of oncology training programs. *J Cancer Educ* 2004;19:220–224.
14. **Baile WF, Buckman R, Lenzi R, Glober G, Beale EA, Kudelka AP.** SPIKES-A six-step protocol for delivering bad news: application to the patient with cancer. *Oncologist* 2000;5:302–311.
15. **Wallace J, Hlubocky FJ, Daugherty CK.** Emotional responses of oncologists when disclosing prognostic information to patients with terminal disease; results of qualitative data from a mailed survey to ASCO members. *J Clin Oncol* 2006 ASCO Annual Meeting Proceedings Part 1. Vol 24(8S):8520.
16. **Taylor KM.** "Telling bad news": physicians and the disclosure of undesirable information. *Sociol Health Din* 1988;10:109–132.
17. **Maguire P, Pitceathly C.** Key communication skills and how to acquire them. *BMJ* 2002;325:697–700.
18. **Harrington SE, Smith TJ.** The role of chemotherapy at the end of life: "when is enough, enough?" *JAMA* 2008;299: 2667–2678.
19. **Garg A, Buckman R, Kason Y.** Teaching medical students how to break bad news. *CMAJ* 1997;6:1159–1164.
20. **Baile WB, Kudelka AP, Beale EA, Glober GA, Myers EG, Greisinger AJ, et al.** Communication skills training in oncology: description and preliminary outcomes of workshops on breaking bad news and managing patient reactions to illness. *Cancer* 1999;86: 887–897.
21. **Maguire P, Faulkner A.** Improve the counselling skills of doctors and nurses in cancer care. *BMJ* 1999;297:847–849.
22. **Simpson M, Buckman R, Stewart M, Maguire P, Lipkin M, Novack D, et al.** Doctor-patient communication: the Toronto consensus statement. *BMJ* 1991;393:1985–1987.

23. **Back AL, Arnold RM, Baile WF, Fryer-Edwards KA, Alexander SC, Barley GE, et al.** Efficacy of communication skills training for giving bad news and discussing transitions to palliative care. *Arch Intern Med* 2007;167:453–460.

24. **Buckman R, Kason Y.** *How to break bad news: a guide for health care professionals.* Baltimore: Johns Hopkins University Press, 1992.

25. **Baile W, Buckman R.** *The pocket guide to communication skills in clinical practice.* Toronto: Medical Audio-Visual Communications, 1998.

26. **Buckman R, Baile W, Korsch B.** *A practical guide to communication skills in clinical practice.* CD-ROM or video set. Toronto: Medical Audio-Visual Communications, 1998.

27. **Baile WB, Glober GA, Lenzi R, Beale EA, Kudelka AP.** Discussing disease progression and end-of-life decisions. *Oncology* 1999;13:1021–1031.

28. **Hall ET.** *The hidden dimension.* New York: Doubleday, 1966.

29. **Older J.** Teaching touch at medical school. *JAMA* 1984;252:931–933.

30. **Buis C, De Boo T, Hull R.** Touch and breaking bad news. *Earn Pract* 1991;8:303–304.

31. **Lipkin M, Quill TE, Napodano J.** The medical interview: a core curriculum for residencies in internal medicine. *Ann Intern Med* 1984;100:277–284.

32. **Frankel RM, Beckman HB.** The pause that refreshes. *Hosp Pract* 1988;23:62–67.

33. **Ptacek JT, Eberhardt L.** The patient-physician relationship: breaking bad news. A review of the literature. *JAMA* 1996;276:496–502.

34. **Billings AJ.** *Outpatient management of advanced cancer: symptom control, support, and hospice-in-the-home.* Philadelphia: JB Lippincott, 1985:236–259.

35. **Buckman R.** Breaking bad news: why is it still so difficult? *BMJ* 1984;288:1597–1599.

36. **Maynard DW.** On clinicians co-implicating recipients perspective in the delivery of bad news. In: **Drew P, Heritage J, eds.** *Talk at work: social interaction in institutional settings.* Cambridge, UK: Cambridge University Press, 1992:331–358.

37. **Oken D.** What to tell cancer patients: a study of medical attitudes. *JAMA* 1961;175:86–94.

38. **Novack DH, Plumer R, Smith RL, Ochitill H, Morrow GR, Bennett JM.** Changes in physicians' attitudes toward telling the cancer patient. *JAMA* 1979;241:897–900.

39. **Jones JS.** Telling the right patient. *BMJ* 1981;283:291–292.

40. **Meredith C, Symonds P, Webster L, Lamont D, Pyper E, Gillis CR, et al.** Information needs of cancer patients in west Scotland: cross-sectional survey of patients' views. *BMJ* 1996;313:724–726.

41. **Benson J, Britten N.** Respecting the autonomy of cancer patients when talking with their families: qualitative analysis of semi-structured interviews with patients. *BMJ* 1996;313:729–731.

42. **Northouse PG, Northouse LL.** Communication and cancer: issues confronting patients, health professionals and family members. *J Psychosocial Oncol* 1988;5:17–45.

43. **Baile WF, Lenzi R, Parker PA, Buckman R, Cohen L.** Oncologists' attitudes toward and practices in giving bad news: an exploratory study. *J Clin Oncol* 2002;20:2189–2196.

44. **Von Roenn JH, von Gunten CF.** Setting goals to maintain hope. *J Clin Oncol* 2003;21:570–574.

45. **Back AL, Arnold RM, Quill TE.** Hope for the best, and prepare for the worst. *Ann Intern Med* 2003;138:439–443.

46. **Buckman R.** Communication in palliative care: a practical guide. In: **Doyle D, Hanks GWC, MacDonald N, eds.** *Oxford textbook of palliative care.* Oxford: Oxford University Press, 1998:141–156.

24 Symptom Relief and Palliative Care

Jennifer A. M. Philip
J. Norelle Lickiss

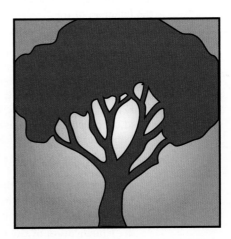

Comprehensive care of a woman with gynecologic cancer involves anticancer treatment (directed at either cure or control of the cancer), good symptom relief, and personal and family support. **In the setting of progressive disease, the priorities for care, from the patient's perspective, must be clarified.** Such priorities may reflect the preferred place of care when dependency increases, the use of time for important tasks, and the personal issues involved in preparation for death. **These matters should not be suddenly raised at time of crisis.** Rather, discussion, elucidation, and realization of such priorities should occur over time and multiple clinical encounters. There is no dichotomy between care concerned with cure or control of cancer and care when disease is irreversibly progressive; all is concerned with enhancement of life (1).

The concept of "*mixed management*" or what may be better called **"parallel care,"** implies attention to the principles of palliative care (personal and family support, symptom relief, and care planning/death preparation) from the time of diagnosis of a disease that is likely to prove to be an eventually fatal illness, e.g., advanced ovarian cancer. **The deficiencies associated with introducing palliative care and symptom relief only when anticancer treatments have failed have been well documented.** Instead, the provision of palliative care concurrent with anticancer treatment is widely advocated (2,3).

The goals of palliative care should be to facilitate comfort, autonomy, dignity, as well as personal rehabilitation and development, especially in the face of an incurable illness. **Efforts must be directed at assisting the patient to have realistic expectations and well-grounded hope in what will not fail her, notably in the fidelity of her caregivers, and a recognition of her own unique value as a person, come what may.** The patient's quality of life will be determined by many aspects of her life including her values, her relationships, her sense of self-worth as well as health related matters. A woman can achieve much and indeed may report "quality" in a number of areas, even in the face of progressive illness. The challenge for health caregivers is to create a climate in which such achievements may emerge.

The last phase of life is crucial to the completion of a human life. Patients report that important issues at the conclusion of a fulfilled life include relief of pain and other symptoms, clear decision making by professionals, preparation for death, being able to contribute to others, and being affirmed as a whole person (4,5). **During this final phase, whether it be months, weeks, or days, it is the responsibility of the medical and nursing professions, through careful symptom relief, good communication, and a supportive relationship, to facilitate maximum autonomy and dignity.** The attitude of the physician to this last phase of life and to death itself may color clinical judgment. In general, it is crucial for the bond between the patient and her primary care physician to be strengthened at this time, and a continuity of professional relationships is desirable (6).

Practical Aspects of Palliative Care

The palliative care of a woman with advanced gynecologic malignancy involves several components: assessment, clarification and delineation of therapeutic options, implementation of treatment, evaluation of outcome, continuing review and reassessment, and prognostication. Attention to each of these clinical tasks is necessary for a woman to maximize her possibilities in the final part of life.

Assessment

It is essential to make a comprehensive assessment, which includes listening to the patient's experience with her cancer, from the prediagnostic phase to the current time. There should be detailing of responses to treatments, side effects experienced, hopes realized and conversely, disappointments encountered. The narrative of the illness experience will give information on not only the patient's responses, but also her vulnerabilities and her supports. It also establishes a shared understanding of what has gone before, and as such is a much more useful therapeutic tool than a checklist approach.

A comprehensive assessment involves at least:

1. **Ascertainment of the patient's current symptoms and other problems,** in her order of priorities, because only the woman herself can determine that which is affecting her quality of life and requiring attention.

2. **Clarification of the nature and the extent of the neoplastic process,** with careful consideration of any other pathologic process that may be contributing to the current problems, or may be likely to contribute in the near future.

3. **Clarification of her understanding of her illness and the treatment goals.**

4. **Delineation of the personal and social context within which the patient is living** and from which she may draw support.

5. **Elucidation of her current goals**—the delineation of such goals and discussion concerning their achievability can do much to enhance a person's sense of self and hence quality of life.

An adequate assessment may involve interaction not only with the patient, but also with family members and friends, though the extent of this interaction will be subject to the woman's wishes. The assessment should be regarded as a continuous process, as both the circumstances of the illness and the woman's priorities are constantly changing.

Clinical Decision Making

On the basis of a comprehensive assessment, with or without further investigations to elucidate the mechanism of troublesome symptoms, it is normally possible to delineate the reasonable therapeutic possibilities.

The choice between therapeutic options should reflect the patient's priorities. In general, alternatives involving the least dependence on medical facilities and the least use of the patient's time, resources, and personal energy should be recommended. For example, it is inappropriate to resort to intravenous (or spinal) techniques for pain relief if oral, transcutaneous, or subcutaneous techniques have not been adequately explored. **When shared decision making serves to realize a woman's nominated priorities, quality of life is often improved.** For example, the realization of a goal to return home may be more important to some than a minor extension of life from a further course of antibiotics.

Careful consideration of relevant antitumor measures (surgery, radiation therapy, or chemotherapy) is always mandatory because control of the neoplastic process usually offers the best chance of alleviating symptoms. **Factors that should be considered when evaluating therapy include** (7):

1. **the stage of disease**

2. **the likely natural history of the illness** with and without intervention, including the likely symptom patterns

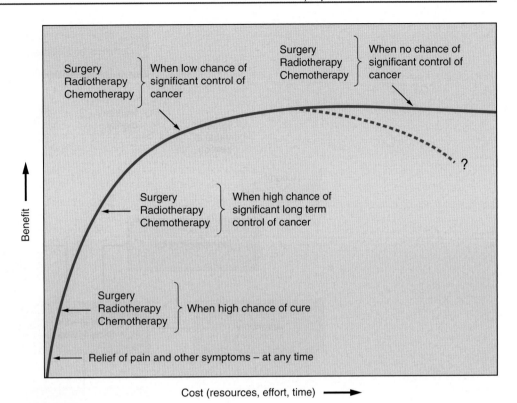

Figure 24.1   **Factors to be taken into account when considering further anticancer therapy: benefit vs. cost.**

3. **the burden of investigation and treatment**
4. **the likely success of the intervention**
5. **the potential for rehabilitation** (physical, psychological, social, or spiritual)
6. **the patient's goals and priorities**

If cost-benefit issues are considered, **it is essential to avoid "flat of the curve" medicine.** Good symptom relief is almost always high in benefit in relation to cost (broadly considered), whereas anticancer measures may vary in benefit. These matters, represented simply in Fig. 24.1, justify reflection by clinicians as well as administrators.

Clinical decision making is always undertaken in a context of prevailing values, much influenced by culture, social circumstances, and facts (legal, medical, and resource limitations). This is portrayed schematically in Fig. 24.2. **Ethical principles such as autonomy, beneficence, non-malfeasance, and justice must be kept in mind.** They need to be appropriately understood: a balance between sometimes competing principles may need to be struck after careful consideration of each. The discussion will usually involve input not only from the patient and her significant other, but also from the professional team involved in her care. However, if clinical wisdom is brought to bear, an appropriate recommendation will emerge to a conscientious clinician.

Decisions concerning treatment should usually involve the patient, who should be adequately informed about the advantages and disadvantages of the various options. Such involvement may help the patient to regain control at a potentially chaotic time in her life. **Although the patient should share in decision making, her attending clinician should indicate the course of action he or she favors,** and ultimately take the responsibility for any intervention, so that a distressing outcome does not engender guilt in the patient and her family. This being said, the physician should not compromise his or her better judgment or conscience in the face of patient or family pressure.

The burden of decision making is considerable, and ways of reaching decisions vary according to social, cultural, economic, and medical contexts. When disagreements arise between

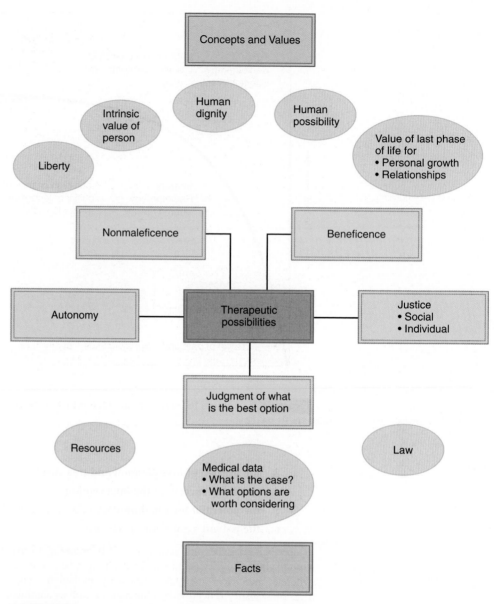

Figure 24.2   **The context of clinical decision-making.**

patients (or their families) and clinicians regarding clinical decisions, it is often useful to consult within the treating team to determine if a range of views exists among clinicians. **A negotiated position between patient and clinician can almost always be reached.** If not, a second opinion or a perceived "independent broker" may be useful (8).

There are no circumstances that justify a physician's declaring that "there is nothing more that can be done." A decision not to pursue anticancer treatments, but to focus solely on symptomatic measures, does not indicate nihilism or inactivity. It may reflect authentic clinical wisdom with clear goals of comfort and dignity.

Evaluation of Outcomes

Evaluation of palliative interventions is best performed by the informed patient, although the observations of the medical and nursing staff are also important. Evaluations should be performed regularly, at intervals consistent with the clinical goal. Pain measurements may, for example, be appropriately performed each time observations such as blood pressure and temperature are undertaken. For patients with advanced disease when the goals of care are centered on comfort and dignity, monitoring only of those parameters that serve these goals is justified. Formal outcome measures based on subjective criteria, of which there are many examples (9–12), should ideally be introduced into routine clinical practice, with outcomes to be measured commensurate with the patient's priorities for comfort and for personal objectives.

Discussing Prognosis

Mention should be made of the art of prognostication, because estimates of survival underlie much of the clinical decision making. There is a considerable body of literature to guide the clinician when formulating a prognosis (13–15). **Factors to be considered** in such a formulation for patients with advanced cancer include: **performance status, symptoms of the cancer cachexia syndrome,** and **patient-rated quality of life,** while **the presence of a leukocytosis or lymphopenia also appear to be important.** Notably, these factors differ from those considered in a newly diagnosed cancer, such as tumor size and grade (15).

While it may be possible to determine a probability of survival for a particular patient, the communication of this information to the patient and her family requires thought and care. Such a discussion should occur in the context of a supportive relationship, and when the clinician has sufficient time to devote to the task. If the discussion has been prompted by a question, it is important to clarify what the patient has asked, and what has motivated her to ask it. The patient's understanding of her current situation should be ascertained. It is often helpful to ask the patient what she believes her prognosis to be. The uncertainty of prognostic elements must be explained, and information should be given slowly, at a pace dictated by the patient (16).

A reasonable approach for many patients in the face of a question concerning prognosis, **is to offer some time boundaries within which death is likely to occur.** Such boundaries are useful for determining priorities and for planning medical care to best serve those priorities. Time boundaries do not give a patient or her family an agonizing date around which to focus, nor do they suggest that what is still somewhat uncertain can be predicted precisely (17).

Symptoms and Their Relief

In general, **effective anti-disease therapy offers the best chance of good symptom relief if the patient is a "responder,"** but the quality of life of a "non-responder" to chemotherapy may be worse than that of an untreated patient. Expertise in palliative therapeutics should be made available alongside surgery, chemotherapy, and radiation therapy, and delivered according to clinical needs, not prognosis (3).

Symptoms are subjective, and their presence and severity is not necessarily apparent to the observer. A patient in severe pain may show no signs of distress, yet she may admit upon careful questioning that the pain is almost unbearable. Her expressions of pain will be influenced by cultural and environmental factors, as well as by personal and interpersonal relationships. Accurate assessment of symptoms requires skill, patience, and active, supportive listening. **Symptoms vary in their significance for the patient,** and anxiety or distress associated with the development of a particular symptom will inevitably have a psychological impact. **It is important to give the patient a chance to express her fears and to offer some simple explanation for the symptom,** because this will at least reduce uncertainty.

Symptoms may arise from the tumor itself, from the treatment, and/or from unrelated causes. **Symptoms may precede signs or objective evidence (x-ray or scans) of disease.** An example is the development of leg pain from lumbosacral plexus infiltration, which may herald recurrent cervical cancer. Imaging may fail to demonstrate a lesion suspected on the basis of symptoms, but the pain needs treatment even while awaiting a definitive diagnosis. Waiting for objective signs may be disastrous in certain circumstances, such as in the early diagnosis of remediable spinal cord compression.

There is now considerable literature concerning the understanding and therapy of major symptoms in cancer, and attention is given here to those seen more commonly, with emphasis on practical considerations.

Pain Management

Pain has been defined by the International Association for the Study of Pain as "an unpleasant sensory and emotional experience associated with actual or potential tissue damage or described in terms of such damage." Thus pain is subjective: All pain is "in the mind." Psychological factors influence the perception of pain in all women: Pain is the experience of a person, not a part of the body, and changing the experience of a person is a major challenge. Effective pain management is dependent upon understanding and delineating the

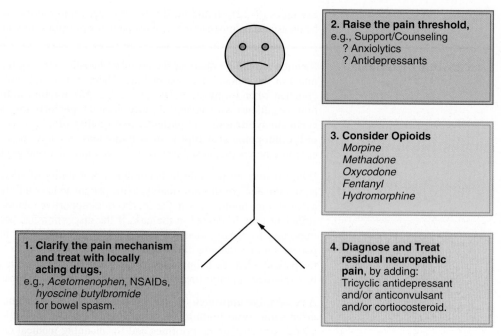

2. Raise the pain threshold,
e.g., Support/Counseling
    ? Anxiolytics
    ? Antidepressants

3. Consider Opioids
Morpine
Methadone
Oxycodone
Fentanyl
Hydromorphine

**1. Clarify the pain mechanism
and treat with locally
acting drugs,**
e.g., *Acetomenophen*, NSAIDs,
hyoscine butylbromide
for bowel spasm.

**4. Diagnose and Treat
residual neuropathic
pain,** by adding:
Tricyclic antidepressant
and/or anticonvulsant
and/or cortiocosteroid.

Figure 24.3   **Schema for the approach to pain management.** NSAIDs, non-steroidal anti-inflammatory drugs

pain mechanisms involved, and prescribing medication based upon these mechanisms. Controversies relevant to gynecological practice remain, not least being the global inequity in access to pain relief for women with gynecological cancer (18).

Pain in gynecological cancer presents in many forms and may occur at any stage in the illness. It may be caused by both the disease and its treatment. Pain caused by treatment (e.g., radiation therapy) requires as close attention as that caused by tumor. Many guidelines for the assessment and treatment of cancer pain have been published, including those by the American Society of Clinical Oncology (19–21). The following simple steps provide a practical approach in the face of the complexity of recent research and practice (22).

Pain management may be considered to have four steps (Fig. 24.3):

1. **Reduce the noxious stimulus at the periphery.**
2. **Raise the pain threshold.**
3. **Consider and use appropriate doses of opioid drugs.**
4. **Recognize residual neuropathic pain and treat it correctly.**

Such steps should be considered in order, but measures relating to all four steps may be instituted simultaneously if the clinical circumstances dictate.

**Step One: Reduce the
Noxious Stimulus
at the Periphery**

This step demands an adequate understanding of the mechanism of the pain stimulus in the individual patient. Pain in patients with gynecologic cancer is most commonly due to soft tissue infiltration, bone involvement, neural involvement, muscle spasm (e.g., psoas spasm), infection within or near tumor masses, or intestinal colic. **Pain felt in the back needs particularly careful consideration, because the causes are many and the treatments are diverse.**

The mechanism of pain can usually be diagnosed clinically. The history should include the mode of onset, characteristics, distribution, aggravating factors, trends over time, and response to therapeutic endeavors thus far. Therapeutic approaches vary according to the mechanism that is operative. Peripherally acting drugs should be used irrespective of specific therapeutic measures (e.g., radiation therapy, chemotherapy, antibiotics, or surgery), which may be required.

Bone metastases frequently cause inflammatory changes with release of inflammatory mediators, including prostaglandins. When the pain is clearly arising from bone metastases, the use of drugs that interfere with prostaglandin synthesis (e.g., non-steroidal anti-inflammatory drugs [NSAIDs]) is logical. These drugs should be avoided or used with caution in patients who have a history of peptic ulceration, excessive alcohol consumption, bleeding diathesis, renal impairment, or known allergies to aspirin or related drugs. **Where the use of NSAIDs is precluded, *acetaminophen (paracetamol)* is a useful alternative.** While its mechanism of action is yet to be fully elucidated, clinical utility suggests some peripheral action, although not a direct anti-inflammatory effect. *Acetaminophen* is fairly well tolerated and safe, but it should be used in reduced dosage in patients with impaired liver function.

Peripherally acting drugs such as *acetaminophen* and NSAIDs are also useful for pain arising in non-osseous sites and for postoperative pain. They should rarely be omitted from analgesic regimens, even in moribund patients. Rectal preparations may prove useful in patients who are unable to take oral drugs.

Muscle spasm requires muscle relaxants, as well as gentle massage. Psoas muscle spasm, usually resulting from direct tumor infiltration, is not infrequent in gynecologic cancer (23). Psoas muscle infiltration should be suspected if there is pain in a lumbosacral plexus distribution associated with difficulty achieving full extension of the hip. While radiation therapy is being considered or applied, relief can usually be achieved by careful adherence to the outlined principles, but will not be adequately managed by opioids alone. ***Acetaminophen* and/or NSAIDs, an oral opioid (such as *oxycodone*),** and a laxative must be supplemented by a drug that is active against spasm in skeletal muscle, such as ***diazepam*. Steroids should also be given (e.g., *dexamethone* 2–4 mg daily). Polypharmacy is justified to relieve pain in the malignant psoas syndrome.** If the pain does not respond to these measures, specialist help must be sought (24). No patient should die with intractable pain.

Experience at the Royal Hospital for Women in Sydney would suggest that **pain associated with subacute and chronic radiation toxicity** (e.g., vulvovaginal ulceration) **may benefit from hyperbaric oxygen treatment.**

Regional blockade with a local anesthetic and neurolytic techniques may be worthy of consideration if the area of pain is circumscribed and attributable to an accessible peripheral nerve, such as pain in the intercostal region.

Step Two: Raise the Pain Threshold	**All persons should be considered to have a threshold** above which they will be troubled by pain. It is useful to consider the threshold as "one's sense of mastery of a situation." **Such a threshold is dynamic,** and may be influenced by many factors. The threshold for pain may be **raised by explanation, comfort, care, concern, diversion, and various forms of relaxation.** Similarly, the threshold will be **lowered,** or a patient's sense of mastery will be affected negatively **by depression, anxiety, uncertainty, loneliness, and isolation.** Threshold issues in general require a nonpharmacological approach.

A wide range of strategies exist to facilitate coping with pain, and simple **measures, such as explanation** of, for example, the likely cause of pain, **should be tried initially.** The diagnosis of a disturbed threshold in an individual patient is difficult, but the narrative approach to assessment of the patient gives clues. As the patient tells the story of her diagnosis, treatment, and the pattern of her pain, she imparts information not only about the cancer but also about herself, and **excessive distress can be readily perceived.** Many complementary therapies, such as massage and meditation, assist in the relief of pain, and it is likely that their benefits stem from enhancing a patient's sense of mastery.

Occasionally, anxiety and depression are so marked that the patient is impeded in her attempts to relate to her loved ones and to come to terms with her disease. In such circumstances, a formal psychiatric consultation may be of assistance and anxiolytics or antidepressants may prove helpful. In general, **threshold issues, including extreme anguish, feelings of futility, loss of sense of meaning, personal guilt, and other forms of spiritual pain, require a different approach, with help from skilled counselors, pastors, and, above all, those people who are close to the patient.**

Pain and suffering are related but distinct (25). Suffering has been described as a sense of impending personal disintegration (26). In common parlance, there may be a sense of being about to "go to pieces." Suffering may be triggered by poorly controlled symptoms, perceived loss of dignity, loss of a sense of control or autonomy, fear for the future, and loss of a future. Pain may be the main cause of suffering, or a manifestation (through threshold shifts) of suffering, with the language of suffering expressed through pain. A conscientious clinical oncologist needs to be aware of suffering in a patient and should seek to provide comfort while seeking ways to relieve distress, (which may progress to suffering), by understanding and alleviating the causes (such as pain) and seeking the help of colleagues (27).

If suffering is defined as a sense of impending "personal disintegration," then the response to suffering should be "reintegration." Such reintegration may be most assisted by others who have skills in that dimension of care focused on existential issues that may or may not relate to religious matters. But every doctor has the responsibility and privilege to be aware of such dimensions of care, to provide the "space" for patients to consider their existential concerns (notably ensure that symptoms are well controlled), and to take time to be informed about current reflections on this area (28).

Step Three: Precise and Appropriate Use of Opioid Drugs

There is abundant literature on opioid use to supplement peripherally acting analgesics, with a range of opioids available (29,30). Despite the initiatives of the World Health Organization, there are still difficulties obtaining opioids for medical use in some countries. A variety of opioids is available, and the principles of choice need to be understood (Table 24.1) (31). In practice, low-potency opioids such as *codeine* or *dextropropoxyphene,* or high-potency opioids such as *morphine,* are combined with peripherally acting drugs such as *acetaminophen* or *aspirin*. Low- and high-potency opioids should not be given concurrently, but a change from one opioid to another may be justified (32,33). While at a global level *morphine* remains the preferred initial opioid of high potency, consideration is increasingly given to alternative high-potency opioids if available, such as, *oxycodone, methadone, fentanyl,* and *hydromorphone* (31). It is critical that local availability and affordability inform the choice of opioids: no woman should be deprived of pain relief because expensive, unaffordable drugs have been prescribed if cheaper drugs would have given significant benefit.

Regardless of the choice, opioids should be given at regular intervals in accordance with the half-life of the drug concerned, rather than haphazardly in response to a severe pain stimulus. Doses of opioid drugs should be carefully titrated against response and side effects.

Oral morphine and *oxycodone* are available in two forms: an immediate-release preparation that reaches a peak within 30 minutes of ingestion, and a sustained release preparation that for morphine takes several hours to reach peak concentrations, while for *oxycodone* peak levels are reached within 40 minutes (34). As a general rule, for a patient not previously taking opioids, initial prescribing should involve regular dosing with an immediate-release preparation as a "dose finding" exercise. This allows rapid escalation or reduction of dose according to clinical response.

Some types of pain are only partially responsive to opioids (30,35), including pain caused by nerve irritation, extreme muscle spasm, incident pain (i.e., pain exacerbated by a particular activity such as movement), or pain that is heightened by unaddressed anguish. Even in these circumstances opioids remain "partially effective" and should be introduced and carefully calibrated to ensure that optimum benefit is achieved while minimizing side effects (36).

Morphine

Immediate-release *morphine* is best given every 4 hours, with a double dose (or 1.5 times the standard dose in the frail) at bedtime and a break of approximately 8 hours overnight to permit sleep for both patient and caregivers. A reasonable starting dose of oral *morphine* in a patient with severe pain not already on an opioid drug would be 10 mg in a patient of average size, or 3 to 5 mg in the frail or very elderly patient. The original dose should be repeated in 1 to 2 hours if there has been inadequate relief of pain. Over the next 24 to 48 hours, dose finding is undertaken by prescribing regular doses every 4 hours, together with one or two "breakthrough" doses, equal to the standard dose. The correct dose may range from 2 mg to more than 100 mg every 4 hours, but most patients need less than 50 mg every 4 hours.

Once the daily dose requirement is established, this can be converted to a sustained-release formulation, once again maintaining supplemental breakthrough doses of the immediate release preparation. For example, a patient taking 20 mg oral *morphine sulfate* mixture every 4 hours can be converted to 60 mg sustained-release *morphine* each 12 hours, with additional breakthrough doses of 20 mg of *morphine sulfate* mixture if required.

Sustained-release *morphine* (or other sustained release opioids) should not be used (i) in patients with uncontrolled or unstable pain; (ii) in patients with extensive upper abdominal or retroperitoneal disease that is likely to interfere with gastrointestinal motility; or (iii) when there is fecal loading or impaction. Subcutaneous *morphine* is a better choice in such circumstances.

If parenteral *morphine* is essential, the subcutaneous route is appropriate, either with intermittent injections through an indwelling butterfly needle every 4 hours or with a continuous

Table 24.1 Opioid Analgesics Used for the Treatment of Chronic Pain

| Drug | Dose (mg) Equianalgesic to Morphine 10 mg IM[a] | | Half-Life (hr) | Duration (hr) | Comment |
	PO	IM			
Morphine	20–30[b]	10	2–3	2–4	Standard for comparison
Morphine CR	20–30	10	2–3	8–12	Various formulations are not bioequivalent
Morphine SR	20–30	10	2–3	24	
Oxycodone	20	—	2–3	3–4	
Oxycodone CR	20	—	2–3	8–12	
Hydromorphone	7.5	1.5	2–3	2–4	Potency may be greater; for example, IV Hydromorphone: IV morphine = 3:1 rather than 6.7:1 during prolonged use
Methadone	20	10	12–190	4–12	Although 1:1 IV ratio with morphine was in single-dose study, there is a change with chronic dosing; large dose reduction (75% to 90%) is needed when switching to methadone
Oxymorphone	10 (rectal)	1	2–3	2–4	Available in rectal and injectable formulations
Levorphanol	4	2	12–15	4–6	
Fentanyl	—	—	7–12	—	Can be administered as a continuous IV or SQ infusion; based on clinical experience, 100 μg/hr is roughly equianalgesic to IV morphine 4 mg/hr
Fentanyl TTS	—	—	16–24	48–72	Based on clinical experience, 100 μg/hr is roughly equianalgesic to IV morphine 4 mg/hr; a ratio of oral morphine: transdermal fentanyl of 70:1 may also be used clinically

IM, intramuscular; SQ, subcutaneous; IV, intravenous; CR, controlled release; PO, oral; SR, sustained release.

[a]Studies to determine equianalgesic doses of opioids have used morphine by the IM route. The IM and IV routes are considered to be equivalent. (Note: SQ route is generally used for recurrent dosing in most countries)

[b]Although the PO:IM morphine ratio was 6:1 in a single-dose study, other observations indicate a ratio of 2–3:1 with repeated administration.

From **Derby S, Chin J, Portenoy RK.** Systemic opioid therapy for chronic cancer pain: practical guidelines for converting drugs and routes of administration. CNS Drugs 1998;9:99–109, with permission.

infusion through a battery-driven syringe driver. **When a patient is constipated or has a bowel obstruction, and pain is not well controlled with simple analgesics such as *acetaminophen (paracetamol)*, 4-hourly *morphine* by the subcutaneous route is a useful maneuver** to achieve pain relief and to calibrate the required *morphine* dose. Once her constipation is relieved, the subcutaneous 24-hourly dose may be easily converted to oral *morphine*. **The intramuscular route is rarely advantageous. In general, a parenteral dose of one-half or one-third of the oral dose appears equianalgesic** (37). If oral or subcutaneous *morphine* is efficacious but the side effects are troublesome, the epidural route is occasionally necessary, but a change to another oral or parenteral opioid should normally be tried first.

Intravenous *morphine* **infusions**, although sometimes useful (e.g., in a patient with peripheral circulatory failure), **do not offer significant advantage over the subcutaneous route for most patients** and, because of the need to maintain intravenous access, generally ensure greater complexity and disruption for the patient. In addition, there are anecdotal reports of the **development of tolerance** associated with the intravenous route, which may not always be overcome by the addition of further *morphine* (38). In the setting of rapid dose escalation of intravenous *morphine*, cessation of the infusion and resumption of appropriate subcutaneous doses every 4 hours may be helpful. Simultaneously, it is important to review other aspects of management, such as the possible need for NSAIDs or drugs relevant to neuropathic pain, and to pay appropriate attention to psychological factors.

The efficacy of the regular dosing approach to *morphine* administration may depend on the contribution of an active metabolite (*morphine 6-glucuronide*), which, like *morphine,* is a powerful mu receptor agonist. **Hepatic impairment, if severe, interferes with** *morphine* **metabolism to glucuronides. Renal impairment, even if only moderate, interferes with excretion of the active metabolites. In both of these circumstances, dose reduction is essential.** In a patient with renal impairment, it may be necessary to extend the dose interval from 4–8 or even 12 hours. The use of *morphine* in a patient with marked renal impairment is very complex, and an alternative opioid that does not have active metabolites may be a better choice (39).

Some physicians and nurses, as well as patients, continue to harbor **misconceptions** about the use of *morphine*. When morphine is to be commenced, counseling should address three issues to counteract widely held fears:

1. **The use of** *morphine* **with careful dose finding and monitoring does not, in the vast majority of patients, lead to addiction** (although physical dependence, a separate issue, occurs). However, specialist help is needed to use *morphine* appropriately in current or former intravenous *heroin* users.

2. **The introduction of** *morphine* **does not mean that the patient is actually dying,** but rather that morphine is the most appropriate opioid at that time. It is the type of pain and its severity, not the prognosis of the patient, that dictates whether an opioid should be introduced. *Morphine,* **correctly used, does not hasten death.**

3. Patients and their families need to be reassured that **the introduction of** *morphine* **does not mean that it will be ineffective at a later stage in the illness,** when the situation may be worse. *Morphine* does not lose its effectiveness, but increased doses may be needed later in response to tumor progression.

Use of Alternative Opioids

Other potent opioids should be considered when: (i) **pain persists** despite careful drug calibration; (ii) **unacceptable side effects persist** (e.g., cognitive impairment, nausea) despite careful drug calibration; or (iii) **drowsiness or toxicity occurs** at levels of the drug required to control the pain. In these circumstances, after reconsideration of the pain mechanism and the other analgesic steps, an alternative opioid should be considered. Availability varies from country to country, but gynecologic oncologists should become familiar with a narrow range of opioids (see Table 24.1). In countries where there is wide availability and affordability of opioids, the choice may depend upon preferred route of administration (oral versus transdermal).

Oxycodone (available as immediate-release tablets, suspension, sustained-release preparations, parenteral and suppositories) is somewhat more potent (20% to 50%) than *morphine*: *Oxycodone* is being most often used in a dose of 5 mg to 20 mg every 4 to 6 hours. Some patients tolerate *oxycodone* better than *morphine* at the same dose, and vice versa. **In general terms** however, **the side-effect profile is similar** (40). Anecdotal reports suggest that *oxycodone* may be more effective in neurogenic pain, so may be helpful to relieve leg pain in patients with recurrent cancer of the cervix (41).

Meperidine (pethidine) **is of very little value in palliative care.** It has poor oral bioavailability and a short half-life, requiring frequent administration, approximately every 2 hours. At high doses (>1 g/day) or when renal failure is present, the metabolites lead to neurotoxicity, including delirium, agitation, and seizures. It is also addictive. If a patient is already receiving *meperidine* subcutaneously or intramuscularly, conversion to *morphine* can be achieved with approximately 10% of the *meperidine* dose given as subcutaneous *morphine,* or 30% of the *meperidine* dose given as oral *morphine* every 4 hours.

Methadone is occasionally useful, particularly for those who appear to have pain that is more difficult to control. Its long half-life is sometimes disadvantageous, particularly in the elderly, and its sedative action may outlast its analgesic activity. It has mechanisms of action that differ slightly from those of *morphine,* being reported to have both opioid receptor activity as well as activity on the N-methyl-D-aspartate (NMDA) receptor pathways (42). Therefore, **methadone is occasionally useful when higher doses of other opioids are reached with only partial or inadequate response.** Conversion from *morphine* to *methadone* may be difficult, with subsequent dose reduction frequently required (43,44). *Methadone* has a similar side-effect profile to *morphine.*

Hydromorphone: Like *morphine, hydromorphone* is a mu agonist but with far greater solubility. It can be administered orally, intravenously, and subcutaneously with a duration of action and half-life similar to *morphine.* Its high potency allows smaller volume injections (45).

Fentanyl offers a transdermal route of administration, enabling continuous administration of a short-acting opioid (46). Dose calibration should usually occur with *morphine, oxycodone,* or subcutaneous or intravenous *fentanyl* before transdermal therapeutic system (TTS) *fentanyl* is applied. **The patch forms a depot of drug in the dermis, resulting in a 12- to 48-hour delay before maximum plasma concentration is reached.** After TTS removal, the terminal half-life is approximately 13 to 25 hours (47). In practice, this means that when the patch is applied, the immediate-release drug should be continued for at least 12 hours. If adverse effects develop, they will continue after TTS *fentanyl* removal, and the patient should be monitored closely. When a patient who is using TTS *fentanyl* experiences an increase of pain, a short-acting opioid should be given concurrently and the dose used to calculate the extra opioid requirement, which can then be incorporated into the TTS *fentanyl* dose.

TTS *fentanyl* is an attractive option for many patients because of the convenience of the delivery system and the slightly less troublesome constipation compared with *morphine* (46). Dose escalation is commonly observed, possibly related to the short half-life of the drug. If very rapid dose escalation occurs (without evidence of rapid tumor progression), a change to another opioid may be wise and less expensive. *Fentanyl* may be particularly useful in patients close to death.

The development of transmucosal *fentanyl citrate* provides an immediate-release *fentanyl* formulation for breakthrough pain that offers rapid onset of analgesia and similar or improved response compared with immediate release *morphine* (48,49). Expense may dictate that traditional preparations are still chosen.

When using TTS *fentanyl,* it must be remembered that:

- **It is a delivery system useful for chronic pain only.** It may be hazardous for unstable pain and should not be used after surgery or in rapidly changing pain states.
- **Because of depot formation in the dermis, a delayed response occurs** that is particularly important in toxicity or overdose situations.
- **A short-acting opioid should be available for breakthrough needs** (e.g., immediate-release *morphine,* or transmucosal *fentanyl citrate*).

Side Effects of Opioids

Side effects can be avoided in large part by precise prescribing. Although there are some side effects that are almost invariable, such as constipation, individual variation in side-effect profile may be used to advantage by substituting an alternative opioid.

Constipation occurs in most patients, and prophylactic laxatives should be prescribed. A reasonable laxative prescription would be *senna* and *sodium docusate* tablets twice daily. Fecal impaction, much more likely if opioids are given without a laxative, may cause a variety of distressing symptoms, such as nausea, vomiting, pelvic pain, or confusion. **TTS *fentanyl* is slightly less constipating** than slow-release *morphine* (46).

Nausea and vomiting may occur in association with opioid therapy as a result of gastric stasis, stimulation of the chemoreceptor trigger zone, or constipation. Nausea is particularly common when opioids are commenced or when the dose is changing, but a tolerance to this side effect develops in most patients within 48 hours. Suitable antinauseants such as ***metoclopramide,*** 10 mg four times daily (oral/subcutaneous injection [SQ]), or ***haloperidol,*** 0.5 to 1.5 mg twice daily (oral/SQ), should be available if required. Regular prophylactic antiemetics should be prescribed for at least the first 48 hours if the patient is very anxious or if there is a history of opioid-induced nausea or vomiting. If vomiting persists, an alternative opioid should be substituted. All opioids may cause nausea, but there appears to be individual but unpredictable variability in response between the drugs. The evolving field of pharmacogenetics may in the future provide some ability to predict an individual's response.

The prescription of opioids should be individualized. As with a number of other medications (e.g., *digoxin*), if the dose prescribed is inadequate, there will be no clinical response. If however, the dose is too high, the patient will enter a toxic range and will develop dose-related side effects. **The dose-related side effects of opioids include drowsiness and delirium. At the extreme end of the toxic range is respiratory depression, with reduced respiratory rate,** which is rarely seen in chronic opioid prescribing, and not before the patient has exhibited earlier signs of toxicity such as drowsiness and delirium.

If drowsiness develops and persists for more than 24 hours, the opioid level is probably above the therapeutic range for that patient. Other causes of drowsiness should be excluded, such as sedating drugs or hypercalcemia, and a dose reduction of opioids should be considered.

The development of confusion or hallucinations indicates either excessive dosage or very occasionally, an idiosyncratic reaction. Hydration—either orally, subcutaneously, or intravenously—may assist in eliminating troublesome metabolites while dose reduction is undertaken. If the pain is not well controlled in the presence of drowsiness or confusion, another approach is usually required, such as an alternative opioid or an alternative route of administration (e.g., spinal).

Pruritus is troublesome for a small number of patients taking *morphine* because of its histaminogenic properties. It usually settles within 48 hours and **can be managed with judicious use of *promethazine*.** Pruritus is rarely reported for other opioids. Anticholinergic side effects of opioids are usually not troublesome.

Tolerance to opioids may be a significant clinical problem if the drug is not introduced and calibrated correctly. When opioids are used correctly, increased requirements during the course of an illness usually signify an increase in the noxious stimulus because of disease progression, rather than a reduction in the effectiveness of the analgesic. *Ketamine,* **a drug used traditionally in anesthesia, has been found to reverse opioid tolerance for some patients with pain** (50).

Step Four: Recognize Neuropathic Pain and Treat Correctly

Neuropathic pain is a term used to describe those pain syndromes in which the pathophysiology is related to aberrant somatosensory processes that originate with a lesion in the peripheral or central nervous system. Neuropathic pain is a frequent complication in gynecologic cancer, especially in advanced cancer of the cervix. It may be due to tumor infiltration (notably lumbar plexopathy) or occasionally may result from therapeutic interventions. It may be flashing or burning in nature, but is often an unpleasant ache in an area of altered sensation corresponding to a peripheral dermatome.

When pain is neuropathic in origin, an opioid and a peripherally acting drug should usually be supplemented by **tricyclic antidepressants, anticonvulsants, and/or corticosteroids** (51). In general, medications should be started at low doses and gradually increased as tolerated, but treatment of severe neuropathic pain is a challenge (52).

Other Dimensions of Pain

Ketamine, a drug used in anesthesia, has been found in lower doses to be useful in the management of very complex pain, both somatic and neuropathic in origin. *Ketamine* acts as an antagonist to the N-methyl-D-aspartate (NMDA) receptor system, a system frequently activated in refractory pain states when high doses of opioids appear ineffective. Low doses of infusional subcutaneous *ketamine* can reduce opioid tolerance and improve analgesia (50). It should be used in consultation with palliative medicine or pain specialists because of **side effects such as hallucinations.** However, it has an emerging role in refractory pain states (53).

Spinal analgesia may benefit a carefully selected small group of patients. Anesthetic opinion should be considered for patients who continue to have pain despite an adequate trial of analgesia according to steps one to four, or for those who have very severe incident pain, i.e., pain with a particular activity, such as weight bearing (54). **The ongoing capacity of the care system to support the spinal analgesic delivery devices** (implantable pumps, intrathecally inserted Port-o-cath devices, or other systems) **must be considered prior to implementation.** For some, the

Table 24.2 Edmonton Classification System for Cancer Pain

1. Mechanism of Pain

No—**No** pain syndrome	
Nc—Any **no**ciceptive combination of visceral and/or bone or soft tissue pain	
Ne—**Ne**uropathic pain syndrome with or without any combination of nociceptive pain	
Nx—Insufficient information to classify.	

2. Incident Pain

Io—No incident pain	
Ii—Incident pain present	
Ix—Insufficient information to classify	

3. Psychological Distress

Po—No psychological distress	
Pp—Psychological distress present	
Px—Insufficient information to classify	

4. Addictive Behavior

Ao—No addictive behavior	
Aa—Addictive behavior present	
Ax—Insufficient information to classify	

5. Cognitive Function

Co—No impairment. Patient able to provide accurate present and past pain history unimpaired	
Ci—Partial impairment. Sufficient impairment to affect patientís ability to provide accurate present and/or past pain history	
Cu—Total impairment. Patient unresponsive, delirious or demented to the stage of being unable to provide any present and past pain history	
Cx—Insufficient information to classify	

Reproduced with permission from **Fainsinger RL, Nekolaichuk CLA.** A "TNM" classification system for cancer pain: The Edmonton Classification System for Cancer Pain (ECS-CP). *Support Care Cancer* 2008;16:547–555.

delivery of spinal analgesia requires ongoing hospitalization because community supports are unavailable. Expense may be very significant.

Pain Prognostic Score

The recognition that patients with cancer-related pain vary considerably in their responses to standard analgesic regimes has led to the development of a classification system for pain. Based on the TNM classification system for cancer, this represents an attempt to group pain such that appropriate comparisons and predictions of outcome can be made (Table 24.2) (55). According to this classification, **the presence of particular pain mechanisms, incident pain** (pain during an activity), **psychological distress, addictive behavior,** and **disturbed cognitive function are all associated with increasing complexity of pain management.**

Special Considerations in Pain Management

The Patient with Renal Failure

In patients with renal impairment, NSAIDs should be avoided, as they will frequently worsen renal function, and the use of *morphine* will result in the accumulation of active *morphine* metabolites. Therefore, **if prescribing *morphine*, a dose reduction may be necessary,** and, more importantly, **the interval between doses should be extended.** Use of **an alternative opioid such as *fentanyl* or *methadone*,** which are reported not to have active metabolites, **may be preferable** (39).

Allergy to Opioids

Many patients will report they are allergic to opioids, or have such an allergy recorded on their medical record. A detailed exploration should be undertaken of the event when an allergy was first cited. Frequently, the original event was the development of nausea and vomiting when opioids were administered. Sometimes it is the report of confusional states, particularly in the setting of post-operative analgesia administration. Neither of these constitute a true allergic reaction. **True allergy to opioids is extremely rare.** If it is suspected, palliative care expertise should be sought.

The Patient with Reduced Motility of the Gastrointestinal Tract

The patient who has a hypomotile gastrointestinal tract, most commonly seen in patients with disseminated ovarian cancer, may have not only impaired peristalsis, but also impaired absorption of oral medication.

Motility may be further impaired by drugs such as $5HT_3$ blockers (e.g., *ondansetron*), which, although very effective antinauseants for patients undergoing chemotherapy, may induce constipation. **Consideration should be given to delivering analgesics via an alternative route, such as transdermally** (*fentanyl*) **or,** for the very ill, **subcutaneously.** Similarly, alternative routes of analgesic administration should be sought for the patient with established fecal loading.

The Patient with Cognitive Impairment

The cognitively impaired patient may not complain of pain, but if she does, she should be believed. If the location of the cancer is likely to cause pain, then pain should be assumed to be present. **Facial expression may assist in the diagnosis (unless the pain is chronic), as may the presence of any physiological indicators such as tachycardia (56). Other clues may include restlessness and agitation.** The family should be questioned about any behavioral changes they have observed. **The possibility of painful fecal loading should be considered.** Ultimately, diagnosis may require a therapeutic trial of analgesia and observation of the response.

Particular note should be made of the interaction of the two symptom complexes of pain and delirium, both of which are common in the very ill. Patients with delirium have global cognitive dysfunction, including problems with memory, concentration, alertness, and frequently hallucinations and delusions. It is postulated that **usual inhibitory processes are also affected with consequent "unmasking" and heightened pain complaints.** When the response to such complaints is to unquestioningly escalate opioid doses, this can further exacerbate the situation, since opioids at high doses (beyond the therapeutic range) may be implicated in causing delirium (57,58).

When a patient develops this complex set of clinical problems, the following approach is recommended:

1. **evaluate the likely pain mechanism**(s) and prescribe the analgesic regimes considered most likely to be effective.
2. **evaluate the likely causes of delirium** and correct where possible.
3. **consider medication of the symptoms of delirium** with an appropriate antipsychotic such as haloperidol or olanzapine.
4. **review the opioid dose regularly** and consider, opioid substitution if necessary (59).

Difficult-to-Manage Postoperative Pain

Occasionally, the management of pain in the postoperative setting is difficult. Possible reasons could include the following:

1. **Inappropriate use of the patient-controlled analgesic (PCA) device.** Patients who are cognitively impaired (including those developing delirium postoperatively), those who are anxious or depressed, the very frail, and those for whom the language of explanation is not their mother tongue, may all struggle to use a PCA device effectively. In such patients, a careful estimate of probable dosage requirements may be wiser.
2. **Pre-operative use of opioids.** Patients who have a history of previous opioid abuse, especially intravenous drug users, have a level of tolerance that appears to persist even when they have not used opioids for some years, and usually require significantly larger doses of opioids than would be expected (60). There is little literature to guide this complex clinical problem, but experience suggests the following:
   a. **open discussion** of the concerns with the patient and with other physicians involved in her care. Many former opioid addicts will fear the prescription of opioids for their pain.

    b.   be prepared to **use higher doses** of opioids.

    c.   **ensure a single point of prescription.**

    d.   **prescribe precise amounts of opioids for relatively short periods of time,** such as 1 week.

On the other hand, patients who are taking preoperative opioids as part of their current treatment need to continue equivalent opioid doses, with an additional moiety to cover the operative trauma.

3. **Extreme patient anxiety.** This significantly disturbs pain threshold levels. Care should be taken not to simply continue to escalate opioid doses in the presence of such extreme distress. Instead, **explanation, support, counseling, and anxiolytics** are likely to be more effective, and associated with fewer adverse effects.

Chronic Nonmalignant Pain

While not the focus of this chapter, a word of caution should be made about the management of the patient with chronic non-malignant pain. In general, the pain management approach for these patients has a rehabilitative focus. In common with cancer pain management is the need for diagnosis, repeated assessment, and use of pharmacological agents and interventions according to the pain mechanism involved. **The difference between the management of cancer pain management and nonmalignant pain lies in the cautious use of opioids and the focus upon functional improvement outcomes in chronic nonmalignant pain** (61). There is an extensive body of literature examining this particular clinical challenge (62,63).

Gastrointestinal Symptoms

Gastrointestinal symptoms are common in gynecological cancer, both because of the cancer and because of various aspects of treatment (64).

Anorexia-Cachexia

Anorexia is a common and significant symptom with a multitude of causes and serious nutritional consequences. **The best initial approach to management includes careful preparation of small meals, elimination of reversible gastric stasis or constipation, emotional support, and direct nutritional supplements.** It is helpful to educate both the patient and her family about the importance of these measures. Extensive research has isolated a number of potential therapies, but these remain in trial and developmental phase (65). Until such agents enter clinical practice, **the pharmacological responses available to clinicians include the use of prokinetics, progestational agents, and cautious use of corticosteroids** (65). **Prokinetic agents** will be useful when the symptom of early satiety is present indicating gastric stasis. **Progestational agents** have been demonstrated in randomized, double-blinded, placebo-controlled trials to increase appetite and food intake and to lead to weight gain in a number of patients, without undue side effects (66), but the expense is considerable. **Corticosteroids** have also been shown to improve appetite and daily activity of patients with cancer, but this effect is short lived, usually with a return to baseline responses by 28 days. Because patients must then undergo the problems of corticosteroid withdrawal, patient selection is critical.

Mouth Symptoms

Mouth symptoms, including xerostomia, pain, and altered taste, can be most distressing.

A dry mouth can result from many factors in the critically ill patient: oral candidiasis, previous radiation therapy, mouth breathing, nasal oxygen, and drugs, particularly those with anticholinergic effects. Management of xerostomia may include minimization of contributory nonessential medications, frequent small drinks with a small amount of lemon/orange to stimulate saliva production, use of artificial saliva or *glycerin* preparations, and *pilocarpine* drops to stimulate saliva locally with minimal systemic effects.

Frank pain can occur from treatment-related mucositis and infected ulcers, so mouth care is crucial in very ill patients. **Oral candidiasis is often overlooked.** It responds to antifungal agents such as *nystatin* mouthwashes (every 2 to 3 hours), *amphotericin* lozenges, and, if necessary, a systemic triazole derivative such as *fluconazole*. Pain from mucositis may be relieved by *sucralfate* suspension and by *acetaminophen* with *morphine* (orally or subcutaneously).

Altered taste, a not uncommon symptom in patients with cancer, is hard to relieve. Once all of the above causes of mouth pathology have been excluded, a dietitian may be able to assist in food choice and encouragement.

Nausea and Vomiting

Nausea and vomiting are common in advanced gynecologic cancer, and each symptom requires precise diagnosis so that rational therapy may be applied. Mechanisms of nausea and vomiting are complex (67). **Nausea, with or without vomiting, is mediated finally by the vomiting**

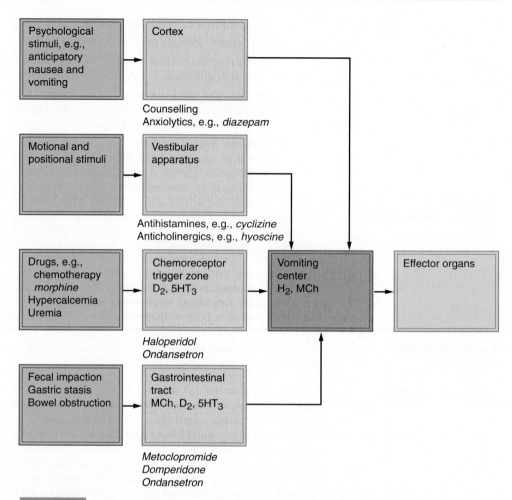

Figure 24.4 Factors that influence nausea and vomiting in the central nervous system and the gastrointestinal tract. Nausea, with or without vomiting, is mediated by the vomiting center. D, dopaminergic; H, histaminic; MCh, muscarinic; 5HT₃, hydroxytryptophan.

center situated in the reticular formation of the medulla oblongata, an area rich in histaminic and muscarinic receptors. The vomiting center is influenced by several connections, each of which can be the causal pathway for nausea (Fig. 24.4 and Table 24.2). The search continues for better understanding and consequently, for better therapeutic approaches.

Causal pathways include:

1. **The cerebral cortex** (e.g., stimulated by anxiety-conditioned responses)
2. **The vestibular center,** which is rich in histaminic (H_1) and muscarinic receptors (e.g., stimulated by cerebral metastases)
3. **The chemoreceptor trigger zone,** which is rich in dopaminergic and serotonergic receptors (e.g., stimulated to by hypercalcemia, uremia, and some drugs, including chemotherapeutic agents)
4. **The gastrointestinal tract** (e.g., stimulated by gastric stasis, intestinal obstruction, fecal impaction, abnormalities of gut motility), which has dopaminergic, muscarinic, and serotonergic receptors.

Once the likely mechanism has been identified by means of a careful history, physical examination, and investigations if indicated, the appropriate antinauseant may be prescribed (Tables 24.3 and 24.4). While the evidence base proving the efficacy of this approach remains scant, it continues to be useful in practice and is recommended as an appropriate approach (68).

When anxiety dominates the scene, anxiolytics may be crucial in reducing the nausea. **When vestibular mechanisms are suspected** or when no specific pathway can be identified,

Table 24.3 Commonly Used Antinauseant Drugs

Drug	Dose	Comment
Metoclopramide	10–20 mg q 4 h (oral or subcutaneous)	Avoid if patient has bowel colic, or high gastrointestinal obstruction.
Haloperidol	1–3 mg bid or tid (oral) 0.5–2mg bid or tid	Lower doses required than when used as a sedative.
Prochlorperazine	5–25 mg bid or tid (oral or rectal)	May be useful if vomiting mechanism is unknown.
Meclozine	10–75 mg/day in divided doses (oral)	Antihistamine with doses that produce minimal sedation.
Cyclizine	25–100 mg/day in divided doses (oral, rectal, or subcutaneous)	Useful if patient has bowel obstruction.
Hyoscine	0.1–0.4 mg q 6–8 h (subcutaneous)	Central nervous system side effects can occur, particularly drowsiness and confusion.
Ondansetron	0.1 mg/kg q 8 h for three doses IV, 4–8 mg tid (oral)	Main use is for chemotherapy-related nausea. Constipation can be troublesome.

q 4 h, every four hours; IV, intravenous; bid, two times a day; tid, three times a day.

See text and manufacturers' information before prescribing; watch for side effects; review frequently; cease ineffective drugs.

relatively less sedating **antihistamines (e.g., *cyclizine*)** that act directly on the vomiting and vestibular centers may be useful. ***Prochlorperazine*** has some affinity for dopaminergic, muscarinic, and histaminic receptors and is moderately useful, although less specific. ***Levomepromazine (methotrimeprazine)*** is a phenothiazine with potent D2- and α1-receptor antagonist and some $5HT_2$-receptor antagonist action. This means it is a broad-spectrum antiemetic, which is most commonly used as a second- or third-line drug when more specific drugs seem ineffective. It is significantly sedating, so is often reserved for patients in the final phase of their life (69).

Nausea clearly related to the chemoreceptor trigger zone requires a drug with high affinity for dopaminergic receptors, such as *haloperidol*. A dose of 1.5 to 3 mg or less at night (orally or subcutaneously) may be sufficient. **Nausea related to chemotherapy or abdominal radiotherapy is usually well controlled with serotonin antagonists such as *ondansetron* or *tropisetron*.** If delayed emesis resulting from chemotherapy is present, the introduction of haloperidol can be a useful adjunct. **Constipation is a potentially distressing side effect of *ondansetron*,** particularly in patients who are prone to bowel obstruction.

Nausea arising from stimuli in the gastrointestinal tract associated with slowing of the gut should respond to **gastrokinetic antinauseants such as *metoclopramide* or *domperidone*,** which promote gastric emptying and increase gut motility. These actions are counterproductive in a patient with a very high gastrointestinal obstruction, when vomiting will be aggravated.

Drugs available by more than one route are advantageous. *Metoclopramide*, *haloperidol*, and *cyclizine* may be used subcutaneously as well as orally.

In addition to the established antinauseant drugs, **corticosteroids,** which act by an unknown mechanism, **are also useful in suppressing nausea,** and are frequently used in premedication programs before chemotherapy. Caution must be exercised if the patient has a history of active peptic ulceration, tuberculosis, diabetes mellitus, psychosis, or severe emotional instability.

Gastrointestinal Hypomotility

A number of women with extensive intraabdominal disease, usually as a result of ovarian cancer, will present with symptoms of gastrointestinal hypomotility. Typically the initial complaints will be of marked constipation requiring increasing doses of laxatives, followed by early satiety, and nausea. Eventually some will progress to develop symptoms of gastrointestinal obstruction. Examination reveals few or absent bowel sounds, and plain abdominal radiographs are frequently normal or may show fecal loading without air-fluid levels. **The**

pathophysiology of this syndrome is not well understood, but probably includes tumor infiltration of the myenteric plexus.

Medication is aimed at increasing bowel peristalsis using infusional *metoclopramide,* 60–90 mg subcutaneously over 24 hours. Our own experience suggests **corticosteroids** (*dexamethasone* 4–8 mg daily) **may also be useful** to improve symptoms of obstruction in this group (70). The clinician should be mindful that gastrointestinal hypomotility will result in reduced absorption of oral medications including analgesics.

Hypomotility or dysmotility of the bowel sometimes follows apparently successful surgery for bowel obstruction. The condition may be temporary and related to the surgery, or it may be longer lasting and related to the underlying malignant infiltration. The difficulty facing the clinician is how best to support such patients nutritionally postoperatively. There is little literature to inform such a decision, and as always, it should be based on the patient's disease status, her performance status, the anticancer options still available, and her personal goals.

Constipation

Constipation, a common symptom, may be due to changing diet, inactivity, opioid use without laxatives, or varying degrees of tumor-induced intestinal obstruction. Constipation can be largely avoided through anticipation and careful prescribing of laxatives. Recent reviews highlight the diversity both of mechanisms leading to constipation and of classes of laxatives (see Table 24.4) (70). **Any prescription of opioids should be accompanied by a laxative as constipation is an inevitable side effect.** In most instances, a combination of a fecal softener and a

Table 24.4 Classification of Laxatives	
I. Bulking or hydrophilic agents	B. Diphenylmethane derivatives
A. Dietary fiber	1. *Phenolphthalein*
B. *Psyllium (plantago)*	2. *Bisacodyl*
C. *Polycarbophil*	3. *Sodium picosulfate*
D. *Methylcellulose, carboxymethylcellulose*	C. Ricinoleic acid (castor oil)
II. Osmotic agents	D. Anthraquinones Anth
A. Poorly absorbed ions	1. *Senna*
1. *Magnesium sulfate (Epsom salt)*	2. *Cascara sagrada*
2. *Magnesium hydroxide (milk of magnesia)*	**IV. Lubricating agent**
3. *Magnesium citrate*	A. Mineral oil
4. *Sodium phosphate*	**V. Neuromuscular agents**
5. *Sodium sulfate (Glauber's salt)*	A. Cholinergic agonists
6. *Potassium sodium tartrate (Rochelle salt)*	1. *Bethanechol*
B. Poorly absorbed disaccharides, sugar alcohols	2. *Neostigmine*
1. *Lactulose*	B. 5-HT$_4$ agonists
2. *Sorbitol, mannitol*	1. *Cisapride*
C. *Glycerin*	2. *Prucalopride*
D. *Polyethylene glycol*	3. *Tegaserod*
III. Stimulant laxatives	C. Prostaglandin agonist
A. Surface-active agents	1. *Misoprostol*
1. *Docusates (dioctyl sulfosuccinate)*	D. *Colchicine*
2. *Bile acids*	E. Opiate antagonists
	1. *Naloxone*
	2. *Naltrexone*

Reproduced with permission from **Schiller LR.** The therapy of constipation (review article). *Aliment Pharmacol Ther* 2001;15:749–763.

peristaltic agent such as *sodium docusate* and *senna* will be adequate to prevent opioid-induced constipation. Care should be taken in the use of bulking agents, because those patients with significant frailty may be unable to ingest the volume of water required for their adequate function.

Severe constipation is a common cause of major symptoms, including nausea, vomiting, spurious diarrhea, pain, and even confusion, especially in the elderly. If unrecognized or untreated, it may result in inadequate absorption of oral medications including analgesics and even, rarely, perforation. **Opioid-induced fecal impaction is usually avoidable, but if present, vigorous local treatment is required.** This includes fecal softeners (e.g., *docusate sodium*), large bowel stimulants (e.g., *senna*), stimulant suppositories, or careful enemas. **Osmotic laxatives (e.g., *lactulose*) may be helpful.** Fecal impaction caused by a holdup at the sigmoid colon (with an empty, dilated rectum) sometimes requires high *docusate sodium* enemas if oral laxatives fail to provide relief.

Drugs other than opioids may also cause constipation. **Drugs commonly implicated** in this population **would include 5HT$_3$ antagonists (e.g., *ondansetron*) and tricyclic antidepressants.** Constipation that is due to mechanical obstruction requires either surgical intervention or acceptance of the problem as an end-stage event.

Medical Management of Intestinal Obstruction

Obstruction may occur at any level of the gastrointestinal tract in patients with gynecologic cancer and frequently involves several different levels. It is a common late-stage problem, particularly in patients with ovarian cancer. Since the ground-breaking work at St. Christopher's Hospice, London (72), there have been several studies, reviews, and recommendations (73–74). The following represents a practical approach for the gynecologist (Table 24.5).

Patients presenting with an acute bowel obstruction should initially be placed on nil by mouth and given intravenous fluids. If there is copious vomiting, nasogastric suction is helpful. **If the obstruction is not relieved within 72–96 hours, a choice needs to be made between surgical intervention and medical management.**

In general, surgery provides the best palliative relief of symptoms, if successful. This is particularly true for the few patients who have a nonmalignant cause for the obstruction, such as adhesions from radiation therapy or previous surgery. Similarly, bowel obstruction in a patient for whom chemotherapeutic options have not been exhausted justifies active surgical intervention. **Stents offer a useful means of bypassing obstruction that is due to a defined tumor mass** and are associated with low morbidity and mortality. Stents have little role, however, in the patient with more than one level of obstruction (75). In patients whose life expectancy is limited to less than 2 months, a noninterventional approach is usually preferable.

One option for conservative management of obstruction at high or low levels is a trial of corticosteroids (e.g., *dexamethasone*, 4–8 mg parenterally daily for 3–5 days) (70,76). This presumably works by decreasing inflammatory edema, thereby improving luminal diameter. It may be repeated in the future. **There is need for caution when using corticosteroids in patients with a history of diabetes mellitus, peptic ulceration, recent infection, impending bowel perforation, significant psychiatric disorder, or tuberculosis.** Corticosteroids are best used in patients considered unsuitable for surgical intervention.

In a patient with high end-stage obstruction, when the aforementioned measures have failed to relieve the problem, **a conservative medical approach may be helpful.** In brief, this approach avoids the use of full intravenous fluid replacement. It relies on careful mouth care, with a little food and drink as desired. **The patient remains mildly dehydrated,** but this is beneficial and decreases the amount of vomiting. Centrally acting antinauseants (e.g., *cyclizine*) are used, if necessary, in combination with low doses of opioid analgesics. Gastrokinetic antinauseants (e.g., *metoclopramide* or *domperidone*) are contraindicated. **For many, gastric drainage via a nasogastric tube or a venting gastrostomy will still be required to ensure comfort.**

Hyoscine butyl bromide **may serve several purposes in patients with bowel obstruction, reducing gastrointestinal secretions and also reducing intestinal tone,** effectively increasing bowel capacity. This alleviates nausea for the patient with complete obstruction and avoids multiple small vomits, although infrequent large-volume vomits continue.

A subcutaneous butterfly needle with or without a battery-driven syringe driver can be used to deliver appropriate doses of antinauseants, such **as *cyclizine* 25–150 mg/day,** as well as

Table 24.5 Management of Gastrointestinal Obstruction in Patients With Gynecological Cancer

1. Is it an obstruction?

Clarify by

   History

   Examination

   Investigation

      Erect abdominal x-ray

      Contrast studies

      CT abdomen

Clarify highest level of obstruction and likely mechanism

   Treat pain – SQ *morphine*

   Treat nausea – SQ *cyclizine*

   Treat conservatively initially with IV fluids and nasogastric suction

2. Is surgery or stenting an option?

Consider the following in making the decision

   Single or multiple levels of obstruction

   Likely prognosis – will the patient live at least 8 weeks?

   Likelihood of a non-malignant cause of obstruction

   Possible anti-cancer treatments available

   Patient performance status

   Patient preferences and goals

   Likely rehabilitative outcome

3. If surgery or stenting not an option:

Consider trial of corticosteroids e.g., *dexamethasone 8 mg/day for 3–5 days*

If clearly end stage, ensure goals of care known to patient, family and treating team.

   Do not check electrolytes.

   Continue to relieve discomfort

   Continue to relieve nausea with *cyclizine* (SQ)

If "high" obstruction

   Decrease fluid intake (negative fluid balance)

   Perform exquisite mouth care

   Decrease GIT fluid production and relax gastrointestinal tract with *hyoscine hydrobromide* or *octreotide* (SQ)

      Will likely require drainage of upper gastrointestinal track using nasogastric tube or venting gastrostomy

If "low" obstruction

   Maintain a light diet if tolerated.

   Consider *metoclopramide* (SQ) to keep upper gastrointestinal tract empty (and reduce vomiting)

hyoscine butyl bromide 10–20 mg every 6 hours. With careful calibration of dose, the patient need not be drowsy. *Morphine* may be given in the same syringe as *hyoscine* if pain is present. If colic is not controlled with *morphine,* additional *hyoscine* may be useful. **Rectal *prochlorperazine,*** 50–100 mg/day, may be tried instead of *cyclizine. Octreotide,* starting at a dose of 50 μg subcutaneously every 8 hours, can provide additional relief of symptoms by further reducing secretions and colic, and has been demonstrated to be superior to *hyoscine hydrobromide,* though it is also more expensive (73). Doses greater than 600 μg per day probably do not afford additional benefit.

Some patients prefer occasional bouts of vomiting to a continuous nasogastric tube. Under all these circumstances, electrolytes should neither be monitored nor corrected. Electrolyte imbalance becomes inevitable and should be allowed to take its course.

Low-bowel obstruction commences with reduced then absent defecation, followed by severe abdominal distention, pain, and later nausea and vomiting. If colostomy or stenting is not to be undertaken, the focus is on relief of discomfort with low-dose opioids. Subcutaneous *morphine* or transdermal *fentanyl* may be the drugs of choice. If nausea occurs, antinauseants are useful. *Metoclopramide* subcutaneously may help keep the stomach empty and may be combined with a centrally acting antinauseant (such as **cyclizine**). A very light diet may be tolerated if the patient wishes to try to eat.

Diarrhea and Tenesmus

Diarrhea in a patient with advanced gynecologic cancer is probably best considered as a sign of fecal impaction until proven otherwise. True irritative diarrhea can occur by tumor involvement of the bowel wall or after radiation therapy. *Loperamide* may be useful in the management of such patients.

When fecal soiling is associated with an enterovaginal or rectovaginal fistula, surgical diversion should be considered if at all possible. If such surgery is not possible, the emphasis is on nursing procedures calculated to keep the vagina and perineum as clean and comfortable as possible, and to support the patient in her distress. Antibiotics, especially *metronidazole,* locally as well as systemically, may reduce some of the distressing odor when necrosis has occurred. A urinary catheter may assist in restoring urinary continence. Cases have been reported of the successful use of *octreotide* **to reduce small bowel fistula drainage** (77). The use of stool bulking agents (e.g., *cellulose*) may reduce the amount of fecal ooze if the fistula is colonic.

Tenesmus usually responds to anticholinergic agents, corticosteroids, and opioids, often in combination. Anecdotal experience has shown that low-dose *ketamine,* followed by very low dose *methadone* may be effective for more refractory cases. Occasionally, resection of tumor as a palliative procedure may be justified. In severe cases, spinal local anesthetics or sacral nerve blocks may be necessary.

Many of the gastrointestinal symptoms (which are such a feature of gynecologic cancer) are disturbances of gastrointestinal motility. This subject is a focus of current research, and the mechanisms involved are being elucidated (78). The gynecologic oncologist needs to recognize the following:

1. **Gastrointestinal motility disturbances,** such as a tendency to constipation and reduced bowel sounds, **may be a feature of gynecologic cancer even before any use of opioid drugs.**
2. **Drugs prone to constipate should be used with caution in such patients.** For example, opioid drugs must always be accompanied by laxatives. The use of 5HT$_3$ blockers as antinauseants in the postoperative period or as premedication for chemotherapy should be minimized if possible.

Ascites

Abdominal distention that is due to intractable ascites can be a major cause of distress. Despite being a common complication of advanced cancer, the optimal approach to management is far from clear. **Paracentesis** has an important role in diagnosis and for the immediate relief of symptoms. It should be performed when there is significant abdominal discomfort and patients should be warned that in the absence of systemic control of the malignancy, ascites will generally reaccumulate. Attempts to reduce the rate of reaccumulation include the institution of diuretics, particularly *spironolactone,* 50–150 mg/day, if necessary coupled with a loop diuretic such as *frusemide.* These may prove helpful initially. If ascites is reaccumulating rapidly, the clinician should anticipate the need for recurrent paracenteses and book clinical reviews accordingly. **Shunting procedures are not reliable** and have been associated with significant morbidity and mortality. **Systemic cytotoxic agents** should be considered, though for the heavily pre-treated patient with advanced disease, their potential is limited. Discomfort is usually controlled with a combination of a drug such as *acetaminophen* and a low dose of an opioid.

Respiratory Symptoms

A clinical history, physical examination, and a chest radiograph should differentiate between dyspnea caused by a pleural effusion, bronchial obstruction, diffuse lung involvement, reduced excursion that is due to massive ascites, bronchial asthma, chronic obstructive airway disease, cardiac failure, and respiratory infection. However, **in advanced cancer, dyspnea may be multifactorial, with anemia, advanced cachexia and resultant muscle asthenia contributing to the situation.** Treatment of contributing comorbidities, such as cardiac failure, should be considered in all patients. **Drainage of a pleural effusion, with early consideration of a pleurodesis, may afford prompt relief of dyspnea, cough, and chest wall discomfort.** Radiation therapy to a bronchial lesion causing hemoptysis, cough, or obstruction may produce prolonged palliation of symptoms.

When the cause of dyspnea is not reversible, the careful use of *morphine* may improve the situation significantly (79). **Oral *morphine*** should be commenced at doses of 2–5 mg every 4 hours and increased until drowsiness develops or until no further benefit is gained. In practice, this usually means doses of approximately 5–10 mg every 4 hours. The mechanism by which *morphine* reduces dyspnea is poorly understood, but includes both central and peripheral actions. If a patient is already receiving *morphine* calibrated correctly for pain relief but becomes dyspneic because of tumor progression, *morphine* may be increased by a further 30% to 50% to give relief.

For the patient with an obstructing bronchial lesion or with carcinomatous lymphangitis, corticosteroids may afford some relief by reducing peritumor edema. This can be achieved with daily doses equivalent to 8–16 mg *dexamethasone*, with reduction to the lowest possible dose when an effect has been achieved. For those with bronchial obstruction, this should be followed by immediate review by a radiation oncologist.

The role of oxygen in dyspneic patients with advanced cancer who are not seriously hypoxic is controversial (80). **Some patients find that oxygen masks or even nasal prongs inhibit communication, restrict their movements, and induce claustrophobia.** These patients may find an open window or a fan to be effective. Other patients appear to obtain benefit from oxygen and feel unable to manage without it. **The use of oxygen should depend upon the patient's report of improvement of dyspnea** and not according to measures of oxygenation. Some patients who have been previously oxygen dependent because of dyspnea can become less so with careful use of *morphine*.

Anxiolytics may be valuable in modest doses. Benzodiazepines (e.g., 2 mg *diazepam* orally or 0.5 mg *lorazepam* sublingually) may have significant benefit for the anxious patient. For the patient who is in the last few days of life, an infusion of subcutaneous *midazolam* at low doses (e.g., 5–15 mg over 24 hours in the patient who is benzodiazepine naive) can afford significant relief of dyspnea.

Urinary Tract Symptoms

Urinary tract symptoms are common in women with far-advanced gynecologic cancer. Bilateral ureteric obstruction, with subsequent infection, pain, and acute renal failure, may justify mechanical measures such as nephrostomy or ureteric stent insertion if the prognosis on other grounds is for at least several good-quality months of life. Although some patients clearly benefit, fine judgment is required in the individual case, and such patients should be managed in consultation with a gynecologic oncologist. **For patients with no reasonable treatment options and problematic symptoms, it is prudent to refrain from mechanical intervention.**

Improved patency of ureters may be achieved by short courses of corticosteroids (e.g., oral *dexamethasone,* 4 mg/day for 3–5 days), but should only be considered if goals are short term, for example, to prolong life for a few weeks (82).

Bladder symptoms may benefit from the use of NSAIDs to reduce detrusor irritability or drugs with an anticholinergic action to reduce bladder contractility. Catheterization may be unavoidable in some circumstances. **Urinary incontinence resulting from fistulae to the vagina or** rectum is usually best managed by urinary diversion if feasible. If not, urinary catheterization may assist in keeping the perineum dry.

Edema

Deep venous thrombosis should be excluded, particularly if other signs such as pain, increased temperature of the affected limb, or superficial venous dilatation are present. Anticoagulation in patients who have a deep venous thrombosis may lead to a reduction of symptoms, but the decision to anticoagulate a patient with advanced cancer must be made in the context of the patient's prognosis and goals.

If the swelling is due to lymphatic obstruction, the management must be individualized. Physical therapies, in experienced hands, are most helpful for moderate to severe lymphedema. Massage, bandaging, and fitting of support garments may add much to a patient's comfort (83). Care should be taken when applying compression bandages to grossly edematous legs to ensure venous circulation is not compromised.

Rarely, a patient who has serious nutritional deficiency (for example, associated with several months of nausea and anorexia) may exhibit severe edema that is due to **thiamine deficiency.** This is classically associated with an increase in jugular venous pressure and a bounding pulse. If recognized, improvement may be dramatic, occurring within 24 to 48 hours of giving thiamine.

Weakness

Weakness or fatigue can be profound when there is a large tumor burden, but there are many reversible causes of this symptom (84). These include nutritional deficiencies, hypotension, hypokalemia, hypoglycemia or hyperglycemia, hypoadrenalism, hypercalcemia, renal failure, infection, and anemia. At least some of these may be readily treated in appropriate circumstances. Anemia *per se* does not require correction in every patient because the benefit may be short lived and not proportionate to the expenditure of resources. A patient who is confined to bed because of advanced disease often tolerates a hemoglobin of 7.0 g/dL or less. However, **if the hemoglobin is low and weakness is a dominant symptom, transfusion may be justified.**

For a number of patients, fatigue remains a dominant symptom without readily correctible contributory factors. For those women who are maintaining some independence, **preliminary evidence suggests that a program which seeks to maintain and increase gentle physical activity improves both fatigue and quality of life** (85).

Hypercalcemia

Hypercalcemia (raised ionized plasma calcium level) **is a recognized complication of malignancy and a potent cause of symptoms, ranging from lethargy; weakness; and constipation to severe nausea; vomiting; confusion; psychotic symptoms (notably paranoia); and exacerbation of bone pain.** In general, treatment of hypercalcemia should be coupled with anticancer therapy directed at removing the cause of the hypercalcemia if still feasible.

Hypercalcemia usually heralds a poor prognosis, and for the relatively asymptomatic or already obtunded patient, aggressive treatment may not be warranted. However, the presence of troublesome symptoms often makes palliative antihypercalcemic therapy worthwhile (86).

Treatment of hypercalcemia depends on its severity. The following measures are necessary in moderate or severe cases:

1. **Modest rehydration with intravenous normal saline** (2–3 L/day or more). **This may be coupled with a loop diuretic** (e.g., *furosemide*) to maintain a diuresis, particularly in older patients.

2. **Infusion of a bisphosphonate** (e.g., *pamidronate* 60–90 mg intravenously in 250 mL of crystalloid over 4-8 hours, or *zolendronic acid* 4 mg given over 15 minutes) (87). The duration of response varies according to the drug given and the clinical circumstances, but may be in the order of 35 days for *pamidronate.*

Improvement of symptoms with these measures can be expected within a few days, as calcium uptake in bone increases. When calcium is extremely high and intravenous bisphosphonate therapy is not causing a rapid reduction, **subcutaneous *calcitonin* administration combined with bisphosphonate therapy may provide a more rapid reduction of calcium levels,** but administration of *calcitonin* always warrants specialist assistance.

Should hypercalcemia recur, the bisphosphonate dose may be repeated. The rate of relapse depends in part on the availability of effective therapy for the underlying tumor, as well as on the biologic characteristics and tempo of the neoplastic process. Therefore the decision to repeat doses of bisphosphonate must take into account these factors, the likely prognosis and the symptoms implicated.

Care of the Patient Close to Death

Good palliative care is concerned with the enrichment of life, even when facing the human task common to all, that of dying **(88). It is important to recognize that a woman is actually dying; this is an important diagnosis with clinical as well as social implications.** What is medically possible at this stage, such as treatment of renal failure, septicemia, or hypercalcemia, may not necessarily be medically wise.

There are many physical indicators that a patient is actually dying, and these are well known to clinicians, although not necessarily to family members. **There may be a change in the tempo of the disease, a manifest change in the function of critical organs, or a rapid deterioration in strength or physical performance in the absence of reversible factors,** such as gross anemia, septicemia, hypercalcemia, or drug interactions.

There are also psychological signs that a patient is dying. An experienced clinician may note the gradual withdrawal of the patient from interest in the wider world, from interest in personal friends, and even the gradual loosening of bonds with those very close. **In some patients, this "cutting of the moorings" is very obvious:** intrapersonal activity may be very intense and expressed only to a trusted few. The patient herself may clearly articulate her awareness that she is now close to death, or she may choose not to speak of it. The essence of clinical response is to respect the mystery of the individual.

The process of dying is fraught with uncertainties. **When it is clear that the patient is dying, the goal is dignity, privacy, peace, and space for the woman** to complete those remaining tasks important to "a life well-lived."

Once recognized that the woman is dying, care should encompass the following domains:

1. **the rigorous treatment of symptoms.**
2. **the discontinuation of those interventions** and treatments (including medications) **that are not involved in maintaining comfort and dignity.**
3. **sensitive communication** and explanation with the patient and her family.
4. **attention to social, psychological and spiritual needs** (88).

Sometimes it is justifiable to offer direct sedation when, in spite of adequate symptom control, distress is extreme and opportunities for verbal communication no longer exist. There are circumstances in which a patient should be able to sleep peacefully as she dies. **This is particularly the case if an agitated delirium is present** after treating any remediable factors such as fecal impaction, urinary retention, or unrelieved pain. If hallucinations are prominent, an antipsychotic may be most useful, whereas if agitation and distress are present, a benzodiazepine should be used, either alone or in combination with an antipsychotic. **Suitable benzodiazepines include** *midazolam* (2–5 mg subcutaneously, intramuscularly, or intravenously stat and 10–50 mg over 24 hours by subcutaneous infusion if distress is protracted) **or** sublingual *lorazepam* (0.5–2.5 mg every 4–6 hours). **Antipsychotics used commonly would include** *haloperidol* (0.5–5 mg twice daily orally or subcutaneously), *risperidone* (0.5–1 mg twice daily orally), or *olanzapine* (2.5–10 mg daily orally or buccal wafer). Some of the older sedating antipsychotic agents (such as *chlorpromazine*) remain useful in this setting.

On rare occasions, distress and agitation may not be relieved with the combination of a benzodiazepine and an antipsychotic. In such circumstances, careful dosing of *phenobarbital* (50–100 mg given 8 hourly orally or subcutaneously) may allow calm in the final part of life. **Large doses of opioids are not appropriate for sedation of the dying.** Ensuring that a patient sleeps most of the time during the last hours (or few days) of her life is not euthanasia.

The development of **"rattling" respirations** indicating pooling of secretions is common in the patient close to death. Management should include repositioning of the patient, and possibly the judicious use of anticholinergic agents (*hyoscine hydrobromide* 0.2–0.4 mg subcutaneously up to 4 hourly) to reduce the production of secretions. The latter must be coupled with measures to keep the mouth moist. Reassurance should be given to families that this is usually not distressing to the patient.

Complex equipment should be avoided if possible, as should tubes of all sorts, to facilitate maximum physical contact with loved ones. Nursing care must remain excellent, with particular emphasis on **pressure care, mouth care, and "grooming."** Teaching family members to assist with the care of their loved one can do much to enhance intimacy and diminish the sense of helplessness many families feel. In the face of imminent death, **respect for individual religious and cultural customs is mandatory.**

It is essential that medical and nursing staff accept and understand the personal significance of the final phase of life. It is a crucial period of personal development and a time for clarifying, reconciling, healing and/or affirming personal relationships—always a complex task at the close of life.

Death serves as the master-test of our journeyman years. It tests the height we have reached, the value of our inner metaphysics; it examines its strength, its utility, durability, and suitability in mobilization and in the most terrible reality: it introduces a factor alien to the subject and thus summons us directly from the subjectively ideal sphere, from the freely suspended realm of ideal self-definitions, to the "cosmic" realm of danger and diffusion, and of the gathering from the bustle of this world of death in which the self finally proves itself after all (89).

It is worthwhile reflecting once again on the issues which patients view as significant in the final part of life, for these must inform all care provided. These are: (i) receiving adequate pain and symptom management; (ii) avoiding inappropriate prolongation of dying; (iii) achieving a sense of control; (iv) relieving the burden on caregivers; and (v) strengthening relationships with loved ones (5,90).

Good care of patients with incurable, progressive disease is concerned with enrichment of remaining life, reduction of relievable distress, and support for personal growth and development, even when facing the human task common to all, that of dying. **The inherent dignity of the dying woman can be maintained and enhanced by the care she receives and the respect afforded to her continued relationships with those she loves** (91).

A Final Note

Mention has been made of the suffering of patients, yet nothing has been said of the distress of the health professionals who care for and journey with these patients. Such distress is often not articulated or shared. The sensitive clinician may take comfort from the words of a French oncologist:

Suffering is something like crossing a sea, traversing a mountain or a desert; it is an experience, painful indeed, in which the person will become more oneself and will discover oneself; it is an experience in which a person will experience evil, and yet, at the same time, will be led to discover and express the deepest meaning of one's life. This is true also for the suffering of the doctor. (92)

However, the burden of distress remains with women with gynecologic cancer, especially in situations of oppression, poverty, and exploitation. Competent as well as compassionate palliative care may salvage dignity and meaning for the individual who is suffering, and in some small way, for the doctor himself. Few doctors have such an opportunity.

References

1. **MacDonald N.** The interface between oncology and palliative medicine. In: **Doyle D, Hanks GW, MacDonald N, eds.** *Oxford textbook of palliative medicine.* Oxford: Oxford University Press, 1993: 11–17.
2. **World Health Organization.** WHO definition of palliative care. Available at: http://www.who.int/cancer/palliative/definition/en. Accessed January 2008.
3. **McDonald N.** Palliative medicine and modern cancer care. In: **Doyle D, Hanks GW, Cherny N, Calman K, eds.** *Oxford textbook of palliative medicine.* Oxford: Oxford University Press, 2003:24–28.
4. **Steinhauser KE, Clipp EC, McNeilly M, Christakis NA, McIntyre L, Tulsky J.** In search of a good death: Observations of patients, families and providers. *Ann Int Med* 2000;132: 825–832.

5. **Steinhauser KE, Christakis NA, Clipp EC, McNelly M, Grambow S, et al.** Preparing for end of life: preferences of patients, families, physicians and other care providers. *J Pain Symptom Manage* 2001;22:727–754.
6. **Finlay I.** End of life care in patients dying of gynecologic cancer. *Hematol Oncol Clin North Am* 1999;13:77–108.
7. **Cowcher K, Hanks GW.** Long-term management of respiratory symptoms in advanced cancer. *J Pain Symptom Manage* 1990;5:705–707.
8. **Philip J, Gold M, Schwarz M, Komesaroff P.** Anger in palliative care: a clinical approach. *Intern Med J* 2007;37:49–55.
9. **Bausewein C, Farquhar M, Booth S, Gysels M, Higginson I.** Measurement of breathlessness in advanced disease: a systematic review. *Respir Med* 2007;101:399–410.

10. **Holen JC, Hjermstad MJ, Loge JH, et al.** Pain assessment tools: is the content appropriate for use in palliative care? *J Pain Symptom Manage* 2006;32:567–580.

11. **Jocham HR, Dassen T, Widdershoven G, Halfens R.** Quality of life in palliative care cancer patients: a literature review. *J Clin Nurs* 2006;15:1188–1195.

12. **Anderson B, Lutgendorf S.** Quality of life as an outcome measure in gynecologic malignancies. *Curr Opin Obstet Gynecol* 2000;12: 21–26.

13. **Glare P.** Clinical predictors of survival in advanced cancer. *J Support Oncol* 2005;3:331–339.

14. **Maltoni M, Caraceni A, Brunelli C, Broeckaert B, Christakis N, Eychmueller S, et al.** Prognostic factors in advanced cancer patients: evidence-based clinical recommendations—a study by the Steering Committee of the European Association for Palliative Care. *J Clin Oncol* 2005;23:6240–6248.

15. **Glare P, Sinclair CT.** Palliative medicine review: prognostication. *J Palliat Med* 2008;11:84–103.

16. **Clayton JM, Hancock KM, Butow PN, Tattersall MH, Currow DC, the Australian and New Zealand Expert Advisory Group, et al.** Clinical practice guidelines for communicating prognosis and end-of life issues with adults in the advanced stages of a life-limiting illness, and their caregivers. *Med J Aust* 2007;186(12 suppl): S77,S79,S83–108.

17. **Glare P, Virik K, Jones M, Hudson M, Eychmuller S, Simes J, et al.** A systematic review of physicians' survival predictions in terminally ill cancer patients. *BMJ* 2003;327:195.

18. **Lickiss JN.** Pain control in patients with gynecologic cancer. In: **Gershenson DM, Gore M, McGuire WP, Thomas G, Quinn MA, eds.** *Gynecologic cancer: controversies in management.* London: Churchill Livingstone, 2004.

19. **Benedetti C, Brock C, Cleeland C, Coyle N, Dubé JE, Ferrell B, et al.** National Comprehensive Cancer Network. NCCN practice guidelines for cancer pain. *Oncology (Williston Park)* 2000;14: 135–150.

20. **Jacox A, Carr D, Payne R.** New clinical practice guidelines for the management of pain in patients with cancer. *New Engl J Med* 1994;330: 651–655.

21. **The Ad Hoc Committee on Cancer Pain of the American Society of Clinical Oncology.** Cancer pain assessment and treatment curriculum guidelines. *J Clin Oncol* 1992;10:1976–1982.

22. **Lickiss JN.** Approaching cancer pain relief. *Eur J Pain* 2001;5(suppl A):5–14.

23. **Stevens MJ, Gonet YM.** Malignant psoas syndrome: recognition of an oncologic entity. *Australas Radiol* 1990;34:150–154.

24. **Portenoy RK, Forbes K, Lussier D, Hanks G.** Difficult pain problems: an integrated approach. In: **Doyle D, Hanks GW, Cherny N, Calman K, eds.** *Oxford textbook of palliative medicine.* Oxford: Oxford University Press, 2003:438–458.

25. **Chapman RC, Gavrin J.** Suffering and its relationship to pain. *J Palliat Care* 1993;9:5–13.

26. **Cassell EJ.** The nature of suffering and the goals of medicine. *N Eng J Med* 1982;306:639–645.

27. **Cassell EJ.** Diagnosing suffering: a perspective. *Ann Int Med* 1999; 131:531–534.

28. **Murata H.** Spiritual pain and its care in patients with terminal cancer: construction of a conceptual framework by philosophical approach. *Palliat Support Care* 2003;1:15–21.

29. **Hanks GW, de Conno F, Cherny N, Hanna K, Kalso E, McQuay HJ.** Morphine and alternative opioids in cancer pain: the EAPC recommendations. *Br J Cancer* 2001;84:587–593.

30. **Mercadante S, Portenoy RK.** Opioid poorly-responsive cancer pain. Part 1: clinical considerations. *J Pain Symptom Manage* 2001;21: 144–150.

31. **Hanks GW, de Conno F, Cherny N, Hanna K, Kalso E, McQuay HJ, et al.** Morphine and alternative opioids in cancer pain: the EAPC recommendations. *Br J Cancer* 2001;84:587–593.

32. **de Stoutz ND, Bruera E, Suarez-Almazor M.** Opioid rotation for toxicity reduction in terminal cancer patients. *J Pain Symptom Manage* 1995;10:378–384.

33. **Indelicato RA, Portenoy RK.** Opioid rotation in the management of refractory cancer pain. *J Clin Oncol* 2002;20:348–352.

34. **Biancofiore G.** Oxycodone controlled release in cancer pain management. *Ther Clin Risk Manage* 2006;2:229–234.

35. **Mercadante S, Portenoy RK.** Opioid poorly-responsive cancer pain. Part 2: basic mechanisms that could shift dose responsive for analgesia. *J Pain Symptom Manage* 2001;21:255–264.

36. **Cherny N, Thaler H, Friedlander-Klar H, Lapin J, Foley KM, Houde R, et al.** Opioid responsiveness of cancer pain syndromes caused by neuropathic or nociceptive mechanisms: a combined analysis of controlled, single-dose studies. *Neurology* 1994;44: 857–861.

37. **Berdine HJ, Nesbit SA.** Equianalgesic dosing of opioids. *J Pain Pall Care Pharmacotherap* 2006;20:79–84.

38. **Portenoy RK, Moulin DE, Rogers A, et al.** IV infusion of opioids for cancer pain: clinical review and guidelines for use. *Cancer Treat Rep* 1986;70:575–581.

39. **Murtagh FE, Chai MO, Donohoe P, Edmonds PM, Higginson IJ.** The use of opioid analgesia in end-stage renal disease patients managed without dialysis: recommendations for practice. *J Pain Pall Care Pharmacotherap* 2007;21:5–16.

40. **Davis MP, Varga J, Dickerson D, Walsh D, LeGrand SB, Lagman R.** Normal release and controlled-release oxycodone: pharmacokinetics, pharmacodynamics and controversy. *Support Care Cancer* 2003;11:84–92.

41. **Niscola P, Perrotti A.P, Del Poeta G, Romani C, Palombi M, Piccioni D, et al.** Case reports: zoster pain in haematological malignancies: effective pain relief with oxycodone in patients unresponsive to other analgesic measures. *Herpes* 2007;14:45–47.

42. **Davis AM, Inturrisi CE.** d-Methadone blocks morphine tolerance and N-methyl-D-Aspartate-induced hyperalgesia. *J Pharmacol Exp Ther* 1999;289:1048–1053.

43. **Plonk WM.** Simplified methadone conversion. *J Palliat Med* 2005;8:478–479.

44. **Zimmerman C, Seccareccia D, Booth CM, Cottrell W.** Rotation to methadone after opioid escalation. *J Pain Pall Care Pharmacotherap* 2005;19:25–31.

45. **Quigley C, Wiffen P.** A systematic review of hydromorphone in acute and chronic pain. *J Pain Symptom Manage* 2003;25:169–178.

46. **Ahmedzai S, Brooks D.** Transdermal fentanyl versus sustained-release oral morphine in cancer pain: preference, efficacy and quality of life. *J Pain Symptom Manage* 1997;16:141–144.

47. **Grond S, Radbruch L, Lehmann KA.** Clinical pharmacokinetics of transdermal opioids: focus on transdermal fentanyl. *Clin Pharmacokinet* 2000;38:59–89.

48. **Taylor DR, Webster LR, Chun SY, Reinking J, Stegman M, Shoemaker S, et al.** Impact of breakthrough pain on quality of life in patients with chronic, noncancer pain: patient perceptions and effect of treatment with oral transmucosal fentanyl citrate. *Pain Med* 2007;8:281–288.

49. **Coluzzi P, Schwartzberg L, Conroy Jr JD, Charapata S, Gay M, Busch MA, et al.** Breakthrough cancer pain: a randomized trial comparing oral transmucosal fentanyl citrate and morphine sulfate immediate release. *Pain* 2001;91:123–130.

50. **McQueen AL, Baroletti SA.** Adjuvant ketamine analgesia for the management of cancer pain. *Ann Pharmacother* 2002;36:1614-1619.

51. **Foley KM.** Opioids and chronic neuropathic pain. *N Eng J Med* 2003;348:1279–1281.

52. **Dworkin RH, O'Connor AB, Backonja M, Farrar J., Finnerup NB, Jensen TS, et al.** Pharmacologic management of neuropathic pain: evidence-based recommendations. *Pain* 2007;132:237–251.

53. **Legge J, Ball N, Elliott DP.** The potential role of ketamine in hospice analgesia: a literature review. *Consult Pharm* 2006;21: 51–57.

54. **Kedlaya D, Reynolds L, Waldman S.** Epidural and intrathecal analgesia for cancer pain. *Best Pract Res Clin Anaesthesiol* 2002;16: 651–665.

55. **Fainsinger RL, Nekolaichuk CLA.** A "TNM" classification system for cancer pain: The Edmonton Classification System for Cancer Pain (ECS-CP). *Support Care Cancer* 2008;16:547–555.

56. **Manfredi PL, Breuer B, Meier DE, Libow L.** Pain assessment in elderly patients with severe dementia. *J Pain Symptom Manage* 2003; 25:48–52.

57. **Daeninck PJ, Bruera E.** Opioid use in cancer pain. Is a more liberal approach enhancing toxicity? *Acta Anaesthesiol Scand* 1999;43: 924–938.

58. **Gagnon B, Lawlor PG, Mancini IL, Pereira JL, Hanson J, Bruera ED.** The impact of delirium on the circadian distribution of

breakthrough analgesia in advanced cancer patients. *J Pain Symptom Manage* 2001;22:826–833.

59. **Moryl N, Kogan M, Comfort C, Obbens E.** Methadone in the treatment of pain and terminal delirium in advanced cancer patients. *Palliat Support Care* 2005;3:311–317.

60. **Scimeca MM, Savage SR, Portenoy RK, Lowinson J.** Treatment of pain in methadone-maintained patients. *Mt Sinai J Med* 2000; 67:412–422.

61. **Scascighini L, Sprott H.** Chronic nonmalignant pain: a challenge for patients and clinicians. *Nat Clin Pract Rheumatol* 2008;4: 74–81.

62. **Portenoy RK.** Opioid therapy for chronic nonmalignant pain: a review of the critical issues. *J Pain Symptom Manage* 1996;11: 203–217.

63. **Passik SD, Kirsh KL, Whitcomb L, Schein JR, Kaplan MA, Dodd SL, et al.** Monitoring outcomes during long-term opioid therapy for noncancer pain: results with the Pain Assessment and Documentation Tool. *J Opioid Manag* 2005;1:257–266.

64. **Marsden DM, Lickiss JN.** Gastrointestinal problems in patients with advanced gynaecological malignancy. *Best Pract Res Clin Obstet Gynaecol* 2000;15:253–263.

65. **Strasser F, Bruera E.** Update on anorexia and cachexia. *Hematol Oncol Clin North Am* 2002;16:589–617.

66. **Loprinzi CL, Ellison N.M, Schaid DJ, Krook JE, Athmann LM, Dose AM, et al.** A controlled trial of megestrol acetate treatment of cancer anorexia and cachexia. *J Nat Cancer Inst* 1990;81: 1127–1132.

67. **Davis MP, Walsh D.** Treatment of nausea and vomiting in advanced cancer. *Support Care Cancer* 2000;6:444–452.

68. **Glare P, Pereira G, Kristjanson LJ, Stockler M, Tattersall M.** Systematic review of the efficacy of antiemetics in the treatment of nausea in patients with far-advanced cancer. *Support Care Cancer* 2004;12:432–440.

69. **Twycross R, Wilcock A, Thorp S.** *Palliative care formulary.* Oxford: Radcliffe Medical Press, 1999.

70. **Philip J, Lickiss JN, Grant PT, Hacker NF.** Corticosteroids in the management of bowel obstruction on a gynecological oncology unit. *Gynecol Oncol* 1999;74:68–73.

71. **Schiller LR.** The therapy of constipation (review article). *Aliment Pharmacol Ther* 2001;15:749–763.

72. **Baines M, Oliver DJ, Carter RL.** Medical management of intestinal obstruction in patients with advanced malignant disease: a clinical pathological study. *Lancet* 1985;2:990–993.

73. **Mercadante S, Casuccio A, Mangione S.** Medical treatment for inoperable malignant bowel obstruction: a qualitative systematic review. *J Pain Symptom Manage* 2007;33:217–223.

74. **Ripamonti C, Twycross R, Baines M, Bozzetti F, Capri S, De Conno F, et al.** Clinical-practice recommendations for the management of bowel obstruction in patients with end-stage cancer. *Support Care Cancer* 2001;9:223–233.

75. **Dionigi G,Villa F, Rovera F, Boni L, Carrafiello G, Annoni M, et al.** Colonic stenting for malignant disease: review of literature. *Surg Oncol* 2007;16(suppl 1):S153–S155.

76. **Feuer DJ, Broadley KE.** Corticosteroids for the resolution of malignant bowel obstruction in advanced gynaecological and gastrointestinal cancer. *Cochrane Database Syst Rev* 2000; CD001219.

77. **Curtin JP, Burt LL.** Successful treatment of small intestine fistula with somatostatin analog. *Gynecol Oncol* 1990;39:225–227.

78. **Hansen MB.** The enteric nervous system II: gastrointestinal functions. *Pharmacol Toxicol* 2003;92:249–257.

79. **Abernethy AP, Currow DC, Frith P, Fazekas BS, McHugh A, Bui C.** Randomised, double blind, placebo controlled crossover trial of sustained release morphine for the management of refractory dyspnoea. *BMJ* 2003;327:523–528.

80. **Philip J, Gold M, Milner A, Di Iulio J, Miller B, Spruyt O.** A randomised, double-blind, cross-over trial of the effect of oxygen on dyspnoea in patients with advanced cancer. *J Pain Symptom Manage* 2006;32:541–550.

81. **Booth S, Wade R, Johnson M, Kite S, Swannick M, Anderson H, for the Expert Working Group of the Scientific Committee of the Association of Palliative Medicine.** The use of oxygen in the palliation of breathlessness. A report of the expert working group of the Scientific Committee of the Association of Palliative Medicine. *Respir Med* 2004;98:66–77.

82. **Chye R, Lickiss JN.** The use of corticosteroids in management of bilateral malignant ureteric obstruction. *J Pain Symptom Manage* 1994;9:537–540.

83. **Twycross R, Jenns K, Todd J.** *Lymphoedema.* Oxford: Radcliffe Medical Press, 2000.

84. **Barnes EA, Bruera E.** Fatigue in patients with advanced cancer: a review. *Int J Gynecol Oncol* 2002;12:424–428.

85. **Radbruch L, Strasser F, Elsner F, Gonçalves JF, Løge J, Kaasa S, et al. for the Research Steering Committee of the European Association for Palliative Care (EAPC).** Fatigue in palliative care patients—an EAPC approach. *Palliat Med* 2008;22:13–32.

86. **Berenson J.** Treatment of hypercalcaemia of malignancy with bisphosphonates. *Semin Oncol* 2002;29:S21–S12.

87. **Berenson J, Hirschberg R.** Safety and convenience of a 15-minute infusion of zoledronic acid. *Oncologist* 2004;9:319–329.

88. **Ellershaw J, Ward C.** Care of the dying patient: the last hours or days of life. *BMJ* 2003;326:30–34.

89. **Bloch E.** Karl Marx, death and the apocalypse. In: **Ashton EB, ed.** *Man on his own.* New York: Herder & Herder, 1970:47.

90. **Singer P, Martin D, Kelner M.** Quality of life care: patients' perspectives. *JAMA* 1999;281:163–168.

91. **Chochinov H.** Dignity and the essence of medicine: the ABC and D of dignity-conserving care. *BMJ* 2007;335:184–187.

92. **Shearer R.** Suffering of the doctor linked with the death of patients. *Palliat Med* 1993;7(suppl):27–37.

25 Psychological Issues

Anna O. Levin
Kristen M. Carpenter
Barbara L. Andersen

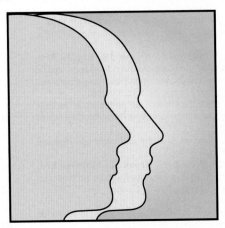

For most women, a diagnosis of gynecologic cancer is a crisis. For the majority, adaptation ensues and emotional distress dissipates with recovery. For others, cancer becomes a chronic stressor, either because the disease has disseminated through the body and can be controlled only with radical treatments, or because a survivor's coping strategies are not adequate. In any case, **management of patients with gynecologic malignancies must consider the psychological and behavioral aspects of the disease.** A review of the data on psychological and behavioral issues relevant to gynecologic cancer is presented, including discussion of sexual morbidity. In addition, practical information that can be used to conceptualize and assist patients' coping is provided.

Pap Screening and Follow-Up

Research suggests that individuals become distressed during medical screening, long before a cancer diagnosis is suggested (1). **In the case of an abnormal screen, many women will experience significant anxiety, distress, and daily life disruptions.** Ideström and colleagues (2) described reactions to abnormal Papanicolaou (Pap) test results in a sample of 242 women. More than half of the women surveyed (59%) reported feelings of worry and anxiety after being informed of their abnormal Pap result, and about a third (30%) of women reported that their daily life was disrupted in the time between the initial Pap result and follow-up tests. A smaller proportion of women (8%) reported sexual dysfunction symptoms. Another large survey of 3,500 women found increased risk for anxiety in response to an abnormal Pap result in women who were younger, had children, were current smokers, or had the highest levels of physical activity (3). Lerman and colleagues (4) reported that women who receive abnormal Pap results worry more about cancer and have significantly more disruptions in mood, daily activities, sexual interest, and sleep patterns when compared to women with normal results. Regarding the initial gynecologic oncology consultation, patients report significantly elevated psychiatric symptoms, with 42% reporting clinical levels of depressive symptoms and 30% reporting moderate to severe anxiety symptoms, regardless of whether the eventual diagnosis is one of cancer or benign gynecologic disease (5).

The relationship between increased psychological distress and nonadherence to screening and treatment recommendations is well documented in cancer patients (e.g., breast cancer [6]). **Possible explanations for noncompliance following an abnormal Pap result include fear of the diagnostic procedures, not wanting to know if something is wrong, fear of a cancer diagnosis, belief that the outcomes will be negative (fatalism), and belief that one is too old for treatment** (7).

Fortunately, nonadherence to follow up recommendations can be addressed through brief, low-cost interventions. For example, Stewart and colleagues (8) prepared a brief psychoeducational brochure for women who were referred for biopsy. Results demonstrated that women who received the brochure were significantly less distressed. Moreover, 75% of women who received the materials complied with treatment and follow-up 18 to 24 months later compared with 46% of women not receiving the materials.

The Stress of Diagnosis

Initial Diagnosis

Severe, acute stress occurs at the time of cancer diagnosis (9,10). In addition to immediate and subsequent psychological effects of stress, **cancer-specific stress triggers biological effects.** For example, following surgery and prior to adjuvant treatment, stress among breast cancer patients is associated with immune down regulation, shown across assays for NK cell cytoxicity (NKCC); the response of NK cells to recombinant interferon gamma (rIFN-g); and T cell responses including proliferative responses to concanavalin A (ConA); phytohemagglutinin (PHA); and a T3 monoclonal antibody (MoAb) (11). **Patients face difficult circumstances throughout their illness,** but the shock of learning the diagnosis is the first. The term **existential plight** has been used to describe this period and the emotional turmoil that continues during treatment (12). **The emotions and sources of distress may include:**

1. **Depression** from life disruption and doubts concerning the future.
2. **Anxiety** anticipating cancer treatment.
3. **Confusion** from dealing with a complex medical environment.
4. **Anger** from the loss of childbearing capacity and the opportunity to choose whether to have children.
5. **Guilt** from concerns that previous sexual activity may have "caused" the cancer. The guilt may be mixed with concerns about how future sexual activity will be disrupted after cancer treatment.

An early study conducted in 1989 compared mood disturbance among those recently diagnosed with a gynecological cancer with two matched groups, one with benign gynecologic disease anticipating surgery and the other with no disease (i.e., healthy women). All completed a self-report inventory on the emotions they experienced during their initial evaluation (13). Findings were as follows:

1. **Only women with cancer described themselves as having negative moods** suggestive of depression.
2. In contrast, **high anxiety was reported by both groups with disease,** whether benign or malignant.
3. There were **no differences in the level of anger** between the groups.
4. **High levels of confusion were reported only by the patients with cancer.**
5. There were **equivalent levels of fatigue among the disease groups.**

Since this early clinical work, consistent data have been reported which underscore the significant distress experienced by many cancer patients. **Mental health disorders among cancer patients are prevalent, largely unrecognized, and usually untreated. It is consistently estimated that 30% to 50% of cancer patients meet criteria for mood or anxiety disorders, with depression being the most common** (14,15). Specifically, estimates for major depressive disorder (MDD) are 22% to 29% for patients with early stage disease (16), 8% to 40% for patients with advanced disease (17), and increase further with recurrence (18). Among breast and gynecologic cancer patients, Zabora et al. found prevalence of MDD to be 33% and 30%, respectively (19). Finally, other morbidity comes with depression, such as comorbid anxiety (20,21), poorer quality of life (21–23), fatigue (25,26), and more distress from physical symptoms (27). Unfortunately, cancer patients with comorbid depression are not readily identified. For example, among 112 women with major depression undergoing cancer treatment, Ell and colleagues found that only 12% were receiving antidepressants and only 5% were receiving psychological therapy (28).

Patients experiencing high levels of distress have many difficulties, including: (i) **problems understanding and remembering all that they have been told,** including both simple

861

information (e.g., what time they are to be admitted) and more complex information (e.g., the organs to be surgically removed and the nature of the side effects); (ii) **difficulty managing personal affairs** (e.g., contacting their insurance company or arranging for child care during recovery); and (iii) **difficulty with being a "patient" and allowing others to care for them.**

Even for those with some knowledge of gynecologic surgeries, cancer treatment is qualitatively different. For example, a woman's mother, sister, or a close friend may have related her experiences with hysterectomy. Even if the surgery involved an abdominal rather than a vaginal approach, the preoperative and postoperative experience for the woman with cancer will be notably different from the patient's expectations (e.g., bowel preparation, length of recovery, vaginal shortening, bladder dysfunction). Thus, it is normal for any patient to experience cognitive, emotional, and behavioral difficulties, and **it is the rare patient who does not require supportive assistance as treatment approaches.**

Finally, the **acute stress associated with a cancer diagnosis may portend later difficulties.** When there is an absence of positive coping, patients subsequently report a loss of meaning in their lives (29). Patients with high levels of diagnostic distress have been also found to have high depressive symptoms during follow-up (30), as well as lower quality of life (30).

Recurrence

Research suggests that patients with recurrent cancer have levels of stress equivalent to that reported when receiving their initial diagnosis. A controlled, prospective study followed 227 women for 8 years after their diagnosis of breast cancer. Among them, 30 were diagnosed with recurrence during follow-up and their reaction to the recurrence was compared to their reaction to their initial diagnosis (31). Women experiencing recurrence reported their stress about cancer to be equivalent to their reports after their initial diagnoses. In contrast, emotional distress and social functioning showed no disruption at recurrence, and was equivalent to that of a disease-free control group.

Another study compared patients with a newly diagnosed recurrence ($n = 69$) to those with an initial breast cancer diagnosis ($n = 113$). Compared to the patients coping with their first diagnosis, patients with a recurrence had significantly lower anxiety and confusion. As expected, physical functioning was poorer among patients with a recurrence, and quality of life improvement was slower during the 12 months following diagnosis (32).

This is not to suggest that women with recurrent gynecologic cancer do not experience difficulties, particularly when disease progresses. Many patients with ovarian cancer, for example, face end-of-life circumstances. In a sample of such patients, Roberts and colleagues (33) found that 39% exhibited acute fears, the most common being **fear of abandonment** (32%) and **fear of social isolation** (17%). Taken together, these results suggest that difficult decisions associated with recurrence are made in a context of emotional distress and physical debilitation.

Psychological Interventions for Diagnostic Distress

Severe emotional distress resulting from a cancer diagnosis and the anticipation of treatments can be reduced with psychological interventions. Many randomized controlled trials (RCTs) have been conducted and show efficacy in patients with newly diagnosed cancer (34–36). While the majority of trials have been conducted with breast cancer patients and have used group treatments, the findings are applicable to gynecologic patients.

Regarding psychological support, crisis or brief therapy (8–10 sessions) is effective. These interventions involve an **assessment of the patient's emotional distress and other difficulties, a focus on the immediate problems facing the patient, and limited therapeutic goals.** The therapist is active in making suggestions for coping and problem management. Therapeutic components may include (i) **distress reduction,** such as providing training in relaxation to lower anxiety and bodily tension and enhance the patient's sense of control; (ii) **information about the disease and treatment;** (iii) **behavioral coping strategies,** e.g., role-playing difficult discussions with family or the medical staff; (iv) **cognitive coping strategies,** such as identifying the patient's troublesome worries and thoughts and providing alternative appraisals; and (v) **provision of social support and comfort,** which acknowledges the difficulty of the situation and provides a context for the patient openly to discuss her fears and anxieties.

Fewer RCT have been conducted with gynecologic cancer patients, but two recent studies have been reported (37,38). Manne and colleagues (38) compared the efficacy of two psychological interventions, **a coping and communication-enhancing intervention (CCI) and a supportive**

counseling (SC) intervention, in reducing depressive symptoms and cancer-specific distress, to a usual care control. Both the CCI and SC courses were seven sessions long. Results showed that, at 6 and 9 months, women who participated in the CCI and SC groups reported equivalent but lower depressive symptoms than patients receiving usual care only (37).

Scott and her colleagues (38) developed an intervention to improve psychological adjustment for patients and their partners with early-stage breast or gynecological cancer. Ninety-four couples, all married, were randomly assigned to couples-based coping training, individual coping training for the patient only, or a medical education control. The couples intervention was associated with significant gains at 6 and 12 months, compared to the other two groups. That is, couples showed significant improvements in supportive communication, sexual adjustment, and psychological distress, and patients demonstrated improved coping skills (38).

Finally, Petersen and Quinlivan tested the efficacy of a counseling and relaxation intervention on psychological symptoms in 50 newly diagnosed patients. Compared to a no-intervention control, women participating in the six-week intervention showed reductions in anxiety and depressive symptoms, including decreased somatization (39).

For patients coping with depression, multiple trials with non cancer patients have tested the relative and comparative efficacy of the two primary treatments (40): medication (41) and/or psychotherapy (42). Among psychotherapies, the most extensively studied and most successful treatment is **Cognitive-Behavioral Therapy (CBT)** (43,44). **In randomized clinical trials, CBT has generally been found to be as effective as anti-depressant medication** (45), even among the severely depressed.

A 2006 report reviewed data on antidepressant medication for patients with cancer and depression (46). The authors found few studies, but concluded that those reported **provided some evidence that antidepressants were effective in reducing depressive symptoms in cancer patients.** Antidepressants may also enhance adherence to recommended treatment regimens.

Psychological Interventions for Treatment Distress

It is most important for a woman to receive information about the treatment plan for her disease. Despite efforts to allay concerns and provide accurate information, misconceptions abound, and anxiety will remain high as patients approach surgery, radiation therapy, or chemotherapy.

Surgery

Although there have been few investigations of patients' psychological reactions to cancer surgery, there are numerous descriptive studies of the reactions of relatively healthy women undergoing surgery for benign conditions (e.g., uterine fibroids). This research suggests a direct relationship between the magnitude of preoperative and postoperative anxiety; that is, **those patients who are the most anxious before surgery are also the most anxious afterward,** albeit less so. In addition, the magnitude of postoperative distress often correlates with behavioral indicants of recovery (e.g., time out of bed, pain reports, days in hospital). In an early study, Gottesman and Lewis noted greater and more lasting crisis feelings and a stronger sense of helplessness among patients with cancer for as long as 2 months after discharge from the hospital compared to patients receiving surgery for benign conditions (47).

Gynecologic cancer surgery may impose unique burdens, with two circumstances being particularly salient. First, **women of childbearing age who are nulliparous or have not yet achieved their desired family size may become distraught if the surgery causes loss of childbearing capability.** Acceptance may not come for months, and in the interim it may be difficult for the woman to socialize with sisters or female friends who are pregnant or who have young children. Because the age of childbearing among women in the United States has risen, the likelihood of this situation occurring for women with gynecologic cancer has increased. Second, **radical surgical procedures, such as radical vulvectomy or pelvic exenteration, which produce genital disfigurement, may produce depression, feelings of isolation, and significant body image concerns** (48,49).

Efforts to reduce distress from surgery or to facilitate recovery are typically informational. Detailed descriptions of the procedure, sensations, or side effects and behavioral coping strategies (e.g., relaxation training or distraction exercises for pain management) have proven effective. **Prepared patients tend to have shorter hospital stays, use fewer medications, and report less severe pain than patients receiving standard hospital care and preoperative nursing information** (50,51). It is hypothesized that this type of preparation reduces stress by helping to build accurate expectations and by enhancing feelings of control and predictability for the patient.

Radiation Therapy

Although there are individual differences, **most patients report confusion and negative emotions regarding radiation treatments. Misinformation is common,** with some patients fearing permanent contamination of themselves or others from treatment, and other patients assuming that radiation attacks only "bad" cells, leaving others unaffected. A patient's prior knowledge of radiation therapy may be based on the experiences of a friend or relative, and if their treatment was unsuccessful or difficult, she may enter treatment believing it will be the same for her (52).

External beam therapy brings fears or uneasiness about the size or the safety of treatment machines, and often, distress from being in a radiation therapy department where other patients, in obvious ill health, may be. For some women, disrobing and exposing the pelvic area is a daily embarrassment, and field-marking tattoos are visible reminders of the cancer. In one study, roughly 80% of patients expressed an unwillingness to discuss these concerns with their physicians (53). This may occur when patients perceive their physicians as too busy, or patients themselves feel they cannot ask "intelligent" questions of their physicians.

As the procedures of radiation therapy become routine, many patients report less emotional distress, but the side effects of fatigue, diarrhea, and anorexia begin. Side effects complicate living, requiring activity reductions and dietary modifications. Previously symptom-free patients may begin to feel and think of themselves as "ill," doubting their positive prognosis. Premenopausal women experience hot flashes, a salient and distressing symptom of the loss of their fertility.

At the termination of treatment, these patients might be expected to report a drop in anxiety and fear, similar to the pattern exhibited by relatively healthy people undergoing surgery. Instead, gynecologic patients (54), as well as other patients with cancer (55), report a different pattern of anxiety responses. Women with high pretreatment anxiety are less anxious on the last treatment day than on the first, although they remain the most distressed. Those with moderate levels of pretreatment distress report little diminution in distress by the last treatment, and surprisingly, those with low levels of anxiety at the onset of treatment report significantly greater anxiety on the last treatment day. As expected, physical symptoms of fatigue, abdominal pain, anorexia, diarrhea, and skin irritation are significant for all patients at the conclusion of treatment.

In contrast to external beam, few patients know of intracavitary radiotherapy. Worries about lengthy isolation and permanent contamination are common, and women may cope with the impending treatment by diverting their attention to less distressing thoughts (56). During treatment, women have significant physical discomfort, even when there has been liberal analgesic medication (54). Gas pains, burning sensations, and lower backache are typical, and emotional distress can be pervasive. Visitation restrictions limit contact with family and friends, and this may be frightening to a patient if it is perceived as isolation from nurses or physicians. It is not surprising that many women are irritable and upset during the treatment. Fortunately, low dose rate brachytherapy has largely been replaced by high dose rate therapy in most Western countries, so lengthy isolation is no longer a problem.

A second radiation application is received by 50% to 75% of women. Whereas physicians may anticipate that this might be an easier experience for patients, it is not. In fact, **women report feeling more anxious during and are more debilitated after their second treatment.** Even women with lower levels of anxiety before their first intracavitary treatment are reported to experience elevated levels of anxiety after their second application (57).

Without assistance, recovery from the physical and psychological distress of radiation therapy is slow. Nail et al. (1986) have documented an incidence of nausea in 5%, anorexia in 15%, diarrhea in 15%, and fatigue in 32% of gynecologic patients treated as long as 3 months previously (58). Complications, such as radiation proctitis or fistulae, can emerge. Decreased lubrication and vaginal tenderness also result in significant sexual disruption during recovery, with lack of sexual interest and dyspareunia being major problems for many women. In fact, a longitudinal study found that sexual dysfunction and adverse vaginal changes persisted 2 years after radiotherapy treatment, with approximately 85% of women reporting low or no sexual interest, and 55% experiencing mild to severe dyspareunia (59).

In view of the commonality, severity, and persistence of sexual dysfunction after radiotherapy, all patients require information on vaginal care and sexuality after radiation treatment. Alterations to the vaginal anatomy, including vaginal shortening and stenosis, begin during the course of radiation treatment (60). **Dyspareunia is the most common symptom,** and it appears to be most severe among women receiving both external and intracavitary radiation, although patients receiving only external beam also report this symptom (61). A regimen of vaginal care is necessary for all patients to reduce pain and maintain, as much as possible, vaginal plasticity. Psychoeducational interventions designed to enhance dilator treatment adherence are described in the following section. Fortunately, the magnitude of pain during intercourse appears to decrease during the months after treatment for women who maintain sexual activity.

Regarding psychological interventions, patients' descriptions of themselves as anxious, confused, and uncomfortable about expressing such concerns, provide targets for intervention. **Patients most vulnerable to distress and most likely to need psychological assistance during treatment may include** (55,57,62):

1. **Those who exhibit relatively little emotional distress before treatment**
2. **Those with a history of emotional problems**
3. **Those with a disease causing chronic discomfort**
4. **Those who are socially isolated**

Several strategies may be useful to address the anxiety-based concerns of the patient. General counseling focused on the patient's problems may be offered. For example, Forester et al. (63) provided weekly sessions in which women receiving external radiation could discuss any topic, although most sessions were supportive and informational. Improved functioning was found when these patients were compared with those receiving no intervention; patients receiving intervention reported lower levels of emotional distress and less severe side effects.

Other interventions have primarily provided information. Topics include simulation, radiation equipment, side effects of radiation, length of recovery, and strategies for managing side effects (e.g., diet modification, skin care, adequate rest). Research on patient preparation suggests that such information needs to be simplified and repeated. Instead of providing all information to patients on one occasion at the start of treatment, an alternative is to repeat portions of it as it becomes more relevant. For example, Israel and Mood (64) provided information about therapeutic procedures early in the treatment, about radiation side effects and their management at the midpoint of treatment, and about emotional issues and the length of recovery toward the end of therapy.

To prevent vaginal stenosis, clinical data suggest patients should use a dilator regularly (e.g., two to three times per week for 10–15 minutes). Intercourse may serve as a substitute, however if the frequency is low (i.e., less than once a week), patients should additionally use a dilator. **Without adequate support, adherence to dilation therapy may be low. Recent trials (65,66) found increased dilator use among women who participated in psychoeducational interventions.** If not contraindicated, topical estrogen cream may promote healing and improve the vaginal epithelium (67). Even with these interventions, pain during intercourse may occur until sufficient healing of the vaginal epithelium has occurred.

Chemotherapy

Patients' reactions to learning that they need chemotherapy can range from extreme negativity (i.e., feeling angry or depressed) **to relief that some kind of treatment is available to them.** This mix of emotions reflects distress at having to undergo a difficult treatment, which many believe is only for "hopeless" cancers, and the fear that it will not control the disease. To allay patients' concerns, medical personnel usually provide descriptions of, and written materials about, the effects and side effects of treatment. In spite of this, as many as 10% of patients report uncertainty and lack of knowledge when beginning treatment (68). Others may approach chemotherapy optimistically and believe that they will belong to the small subset of people who do not experience any side effects.

Once any type of information about chemotherapy has been delivered, patient understanding needs to be assessed, because many patients become confused or forgetful when too much information is given. One way to ensure understanding is to ask the patient to explain in her own words what she has been told, as if she were telling her husband or a close friend. This strategy provides an opportunity to reinforce her understanding and to correct any misconceptions.

Patients experience a significant and constant level of distress throughout chemotherapy. As treatment occupies more and more of a patient's life, worries become intrusive, and the intense and noxious side effects generate stronger feelings of illness. Active coping and seeking social support are associated with lowered anxiety and depression, whereas avoidance is positively correlated with both anxiety and depression (69). In addition, women who attempt to control the side effects and fail become more distressed than those who report that they have coped successfully (68).

Anticipatory nausea and vomiting may complicate the course of chemotherapy for approximately 25% of patients. This refers to nausea and/or vomiting before the administration of chemotherapy. It is hypothesized that this disturbing situation develops because the stimuli surrounding the administration of chemotherapy (e.g., needles and smell of alcohol) become paired with posttreatment nausea and vomiting. With repeated cycles, the stimuli become conditioned and are able to evoke nausea or vomiting before the administration of chemotherapy. Once anticipatory reactions develop, they can become more general (e.g., alcohol-containing substances such as perfume may cause nausea), and they occur progressively earlier (e.g., on entering the hospital, rather than on entering the treatment room).

Factors that place a patient at risk for development of anticipatory nausea and vomiting include (70,71):

1. Age less than 50 years
2. Lengthy infusion and higher doses of chemotherapy
3. Severe posttreatment nausea or vomiting in the early cycles
4. Extreme anxiety and/or depression
5. Previous susceptibility to nausea and/or motion sickness

Additionally, women with higher levels of state anxiety tend to be more susceptible to both anticipatory and post-treatment nausea and vomiting (72).

Another concomitant of some chemotherapy is confusion ("chemo brain"), a distressing symptom for the patient and her family. Pharmacologic effects of chemotherapeutic agents account for some cognitive changes (73), and such changes further emphasize the illness and its consequences to the patient.

In a review of 54 studies investigating the efficacy of behavioral intervention methods, the authors concluded that, in addition to controlling anticipatory nausea and vomiting, interventions integrating several behavioral methods can reduce patients' anxiety and distress concerning other treatments. The review also suggested that, although a variety of behavioral methods have been shown to reduce acute treatment-related pain, hypnotic-like methods, involving relaxation, suggestion, and distracting imagery, hold the greatest promise for pain management (74).

Psychological Outcomes for Gynecologic Oncology Survivors

Cancer survivors may need to cope with the expected but nevertheless troubling permanent sequelae of the disease or its treatment (e.g., menopause, perceived loss of femininity, infertility). This will demand new behaviors or emotional coping methods. From the limited literature on gynecologic cancer survivorship, three trends are evident. First, side effects of treatment (e.g., fatigue, pain, sexual difficulties, and bladder/bowel dysfunction) are common and persistent (8,75–79). Indeed, patients report that physical sequelae from cancer therapy pose the most significant survivorship challenge (80). Second, while overall rates of psychological distress are not exceptional, a significant portion of patients experience psychological maladjustment as survivors (8,76–78,80,81). Third, physical sequelae and psychological adjustment appear to co-vary (75,81,82), and are not necessarily mitigated by time in the years following cancer treatment. Nevertheless, **data indicate that most patients cope successfully; many report renewed vigor in their approach to life, stronger interpersonal relationships, and a "survivor" adaptation** (83,84). Longitudinal data also confirm that, for most, emotions are within the normal range by 6 to 12 months post-treatment (85,86).

A small subset (5% to 10%) may have lingering emotional distress from the trauma of diagnosis, treatment, and more generally, the threat of death. When pronounced, this long-term distress has been likened to posttraumatic stress disorder. In fact, residual distress from the diagnosis and treatment of a life-threatening illness is included as one of the circumstances that may precipitate posttraumatic stress disorder (PTSD) (87). Such reactions are substantial in gynecologic cancer survivors, with symptom rates reported at 19% (76), and may be more common for those undergoing the more difficult of treatment regimens, or those receiving life-altering and/or disfiguring cancer treatments, (e.g., pelvic exenteration). Patients with a prior history of psychiatric treatment and/or traumatic stress are at increased risk for post cancer PTSD (26), as are patients who report greater rates of unmet supportive care needs (76).

Sexual Functioning Morbidity

The long-term impact of gynecologic cancers and cancer treatments on sexual health is well documented (88,89). **While sexual problems may not be a woman's primary concern when she is initially diagnosed, persistent sexual problems are a large concern for most long-term survivors (90). In fact, one study found that women ranked problems with sexual arousal as the most distressing of their cancer treatment-related symptoms (91).**

Most health care professionals are aware of the likelihood of sexual difficulties for their patients. Unfortunately, assessment, treatment, or referral for treatment is uncommon. Stead and colleagues (92) interviewed 43 physicians and nurses regularly treating women with ovarian cancer, and while 98% reported that they felt sexual issues should be discussed with patients, only 21% reported actually doing so. In order to orient readers, a description of unimpaired sexual responding and DSM-IV definitions of sexual dysfunctions are provided. Next, research describing sexual morbidity among gynecologic oncology patients is presented. Finally, an overview of treatments potentially available for patients referred for sexual therapy is given.

Description of Sexual Response Cycle and Sexual Dysfunctions

Sexual Desire

Sexual desire is the least understood of all the phases of the sexual response cycle. It has been conceptualized as a drive or motivation for sexual activity. Androgen is hypothesized as providing the hormonal basis for sexual desire in women, as suggested by experimental studies of women without cancer but undergoing surgically induced menopause (93). Data suggest that exogenous androgen may enhance the intensity of sexual desire and arousal, but estrogen may have no effect.

The diagnosis "inhibited sexual desire" characterizes those people who report that they are usually uninterested in sexual activity. Such an attitude can be manifest by avoidance of sexual contacts, refusal of sexual activity, or infrequent initiation of sexual activity. Inhibited people report an absence or low frequency of sexual fantasy or other pleasant, arousing sexual thoughts. People with sexual desire dysfunction may, however, experience sexual excitement and/or orgasm when engaging in sexual activity. However, disruption in the focus, intensity, or duration of sexual activity is typical with desire disorder, with accompanying disruption of arousal and/or orgasm.

Sexual Excitement

The phase of sexual excitement begins with psychological or physical stimulation. Physiologic responses that occur during the excitement phase include vaginal engorgement and lubrication. Maximal vasocongestion produces a congested orgasmic "platform" in the lower one-third of the vaginal barrel.

Dysfunctional sexual excitement would include insufficient response so that penetration during heterosexual intercourse would be difficult or uncomfortable. Psychologically, a woman may report that she does not feel aroused and/or that her body is not responding. As with desire phase difficulties, subsequent orgasmic disruption could easily result from lowered levels of excitement.

Orgasm

Although the specific neurophysiologic mechanism of orgasm is not known, it has been proposed that orgasm is triggered when a plateau of excitement has been reached (94). Subjectively, a woman's awareness of orgasm typically focuses on pelvic sensations, centered in the clitoris, vagina, and uterus. Orgasm is marked by rhythmic contractions of the uterus, the orgasmic platform, and the rectal sphincter. A woman's awareness of orgasm is reported to be similar, regardless of the manner in which it is achieved (95).

Orgasmic disorder in women (formerly known as inhibited orgasm) is the persistent or recurrent delay in, or absence of, orgasm following a sexual excitement phase. There is great variability amongst women in terms of type and intensity of stimulation that triggers orgasm. Diagnosis should take into account this individual variability, as well as consideration of age, sexual experience, and the adequacy of sexual stimulation.

Resolution

If effective stimulation ends and/or orgasm occurs, the anatomic and physiologic changes that occurred during excitement reverse. The orgasmic platform disappears, the uterus moves back into the true pelvis, and the vagina shortens and narrows. **Such bodily responses after orgasm usually are accompanied by subjective feelings of tension release, relaxation, and contentment. If orgasm does not occur, the same physiologic processes are completed at a slower rate.**

Women with excitement or orgasmic dysfunctions typically report discontentment with the resolution period as well, with symptoms of continued pelvic vasocongestion, residual sexual tension, lack of satisfaction, and/or negative effect. **Complaints with resolution after unimpaired excitement and orgasm are infrequent;** when they occur, they may be prompted by inhibitory affects, such as guilt or marital discord, that are associated with sexual activity generally.

Description of Sexual Morbidity

When queried about sexuality, women with cancer indicate that these are important concerns that need to be addressed (48,49,96,97). This is not surprising as **30% to 90% of patients experience significant sexual disruption.** The physical and physiological changes from cancer treatments may alter a woman's body image, as well as her perception of herself in the sexual domain (sexual self schema). Women may feel that their treatments have caused a loss of femininity, and may also have to deal with early loss of fertility. This may be particularly detrimental for nulliparous women, or those who were planning to have children in the future. Some women may also fear contaminating their partner(s) through intercourse, especially during radiation treatments. They may also fear that sexual activity will make treatments less effective, or cause the cancer to spread (98).

An early comprehensive study of sexual dysfunction in women with gynecologic cancer comes from Andersen et al. (12,13). Women with clinical stage I or II gynecologic cancers ($n = 47$) were compared with two matched comparison groups: women treated for benign gynecologic disease ($n = 18$) and gynecologically healthy women ($n = 57$). All women were assessed after diagnosis but before treatment and then reassessed 4, 8, and 12 months after treatment. The frequency of intercourse declined for women treated for disease, whether malignant or benign. Considering the sexual response cycle, diminution of sexual excitement was pronounced for women with disease; however, the difficulty was more severe and distressing for the women with cancer, possibly because of significant coital and postcoital pain, premature menopause, and/or treatment-related side effects.

Changes in desire, orgasm, and the resolution phase of the sexual response cycle also occurred. **In approximately 30% of the women treated for cancer, a sexual dysfunction was diagnosed.** Table 25.1 provides a summary of the rates of sexual dysfunction 12 months after treatment. In all cases, the rates of dysfunction were 2 to 3 times those found among healthy women. The nature, early timing, and maintenance of sexual functioning morbidity suggest the instrumental role that cancer and cancer treatments play in these deficits (particularly arousal problems).

Gynecologic cancers are treated with some combination of surgery, radiation or chemotherapy. Below is a brief review of the impact of each specific treatment.

Table 25.1	Sexual Dysfunction Diagnoses According to Gynecologic Condition[a]			
	Sexual Dysfunction (% Affected)			
Group	Desire	Excitement	Orgasm	Dyspareunia
Cancer	32%	29%	29%	29%
Benign	13%	20%	14%	14%
Healthy	9%	9%	6%	6%

[a]Twelve months posttreatment. From **Andersen BL, Anderson B, deProsse C.** Controlled prospective longitudinal study of women with cancer: I. sexual functioning outcomes. *J Consult Clin Psychol* 1989;57: 683–691.

Surgical Procedures. **Women with cervical or endometrial cancer may undergo surgery which can shorten the vagina.** For premenopausal patients with ovarian or endometrial cancer, oophorectomy will lead to sexually relevant menopausal symptoms (e.g., vaginal dryness). **Surgical treatment for vulvar cancer drastically changes genital appearance and structure,** which can entail **body image changes.**

Radiotherapy. Radiotherapy, particularly intracavitary radiation, can result in vaginal atrophy, shortening, stenosis, and reduced tissue elasticity. Women undergoing radiation should use a dilator to prevent or ameliorate some of these symptoms. Ovarian failure is also likely.

Chemotherapy. During chemotherapy, loss of sexual desire is common. Chemotherapy can also cause ovarian failure among patients nearing the age of menopause.

Sexual morbidity persists long into gynecologic cancer survivorship. In a recent study, Carpenter et al. (98) examined sexuality in a sample of 175 gynecologic cancer survivors 2 to 10 years after initial treatment. Sexual morbidity was prevalent, with the majority of patients reporting sexual responsiveness scores at least as low as those reported by women seeking treatment for sexual dysfunction. Despite these sexual difficulties, most resumed intercourse at rates comparable to available norms for similarly aged women (100), but sexual satisfaction and responsiveness were significantly impaired following treatment, consistent with prior research (101–104). Taken together, **these data suggest that resumption of sexual intercourse is not necessarily an adequate marker for improved sexual health and that assessment of sexual difficulties following gynecologic cancer treatment requires a more comprehensive approach.**

Assessment of Sexuality/Sexual Functioning

A brief sexual history should be obtained from all patients before treatment. **Obtaining a sexual assessment can achieve three goals:**

1. **It identifies sexuality as an area of well being that the medical team considers important.**
2. **It provides the healthy baseline data** necessary to evaluate any future changes in sexual functioning. Retrospective reports are subject to reporting biases.
3. **It provides an informed context for future discussions about sexuality** between the patient and the medical team.

A pretreatment sexual history is best obtained by questioning the patient directly. Questionnaires can be used to assess such topics as sexual behavior (96,105) or sexual arousal (12). Even for the older woman or the woman who is not currently sexually active, such information is desirable. **The most important determinant of the frequency of sexual activity for a woman is the presence of a healthy and interested sexual partner, not age** (106). Women who are not currently sexually active may wish to be so in the future and need to know how their functioning may be changed. The following areas are important:

1. **Marital status** and **availability of current sexual partner(s)**
2. **Body image concerns**
3. **Frequency of sexual activity** (intercourse or an equivalent intimate activity)

4. **Presence of current female sexual dysfunction** (e.g., lack of desire, orgasmic difficulties)

5. **Presence of current sexual dysfunction in the partner** (e.g., premature ejaculation, erectile difficulties, sexual difficulties secondary to medication usage)

If the sexual problems resulting from gynecologic cancer and its treatments are to be minimized, a significant investment of time, energy, and resources is necessary. **There are at least three components that are essential in a sexual functioning intervention: (i) information about sexuality** (e.g., male and female sexual anatomy, the sexual response cycle, sexual dysfunctions, and potential sources of difficulty after cancer treatment); (ii) **surgical or medical interventions** (e.g., hormonal therapy, reconstructive surgery); and (iii) **specific sexual therapeutic suggestions.** Because institutions differ in the services they are able to provide, a system for intervention development is described.

Preventing Sexual Morbidity: Information

Physicians and nurses need to be familiar with the potential sexual outcomes for patients with gynecologic cancer. In the study by Stead and colleagues (92), reasons clinicians listed for not discussing sexual sequelae included lack of knowledge and experience with such information, embarrassment, and lack of resources to provide support if needed. The acquisition of such knowledge is crucial for the gynecologic oncology service provider; it is best if this information is part of a broad understanding of normal female sexual function and response. **Patients make few inquiries, despite their concerns,** so care providers need to initiate discussion of sexuality topics and provide information to all patients. When questions do arise, an informed and understanding response encourages future discussion.

Departments caring for patients with gynecologic cancer need a plan for providing psychosexual assistance. For the individual patient, **preventive rather than rehabilitative efforts are desirable.** This should include the routine provision of sexual information to patients (81). Longitudinal data indicate that if sexual difficulties develop, most are evidenced in the early months of recovery (107); therefore, **information should be provided before and immediately after treatment, as patients resume sexual activity.**

Information *per se* **is an important component of sexual therapy interventions** (108). Gamel and colleagues provide a review of the nature and timing of information that should be provided to gynecologic cancer patients (109). **At the time of diagnosis and treatment, patients should be well informed of the potential direct effects that the treatments might have on sexuality,** such as changed general health (e.g., chronic fatigue), structural changes to the genitalia, hormonal changes, and interference with the physiologic components of the sexual response cycle. **During extended recovery, health care professionals should discuss the long-lasting sexual complications, and strategies for overcoming them.** Although sexual problems for most patients with gynecologic cancer are more difficult to treat than those of healthy women, such information aids in preventing problems resulting from ignorance or misconception and potentially decreasing the severity of problems that arise from other factors.

Reducing Sexual Morbidity: Medical Therapies

Specific medical interventions may enhance sexual functioning for selected patients (110,111). For example, hormonal medication may be used for menopausal symptoms; a Fenton's operation may be necessary to treat introital stenosis after vulvectomy. **All patients with vaginal dryness should be instructed to use lubricants during vaginal intercourse. Dilator therapy should be prescribed for all patients receiving radiotherapy.** Despite these efforts, certain sexual activities may remain difficult. If vaginal stenosis is severe, patients and partners may need to reorient themselves to a sexual lifestyle that does not include vaginal intercourse.

Treatment for Sexual Morbidity: Behavioral Sexual Therapies

Patients with significant sexual difficulties should be referred to a professional (usually a Ph.D.-level clinical psychologist) who is trained broadly in sexual therapy and familiar with the specific difficulties of the patient with gynecologic cancer. Unfortunately, there have been few clinical (112–114), or empirical (38,109,115,116) reports of sexual therapies for cancer patients. Some interventions have provided brief counseling to patients with gynecologic cancer on a variety of topics, and these often include a sexuality module (115,117). A handful of interventions specifically addressing sexuality have applied strategies from established psychotherapies, such as Cognitive Behavioral Therapy (CBT), mindfulness training (114), sex therapy (112), and couples therapy (38).

Results of these studies have suggested the effectiveness of psychotherapies in ameliorating sexual functioning after gynecologic cancer. **For many patients, behaviorally oriented sex therapy offers the most promise for change.** Behavioral therapies can target the specific sexual problems of the patient. The sections below provide information and examples of the therapies for specific sexual problems.

Problems of Low Sexual Desire

In the treatment of desire problems, a careful determination of cause is important. **Desire problems commonly occur in the earliest months of recovery. Therefore, a lack of desire may not be a problem but, rather, evidence of a normal, prolonged recuperative process.**

Interventions for desire problems include the following:

1. **Determining what conditions for sexual activity are more or less appealing,** and encouraging sexual activity under the most desirable circumstances.
2. **Increasing the frequency and variety of intimate activities** that the woman might find pleasurable.
3. **Increasing the frequency and variety of the woman's sexual fantasies** during sexual activity and on other occasions.

Problems of Low Sexual Arousal

Interventions to enhance arousal include the use of individual and couple body-touching exercises (i.e., sensate focus) and mindfulness training. Graduated steps for sexual activity are suggested to the woman or to the couple, with each stage using more intimate touching and higher levels of arousal. For example, the couple's sensate focus could involve steps that include caressing of hands, arms, and face; caressing the whole body without genitals, breasts, or buttocks; caressing whole body without genital stimulation; caressing the whole body; and, finally, caressing the whole body with focused stimulation.

Individual masturbatory activities can be designed for the patient according to the same principles. Although activities such as these are useful for all couples, they are particularly important for women who are unable to resume intercourse. **Such graduated activities have several potential benefits:**

1. **They can reintroduce relaxing and enjoyable sexual activity to a woman or a couple.** This is important because many patients come to sexual therapy after repeated frustrating, discouraging, or unsatisfactory sexual encounters.
2. **The activities are not strenuous,** which is helpful to the woman who is not fully recovered or who tires easily.
3. **The activities do not focus on a particular area of the body,** and one objective is to find new, previously unexplored areas or methods of stimulation.
4. **Touching an area affected by treatment can be eliminated** or introduced gradually.

Such a strategy can be less anxiety provoking for a woman and her partner. Also, both partners can learn what sensitivity, if any, remains in body areas changed by treatment. Some areas have sensations similar to those present before cancer treatment, whereas others may feel unpleasant to the touch. Some couples may prefer not to explore certain areas. When this is done in the context of sensate focus exercises, other areas remain for touching, and a loving, sexual relationship can prevail, rather than a rejecting or anxiety-provoking one.

It is important that the patient treated for gynecologic cancer be aware that the origin of her sexual difficulties is "in her body" and not "in her head." That is, sexual morbidity is likely to be due to nerve damage or the structural changes imposed. Women report that their bodies do not feel aroused; concurrently, they report few arousing feelings or thoughts (19). Also, normal excitement responses are disrupted with treatment side effects. For example, dyspareunia is a common problem after radiation therapy because of direct damage to the vaginal epithelium, decreased vascular engorgement, and reduced vaginal lubrication. Such causal explanations are important for patients to receive and, thereby, may prevent patients from feeling guilty or responsible for their post cancer sexual difficulties.

Problems of Negative Sexual Reactions/ Responses

Women may, understandably, react negatively to their changed bodies after radical surgery—such as vulvectomy or pelvic exenteration—although the same reactions can occur for any person with cancer (118). Extreme responses may include disgust or anxiety when looking at the site and fear of being seen by others. Many healthy women with sexual difficulties or anxieties have similar feelings. For such women, **treatments for anxiety-reduction, particularly systematic desensitization (119,120), individual sensate focus exercises (121,122), and mindfulness training (90), have proven effective.**

A focus on couples' communication has also been found to significantly enhance patients' perceptions of their partners' acceptance of their bodies (38). Although such interventions may not change a woman's negative body feelings to positive, an attainable goal is for the feelings to become neutral, or at least nondisruptive, to her sexual activities and overall mood.

Resuming Sexual Intercourse

The graduated sexual activities described above provide a relaxing and sensual context in which intercourse can be resumed. Although there is no "correct" intercourse position, there may be positions that are more comfortable for the woman recovering from cancer treatment. If the patient tires easily or needs body support, the male superior position is the least strenuous for the woman. In contrast, if a woman is having pain with intercourse (e.g., after intracavitary radiation), it is important that she have control over the depth of penetration and the rate of thrusting. In this case, the female superior position is often optimal. If this position does not provide relief from pain and a longer period of healing is necessary, couples must be told to wait and enjoy other intimate activities.

Women should be using a vaginal dilator regularly when intercourse is not possible. In addition to keeping the vagina "open," the dilator exercises provide a source of feedback to the woman regarding the degree of persistent vaginal discomfort (66). This information helps her to decide when it might be most comfortable to resume intercourse.

Orgasmic Dysfunction

Among patients with cancer, the typical difficulty is a dramatic decline in frequency of orgasm or a failure of orgasm to occur. This problem is typically accompanied by the excitement difficulties described previously, so that the woman feels she does not become sufficiently aroused to approach the plateau necessary for orgasm.

Orgasmic dysfunction among women after gynecologic treatment is common. The difficulty is typically acute, with disruption occurring immediately after treatment. This difficulty can be pervasive, even to the extent that a woman who was regularly orgasmic with coital activity before treatment becomes nonorgasmic. With this pattern, it is likely that the difficulty is a result of altered structure or innervations. For some women, orgasm may occur intermittently and be more difficult to achieve. Before beginning a treatment program for orgasmic difficulties, it is important that other reasons for orgasmic difficulties be assessed, including insufficient arousal or dyspareunia.

The most successful treatment for nonorgasmic women includes a series of individual sexuality and masturbation exercises. The treatment consists of several graduated exercises extending across several weeks. Activities are body touching, identification of genital anatomy, actual body and genital self-examination to identify pleasurable sensations, and finally, focused genital stimulation. Even though pelvic or genital anatomy after cancer treatment is changed, it is possible that orgasm can still be experienced through other means, because women can experience orgasm without genital stimulation or without specific organs such as the clitoris, once believed critical to the response.

If the woman is motivated to undertake treatment, the exercises are completed with conscientious effort, and orgasm does not occur, the change in orgasmic ability may be long-standing. Even in this case, the exercises may help the woman to take a more active role in her sexuality, give her an improved body concept, and allow her to discover new modes of experiencing sexual pleasure (51,123).

Problems During Resolution Phase

Sexual dysfunction or difficulty during resolution is seldom noted in healthy women. However, disruption during this phase is common among women with gynecologic cancer. **Sources of difficulty may include residual pain if there has been dyspareunia or continued arousal from lack of orgasm.** The most straightforward remedy to such problems is enhanced functioning during earlier phases of the sexual response cycle so that the resolution period is satisfactory. However, for those women with permanent sexual changes, efforts should be made to counteract feelings of discouragement, "letdown," or continued tension that might predominate a woman's view of her sexual functioning during the resolution phase. The woman should be reoriented to focus on the positive aspects of her sexual life, such as the continued ability to engage in sexual activity, the experience of physical closeness and intimacy with her partner, and the sharing of alternative sexual activities with her partner.

New Sex Therapy Techniques

In addition to those discussed here, **new treatments are needed.** For example, a 2006 study found **mindfulness training** to be effective in treating sexual dysfunction in gynecological cancer patients (90,114). Also, **biofeedback** has had some utility in the treatment of sexual dysfunctions and has been important in the area of physical rehabilitation. It has been used to enhance sexual arousal in healthy women (124) and sexually dysfunctional women (125), and as a treatment for dyspareunia (126). For gynecologic cancer patients, it might have some role, for example, in providing feedback during masturbatory treatment of women who have had radical genital surgery. Structural or neural changes may be such that women are not able to perceive the low level of genital sensation generated, and biofeedback may provide the necessary amplification.

References

1. **Wardle J, Pope R.** The psychological costs of screening for cancer. *J Psychosom Res* 1992;36:609–624.
2. **Ideström M, Milsom I, Andersson-Ellström A.** Women's experience of coping with a positive Pap smear: a register-based study of women with two consecutive Pap smears reported as CIN 1. *Acta Obstet Gynecol Scand* 2003;82:756–761.
3. **Gray N, Sharp L, Cotton S, Masson L, Little J, Walker L, et al. for the TOMBOLA group.** Psychological effects of a low-grade abnormal cervical smear test result: anxiety and associated factors. *Br J Cancer* 2006;94:1253–1262.
4. **Lerman C, Miller SM, Scarborough R, Hanjani P, Nolte S, Smith D.** Adverse psychologic consequences of positive cytologic cervical screening. *Am J Obstet Gynecol* 1991;165:658–662.
5. **Fowler JM, Carpenter KM, Gupta P, Golden-Kreutz DM, Andersen BL.** The gynecologic oncology consult: symptom presentation and concurrent symptoms of depression and anxiety. *Obstet Gynecol* 2004;103:1211–1217.
6. **Andrykowski MA, Carpenter JS, Studts JL, Cordova MJ, Cunningham LLC, Mager W, et al.** Adherence to recommendations for clinical follow-up after benign breast biopsy. *Breast Cancer Res Treat* 2001;69:165–178.
7. **Yabroff KR, Kerner JF, Mandelblatt JS.** Effectiveness of interventions to improve follow-up after abnormal cervical cancer screening. *Prev Med* 2000;31:429–439.
8. **Stewart DE, Lickrish GM, Sierra S, Parkin H.** The effect of educational brochures on knowledge and emotional distress in women with abnormal Papanicolaou smears. *Obstet Gynecol* 1993;81:280–282.
9. **Epping-Jordan JE, Compas BE, Osowiecki DM, Oppedisano G, Gerhardt C, Primo K, Krag DN.** Psychological adjustment in breast cancer: processes of emotional distress. *Health Psychol* 1999;18:315–326.
10. **Stanton AL, Danoff-Burg S, Huggins ME.** The first year after breast cancer diagnosis; hope and coping strategies as predictors of adjustment. *Psychooncology* 2002;11:93–102.
11. **Andersen BL, Farrar WB, Golden-Kreutz D, Kutz LA, MacCallum R, Courtney ME, Glaser R.** Stress and immune responses following surgical treatment of regional breast cancer. *J Natl Cancer Inst* 1998;90:30–36.
12. **Andersen BL, Anderson B, DeProsse C.** Controlled prospective longitudinal study of women with cancer: I. Sexual functioning outcomes. *J Consult Clin Psychol* 1989;57:683–691.
13. **Andersen BL, Anderson B, DeProsse C.** Controlled prospective longitudinal study of women with cancer: II. Psychological outcomes. *J Consult Clin Psychol* 1989;57:692–697.
14. **Massie MJ.** Prevalence of depression in patients with cancer. *J Natl Cancer Inst Monogr* 2004:57–71.
15. **van't Spijker A, Trijsburg RW, Duivenvoorden HJ.** Psychological sequelae of cancer diagnosis: a meta-analytical review of 58 studies after 1980. *Psychosom Med* 1997;59:280–293.
16. **Raison CL, Miller AH.** Depression in cancer: new developments regarding diagnosis and treatment. *Biol Psychiatry* 2003;54:283–294.
17. **Hotopf M, Chidgey J, Addington-Hall J, Ly KL.** Depression in advanced disease: a systematic review Part 1. Prevalence and case finding. *Palliat Med* 2002;16:81–97.
18. **Burgess C, Cornelius V, Love S, Graham J, Richards M, Ramirez A.** Depression and anxiety in women with early breast cancer: five-year observational cohort study. *BMJ* 2005;330:1–4.
19. **Zabora J, Brintzenhofeszoc K, Curbow B, Hooker C, Piantadosi S.** The prevalence of psychological distress by cancer site. *Psychooncology* 2001;10:19–28.
20. **Dausch BM, Compas BE, Beckjord E, Luecken L, Anderson-Hanley C, Sherman M, et al.** Rates and correlates of DSM-IV diagnoses in women newly diagnosed with breast cancer. *J Clin Psych Med Set* 2004;11:159–169.
21. **Schwartz L, Drotar D.** Posttraumatic stress and related impairment in survivors of childhood cancer in early adulthood compared to healthy peers. *J Pediatr Psychol* 2006;31:356–366.
22. **Deshields T, Tibbs T, Fan M-Y, Taylor M.** Differences in patterns of depression after treatment for breast cancer. *Psychooncology* 2006;15:398–406.
23. **Peters L, Sellick K.** Quality of life of cancer patients receiving inpatient and home-based palliative care. *J Adv Nurs* 2006;53:524–533.
24. **Yen J-Y, Ko C-H, Yen C-F, Yang M-J, Wu C-Y, Juan C-H, et al.** Quality of life, depression, and stress in breast cancer women outpatients receiving active therapy in Taiwan. *Psychiatry Clin Neurosci* 2006;60:147–153.
25. **Sadler IJ, Jacobsen PB, Booth-Jones M, Belanger H, Weitzner MA, Fields KK.** Preliminary evaluation of a clinical syndrome approach to assessing cancer-related fatigue. *J Pain Symptom Manage* 2002;23:406–416.
26. **Smith EM, Gomm SA, Dickens CM.** Assessing the independent contribution to quality of life from anxiety and depression in patients with advanced cancer. *Palliat Med* 2003;17:509–513.
27. **Mystakidou K, Tsilika E, Parpa E, Katsouda E, Galanos A, Vlahos L.** Assessment of anxiety and depression in advanced cancer patients and their relationship with quality of life. *Qual Life Res* 2005;14:1825–1833.
28. **Ell K, Sanchez K, Vourlekis B, Lee P-J, Dwight-Johnson M, Lagomasino I, et al.** Depression, correlates of depression, and receipt of depression care among low-income women with breast or gynecologic cancer. *J Clin Oncol* 2005;23:3052–3060.
29. **Jim HS, Richardson SA, Golden-Kreutz DM, Andersen BL.** Strategies used in coping with a cancer diagnosis predict meaning in life for survivors. *Health Psychol* 2006;25:753–761.
30. **Golden-Kreutz DM, Andersen L.** Depressive symptoms after breast cancer surgery: relationships with global, cancer-related, and life event stress. *Psychooncology* 2004;13:211–220.
31. **Andersen BL, Shapiro CL, Farrar WB, Crespin TR, Wells-Di Gregorio SM.** Psychological responses to cancer recurrence: a controlled prospective study. *Cancer* 2005;104:1540–1547.

32. **Yang H-C, Thornton LM, Shapiro CL, Andersen BL.** Surviving recurrence: psychological and quality of life recovery. *Cancer* 2008;112:1178–1187.

33. **Roberts JA, Brown D, Elkins T, Larson DB.** Factors influencing view of patients with gynecologic cancer about end-of-life decisions. *Am J Obstet Gynecol* 1997;176:166–172.

34. **Andersen BL.** Psychological interventions for cancer patients to enhance the quality of life. *J Consult Clin Psychol* 1992;60:552–568.

35. **Blake-Mortimer J, Gore-Felton C, Kimerling R, Turner-Cobb JM, Spiegel D.** Improving the quality and quantity of life among patients with cancer: a review of the effectiveness of group psychotherapy. *Eur J Cancer* 1999;35:1581–1586.

36. **Fawzy FI.** Psychosocial interventions for patients with cancer: what works and what doesn't. *Eur J Cancer* 1999;35:1559.

37. **Manne SL, Rubin S, Edelson M, Rosenblum N, Bergman C, Hernandez E, et al.** Coping and communication-enhancing intervention versus supportive counseling for women diagnosed with gynecological cancers. *J Consult Clin Psychol* 2007;75:615–628.

38. **Scott JL, Halford WK, Ward BG.** United we stand? The effects of a couple-coping intervention on adjustment to early stage breast or gynecological cancer. *J Consult Clin Psychol* 2004;72:1122.

39. **Petersen RW, Quinlivan JA.** Preventing anxiety and depression in gynaecological cancer: a randomised controlled trial. *BJOG* 2002;109:386–394.

40. **Marangell LB.** Augmentation of standard depression therapy. *Clin Ther* 2000;22(suppl A):A25.

41. **Rapaport MH, Gharabawi GM, Canuso CM, Mahmoud RA, Keller MB, Bossie CA, et al.** Effects of risperidone augmentation in patients with treatment-resistant depression: results of open-label treatment followed by double-blind continuation. *Neuropsychopharmacology* 2006;31:2505–2513.

42. **Pedro L, Delgado, Zarkowski P.** Treatment of mood disorders. In: **Panksepp J, ed.** *Textbook of biological psychiatry.* Hoboken, NJ: Wiley-Liss, 2003;231–266.

43. **Butler AC, Chapman JE, Forman EM, Beck AT.** The empirical status of cognitive-behavioral therapy: a review of meta-analyses. *Clin Psychol Rev* 2006;26:17–31.

44. **Hollon SD, Stewart MO, Strunk D.** Enduring effects for cognitive behavior therapy in the treatment of depression and anxiety. *Annu Rev Psychol* 2006;57:285–315.

45. **Strunk DR, DeRubeis RJ.** Cognitive therapy for depression: a review of its efficacy. *J Cognit Psychother* 2001;15:289–297.

46. **Williams S, Dale J.** The effectiveness of treatment for depression/depressive symptoms in adults with cancer: a systematic review. *Br J Cancer* 2006;94:372–390.

47. **Gottesman D, Lewis MS.** Differences in crisis reactions among cancer and surgery patients. *J Consult Clin Psychol* 1982;50:381–388.

48. **Andersen BL, Hacker NF.** Treatment for gynecologic cancer: a review of the effects on female sexuality. *Health Psychol* 1983;2:203–221.

49. **Andersen BL, Hacker NF.** Psychosexual adjustment after vulvar surgery. *Obstet Gynecol* 1983;62:457–462.

50. **Hayward JES.** *Information: a prescription against pain.* London: Royal College of Nursing, 1975.

51. **Wallace DH, Barbach LG.** Preorgasmic group treatment. *J Sex Marital Ther* 1974;1:146–154.

52. **Peck A, Boland J.** Emotional reactions to radiation treatment. *Cancer* 1977;40:180–184.

53. **Mitchell GW, Glicksman AS.** Cancer patients: knowledge and attitudes. *Cancer* 1977;40:61–66.

54. **Andersen BL.** Psychological aspects of gynaecological cancer. In: **Broome AK, Wallace L, eds.** *Psychology and gynaecological problems,* London: Tavistock/Routledge, 1984:117–141.

55. **Andersen B, Tewfik H.** Psychological reactions to radiation therapy: reconsideration of the adaptive aspects of anxiety. *J Pers Soc Psychol* 1985;48:1024–1032.

56. **Karlsson JA, Andersen BL.** Radiation therapy and psychological distress in gynecologic oncology patients: outcomes and recommendations for enhancing adjustment. *J Psychosom Obstet Gynecol* 1986;5:283–294.

57. **Mages NL, Mendelsohn GA.** Effect of cancer on patients' lives: a personological approach. In: **Stone GC, Cohen F, Adler NE, eds.** *Health psychology.* San Francisco: Jossey-Bass, 1979:255–284.

58. **Nail LM, King KB, Johnson JE.** Coping with radiation treatment for gynecologic cancer: mood and disruption in usual function. *J Psychosom Obstet Gynaecol* 1986;5:271–281.

59. **Jensen PT, Groenvold M, Klee MC, Thranov I, Petersen MA, Machin D.** Longitudinal study of sexual function and vaginal changes after radiotherapy for cervical cancer. *Int J Radiat Oncol Biol Phys* 2003;56:937–949.

60. **Katz RC, Flasher L, Cacciapaglia H, Nelson S.** The psychosocial impact of cancer and lupus: a cross validation study that extends the generality of "benefit finding" in patients with chronic disease. *J Behav Med* 2001;24:561–571.

61. **Andersen B, Anderson B, DeProsse C.** Controlled prospective longitudinal study of women with cancer: II. Psychological outcomes. *J Consult Clin Psychol* 1989;57:692–697.

62. **Andersen BL, Jochimsen PR.** Sexual functioning among breast cancer, gynecologic cancer, and healthy women. *J Consult Clin Psychol* 1985;53:25–32.

63. **Forester B, Kornfield DS, Fleiss JL.** Psychotherapy during radiotherapy: effects on emotional and physical distress. *Am J Psychiatry* 1985;142:22–27.

64. **Israel MJ, Mood DW.** Three media presentations for patients receiving radiation therapy. *Cancer Nurs* 1982;5:57–63.

65. **Jeffries SA, Robinson JW, Craighead PS, Keats MR.** An effective group psychoeducational intervention for improving compliance with vaginal dilation: a randomized controlled trial. *Int J Radiat Oncol Biol Phys* 2006;65:404–411.

66. **Robinson JW, Faris PD, Scott CB.** Psychoeducational group increases vaginal dilation for younger women and reduces sexual fears for women of all ages with gynecological carcinoma treated with radiotherapy. *Int J Radiat Oncol Biol Phys* 1999;44:497–506.

67. **Pitkin RM, VanVoorhis LW.** Postirradiation vaginitis. An evaluation of prophylaxis with topical estrogen. *Radiology* 1971;99:417–421.

68. **Leventhal H, Easterling DV, Coons HL, Luchterhand CM, Love RR.** Adaptation to chemotherapy treatments. In: **Andersen BL, ed.** *Women with cancer: psychological perspectives.* New York: Springer-Verlag, 1986:192–193.

69. **Lutgendorf SK, Anderson B, Sorosky JI, Buller RE, Lubaroff DM.** Interleukin-6 and use of social support in gynecologic cancer patients. *Int J Behav Med* 2000;7:127–142.

70. **Andrykowski MA.** Defining anticipatory nausea and vomiting: differences among cancer chemotherapy patients who report pretreatment nausea. *J Behav Med* 1988;11:59–69.

71. **Carey MP, Burish TG.** Etiology and treatment of the psychological side effects associated with cancer chemotherapy: a critical review and discussion. *Psychol Bull* 1988;104:307–325.

72. **Andrykowski MA.** The role of anxiety in the development of anticipatory nausea in cancer chemotherapy: a review and synthesis. *Psychosom Med* 1990;52:458–475.

73. **Silberfarb PM, Maurer LH, Crouthamel CS.** Psychosocial aspects of neoplastic disease: I. functional status of breast cancer patients during different treatment regimens. *Am J Psychiatry* 1980;137:450–455.

74. **Redd WH, Montgomery GH, DuHamel KN.** Behavioral intervention for cancer treatment side effects. *J Natl Cancer Inst* 2001;93:810–823.

75. **Carlsson M, Strang P, Bjurström C.** Treatment modality affects long-term quality of life in gynaecological cancer. *Anticancer Res* 2000;20:563–568.

76. **Hodgkinson K, Butow P, Hunt GE, Wyse R, Hobbs KM, Wain G.** Life after cancer: couples' and partners' psychological adjustment and supportive care needs. *Support Care Cancer* 2007;15:405–415.

77. **Li C, Samsioe G, Iosif C.** Quality of life in long-term survivors of cervical cancer. *Maturitas* 1999;32:95–102.

78. **Li C, Samsioe G, Iosif C.** Quality of life in endometrial cancer survivors. *Maturitas* 1999;31:227–236.

79. **Matthews AK, Aikens JE, Helmrich SP, Anderson DD, Herbst AL, Waggoner SE.** Sexual functioning and mood among long term survivors of clear cell adenocarcinoma of the vagina or cervix. *J Psychosoc Oncol* 1999;17:27–45.

80. **Wenzel L, Huang HQ, Monk BJ, Rose PG, Cella D.** Quality-of-life comparisons in a randomized trial of interval secondary cytoreduction in advanced ovarian carcinoma: a Gynecologic Oncology Group Study. *J Clin Oncol* 2005;23.

81. Wenzel LB, Donnelly JP, Fowler JM, Habbal R, Taylor TH, Aziz N, Cella D. Resilience, reflection, and residual stress in ovarian cancer survivorship: a gynecologic oncology group study. Psychooncology 2002;11:142–153.
82. Miller BE, Pittman B, Case D, McQuellon RP. Quality of life after treatment for gynecologic malignancies: a pilot study in an outpatient clinic. Gynecol Oncol 2002;87:178–184.
83. Andersen BL, Andersen B. Psychosomatic aspects of gynecologic oncology: present status and future directions. J Psychosom Obstet Gynaecol 1986;5:233–244.
84. Taylor SE. Adjustment to threatening events: a theory of cognitive adaptation. Am Psychol 1983;38:1161–1173.
85. Klee M, Thranov I, Machin Prof D. The patients' perspective on physical symptoms after radiotherapy for cervical cancer. Gynecol Oncol 2000;76:14–23.
86. Smith TW, Nealey JB, Hamann HA. Health psychology. In: Snyder CR, Ingram RE, eds. Handbook of psychological change: psychotherapy processes & practices for the 21st century. Hoboken, NJ: Wiley, 2000:562–590.
87. American Psychiatric Association. Diagnostic and statistical manual of mental disorders, 4th ed. Washington: American Psychiatric Association, 1994.
88. Bodurka DC, Sun CC. Sexual function after gynecologic cancer. Obstet Gynecol Clin North Am 2006;33:621–630, ix.
89. Stead ML, Fallowfield L, Selby P, Brown JM. Psychosexual function and impact of gynaecological cancer. Best Pract Res Clin Obstet Gynaecol 1997;21:309–320.
90. Brotto LA, Heiman JR. Mindfulness in sex therapy: applications for women with sexual difficulties following gynecologic cancer. J Sex Relationship Ther 2007;22:3–11.
91. Bergmark K, Avall-Lundqvist E, Dickman PW, Henningsohn L, Steineck G. Patient-rating of distressful symptoms after treatment for early cervical cancer. Acta Obstet Gynecol Scand 2002;81:443–450.
92. Stead ML. Sexual dysfunction after treatment for gynaecologic and breast malignancies. Curr Opin Obstet Gynecol 2003;15:57–61.
93. Sherwin B, Gelfand M, Brender W. Androgen enhances sexual motivation in females: a prospective, crossover study of sex steroid administration in the surgical menopause. Psychosom Med 1985;47:339–351.
94. Masters WH, Johnson VE. Human sexual response. New York: Bantam Books, 1966.
95. Newcomb MD, Bentler PM. Dimensions of subjective female orgasmic responsiveness. J Person Soc Psych 1983;44:862–873.
96. Andersen BL, Broffitt B. Is there a reliable and valid self-report measure of sexual behavior? Arch Sex Behav 1988;17:509–525.
97. Wright EP, Kiely MA, Lynch P, Cull A, Selby PJ. Social problems in oncology. Br J Cancer 2002;87:1099–1104.
98. Lagana L, Classen C, Caldwell R, McGarvey EL, Baum LD, Cheasty E, et al. Sexual difficulties of patients with gynecological cancer. Prof Psychol Res Pract 2005;36:391–399.
99. Carpenter KM, Andersen BL, Fowler JM, Maxwell GL. Sexual self schema as a moderator of sexual and psychological outcomes for gynecologic cancer survivors. Arch Sex Behav 2008 Apr 17. [Epub ahead of print]
100. Laumann EO, Gagnon JH, Michael RT, Michaels S. The social organization of sexuality: sexual practices in the United States. Chicago: University of Chicago Press, 1994.
101. Gershenson DM, Miller AM, Champion VL, Monahan PO, Zhao Q, Cella D, et al. Reproductive and sexual function after platinum-based chemotherapy in long-term ovarian germ cell tumor survivors: a Gynecologic Oncology Group Study. J Clin Oncol 2007;25:2792–2797.
102. Hawighorst-Knapstein S, Fusshoeller C, Franz C, Trautmann K, Schmidt M, Pilch H, et al. The impact of treatment for genital cancer on quality of life and body image—results of a prospective longitudinal 10-year study. Gynecol Oncol 2004;94:398–403.
103. Lindau ST, Gavrilova N, Anderson D. Sexual morbidity in very long-term survivors of vaginal and cervical cancer: a comparison to national norms. Gynecol Oncol 2007;106:413–418.
104. Weijmar-Schultz WCM, Wiel HBMVD, Bouma J, Lappohn RE. Gynaecological conditions and sexual dysfunction. Sex Marital Ther 1991;6:177–194.
105. Derogatis LR, Melisaratos N. The DFSI: a multidimensional measure of sexual functioning. J Sex Marital Ther 1979;5:244–281.
106. Bachmann GA, Leiblum SR, Kemmann E, Colburn DW, Swartzman L, Shelden R. Sexual expression and its determinants in the post-menopausal woman. Maturitas 1984;6:19–29.
107. Andersen BL. Predicting sexual and psychologic morbidity and improving the quality of life for women with gynecologic cancer. Cancer 1993;71(Feb 15):1678–1690.
108. Kilmann P, Mills K, Bella B, Caid C, Davidson E, Drose G, et al. The effects of sex education on women with secondary orgasmic dysfunction. J Sex Marital Ther 1983;9:79–87.
109. Gamel C, Hengeveld M, David B. Informational needs about the effects of gynaecological cancer on sexuality: a review of the literature. J Clin Nurs 2000;9:678–688.
110. Berek JS, Andersen BL. Sexual rehabilitation: surgical and psychological approaches. In: Hoskins WJ, Perez CA, Young RC, eds. Gynecologic oncology: principles and practice. Philadelphia: JB Lippincott, 1992:401–416.
111. Denton AS, Maher EJ. Interventions for the physical aspects of sexual dysfunction in women following pelvic radiotherapy. Cochrane Database Syst Rev 2003:CD003750.
112. Caldwell R, Classen C, Lagana L, McGarvey E, Baum L, Duenke SD, et al. Changes in sexual functioning and mood among women treated for gynecological cancer who receive group therapy: a pilot study. J Clin Psychol Med Sett 2004;10:149–159.
113. Witkin MH. Helping husbands adjust to their wives' mastectomies. Med Aspects Hum Sex 1978;12:93–94.
114. Brotto LA, Heiman JR, Goff B, Greer B, Lentz GM, Swisher E, et al. A psychoeducational intervention for sexual dysfunction in women with gynecologic cancer. Arch Sex Behav 2008;37:317–329.
115. Capone MA, Good RS, Westie KS, Jacobson AF. Psychosocial rehabilitation of gynecologic oncology patients. Arch Phys Med Rehabil 1980;61:128–132.
116. Christensen DN. Postmastectomy couple counseling: an outcome study of a structured treatment protocol. J Sex Marital Ther 1983;9:266–275.
117. Cain EN, Kohorn EI, Quinlan DM. Psychosocial benefits of a cancer support group. Cancer 1986;57:183–189.
118. Steinberg MD, Juliano MA, Wise L. Psychological outcome of lumpectomy versus mastectomy in the treatment of breast cancer. Am J Psychiatry 1985;142:34–39.
119. Jones WJ, Park PM. Treatment of single-partner sexual dysfunction by systematic desensitization. Obstet Gynecol 1972;39:411–417.
120. Lazarus A. The treatment of chronic frigidity by systematic desensitization. J Nerv Ment Dis 1963;136:272–276.
121. Fichten CS, Libman E, Brender W. Methodological issues in the study of sex therapy: effective components in the treatment of secondary orgasmic dysfunction. J Sex Marital Ther 1983;9:191–202.
122. Sarwer DB, Durlak JA. A field trial of the effectiveness of behavioral treatment for sexual dysfunctions. J Sex Marital Ther 1997;23:87–97.
123. Cotten-Huston AL, Wheeler KA. Preorgasmic group treatment: assertiveness, marital adjustment and sexual function in women. J Sex Marital Ther 1983;9:296–302.
124. Cerny JA. Biofeedback and the voluntary control of sexual arousal in women. Behav Ther 1978;9:847–855.
125. Palace EM. Modification of dysfunctional patterns of sexual response through autonomic arousal and false physiological feedback. J Consult Clin Psychol 1995;63:604–615.
126. Bergeron S, Binik YM, Khalifé S, Pagidas K, Glazer HI, Meana M, et al. A randomized comparison of group cognitive-behavioral therapy, surface electromyographic biofeedback, and vestibulectomy in the treatment of dyspareunia resulting from vulvar vestibulitis. Pain 2001;91:297–306.

Index